ENCYCLOPEDIA OF THE ALKALOIDS

Volume 1 (A-H)

ENCYCLOPEDIA OF THE ALKALOIDS

Volume 1 (A-H)

John S. Glasby

ICI (Organics Division) Ltd.
Ayrshire, Scotland

PLENUM PRESS • NEW YORK AND LONDON

Library of Congress Cataloging in Publication Data

Glasby, John Stephen.
  Encyclopedia of the alkaloids.

  Includes bibliographical references.
  1. Alkaloids — Dictionaries. I. Title.
QD421.G54   547'.72'03   75-17753
ISBN 0-306-30845-2

© 1975 Plenum Press, New York
A Division of Plenum Publishing Corporation
227 West 17th Street, New York, N.Y. 10011

United Kingdom edition published by Plenum Press, London
A Division of Plenum Publishing Company, Ltd.
Davis House (4th Floor), 8 Scrubs Lane, Harlesden, London, NW10 6SE, England

Printed in the United States of America

Preface

In many respects the plant alkaloids are among the most important and interesting of all naturally-occurring compounds. Not only are their structures often extremely complex but their marked physiological action makes them of great importance in medicine. In addition, their undoubted toxic properties often bring them to the attention of veterinary and forensic scientists.

A voluminous literature has now accumulated regarding the discovery of new alkaloids, their occurrence, structures, physiological properties, synthesis and biosynthesis, and in compiling these volumes the author has kept in view these various aspects of the subject. Wherever possible, the original papers have been consulted and references to these are given for each alkaloid listed. A number of these bases have not yet been characterized, nor have they been given trivial names, and in these cases the presently accepted nomenclature has been followed, namely assigning them the initial letters of the name of the plant in which they were first discovered followed by a letter or number. In any case of doubt the identity of the alkaloid may be ascertained by reference to the original paper.

In a field as large as this, where new alkaloids are being discovered in increasing numbers every year, there will inevitably be some omissions and for these the author bears full responsibility. It is hoped, however, that the encyclopedia will prove useful as a reference work for all chemists and biochemists working in the field of natural products.

Stevenston   J. S. GLASBY
May, 1975

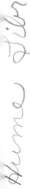

Contents

A

ABRASINE

$C_{18}H_{21}O_3N_3$

M.p. 218–220°C

The dried roots of *Abrus precatorius* L. yield this alkaloid which occurs together with Precasine (q.v.). The base yields a crystalline hydrochloride, m.p. 226–7°C, prepared by passing HCl through a solution of the alkaloid in MeOH. The infrared spectrum indicates the presence of an amide group and unsaturation.

Khaleque, Aminuddin, Azim-Ul-Mulk., *Sci. Res.*, (Dacca), **3**, 203 (1966)

(+)-ABRINE

$C_{12}H_{14}O_2N_2$

M.p. 295°C (*dec.*).

This alkaloid is present in the seeds of *Abrus precatorius* L. and forms colourless prisms when crystallized from H_2O. It is dextrorotatory with $[\alpha]_D^{25} + 62.4°$ (0.5 N/NaOH) or $+ 46°$ (0.5 N/HCl). The betaine corresponding to (+)-methyl-abrine is identical with Hypaphorine (q.v.). As a growth-promoting substance in rats, (+)-abrine is more effective than the optically inactive form but less so than (−)-tryptophan. The following salts and derivatives of the alkaloid are known: hydrochloride, m.p. 221.5°C (*dec.*); nitrate, colourless needles from H_2O, m.p. 143°C (*dec.*); picrate, orange-red prisms, m.p. 194°C (*dec.*); N-acetyl derivative, a colourless crystalline solid from aqueous EtOH, m.p. 286–7°C and the N-nitroso compound, m.p. 121°C. The alkaloid must not be confused with abrin, the toxic albuminoid compound isolated from the same source.

Ghatak, Kaul., *J. Ind. Chem. Soc.*, **9**, 383 (1932)
Ghatak., *Bull. Acad. Sci. U.P. India*, **3**, 295 (1934)
Ghatak., *Chem. Zentr.*, **I**, 576 (1935)
Hoshino, *Annalen*, **520**, 31 (1935)
Cahill, Jackson., *J. Biol. Chem.*, **226**, 29 (1938)
Synthesis:
Gordon, Jackson., *J. Biol. Chem.*, **110**, 151 (1935)
Miller, Robson., *J. Chem. Soc.*, 1910 (1938)

ABROMINE

$C_6H_{13}O_2N$

M.p. 283–5°C (*dec.*).

The dried, powdered roots of *Abroma augusta* have been shown to contain this alkaloid, the structure of which has not yet been determined. The salts which

1

have been prepared to characterize the base include the hydrochloride, m.p. $230°C$; the picrate, m.p. $176–8°C$ and the reineckate, m.p. $146°C$ (*dec.*).

Srivastava, Basu., *Ind. J. Pharm.*, **18**, 472 (1956)

ABROTINE

$C_{21}H_{22}ON_2$

A crystalline, ditertiary base isolated from *Artemesia abrotanum* L., the structure of this alkaloid has not yet been elucidated, nor does it appear to have been investigated further since its discovery almost a century ago. It is stated to form a crystalline sulphate and platinichloride.

Giacosa., *Jahresb.*, 1356 (1883)

(+)-ACANTHOIDINE

$C_{16}H_{26}O_2N_4$

CH₃O
CH₃O — CH₂CH₂CHCH₂CH₂CH₂
             NH   NH
             CH   CH
             NH   NH

This alkaloid has been isolated from the dried stalks of *Carduus acanthoides* L. and characterized as the dihydrochloride which yields fine, colourless needles from EtOH, m.p. $250–1°C$; $[\alpha]_D^{29} + 6.8° \pm 1.5°$ (c 0.4, H_2O). This salt is hygroscopic but can be kept without decomposition. It is less soluble than the corresponding salt of Acanthoine (q.v.) in most organic solvents. The dihydrochloride of the optically inactive form has been prepared as colourless needles with m.p. $234–5°C$. The alkaloid exhibits some hypertensive activity.

Wall *et al.*, *J. Amer. Pharm. Soc.*, **48**, 695 (1959)
Frydman, Deulofeu., *Tetrahedron,* **18**, 1063 (1962)

(+)-ACANTHOINE

$C_{16}H_{22}O_2N_4$

CH₃O
CH₃O — CH:CHCHCH:CHCH₂
             NH   NH
             CH   CH
             NH   NH

Also present in *Carduus acanthoides* L., this unstable base forms a crystalline dihydrochloride hemihydrate as yellow needles from *iso*propanol, m.p. $221°C$; $[\alpha]_D^{29} + 7.1° \pm 1.2°$ (c 0.4, H_2O). This salt is hygroscopic and decomposes on standing to give unidentified, coloured compounds. It is very soluble in H_2O, EtOH, MeOH and Me_2CO but insoluble in C_6H_6 and Et_2O. On alkaline hydrolysis, the salt yields two moles of NH_3, 2 moles of formic acid and an optically active base, $C_{14}H_{20}O_2N_2$. Oxidation of this base with $KMnO_4$ furnishes veratric acid, aminomalonic acid and glycine. Like the previous alkaloid, this base shows hypertensive activity.

Wall *et al.*, *J. Amer. Pharm. Soc.*, **48**, 695 (1959)

Frydman, Deulofeu., *Tetrahedron*, **18**, 1063 (1962)

6-ACETONYLDIHYDROSANGUINARINE

$C_{23}H_{19}O_5N$

M.p. 194–195.5°C

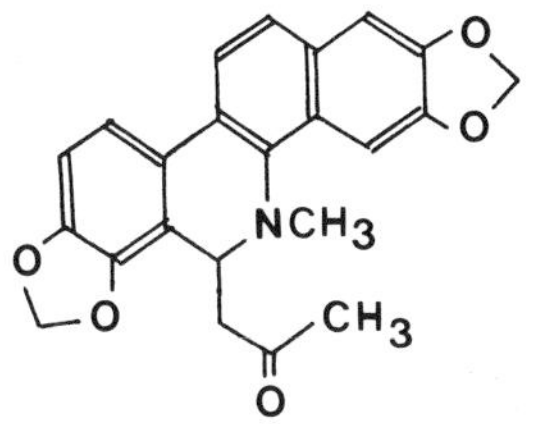

This alkaloid occurs in the callus tissue of *Papaver somniferum* and forms yellow needles when crystallized from $CHCl_3$-MeOH. The structure given above has been confirmed by synthesis.

Furuya, Ikuta, Syonok., *Phytochem.*, **11**, 3041 (1972)

3-β-ACETOXY-7-β-HYDROXY-N-(2-HYDROXYETHYL)-N-METHYL-(E)-CASS-13(15)-EN-16-AMIDE

$C_{26}H_{39}O_5N$

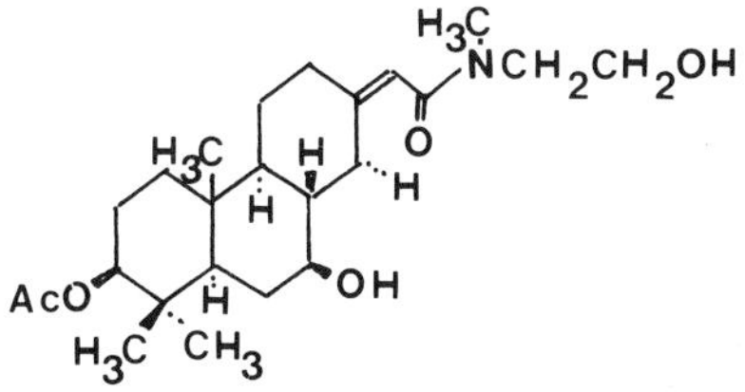

A recently discovered alkaloid, this base occurs in the bark of *Erythrophleum suaveolens*. The structure has been determined from chemical and spectroscopic evidence, particularly from mass spectral data.

Cronlund., *Acta. Pharm. Suic.*, **10**, 333 (1973)

7β-ACETOXY-1-METHOXYMETHYL-1:2-DEHYDRO-8α-PYRROLIZIDINE

$C_{11}H_{17}O_3N$

B.p. 61°C/0.03 mm.

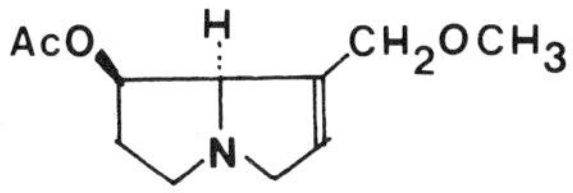

A liquid alkaloid present in *Crotalaria aridicola* Domin., this base is dextrorotatory with $[\alpha]_D^{24} + 15.2°$ (c 3.6, EtOH). It forms a picrate as minute yellow needles, m.p. 153–153.5°C. The alkaloid may be partially synthesized from commonly available amino alcohols.

Culvenor, O'Donovan, Smith., *Austral. J. Chem.*, **20**, 757 (1967)

1-ACETOXYMETHYL-2-PROPYL-4-QUINOLONE

$C_{15}H_{17}O_3N$

M.p. 112°C

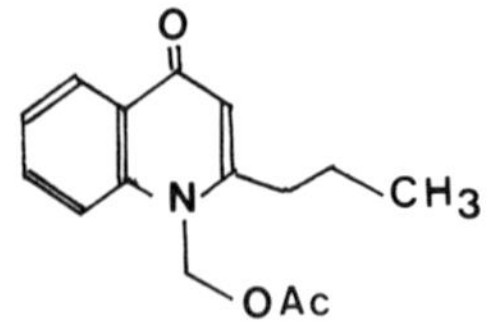

A minor Rutaceous alkaloid, this base has been obtained from *Boronia ternata* Endl. The alkaloid forms colourless prisms when recrystallized from C_6H_6-light petroleum and on alkaline hydrolysis it furnishes 2-propyl-4-quinolone, m.p. 166–8°C which may be characterized as the crystalline picrate, m.p. 214–6°C.

Duffield, Jefferies., *Austral. J. Chem.*, 16, 292 (1963)

3β-ACETOXYTROPANE

$C_{10}H_{17}O_2N$

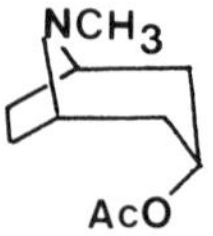

This simple tropane alkaloid was first isolated from the leaves and stems of *Datura sanguinea*. It has subsequently been found in various species of *Solandra* and in the roots of *Datura Metel* var. *fastuga* grown in Bangladesh.

Evans, Major., *J. Chem. Soc., C*, 1621 (1966)
Evans, Ghani, Woolley., *Phytochem.*, 11, 470 (1972)
Anwar, Ghani., *Bangladesh Pharm. J.*, 2, 25 (1973)

17-ACETYLAJMALINE

$C_{22}H_{28}O_3N_2$

M.p. 153–5°C

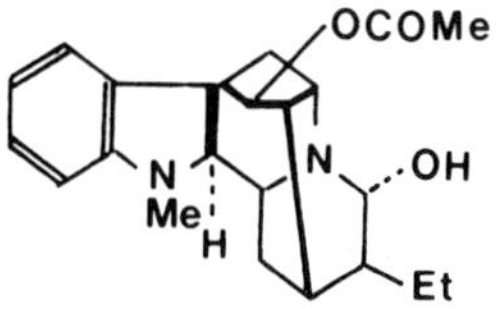

A novel dihydroindole alkaloid, this base occurs in the roots of *Rauwolfia vomitora* and has $[\alpha]_{5780}^{20}$ + 53° (c 0.96, $CHCl_3$). The above structure has been assigned on the basis of infrared, ultraviolet and NMR comparison with ajmaline, 21-deoxyajmaline and dihydroajmaline. The alkaloid has been partially synthesized from ajmaline by treatment with Ac_2O at 100°C for 2 hours to form the 17:21-diacetylajmaline, the hydrochloride of which is then boiled in H_2O for 3 hours and the resulting mixture of products chromatographed to achieve separation.

Bombardelli, Bonati, Russo., *Fitoterapia*, 38, 126 (1967)
Muquet, Pousset, Poisson., *Compt. Rend.*, 266C, 1542 (1968)

4

1-ACETYLASPIDOALBINE

$C_{21}H_{26}O_2N_2$

M.p. 173–4°C

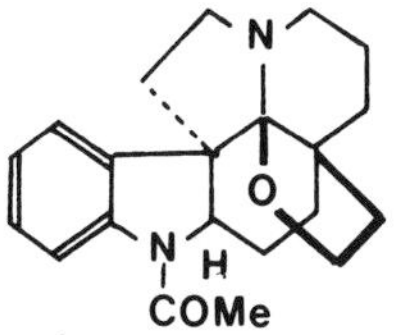

This indolizidinocarbazole alkaloid occurs in *Vallesia dichotoma* Ruiz et Pav. and forms colourless needles from $CHCl_3$. It is dextrorotatory with $[\alpha]_D + 46°$ ($CHCl_3$) and the ultraviolet spectrum shows absorption maxima at 212 and 253 mμ, typical of this type of alkaloid. Acid hydrolysis gives aspidoalbine, m.p. 180°C.

Brown, Budzikiewicz, Djerassi., *Tetrahedron Lett.*, 1731 (1963)

ACETYLCARANINE

$C_{18}H_{19}O_4N$

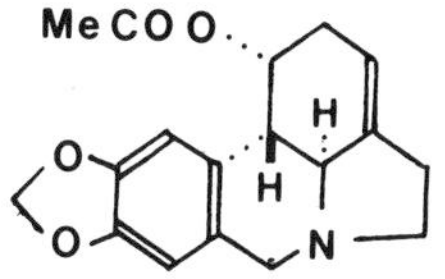

A minor alkaloid of *Crinum macrantherum*, the structure of this base is confirmed by its hydrolysis to acetic acid and Caranine (q.v.).

Hauth, Stauffacher., *Helv. Chim. Acta,* **47**, 185 (1964)

ACETYLCEPHALOTAXINE

$C_{20}H_{23}O_5N$

M.p. 141–3°C

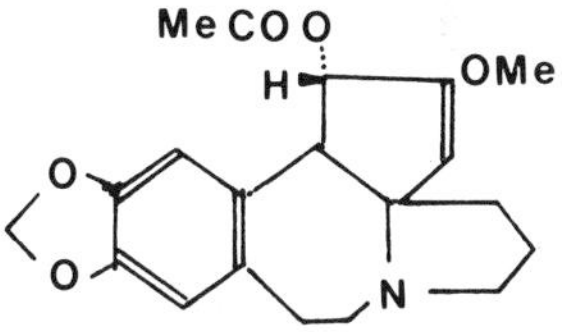

One of several minor alkaloids obtained from *Cephalotaxus fortunei*, this base has been assigned the above structure on the basis of interconversion with Cephalotaxine (q.v.).

Paundler, McKay., *J. Org. Chem.*, **38**, 2110 (1973)

ACETYLCHOLINE

$C_7H_{17}O_3N$

This trimethylammonium base is found in the mycelium of *Claviceps purpurea* together with the ergot alkaloids. Like other simple bases and aminoacids, it is probably formed in the fungus from the proteins of the host plant.

Ewins., *Biochem. J.*, **8**, 44, 366 (1914)

5

ACETYLCORYNOLINE

$C_{23}H_{26}O_6N$

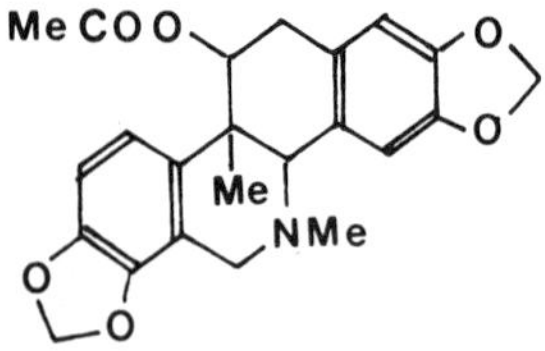

A minor alkaloid present in *Corydalis incisa*, this base has been recently isolated. No salts or derivatives have yet been reported and the above structure has been assigned on the basis of chemical and spectroscopic evidence.

Nonaka *et al.*, *J. Pharm. Soc., Japan*, **93**, 87 (1973)

N-ACETYLCYLINDROCARPINOL

$C_{22}H_{30}O_3N_2$

M.p. 211–5°C

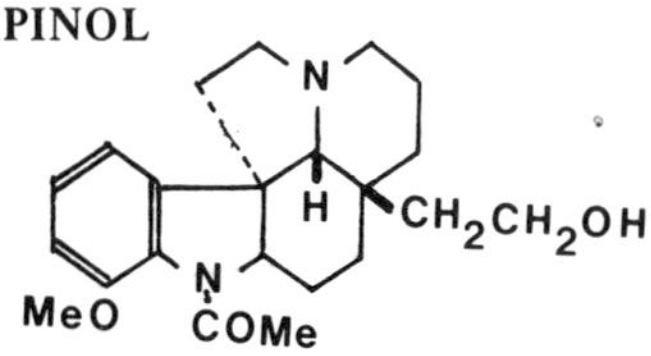

Aspidosperma cylindrocarpon yields this minor alkaloid which is obtained in the form of colourless needles. The structure has been confirmed by interconversion with Cylindrocarpinol (q.v.).

Milborrow, Djerassi., *J. Chem. Soc., C*, 417 (1969)

C-ACETYLCYPHOLOPHINE

$C_{20}H_{28}O_4N_2$

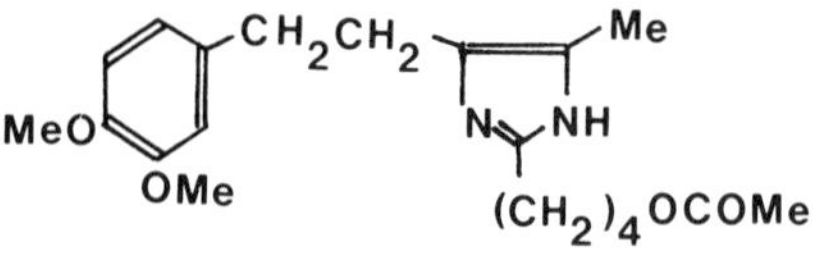

The minor constituent of *Cypholophus friesianus* (family Urticaceae), this base has the structure given above which has been confirmed by synthesis. Two methoxyl groups, a methyl group and an imino group are present, the second nitrogen atom being tertiary in character.

Hart *et al.*, *J. Chem. Soc., D*, 441 (1970)
Hart *et al.*, *Austral. J. Chem.*, **24**, 857 (1971)

ACETYLDEBENZOYLALOPECURINE

$C_{18}H_{27}O_3N$

M.p. 238–240°C

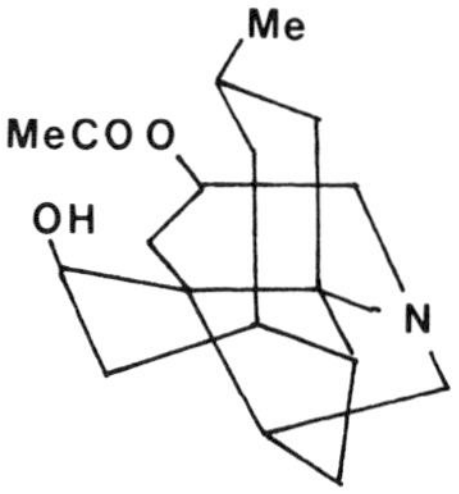

Lycopodium alopecuroides is particularly rich in alkaloids and this minor base is one of many which have been isolated from it. On acid hydrolysis, the alkaloid furnishes acetic acid and debenzoylalopecurine.

Ayer *et al., Can. J. Chem.*, **47**, 2449 (1969)

N-ACETYL-17-DEMETHOXYCYLINDROCARINE

$C_{22}H_{28}O_3N_2$

M.p. 160–2°C

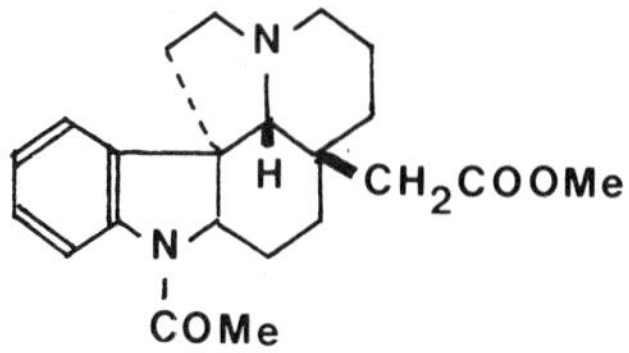

A further minor constituent of *Aspidosperma cylindrocarpon*, this alkaloid crystallizes as colourless needles which, in MeOH solution possesses the following specific rotations: $[\alpha]_D^{20} \pm 0°$ (c 0.001, MeOH); $[\alpha]_{300} - 800°$, $[\alpha]_{265} - 5400°$ and $[\alpha]_{240} + 8400°$. The ultraviolet spectrum is characteristic of the alkaloids having an indolizidinocarbazole structure with absorption maxima at 212, 250, 278 and 288 mμ. No salts or derivatives have been described.

Milborrow, Djerassi., *J. Chem. Soc.*, C, 417 (1969)

N-ACETYL-N-DEPROPIONYLASPIDOALBINE

$C_{23}H_{30}O_5N_2$

M.p. 194–5°C

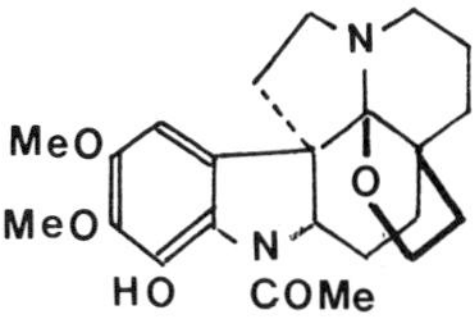

This alkaloid has been isolated from the stem bark of both *Aspidosperma album* and *A. spruceanum*. When recrystallized from $CHCl_3$ it forms colourless prisms and is strongly dextrorotatory with $[\alpha]_D + 174°$ (c 1.93, $CHCl_3$).

Ferrari, Marion, Palmer., *Can. J. Chem.*, **41**, 1531 (1963)
Gilbert *et al., Tetrahedron*, **21**, 1141 (1965)

ACETYLEVOXINE

$C_{20}H_{23}O_7N$

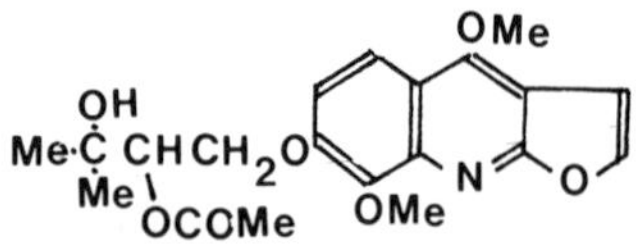

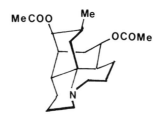

A recently isolated alkaloid, this base accompanies Evoxine (q.v.) in *Haplophyllum hispanicum*. The structure has been established by comparison with the already known Evoxine (q.v.).

Gonzalez *et al., An. Quim.*, **68**, 1133 (1972)

ACETYLFAWCETTIINE

$C_{20}H_{31}O_4N$

M.p. 116–7°C

This alkaloid is a minor constituent of *Lycopodium fawcettii* and forms colourless crystals from EtOH. Two acetyl groups are present in the molecule.

Burnell, *J. Chem. Soc.*, 3091 (1959)
Burnell, Mootoo, Taylor., *Can. J. Chem.*, **38**, 1927 (1960)
Burnell, Mootoo, Taylor., *ibid*, **39**, 1090 (1961)

17-ACETYLHENNINGSOLINE

$C_{24}H_{28}O_6N_2$

M.p. 280–2°C (*dec.*).

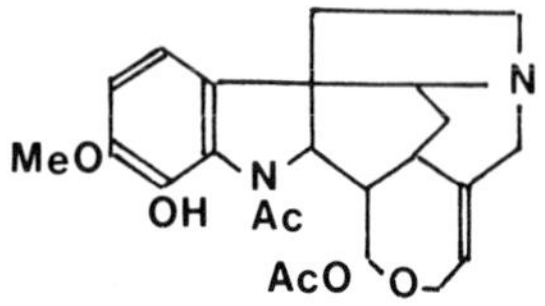

An alkaloid present in *Strychnos henningsii* Gilg., this base is laevorotatory with $[\alpha]_D^{23} - 190°$ (c 1.0, $CHCl_3$). The ultraviolet spectrum in EtOH exhibits absorption maxima at 208, 266 and 285 mμ.

Spiteller-Friedmann, Spiteller., *Annalen*, **712**, 179 (1968)

1-ACETYL-17-HYDROXYASPIDOALBINE

$C_{21}H_{26}O_3N_2$

M.p. Indefinite

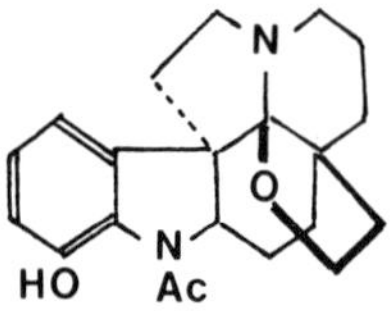

This amorphous alkaloid occurs in *Vallesia dichotoma* Ruiz et Pav and has no definite melting point. The ultraviolet spectrum in ethanol shows absorption maxima at 219, 257 and 290 mμ. The base may be characterized as the O-methyl ether which is crystalline with m.p. 237–9°C and $[\alpha]_D$ + 6° (CHCl$_3$).

Brown, Budzikiewicz, Djerassi., *Tetrahedron Lett.*, 1731 (1963)

N-ACETYL-11-HYDROXYASPIDOSPERMATIDINE

$C_{20}H_{24}O_2N_2$

M.p. Indefinite

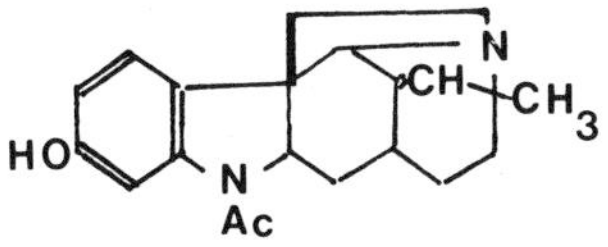

A minor constituent of *Aspidosperma compactinervium* Kuhlmann, this base is a non-crystallizable amorphous solid with no definite melting point. The characteristic ultraviolet spectrum shows four absorption maxima at 218, 252, 294 and 300 mμ.

Gilbert *et al.*, *Tetrahedron*, **21**, 1141 (1965)

ACETYLINDICINE

$C_{17}H_{26}O_5N$

M.p. Indefinite

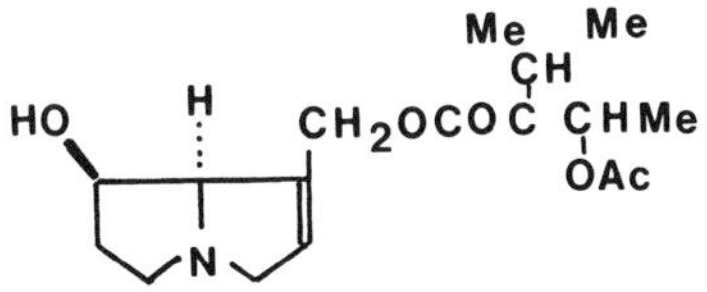

This alkaloid occurs in small amounts in *Heliotropium indicum* L. It is laevo-rotatory with $[\alpha]_D$ − 14.8° (EtOH). Two hydroxyl groups are present. The monoacetate is a colourless gum giving a crystalline picrate, m.p. 151–2°C and the diacetate is also non-crystallizable but forms a crystalline picrate, m.p. 131–2°C.

Mattocks., *J. Chem. Soc.*, C, 329 (1967)

ACETYLISOCORYNOLINE

$C_{23}H_{26}O_6N$

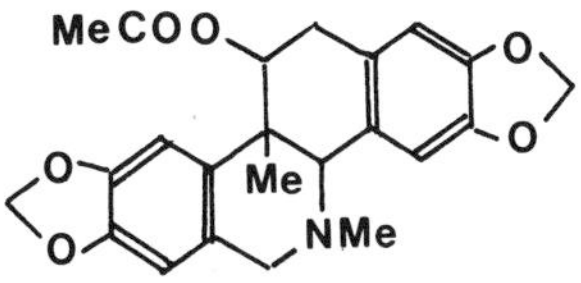

A further recently discovered minor alkaloid from *Corydalis incisa*, this alkaloid has been obtained only in small quantities and the structure determined by chemical and spectroscopic methods. No derivatives have yet been recorded.

Nonaka *et al.*, *J. Pharm. Soc., Japan*, **93**, 87 (1973)

N_a-ACETYLISOSTRYCHNOSPLENDINE

$C_{21}H_{26}O_3N_2$

M.p. 190–2°C

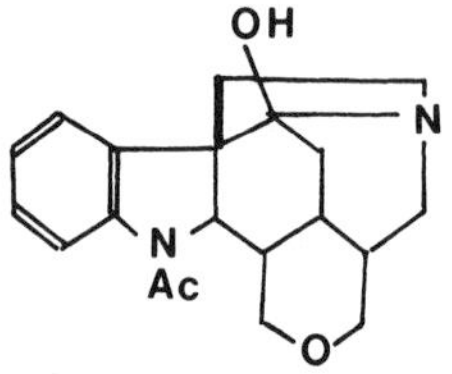

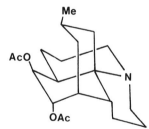

A minor alkaloid of *Strychnos splendens,* this base is obtained by extraction of the bark with a 3:1 Et_2O-$CHCl_3$ mixture. It is dextrorotatory with $[\alpha]_D^{20} + 125°$ (c 1.0, EtOH) and gives an ultraviolet spectrum having an absorption maximum at 250 mμ and a shoulder at 277 mμ. The structure has been determined mainly from the infrared and mass spectra of the small quantity of material available for examination.

Koch *et al., Bull. Soc. Chim. Fr.,* 8, 3250 (1968)

ACETYLLABURNINE

$C_{10}H_{17}O_2N$

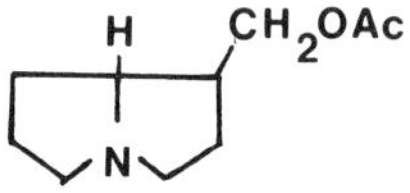

This alkaloid occurs in *Vanda cristata* and has been identified by comparison with a synthetic specimen. The alkaloid is stable and may be gas chromatographed without decomposition unlike the parent pyrrolizidine carbinol which is extremely sensitive to these conditions.

Lindstrom, Lüning., *Acta Chem. Scand.,* 23, 3352 (1969)

ACETYLLYCOCLAVINE

$C_{19}H_{31}O_4N$

M.p. 144–5°C

First isolated from *Lycopodium clavatum* var. *megastachyon* Fern. et Bissel, this alkaloid also occurs in other *Lycopodium* species as a minor component. It yields colourless crystals from light petroleum and contains two acetyl groups and a methyl group.

Ayer, Law., *Can. J. Chem.,* 40, 2088 (1962)

O-ACETYLLYCOFAWCINE (*Base O*)

$C_{20}H_{31}O_5N$

M.p. 181–2°C

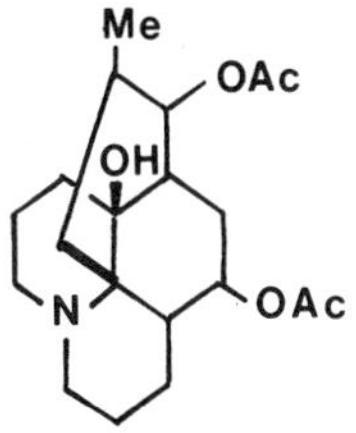

One of several alkaloids present in *Lycopodium fawcettii*, the base contains two acetyl groups and a tertiary hydroxyl group in the molecule. The structure has been established from spectroscopic evidence, particularly the mass spectral fragmentation pattern.

Burnell, Mootoo, Taylor., *Can. J. Chem.*, **38**, 1927 (1960)
Burnell *et al., ibid*, **41**, 3091 (1963)
Structure:
Ayer *et al., Can. J. Chem.*, **43**, 328 (1965)

7-ACETYLLYCOFOLINE (*Base M*)

$C_{18}H_{27}O_3N$

M.p. Indefinite

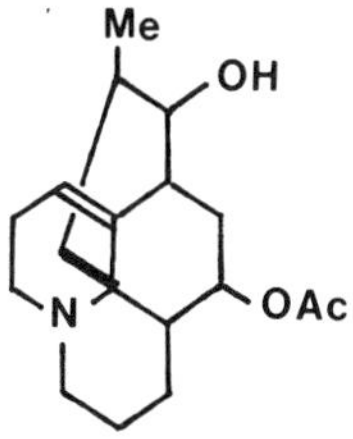

An amorphous alkaloid found in *Lycopodium fawcettii,* this base is laevorotatory with $[\alpha]_D - 61°$ (c 1.1, EtOH). An acetyl group, a methyl group and a secondary hydroxyl group have been shown to be present.

Anet, Khan., *Can. J. Chem.*, **37**, 1589 (1959)
Anet *et al., ibid*, **40**, 236 (1962)

O-ACETYLMACRANTHINE

$C_{18}H_{21}O_6N$

M.p. 222–4°C

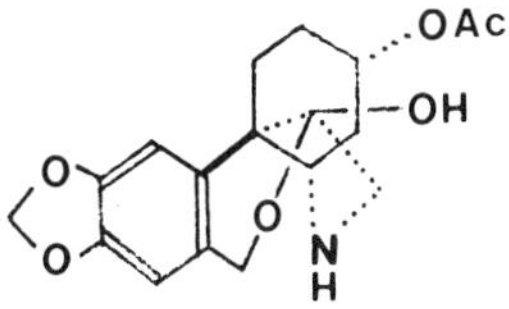

A minor base of *Crinium macrantherum* Engl., this alkaloid yields colourless crystals from Me CO and has $[\alpha]_D^{22} - 26°$ (c 0.213, CHCl$_3$) or $+ 18°$ (c 0.213, EtOH). The structure has been determined from the infrared, ultraviolet and mass spectra and comparison with Macranthine (q.v.).

Hauth, Stauffacher., *Helv. Chim. Acta.*, **47**, 185 (1964)

N-ACETYLMESCALINE

$C_{13}H_{19}O_4N$

M.p. 93–4°C

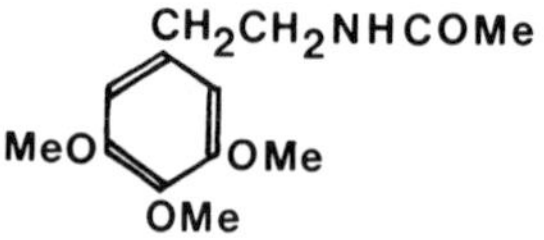

CH₂CH₂NHCOMe structure: CH$_2$CH$_2$NHCOMe on benzene ring with MeO, OMe, OMe substituents

One of several closely related alkaloids found in *Anhalonium Lewinii* Hennings, this base possesses hallucinogenic properties similar to those of Mescaline (q.v.).

Späth, Brück., *Monatsh.*, **71**, 1275 (1938)

O-ACETYLMESEMBRENOL

$C_{19}H_{25}O_3N$

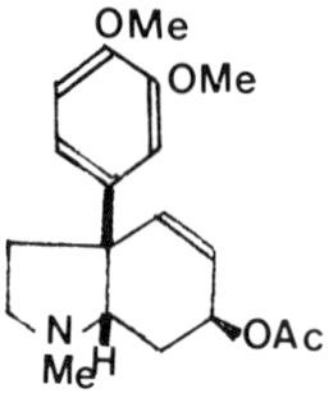

Sceletium strictum yields a number of minor alkaloids having similar structures. This base has been shown to possess the above structure from spectroscopic techniques, particularly from the NMR spectrum.

Jeffs *et al.*, *J. Org. Chem.*, **35**, 3512 (1970)

1-ACETYL-16-METHYLASPIDOSPERMIDINE

$C_{22}H_{30}ON_2$

M.p. Indefinite

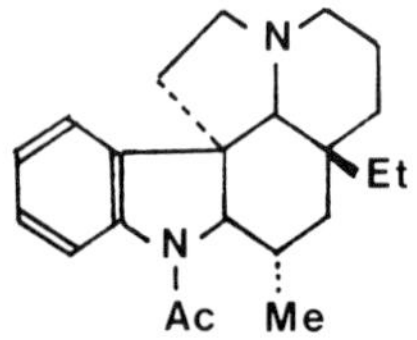

This alkaloid occurs only in minute traces in the bark extract of *Aspidosperma compactinervium* Kuhlmann. It forms a transparent glassy mass with no sharp melting point. All attempts to crystallize the material have so far failed. The following salts and derivatives have been prepared to characterize the base: perchlorate, m.p. 286–7°C (*dec.*); picrate, m.p. 235–6°C (*dec.*); 4-methiodide, m.p. 262–4°C (*dec.*) and the 4-methopicrate, m.p. 239–240°C (*dec.*). The crystal structure of the 4-methiodide has been determined by means of single-crystal X-ray analysis.

Barton, Harley-Mason., *Chem. Commun.*, 298 (1965)
Crystal structure:
Kennard *et al.*, *ibid*, 1286 (1967)

O-ACETYLMONTANINE

$C_{19}H_{19}O_5N$

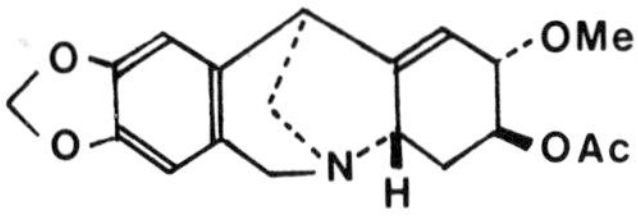

A trace constituent of the bulbs of *Rhodophiala bifida,* this alkaloid yields a crystalline hydrochloride, m.p. 210–3°C. Mild hydrolysis of the free base furnishes acetic acid and Montanine (q.v.).

Wildman *et al., Pharmazie,* **22**, 725 (1967)

3-ACETYLNERBOWDINE

$C_{18}H_{23}O_6N$

M.p. 207–9°C

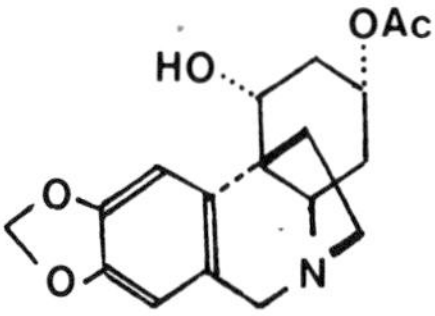

This isoquinoline alkaloid occurs in *Buphane disticha* (L.F.) Herb. It forms colourless needles when recrystallized from Et_2O and is laevorotatory with $[\alpha]_D^{21} - 116°$ (c 0.4, $CHCl_3$) or $- 45°$ (c 0.4, EtOH).

Hauth, Stauffacher., *Helv. Chim. Acta,* **44**, 491 (1961)
Hauth, Stauffacher., *ibid,* **46**, 810 (1963)

ACETYLPLATYDESMINE

$C_{17}H_{19}O_4N$

M.p. 126–7°C

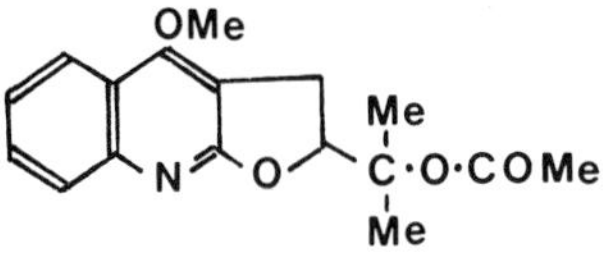

The milled, dried leaves of *Geijera salicifolia* Schutt. yield this base which forms colourless needles from $CHCl_3$. It has $[\alpha]_D + 23°$ (c 1.8, $CHCl_3$) and gives a picrate as yellow needles from EtOH with m.p. 150–1°C. Alkaline hydrolysis furnishes acetic acid and Platydesmine (q.v.).

Johns, Lamberton., *Austral. J. Chem.,* **19**, 1991 (1966)
Boyd, Grundon., *Tetrahedron Lett.,* 2637 (1967)

ACETYLPORANTHERICINE

$C_{17}H_{29}O_2N$

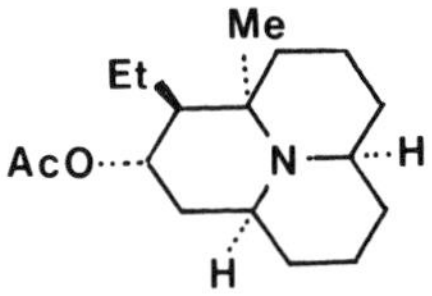

This alkaloid from *Poranthera corymbosa* is a colourless oil which is only slightly dextrorotatory with $[\alpha]_D + 2°$ (c 1.6, $CHCl_3$). An ethyl group and a bridge methyl group are present as substituents in the molecule in addition to the acetyl group.

Dernie *et al.*, *Tetrahedron Lett.*, 1767 (1972)

ACETYLSENKIRKINE

$C_{21}H_{29}O_7N$

M.p. 195–6°C

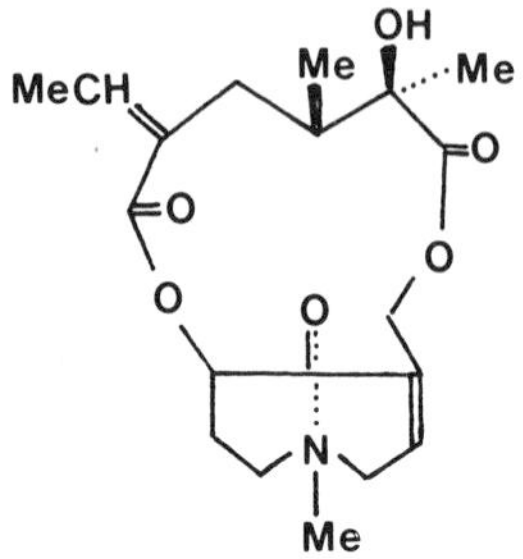

In addition to Senkirkine (q.v.), the leaves of *Senecio kirkii* yield this alkaloid which forms colourless needles from AcOEt-Me$_2$CO. The base has $[\alpha]_D^{25} - 34°$ (c 0.44, MeOH) and the ultraviolet spectrum has a single absorption maximum at 218 mμ. The aurichloride has m.p. 108–9°C; picrate, m.p. 208–9°C and the picrolonate, m.p. 222°C.

Briggs, Mangan, Russell., *J. Chem. Soc.*, 1891 (1948)
Danilova, Konovalova., *J. Gen. Chem., USSR,* **20,** 1921 (1961)
Briggs *et al., J. Chem. Soc.,* 2492 (1965)

ACETYLTABASCANINE

$C_{26}H_{34}O_7N_2$

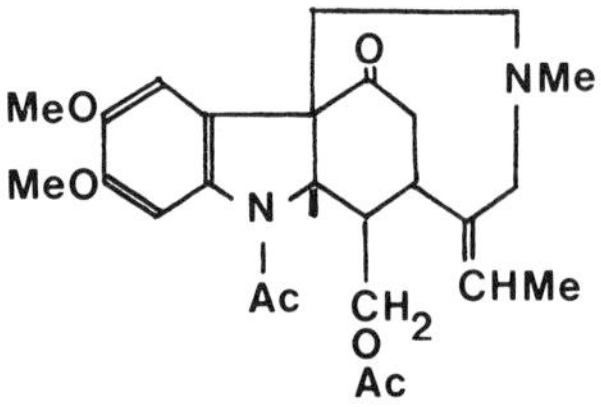

This alkaloid has recently been isolated from *Strychnos tabascana*. The structure has been determined by chemical and spectroscopic means.

Galeffi *et al., Farmaco, Ed. Sci.,* **26,** 1100 (1971)

O-ACETYLYOHIMBINE

$C_{23}H_{28}O_4N_2$

M.p. 150°C

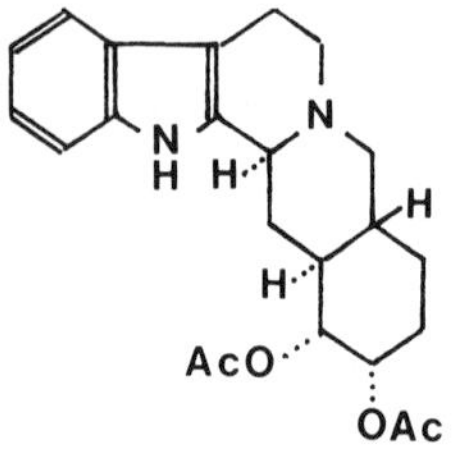

This derivative of yohimbine was prepared synthetically before its discovery as a naturally-occurring alkaloid in *Aspidosperma excelsum*. The base is freely soluble in EtOH, Et_2O and $CHCl_3$ and exhibits a green fluorescence in solution.

Benoin, Burnell, Medina., *Can. J. Chem.*, **45**, 725 (1967)

ACHILLEINE

The presence of this alkaloid in *Achillea millefolium* and *A. moschata* has been reported. It is stated to be an amorphous solid which, on alkaline hydrolysis yields achilletine, $C_{11}H_{17}O_4N$, also amorphous, NH_3 and a reducing sugar.

Zanon., *Annalen.*, **58**, 21 (1846)
von Planta., *ibid*, **155**, 153 (1870)

ACONIFINE

$C_{33}H_{47}O_{10}N$

This aconite alkaloid has only recently been isolated from *Aconitum karakolicum* together with the allied alkaloids karakoline and karakolidine (q.v.). The structure has been determined primarily on the basis of mass spectrometry and NMR evidence.

Sultankhodzaev, Yusunov, Yusunov., *Khim. Prir. Soedin.*, **9**, 127 (1973)

ACONITINE

$C_{34}H_{47}O_{11}N$

M.p. 202–4°C

This base is the most important and one of the most complex of all the aconite alkaloids. It is found in *A. Fauriei, A. grossedentatum, A. hakusanense, A. ibukiense, A. Majimai, A. mokchangense, A. Napellus* L., *A. sachaliense, A. subcuneatum, A. tianchicum, A. tortuosum* and *A. Zuccarini*. From $CHCl_3$, the base crystallizes in rhombic prisms (a:b:c = 0.54491:1:0.38917); $[\alpha]_D + 14.61°$ ($CHCl_3$). It is freely soluble in $CHCl_3$ or C_6H_6, less so in EtOH or Et_2O and virtually insoluble in H_2O or light petroleum.

15

All of the salts are laevorotatory. The hydrochloride (3.5 H_2O) has m.p. 149°C or 194–5°C (*dry*); the hydrobromide (2.5 H_2O) forms hexagonal tablets from H_2O, m.p. 207°C after drying at 120°C or clusters of fine needles with 0.5 H_2O from Et_2O, m.p. 206–7°C; the hydriodide, m.p. 226°C; the perchlorate, m.p. 216–222°C and the aurichloride which, according to Jowett, exists in three modification with m.p. 135°C (*dec.*), 152°C and 176°C respectively.

Hydrolysis of the base with dilute acids yields acetic acid and benzoylaconine, $C_{32}H_{45}O_{10}N$, m.p. 130°C which also forms crystalline salts, e.g. the hydrochloride, two forms m.p. 217°C and 270°C; the hydrobromide, m.p. 273°C and the hydriodide, m.p. 205°C.

Alkaline hydrolysis gives acetic and benzoic acids and aconine, $C_{25}H_{41}O_9N$, m.p. indefinite. The salts of aconine are not only difficult to crystallize but also hygroscopic; hydrochloride, m.p. 176°C and hydrobromide, m.p. 225°C.

Oxidation of aconitine with $KMnO_4$ furnishes acetaldehyde and oxonitine, $C_{34}H_{45}O_{12}N$, m.p. 279–284°C together with oxoaconitine, $C_{34}H_{43}O_{12}N$, m.p. ·266–272°C. With chromic acid, the alkaloid yields aconitoline, $C_{33}H_{41}O_{10}N$, m.p. 220°C and aconitinone, $C_{33}H_{41}O_{10}N$, m.p. 150°C (*dec.*). The action of fuming HNO_3 on aconitine gives mainly the nitronitroso-derivative, $C_{31}H_{35}O_{13}N_3$, m.p. 268°C (*dec.*).

Distillation of the alkaloid with $Ba(OH)_2$ or Zn dust gives a nitrogen-free product, $C_{19}H_{24}O$, b.p. 215–220°C.

Geiger, Hesse., *Annalen, 7*, 276 (1833)
von Planta., *ibid, 74*, 257 (1850)
Groves., *Pharm. J., 8*, 121 (1860)
Jowett., *J. Chem. Soc., 63*, 994 (1893)
Schultz., *Arch. Pharm., 246*, 281 (1908)
Carr., *J. Chem. Soc., 101*, 2241 (1912)
Jacobs, Elderfield., *Tetrahedron Lett., 58*, 1059 (1936)
Lawson., *J. Chem. Soc., 80* (1936)
Jacobs, Elderfield, Craig., *J. Biol. Chem., 128*, 439 (1939)
Konovalova, Orekhov., *Bull. Soc. Khim., 7*, 95 (1940)
Jacobs, Craig., *J. Biol. Chem., 136*, 323 (1940)
Majima, Tamura., *Annalen, 545*, 1 (1940)
Edwards, Marion., *Can. J. Chem., 20*, 627 (1952)
Jacobs, Pelletier., *J. Amer. Chem. Soc., 76*, 4048 (1954)
Wiesner *et al., Tetrahedron Lett., 2*, 15 (1959)
Przybylska, Marion., *Can. J. Chem., 37*, 1116 (1959)
Przybylska, Marion., *ibid, 37*, 1843 (1959)
Bachelor, Brown, Büchi., *Tetrahedron Lett., 10*, 1 (1960)

ACONOSINE

$C_{22}H_{35}O_4N$

M.p. 148°C

One of the minor aconite alkaloids, this base occurs in *Acotinum nasutum*. It is laevorotatory with $[\alpha]_D^{20} - 21°$ (c 1.0, MeOH). No salts or derivatives have yet been prepared.

Murav'eva, Plakhanova, Yusunov., *Khim. Prir. Soedin., 8*, 128 (1972)

ACRIFOLINE (*Alkaloid L-27*)

$C_{16}H_{25}O_2N$

M.p. 97–104°C

One of the numerous family of the *Lycopodium* alkaloids, this base occurs in *L. acrifolium* and *L. annotinum* var. *acrifolium* Fern. The alkaloid yields colourless needles and gives crystalline salts including the hydriodide, m.p. 259°C (*dec.*); nitrate, m.p. 236°C (*dec.*); perchlorate, m.p. 266°C and the methiodide, m.p. 281°C.

Manske, Marion., *J. Amer. Chem. Soc.*, 69, 2126 (1947)

ACRONIDINE

$C_{18}H_{17}O_4N$

M.p. 151–3°C

One of the alkaloids of the leaves of *Acronychia baueri*, this base is optically inactive in $CHCl_3$. It forms a crystalline hydrochloride, m.p. 320°C (*dec.*) and a picrate, m.p. 216–8°C. Oxidation with $KMnO_4$ gives α-hydroxy*iso*butyric acid. When refluxed with alcoholic HCl it furnishes *nor*acronidine, $C_{17}H_{17}O_4N$, m.p. 256–7°C, giving an acetyl derivative, m.p. 212–4°C. Hydrogenation with Raney Ni yields the tetrahydro derivative, m.p. 192.5–194.5°C and a dihydro compound shown to be a dihydropyranoquinoline, m.p. 225–7°C.

Lamberton, Price., *Austral. J. Chem.*, 6, 66 (1953)

ACRONYCIDINE

$C_{15}H_{15}O_5N$

M.p. 136.5–137.5°C

A furoquinoline alkaloid present in the bark of *Melicope fareana*, the base is obtained as colourless prisms or needles when crystallized from MeOH. It may be characterized as the hydrochloride, m.p. 120–1°C or the picrate, m.p. 181–182.5°C. The structure has been shown, by spectroscopic methods, to be 4:5:7:8-tetramethoxyfuro-2,3-b-quinoline.

Hughes *et al., Nature*, 162, 223 (1948)
Lahey, Lamberton, Price., *Austral. J. Sci. Res.*, 3A, 155 (1950)

ACRONYCINE

$C_{20}H_{19}O_3N$

M.p. 175°C

A further base found in *Acronychia baueri,* the alkaloid forms light yellow needles from absolute EtOH. It is readily soluble in most organic solvents but insoluble in H_2O. The salts, which are all coloured, are readily obtained in a crystalline form and include the hydrochloride, red needles from H_2O, m.p. 125–130°C (*dec.*); sulphate as masses of small red crystals, m.p. 158–9°C; picrate, orange crystals, m.p. 150–4°C and the mononitro derivative, pale yellow plates from EtOAc, m.p. 222°C. Two possible structures have been proposed for this alkaloid, the linear and angular forms, of which the latter has been shown to be correct by synthesis by three interrelated routes. The base possesses a broad-spectrum antitumour activity against experimental neoplasts.

Brown *et al., Austral. J. Sci. Res.,* **A2**, 622 (1949)
Drummond, Lahey., *ibid,* **A2**, 630 (1949)
Structure:
MacDonald, Robertson, *Austral. J. Chem.,* **19**, 275 (1966)
Govindachari, Pai, Subramaniam, *Tetrahedron,* **22**, 3245 (1966)
Synthesis:
Beck *et al., J. Amer. Chem. Soc.,* **89**, 3934 (1967)
Beck *et al., ibid,* **90**, 4706 (1968)
Antitumour activity:
Svoboda *et al., J. Pharm. Sci.,* **55**, 758 (1966)

ACROPHYLLIDINE

$C_{17}H_{19}O_4N$

M.p. 177–8°C

One of two closely-related alkaloids isolated from the bark of *Acronychia haplophylla,* this furoquinoline base yields colourless needles from EtOH and exhibits absorption maxima in the ultraviolet spectrum typical of these alkaloids at 227, 261.5 and 320–325 mμ. There are also conspicuous shoulders present at 253, 257.5 and 290 mμ.

Lahey, McCamish., *Tetrahedron Lett.,* **12**, 1525 (1968)
Lahey, McCamish, McEwan., *Austral. J. Chem.,* **22**, 447 (1969)

ACROPHYLLINE

$C_{17}H_{17}O_3N$

M.p. 120°C

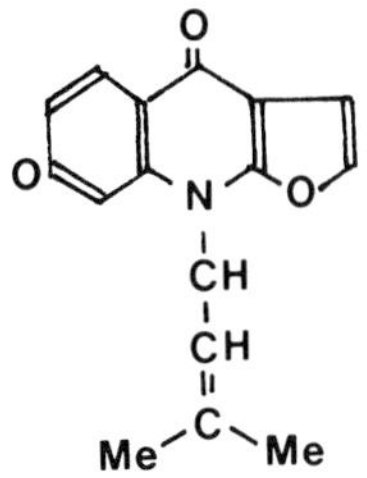

This alkaloid has also been isolated from the bark of *Acronychia haplophylla* and has a furoquinolone structure similar to the preceding base. It forms a crystalline hydrochloride, m.p. 195–6°C and a picrate, m.p. 180–2°C. The ultraviolet spectrum in EtOH is almost identical with that of acrophyllidine with absorption maxima at 261 and 320–325 mμ and shoulders at 253, 257.5 and 290 mμ. In 0.2 N-HCl solution, the peak at 320 mμ remains but a new peak appears at 249 mμ. Reduction of the base with PtO$_2$ gives hexahydroacrophylline, m.p. 174°C which has also been synthesized from *m*-anisidine.

Lahey, McCamish., *Tetrahedron Lett.*, 1525 (1968)
Lahey, McCamish, McEwan., *Austral. J. Chem.*, 22, 447 (1969)
Prabhakar, Pai, Ramachandran., *Ind. J. Chem.*, 8, 857 (1970)

ACTINIDINE

$C_{10}H_{13}N$

B.p. 100–3°C/9 mm.

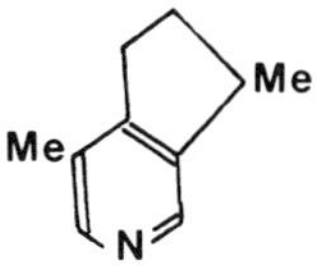

From the leaves and gall of *Actinidia polygama*, this base is obtained as an oil with $[\alpha]_D^{11} - 7.2°$ (c 17.54, CHCl$_3$). The crystalline picrate forms colourless needles, m.p. 143°C. (±)-actinidine may be crystallized and has m.p. 142–3°C; b.p. 100–3°C/12 mm. The picrate of this base forms needles from Et$_2$O with m.p. 139–140°C.

Sakan *et al.*, *Bull. Chem. Soc. Japan*, 32, 315 (1959)
Sakan *et al.*, *ibid*, 32, 1155 (1959)
Djerassi *et al.*, *Chem. & Ind.*, 210 (1961)

(+)-ACTINODAPHNINE

$C_{18}H_{17}O_4N$

M.p. 210–1°C

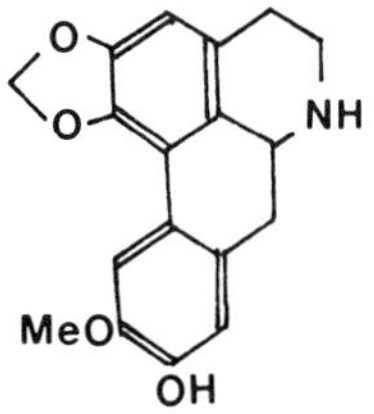

The dextrorotatory form of this aporphine alkaloid is found in the bark of

Actinodaphne hookeri and forms colourless needles from EtOH. It is freely soluble in most organic solvents although only moderately so in ether and insoluble in H_2O. It has $[\alpha]_D^{20} + 32.77°$ (EtOH). Several crystalline salts and derivatives have been prepared: hydrochloride, fine needles from Et_2O/EtOH, m.p. 280–1°C (*dec.*); $[\alpha]_D^{20} + 8.75°$ (H_2O); hydriodide, colourless needles when crystallized from EtOH, m.p. 264–5°C (*dec.*); sulphate (trihydrate) as colourless needles from aqueous EtOH, m.p. 249–250°C (*anhyd., dec.*); picrate (mono-hydrate) as fine needles from aqueous EtOH, m.p. 220–2°C (*dec.*); methiodide, m.p. 243–4°C; benzoyl derivative, m.p. 232–3°C and the acetate, colourless prisms from ethyl acetate, m.p. 229–230°C.

(±)-actinodaphnine has been characterized as the crystalline methyl ether, m.p. 114–5°C.

Krishna, Ghose., *J. Ind. Chem. Soc.*, **9**, 429 (1932)
Ghose, Krishna, Schlittler., *Helv. Chim. Acta.*, **17**, 919 (1934)
Hey, Lobo., *J. Chem. Soc.*, 2246 (1954)

ACUTINE

$C_{16}H_{19}ON$

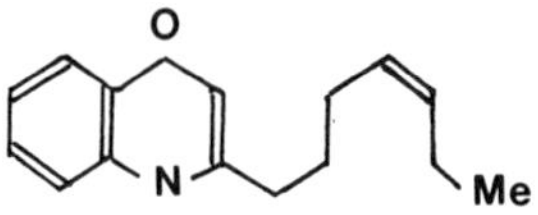

This alkaloid is present in the above ground parts of *Haplophyllum acutifolium*. The above structure has been determined by infrared, ultraviolet, NMR and mass spectroscopy. Hydrogenation gives the dihydro-derivative, $C_{16}H_{21}ON$ which has been synthesized by the acid catalyzed condensation of $CH_3.(CH_2)_6.COCH_2CO.OCH_3$ with aniline followed by subsequent ring closure in refluxing diphenyl ether.

Razzakova, Bessonova, Yunusov, Yu., *Khim. Prir. Soedin.*, 206 (1973)

ACUTUMIDINE

$C_{18}H_{22}O_6NCl$

M.p. 239–241°C (*dec.*).

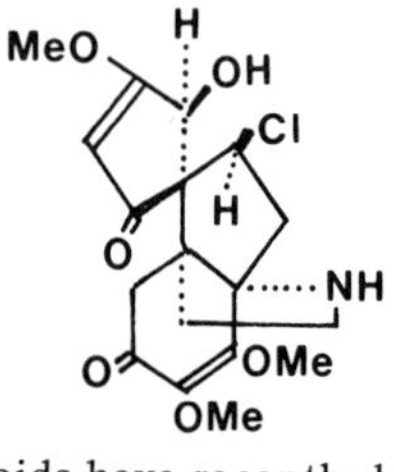

Three chlorine-containing alkaloids have recently been isolated from the leaves of *Menispermum dauricum* and *Sinomenium acutum* Rehd et Wils, of which acutumidine is one. The base is laevorotatory, $[\alpha]_D - 212°$ (pyridine). It contains three methoxyl groups and one hydroxyl group. The structure and absolute configuration have been determined from NMR, infrared, ultraviolet and mass spectroscopy.

Tomita, Okamoto, Kiluchi, Osaki, Nishikawa, Kamiya, Sasaki, Matoba, Goto., *Tetrahedron Lett.*, 2421, 2425 (1967)
Tomita, Okamoto, Kilichi, Osaki, Nishikawa, Kamiya, Sasaki, Matoba, Goto., *ibid*, 769 (1968)

ACUTUMINE (*N-Methylacutumidine*)

$C_{19}H_{24}O_6NCl$

M.p. 238–240°C (*dec.*).

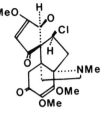

A second base obtained from the leaf extract of *Menispermum dauricum* and *Sinomenium acutum* Rehd. et Wils, this alkaloid is also laevorotatory with $[\alpha]_D - 206°$ (pyridine). A solution of the alkaloid in EtOH gives an ultraviolet spectrum with absorption maxima at 245 and 270 mμ.

Goto, Sudzuki., *Bull. Chem. Soc. Japan*, 4, 220 (1929)
Biosynthesis:
Barton, Kirby, Kirby., *J. Chem. Soc., C*, 929 (1968)
Crystal structure:
Tomita, Okamoto, Kiluchi, Osaki, Matoba, Nishikawa, Kamiya, Sasaki, Goto., *Tetrahedron Lett.*, 2421, 2425 (1967)
Tomita, Okamoto, Kiluchi, Osaki, Nishikawa, Kamiya, Sasaki, Matoba, Goto., *ibid*, 769 (1968)
Nishikawa, Kamiya, Tomita, Okamoto, Kiluchi, Osaki, Tomiie, Nitta, Goto., *J. Chem. Soc., B*, 652 (1968)

ACUTUMININE

$C_{19}H_{24}O_5NCl$

M.p. 175–177.5°C

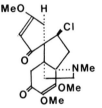

The third chlorine-containing alkaloid is found in the leaves of *Menispermum dauricum* and, like the two preceding bases, is laevorotatory with $[\alpha]_D - 110°$ (CHCl$_3$). The ultraviolet spectrum is almost identical with that of Acutumine, with absorption maxima occurring at 246 and 272 mμ. Information from the NMR, infrared, ultraviolet and mass spectra have provided the above structure.

Okamoto *et al.*, *Tetrahedron Lett.*, 1933 (1969)

ADALINE

$C_{13}H_{23}ON$

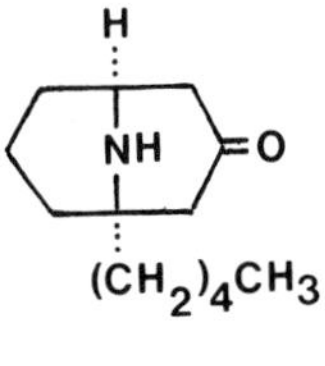

This novel alkaloid has been isolated from the arthropod *Adalia bipunctata* (family Coccinellidae). The structure had been determined from chemical and spectroscopic data and confirmed by synthesis and X-ray analysis of the crystalline hydrochloride. The crystals of the latter have space group $P2_1$ with $a = 11.20$, $b = 8.90$, $c = 7.60$ Å and $109.9°$

Tursch *et al.*, *Tetrahedron Lett.*, 201 (1973)

Synthesis:

Tursch *et al.*, *Bull. Soc. Chim. Belg.*, **82**, 699 (1973)

(+)-ADENOCARPINE (*Teidine*)

$C_{19}H_{24}ON_2$

M.p. Indefinite

The presence of unidentified alkaloids has been recorded in *Adenocarpus hispanicus* and *A. intermedius* but it is only comparatively recently that this base and the optically inactive form have been isolated and characterized as major components of several *Adenocarpus* species. (+)-Adenocarpine is obtained in the form of a viscous oil which slowly solidifies without crystallization. It has $[\alpha]_D^{18} + 29.3°$ (EtOH) and may be hydrolyzed by dilute H_2SO_4 to *trans*-cinnamic acid. Several crystalline salts and derivatives have been prepared including the hydrochloride, m.p. 203–4°C; $[\alpha]_D^{20} + 56.2°$ (EtOH); hydrobromide, obtained as the dihydrate from H_2O, m.p. 192°C and anhydrous from MeOH, m.p. 205°C; hydriodide, m.p. 204°C; perchlorate, m.p. 159–160°C; picrate, m.p. 213°C and the N-*p*-toluenesulphonyl derivative which forms pale yellow needles from EtOH, m.p. 169–170°C. Reaction with bromine shows the presence of unsaturation in the molecule. The (−)- form of the base is also a resin with $[\alpha]_D^{18} - 30.0°$ (EtOH), forming a hydrochloride as colourless crystals, m.p. 204–5°C; $[\alpha]_D^{20} - 53.3°$ (EtOH).

Santos Ruiz, Llorente., *Anales, real. soc. espan. fis. y chim.*, **37**, 624 (1941)
Rivas, *ibid*, **38**, 197 (1942)
Rivas, Talarid., *Mon. farm. y terap.* (Madrid), **56**, 377 (1950)
Gonzales, Gonzales, Cartaya., *Anales, real. soc. espan. fis. y chim.*, **49B**, 783 (1953)
Rivas, Mendez., *ibid*, **51B**, 55 (1955)

(±)-ADENOCARPINE (*Orensine*)

$C_{19}H_{24}ON_2$

M.p. Indefinite

This base has only been found in *Adenocarpus commutatus* and is also resinous, all attempts to obtain it in a crystalline form having failed. The salts, however, are crystalline, e.g. the hydrochloride which forms a dihydrate, m.p. 82–3°C, the anhydrous form having m.p. 208–210°C. A crystalline hydriodide monohydrate is also known, m.p. 133–4°C and the picrate, m.p. 210–1°C.

Rivas, Costa., *Ann. pharm. franc.*, **10**, 54 (1952)
Schöpf, Kreibich., *Naturwiss.*, **41**, 335 (1954)

ADIANTIFOLINE

$C_{42}H_{50}O_9N_2$

M.p. 143.5–144°C

This alkaloid is of the bisbenzyl*iso*quinoline type and forms yellow needles from absolute EtOH. It is isolated from the non-phenolic tertiary alkaloidal fraction of the root and aerial portions of *Thalictrum minus* var. *adiantifolium*. The base is dextrorotatory with $[\alpha]_D^{28} + 90°$ (c 0.11, MeOH) and has an ultraviolet spectrum which is virtually identical with that of Thalicarpine (q.v.), of which it is the O-methyl ether. This structure is confirmed by the NMR spectrum in deutero-chloroform which is similar to that of thalicarpine except for the presence of an additional methoxyl group and the absence of one aromatic proton.

Doskotch, Schiff, Beal., *Tetrahedron Lett.*, **48**, 4999 (1968)

ADIFOLINE

$C_{22}H_{20}O_7N_2$

M.p. 350°C

The original formula proposed for this alkaloid of $C_{22}H_{20}O_8N_2$ has recently been revised to that given above. The base is present in the heartwood of Adina cordifolia and forms yellow prisms or needles from AcOH or EtOH respectively. On methylation, the alkaloid yields trimethyladifoline, $C_{25}H_{26}O_7N_2$, while acetylation furnishes the diacetate which can be further methylated to yield methyladifoline diacetate indicative of the presence of two phenolic or enolic groups and a carboxylic acid group in the molecule. The base also readily undergoes dehydration to give anhydroadifoline, $C_{22}H_{18}O_6N_2$, m.p. 198–200°C which, with CH_2N_2, furnishes dimethylanhydroadifoline. The relative configuration of the alkaloid has been determined from the study of the NMR coupling constants by comparison with calculated dihedral angles from Dreiding models.

Cross, King, King., *J. Chem. Soc.*, 2714 (1961)
Brown *et al.*, *Chem. Commun.*, 350 (1968)

ADIRUBINE

$C_{22}H_{28}O_5N_2$

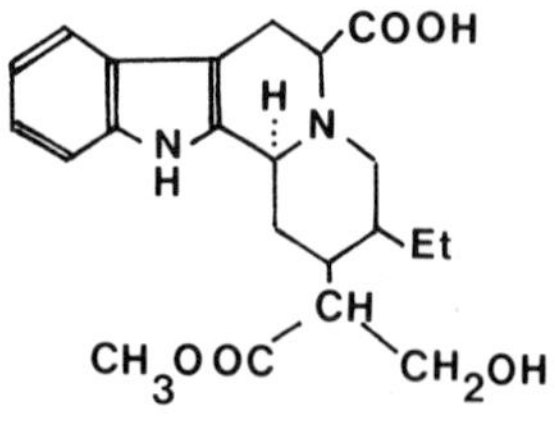

This base has recently been isolated from *Adina rubescens* and is characterized by the crystalline acetate, m.p. 151–4°C; $[\alpha]_D^{25} - 19°$ (CHCl$_3$). The presence of a carboxylic acid group is indicated by the infrared spectrum.

Brown, Chapple, Lee., *Chem. Commun.*, 1007 (1972)

ADLUMICEINE

$C_{22}H_{25}O_7N$

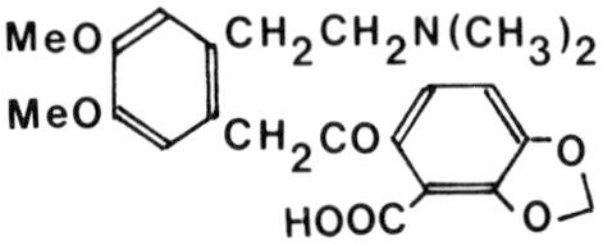

An alkaloid of *Corydalis sempervirens* and *Papaver rhoeas*, this base has the structure given above as determined by infrared, NMR and mass spectrometry.

Preininger *et al.*, *Phytochem.*, **12**, 2513 (1973)

ADLUMINE

$C_{21}H_{21}O_6N$

M.p. 180°C

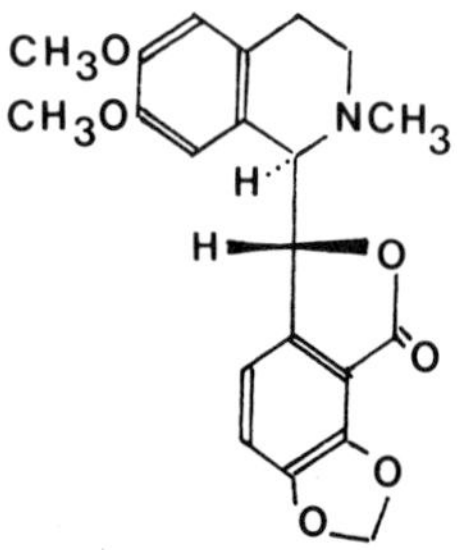

In 1900, Schlotterbeck isolated an alkaloid from *Adlumia cirrhosa* Rap, $C_{39}H_{41}O_{12}N$, m.p. 188°C to which the name Adlumine was given. This base was subsequently shown by Manske to be possibly a mixture of adlumine and Bicucculine (q.v.). Adlumine is present in *A. fungosa* Greene which is almost certainly identical with *A. cirrhosa*. The alkaloid has $[\alpha]_D^{22} + 42.5°$ (CHCl$_3$). Oxidation with HNO$_3$ yields 2-carboxy-3:4-methylenedioxybenzaldehyde and 4:5-dimethoxy-2α-methylaminobenzaldehyde.

Schlotterbeck., *Amer. Chem. J.*, **24**, 249 (1900)
Manske., *Can. J. Chem.*, 8, 210, 404 (1933)
Manske., *ibid*, **16B**, 89 (1938)

24

ADLUMIDINE

$C_{19}H_{15}O_6N$

M.p. 238°C

The adlumidine obtained by Schlotterbeck from *Adlumia cirrhosa* Rap. with the formula $C_{30}H_{29}O_9N$, m.p. 234°C has been stated by Manske to be identical with the present base which occurs in *Corydalis thalictrifolia* Franch as well as in *A. cirrhosa* Rap. No methoxyl groups are present in this alkaloid.

Schlotterbeck., *Amer. Chem. J.*, **24**, 249 (1900)
Manske., *Can. J. Chem.*, **8**, 210, 404 (1933)
Manske., *ibid*, **16B**, 89 (1938)

ADOUETIN X (*Ceanothamine B*)

$C_{28}H_{44}O_4N_4$

M.p. 277–9°C

This alkaloid is a member of the peptide class of bases and occurs in *Waltheria americana*. It yields clusters of colourless crystals when recrystallized from dioxan and is strongly laevorotatory having $[\alpha]_D - 316°$ (CHCl$_3$). It has recently been shown to be identical with Ceanothamine B which is present in the root bark of *Ceanothus americanus*. According to Warnhoff and his colleagues, the latter base forms slender colourless needles from CH$_2$Cl$_2$-AcOEt, m.p. 279–280.5°C; $[\alpha]_D^{25} - 370°$ (c 0.205, CHCl$_3$).

Warnhoff, Pradham, Ma., *Can. J. Chem.*, **43**, 2594 (1965)
Servis, Kosak., *J. Amer. Chem. Soc.*, **90**, 4179, 6895 (1968)
Pais *et al.*, *Bull. Soc. Chim. Fr.*, 1145 (1968)

ADOUETIN Y

$C_{34}H_{40}O_4N_4$

M.p. 292°C

The second of the four closely-related peptide alkaloids isolated from *Waltheria americana*, this base is also laevorotatory with $[\alpha]_D - 230°$ (1:9 MeOH-CHCl$_3$). It crystallizes as colourless crystals from MeOH.

Pais *et al.*, *Bull. Soc. Chim. Fr.*, 1145 (1968)

ADOUETIN Y'

$C_{31}H_{42}O_4N_4$

M.p. 289–290.5°C

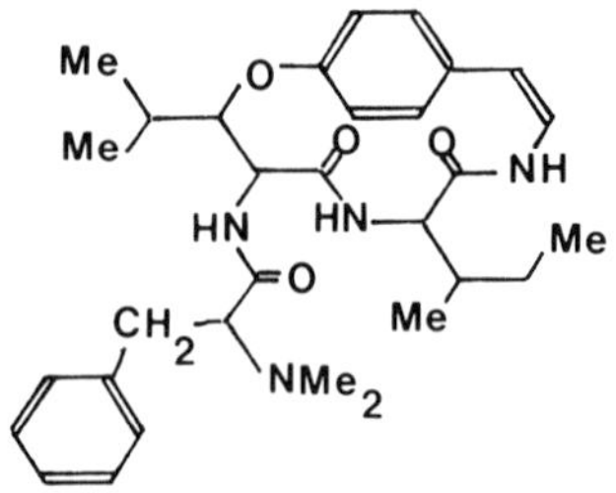

Also present in *Waltheria americana*, this base forms white needles when crystallized from a mixture of $CHCl_3$ and Et_2O. The alkaloid differs from the preceding base only in the substitution of an *iso*propyl group for a phenyl group in the peptide chain.

Pais *et al.*, *Bull. Soc. Chim. Fr.*, 1145 (1968)

ADOUETIN Z

$C_{42}H_{45}O_5N_5$

M.p. 140–5°C

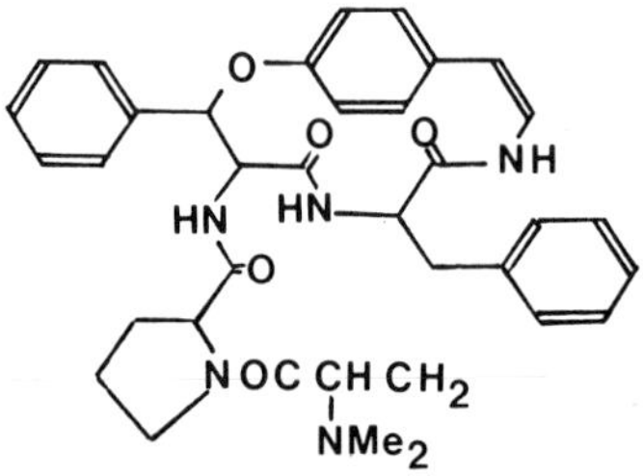

The most complex of the four alkaloids isolated from *Waltheria americana*, this base forms colourless crystals from cyclohexane, $[\alpha]_D - 184°$ ($CHCl_3$). On reduction, the alkaloid yields a dihydro derivative, m.p. 221°C; $[\alpha]_D - 87°$ ($CHCl_3$).

Pais *et al.*, *Bull. Soc. Chim. Fr.*, 1145 (1968)

AEGELINE

$C_{18}H_{19}O_3N$

M.p. 173–5°C

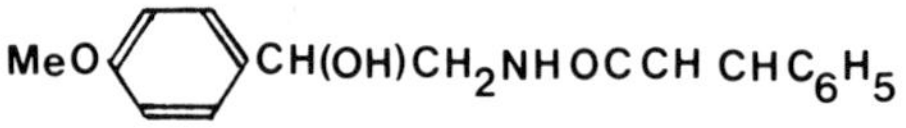

This amide alkaloid occurs in *Aegele marmelos* Correa and may be readily crystallized from several solvents including EtOH, Me_2CO or AcOEt. It forms colourless crystals and is optically inactive although both the (+)- and (−)- forms have been obtained. The base may be characterized as the crystalline acetate, m.p. 159–160°C from AcOEt. Degradative and spectroscopic studies show the base to be N-(-hydroxy-4-methoxyphenyl)-cinnamide.

Chatterjee, Bose., *J. Ind. Chem. Soc.*, **29**, 425 (1952)
Albonico, Kuck, Deulofeu., *J. Chem. Soc.*, C, 1327 (1967)
Synthesis:
Chakravarti, Dasgupta., *Chem. & Ind.*, 1632 (1955)

26

AFFININE

$C_{20}H_{24}O_2N_2$

M.p. 265°C (dec.).

Peschiera affinis (Muell. Arg) Miers contains this dihydroindole type alkaloid which crystallizes as colourless rhombs. The ultraviolet spectrum has absorption maxima at 238 and 318 mμ. The hydrochloride has m.p. 267–9°C; $[\alpha]_D^{20}$ – 105.4° (c 0.5, MeOH) and the acetate m.p. 95–115°C containing Me_2CO which is difficult to remove.

Weisbach *et al., J. Pharm Sci.*, **52**, 350 (1963)
Cava *et al., Chem. & Ind.*, 1193 (1964)

16-epi-AFFININE

$C_{20}H_{24}O_2N_2$

M.p. 152–4°C

From the root and stem bark of *Pleiocarpa talbotii* Wernham, Naranjo *et al* have obtained this epimer of affinine. The base forms colourless crystals from an ether-pentane mixture, $[\alpha]_D^{23}$ – 190° (c 0.95, CHCl$_3$). The ultraviolet spectrum is very like that of affinine itself with absorption maxima at 209, 238 and 318 mμ.

Naranjo, Pinar, Hesse, Schmid., *Helv. Chim. Acta.*, **55**, 752 (1972)

AFFINISINE

$C_{20}H_{24}ON_2$

M.p. 194–6°C

A second alkaloid present in *Peschiera affinis* (Muell. Arg) Miers, this base is also found in *Tabernaemontana fuchsiaefolia*. Affinisine is dextrorotatory with $[\alpha]_D^{30}$ + 19° (c 0.778, CHCl$_3$). Like the two preceding bases it contains a primary hydroxyl group which yields an O-acetyl derivative, m.p. 179–180°C; $[\alpha]_D^{30}$ + 8° (c 0.82, CHCl$_3$). The alkaloid is related to sarpagine (q.v.) being N(β)-methyldesoxysarpagine.

Gosset, LeMen, Janot., *Bull. Soc. Chim. Fr.*, 1033 (1961)
Defay, Kaisen, Pecher, Martin., *Bull. Soc. Chim. Belg.*, **70**, 475 (1961)
Cava, Talapatra, Weisbach, Douglas, Raffauf, Ribeiro., *Chem. & Ind.*, 1193 (1964)

Bartlett, Sklar, Taylor, Schlittler, Amal, Beak, Bringi, Wenkert., *J. Amer. Chem. Soc.*, **84**, 622 (1962)

Achenbach., *Tetrahedron Lett.*, 4405 (1966)

AGROCLAVINE

$C_{16}H_{18}N_2$

M.p. 203°C (*dec.*).

One of the ergot alkaloids, isolated from the mycelium of *Claviceps purpurea*, this base crystallizes as long tablets from Et_2O. When Me_2CO is used as the crystallizing solvent it forms slender, colourless needles. The alkaloid is laevo-rotatory with $[\alpha]_D^{30} - 142°$ ($CHCl_3$). The base may be reduced to the dihydro-derivative, m.p. $233-7°C$; $[\alpha]_D^0 + 66°$ ($CHCl_3$).

Abe., *J. Agric. Chem. Soc. Japan*, **22**, 2, 61 (1948)

Abe., *ibid*, **27**, 18 (1953)

Hoffmann *et al.*, *Helv. Chim. Acta*, **40**, 1358 (1957)

AJACINE (*Acetylanthraniloyllycoctonine*)

$C_{33}H_{48}O_9N_2$

M.p. 154°C

One of the aconite alkaloids, this base occurs in the seeds of *Delphinium ajacis* L and may be obtained in the crystalline form from Et_2O; $[\alpha]_D^{22} + 49.5°$ (EtOH) or $+ 30.8°$ (0.2 N/HCl). The alkaloid also crystallizes from 70 percent EtOH as slender needles. Acid hydrolysis yields acetic acid and anthraniloyllycoctonine, $C_{31}H_{46}O_8N_2$ (q.v.), m.p. $160-165.5°C$ which also occurs naturally in *Delphinium barkeyi*. Alkaline hydrolysis, on the other hand, gives acetylanthranilic acid and lycoctonine. The earlier formula for ajacine, $C_{34}H_{46}O_9N_2.2H_2O$, must clearly be revised to that given above based upon the presently accepted structure of anthraniloyllycoctonine.

Keller, Völker., *Arch. Pharm.*, **251**, 209 (1913)

Hunter., *Pharm. J.*, **152**, 82, 95 (1943)

Hunter., *Quart. J. Pharm.*, **17**, 302 (1944)

Goodson., *J. Chem. Soc.*, 108 (1944)

Goodson., *ibid*, 245 (1945)

AJACININE

$C_{22}H_{35}O_6N$

M.p. 210–1°C

First isolated by Keller and Völker from the seeds of *Delphinium ajacis* L, this base has also been investigated by Hunter. The alkaloid crystallizes from EtOH and has $[\alpha]_D^{17} + 52°$ (CHCl₃). The following salts have been prepared: hydrobromide, not crystallized, m.p. 154–160°C; hydriodide, colourless crystals, m.p. 169–170°C; acid oxalate, needles from H_2O, m.p. 195°C (*dec.*) and the picrate, m.p. 99–103°C not obtained in the crystalline form.

Keller, Völker., *Arch. Pharm.*, **251**, 209 (1913)
Hunter., *Pharm. J.*, **152**, 82, 95 (1943)
Hunter., *Quart. J. Pharm.*, **17**, 302 (1944)

AJACINOIDINE

$C_{38}H_{56}O_{12}N_2$

M.p. 120–6°C

This amorphous alkaloid is also present in the seeds of *Delphinium ajacis* L. It has $[\alpha]_D^{16} + 46°$ (CHCl₃). The picrate is also amorphous, m.p. 125–130°C.

Hunter., *Pharm. J.*, **152**, 82, 95 (1943)

AJACONINE

$C_{22}H_{33}O_3N$

M.p. 172°C

The presence of this alkaloid in the seeds of *Delphinium ajacis* L was demonstrated by Keller and Völker and by Hunter. The latter assigned the formula $C_{21}H_{31}O_3N$ to the base, this being revised by Goodson. The optical rotation has been given as $[\alpha]_D^{18} - 119°$ (EtOH) by Goodson and $[\alpha]_D^{17} - 133°$ (CHCl₃) by Hunter. Some crystalline salts and derivatives are known: the sulphate (7 H_2O) from aqueous Me_2CO, m.p. 113°C; the anhydrous form having m.p. 231°C (*dec.*); $[\alpha]_D^{25} + 5.5°$ (c 2.0, H_2O). The acid oxalate is also crystalline, m.p. 234–5°C but the picrate is amorphous, m.p. 95–8°C. A methiodide, m.p. 134°C is also known. Ajaconine is an N-methyl base and contains no methoxyl groups. It absorbs one mole of hydrogen in the presence of Pd to form the dihydro-derivative which is identical with dihydroatisine and dihydroatidine.

Keller, Völker., *Arch. Pharm.*, **251**, 209 (1913)
Hunter., *Chemist & Druggist*, **139**, 304 (1943)
Goodson., *J. Chem. Soc.*, 245 (1945)

Hunter., *Quart. J. Pharm. Pharmacol.*, **17**, 302 (1947)
Pelletier., *Chem. & Ind.*, 1670 (1957)
Dvornik, Edwards., *Chem. & Ind.*, 952 (1957)
Dvornik, Edwards., *ibid*, 623 (1958)
Dvornik, Edwards., *Can. J. Chem.*, **35**, 860 (1957)
Dvornik, Edwards., *Proc. Chem. Soc.*, **280**, 305 (1958)
Dvornik, Edwards., *Tetrahedron*, **14**, 54 (1961)
Absolute configuration:
Pelletier., *J. Amer. Chem. Soc.*, **87**, 799 (1965)
Mass spectrum:
Sastry, Waller., *Chem. & Ind.*, 381 (1972)

AJMALIDINE

$C_{20}H_{24}O_2N_2$

M.p. 241–2°C

A minor constituent of *Rauwolfia sellowii* Muell., the alkaloid is isolated from
the alkaloidal mixture on a chromatographic column using dimethylformamide
as the eluting agent. The structure has been deduced mainly from the ultraviolet
spectrum and mass spectrometry.

Pakrashi *et al.*, *J. Amer. Chem. Soc.*, **77**, 6687 (1955)
Bartlett *et al.*, *ibid*, **84**, 622 (1962)
Mass spectrum:
Biemann, Bommer, Burlingame, McMurray., *Tetrahedron Lett.*, 1963 (1969)

AJMALINE

$C_{20}H_{26}O_2N_2$

M.p. 205–7°C

This alkaloid occurs chiefly in *Rauwolfia serpentina* Benth. but is also found in
R. vomitoria Afz. (sample from French Guinea). From aqueous AcOEt, the base
forms yellow plates (3.5 H_2O), m.p. 159–160°C; $[\alpha]_D^{20} + 144°$ (CHCl$_3$),
$[\alpha]_D^{33} + 128°$ (CHCl$_3$). The hydrate is completely dehydrated only at 200°C and
when heated at this temperature or boiled with alcoholic KOH, the base is
isomerized to *iso*ajmaline, m.p. 265–6°C; $[\alpha]_D^{35} + 72.8°$ (EtOH), which behaves
as a diacidic base. Several crystalline salts and derivatives have been prepared:
hydrochloride (2 H_2O), m.p. 133–4°C or 253–5°C (*dry*), $[\alpha]_D^{40} + 84.6°$ (H_2O);
dihydrochloride, colourless plates from H_2O, m.p. 305–6°C (*dec.*); platinichloride, m.p. 217–8°C; oxime, m.p. 218°C; picrate, m.p. 126–7°C or 223°C
(*dry*); methochloride, m.p. 288–290°C (*dec.*); methiodide, m.p. 229°C (*dec.*);
methohydroxide, m.p. 124°C; benzoyl derivative, colourless needles from C_6H_6,
m.p. 214–6°C; diacetate, two modifications, a metastable form as needles from

light petroleum, m.p. 132°C and colourless rods from EtOH, m.p. 187−9°C.
Bromine reacts with the base to form the dibromo-derivative, m.p. 230°C (*dec.*) while HNO_3 yields a trinitro-derivative, m.p. 238−258°C (*dec.*) Methyl iodide converts the base into methylajmaline hydriodide, $C_{21}H_{28}O_2N_2.HI$, m.p. 230−1°C. The structure of the alkaloid has been confirmed by synthesis.

Siddiqui, Siddiqui., *J. Ind. Chem. Soc.*, **8**, 667 (1931)
Siddiqui, Siddiqui., *ibid*, **9**, 539 (1932)
Siddiqui, Siddiqui., *ibid*, **12**, 37 (1935)
Paris., *Ann. Pharm. franc.*, **1**, 138 (1943)
Mukherji, Robinson, Schlittler., *Experientia*, **5**, 215 (1949)
Anet *et al., Chem. & Ind.*, **20**, 442 (1952)
Robinson *et al., J. Chem. Soc.*, 1242 (1954)
Chatterjee, Bose., *J. Ind. Chem. Soc.*, **31**, 17 (1954)
Saxton., *Quart. Rev.*, **10**, 138 (1956)
Woodward., *Angew. Chem.*, **68**, 13 (1956)

Synthesis:
Masamune, Ang, Egli, Nakatsuka, Sarkar, Yasunari., *J. Amer. Chem. Soc.*, **89**, 2506 (1967)
Masamune, Ang, Egli, Nakatsuka, Sarkar, Yasunari., *ibid*, **90**, 1680 (1968)

AJMALININE

$C_{20}H_{26}O_3N_2$

M.p. 180−1°C

This Rauwolfia alkaloid also occurs both in *R. serpentina* Benth. and *R. vomitoria* Afz. It forms hexagonal prisms when crystallized from moist AcOEt; $[\alpha]_D − 97°$ ($CHCl_3$). Heating at 210°C converts the alkaloid into *apo*ajmalinine, $C_{13}H_{17}O_3N$, rectangular plates, m.p. 270−2°C; $[\alpha]_D ± 0°$. One methoxyl group is present in the molecule. The alkaloid may be characterized by means of the following salts and derivatives: hydrochloride, a doubtfully crystalline powder, m.p. 240−5°C (*dec.*); $[\alpha]_D^{40} − 44°$ (H_2O); platinichloride, an amorphous powder, m.p. 254−8°C (*dec.*); methiodide, m.p. 233−4°C (*dec.*); picrate, yellow powder, m.p. 200−5°C; O-benzoyl derivative, m.p. 140−150°C (*decomposing from 100°C*).

Siddiqui, Siddiqui., *J. Ind. Chem. Soc.*, **8**, 667 (1931)
Siddiqui, Siddiqui., *ibid*, **9**, 539 (1932)
Siddiqui, Siddiqui., *ibid*, **12**, 37 (1935)

AKNADICINE

$C_{19}H_{23}O_5N$

M.p. 156°C

The roots and rhizomes of *Stephania hernandifolia* Willd. yield two closely related alkaloids, aknadicine and aknadinine (q.v.). Aknadicine crystallizes as colourless plates from MeOH, $[\alpha]_D^{27} - 200°$ (c 0.55, EtOH). The ultraviolet spectrum of the base in EtOH shows one absorption maximum at 266 mμ. Methylation of the hydroxyl group with $CH_2N_2/MeOH$ gives O-methylaknadicine characterized by the crystalline hydrochloride, m.p. 229°C and hydrobromide, m.p. 222.5°C. N-methylation with $CH_2O/H.COOH$ yields aknadinine (q.v.). The relation to the *Stephania* alkaloid stephanoline is confirmed by the action of MeI/MeONa on the base when homostephanoline is formed.

Moza, Basu., *Ind. J. Pharm.*, **28**, 338 (1966)
Moza, Bhaduri, Basu., *Chem. & Ind.*, 1178 (1969)

AKNADILACTAM

$C_{20}H_{23}O_6N$

M.p. Indefinite

This base occurs in the roots of *Stephania sasakii* Hayata and is an amorphous solid which resists attempts at crystallization. It has $[\alpha]_D - 212°$ (CHCl$_3$) and exhibits a broad absorption maximum in the ultraviolet spectrum (in EtOH) at 267 mμ together with a shoulder at 232 μ.

Kunimoto, Okamoto, Yuge, Nagai., *Tetrahedron Lett.*, 3287 (1969)

AKNADININE

$C_{20}H_{25}O_5N$

M.p. 66–70°C

Aknadinine accompanies aknadicine in the roots and rhizomes of *Stephania hernandifolia* Willd. The alkaloid is an amorphous, low-melting solid with $[\alpha]_D^{27} - 280°$ (c 1.0, EtOH). The ultraviolet spectrum in ethanol solution is identical in most respects with that of aknadicine with an absorption maximum at 266 mμ. The following crystalline salts have been prepared: hydrobromide, m.p. 215°C; perchlorate, slender needles from Et$_2$O/CHCl$_3$, m.p. 229–230°C; $[\alpha]_D^{32} - 145°$ (c 0.51, MeOH); oxalate, m.p. 198–9°C; $[\alpha]_D^{32} - 123°$ (c 3.46, MeOH); styphnate, m.p. 207°C. Methylation of the alkaloid yields the O-methyl derivative which is identical with hasubanonine (q.v.). EtI/NaOEt gives the O-ethyl derivative, hydrobromide, m.p. 196.5°C.

Moza, Basu., *Ind. J. Pharm.*, **28**, 338 (1966)
Moza, Bhaduri, Basu., *Chem. & Ind.*, 1178 (1969)

AKUAMMENINE

$C_{20}H_{22}O_4N_2$

The Apocynaceous species *Picralima klaineana* Pierre is widely, although sparsely, distributed throughout tropical Africa and is especially rich in alkaloids of which akuammenine and the following eight bases have been isolated and characterized. Akuammenine has, as yet, only been obtained as the picrate, scarlet needles, m.p. 225°C. The alkaloid contains one methoxyl group.

Henry, Sharp., *J. Chem. Soc.*, 1950 (1927)
Henry., *ibid*, 2759 (1932)
Clinquart., *J. Pharm. Belg.*, **9**, 187 (1927)

(−)-AKUAMMICINE

$C_{20}H_{22}O_2N_2$

M.p. 177.5°C

CH CH$_3$
N
H
CO OMe

The earlier formula for this alkaloid, $C_{19}H_{20}O_2N_2$ has been revised to that given above. The base forms plates from EtOH; $[\alpha]_D^{19} - 737.5°$ (EtOH or CHCl$_3$). It occurs to the extent of only 0.0064 percent in the seeds of *Picralima klaineana* Pierre. Several crystalline derivatives and salts are known: hydrochloride (2 H$_2$O), colourless prisms from EtOH or H$_2$O, m.p. 144°C or 171°C (*dry*); $[\alpha]_D^{16} + 626.6°$ (EtOH); hydriodide (2 H$_2$O), m.p. 128°C; nitrate, colourless needles, m.p. 182.5°C; sulphate, cubic crystals with 1 H$_2$O, m.p. 161°C; $[\alpha]_D^{14} - 594°$ (H$_2$O); perchlorate (2 H$_2$O), m.p. 134−6°C; picrate, light yellow needles, m.p. 169°C; methiodide, light yellow prisms from H$_2$O, m.p. 252°C. With concentrated HNO$_3$, the alkaloid gives a bright green colouration which becomes blue on dilution with H$_2$O. With piperonal and HCl the colour is first magenta, changing to ultramarine on standing. (+)-akuammicine melts at 181−182.5°C and has $[\alpha]_D^{20} + 720°$ (c 0.24, MeOH).

Clinquart., *J. Pharm. Belg.*, **9**, 187 (1927)
Henry, Sharp., *J. Chem. Soc.*, 1950 (1927)
Aghoramurthy, Robinson., *Tetrahedron*, **1**, 172 (1957)
Edwards, Smith., *J. Chem. Soc.*, **152**, 1458 (1961)
Edwards, Smith., *Proc. Chem. Soc.*, 215 (1960)

(±)-AKUAMMICINE (*ψ-Akuammicine*)

$C_{20}H_{22}O_2N_2$

M.p. 187.5°C

CH CH$_3$
N
H
CO OMe

A minor constituent of *Picralima klaineana* Pierre where it occurs to the extent of only 0.0037 percent in the seeds, this alkaloid crystallizes from EtOH as colourless plates and yields a crystalline hydrochloride, m.p. of monohydrate 216°C and a picrate, m.p. 196°C.

Clinquart., *J. Pharm. Belg.*, **9**, 187 (1927)
Henry, Sharp., *J. Chem. Soc.*, 1950 (1927)
Aghoramurthy, Robinsob., *Tetrahedron*, **1**, 172 (1957)
Edwards, Smith., *J. Chem. Soc.*, **152**, 1458 (1961)
Edwards, Smith., *Proc. Chem. Soc.*, 215 (1960)

AKUAMMIDINE (*Rhazine*)

$C_{21}H_{24}O_3N_2$

M.p. 248.5°C

One of the major alkaloids of both *Picralima klaineana* Pierre and *Rhazya stricta* Decaisne, the base crystallizes as the monohydrate in colourless needles, $[\alpha]_D^{20} +$ 21° (EtOH) or + 70.2° (0.1 N/HCl). It is soluble in most organic solvents with the exception of C_6H_6. The salts are readily crystallized: hydriodide, colourless prisms of the trihydrate from aqueous EtOH, m.p. 90°C or 238°C (*dry*); perchlorate, m.p. 110°C; picrate, yellow spherical crystals from EtOH, m.p. 215°C; methiodide, colourless prisms of the monohydrate from aqueous MeOH, m.p. 195°C or 233°C (*dry*); O-benzoyl derivative, slender needles from EtOH, m.p. 219°C. In concentrated HNO_3, the alkaloid gives an intense yellow colouration.

Clinquart., *J. Pharm. Belg.*, **9**, 187 (1927)
Henry, Sharp., *J. Chem. Soc.*, 1950 (1927)
Henry., *ibid*, 2759 (1932)
Hamet., *Compt. rend.*, **221**, 699 (1945)
Levy, LeMan, Janot., *ibid*, **253**, 131 (1961)
Chatterjee *et al.*, *Chem. & Ind.*, 1034 (1961)
Silvers, Tulinsky., *Tetrahedron Lett.*, **8**, 339 (1962)

AKUAMMIDINE ALDEHYDE

$C_{21}H_{22}O_3N_2$

M.p. 231–2°C

A carboline alkaloid, this base occurs in *Aspidosperma dasycarpon*. The structure has been determined from chemical degradation and spectroscopic evidence.

Joule *et al.*, *Tetrahedron*, **21**, 1717 (1965)

AKUAMMIGINE

$C_{21}H_{24}O_3N_2$

M.p. 113°C

This base is present in the seeds of *Picralima klaineana* Pierre, the original formula of $C_{22}H_{26}O_3N_2$ being changed to that given above. The alkaloid forms yellow tablets of the monohydrate when crystallized from aqueous EtOH and has $[\alpha]_D^{20} - 44.4°$ (EtOH). In concentrated HNO_3 the base yields a bright yellow colour while with piperonal and HCl, the colour is first pink, becoming amethyst on standing. Several salts are known: the hydrochloride, prisms from either EtOH or H_2O, m.p. 287°C; $[\alpha]_D^{20} - 37.8°$ (MeOH); hydrobromide, m.p. 248–250°C; nitrate, colourless prisms from aqueous EtOH, m.p. 261°C; perchlorate monohydrate, m.p. 75°C or 204°C (*dec. dry*); picrate as garnet-red crystals of the monohydrate, m.p. 173°C or 240°C (*dry*). The base yields a monobenzoyl derivative which is neutral in reaction and insoluble in acids indicating that the entering acyl group is attached to the nitrogen atom. So far, however, this compound has not been obtained in a form suitable for analysis.

Clinquart., *J. Pharm. Belg.*, **9**, 187 (1927)
Henry, Sharp., *J. Chem. Soc.*, 1950 (1927)
Henry., *ibid*, 2759 (1932)
Hamet., *Compt. rend.*, **221**, 699 (1945)
Robinson, Thomas., *J. Chem. Soc.*, 3479 (1954)
Stereochemistry:
Shamma, Richey., *J. Amer. Chem. Soc.*, **85**, 2507 (1963)
Synthesis:
Gutzwiller *et al.*, *J. Amer. Chem. Soc.*, **93**, 5907 (1971)

ψ-AKUAMMIGINE

$C_{22}H_{26}O_3N_2$

M.p. 165°C

This alkaloid is present to the extent of 0.017 per cent in the seeds of *Picralima klaineana* Pierre and forms colourless prisms which are laevorotatory with $[\alpha]_D^{20} - 53.8°$ ($CHCl_3$) or $- 35°$ (EtOH). In concentrated HNO_3 the alkaloid gives a brown colour initially changing to yellow while with piperonal in HCl the colour is pink turning to amethyst on standing. The hydrochloride forms a crystalline monohydrate from aqueous EtOH, m.p. 183°C or 218°C (*dry*); methiodide, m.p. 275°C and the picrate, m.p. 223°C.

Henry, Sharp., *J. Chem. Soc.*, 1950 (1927)
Henry, Sharp., *ibid*, 2759 (1932)
Robinson, Thomas., *ibid*, 3522 (1954)
Levy, LeMen, Janot., *Bull. Soc. Chim. Fr.*, 1658 (1961)
Oliver *et al.*, *ibid*, 646 (1963)
Britten *et al.*, *Chem. & Ind.*, 1120 (1963)

(4R)-AKUAMMIGINE N-OXIDE

$C_{22}H_{26}O_4N_2$

The stems of various *Uncaria* species yield this and the following alkaloid. The structure has been determined from chemical and spectroscopic data. The base may also be prepared synthetically by oxidation of Akuammigine with a peracid.

Merlini, Nasini, Phillipson., *Tetrahedron,* **28,** 5971 (1972)

(4S)-AKUAMMIGINE N-OXIDE

$C_{22}H_{26}O_4N_2$

Also present in the alkaloidal extract from the stems of *Uncaria* species, this base may also be prepared by the peracid oxidation of Akuammigine.

Merlini, Nasini, Phillipson., *Tetrahedron,* **28,** 5971 (1972)

AKUAMMILINE

$C_{22}H_{24}O_4N_2$

M.p. 160°C

A minor alkaloid from the seeds of *Picralima klaineana* Pierre, this base is also found in *Conopharyngia durissima.* It is readily soluble in EtOH, Et$_2$O, CHCl$_3$ and warm C$_6$H$_6$. The alkaloid gives no colour reaction with concentrated HNO$_3$ but with piperonal and HCl gives a pink colour changing to amethyst on standing. The hydrochloride crystallizes from EtOH or H$_2$O as the monohydrate, m.p. 196°C; $[\alpha]_D^{20} - 29.6°$ (H$_2$O); hydriodide as slender, colourless needles from aqueous EtOH, m.p. 210°C; nitrate, m.p. 204°C and the methiodide, clusters of fine needles from H$_2$O, m.p. 233°C; $[\alpha]_D^{20} - 83.3°$ (EtOH). The base also forms a neutral benzoyl derivative showing that the acyl group is on the nitrogen atom. Reduction with LiAlH$_4$ yields picralinol.

Clinquart., *J. Pharm. Belg.,* **9,** 187 (1927)
Henry, Sharp., *J. Chem. Soc.,* 1950 (1927)
Henry,, *ibid,* 2759 (1932)

Dugan et al., *Helv. Chim. Acta*, **52**, 701 (1969)

Structure:

LeMen., *Lloydia*, **27**, 456 (1964)

AKUAMMINE (*Vincamajoridine*)

$C_{22}H_{26}O_4N_2$

M.p. 255°C

The major alkaloid present in the seeds of *Picralima klaineana* Pierre, this base crystallizes from EtOH as slender needles which are freely soluble in $CHCl_3$ but only sparingly so in Et_2O or EtOH. The alkaloid has $[\alpha]_D^{20} - 73.4°$ ($CHCl_3$). In concentrated HNO_3 it gives a blood-red colour and with piperonal and HCl the colour is first pink and then amethyst on standing. Several crystalline salts and derivatives have been prepared including the hydrochloride monohydrate, m.p. 227°C; $[\alpha]_D^{22} - 26.6°$ (H O); hydrobromide monohydrate, m.p. 228°C; $[\alpha]_D^{20} - 26.1°$ (H_2O); hydriodide, steel-grey needles of the monohydrate, m.p. 226°C; dinitrate, m.p. 224°C; sulphate, colourless needles, m.p. 221°C; $[\alpha]_D^{19} - 40.3°$ (H_2O); picrate, yellow needles from EtOH, m.p. 199°C; picrolonate, small yellow needles, m.p. 194°C and the methiodide, m.p. 274°C.

Clinquart., *J. Pharm. Belg.*, **9**, 187 (1927)
Henry, Sharp., *J. Chem. Soc.*, 1950 (1927)
Henry., *ibid*, 2759 (1932)
Millson, Robinson, Thomas., *Experientia*, **9**, 89 (1953)
Janot et al., *ibid*, **11**, 343 (1955)
Gimenez., *Anales univ. Murcia.*, **16**, C239 (1957–8)
Asatinani et al., *Soobshch. Akad. Nauk. Gruz. SSR*, **64**, 341 (1971)

AKUAMMINE HYDRATE

$C_{22}H_{28}O_5N_2$

This base is prepared by treatment of akuammine with alkali in hot EtOH but also occurs naturally in the seeds of *Picrilima klaineana* Pierre. It forms a crystalline methiodide, m.p. > 300°C.

Henry, Sharp., *J. Chem. Soc.*, 1950 (1927)
Henry., *ibid*, 2759 (1932)

ALAFINE

A pyrrolizidine alkaloid, this base has recently been isolated from *Alafia multiflora*. It has been partially identified as an ester of syringic acid and trachelanthamidine.

Paris et al., *Ann. Pharm. Fr.*, **29**, 57 (1971)

ALANGICINE

$C_{28}H_{36}O_5N_2$

M.p. 147–8°C

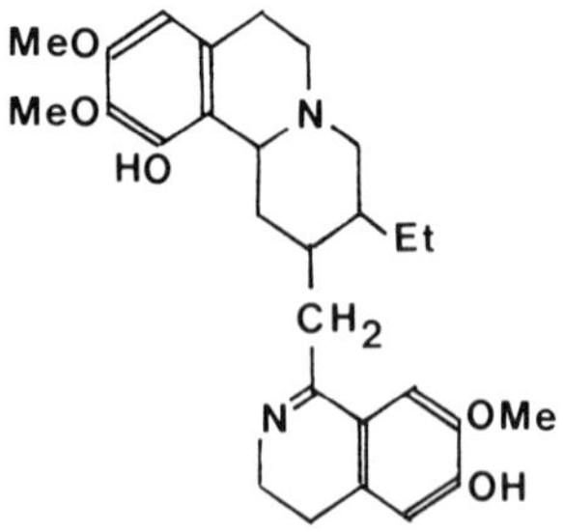

The root bark of *Alangium lamarckii* Thw. contains this alkaloid which may be purified by chromatography over silica gel, followed by recrystallization from EtOH when it forms yellow granules. It is dextrorotatory with $[\alpha]_D + 64.1°$ (c 0.26, MeOH). In EtOH solution, the ultraviolet spectrum shows absorption maxima at 275, 312 and 408 mμ, while in alkaline solution, (0.1 N/NaOH), the maxima occur at 238, 292 and 328 mμ.

Pakrashi, Ali., *Tetrahedron Lett.*, 2143 (1967)

ALANGIMARCKINE

$C_{29}H_{37}O_3N_3$

M.p. 184–6°C

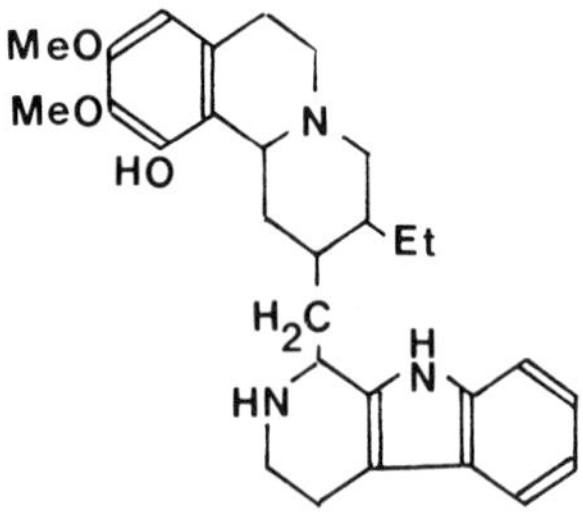

This alkaloid has been isolated from the leaves of *Alangium lamarckii* Thw. It is laevorotatory with $[\alpha]_D^{25} - 67.7°$ (pyridine). The base differs from the preceding alkaloid in having a carboline type constituent in place of the *iso*quinoline nucleus.

Battersby *et al.*, *Tetrahedron Lett.*, 4965 (1966)

ALANGINE

$C_{19}H_{25}O_2N$

M.p. 205–8°C (*dec.*).

The bark of *Alangium lamarckii* Thw. is stated to contain this alkaloid which has $[\alpha]_D + 9°$ (EtOH). Among the salts which have been prepared are the hydrochloride, m.p. 264°C; picrate, m.p. 84°C and the methiodide, m.p. 201°C (*dec.*). The base is monoacidic, tertiary and contains one methoxyl and possibly an alcoholic hydroxyl group but no methylimino group.

Chopra, Chowham., *Ind. J. Med. Res.*, **21**, 507 (1934)
Parihar, Dutt., *Proc. Ind. Acad. Sci.*, **23A**, 325 (1946)

ALANGINE A

$C_{21}H_{24-26}O_3N_2$

M.p. $219-220°C$

This, and the following alkaloid, have been isolated from the root bark of *Alangium lamarackii* Thw. The base crystallizes from C_6H_6 and is soluble in most organic solvents although only sparingly so in Et_2O and hot C_6H_6. It is insoluble in cold C_6H_6 and in H_2O. The alkaloid is only moderately stable and darkens slowly on exposure to light.

Singh, Tewari., *Proc. Nat. Acad. Sci., India,* 17, 1 (1948)

ALANGINE B

$C_{21}H_{24-26}O_3N_2$

From the root bark of *Alangium lamarckii* Thw. this alkaloid is obtained as an amorphous yellow powder with no definite melting point. It is soluble in most organic solvents but even more unstable than Alangine A to light, darkening quite rapidly.

Singh, Tewari., *Proc. Nat. Acad. Sci., India,* 17, 1 (1948)

ALATAMINE

$C_{41}H_{44}O_{18}N$

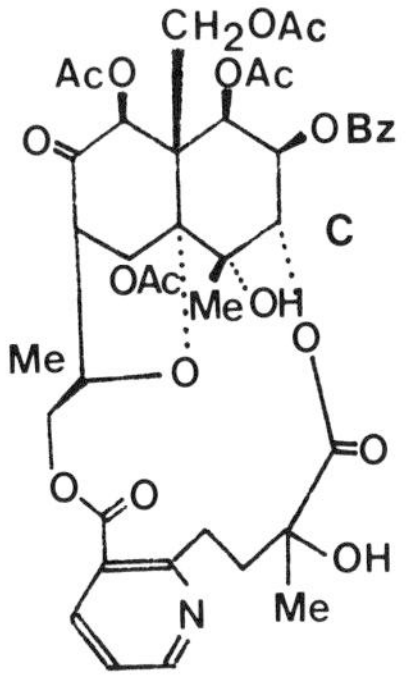

This macrocyclic alkaloid has recently been obtained from *Euonymus alatus* f. *striatus.* The highly-substituted and acetylated structure has been determined from chemical and spectroscopic data.

Shizuri, Yamada, Hirata., *Tetrahedron Lett.,* 741 (1973)

ALBERTINE

$C_{15}H_{22}O_2N_2$

M.p. $161°C$

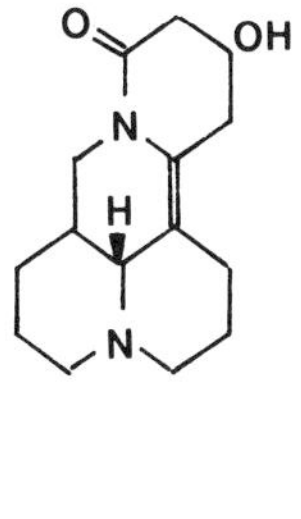

This alkaloid occurs in the areial parts of *Leontice albertii*. The base crystallizes as colourless prisms from Me_2CO and is laevorotatory with $[\alpha]_D^{21} - 101.5°$ (c 2.03, EtOH). It forms a crystalline perchlorate, m.p. $228-9°C$ and a methiodide, m.p. $285°C$. The base also furnishes an *o*-tosylate, m.p. $155-6°C$. Catalytic hydrogenation in AcOH over Pt at $70-80°C$ gives the dihydro derivative, m.p. $170°C$ while reduction with $LiAlH_4$ furnishes the deoxy compound, forming a diperchlorate, m.p. $190°C$. When treated with P_2O_5 at $200-210°C$ for 5 hours, albertine yields the anhydro base, m.p. $163-4°C$; $[\alpha]_D - 90°$ which proves to be identical with sophoramine. Infrared, ultraviolet and NMR spectroscopy shows the structure to be 13-hydroxy-7:11-dehydromatrine.

Iskandarov, Nuriddinov, Yunusov., *Khim. Prir. Soedin.*, **3**, 26 (1967)
Iskandarov, Yunusov., *ibid*, **4**, 137 (1968)
Iskandarov, Kamalitdinov, Yunusov., *ibid*, **5**, 628 (1972)

ALBOMACULINE

$C_{19}H_{23}O_5N$

M.p. $180-1°C$

One of the Amaryllidaceous alkaloids, this base occurs to the extent of 0.004 per cent in the bulbs of *Haemanthus albomaculatus*. It is dextrorotatory with $[\alpha]_D + 71.1°$ $(CHCl_3)$. The perchlorate forms colourless prisms from MeOH, m.p. $285-9°C$ (*dec.*); the picrate, colourless crystals from EtOH, m.p. $189-198°C$ and the methopicrate, yellow prisms from aqueous EtOH, m.p. $244-6°C$ (*dec.*). Reduction of the alkaloid yields the dihydro derivative as an oil which appears to consist of two isomers since no constant melting derivative can be obtained. More vigorous reduction furnishes a tetrahydro derivative which is also an oil that is not crystallizable.

Briggs *et al.*, *J. Amer. Chem. Soc.*, **78**, 2899 (1956)
Boit, Ehmke., *Chem. Ber.*, **90**, 57 (1957)
Jeffs, Toube., *J. Org. Chem.*, **31**, 189 (1966)

ALBORINE

$C_{22}H_{22}O_6N^+$

M.p. $238-240°C$

This quaternary alkaloid is present in *Papaver alborosum* Hulten as the hydroxyide of the protoberberine base and is separated from the accompanying Oreophiline (q.v.) by extraction of the $CHCl_3$ extract with MeOH after chromatography on an alumina column. It yields colourless crystals from Et_2O having the above melting point. When crystallized from MeOH, however, the crystals darken at 240°C and do not melt up to 360°C. As with the majority of these quaternary alkaloids, the hydroxyl ion may be replaced by halogen to yield characteristic salts, e.g. the chloride, obtained as pale yellow crystals, and the iodide, also as yellow crystals. Both salts have m.p. > 360°C.

Pfeifer, Thomas., *Pharmazie.*, **21**, 701 (1966)

ALCHORNEINE

$C_{12}H_{19}ON_3$

M.p. 43°C

A low-melting tetrahydroimidazopyrimidine alkaloid, this base occurs in *Alchornea floribunda* and *A. hirtella* (African Euphorbiaceae). It is a laevorotatory alkaloid with $[\alpha]_D - 105°$ (CHCl$_3$). Both spectroscopic and chemical analysis have been used to confirm the structure. Treatment with NaOMe opens the pyrimidine ring while acid hydrolysis furnishes an imidazolidinone.

The tartrate exhibits strong vagolytic action and inhibition of intestinal peristalsis in dogs and also shows ganglioplegic parasympathy.

Khuong-Huu-Laine, Leforestier, Maillard, Goutarel., *Compt. rend.*, **270C**, 2070 (1970)
Khuong-Huu-Laine, Leforestier, Maillard, Goutarel., *Tetrahedron*, **28**, 5207 (1972)
Crystal structure:
Cesario, Guilhem., *Acta Cryst.*, **28B**, 151 (1972)

ALCHORNEINONE

$C_{12}H_{20}O_3N_2$

This imidazole-type alkaloid is present in the leaves of *Alchornea floribunda*. The free base is an oily liquid.

Khuong-Huu-Laine, Leforestier, Goutarel., *Tetrahedron*, **28**, 5207 (1972)

ALCHORNIDINE

$C_{16}H_{23}O_2N_3$

M.p. 96–7°C

From another species of Euphorbiaceae, *Alchornea javanensis,* Hart *et al* have isolated this imidazopyrimidine alkaloid. The base has $[\alpha]_D - 18°$ (CHCl$_3$). The structure has been confirmed by chemical analysis and spectroscopic investigation.

Hart, Johns, Lamberton., *Chem. Commun.,* 1484 (1969)
Hart, Johns, Lamberton, Willing., *Austral. J. Chem.,* **23,** 1679 (1970)

ALCHORNINE

$C_{11}H_{17}ON_3$

M.p. 134–5°C

This second alkaloid obtained from *Alchornea javanensis* has $[\alpha]_D + 74°$ (CHCl$_3$) and forms a crystalline picrate, m.p. 275–8°C.

Hart, Johns, Lamberton., *Chem. Commun.,* 1484 (1969)
Hart *et al., Austral. J. Chem.,* **23,** 1679 (1970)

α-ALDOTRIPIPERIDEINE

$C_{15}H_{27}N_3$

M.p. 115–8°C

A tetracyclic alkaloid, this base has recently been isolated from *Coelidium fourcadei.* The structure, containing two imino groups, has been determined on the basis of spectropic studies, particularly the mass spectrum fragmentation pattern.

Arndt, Du Plessis., *J. S. Afr. Chem. Inst.,* **21,** 54 (1968)

ALGININE

$C_{23}H_{29}O_3N$

M.p. 271–2°C

Isolated from *Fritillaria sewerzowii* Rgl., this base has $[\alpha]_D + 108.5°$ (EtOH). It yields a crystalline hydrochloride, m.p. 323–5°C and a methiodide, m.p. 310–1°C. The nitrogen atom is tertiary and there are three hydroxyl groups in the molecule. According to Zolotukhina, the alkaloid is notably a local anaesthetic and also shows some mydriatic activity.

Yunusov, Konovalova, Orekhov., *J. Gen. Chem., USSR,* **9,** 1911 (1939)
Zolotukhina., *Pharmacol & Toxicol.,* **7,** 51 (1944)
Zolotukhina., *ibid,* **8,** 15 (1945)

ALKALOID AA-1

$C_{16}H_{28}O_2N_2$

M.p. 80–1°C

This alkaloid has been found in the seeds of *Anabasis aphylla* and is separated from the following base by paper chromatography. It forms colourless crystals when recrystallized from MeOH and gives a hydrochloride, m.p. 249–250°C; hydrobromide, m.p. 256–8°C; hydriodide, m.p. 240–1°C and the picrate, m.p. 219–220°C. Reduction with LiAlH$_4$ gives aphyllic alcohol, m.p. 151–2°C; $[\alpha]_D$ + 19.4° and boiling with H$_2$SO$_4$ yields aphyllic acid, m.p. 225–7°C and MeOH, thereby establishing the structure as methyl aphyllate. This has been further confirmed by comparison with an authentic specimen when no depression of melting point was observed.

Aslanov, Mukhamedzhanov, Sadykov., *Nauch. Tr., Tashkent. Gos. Univ.*, No. 286, 71 (1966)

ALKALOID AA-2

$C_{17}H_{21}N_3$

M.p. 65–6°C

A second alkaloid isolated from the pulverized, defatted seeds of *Anabasis aphylla,* the base yields colourless crystals from EtOH and yields a hydrochloride, m.p. 265–6°C; hydrobromide, m.p. 292–3°C and the picrate, m.p. 88–90°C. The structure has not yet been determined.

Aslanov, Mukhamedzhanov, Sadykov., *Nauch. Tr., Tashkent. Gos. Univ.*, No. 286, 71 (1966)

ALKALOID AA-I

$C_{19}H_{21}O_2N$

This oily base occurs in the basic fraction obtained from the roots of *Aristolchia argentina*. It has been isolated as the crystalline oxalate, m.p. 176–7°C and also yields a picrate, m.p. 235–6°C. The free alkaloid gives an NMR spectrum indicative of a 1-dimethylaminoethylphenanthrene structure. The structure and substitution pattern have been confirmed by preparation of the methoxy derivative by treatment with CH$_2$N$_2$, the hydriodide of which is identical with that formed from 1-dimethylamino-3:4-dimethoxyphenanthrene.

Priestap *et al.*, *Chem. Commun.*, 754 (1967)

ALKALOID AC-1

$C_{19}H_{15}O_4N$

M.p. 252–4°C

This alkaloid has recently been reported as present in the bark of *Atalanta ceylanica*. The base yields red needles from Et₂O-light petroleum and is obtained in 0.04 per cent yield. The ultraviolet spectrum in EtOH has absorption maxima at 238, 267 and 284 mμ with a shoulder at 293 mμ. In EtOH-NaOMe solution, the maxima occur at 237, 281, 343 and 456 m with a shoulder at 293 mμ and in EtOH-AlCl₃ solution, they are at 276, 293, 304, 365 and 480 mμ with shoulders present at 272 and 330 mμ. Treatment with CH₂N₂ gives the 11-O-methyl ether as orange needles, m.p. 155–7°C while methyl iodide in Me₂CO furnishes the 6:11-dimethyl ether, m.p. 97–8°C. Ac O in pyridine gives the 6:11-diacetate as colourless prisms, m.p. 178–181°C confirming the presence of two phenolic hydroxyl groups. A *gem*-dimethyl group is also present in the molecule.

Fraser, Lewis., *J. Chem. Soc., Perkin I,* 1173 (1973)

ALKALOID AC-2

$C_{24}H_{23}O_4N$

M.p. 190–191.5°C

A second anthraquinone alkaloid isolated from the bark of *Atalantia ceylanica*, this base also forms red needles from Et₂O-light petroleum. The ultraviolet spectrum in EtOH has absorption maxima at 239, 272, 347 and 436 mμ with a shoulder af 323 mμ. In EtOH-NaOMe solution, the maxima are present at 244, 283 and 460 mμ with shoulders at 299, 308 and 341 mμ; and in EtOH-AlCl₃ solution, they occur at 270, 308, 367 and 482 mμ. Treatment with CH₂N₂ in MeOH gives the 11-methyl ether, m.p. 126.5°C.

Fraser, Lewis., *J. Chem. Soc., Perkin I,* 1173 (1973)

ALKALOID AC-A

$C_{19}H_{18}ON_2$

An *iso*pentylhalfordinol ether, this alkaloid occurs in the fruit of *Aeglopsis chevalieri* and is isolated by chromatography on alumina followed by recrystallization from EtOH.

Dreyer.; *J. Org. Chem.,* **33**, 3658 (1968)

ALKALOID AC-B

$C_{19}H_{18}ON_2$

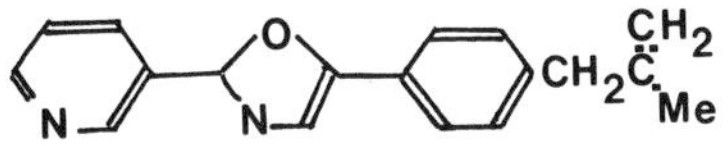

This alkaloid from the fruit of *Aeglopsis chevalieri* is isomeric with the preceding base from which it is isolated by column chromatography on alumina and purified by recrystallization from MeOH. The structure has been determined by chemical and spectroscopic investigation.

Dreyer., *J. Org. Chem.*, **33**, 3658 (1968)

ALKALOID AL-A

$C_{10}H_{12}O_3N_4$

M.p. 216–7°C

An alkaloid obtained from *Asteracantha longifolia* (Syn. *Hygrophilia spinosa*), this base yields a crystalline sulphate, m.p. 210–1°C and an oxalate, m.p. 221–2°C.

Basu, Lal., *Quart. J. Pharmacol.*, **20**, 38 (1947)

ALKALOID AM-A

M.p. 172–3°C

This uncharacterized alkaloid is present in *Aegle marmelos*. It has been shown to be different from Rutacine (q.v.).

Khaleque *et al.*, *Sci. Res.*, (Dacca), **7**, 122 (1970)

ALKALOID AM-B

M.p. 136–7°C

A second unidentified alkaloid occurring in *Aegle marmalos*. No salts or derivatives have yet been prepared to characterize the base.

Khaleque *et al.*, *Sci. Res.*, (Dacca), **7**, 122 (1970)

ALKALOID AM-I

M.p. 238–240°C

One of three minor alkaloids isolated from *Androcymbium melanthoides* var. *stricta*. This base is laevorotatory with $[\alpha]_D^{23} - 291° \pm 4°$ (c 0.550, MeOH).

Pijewska *et al.*, *Collect. Czech. Chem. Commun.*, **32**, 158 (1967)

ALKALOID AM-II

M.p. 270–3°C (*dec.*).

A second uncharacterized minor constituent of *Androcymbium melanthoides* var. *stricta*. No salts or derivatives have been prepared owing to the small amount of material available for study.

Pijewska *et al.*, *Collect. Czech. Chem. Commun.*, **32**, 158 (1967)

ALKALOID AM-III

M.p. 143–5°C and 160°C

This minor alkaloid of *Androcymbium melanthoides* var. *stricta* forms colourless crystals with a double melting point. It is slightly dextrorotatory with $[\alpha]_D^{23}$ + 9.5° (c 0.631, $CHCl_3$-MeOH).

Pijewska *et al.*, *Collect. Czech. Chem. Commun.*, **32**, 158 (1967)

ALKALOID AM-1

$C_{19}H_{15}O_4N$

M.p. 190°C

The seeds of *Argemone mexicana* L. yield this minor alkaloid which is soluble in EtOH, the solution possessing a marked blue fluorescence. It does not give the colour reactions of Protopine (q.v.) which is also present in these seed oils and this base is regarded as forming part of the complex molecule of the still undiscovered toxic principle.

Mukherjee, Lal, Mathur., *Ind. J. Med. Res.*, **29**, 361 (1941)

ALKALOID AP-A

M.p. 88°C

This uncharacterized alkaloid has been reported as being present in the leaves of *Aderanthera pavonina*. No salts or derivatives have been recorded.

Patel, Shah, Parikh., *Curr. Sci.*, **16**, 346 (1947)

ALKALOID AS-1

$C_{34}H_{47}O_{12}N$

A toxic aconitine alkaloid isolated from *Aconitum sachalinense*, the base is obtained as the crystalline perchlorate. Alkaline hydrolysis with methanolic KOH furnishes p-methoxybenzoic acid, acetic acid and an amorphous alkamine which yields a pentaacetyl derivative, $C_{34}H_{39}O_{14}N$. It has been suggested that the alkaloid is an epimer of mesaconiine.

Ichinohe, Yamaguchi., *Bull. Chem. Soc. Japan,* **42**, 3038 (1969)

ALKALOID AS-A

$C_{43}H_{50}O_{12}N_3$

The roots of *Aconitum septentionale* contain several minor alkaloids which have been isolated and characterized by Marion and his colleagues. This base is the major component of these minor alkaloids and is a double ester consisting of an alkamine which is esterified with the methyl ester of N-succinoylanthranilic acid.

Marion *et al., Can. J. Chem.,* **45**, 969 (1967)

ALKALOID AS-B

$C_{17}H_{25}O_2N$

A further minor alkaloid isolated from the roots of *Aconitum septentrionale.* This base has not been examined further since its isolation.

Marion *et al., Can. J. Chem.,* **45**, 969 (1967)

ALKALOID AS-C

$C_{23}H_{37}O_3N$

Also present in small quantities in the root extract of *Aconitum septentrionale,* this alkaloid has not yet been fully characterized.

Marion *et al., Can. J. Chem.,* **45**, 969 (1967)

ALKALOID AS-D

$C_{30}H_{42}O_7N_2$

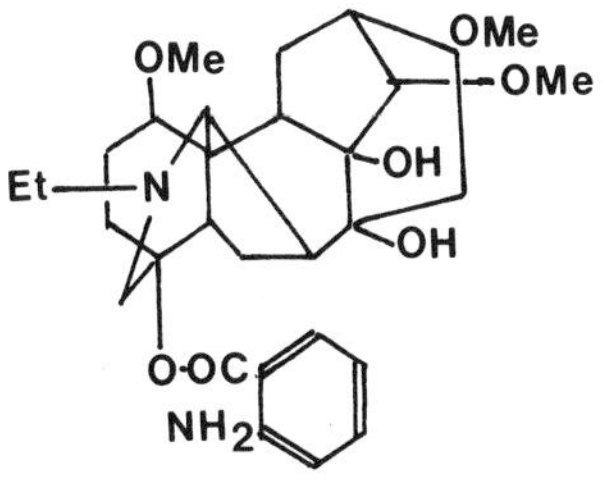

This minor base obtained from the roots of *Aconitum septentrionale* has been shown to be identical with deacetyllappaconitine.

Marion *et al., Can. J. Chem.,* **45**, 969 (1967)

ALKALOID AS-E

$C_{37}H_{54}O_7N$

A further minor base present in the root extract of *Aconitum septentrionale,* the alkaloid has been shown to possess no ester group in the molecule.

Marion *et al., Can. J. Chem.,* **45**, 969 (1967)

ALKALOID AS-F

$C_{19}H_{29}O_6N$

Also occurring in small quantities in the roots of *Aconitum septentrionale,* this alkaloid probably belongs to the atisine group of bases.

Marion *et al., Can. J. Chem.,* **45**, 969 (1967)

ALKALOID AS-I

$C_{20}H_{19}O_3N_3$

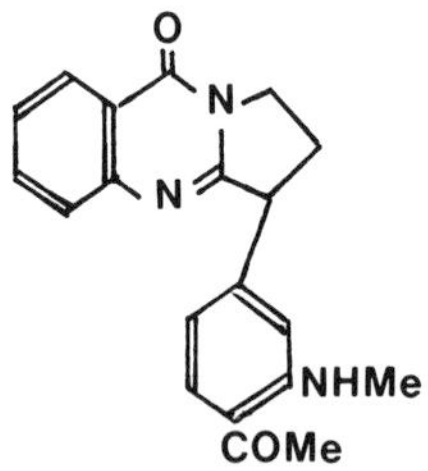

Anisotes sessiliflorus yields a number of alkaloids, including five closely related 4-quinazolone bases described here. The structure of this alkaloid has been determined by the extensive use of spectroscopic techniques and some selected chemical reactions.

Arndt, Eggers, Jordaan., *Tetrahedron,* **23**, 3521 (1967)

ALKALOID AS-II

$C_{20}H_{19}O_3N_3$

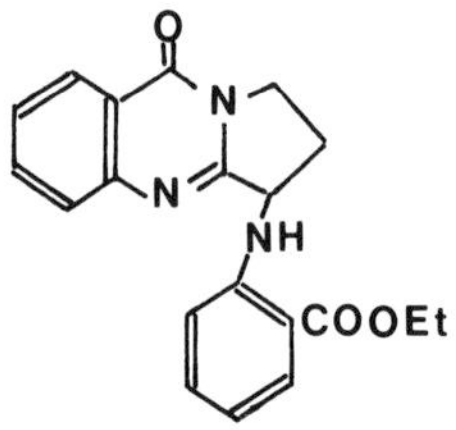

This alkaloid from *Anisotes sessiliflorus* is isomeric with the preceding base and also contains the 4-quinazolone skeleton. Its structure has also been elucidated by means of spectroscopic determinations.

Arndt, Eggers, Jordaan., *Tetrahedron,* **23**, 3521 (1967)

ALKALOID AS-III

$C_{20}H_{21}O_3N_3$

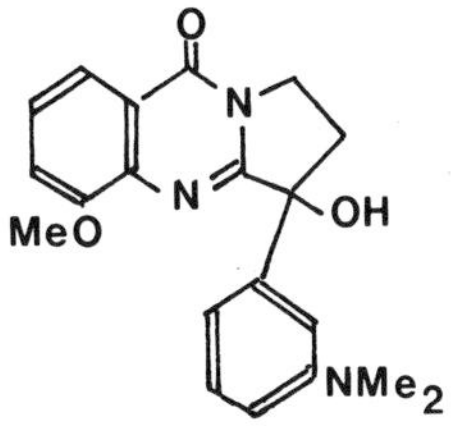

Also present in *Anisotes sessiliflorus,* this base has the structure given above based upon infrared, ultraviolet, NMR and mass spectrometry.

Arndt, Eggers, Jordaan., *Tetrahedron,* **23,** 3521 (1967)

ALKALOID AS-IV

$C_{20}H_{21}O_2N_3$

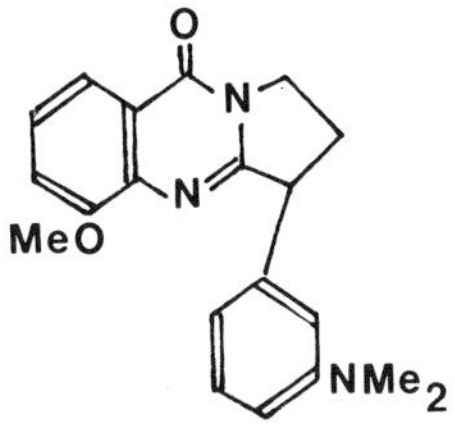

A further 4-quinazolone alkaloid obtained from *Anisotes sessiliflorus,* the base is the dehydroxy analogue of the foregoing alkaloid as shown by spectroscopic and chemical determinations.

Arndt, Eggers, Jordaan., *Tetrahedron,* **23,** 3521 (1967)

ALKALOID AS-V

$C_{19}H_{19}O_2N_3$

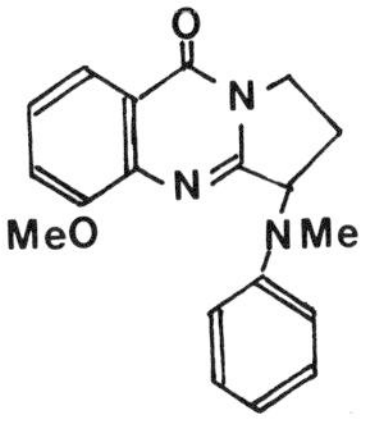

The fifth 4-quinazolone alkaloid isolated from *Anisotes sessiliflorus,* this base has been demonstrated to possess the structure given above on the basis of spectroscopic investigations coupled with selected chemical reactions.

Arndt, Eggers, Jordaan., *Tetrahedron,* **23,** 3521 (1967)

ALKALOID AT-A

M.p. 229–230°C

The plant *Amsonia tabernaemontana* contains four uncharacterized minor alkaloids which have been isolated and separated by column chromatography on alumina. This base yields colourless crystals from EtOH. No salts or derivatives have been reported.

Zabolotnaya et al., Med. Prom. SSSR, 18, 28 (1964)

ALKALOID AT-B

M.p. 246–247.5°C

A further constituent of the alkaloidal extract of *Amsonia tabernaemontana*, this alkaloid is obtained as colourless needles having the melting point given above.

Zabolotnaya et al., Med. Prom. SSSR, 18, 28 (1964)

ALKALOID AT-G

M.p. 115–116.5°C

This alkaloid obtained from *Amsonia tabernaemontana* is crystalline and is probably a dihydroindole base. No salts or derivatives have been prepared owing to the small amount of material available for study.

Zabolotnaya et al., Med. Prom. SSSR, 18, 28 (1964)

ALKALOID AT-V

M.p. 224–5°C (*dec.*).

A fourth minor constituent of *Amsonia tabernaemontana*, this alkaloid yields colourless crystals from EtOH. It has not been characterized further.

Zabolotnaya et al., Med. Prom. SSSR, 18, 28 (1964)

ALKALOID AU-I

$C_{21}H_{25}O_2N_3$

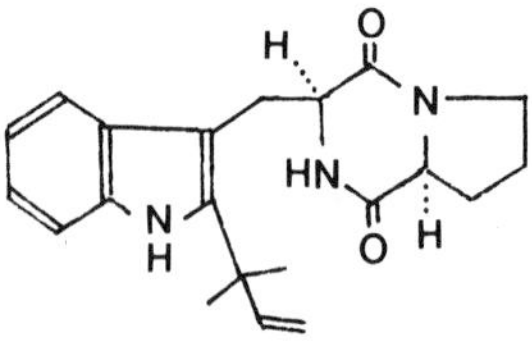

This dioxopiperazine base has been obtained from *Aspergillus ustus* and, although not an alkaloid in the strict sense of the word, it does possess the basic indole moiety and is included here for completeness. The absolute configuration of the base has been determined from chemical and spectroscopic data.

Steyn., Tetrahedron, 29, 107 (1973)

ALKALOID AU-II

$C_{21}H_{23}O_2N_3$

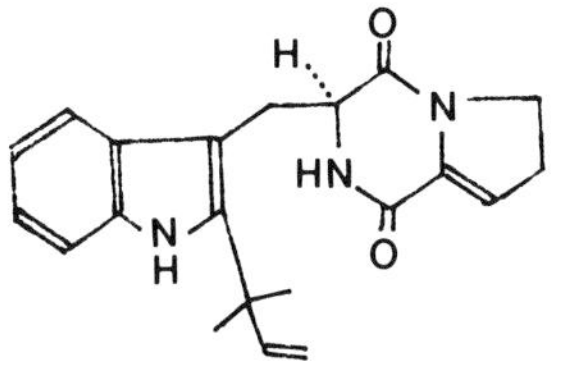

A further dioxopiperazine base obtained from *Aspergillus ustus*, the structure has been shown to be the 12:13-dehydro analogue of the preceding base.

Steyn., *Tetrahedron*, **29**, 107 (1973)

ALKALOID AU-III

$C_{21}H_{21}O_2N_3$

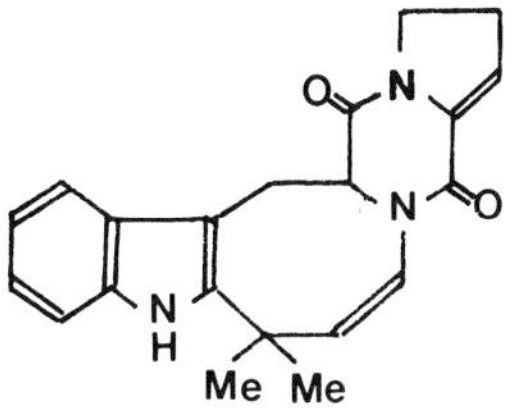

This pentacyclic indole also occurs in *Aspergillus ustus*. It has been suggested as a probable precursor of Austamide (q.v.).

Steyn., *Tetrahedron*, **29**, 107 (1973)

ALKALOID AV-1

$C_{22}H_{35}O_3N$

M.p. 145–7°C

An alkaloid obtained from the aerial parts of *Aconitum variegatum*, the base appears to be either an atisine or a garryine type alkaloid. It yields clusters of small, colourless crystals when recrystallized from Me_2CO.

Shpanov., *Med. Prom. SSSR*, **18**, 21 (1964)

ALKALOID BC-1

$C_{15}H_{21}O_3N$

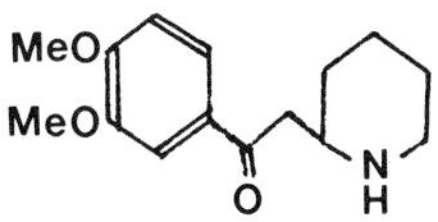

This substituted piperidine type alkaloid occurs, together with Cryptopleurine (q.v.) in the $CHCl_3$ extract of *Boehmeria cylindrica* fruiting plants. Infrared, ultraviolet, NMR and mass spectrometry have shown the structure to be that given above. No derivatives have been reported.

Farnsworth *et al.*, *Austral. J. Chem.*, **22**, 1805 (1969)

ALKALOID BC-2

$C_{23}H_{27}O_4N$

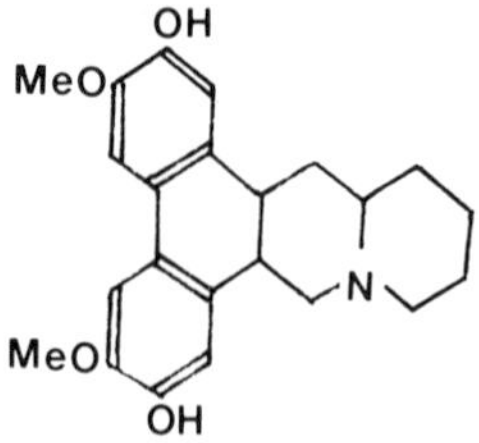

This alkaloid has been reported from the fruiting plant *Boehmeria cylindrica* using a modified procedure to that employed above in the isolation of the preceding base. Structurally, the alkaloid is related to Cryptopleurine (q.v.).

Farnsworth *et al.*, *Austral. J. Chem.*, **22**, 1805 (1969)

ALKALOID BC-3

$C_{24}H_{29}O_3N$

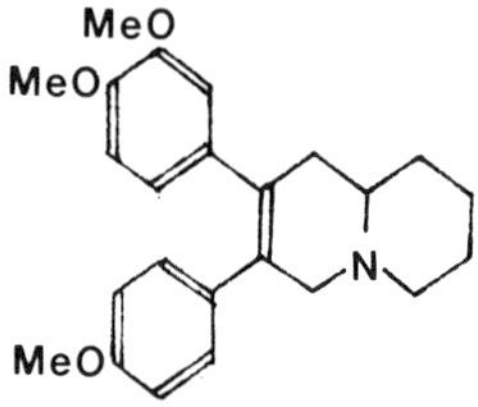

Isolated together with Alkaloid BC-2 from *Boehmeria cylindrica*, this base has been shown to be 2-(3:4-dimethoxyphenyl)-3-(*p*-methoxyphenyl)-2:3-dehydro-quinolizidine.

Farnsworth *et al.*, *Austral. J. Chem.*, **22**, 1805 (1969)

ALKALOID BC-A

M.p. 180–2°C

An uncharacterized alkaloid obtained by chromatographic separation of the basic fraction of *Bocconia cordata,* this base gives an ultraviolet spectrum having two absorption maxima at 236 and 285.5 mμ.

Kiryakov, Kitova, Georgieva., *Compt. Rend. Acad. Bulg.*, **20**, 189 (1967)

ALKALOID BC-B

M.p. 286–8°C

The protopine fraction obtained during the chromatography of the bases from *Bocconia cordata* contains this novel alkaloid which has an ultraviolet spectrum exhibiting absorption maxima at 242 and 290 mμ.

Kiryakov, Kitova, Georgieva., *Compt. Rend. Acad. Bulg.*, **20**, 189 (1967)

ALKALOID BP-1

$C_{24}H_{31}O_4N$

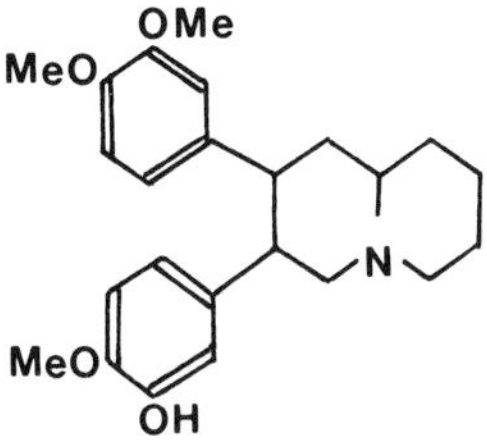

This quinolizidine alkaloid occurs in *Boehmeria platyphylla* as a minor constituent. The structure has been deduced from chemical degradation and spectroscopic data.

Hart, Johns, Lamberton., *Austral. J. Chem.*, **21**, 2579 (1968)

ALKALOID B-387

M.p. 188–9°C

A recently discovered alkaloid from *Buxus microphylla* var. *sinica*, the base has not yet been fully characterized.

Bauerova, Voticky., *Pharmazie*, **28**, 212 (1973)

ALKALOID C-A

An unidentified alkaloid found in various species of *Corydalis* grown in Korea. It occurs in the last fraction during chromatographic analysis of the alkaloidal extract and decomposes above 250°C. From its close association with the quaternary bases of these plants, it seems possible that it is a quaternary alkaloid.

Kaneko, Naruto, Ikeda., *J. Pharm. Soc., Japan*, **88**, 235 (1968)

ALKALOID CA-II

$C_{15}H_{24}O_2N_2$

This uncharacterized alkaloid occurs in the leaves of *Cadia purpurea*. No salts or derivatives have yet been described.

van Eijk, Radena., *Pharm. Weekbl.*, **107**, 13 (1972)

ALKALOID CA-IV

$C_{20}H_{27}O_3N_3$

Also present in the leaves of *Cadia purpurea*, this base may be identical with Calpurnine (q.v.) or one of its isomers.

van Eijk, Radena., *Pharm. Weekbl.*, **107**, 13 (1972)

ALKALOID CA-A

M.p. 240°C

One of two minor constituents of *Ceanothus americana* L., this alkaloid forms colourless crystals. Its presence has been confirmed by several workers but the quantities available for examination are very small and the structure is not yet known.

Gordin., *Pharm. Ber.*, **18**, 266 (1900)
Clark., *Amer. J. Pharm.*, **98**, 147 (1926)
Clark., *ibid*, **100**, 240 (1928)
Bertho, Liang., *Arch. Pharm.*, **271**, 273 (1933)

ALKALOID CA-B

M.p. 183°C

This alkaloid occurs with the preceding base in the alkaloid extract from *Ceanothus americana* L. No salts or derivatives have been reported.

Gordin., *Pharm. Ber.*, **18**, 266 (1900)
Clark., *Amer. J. Pharm.*, **98**, 147 (1926)
Clark., *ibid*, **100**, 240 (1928)
Bertho, Liang., *Arch. Pharm.*, **271**, 273 (1933)

ALKALOID CA-B

$C_{21}H_{23}O_6N$

M.p. 264–7°C

This minor alkaloid from *Colchicum autumnale* must not be confused with the preceding base. It forms yellow pyramids from EtOH and is laevorotatory with $[\alpha]_D^{22} - 171.2°$ (c 1.0863, $CHCl_3$). Four methoxyl groups have been shown to be present and the alkaloid is characterized as the dibromo derivative, m.p. 144–7°C.

Santavy, Reichstein., *Helv. Chim. Acta*, **33**, 1606 (1950)
Santavy., *Collect. Czech. Chem. Commun.*, **15**, 552 (1950)

ALKALOID CA-C

$C_{21}H_{23}O_6N$

M.p. 176–182°C

Also present in *Colchicum autumnale*, this alkaloid crystallizes as yellow plates from EtOH and has $[\alpha]_D^{21} - 130.7°$ (c 2.0118, $CHCl_3$). Three methoxy groups are present.

Santavy, Reichstein., *Helv. Chim. Acta*, **33**, 1606 (1950)
Santavy., *Collect. Czech. Chem. Commun.*, **15**, 552 (1950)

ALKALOID CA-D

$C_{21}H_{23}O_6N$

M.p. 235–7°C

This minor alkaloid has been isolated from *Colchicum autumnale* and yields colourless needles from MeOH. It is dextrorotatory with $[\alpha]_D^{18} + 294°$ (c 1.0, CHCl$_3$). The oxime has been prepared as colourless crystals with m.p. 300–1°C; $[\alpha]_D + 320°$ (c 0.731, MeOH); the acetyl derivative, m.p. 230–2°C; $[\alpha]_D + 283°$ (c 0.558, CHCl$_3$) and the ethyl ether with m.p. 232–4°C; $[\alpha]_D^{23} - 136°$ (c 0.744, CHCl$_3$).

Santavy, Reichstein., *Helv. Chim. Acta,* **33**, 1606 (1950)
Santavy., *Collect. Czech. Chem. Commun.,* **15**, 552 (1950)

ALKALOID CA-E

$C_{21}H_{23}O_6N$?

M.p. 178–180°C

A further minor constituent of *Colchicum autumnale,* this alkaloid forms light yellow plates from MeOH and has $[\alpha]_D - 129.2°$ (c 0.927, CHCl$_3$). The empirical formula given above is only tentative at the moment.

Santavy, Reichstein., *Helv. Chim. Acta,* **33**, 1606 (1950)
Santavy., *Collect. Czech. Chem. Commun.,* **15**, 552 (1950)

ALKALOID CA-E$_1$

$C_{21}H_{23}O_6N$

M.p. 140–180°C

Also present in small quantities in the alkaloidal extract of *Colchicum autumnale,* this base yields pale yellow crystals which melt gradually over a very wide temperature range. It is laevorotatory having $[\alpha]_D^{19} - 133°$ (c 1.0233, CHCl$_3$). The acetyl derivative has been prepared and has m.p. 192–4°C; $[\alpha]_D - 126°$ (c 0.981, CHCl$_3$). With CH_2N_2, the alkaloid furnishes an oily ether ether and not the expected methyl ether.

Santavy., *Collect. Czech. Chem. Commun.,* **15**, 552 (1950)

ALKALOID CA-E$_2$

$C_{21}H_{23}O_6N$

M.p. 140–180°C

This constituent of *Colchicum autumnale* has the same melting point range as the previous base but differs from it in specific rotation, this being $[\alpha]_D - 110°$ (c 1.6873, CHCl$_3$).

Santavy., *Collect. Czech. Chem. Commun.,* **15**, 552 (1950)

ALKALOID CA-F

$C_{21}H_{23}O_5N$

M.p. 184–6°C

A further minor base isolated from *Colchicum autumnale,* this alkaloid forms colourless prisms from MeOH and has $[\alpha]_D^{22} - 122°$ (c 1.032, $CHCl_3$). It is freely soluble in $CHCl_3$ and EtOH, less so in AcOEt, Me_2CO, C_6H_6 or H_2O, slightly soluble in Et_2O and insoluble in petroleum ether. The acetyl derivative has m.p. 228–230°C; $[\alpha]_D - 140°$. The base yields mixed crystals with Colchicine (q.v.), m.p. 187–9°C; $[\alpha]_D^{20} - 141°$.

Santavy., *Collect. Czech. Chem. Commun.,* **15**, 552 (1950)
Santavy, Reichstein., *Helv. Chim. Acta,* **33**, 1606 (1950)
Santavy, Talas., *Chem. Listy.,* **47**, 232 (1953)
Santavy, Talas., *Collect. Czech. Chem. Commun.,* **19**, 141 (1954)

ALKALOID CA-G

$C_{22}H_{25}O_6N$?

M.p. 187–9°C

Also present in *Colchicum autumnale,* this alkaloid is obtained as a colourless powder and is laevorotatory with $[\alpha]_D^{19} - 139.2°$ (c 0.927, $CHCl_3$).

Santavy., *Collect. Czech. Chem. Commun.,* **15**, 552 (1950)
Santavy, Reichstein., *Helv. Chim. Acta,* **33**, 1606 (1950)

ALKALOID CA-I

$C_{22}H_{25}O_6N$?

M.p. 184–6°C

This alkaloid of *Colchicum autumnale* crystallizes as colourless needles from MeOH and has $[\alpha]_D^{23} + 307°$ (c 0.894, $CHCl_3$). It yields a crystalline oxime, m.p. 273–6°C with $[\alpha]_D + 294°$ (c 0.578, MeOH).

Santavy., *Collect. Czech. Chem. Commun.,* **15**, 552 (1950)
Santavy, Reichstein., *Helv. Chim. Acta,* **33**, 1606 (1950)

ALKALOID CA-S

$C_{22}H_{25}O_6N$

M.p. 136–8°C

A further alkaloid isolated from *Colchicum autumnale,* this base is laevorotatory having $[\alpha]_D^{25} - 119°$. It occurs mainly in the basic $CHCl_3$ extract of the seeds and is soluble in $CHCl_3$ and H_2O, less so in MeOH or Me_2CO, slightly soluble in

Et$_2$O and virtually insoluble in petroleum ether. The acetyl derivative has m.p. 200–2°C and $[\alpha]_D^{26}$ − 218°. Four methoxyl groups have been shown to be present.

Santavy, Talas., *Chem. Listy.*, **47**, 232 (1953)

Santavy, Talas., *Collect. Czech. Chem. Commun.*, **19**, 141 (1954)

ALKALOID CA-1

$C_{22}H_{33}O_3N_3$

M.p. 155–6°C

One of a group of three alkaloids from *Cynometra ananta* which have spasmolytic, but weak central depressive activity; marked analgaesic action, but no secondary effect.

Belg. Patent, 780,935 17 June 1972

ALKALOID CA-2

$C_{16}H_{19}O_2N_3$

M.p. 212°C

Also present in *Cynometra ananta*, this alkaloid possesses similar pharmacological properties to those of the preceding base.

Belg. Patent, 780,935 17 June 1972

ALKALOID CA-3

$C_{15}H_{15}ON_3$

M.p. 200°C (*dec.*).

A third alkaloid which has been obtained from *Cynometra ananta*, the base also has spasmolytic and weak central depressive activity and a pronounced analgaesic action with no secondary effect.

Belg. Patent, 780,935 17 June 1972

ALKALOID CC-A

M.p. 211°C

This alkaloid occurs in the non-phenolic portion of the alkaloidal extract from *Cryptocarya chinensis*, a Lauraceous plant indigenous to Formosa. It forms colourless crystals from Me$_2$CO and has $[\alpha]_D^{12}$ − 103.7° (c 1.0, CHCl$_3$).

Lu, Lan., *J. Pharm. Soc., Japan,* **86**, 177 (1966)

ALKALOID CC-B

A second minor constituent of *Cryptocarya chinensis,* this base also occurs in the non-phenolic portion of the alkaloidal extract. It has been characterized as the crystalline picrate, m.p. 164–8°C.

Lu, Lan., *J. Pharm. Soc., Japan,* 86, 177 (1966)

ALKALOID CC-2

$C_{21}H_{27}O_5N$

M.p. 170°C

This alkaloid was first isolated from the corms of *Colchicum cornigerum* collected on the Sinai peninsula. It crystallizes as colourless prisms from a mixture of Et_2O and AcOEt and is dextrorotatory with $[\alpha]_D^{20} + 38°$ ($CHCl_3$). The molecular structure and absolute stereochemistry given above have been determined by X-ray analysis of the crystalline methiodide. The rhombic crystals of this derivative have space group $P2_12_12_1$ and a = 7.75, b = 14.57 and c = 21.55 Å with Z = 4.

El-Hamidi, Santavy., *Collect. Czech. Chem. Commun.,* 27, 2111 (1962)
Structure:
Cameron, Hannaway., *J. Chem. Soc., Perkin 2,* 1002 (1973)

ALKALOID CC-3

$C_{20}H_{25}O_5N$

M.p. 195°C

A non-tropolone alkaloid obtained from the corms of *Colchicum cornigerum* from Formosa, this base crystallizes from Et_2O-AcOEt in colourless crystals. It has $[\alpha]_D^{22} + 155° \pm 3°$ (c 0.76, $CHCl_3$). The Oberlin-Zeisel test is negative for this alkaloid.

El-Hamidi, Santavy., *Collect. Czech. Chem. Commun.,* 27, 2111 (1962)

ALKALOID CC-4

M.p. 126°C

Also present in the corms of Formosan *Colchicum cornigerum,* the structure of this non-tropolone alkaloid has not yet been determined.

El-Hamidi, Santavy., *Collect. Czech. Chem. Commun.,* 27, 2111 (1962)

ALKALOID CC-6

This alkaloid of *Colchicum cornigerum* has been isolated as the acetyl derivative, m.p. 180°C which yields colourless crystals from Et_2O-AcOEt. This alkaloid gives a positive Oberlin-Zeisel reaction.

El-Hamidi, Santavy., *Collect. Czech. Chem. Commun.*, **27**, 2111 (1962)

ALKALOID CC-12

$C_{19}H_{21}O_6N$

M.p. 197–9°C

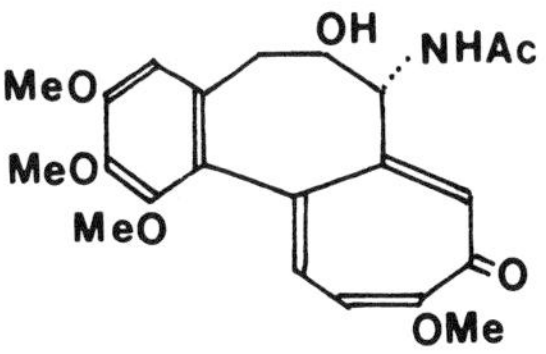

A colchicine type alkaloid present in *Colchicum cornigerum*, the base is laevo-rotatory with $[\alpha]_D^{22} - 45°$ and has the structure given above since NMR spectroscopy shows the hydroxyl group to be adjacent to the methylamino group.

Cross *et al.*, *Collect. Czech. Chem. Commun.*, **31**, 374 (1966)

ALKALOID CF-A

$C_{19}H_{21}O_4N$

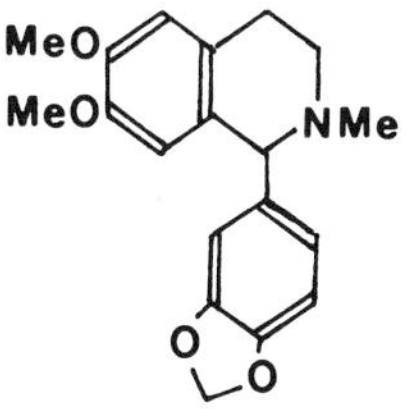

One of three tetrahydro*iso*quinoline alkaloid isolated from *Cryptostylis fulva*. The structure has been assigned by spectroscopic methods and confirmed by synthesis.

Leander, Luning., *Acta Chem. Scand.*, **23**, 244 (1969)

ALKALOID CF-B

$C_{20}H_{25}O_4N$

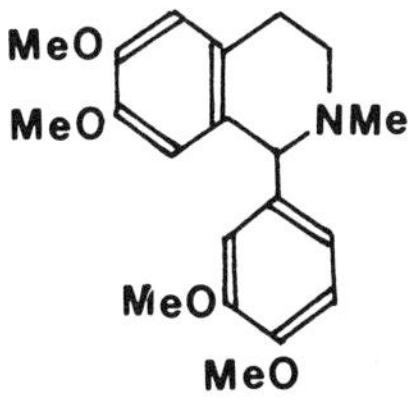

A further alkaloid of the *iso*quinoline type obtained from *Cryptostylis fulva*. The base differs from the preceding and following alkaloid only in the substitution pattern of the phenyl ring. The structure has also been confirmed by synthesis.

Leander, Luning., *Acta Chem. Scand.*, **23**, 244 (1969)

ALKALOID CF-C

$C_{21}H_{27}O_5N$

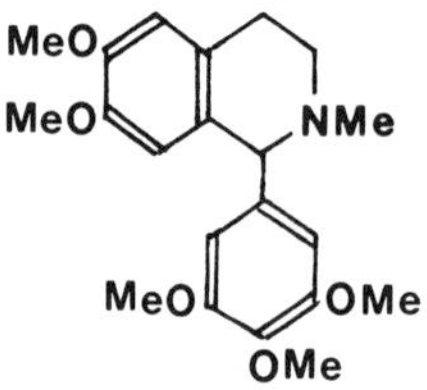

The third isoquinoline base isolated from *Cryptostylis fulva,* this alkaloid has been shown by spectroscopic examination and synthesis to be the 3:4:5-trimethoxyphenyl derivative.

Leander, Luning., *Acta Chem. Scand.*, **23**, 244 (1969)

ALKALOID CF-D

M.p. 138–9°C

An uncharacterized alkaloid obtained from *Coelidium fourcadei,* the base forms colourless crystals and yields a dihydro derivative when reduced with $NaBH_4$.

Arndt, Du Plessis., *J. S. Afr. Chem. Inst.*, **21**, 54 (1968)

ALKALOID CF-E

M.p. 148–9°C

The second base found in *Coelidium fourcadei,* this alkaloid is isomeric with the preceding base, as is also the dihydro derivative formed by treatment with $NaBH_4$. No salts or derivatives have been prepared.

Arndt, Du Plessis., *J. S. Afr. Chem. Inst.*, **21**, 54 (1968)

ALKALOID CG-A$_2$

$C_{18}H_{25}O_6N$

M.p. 160–1°C

The powdered seeds of *Crotalaria grahamiana,* after defatting with petroleum ether and extraction with EtOH yield Monocrotaline (q.v.) and this minor component which forms slender, colourless rods and having $[\alpha]_D + 125.7°$ (EtOH). It forms a crystalline methiodide, m.p. 240–1°C and has no methoxyl groups but contains three methyl groups. Hydrolysis with $Ba(OH)_2$ gives a necic acid which has been identified as retronecine from paper chromatography.

Gandhi, Rajagopalan, Seshardi., *Curr. Sci.*, **35**, 514 (1966)

ALKALOID CL-1

$C_{20}H_{26}O_2N_2$

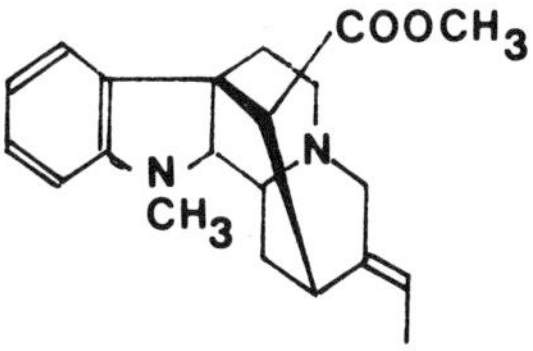

A minor constituent of *Carathanthus longifolus*, the structure of this base has been determined by chemical correlation with the akuammiline analogue.

Rasonaivo *et al.*, *Tetrahedron Lett.*, 1425 (1973)

ALKALOID CL-A

$C_{36}H_{38}O_6N_2$

M.p. 273–298°C (*dec.*).

A minor constituent of *Chondrodendron limacifolium*, this alkaloid contains two methoxyl groups and furnishes a sulphate obtained as a mixture of colourless rhombs and hexagonal plates, m.p. 289°C with effervescence.

Barltrop, Jeffreys., *J. Chem. Soc.*, 159 (1954)

ALKALOID CL-B

$C_{35}H_{33}O_8N_2$

M.p. 230°C (*dec.*).

A further minor alkaloid present in *Condrodendron limacifolium*, the base is dextrorotatory with $[\alpha]_D^{20} + 31.1°$ (c 0.5, CHCl$_3$). It has been shown to contain three methoxyl groups in the molecule.

Barltrop, Jeffreys., *J. Chem. Soc.*, 159 (1954)

ALKALOID CL-C

$C_{12}H_{22}ON_2$

M.p. 128–9°C

This alkaloid occurs in *Cytisus laburnum* and is slightly dextrorotatory with $[\alpha]_D^{19} + 18.6°$ (EtOH). It is characterized as the crystalline picrate, m.p. 204–5°C.

Galovinsky, Vogel, Nasvadba., *Scientia Pharm.*, **21**, 256 (1953)

ALKALOID CL-I

M.p. 216–7°C

An alkaloid of *Cocculus laurifolius,* this crystalline base yields a hydrobromide, m.p. 266°C. It has been shown to be a phenolic, tertiary base.

Tomita, Kusuda., *Pharm. Bull.,* 1, 1 (1953)

ALKALOID CM-A

This alkaloid from *Calligonum minimum* has been studied by Abdusalamov and Sadykov who have shown it to be a triacetoneamine probably formed during the isolation of the associated alkaloids.

Abdusalamov, Sadykov., *Uzbeksk. Khim. Zh.,* 6, No. 4, 79 (1962)

ALKALOID CP-P

$C_6H_{11}ON$

Corydalis pallida var. *tenuis* yields this simple alkaloid which has been shown to be 3-ethyl-2-pyrrolidone. Pharmacologically it has proved to be an effective anti-ulcer drug.

Kametani., Jap. Patent, 73 08 484

ALKALOID CR-A

$C_{15}H_{16}O_5N_2$

M.p. 171.5–173°C

This alkaloid occurs with Sparteine (q.v.) in the aerial parts of Cytisus ruthenicus. The base has $[\alpha]_D^{18} - 15.26°$ (Me_2CO) and is readily soluble in Me CO but insoluble in C_6H_6, Et_2O or H_2O. Crystalline salts have been prepared including the hydriodide, m.p. 231–3°C; perchlorate, m.p. 198–200°C and the dipicrate, m.p. 199–201°C. No methoxyl groups or methyl groups are present but the alkaloid contains one methylimino group.

Alekseev, Todoshchenko, Ban'kovs'kii., *Farm. Zh.,* (Kiev), 22, 59 (1967)

ALKALOID CS-A

$C_{14}H_{19}O_3N$

A highly toxic alkaloid, this base is a minor constituent of *Cassia siamea* Linn. Only small quantities have been isolated and no salts or derivatives have been reported.

Wells., *Philipp. J. Sci.,* 14, 1 (1919)

ALKALOID CV-A

$C_{23}H_{26}O_4N_2$

M.p. 270°C (*dec.*).

This alkaloid has been described as occurring in *Ceanothus velutinus* Dougl. Apart from the empirical formula and melting point, no other details have been recorded.

Richards, Lynn., *J. Amer. Pharm. Assoc.*, **28**, 332 (1934)

ALKALOID CW-A

$C_{18}H_{19}O_4N$

M.p. 235–7°C

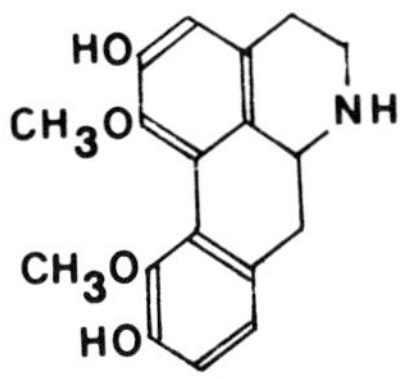

One of five closely related aporphine alkaloids isolated from *Croton wilsonii* by countercurrent techniques, this base is dextrorotatory with $[\alpha]_D^{18} + 142°$ (c 0.52, pyridine). The N-methyl derivative is amorphous but gives a crystalline hydrochloride, m.p. 244–5°C; $[\alpha]_D^{23} + 209°$ (c 0.55, MeOH) which is identical with the hydriodide of Alkaloid CW-B (q.v.). The structure of the alkaloid has been confirmed by comparison with an authentic specimen prepared synthetically.

Stuart, Chambers., *Tetrahedron Lett.*, 4135 (1967)

ALKALOID CW-B

$C_{19}H_{21}O_4N$

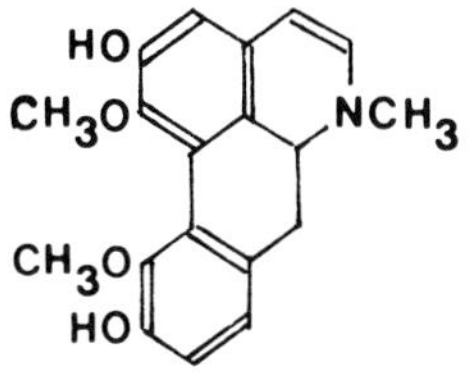

This aporphine alkaloid from *Croton wilsonii* is the N-methyl derivative of the preceding base and gives a crystalline hydrochloride, m.p. 244–5°C; $[\alpha]_D^{23} + 209°$ (c 0.55, MeOH). The structure has been established by correlation with Alkaloid CW-A.

Stuart, Chambers., *Tetrahedron Lett.*, 4135 (1967)

ALKALOID CW-C

$C_{19}H_{21}O_4N$

M.p. 157–8°C

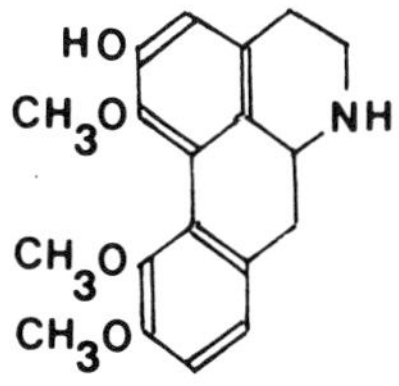

Isolated by countercurrent techniques from *Croton wilsonii*, the structure has been established by treatment with CH_2N_2 to give the O-methyl derivative which proves to be identical with Catalpifoline (q.v.).

Stuart, Chambers., *Tetrahedron Lett.*, 4135 (1967)

ALKALOID CW-D

$C_{20}H_{23}O_4N$

M.p. 218–9°C

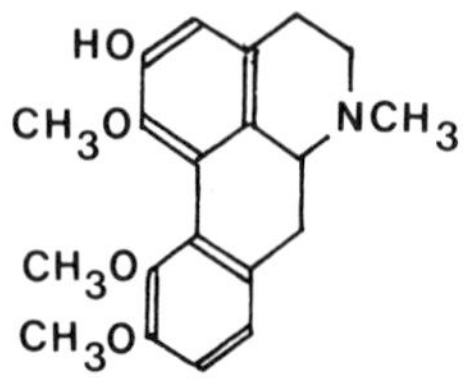

A fourth aporphine alkaloid present in *Croton wilsonii*, this base is dextro-rotatory with $[\alpha]_D^{23} + 139°$ (c 0.51, MeOH). The structure has been determined by treatment with CH_2N_2 and reaction of the resulting O-methyl ether with methyl iodide to yield O,O-dimethylmagniflorine iodide, m.p. 242–4°C.

Stuart, Chambers., *Tetrahedron Lett.*, 4135 (1967)

ALKALOID CW-E

$C_{19}H_{21}O_4N$

M.p. 211–3°C

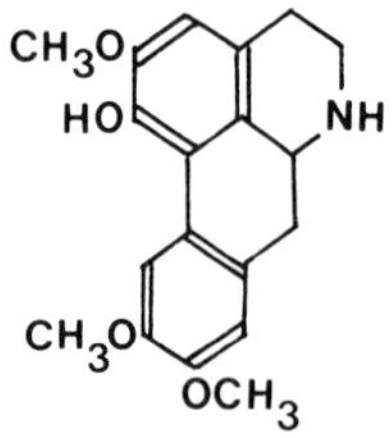

A further aporphine alkaloid isolated from *Croton wilsonii*, the base yields a neutral diacetate, m.p. 229–231°C; $[\alpha]_D^{23} + 56°$ (c 0.59, MeOH). The structure follows from the identity of the O-methyl ether with O-methylisoboldine.

Stuart, Chambers., *Tetrahedron Lett.*, 4135 (1967)

ALKALOID C1

$C_{15}H_{22}ON_2$

This minor alkaloid has recently been isolated from the leaves of *Cadia purpurea*. The structure is not yet known with certainty.

van Eijk, Radena., *Pharm. Weekbl.*, **107**, 13 (1972)

ALKALOID DA-A

$C_{28}H_{36}O_{13}N$

A minor aconitine alkaloid, this base is present in *Delphinium* araraticum. No salts or derivatives have been prepared to characterize the base.

Namedor., *Aptechn. Delo.*, **14**, 26 (1965)

ALKALOID DB-A

$C_{24}H_{37}O_6N$

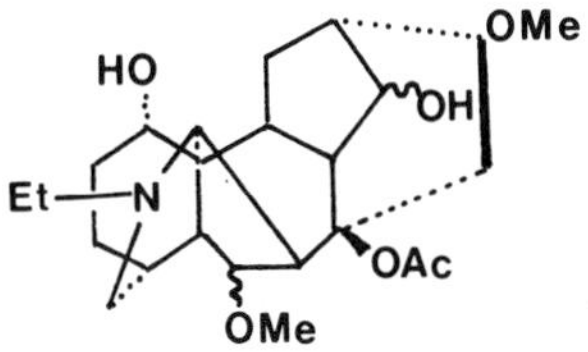

A recently discovered atisine alkaloid from *Delphinium bicolor,* the stereochemistry and structure of the base have been established by chemical and spectroscopic techniques.

Jones, Benn., *Tetrahedron Lett.*, 4351 (1972)

ALKALOID DB-B

$C_{21}H_{33}O_5N$

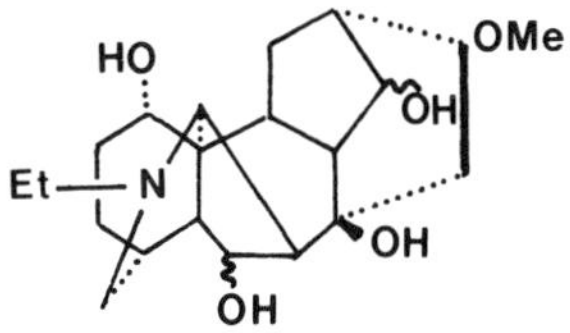

A further atisine alkaloid found in *Delphinium bicolor,* this base is the demethyl-deacetyl derivative of the preceding alkaloid, the stereochemistry also being determined by means of infrared, NMR and mass spectrometry.

Jones, Benn., *Tetrahedron Lett.*, 4351 (1972)

ALKALOID DD-1

$C_{13}H_{21}O_2N$

M.p. Indefinite

This alkaloid obtained from *Dioscorea dumetorum* yields an amorphous solid which cannot be crystallized. When injected into mice it causes convulsions which are, at first, clonic but become tonic and sometimes result in death. Concentrations of 10^{-5} reduce the response to acetylcholine of isolated guinea-pig ileum and rabbit duodenum preparations.

Bevan, Broadbent, Hirst., *Nature,* **177**, 935 (1956)

ALKALOID DF-A

$C_{18}H_{30}O_5N$

M.p. 85–6°C

This minor constituent of *Delphinium foetidum* is one of three bases isolated by Zolotnitskaya. It forms colourless crystals which are readily soluble in $CHCl_3$, EtOH and Me_2CO but insoluble in H_2O.

Zolotnitskaya., *Dokl. Akad. Nauk. Arm. SSR.*, 37, 95 (1963)

ALKALOID DF-B

$C_{15}H_{23}O_4N$

M.p. 143°C

A second base obtained from *Delphinium foetidum,* this alkaloid also forms colourless crystals. It is soluble in $CHCl_3$ and MeOH, insoluble in Me_2CO or H_2O.

Zolotnitskaya., *Dokl. Akad. Nauk. Arm. SSR.*, 37, 95 (1963)

ALKALOID DF-C

$C_{29}H_{46}N_2$

This alkaloid from *Delphinium foetidum* has no definite melting point. It dissolves readily in $CHCl_3$, EtOH and Et_2O but is insoluble in H_2O.

Zolotnitskaya., *Dokl. Akad. Nauk. Arm. SSR.*, 37, 95 (1963)

ALKALOID DF-1

$C_{35}H_{54}O_8N_2$

M.p. 166°C

One of a series of minor bases isolated from *Delphinium* species, this alkaloid occurs in *D. flexosum.* It is freely soluble in $CHCl_3$ but soluble only with difficulty in EtOH, Et_2O, Me_2CO or H_2O.

Zolotnitskaya *et al., Biol. Zh. Armenia,* 20, 11 (1967)

ALKALOID DF-2

$C_{18}H_{29}O_7N$

M.p. 201–2°C

This minor alkaloid of *Delphinium flexosum* is present in the $CHCl_3$ extract. It dissolves freely in MeOH or Me_2CO but is only sparingly soluble in EtOH, Et_2O, $CHCl_3$ or H_2O. It is stated to exert a powerful bactericidal effect.

Zolotnitskaya *et al., Biol. Zh. Armenia,* 20, 11 (1967)

ALKALOID DF-3

M.p. 113–5°C

An uncharacterized alkaloid obtained from *Delphinium flexosum*, the base forms colourless needles when recrystallized from MeOH. It is present only in minute quantities and insufficient material has been isolated for the empirical formula to be determined.

Zolotnitskaya *et al., Biol. Zh. Armenia,* **20**, 11 (1967)

ALKALOID DF-4

$C_{18}H_{30}O_5N$

M.p. 110°C

This alkaloid occurs in *Delphinium foetidum* and crystallizes from EtOH as white needles. It is soluble in $CHCl_3$, Me_2CO or EtOH but insoluble in H_2O.

Zolotnitskaya *et al., Biol. Zh. Armenia,* **20**, 11 (1967)

ALKALOID DF-5

$C_{15}H_{23}O_4N$

M.p. 153–4°C

A further minor constituent of *Delphinium foetidum,* this base is soluble in Et_2O and $CHCl_3$ but only sparingly so in Me_2CO, EtOH or H_2O.

Zolotnitskaya *et al., Biol. Zh. Armenia,* **20**, 11 (1967)

ALKALOID DI-V

$C_{45}H_{72}O_{14}N_2$

M.p. 192.5–193°C

This alkaloid is present as a minor constituent of *Delphinium iliense* and forms colourless needles when recrystallized from a mixture of Me_2CO and Et_2O. The structure has not yet been determined but the base appears to be a complex aconite alkaloid of the ester type.

Brutko, Massagetov., *Khim. Prir. Soedin.,* **3**, 21 (1967)

ALKALOID DL-A

$C_{13}H_{23}O_2N$

Present in *Duboisia leuchhardtii,* the alkaloid has been characterized as the crystalline hydrobromide, m.p. 206–7°C. It also forms an aurichloride as yellow needles, m.p. 98–100°C and a picrate, m.p. 219–220°C. The alkaloid has been identified as (±)-2-methylbutyryltropine.

Deckers, Maier., *Chem. Ber.,* **86**, 1423 (1953)

ALKALOID DL-B

$C_{12}H_{21}O_2N$

Also isolated from *Duboisia leuchhardtii,* the base forms a crystalline hydrobromide as colourless needles, m.p. 218–9°C; an aurichloride, m.p. 129°C and a picrate, m.p. 211°C. Chemical investigation has shown the alkaloid to be isobutyryltropine.

Deckers, Maier., *Chem. Ber.,* **86**, 1423 (1953)

ALKALOID DM-A

$C_{15}H_{18}N_2$

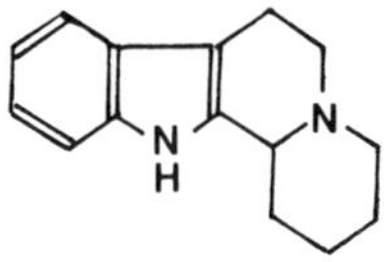

An indoloquinolizine alkaloid, this base is the major alkaloid of *Dracontomelum mangiferum.* Chemical and spectroscopic evidence has shown it to be (−)-1:2:3:4:6:7-hexahydro-12H-indolo[2,3-a]quinolizine, a base not found previously in nature although the optically inactive form had been synthesized earlier.

Johns, Lamberton, Occolowitz., *Austral. J. Chem.,* **19**, 1951 (1966)

ALKALOID DM-1

$C_{30}H_{47}O_5N$

This alkaloid has been obtained from *Daphniphyllum macropodum* as the crystalline iodomethylate, $C_{31}H_{50}O_5NI$ with m.p. 286–7°C. The complete structure has not yet been elucidated.

Kamijo *et al., Tetrahedron Lett.,* 2889 (1966)

ALKALOID DM-2

$C_{31}H_{53}O_3N$

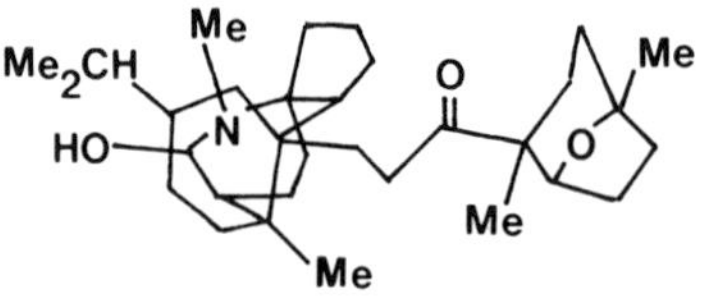

The bark of *Daphniphyllum macropodum* also yields this novel alkaloid, isolated as the iodomethylate, m.p. 306–7°C. The structure given above has been deduced from computer-assisted evaluation of X-ray data and confirmed by conventional analysis.

Kamijo *et al., Tetrahedron Lett.*, 2889 (1966)

ALKALOID DM-3

A third complex alkaloid from the bark of *Daphniphyllum macropodum,* this base has also been obtained as the crystalline iodomethylate, m.p. 264–5°C. The structure is still unknown.

Kamijo *et al., Tetrahedron Lett.*, 2889 (1966)

ALKALOID DR-A

$C_{21}H_{31}O_4N$

One of two minor bases isolated from *Delphinium rugulosum,* this alkaloid is stated to possess curare-like activity. No further details have been given.

Namedov., *Aptechn. Delo.*, **14**, 26 (1965)

ALKALOID DR-B

$C_{19}H_{29}O_4N$

Also present in *Delphinium rugulosum,* this base resembles the preceding alkaloid is possessing curare-like activity. The structure has not yet been elucidated.

Namedov., *Aptechn. Delo.*, **14**, 26 (1965)

ALKALOID DS-A

M.p. 245–7°C

The leaves of *Doryphora sassafras* yield four closely-related alkaloids which have been isolated by Gharbo and his colleagues. This particular base forms colourless needles and is soluble in MeOH but insoluble in Et_2O. The ultraviolet spectrum has a single absorption maximum at 234 mμ. No analysis of the alkaloid has yet been carried out.

Gharbo *et al., Lloydia,* **28**, 237 (1965)

ALKALOID DS-B

This minor constituent of the leaf extract of *Doryphora sassafras* has been characterized as the crystalline hydriodide, m.p. 190–2°C. The ultraviolet spectrum is similar to that of the preceding base with an absorption maximum at 251 mμ.

Gharbo *et al., Lloydia,* **28**, 237 (1965)

ALKALOID DS-C

M.p. 249–251°C

This alkaloid, present in the leaves of *Doryphora sassafras*, forms light tan needles and is readily soluble in MeOH and only slightly so in Me_2CO. The ultraviolet spectrum in ethanol has a single absorption maximum at 250 mμ.

Gharbo *et al.*, *Lloydia*, **28**, 237 (1965)

ALKALOID DS-D

The fourth alkaloid isolated from *Doryphora sassafras* leaves forms colourless prisms and gives an ultraviolet spectrum in EtOH with an absorption maximum at 234 mμ.

Gharbo *et al.*, *Lloydia*, **28**, 237 (1965)

ALKALOID DS-1

$C_{15}H_{23}O_4N$

M.p. 157–8°C

A minor alkaloid found in *Delphinium semibarbatum*, this base forms colourless prisms from a mixture of EtOH and Me_2CO. The structure has not yet been elucidated.

Brutko, Massagetov., *Khim. Prir. Soedin.*, **3**, 21 (1967)

ALKALOID DS-2

$C_{20}H_{25}O_7N$

M.p. 153–4°C

Also present in small amounts in *Delphinium semibarbatum*, this base yields colourless crystals from Me_2CO. Like the preceding alkaloid, the structure has not been determined.

Brutko, Massagetov., *Khim. Prir. Soedin.*, **3**, 21 (1967)

ALKALOID DT-A

M.p. 215–220°C (*dec.*).

An alkaloid of *Dipidax triquetra*, this base forms colourless crystals from a mixture of $CHCl_3$ and MeOH. Insufficient of the material has been obtained for a chemical analysis.

Pihewska *et al.*, *Collect. Czech. Chem. Commun.*, **32**, 158 (1967)

ALKALOID EC-b

M.p. 238–9°C

This tertiary base has been isolated from *Eschscholtzia californica* and crystallizes as colourless needles from EtOH. No chemical analysis has yet been made and no salts or derivatives have been described.

Gertig., *Acta Polon. Pharm.*, **22**, 271 (1965)

ALKALOID EE-1

$C_{29}H_{37}O_{13}N$?

M.p. 258–260°C

A complex alkaloid present in *Euonymus europeus,* this base is dextrorotatory with $[\alpha]_D + 21°$ (CHCl$_3$). The structure is unknown and no salts or derivatives have been reported.

Doebel, Reichstein., *Helv. Chim. Acta*, **32**, 592 (1949)

ALKALOID EE-2

$C_{27}H_{35}O_{12}N$?

M.p. 288–290°C

Also present in *Euonymus europeus,* this base has a specific rotation similar to that of the preceding alkaloid with $[\alpha]_D + 14°$ (CHCl$_3$).

Doebel, Reichstein., *Helv. Chim. Acta*, **32**, 592 (1949)

ALKALOID EE-3

$C_{31}H_{39}O_{14}N$?

M.p. 164–8°C

Euonymus europeus also contains this complex alkaloid as a minor constituent. It is slightly dextrorotatory with $[\alpha]_D + 8°$ (CHCl$_3$).

Doebel, Reichstein., *Helv. Chim. Acta.*, **32**, 592 (1949)

ALKALOID EF-A

M.p. 115°C

An alkaloid from *Emilia flammea,* this base yields ochonecine on alkaline hydrolysis indicating that it is a diester of this necine. The structure has not yet been determined.

Kohlmuenzer, Tomceyk., *Diss. Pharm. Pharmacol.*, **21**, 433 (1969)

ALKALOID EF-B

M.p. 128–130°C

Emilia flammea also yields this uncharacterized alkaloid. As yet, the structure is unknown and no salts or derivatives have been described.

Kohlmuenzer, Tomceyk., *Diss. Pharm. Pharmacol.*, **21**, 433 (1969)

ALKALOID EG-A

$C_{25}H_{39}O_6N$

M.p. 147–9°C

One of the number of alkaloid obtained from *Erythrophleum guineense*, this base has $[\alpha]_D - 60°$ (95% EtOH) and is characterized as the crystalline picrate, m.p. 182–5°C.

Engel, Tondeur., *Experientia*, **4**, 430 (1948)

ALKALOID EG-B

$C_{25}H_{39}O_5N$

M.p. 84–5°C

A further laevorotatory alkaloid found in *Erythrophleum guineense*, the base has $[\alpha]_D - 56°$ (95% EtOH). It gives a crystalline hydrochloride, m.p. 212–5°C; $[\alpha]_D - 48°$ (H_2O); perchlorate, m.p. 189–192°C; $[\alpha]_D - 50°$ (50% EtOH) and a bisulphate, m.p. 198–208°C; $[\alpha]_D - 49.5°$ (H_2O).

Engel, Tondeur., *Experientia*, **4**, 430 (1948)

ALKALOID ET-1

A glycoalkaloid found in *Erythrina thollonia*, this base possesses curare-like activity. On acid hydrolysis it furnishes glucose and an erythroalkaloid, m.p. 196°C.

Lapiere., *Bull. Soc. Chim. Biol.*, **31**, 862 (1949)

ALKALOID ET-A

M.p. 187°C

An alkaloid obtained from *Euphorbia thymifolia*, this base contains a secondary amino group and is actively unsaturated. It has been found to inhibit the growth of *Eschscherischia coli* and *Bacillus subtilis* but not that of *B. cereus* or *Staphylococcus aureus*.

Jabbar, Khan., *Pakistan J. Sci. Ind. Res.*, **8**, 293 (1965)

ALKALOID ET-B

A further minor constituent of *Euphorbia thymifolia*, this alkaloid differs from the two accompanying bases in being inactive against both *Bacillus subtilies* and *Eschscherischia coli.*

Jabbar, Khan., *Pakistan J. Sci. Ind. Res.,* 8, 293 (1965)

ALKALOID ET-C

Also present in *Euphorbia thymifolia,* this alkaloid resembles Alkaloid ET-A in inhibiting the growth of *Eschscherischia coli* and *Bacillus subtilis.*

Jabbar, Khan., *Pakistan J. Sci. Ind. Res.,* 8, 293 (1965)

ALKALOID FI-1

M.p. $145-6°C$

An alkaloid isolated from the corms of *Fritillaria imperialis,* this base crystallizes from EtOH in colourless prisms and is laevorotatory with $[\alpha]_D - 14°$.

Suri, Ram., *Ind. J. Chem.,* 7, 1057 (1969)

ALKALOID FI-A

$C_{15}H_{18}O_2N$

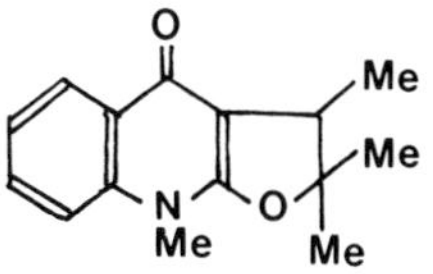

Flindersia ifflaiana contains this furoquinoline alkaloid as a minor constituent. The structure has been confirmed by synthesis from 1-methyl-4-β(3-methyl-2-butenyl)oxy-2-quinolone.

Grundon, Chamberlain., *J. Chem. Soc., C,* 901 (1971)

ALKALOID FO-A

$C_{21}H_{23}O_5N$

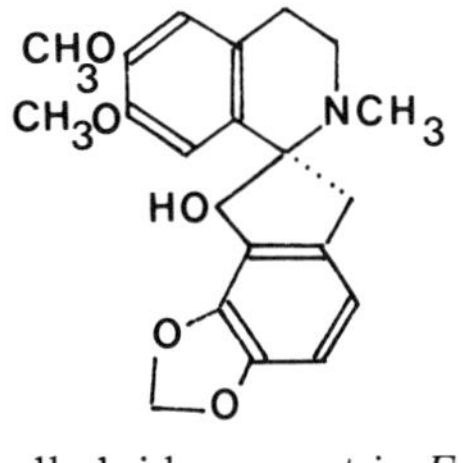

One of three spiro*iso*quinoline alkaloids present in *Fumaria officinalis.* The proposed structure, based upon chemical and spectroscopic data, contains two methoxyl groups, a methylenedioxy group and a methylimino group.

Saunders *et al., Can. J. Chem.,* 46, 2873 (1968)

ALKALOID FO-B

$C_{20}H_{21}O_5N$

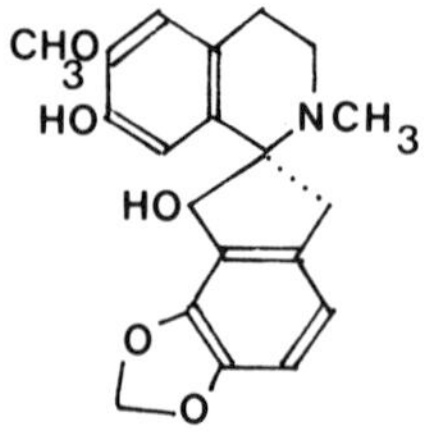

A second spiro*iso*quinoline alkaloid isolated from *Fumaria officinalis*, this base has the structure given above on the basis of chemical analysis and infrared, NMR and mass spectrometry.

Saunders *et al., Can. J. Chem.*, **46**, 2873 (1968)

ALKALOID FO-C

$C_{21}H_{21}O_5N$

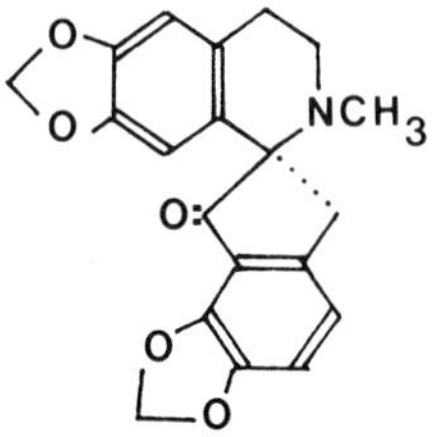

Also present in *Fumaria officinalis*, this spiro*iso*quinoline alkaloid is the dehydro analogue of Alkaloid FO-A. Two methoxyl groups, a methylenedioxy group a keto group and a methyimino group are present in the molecule.

Saunders *et al., Can. J. Chem.*, **46**, 2873 (1968)

ALKALOID FP-1

The root bark of *Fagara parvifolia* A. Chev. yields four alkaloids which have been investigated by Paris and his co-workers. This particular base has m.p. 200–2°C and yields a hydrochloride as pale yellow crystals, m.p. 220–2°C.

Paris, Moyse, Mignon., *Ann. Pharm. Fr.*, **6**, 409 (1948)

ALKALOID FP-2

M.p. 268–270°C

Also present in *Fumaria parvifolia* A. Chev., this alkaloid yields a crystalline hydrochloride as orange-yellow crystals, m.p. 260–2°C and a picrate, m.p. 222–3°C.

Paris, Moyse, Mignon., *Ann. Pharm. Fr.*, **6**, 409 (1948)

ALKALOID FP-3

M.p. 208–210°C

Isolated from *Fumaria parvifolia* A. Chev., this alkaloid crystallizes from EtOH as white crystals. No salts have been reported.

Paris, Moyse, Mignon., *Ann. Pharm. Fr.*, **6**, 409 (1948)

ALKALOID FP-4

M.p. 218–220°C

This alkaloid from *Fumaria parvifolia* A. Chev. also forms white crystals from EtOH. As in the case of the preceding base, no salts have yet been described.

Paris, Moyse, Mignon., *Ann. Pharm. Fr.*, **6**, 409 (1948)

ALKALOID FR-1

$C_{21}H_{26}O_4N$

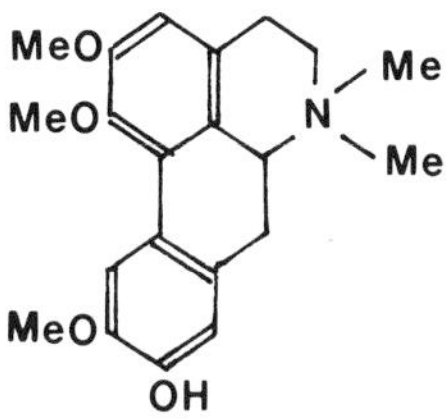

The bark of *Fagara rhoifolia* yields α-Allocryptopine (q.v.) as the major alkaloid but the butanol soluble fraction also contains this base, shown to be 6-hydroxy-2:3:5-trimethoxy-N,N-dimethylaporphinium chloride, m.p. 218–220°C; $[\alpha]_D^{22}$ + 29.6°. The quaternary base yields an iodide, m.p. 228–9°C; picrate, m.p. 147–9°C and the 6-acetyl derivative, m.p. 234–6°C.

Calderwood, Fish., *Chem. Ind.*, **6**, 237 (1966)

ALKALOID FR-5

M.p. 245–7°C

A minor alkaloid of the tubers of *Fritillaria raddeana*, this uncharacterized base is found in the mother liquors. An insufficient amount of material has been obtained for a chemical analysis to be carried out.

Aslanov, Sadykov., *J. Gen. Chem., USSR*, **26**, 579 (1956)

ALKALOID FR-6

A further minor constituent obtained from the tubers of *Fritillaria raddeana*, this base is characterized as the crystalline hydrochloride, m.p. 197–9°C.

Aslanov, Sadykov., *J. Gen. Chem., USSR*, **26**, 579 (1956)

ALKALOID FV-A

A non-crystallizable base present in *Fagara viridis* A. Chev., this alkaloid yields a crystalline hydrochloride as yellow prisms, m.p. 245°C. No further salts or derivatives have been prepared.

Paris, Moyse-Mignon., *Ann. Pharm. Fr.,* **6**, 409 (1948)

ALKALOID FV-1

$C_{21}H_{21}O_5N$

M.p. 171–2°C

This alkaloid from *Fumaria vaillantii* forms colourless prisms from EtOH. The structure has not yet been elucidated.

Kiryakov, Panov., *Dokl. Bolg. Akad. Nauk.,* **24**, 1191 (1971)

ALKALOID FV-2

$C_{20}H_{19}O_5N$

M.p. 118–120°C

A second base found in *Fumaria vaillantii,* this alkaloid also forms colourless prisms from EtOH. Reaction with CH_2N_2 gives the preceding alkaloid.

Kiryakov, Panov., *Dokl. Bolg. Akad. Nauk.,* **24**, 1191 (1971)

ALKALOID GA-IIIa

One of two alkaloids from *Gentiana asclepiadea* described by Marekov and his colleagues. This base is stable to air and light and is somewhat more polar than the accompanying base. The infrared spectrum shows the presence of an absorption due to a double bond at 1645 cm^{-1}. The structure is unknown.

Marekov, Mollov, Popov., *Compt. Rend. Acad. Bulg. Sci.,* **18**, 999 (1965)

ALKALOID GA-IIIb

The second polar alkaloid isolated from *Gentiana asclepiadea,* this base is also stated to be stable to air and light. Its structure is not yet known with certainty.

Marekov, Mollov, Popov., *Compt. Rend. Acad. Bulg. Sci.,* **18**, 999 (1965)

ALKALOID GA-A

M.p. 249–252°C

This alkaloid is also present in *Gentiana* species, notably in *G. asclepiadea.* The structure is believed to contain a gentioflavine moiety linked to another group through a vinyl group.

Marekov, Popov., *Compt. Rend. Acad. Bulg. Sci.*, 575 (1970)

ALKALOID GB-III

Gentiana bulgarica contains this minor alkaloid which is stable to light and air and gives an infrared spectrum similar to that of Alkaloid GA-IIIa (q.v.).

Marekov, Mollov, Popov., *Compt. Rend. Acad. Bulg. Sci.*, **18**, 999

ALKALOID GC-III

This alkaloid, found in *Gentiana cruciata,* differs from the minor bases isolated from *G. asclepiadea* and *G. bulgarica* in undergoing a rapid change on keeping. The structure is unknown.

Marekov, Mollov, Popov., *Compt. Rend. Acad. Bulg. Sci.*, **18**, 999 (1965)

ALKALOID GC-IVb

M.p. 138–140°C

The aerial portions of *Gentiana cruciata* yield this alkaloid, the structure of which has not yet been determined. It occurs only in small quantities in the plant.

Marekov, Mollov, Popov., *Compt. Rend. Acad. Bulg. Sci.*, **18**, 999 (1965)

ALKALOID GC-1

M.p. 214°C

This alkaloid from *Galanthus caucasicus* forms colourless crystals from H_2O and is dextrorotatory with $[\alpha]_D^{20} + 94.3°$ (c 0.71, MeOH). The structure is unknown.

Abdusamtov, Yunusov., *Khim. Prir. Soedin.*, **5**, 331 (1969)

ALKALOID GF-A

M.p. 182–3°C

Glaucium flavum var. *leocarpum* yields three alkaloids which have been examined by Kiryakov and Panov. This base forms colourless crystals from EtOH and gives an ultraviolet spectrum with two absorption maxima at 236 and 285.5 mμ.

Kiryakov, Panov., *Dokl. Bolg. Akad. Nauk.*, **22**, 1019 (1969)

ALKALOID GF-B

M.p. $23°C$

A low-melting alkaloid found in *Glaucium flavum* var. *leocarpum*. The base yields clusters of small crystals from a mixture of EtOH and $CHCl_3$.

Kiryakov, Panov., *Dokl. Bolg. Akad. Nauk.*, **22**, 1019 (1969)

ALKALOID GF-C

M.p. $128°C$

The third minor constituent of *Glaucium flavum* var. *leocarpum* has been obtained only in small quantities. It forms colourless crystals from EtOH but, as in the case of the two preceding bases, insufficient material is available for a chemical analysis.

Kiryakov, Panov., *Dokl. Bolg. Akad. Nauk.*, **22**, 1019 (1969)

ALKALOID GP-IIIa

This alkaloid has been isolated from *Gentiana punctata*. When treated with dry HCl in MeOH it yields Centiamine (q.v.).

Marekov, Mollov, Popov., *Compt. Rend. Acad. Bulg. Sci.*, **18**, 999

ALKALOID GP-IIIb

The aerial parts and roots of *Gentiana punctata* contain this alkaloid which is stated to be different in character from the other minor alkaloid of *Gentiana* species. No structure has yet been put forward for this base.

Marekov, Mollov, Popov., *Compt. Rend. Acad. Bulg. Sci.*, **18**, 999

ALKALOID GP-IV

From the roots of *Gentiana punctata*, Marekov and his colleagues have obtained this minor constituent. It is accompanied by the following alkaloid.

Marekov, Mollov, Popov., *Compt. Rend. Acad. Bulg. Sci.*, **18**, 999

ALKALOID GP-IVa

This alkaloid occurs in trace amounts in admixture with the preceding base, occurring in the roots of *Gentiana punctata*. So far, it has not been characterized.

Marekov, Mollov, Popov., *Compt. Rend. Acad. Bulg. Sci.*, **18**, 999

ALKALOID GPZ-1

$C_{12}H_{17}ON_2$

The major alkaloid of *Gymnacranthera paniculata* var. *zippeliana* has been obtained as colourless crystals and identified by chemical and spectroscopic methods as 1:5-dimethoxy-3-(dimethylaminoethyl)-indole.

Johns, Lamberton, Occolowitz., *Austral. J. Chem.*, **20**, 1737 (1967)

ALKALOID GPZ-2

$C_{12}H_{14}N_2$

Gymnacranthera paniculata var. *zippeliana* yields this carboline alkaloid as a minor constituent. The structure has been established by chemical analysis and spectroscopic investigation.

Johns, Lamberton, Occolowitz., *Austral. J. Chem.*, **20**, 1737 (1967)

ALKALOID GT-A

$C_9H_{11}O_2N$

M.p. 161.5°C

This pyridine alkaloid occurs in the roots of *Gentiana tibetica*. Oxidiation with chromic acid yields the corresponding lactone. The structure has been determined by infrared, ultraviolet, NMR and mass spectrometry.

Rulko *et al., Rocz. Chem.*, **41**, 567 (1967)

ALKALOID GW-1

M.p. 126–7°C

An alkaloid present in the tubers of *Galanthus woronowi*, this base is obtained as colourless crystals from H_2O. It is laevorotatory with $[\alpha]_D - 188.8°$ (EtOH) and gives a series of crystalline salts and derivatives including the hydrochloride, m.p. 256–7°C; $[\alpha]_D - 93.1°$ (H_2O); nitrate, m.p. 224–5°C; perchlorate, m.p. 223–4°C; platinichloride, m.p. 216–7°C and the methiodide, m.p. 279°C; $[\alpha]_D - 94.5°$ (EtOH). Catalytic hydrogenation over PtO_2 gives the dihydro derivative, m.p. 116–8°C, forming a crystalline hydrobromide, m.p. 221.5–223°C.

Proskurnina, Yakovleva., *J. Gen. Chem. USSR*, **22**, 1899 (1952)

ALKALOID HA-1

$C_{16}H_{19}ON$

M.p. 122–3°C

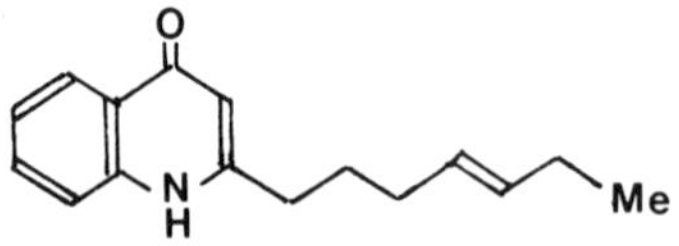

A pyridone alkaloid present in the green parts of *Haplophyllum acutifolium,* the base has been assigned the tentative structure given above. No salts or derivatives have yet been reported.

Gulyamova, Bessonova, Yunusov., *Khim. Prir. Soedin.,* 7, 850 (1971)

ALKALOID HA-A

This base is obtained from *Hedyotis auricularia* Linn and has been characterized only as the crystalline hydriodide, m.p. 215–220°C (*dec.*). No further physical or chemical constants have been recorded.

Ratnagiriswaran, Venkatachalam., *J. Ind. Chem. Soc.,* 19, 389 (1942)

ALKALOID HE-A

$C_8H_{12-14}N_2$

Isolated from *Helvella esculenta,* this alkaloid is a volatile liquid which yields a crystalline picrate as light yellow needles with m.p. 145–150°C.

Aye., *Arch. Pharm.,* 271, 537 (1933)

ALKALOID HE-I

$C_{24}H_{37}O_6N_2{}^+$

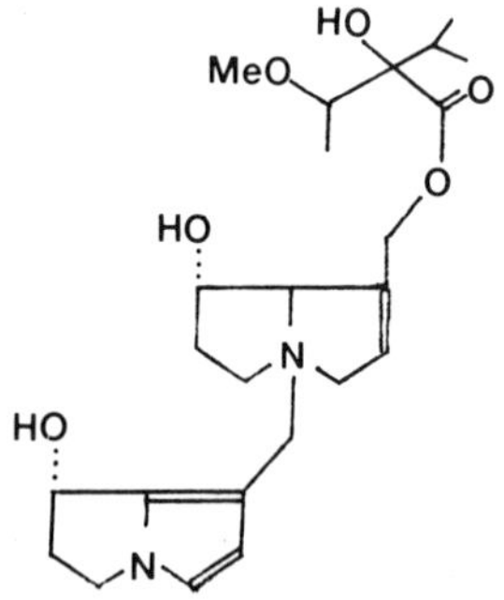

This quaternary alkaloid occurs in *Heliotropium europaeum,* mainly in the seeds and is isolated from a countercurrent distribution fraction which also contains Heliotrine (q.v.). The presence of a pyrrole ring is shown by the intense mauve colour produced with Ehrlich reagent and the structure has been established as the N-dihydropryyolizinomethyl derivative of heliotrine by synthesis. The dimeric structure also explains the cleavage of the alkaloid to heliotrine by reduction with Zn and HCl and the formation of a heliotrine ion by electron impact.

Culvenor, Smith., *Tetrahedron Lett.*, 3603 (1969)

ALKALOID HE-1

The root and stem bark of *Hunteria eburnea* yield a crude extract which exhibits marked hypotensive properties, not shown by any of the alkaloids earlier obtained in a pure form from the plant. By using a fractional precipitation method which eliminated any atmospheric oxidation during isolation, Renner has obtained the active alkaloid as the crystalline perchlorate, m.p. 279–281°C (*dec.*); $[\alpha]_D$ + 29.4° (c 1.0, MeOH). This salt gives an ultraviolet spectrum having absorption maxima at 222 and 280 mμ and pronounced shoulders at 293, 305 and 315 mμ. The hydrochloride, prepared by passing the perchlorate through a chloride exchange column, crystallizes from MeOH-Me$_2$CO with m.p. 310–315°C (*dec.*); $[\alpha]_D$ + 27.5° (c 1.0, MeOH).

Renner., *German Patent*, 1,137,031 27 September 1962

ALKALOID HF-1

$C_{17}H_{17}O_2N$

M.p. 201–2°C

An alkaloid of *Hunnemannia fumariaefolia*, this base yields colourless crystals from EtOH or Et$_2$O and has $[\alpha]_D^{23}$ – 356° ± 3° (c 0.5, CHCl$_3$). The hydrochloride is also crystalline with m.p. 266–8°C. Methylation with CH$_2$N$_2$ gives (–)-Tetrahydropalmatine (q.v.), m.p. 141–2°C. The structure of the alkaloid has been established as (–)-bis-O,O′-didemethyltetrahydropalmatine.

Slavikova, Slavik., *Collect. Czech. Chem. Commun.*, 31, 1355 (1966)

ALKALOID HS-3

$C_{15}H_{17}ON_3$

M.p. 105–7°C

One of two minor alkaloids obtained from *Haloxylon salicornicum*, this base crystallizes from EtOH in colourless needles. No derivatives have been described.

Michel *et al.*, *Acta Pharm. Suecica*, **4**, 97 (1967)

ALKALOID HS-S

$C_{15}H_{27}ON_3$

M.p. 135–6°C

The second minor constituent of *Haloxylon salicornicum* also forms colourless needles when recrystallized from EtOH. As in the case of the preceding base, no salts or derivatives are yet known.

Michel *et al., Acta Pharm. Suecica.,* **4**, 97 (1967)

ALKALOID HV-V

$C_{25}H_{43}O_6N$

M.p. 267–8°C (*dec.*).

This alkaloid is found in *Helleborus viridis* L., forming colourless needles from EtOH. It is a weak base and no derivatives have been reported.

Keller, Schöbel., *Arch. Pharm.,* **265**, 238 (1927)
Keller, Schöbel., *ibid,* **266**, 545 (1928)

ALKALOID IL-A

M.p. 190°C

The Peruvian plant *Isotoma longiflora* yields this alkaloid which has been characterized as the crystalline hydrochloride, m.p. 160°C. It has been suggested that the alkaloid may be a lobeline derivative.

Sanchez., *Rev. Med. explt.,* (Peru), **4**, 284 (1945)

ALKALOID K-B

$C_{21}H_{25}O_6N$

M.p. 287–8°C

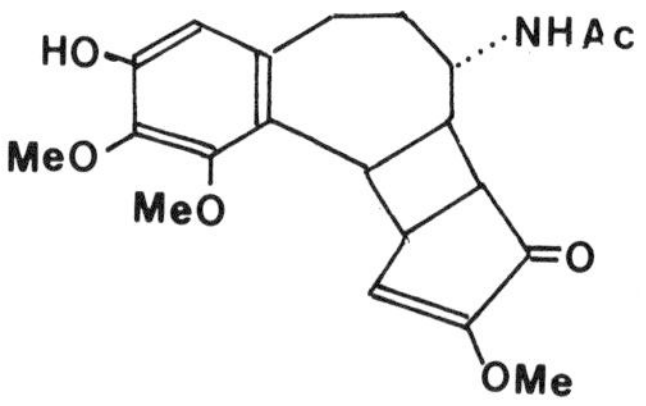

An alkaloid obtained from the corms of *Colchicum kesselringii,* the base is strongly laevorotatory with $[\alpha]_D - 420°$ (CHCl$_3$). The structure has been established from spectroscopic data and comparison with similar *Colchicum* alkaloids.

Turdikulov *et al., Khim. Prir. Soedin.,* **8**, 502 (1972)

ALKALOID K-3

$C_{22}H_{25}O_6N$

M.p. $255-7°C$

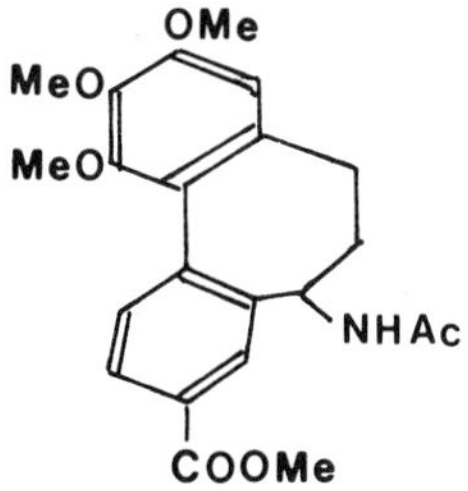

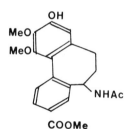

Isolated from various species of *Colchicum*, this alkaloid is hydrolyzed by NaOH to colchicinoic acid, m.p. $260-2°C$ which, with CH_2N_2, reverts to the original base. The alkaloid is therefore established as methyl colchicinoate.

Yusupov, Sadykov., *J. Gen. Chem., USSR,* **34**, 1677 (1954)

ALKALOID K-4

$C_{21}H_{23}O_6N$

M.p. $238-240°C$

This alkaloid of *Colchicum* species is closely related to the preceding base. When treated with CH_2N_2 it yields Alkaloid K-3, while alkaline hydrolysis with 3 per cent NaOH gives 2-demethylcolchicinoic acid. The base is therefore the methyl ester of 2-demethylcolchicinoic acid.

Yusupov, Sadykov., *J. Gen. Chem., USSR,* **34**, 1677 (1954)

ALKALOID KD-1

$C_{17}H_{23}O_2N$

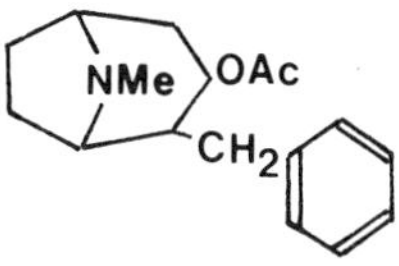

The leaves of *Knightia deplanchei* have recently been shown to contain four new alkaloids of the tropane type. The structure of this base has been determined from analysis of the mass spectral fragmentation pattern.

Kan-Fan, Lounasmaa., *Acta Chem. Scand.,* **27**, 1039 (1973)

ALKALOID KD-2

$C_{23}H_{27}O_2N$

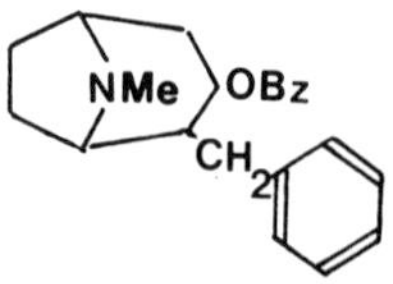

A second tropane base present in the leaf extract of *Knightia deplanchei,* the alkaloid contains a benzoyl and benzyl group in the molecule.

Kan-Fan, Lounasmaa., *Acta. Chem. Scand.,* **27,** 1039 (1973)

ALKALOID KD-3

$C_{23}H_{27}O_2N$

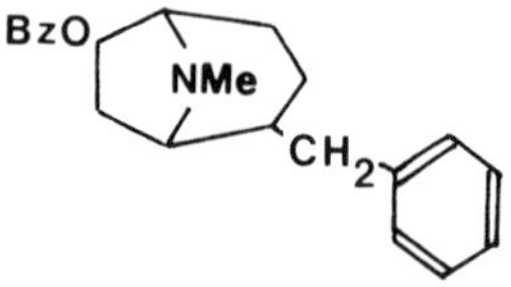

This tropane alkaloid from the leaves of *Knightia deplanchei* is isomeric with the foregoing base. The structure has been determined on the basis of the mass spectrum fragmentation pattern.

Kan-Fan, Lounasmaa., *Acta. Chem. Scand.,* **27,** 1039 (1973)

ALKALOID KD-4

$C_{24}H_{27}O_3N$

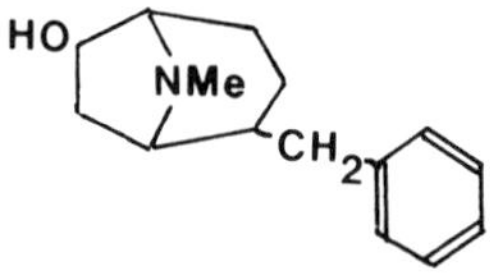

Also present in the leaves of *Knightia deplanchei,* this base has the tropane skeleton but differs from the preceding bases in containing a hydroxyl group and a cinnamyl group in the molecule. Hydrogenation yields the dihydro derivative. As in the case of the three preceding alkaloids, the structure has been established from the mass spectrum.

Kan-Fan, Lounasmaa., *Acta Chem. Scand.,* **27,** 1039 (1973)

ALKALOID LA-1

M.p. 180–3°C

The upper parts of *Leontice albertii* have been shown to contain methylcytisine as the major alkaloid accompanied by this minor constituent which may be isolated by column chromatography followed by recrystallization from EtOH when the base yields colourless crystals. It has been further characterized as the crystalline picrate with m.p. 168–171°C (*dec.*).

Yunusov, Sorokina., *J. Gen. Chem. USSR,* **19,** 1955 (1949)

ALKALOID L-5

$C_{20}H_{21}O_5N$

M.p. 179–183°C

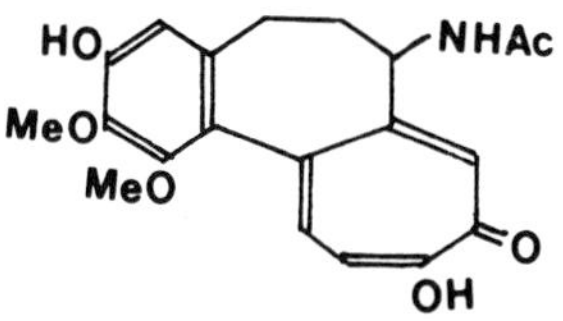

The bulbs of *Colchicum luteum* have been found to contain this alkaloid which has been shown to be 2-demethylcolchicine by chemical and spectroscopic investigation.

Chommadov, Yusupov, Sadykov., *Khim. Prir. Soedin.*, **6**, 82 (1970)

ALKALOID L-6

$C_{21}H_{21}O_6N$

M.p. 291–3°C

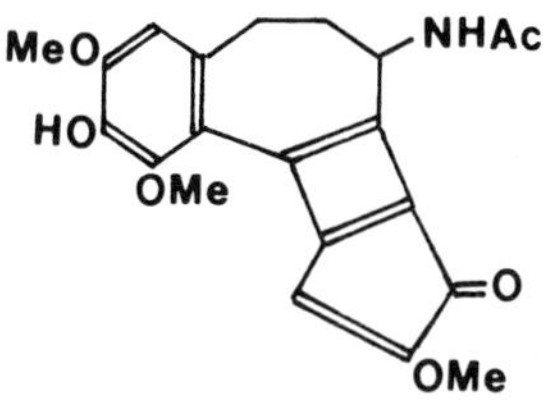

From the phenolic fraction of the alkaloidal extract of the bulbs of *Colchicum luteum,* this base is obtained as colourless crystals from Me_2CO. It is laevo-rotatory with $[\alpha]_D - 410°$ (c 0.88, MeOH) and on methylation it furnishes β-lumicolchicine. The structure of the alkaloid as 3-demethyl-β-lumicolchicine has been determined on the basis of infrared, ultraviolet, NMR and mass spectrometry of the free base, its methyl ether and the acetyl derivative.

Chommadov, Yusupov, Sadykov., *Khim. Prir. Soedin.*, **6**, 82 (1970)
Chommadov *et al., Izv. Akad. Nauk. Turkm. SSR, Ser. Fiz-Tekh., Khim. Geol. Nauk.*, 111 (1970)

ALKALOID L-9

This base has been shown to be a complex of O-acetyllofoline and lycopodine.

Manske, Marion., *Can. J. Chem.*, **21B**, 92 (1943)
Ayer, Hogg, Soper., *ibid*, **42**, 949 (1964)

ALKALOID L-28

$C_{17}H_{27}O_2N$

An alkaloid of *Lycopodium annotinum* var. *acrifolium* Fern, the free base is non-crystallizable but the perchlorate forms colourless crystals, m.p. 211°C.

Manske, Marion., *J. Amer. Chem. Soc.*, **69**, 2126 (1947)

ALKALOID L-30

$C_{16}H_{25}O_2N$

M.p. 178°C

This base, obtained from *Lycopodium annotinum* var. *acrifolium* Fern crystallizes from Et_2O-hexane in nacreous plates and yields a crystalline perchlorate, m.p. 311°C (*dec.*).

Manske, Marion., *J. Amer. Chem. Soc.*, **69**, 2126 (1947)

ALKALOID L-31

$C_{20}H_{29}O_4N$

A further alkaloid found in *Lycopodium annotinum* var. *acrifolium* this base yields a perchlorate, obtained as the crystalline monohydrate, m.p. 132°C or 217°C (*dry*).

Manske, Marion., *J. Amer. Chem. Soc.*, **69**, 2126 (1947)

ALKALOID L-34

$C_{16}H_{25}O_2N$

M.p. 236°C

An alkaloid present in *Lycopodium densum* Labill., the base crystallizes in colourless prisms from Et_2O-hexane.

Manske., *Can. J. Chem.*, **31**, 894 (1953)

ALKALOID L-35

$C_{14}H_{21}ON$

M.p. 133°C

Also present in *Lycopodium densum* Labill., this base forms colourless polyhedra. No salts or derivatives have been reported.

Manske., *Can. J. Chem.*, **31**, 894 (1953)

ALKALOID LB-1

M.p. 220°C

This minor constituent of *Lunaria biennis* Mnch. (Syn. *L. annua*) has been described by Harris. No further investigation appears to have been carried out since its isolation.

Harris., *Bull. Acad. Roy. Belg.*, 1042 (1909)

ALKALOID LBX

$C_{26}H_{31}O_4N_3$

M.p. 250°C (*dec.*).

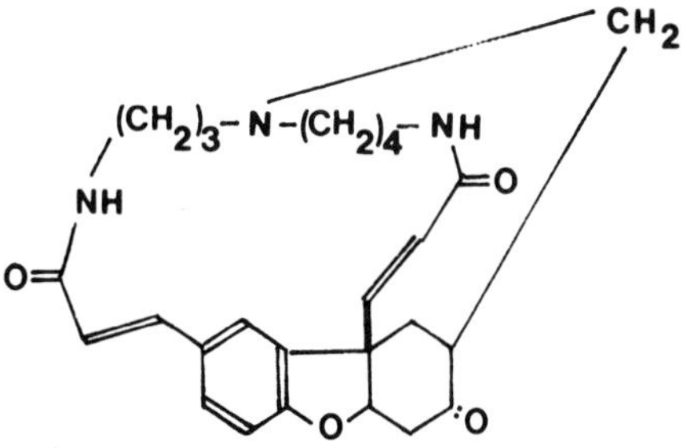

The seeds of *Lunaria biennis* Mnch. have also been found to contain three very similar alkaloids, so far only identified by the letters LBX, LBY and LBZ. This particular base forms colourless crystals from MeOH-Et$_2$O and has $[\alpha]_D$ + 201° (c 0.6, CHCl$_3$). The structure has recently been revised to that given above.

Poupat *et al.*, *Compt. rend.*, **269**, 335 (1969)

Revised structure:
Doskotch, Fairchild, Kubelka., *Experientia*, **28**, 382 (1972)
Poupat *et al.*, *Tetrahedron*, **28**, 3087 (1972)

ALKALOID LBY

$C_{25}H_{33}O_4N_3$

M.p. 268–273°C

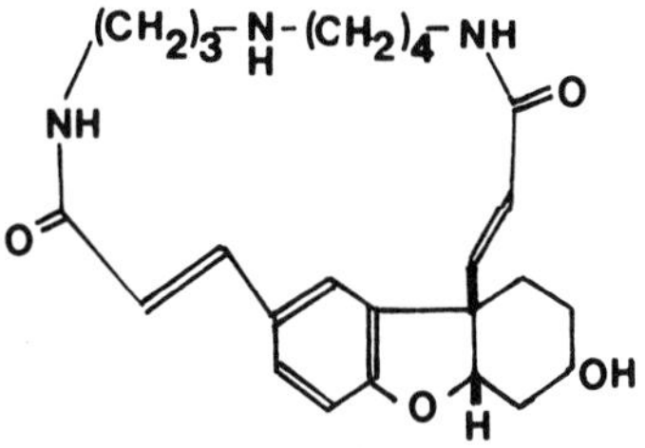

This base from the seeds of *Lunaria biennis* Mnch., a species of Cruciferae, crystallizes as the monohydrate with $[\alpha]_D^{20}$ + 108° (c 0.43, EtOH). Unlike the other two alkaloids of this small group, it appears to have a linear structure in the macrocyclic ring.

Poupat *et al.*, *Compt. rend.*, **269**, 335 (1969)
Doskotch, Fairchild, Kubelka., *Experientia*, **28**, 382 (1972)
Poupat *et al.*, *Tetrahedron*, **28**, 3087 (1972)

ALKALOID LBZ

$C_{26}H_{33}O_4N_3$

M.p. Indefinite

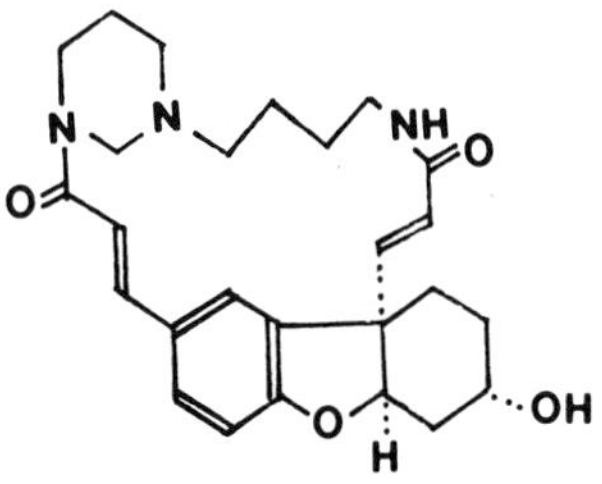

The third alkaloid of this group to be obtained from the seeds of *Lunaria biennis* Mnch. has not been obtained in the crystalline form. Like Alkaloid LBX its structure has recently been revised to that given above.

Poupat *et al., Compt. rend.,* **269**, 335 (1969)

Doskotch, Fairchild, Kubelka., *Experientia,* **28**, 382 (1972)

ALKALOID LC-1

M.p. $52-3°C$

The dried roots of *Lycichitium cantschatiense* var. *japonicum* yield this low-melting alkaloid which forms colourless crystals from a mixture of Et_2O and hexane. The base is separated from accompanying alkaloid by column chromatography and gives an ultraviolet spectrum in EtOH with absorption maxima at 225, 270, 305 and 318 mμ.

Katsui *et al., Tetrahedron Lett.,* 6257 (1966)

ALKALOID LF-K

M.p. $117°C$

One of the numerous *Lycopodium* alkaloids, this base occurs in *L. fawcettii.* On alkaline hydrolysis it forms deacetylfawcettiine.

Burnell, Mootoo, Taylor., *Can. J. Chem.,* **38**, 1927 (1960)

ALKALOID LF-M

A further alkaloid isolated from *Lycopodium fawcettii,* this base has been characterized as the crystalline perchlorate, yielding colourless needles from H_2O, m.p. $280-2°C$.

Burnell, Mootoo, Taylor., *Can. J. Chem.,* **38**, 1927 (1960)

ALKALOID LF-O

$C_{20}H_{31}O_5N$

M.p. $181-2°C$

A minor constituent of *Lycopodium fawcettii,* the alkaloid crystallizes from EtOH as colourless prisms with the above melting point. No salts or derivatives have been reported for this base.

Burnell, Mootoo, Taylor., *Can. J. Chem.,* **38**, 1927 (1960)

ALKALOID LP-1

$C_{21}H_{23}O_3N_2$

M.p. 115–6°C

This alkaloid has been obtained from the leaves of *Lobelia portoricensis*. It yields a series of crystalline salts including the hydrochloride, m.p. 187–8°C; perchlorate, m.p. 156–8°C and the picrate, m.p. 175–6°C.

Melendez, Carreras, Gijon., *J. Pharm. Sci.*, **56**, 1677 (1967)

ALKALOID LU-A

M.p. 202–4°C

From *Lobelia urens*, this minor alkaloid has been isolated as bright rose needles. It occurs together with (–)-Lobeline (q.v.) and Lobelanidine (q.v.). The structure has not yet been elucidated.

Steinegger, Grütter., *Pharm. Acta Helv.*, **25**, 49 (1950)

ALKALOID MA-1

$C_{41}H_{46}O_3N_4$

Melodinus australis yields a series of minor alkaloids which have been isolated and examined by Linde. This complex base sinters at 220°C and carbonizes before melting. It is dextrorotatory with $[\alpha]_D^{23}$ + 54° (c 0.830, CHCl$_3$). The structure has not been established but from comparison with the accompanying alkaloids it may possibly be a dimeric imidazolidinocarbazole base.

Linde., *Helv. Chim. Acta*, **48**, 1822 (1965)

ALKALOID MA-2

M.p. 186–195°C

This alkaloid from *Melodinus australis* occurs only in minute traces and only a small quantity of material has been obtained, insufficient for a chemical analysis. It is dextrorotatory with $[\alpha]_D^{24}$ + 112.2° (c 0.401, CHCl$_3$).

Linde., *Helv. Chim. Acta*, **48**, 1822 (1965)

ALKALOID MA-3

$C_{20}H_{24}O_2N_2$

M.p. 170–5°C

A further alkaloid isolated from *Melodinus australis*, this base forms colourless prisms from Et$_2$O and has $[\alpha]_D^{23}$ + 177° (c 1.075, CHCl$_3$). While the structure is not yet fully determined, it appears to belong to the imidazolinocarbazole class.

Linde., *Helv. Chim. Acta*, **48**, 1822 (1965)

ALKALOID MA-4

$C_{19}H_{22}ON_2$

M.p. 214–6°C

A fourth alkaloid from *Melodinus australis,* this compound crystallizes in colourless prisms from a mixture of Et_2O and $CHCl_3$. It is laevorotatory with $[\alpha]_D^{24} - 421°$ (c 0.973, $CHCl_3$).

Linde., *Helv. Chim. Acta,* **48**, 1822 (1965)

ALKALOID MA-5

$C_{21}H_{22}O_4N_2$

M.p. 245–8°C

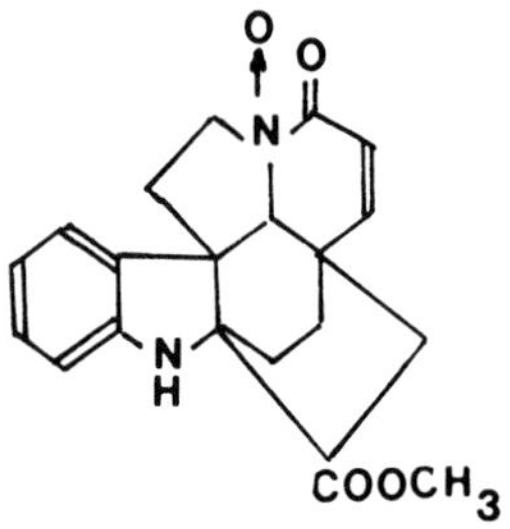

This imidazolinocarbazole alkaloid from *Melodinus australis* crystallizes as colourless needles from $CHCl_3$-Et_2O. It is laevorotatory with $[\alpha]_D^{24} - 48.4°$ (c 0.223, $CHCl_3$) and $-55.1°$ (c 0.49, $CHCl_3$). Its structure has been established as the N-oxide given above on the basis of chemical and spectroscopic evidence.

Linde., *Helv. Chim. Acta,* **48**, 1822 (1965)

ALKALOID MA-6

$C_{21}H_{22}O_3N_2$

M.p. 227–231°C

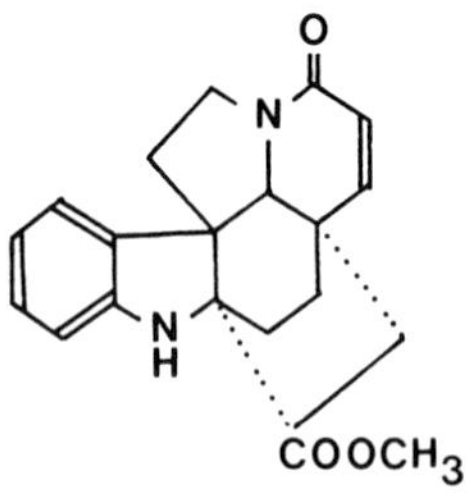

Also present in *Melodinus australis,* this imidizolidinocarbazole base has the structure given above. It forms colourless prisms from Et_2O-$CHCl_3$ and has $[\alpha]_D^{20} - 99°$ (c 0.699, $CHCl_3$).

Linde., *Helv. Chim. Acta,* **48**, 1822 (1965)

ALKALOID MA-7

$C_{21}H_{26}O_3N_2$

M.p. $190-7°C$

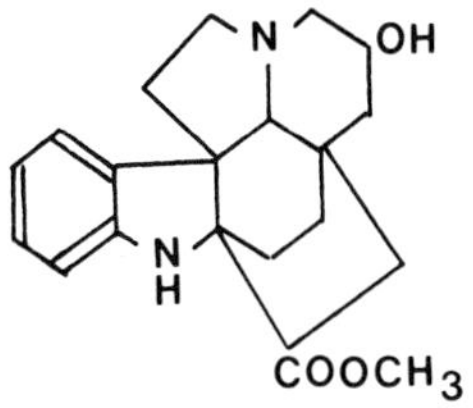

A further imidazolinocarbazole base found in *Melodinus australis,* this alkaloid is laevorotatory with $[\alpha]_D^{23} - 62°$ (c 1.142, $CHCl_3$) and has the structure given. One non-phenolic hydroxyl group and one methoxylcarbonyl group are present in the molecule.

Linde., *Helv. Chim. Acta,* **48**, 1822 (1965)

ALKALOID MA-8

$C_{21}H_{26}O_3N_2$

M.p. $187-192°C$

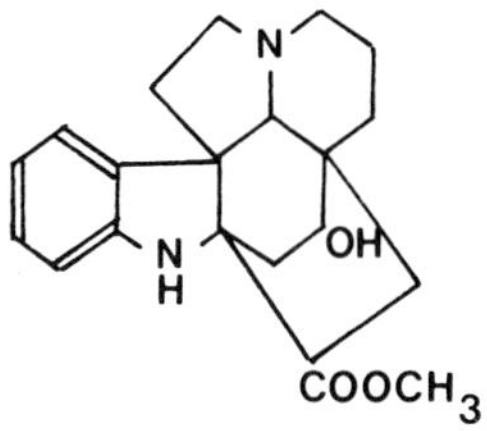

This alkaloid, isomeric with the preceding base, also occurs in *Melodinus australis.* It has a specific rotation almost identical with that of Alkaloid MA-7, with $[\alpha]_D^{23} - 63°$ (c 1.037, $CHCl_3$). The structure has been determined mainly from the NMR and mass spectra.

Linde., *Helv. Chim. Acta,* **48**, 1822 (1965)

ALKALOID MA-A

M.p. $220-1°C$

An uncharacterized alkaloid present in small quantities in the root wood of *Machilus acuminatissimus.* The base is obtained as pale brown crystals from MeOH-EtOH, the structure of which is unknown.

Lu., *J. Pharm. Soc., Japan,* **87**, 1278 (1967)

ALKALOID MJ-1 (*Jolantamine*)

M.p. $215-6°C$

The major alkaloid of *Merendera jolanta,* this alkaloid forms colourless crystals from $CHCl_3$. It is dextrorotatory with $[\alpha]_D^{20} + 112°$ (c 0.95, $CHCl_3$). The base contains a hydroxyl group, a methoxyl group, a keto group and one methimino group in the molecule.

Zuparova *et al.*, *Khim. Prir. Soedin.*, 8, 487 (1972)

ALKALOID MJ-2

M.p. 179–182°C

A minor, uncharacterized alkaloid present in *Merendera jolanta,* this base forms colourless crystals but has not been isolated in sufficient quantity for a chemical analysis to be carried out.

Zuparova *et al.*, *Khim. Prir. Soedin.*, 8, 487 (1972)

ALKALOID MJ-3

M.p. 268–270°C

This base also occurs in *Merendera jolanta* as a minor constituent. At present, insufficient material has been obtained to enable the empirical formula to be ascertained.

Zuparova *et al.*, *Khim. Prir. Soedin.*, 8, 487 (1972)

ALKALOID MJ-4

This minor constituent of *Merendera jolanta* has not yet been characterized. It occurs only in minute traces in the plant.

Zuparova *et al.*, *Khim. Prir. Soedin.*, 8, 487 (1972)

ALKALOID ML-A

M.p. 260–2°C

The bark of *Magnolia leliflora* yields two minor alkaloids. This base is tertiary in character and, as yet, no salts or derivatives have been prepared.

Nakuno., *Pharm. Bull.* (Tokyo), 1, 29 (1953)

ALKALOID ML-B

M.p. 254°C

A second minor constituent of *Magnolia leliflora* bark, this alkaloid is present only in minute quantities and insufficient has been obtained for any salts or derivatives to be prepared.

Nakuno., *Pharm. Bull.*, (Tokyo), 1, 29 (1953)

ALKALOID ML-1

$C_{17}H_{19}O_3N_3$

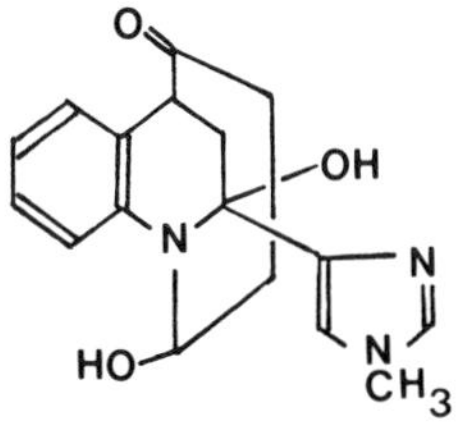

One of three tetrahydroquinolylimidazole alkaloids present in *Macrorungia longistrobus*, the structure has been demonstrated to be that shown above.

Arndt, Eggers, Jordaan., *Tetrahedron*, **25**, 2767 (1969)

ALKALOID ML-2

$C_{17}H_{19}ON_3$

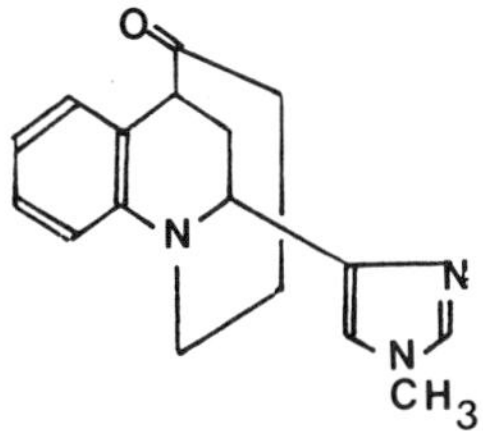

Also present in *Macrorungia longistrobus*, this alkaloid has a similar structure to the preceding base. No salts or derivatives have been recorded.

Arndt, Eggers, Jordaan., *Tetrahedron*, **25**, 2767 (1969)

ALKALOID ML-3

$C_{17}H_{17}O_3N_3$

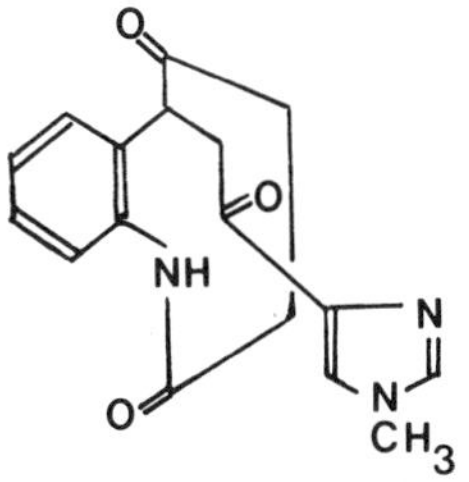

A third tetrahydroquinolylimidazole alkaloid isolated from *Macrorungia longistrobus*, the structure given above has been confirmed by spectroscopic data.

Arndt, Eggers, Jordaan., *Tetrahedron*, **25**, 2767 (1969)

ALKALOID MT-A

M.p. 260°C

An uncharacterized alkaloid present in *Menyanthes trifoliata*, this base occurs mainly in the leaves of the plant. The structure is unknown.

Rulko., *Rocz. Chem.*, **43**, 1831 (1969)

ALKALOID MT-B

M.p. 143–4°C

Also isolated from the leaves of *Menyanthes trifoliata,* this alkaloid forms colourless crystals. Insufficient material has been obtained for a chemical analysis to be carried out.

Rulko., *Rocz. Chem.*, **43**, 1831 (1969)

ALKALOID MT-C

This minor constituent of *Menyanthes trifoliata* is a colourless oil which cannot be crystallized. As in the case of the two preceding bases, insufficiency of material makes it impossible for an empirical formula to be given at the present time.

Rulko., *Rocz. Chem.*, **43**, 1831 (1969)

ALKALOID ND-305B

$C_{19}H_{19}ON_3$

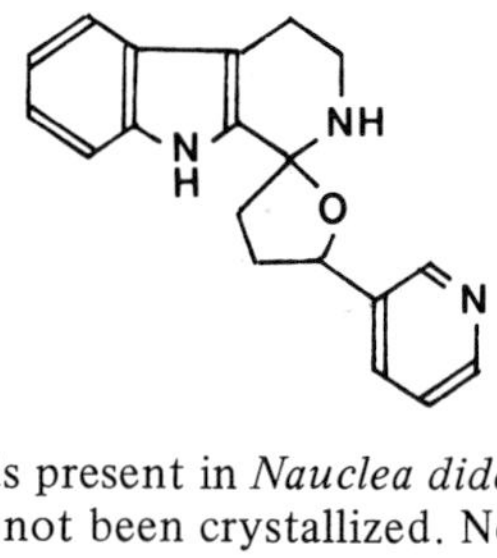

One of three related alkaloids present in *Nauclea diderrichii,* this base is obtained as a syrup which has, as yet, not been crystallized. No derivatives have been reported.

Murray, Szalokcai, McLean., *Can. J. Chem.,* **50**, 1486 (1972)
Murray, McLean., *ibid,* **50**, 1496 (1972)

ALKALOID ND-363C

$C_{21}H_{21}O_3N_3$

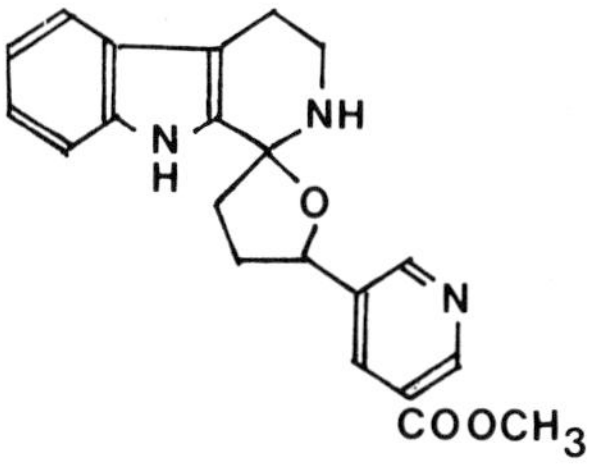

This syrupy base also occurs in *Nauclea diderrichii* and differs from the foregoing alkaloid only in the presence of an acetoxy group in the pyridine ring.

Murray, Szalokcai, McLean., *Can. J. Chem.*, **50**, 1486 (1972)
Murray, McLean., *ibid*, **50**, 1496 (1972)

ALKALOID ND-370

$C_{21}H_{26}O_4N_2$

M.p. 203–9°C

This third alkaloid obtained from *Nauclea diderrichii* forms colourless crystals from MeOH after separation from the accompanying bases by countercurrent distribution techniques.

Murray, McLean., *Can. J. Chem.*, **50**, 1496 (1972)

ALKALOID NLM-A

$C_{30}H_{42}O_4N_2$

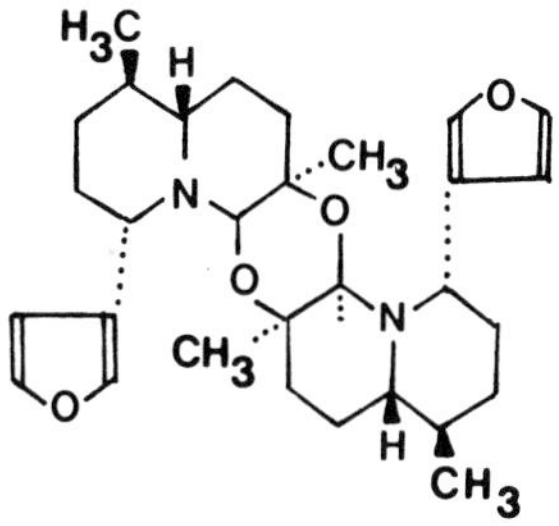

A dimeric alkaloid of *Nuphar luteum* subsp. *macrophyllum*, the structure given has been elucidated by chemical and spectroscopic means and confirmed by transformation of Δ^6-dehydrodeoxynupharidine into the corresponding C_{30} diol.

LaLonde, Wong, Das., *J. Amer. Chem. Soc.*, **94**, 8522 (1972)

ALKALOID OC-A

$C_{15}H_{22}O_2N_2$

A laevorotatory alkaloid occurring in *Ostryoderis chevalieri* Dunn, this base has $[\alpha]_D - 75°$. No further investigation of this alkaloid appears to have been carried out since its discovery.

Balansard, Martini., *Bull. Sci. Pharmacol.*, **46**, 268 (1939)

ALKALOID OGG-3

An alkaloid from *Ornithoglossum glaucum* var. *grandiflora,* the structure of this base is still unknown although it probably has a homoproaporphine structure containing four six-membered rings similar to Bulbocodine (q.v.).

Reichstein, Snatzke, Santavy., *Planta Med.,* **16**, 357 (1968)

ALKALOID OP-1

$C_{16}H_{17}O_3N$

M.p. 140°C

The bark of *Ocotea puberula* contains this minor alkaloid which forms mono-clinic, colourless crystals. The base is soluble in most organic solvents and yields crystalline salts and derivatives, e.g. the hydrochloride as colourless needles, m.p. 265–7°C (*dec.*); picrate, m.p. 169°C and the methiodide as colourless crystals, m.p. 221–2°C (*dec.*).

Iacobuca., *Cienc. e invest.,* (Buenos Aires), 7, 48 (1951)

ALKALOID Pa-6

$C_{19}H_{15}O_2N_3$?

M.p. 238–240°C

The alkaloid has been isolated from the leaves of *Mitragyna javanica* var. *microphylla* and appears to have a different structure from the other alkaloids found in *Mitragyna* species. The crystalline perchlorate has m.p. 234°C.

Shellard *et al., Planta Med.,* **15**, 245 (1967)

ALKALOID PA-A

$C_{20}H_{27}O_5N$

A pyrrolizidine alkaloid present in *Phalaenopsis amabilis,* the base has the structure given. Acid methanolysis gives (−)-dimethyl-2-benzylmalate and trachelanthamidine. The alkaloid is a diasterioisomer of Alkaloid PM-A.

Brandange, Luning., *Acta. Chem. Scand.,* **23**, 1151 (1969)

ALKALOID PA-1

$C_{15}H_{10}O_2N_2$

M.p. 241.5–242°C

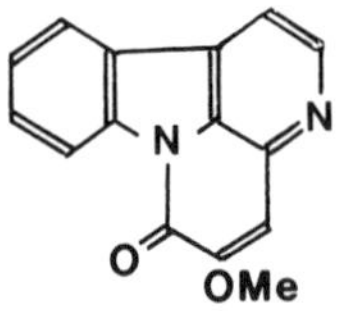

This base has been isolated from the leaves of *Pentaceras australis* and shown to have the structure of 5-methoxy-canthin-6-one. The hydrochloride forms colourless crystals, m.p. 206–7°C; the picrate, m.p. 242–4°C and the methiodide, m.p. 308–9°C.

Haynes, Nelson, Price., *Austral. J. Sci. Res.,* **5A**, 387 (1952)
Haynes, Nelson, Price., *ibid*, **5A**, 563 (1952)

ALKALOID PA-2

$C_{15}H_{10}ON_2S$

M.p. 252.5–253.5°C

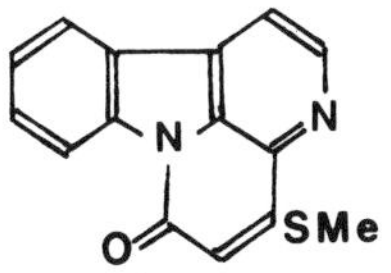

Also present in *Pentaceras australis,* but this time in the bark, this alkaloid contains sulphur, the structure being 4-methylthiocanthin-6-one.

Nelson, Price., *Austral. J. Sci. Res.,* **5A**, 768 (1952)

ALKALOID PA-I

$C_{14}H_{18}ON_2$

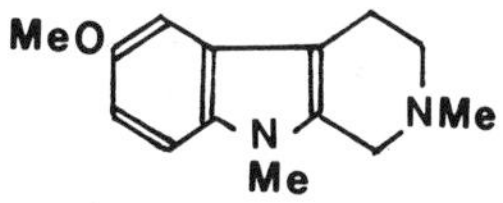

This carboline alkaloid occurs in *Phalaris arundinacea* and is separated from the accompanying alkaloids, hordenine and gramine, by countercurrent distribution methods followed by column chromatography on an alumina column. The structure has been elucidated by the use of infrared, NMR and mass spectrometry.

Audette *et al., Can. J. Chem.,* **48**, 149 (1970)

ALKALOID PA-II

$C_{21}H_{28}O_3N_2$

M.p. 216°C

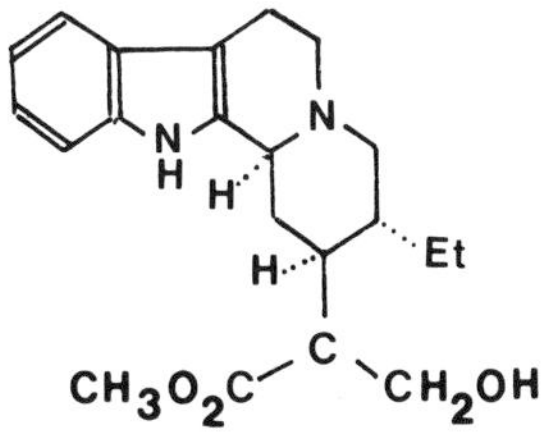

An alkaloid of *Pausinystalia angolensis,* this yohimbine type base crystallizes in colourless prisms from Me_2CO and is laevorotatory with $[\alpha]_D^{20} - 84°$ (c 1.0, pyridine). Selenium dehydrogenation yields alstyrine, m.p. 98°C. The structure has been determined by chemical and spectroscopic methods.

Can der Meulen, van der Kerk., *Rev. Trav. Chim.,* **83**, 141, 148 (1964)

ALKALOID PB-A

$C_{16}H_{21}O_3N$

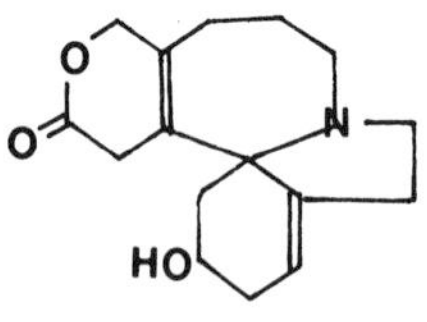

Phelline billardieri yields two minor alkaloids of the homoerythrina type. This base yields colourless crystals and has been assigned the partial structure shown above on the basis of spectroscopic data.

Hoang Nhu Mai *et al., Compt. Rend.,* **270C**, 2154 (1970)

ALKALOID PB-B

$C_{17}H_{23}O_3N$

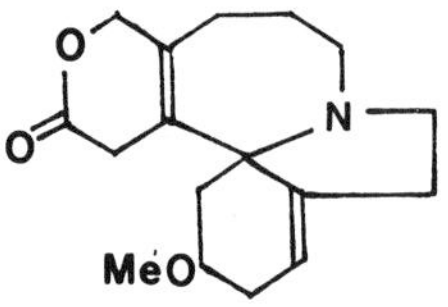

This homoethryine type alkaloid from *Phelline billardieri* is the O-methyl ether of the preceding base, the structure. No salts or derivatives have been reported.

Hoang Nhu Mai *et al., Compt. Rend.,* **270C**, 2154 (1970)

ALKALOID PB-E

$C_{22}H_{27}O_6N$

M.p. 135°C

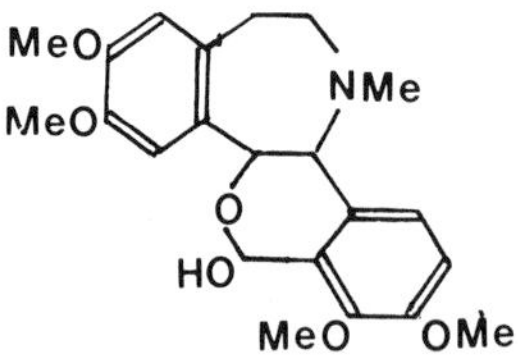

A major alkaloid of *Papaver bracteatum,* this base is strongly dextrorotatory with $[\alpha]_D^{22} + 306°$ (c 1.084, MeOH). It forms a crystalline hydrochloride, m.p. 161–3°C (*dec.*); $[\alpha]_D^{20} + 210°$ (c 0.796, MeOH) and a methyl ether, m.p. 105°C; $[\alpha]_D^{20} + 302°$ (c 0.511, MeOH). Oxidation with hydrogen peroxide yields the N-oxide, m.p. 167–9°C. NMR shows the presence of four methoxyl groups and a methylimino group and the ultraviolet spectrum is similar to that of Rhoeadine (q.v.), while the infrared spectrum shows both free and bonded hydroxyl absorptions and no carboxyl. The structure has been established as 18-hydroxy-8:9:15:16-tetramethoxy-1:2:4:5:18-pentahydro-3H-N-methyl-2-benzopyrano 3,4,6-3-benzazepine.

Guggisberg *et al., Helv. Chim. Acta.,* **50**, 621 (1967)

ALKALOID PC-1

M.p. 206°C

This uncharacterized non-phenolic alkaloid occurs in *Papaver commutatum*. No salts or derivatives have so far been prepared.

Slavik, Appelt, Slavikova., *Collect. Czech. Chem. Commun.*, **30**, 3961 (1965)

ALKALOID PC-2

M.p. 230°C

A further unidentified non-phenoloc alkaloid present in *Papaver commutatum*, this minor constituent forms colourless crystals and has been separated from the accompanying bases by means of column chromatography.

Slavik, Appelt, Slavikova., *Collect. Czech. Chem. Commun.*, **30**, 3961 (1965)

ALKALOID PC-3

M.p. 195°C

Also present in *Papaver commutatum*, this non-phenolic alkaloid occurs only in trace amounts and is so far unidentified.

Slavik, Appelt, Slavikova., *Collect. Czech. Chem. Commun.*, **30**, 3961 (1965)

ALKALOID PC-A

M.p. 222–6°C

An unidentified alkaloid isolated from *Papaver caucasicum*, this base in non-phenolic in character and gives an ultraviolet spectrum in MeOH with absorption maxima at 248, 282 and 295 mμ. The crystalline methiodide has m.p. 274–6°C.

Pfeifer, Kuehn., *Pharmazie*, **23**, 199 (1968)

ALKALOID PC-B

M.p. 142–4°C

A further non-phenolic alkaloid found in *Papaver caucasicum*, this base crystallizes from a mixture of Et_2O, $CHCl_3$ and *n*-heptane and is characterized as the crystalline methiodide, m.p. 193–5°C (*dec.*).

Pfeifer, Kuehn., *Pharmazie*, **23**, 199 (1968)

ALKALOID PC-C

M.p. $221-2°C$

A third non-phenolic alkaloid which has been obtained from *Papaver caucasicum*. No derivatives of this base have been recorded.

Pfeifer, Kuehn., *Pharmazie*, **23**, 199 (1968)

ALKALOID PC-D

M.p. $175-7°C$

Papaver caucasicum also contains this minor alkaloid which, like the three preceding bases in non-phenolic in character. No salts or derivatives have yet been prepared.

Pfeifer, Kuehn., *Pharmazie*, **23**, 199 (1968)

ALKALOID PC-I

$C_{19}H_{23}O_3N$

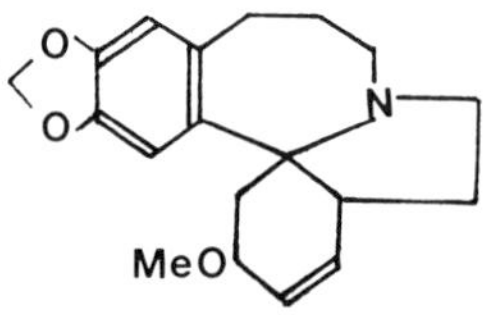

A homoerythrina type alkaloid isolated from *Phelline comosa* Labill, this base is dextrorotatory with $[\alpha]_D + 75°$ (c 1.5, $CHCl_3$). The ultraviolet spectrum exhibits two absorption maxima at 242 and 291 mμ. On catalytic hydrogenation, the base yields the dihydro derivative, characterized as the crystalline picrate, m.p. $186-8°C$. The structure has been determined from the spectroscopic data.

Langlois *et al.*, *Bull. Soc. Chim. Fr.*, **10**, 3535 (1970)

ALKALOID PC-II

$C_{20}H_{27}O_3N$

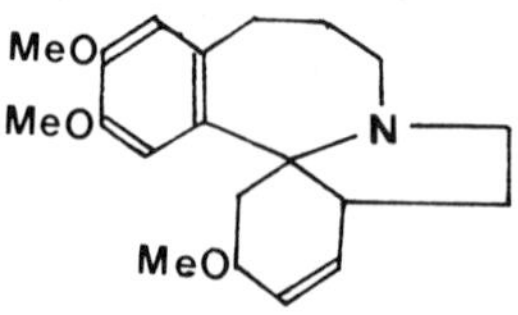

A second homoerythrina type alkaloid found in *Phelline comosa* Labill, the base has $[\alpha]_D + 72°$ (c 0.7, $CHCl_3$). The ultraviolet spectrum has absorption maxima at 236 and 283 mμ. A picrate has been prepared as light yellow crystals, m.p. $143-5°C$ and catalytic hydrogenation gives the dihydro derivative which has $[\alpha]_D + 20°$ (c 0.8, $CHCl_3$).

Langlois *et al.*, *Bull. Soc. Chim. Fr.*, **10**, 3535 (1970)

100

ALKALOID PC-III

$C_{19}H_{23}O_4N$

M.p. 184–5°C

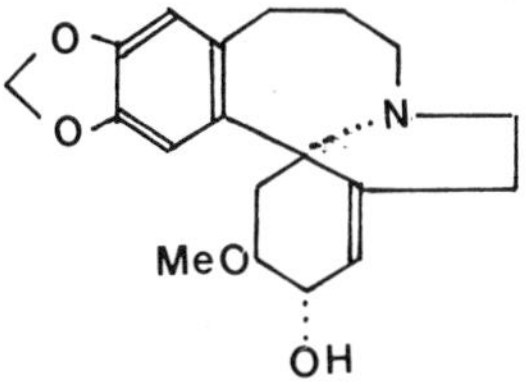

Phelline comosa Labill. also yields this homoerythrina alkaloid. The base is dextrorotatory with $[\alpha]_D + 172°$ (c 1.4, $CHCl_3$). It gives an ultraviolet spectrum with two absorption maxima occurring at 238 and 294 mμ. The structure has been determined on the basis of spectroscopic evidence.

Langlois *et al., Bull. Soc. Chim. Fr.,* **10,** 3535 (1970)

ALKALOID PC-IV

$C_{19}H_{23}O_3N$

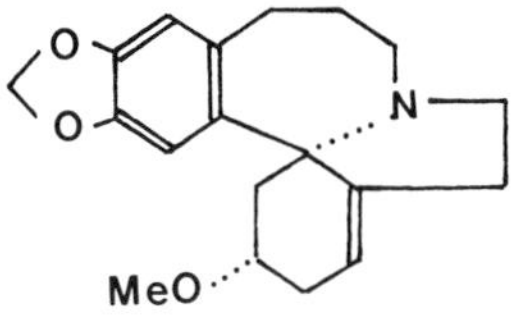

Also obtained from *Phelline comosa* Labill., this base has $[\alpha]_D + 122°$ (c 1.0, $CHCl_3$). It is suggested that the alkaloid may be identical with Schelhemmericine (q.v.).

Langlois *et al., Bull. Soc. Chim. Fr.,* **10,** 3535 (1970)

ALKALOID PC-V

$C_{21}H_{29}O_4N$

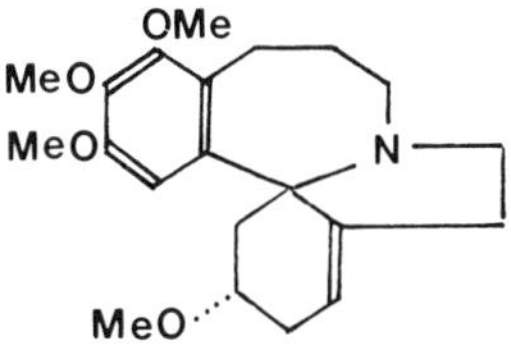

A fifth homoerythrina type alkaloid of *Phelline comosa* Labill, this base is also dextrorotatory with $[\alpha]_D + 91°$ (c 1.5, $CHCl_3$). The ultraviolet spectrum consists of three absorption maxima at 224, 275 and 282 mμ. Four methoxyl groups are present in the molecule, the structure of which has been established on the basis of spectroscopic techniques.

Langlois *et al., Bull. Soc. Chim. Fr.,* **10,** 3535 (1970)

ALKALOID PC-VI

$C_{19}H_{21}O_4N$

M.p. 126°C

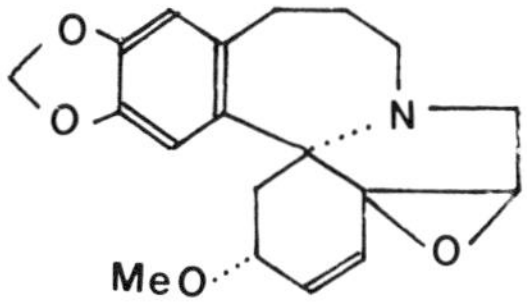

This alkaloid from *Phelline comosa* Labill. forms colourless crystals from Me_2CO and has $[\alpha]_D + 63°$ (c 1.8, $CHCl_3$). The ultraviolet spectrum contains two absorption maxima at 243 and 292 mμ. The alkaloid contains a methoxyl group, a methylenedioxy group and an epoxy group. A crystalline hydrochloride has been prepared with m.p. 218–9°C; $[\alpha]_D + 71°$ (c 1.6, EtOH).

Langlois *et al.*, *Bull. Soc. Chim. Fr.*, **10**, 3535 (1970)

ALKALOID PC-VII

$C_{20}H_{25}O_4N$

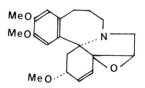

This homoerythrina alkaloid from *Phelline comosa* Labill., gives an ultraviolet spectrum with absorption maxima at 234 and 283 mμ. It yields a crystalline hydrochloride, m.p. 244°C; $[\alpha]_D + 82°$ (c 1.0, EtOH). Three methoxyl groups and an epoxy group are present in the molecule.

Langlois *et al.*, *Bull. Soc. Chim. Fr.*, **10**, 3535 (1970)

ALKALOID PE-A

M.p. 26–7°C

An amorphous alkaloid occurring in *Piscidia erythrina* L., this low-melting base yields a crystalline hydrochloride, m.p. 124°C. No other salts have been described.

Danckworth, Schütte., *Arch. Pharm.*, **272**, 701 (1934)

ALKALOID PI-1

$C_{12}H_{10}N_2$

M.p. 237–8°C

Passiflora incarnata yields this crystalline alkaloid which slowly distils with steam. The crystals exhibit a bright blue fluorescence in ultraviolet light. The hydrochloride is also crystalline and the base may be characterized as the aurichloride, m.p. 191–3°C. As yet, the structure has not been elucidated.

Neu., *Arzneimittel-Forsch.*, **4**, 601 (1954)

ALKALOID PM-A

$C_{20}H_{27}O_5N$

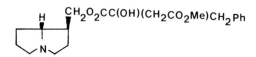

A pyrrolizidine alkaloid found in *Phalaenopsis mannii*, the base is diastereo-isomeric with Alkaloid PA-A (q.v.). Acid methanolysis gives (−)-dimethyl-2-benzylmalate and Laburnine (q.v.).

Brandange, Luning., *Acta Chem. Scand.*, **23**, 1151 (1969)

ALKALOID PN-A

$C_{12}H_{13}O_2N$

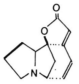

An alkaloid obtained from *Phyllanthus niruri*, the base is dextrorotatory with $[\alpha]_D + 213°$ (CHCl$_3$), gives an ultraviolet spectrum with a single absorption maximum at 256 mμ, and has proved to be the enantiomer of norsecurinine.

Rouffiac, Parello., *Plant. Med. Phytother.*, **3**, 220 (1969)

ALKALOID PO-A

$C_{22}H_{23}O_6N$

This alkaloid has been isolated from *Papaver orientale* and occurs, along with isothebaine, in the crude alkaloid extract obtained from the plant during, or shortly after, the flowering period. The ultraviolet spectrum confirms its tetrahydroprotoberberine character.

Nemeckova, Preininger, Santavy., *Abh. Deut. Akad. Wiss. Berlin, Kl. Chem. Geol. Biol.*, 319 (1966)

ALKALOID PO-B

$C_{19}H_{21}O_7N$

Also present in *Papaver orientale* during the flowering season, this alkaloid has been shown to be a 13-methyltetrahydroprotoberberine derivative.

Nemeckova, Preininger, Santavy., *Abh. Deut. Akad. Wiss. Berlin, Kl. Chem. Geol. Biol.*, 319 (1966)

ALKALOID PO-3

$C_{19}H_{16}O_4N^+$

M.p. 252°C

This quaternary alkaloid occurs in *Papaver orientale* and has been separated by column chromatography from the accompanying bases. The crystalline tartrate has m.p. 281°C.

Preininger, Santavy., *Acta Univ. Palacki, Olomuc., Fac. Med.*, **43**, 5 (1966)

ALKALOID PO-4

$C_{22}H_{20}O_6N^+$

M.p. $300°C$

A protoberberine alkaloid present in *Papaver* species, particularly *P. orientale,* this quaternary base is obtained as the crystalline hydrochloride, m.p. $> 300°C$. This salt has $[\alpha]_D^{22}$ $0°$ (c 0.228, EtOH) and forms colourless crystals from a mixture of MeOH and Et_2O. It has been assigned the protoberberine structure on the basis of ultraviolet, NMR spectra and chemical evidence.

Preininger, Santavy., *Acta Univ, Palacki, Olomuc., Fac. Med.,* **43**, 5 (1966)
Preininger *et al., Collect. Czech. Chem. Commun.,* **35**, 124 (1970)

ALKALOID PO-5

$C_{22}H_{22}O_6N^+$

Like the two preceding bases, this quaternary alkaloid occurs in *Papaver orientale* and other *Papaver* species. The chloride crystallizes from EtOH and has m.p. $> 300°C$; $[\alpha]_D^{22}$ $0°$ (c 0.345, EtOH). Hydrogenation over PtO_2 in AcOH gives optically inactive Mecambridine (q.v.).

Preininger, Santavy., *Acta Univ. Palacki, Olomuc., Fac. Med.,* **43**, 5 (1966)
Preininger *et al., Collect. Czech. Chem. Commun.,* **35**, 124 (1970)

ALKALOID PT-1

M.p. $239-241°C$

This uncharacterized alkaloid has been isolated from *Ptelea trifoliata.* No salts or derivatives have been reported, nor has a chemical analysis been carried out.

Kowalska, Borkowski., *Acta Polon. Pharm.,* **23**, 295 (1966)

ALKALOID P2

This base occurs in *Baptisia australis* and *B. perfoliata,* being found with Baptifoline (q.v.) in the mother liquor. It forms a picrate as pale yellow needles, m.p. $241°C$.

Marion, Turcotte., *J. Amer. Chem. Soc.,* **70**, 3254 (1948)

ALKALOID Q

$C_{32}H_{53}O_4N$

M.p. 209–210°C

A steroidal alkaloid obtained from *Veratrum californicum*, this base is laevo-rotatory with $[\alpha]_D^{25} - 95°$ (c 1.0, EtOH-CHCl$_3$). The structure has not yet been elucidated.

Keeler., *Phytochem.*, **7**, 303 (1968)

ALKALOID RH-1

M.p. 23°C

A low-melting alkaloid found in *Roemeria hybrida*. The structure has not yet been determined and very little pure base has been obtained for examination. No chemical analysis has been carried out.

Platonova *et al., J. Gen. Chem.*, USSR, **26**, 181 (1956)

ALKALOID RL-A

$C_{10}H_{18}O_2N_2$

This oily alkaloid occurs in *Rhizoctonia leguminicola* and has been purified through the crystalline picrate which forms yellow needles from H$_2$O, m.p. 178–183°C. With Ac$_2$O in pyridine, the N-acetyl derivative is formed which, on treatment with methyl iodide gives two stereoisomeric methiodide, m.p. 182–3°C and 258–260°C respectively.

Whitlock *et al., Tetrahedron Lett.*, 3819 (1966)

ALKALOID RO-A

$C_{20}H_{27}O_4N$

M.p. 197–8°C (*dec.*).

This alkaloid has been isolated from the CHCl.CHCl-NH$_3$ extract of *Rosmarinus officinalis* after the removal of Rosmaricine (q.v.). The base is dextrorotatory with $[\alpha]_D^{20} + 36°$ (dioxan) and yields a crystalline hydrochloride as colourless needles from H$_2$O, m.p. 214–6°C (*dec.*); the sulphate as crystals from aqueous MeOH, m.p. 188–190°C (*dec.*); and contains four active hydrogen atoms, a methyl group and a γ-lactone group. Treatment with Ac$_2$O furnishes the O,O,N-triacetyl derivative which crystallizes from MeOH, m.p. 291–2°C (*dec.*), while nitrous acid gives a compound, $C_{20}H_{26}O_5$, m.p. 178–180°C (*dec.*). Dehydrogenation with Se at 340°C yields 6-hydroxy-1-methyl-7-*iso*propyl-phenanthrene. When the plant is extracted with sodium carbonate, no alkaloids are obtained, indicating that this base is a transformation product arising from unstable diterpenoid compounds during the extraction in the presence of NH_3.

Yakhontova, Kuzuvkov., *Khim. Prir. Soedin.*, **3**, 140 (1967)

ALKALOID RP-1

M.p. 140–4°C

This alkaloid of *Rauwolfia perakensis* is amorphous. It gives a green colour with Keller reagent and a yellow colour with concentrated HNO_3 or H_2SO_4. It furnishes a crystalline hydrochloride, m.p. 192–4°C (*dec.*) crystallizing from aqueous MeOH; a nitrate as colourless prisms, m.p. 240–2°C (*dec.*) and a picrate as yellow needles, m.p. 204–5°C.

Kiang, Wan., *J. Chem. Soc.*, 1394 (1960)

ALKALOID RP-2

M.p. 76–80°C

A second amorphous alkaloid from *Rauwolfia perakensis*, this base occurs mainly in the roots. It has been characterized as the crystalline picrate, yellow needles from EtOH, m.p. 136–8°C.

Kiang, Wan., *J. Chem. Soc.*, 1394 (1960)

ALKALOID RP-3

M.p. 110–4°C

Also present in *Rauwolfia perakensis* roots, this alkaloid is amorphous but gives a crystalline picrate from aqueous EtOH, m.p. 167–8°C. The free base gives a wine colour with Fröhde's reagent, a yellow colour with concentrated H_2SO_4 and with concentrated HNO_3 a brown colour changing to orange.

Kiang, Wan., *J. Chem. Soc.*, 1394 (1960)

ALKALOID RP-7

$C_{21}H_{22}O_2N_2$

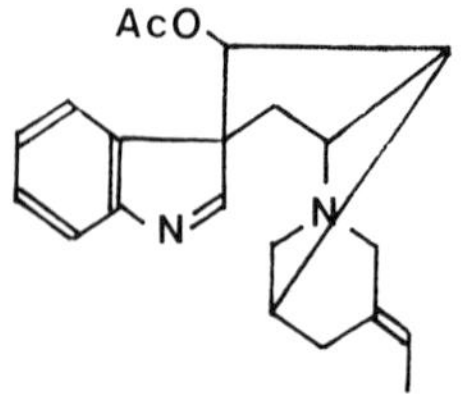

Rauwolfia perakensis has been shown to contain this alkaloid of the carboline type containing a vinyl group and an acetyl group. The structure has been confirmed by partial synthesis from Tetraphyllicine (q.v.).

Kiang *et al.*, *Tetrahedron*, **22**, 3293 (1966)

ALKALOID RS-A

$C_{21}H_{26}O_3N_2$

M.p. $125-8°C$ and $181-3°C$

This crystalline alkaloid from *Rauwolfia serpentina* is dimorphic and has the two melting points given above. The ultraviolet spectrum in EtOH has absorption maxima at 226, 282 and 290 mμ. The hydrochloride has m.p. $235-240°C$ (*dec.*); $[\alpha]_D^{20} - 75°$ (H_2O); the methiodide, m.p. $233-6°C$ (*dec.*); the monoacetate, m.p. $180-1°C$; $[\alpha]_D^{26} - 124°$ (pyridine); the diacetate, m.p. $193-5°C$; $[\alpha]_D^{26} - 102°$; the benzoate, m.p. $230-1°C$, giving a hydrochloride, m.p. $246-8°C$ and the hydrazide, m.p. $288-295°C$; $[\alpha]_D^{26} - 93°$ (pyridine). Structurally, the alkaloid is an isomer of Yohimbine (q.v.).

Bader *et al.*, *Experientia*, **10**, 298 (1954)

ALKALOID RS-C

$C_{22}H_{26}O_4N_2$

M.p. $240°C$ (*dec.*).

A further alkaloid obtained from *Rauwolfia serpentina*, this base has $[\alpha]_D^{20} - 127°$ (c 0.5, $CHCl_3$). It yields a crystalline hydrochloride, m.p. $263-4°C$ and is possibly 11-methoxy-δ-yohimbine.

Hofmann., *Helv. Chim. Acta*, **37**, 849 (1954)

ALKALOID RS-1

$C_{22}H_{26}O_4N_2$

M.p. $228°C$

Rauwolfia serpentina also contains this alkaloid which crystallizes as four-cornered leaflets. The base occurs mainly in the reserpine fraction of the alkaloidal extract. It is laevorotatory with $[\alpha]_D^{20} - 127°$ ($CHCl_3$) and gives an ultraviolet spectrum in EtOH with two absorption maxima at 228–230 and 298 mμ. The hydrochloride has m.p. $258-263°C$.

Popelak, Spingler, Kaiser., *Naturwiss.*, **40**, 625 (1953)

ALKALOID RS-2

$C_{21}H_{25}O_3N_2$

M.p. 247–8°C

A second alkaloid present in *Rauwolfia serpentina*, this base is also laevorotatory with $[\alpha]_D^{20} - 61°$ (CHCl$_3$). It crystallizes from EtOH in colourless prisms and gives an ultraviolet spectrum with absorption maxima at 226 and 282 mμ.

Popelak, Spingler, Kaiser., *Naturwiss.*, **40**, 625 (1953)

ALKALOID SA-1

M.p. 94–7°C

An alkaloid of *Sinomenium acutum*, this base crystallizes from a mixture of Et$_2$O and EtOH as colourless columnar crystals. It is laevorotatory with $[\alpha]_D^{18} - 74.1°$ (c 1.0, CHCl$_3$).

Sasaki, Onji., *J. Pharm. Soc., Japan*, **88**, 1286 (1968)

ALKALOID SD-1

$C_{18}H_{19}O_3N$

M.p. 285°C

This alkaloid is found in *Stephania dinkelagei* and is laevorotatory with $[\alpha]_D - 24.4°$ (c 0.7, CHCl$_3$). It is slightly soluble in C$_6$H$_6$ and readily so in Et$_2$O or CHCl$_3$. The ultraviolet spectrum in EtOH has an absorption maximum at 275 mμ with an inflexion at 225 mμ; while that in alkaline solution has absorption maxima at 230 and 277 mμ. The base contains two methoxyl groups and has a low toxicity, exhibiting a relaxing action on rabbit uterus in spasm with acetylcholine or barium chloride.

Paris, LeMen., *Ann. Pharm. Fr.*, **13**, 200 (1955)

ALKALOID SF-1

M.p. 212–3°C

This alkaloid has been reported as occurring in *Sternbergia fischeriana* and is stated to form a green viscous mass. It has been characterized as the crystalline hydrobromide, m.p. 174–5°C and the picrate, pale yellow needles, m.p. 217–9°C. Insufficient material has been obtained for a chemical analysis to be carried out on the base or its salts.

Proskurnina, Ismailov., *J. Gen. Chem. USSR*, **23**, 2056 (1953)

ALKALOID SG-1

$C_{23}H_{26}O_3N_4$

M.p. 260°C

The $CHCl_3$ extract of the upper parts of *Sophora griffithii* contains this alkaloid which forms colourless crystals when recrystallized from EtOH-Et_2O. It is strongly laevorotatory with $[\alpha]_D - 305°$ (c 3.28, EtOH) and contains a 2(1*H*)-pyridone ring and two lactam groups. Hydrogenation over Raney Ni furnishes the octahydro derivative, m.p. 208–9°C and $[\alpha]_D - 143°$ (c 0.81, EtOH).

Primukhamedov, Aslanov, Sadykov., *Nauch. Tr., Tashkent. Gos. Univ.,* No. 341, 128 (1968)

ALKALOID SG-A

$C_{19}H_{18}O_2N$

M.p. 79–81°C

One of a number of alkaloids isolated from *Stephania glabra,* this base crystallizes in colourless needles from Et_2O and has $[\alpha]_D - 88°$ (c 1.0, EtOH). The ultraviolet spectrum has two absorption maxima at 233 and 316 mμ. The hydrochloride is crystalline with m.p. 252–3°C and the base also yields an N-acetyl derivative, m.p. 146°C.

Fadeeva, Il'inskaya., *Khim. Prir. Soedin., Akad. Nauk. Uzbek SSR,* 6, 392 (1965)

ALKALOID SG-C

$C_{21}H_{25}O_4N$

M.p. 182–3°C

Stephania glabra also furnishes this crystalline alkaloid which forms colourless crystals from Me_2CO. The alkaloid is strongly dextrorotatory with $[\alpha]_D + 259°$ (c 1.0, EtOH) and contains three methoxyl groups and one methylimino group. It yields a crystalline hydrochloride with m.p. 230–2°C.

Fadeeva, Il'inskaya., *Khim. Prir. Soedin., Akad. Nauk. Uzbek SSR,* 6, 392 (1965)

ALKALOID SG-D

$C_{20}H_{25}O_4N$

M.p. 153–4°C

A further alkaloid which has been isolated from *Stephania glabra,* the base crystallizes from C_6H_6 and has $[\alpha]_D - 72°$ (c 1.0, EtOH). It contains two methoxyl groups and one methylimino group in the molecule. The hydrochloride has m.p. 227–8°C and the hydrobromide, m.p. 229–230°C. Hydrogenation over PtO_2 furnishes the tetrahydro derivative, m.p. 155–6°C.

Fadeeva, Il'inskaya., *Khim. Prir. Soedin., Akad. Nauk. Uzbek SSR,* **6,** 392 (1965)

ALKALOID SH-C

M.p. 236–8°C

This alkaloid has been obtained from *Salcornia herbacea* and characterized as the crystalline perchlorate, m.p. 210–2°C. A crystalline picrate is also known, m.p. 117°C. The ultraviolet spectrum of the free base consists of two absorption maxima at 240 and 280 mμ.

Borkowski, Drost., *Pharmazie,* **20,** 390 (1965)

ALKALOID SH-D

M.p. 178–180°C

A second uncharacterized alkaloid present in *Salcornia herbacea,* the base has been obtained in insufficient quantity for a chemical analysis to be carried out and no salts or derivatives have been reported.

Borkowski, Drost., *Pharmazie,* **20,** 390 (1965)

ALKALOID SJ-1

M.p. 135°C

One of three uncharacterized minor constituents of *Stephania japonica,* the base yields colourless crystals and is separated from the accompanying alkaloids by chromatography. The structure is unknown.

Tomita *et al., J. Pharm. Soc., Japan,* **76,** 686 (1956)

ALKALOID SJ-2

M.p. 165°C

This alkaloid of *Stephania japonica* occurs in the tertiary non-phenolic extract of the plant and is separated by chromatography on an alumina column.

Tomita *et al., J. Pharm. Soc., Japan,* **76,** 686 (1956)

110

ALKALOID SJ-3

M.p. 207–8°C

A further alkaloid of *Stephania japonica*, this base is found in the phenolic fraction following column chromatography. The structure has not yet been determined.

Tomita *et al.*, *J. Pharm. Soc., Japan*, **76**, 686 (1956)

ALKALOID SM-1

M.p. 278–9°C

A steroidal alkaloid present in *Solanum mammosum*, this base has $[\alpha]_D^{25} - 103°$ (MeOH). On alkaline hydrolysis it yields solasodine, two moles of glucose and one mole of rhamnose.

Saelkoff., *Arch. Pharm.*, **301**, 111 (1968)

ALKALOID SM-2

M.p. 269–270°C

A further steroidal, glycosidic alkaloid obtained from the fruit of *Solanum mammosum*, this base is also laevorotatory with $[\alpha]_D^{23} - 79.3°$ (dimethylformamide). Hydrolysis furnishes solasodine, two moles of glucose, one mole of rhamnose and one mole of galactose.

Saelkoff., *Arch. Pharm.*, **301**, 111 (1968)

ALKALOID SN-A

M.p. 213–5°C (*dec.*).

A hepatotoxic alkaloid isolated from *Senecio nudicaulis*, this base has $[\alpha]_D - 103.4°$ (CHCl$_3$). It yields a crystalline nitrate, m.p. 205–7°C; perchlorate, m.p. 240–2°C and the methiodide, m.p. 226–8°C (*dec.*).

Aghoranurti, Rajagopalam, Seshadri., *Curr. Sci.*, **33**, 80 (1964)

ALKALOID SN-1

M.p. 320–5°C

This steroidal alkaloid occurs in *Solanum nigrum* and has been obtained as colourless crystals from MeOH. The structure is not yet known and no derivatives have been reported.

Aslanov., *Khim. Prir. Soedin.*, **5**, 674 (1971)

ALKALOID SP-1

$C_{45}H_{73}O_{16}N$

M.p. 270–280°C (dec.).

This glycoalkaloid of *Solanum panduraeforme* crystallizes as the hemihydrate and is laevorotatory with $[\alpha]_D^{23} - 73°$. It forms a picrate, yellow crystals from Me_2CO, m.p. 180–5°C and the picrolonate pentahydrate, m.p. 200–1°C (*dry*). Acid hydrolysis furnishes L-rhamnose, D-glucose, D-galactose and a crystalline aglycone, $C_{27}H_{43}O_7N$, m.p. 250–2°C (*dec.*); $[\alpha]_D^{30} - 40.5°$, giving a sulphate, m.p. 275°C; picrate, m.p. 145°C and picrolonate, m.p. 218–220°C. Dehydration with dry HCl in MeOH gives a diene, m.p. 218–223°C (*dec.*) characterized as the hydrochloride, m.p. 251–4°C.

Veldsman, Louw., *J. S. Afr. Chem. Inst.*, 2, 119 (1949)

ALKALOID SP-A

$C_{19}H_{23}O_3N$

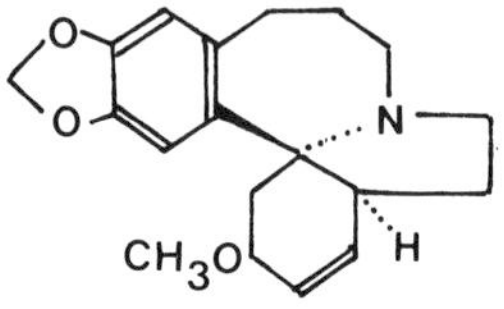

One of a number of closely related homoerythrina alkaloids which have been isolated from *Schelhammera pedunculata*. The structure of this base has been deduced on the basis of infrared, ultraviolet, NMR and mass spectrometry.

Johns, Lamberton, Sioumis., *Austral. J. Chem.*, 22, 2219 (1969)

ALKALOID SP-B

$C_{19}H_{25}O_3N$

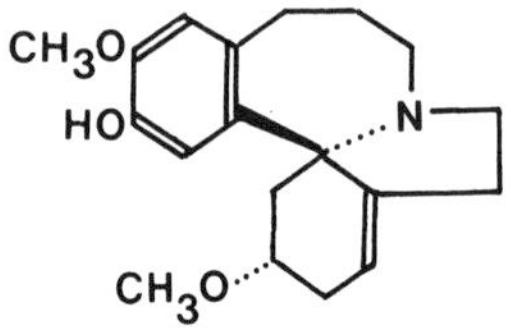

Also present in *Schelhammera pedunculata,* this alkaloid is the dehydro base corresponding to the preceding alkaloid. The structure has been established as that given above from spectroscopic evidence.

Johns, Lamberton, Sioumis., *Austral. J. Chem.*, 22, 2219 (1969)

ALKALOID SP-E

$C_{19}H_{23}O_3N$

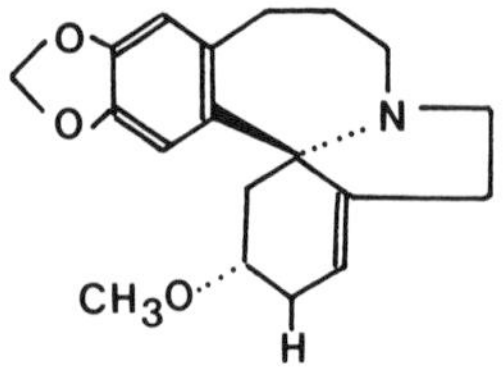

This alkaloid from *Schelhammera pedunculata* has also been obtained as the major constituent of *S. multiflora* and is also identical with Alkaloid PC IV (q.v.).

Johns, Lamberton, Sioumis., *Austral. J. Chem.*, **22**, 2219 (1969)

ALKALOID SP-G

$C_{19}H_{21}O_3N$

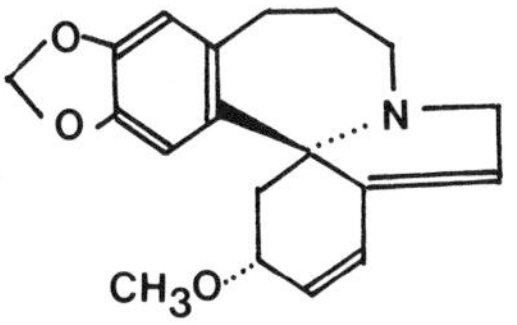

A fourth homoerythrina base from *Schelhammera pedunculata,* the structure is that given above. One methoxyl group and one methylenedioxy group are present.

Johns, Lamberton, Sioumis., *Austral. J. Chem.*, **22**, 2219 (1969)

ALKALOID SP-H

$C_{20}H_{25}O_4N$

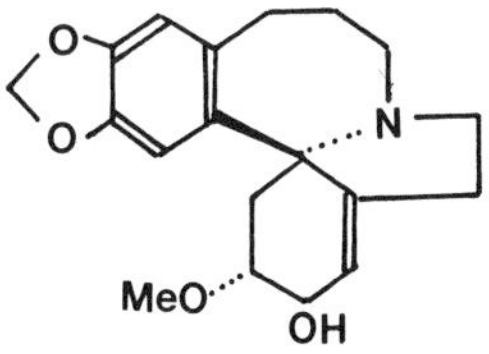

Schelhammera pedunculata yields this homoerythrina alkaloid which contains two methoxyl groups and a methylenedioxy group. The structure has been established from the infrared, ultraviolet, NMR and mass spectra.

Johns, Lamberton, Sioumis., *Austral. J. Chem.*, **22**, 2219 (1969)

ALKALOID SP-J

$C_{19}H_{21}O_4N$

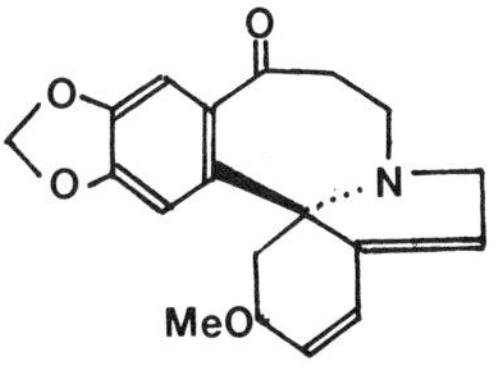

One of two isomeric homoerythrina alkaloids from *Schelhammera pedunsulata,* this base contains a methoxyl group, a methylenedioxy group and a keto group in the molecule.

Johns, Lamberton, Sioumis., *Austral. J. Chem.*, **22**, 2219 (1969)

ALKALOID SP-K

$C_{19}H_{21}O_4N$

The second isomeric homoerythrina alkaloid of *Schelhammera pedunculata,* this base differs from the preceding alkaloid only in the position of the keto group.

Johns, Lamberton, Sioumis., *Austral. J. Chem.*, **22**, 2219 (1969)

ALKALOID SP-I

$C_{17}H_{24}ON_2$

M.p. 174–5°C

The distillation residues of *Sophora pachycarpa,* after removal of Pachycarpine and Matrine (q.v.), on extraction with Et_2O, yield four minor alkaloids. This particular base has $[\alpha]_D^{20} - 104.4°$ and yields a hydriodide, m.p. 207–8°C; perchlorate, m.p. 244–5°C; $[\alpha]_D^{20} - 55°$ and a picrate, m.p. 210–1°C.

Sadykov, Kushmuradov., *J. Gen. Chem., USSR,* **32**, 1345 (1962)

ALKALOID SP-II

$C_{17}H_{19}ON_2$

M.p. 132–3°C

A second minor constituent of *Sophora pachycarpa,* the alkaloid has $[\alpha]_D^{20} +$ 30.6° and gives a hydriodide, m.p. 260–2°C; $[\alpha]_D^{20} + 28.5°$; perchlorate, m.p. 256–7°C and a picrate, m.p. 195–6°C. Catalytic hydrogenation with Raney Ni gives the dihydro derivative, m.p. 196–7°C; $[\alpha]_D^{20} + 14.85°$ and characterized as the crystalline picrate, m.p. 204–5°C. With $LiAlH_4$ the dihydro compound yields the deoxy base, $C_{13}H_{23}N_2$, m.p. 197–8°C; $[\alpha]_D^{20} - 14.59°$, also giving crystalline salts, e.g. the hydrochloride decomposing at 310–2°C; $[\alpha]_D^{20} - 40°$; hydrobromide, decomposing at 308–310°C; $[\alpha]_D^{20} - 8.3°$; perchlorate, m.p. 256–8°C and the picrate which decomposes at 210–2°C.

Sadykov, Kushmuradov., *J. Gen. Chem., USSR,* **32**, 1345 (1962)

ALKALOID SP-III

$C_{15}H_{20}ON_2$

M.p. 143–4°C

This alkaloid from *Sophora pachycarpa* is dextrorotatory with $[\alpha]_D^{20} + 52.3°$ and is characterized as the crystalline hydrochloride, m.p. 335–6°C; $[\alpha]_D^{20} + 56°$.

Sadykov, Kushmuradov., *J. Gen. Chem., USSR,* **32**, 1345 (1962)

ALKALOID SP-IV

M.p. 108–9°C

An uncharacterized alkaloid from *Sophora pachycarpa,* this base has $[\alpha]_D^{20} +$ 65.3°. No salts or derivatives have been prepared.

Sadykov, Kushmuradov., *J. Gen. Chem., USSR,* 32, 1345 (1962)

ALKALOID SS-A

$C_{25}H_{44}ON$

M.p. 136–7°C

Sarcococca saligna furnishes this alkaloid in 0.05 per cent yield as white, needle-shaped crystals from the cold EtOH extract of the leaves of the plant. The base is dextrorotatory with $[\alpha]_D^{25} + 64°$ (MeOH). The structure is not yet known.

Kiamuddin, Haque., *Pakistan. J. Sci. Ind. Res.,* 9, 103 (1966)

ALKALOID ST-1

$C_{20}H_{21}N_2Cl$

M.p. 239–243°C

A calabash curare alkaloid from *Strychnos toxifera,* this quaternary base is obtained as the chloride which forms colourless crystals. It has $[\alpha]_D^{20} - 13.4°$ (c 0.8955, H_2O) and gives an ultraviolet spectrum with an absorption maximum at 270 mμ.

Wieland, Merz., *Chem. Ber.,* 85, 731 (1952)

ALKALOID SV-1

$C_{18}H_{25}O_5N$

One of three minor constituents of *Senecio vernalis,* the alkaloid occurs in the basic fraction of the MeOH extract and is separated by column chromatography. A crystalline nitrate and picrate have been described.

Rulko, Witkiewicz., *Rocz. Chem.,* 47, 71 (1973)

ALKALOID SV-2

$C_{19}H_{27}O_6N$

Also present in the basic fraction of the EtOH extract from *Senecio vernalis,* this alkaloid has been characterized as the crystalline nitrate and picrate.

Rulko, Witkiewicz., *Rocz. Chem.,* 47, 71 (1973)

ALKALOID SV-3

$C_{18}H_{25}O_5N$

The third pyrrolizidine alkaloid to be isolated from the EtOH portion of *Senecio vernalis*. The structure is not yet known.

Rulko, Witkiewicz., *Rocz. Chem.*, **47**, 71 (1973)

ALKALOID T

$C_{38}H_{44-46}O_6N_2$

M.p. 218–220°C

This alkaloid has been isolated from the root bark of *Triclisia patens*. It has been characterized as the methochloride, m.p. 296°C and the methiodide, m.p. 227–9°C. Pharmacologically, the base acts as a curarizing agent.

French Patent, Fr. M2437 27 April 1964

ALKALOID TB-1

$C_{33}H_{43}O_{14}N_2$

M.p. 112–3°C

The leaves of *Taxus baccata* (English yew) yield this complex alkaloid which is obtained from the Et_2O extract as a white, amorphous powder. No salts or derivatives have been described and the structure is unknown.

Mirzoev., *Azerb. Khim. Zh.*, **1**, 73 (1971)

ALKALOID TI-A

An uncharacterized minor constituent of *Tylophora indica*, this base has been isolated chromatographically. No further details are available.

Rao, Wilson, Cummings., *J. Pharm. Sci.*, **60**, 1725 (1971)

ALKALOID TI-B

A further alkaloid from *Tylophora indica* and also present in *T. dalzellii*, this base has been shown to be demethyltylophorinine. It exhibits a pronounced anti-leukaemic activity.

Rao, Wilson, Cummings., *J. Pharm. Sci.*, **60**, 1725 (1971)

116

ALKALOID TL-A$_1$

One of two minor alkaloids found in the powdered seeds of *Thermopsis lanceolata*. The base occurs only in trace amounts and insufficient material has been obtained for a chemical analysis to be carried out.

Orazgel'diev, Aslanov, Sadykov., *Izv. Akad. Nauk. Turkm SSR, Ser. Fiz-Tekh. Khim. Geol. Nauk.*, **6**, 119 (1967)

ALKALOID TL-A$_2$

Also present in the powdered seeds of *Thermopsis lanceolata,* this alkaloid has been characterized as the picrate, pale yellow crystals, m.p. 159−160°C. No further salts or derivatives have been reported.

Orazgel'diev, Aslanov, Sadykov., *Izv. Akad. Nauk. Turkm. SSR, Ser. Fiz-Tekh. Khim. Geol. Nauk.*, **6**, 119 (1967)

ALKALOID TM-A

$C_{32}H_{46}O_6N_2$

M.p. 125−7°C

An alkaloid of *Trianthema monogyna* L., this base forms colourless crystals from MeOH and yields well crystalline salts including the sulphate, m.p. 110−1°C; oxalate, m.p. 138°C; aurichloride, m.p. 150−3°C and the picrate, m.p. 112°C.

Basu, Sharma., *Quart. J. Pharm.*, **20**, 39 (1947)
Chopra *et al., Ind. J. Med. Res.*, **28**, 475 (1940)

ALKALOID TN-4

An uncharacterized alkaloid recently discovered in *Corydalis incisa.* No salts or derivatives have yet been reported.

Nonaka *et al., J. Pharm. Soc., Japan,* **93**, 87 (1973)

ALKALOID TN-5

Also present on *Corydalis incisa,* this base has been obtained by countercurrent distribution methods. As yet it has not been characterized.

Nonaka *et al., J. Pharm. Soc., Japan,* **93**, 87 (1973)

ALKALOID TN-12

A further uncharacterized alkaloid present in *Corydalis incisa* this base is, like the other four closely related alkaloids, present only in small amounts in the total alkaloidal extract.

Nonaka *et al., J. Pharm. Soc., Japan,* **93**, 87 (1973)

ALKALOID TN-21

A fourth minor constituent of *Corydalis incisa,* the alkaloid occurs in minute amounts in the alkaloidal extract.

Nonaka *et al., J. Pharm. Soc., Japan,* **93**, 87 (1973)

ALKALOID TN-23

This uncharacterized alkaloid has also been isolated from *Corydalis incisa* and is, like the remaining four bases, still under investigation.

Nonaka *et al., J. Pharm. Soc., Japan,* **93**, 87 (1973)

ALKALOID TR-A

A minor constituent of the phenolic alkaloids present in the roots of *Thalictrum rochebrunianum,* a plant of the Ranunculaceae indigenous to Japan. The alkaloid is still uncharacterized and occurs together with Hernandezine and Thalibrunine (q.v.).

Fong, Beal, Cava., *Lloydia,* **29**, 94 (1966)

ALKALOID UE-1

This alkaloid has been obtained from the weak base fraction of the alkaloid extract from *Ulex europeus.* It has been characterized as the crystalline picrate, m.p. 80–5°C.

Ribas, Basanta., *Anales. real. soc. espan. fis. y quim.,* **48B**, 161 (1952)

ALKALOID UE-2

A further weak base present in *Ulex europeus,* this alkaloid is separated from the foregoing base by column chromatography. It yields a crystalline picrate, m.p. 175°C.

Ribas, Basanta., *Anales. real. soc. espan. fis. y quim.,* **48B**, 161 (1952)

ALKALOID VA-A

$C_8H_{11}N$

Isolated from *Viscium album* L., this liquid alkaloid has been characterized as the platinichloride which forms pale yellow crystals from EtOH, m.p. 250°C (*dec.*). No other salts or derivatives have been described.

LePrince., *Compt. rend.,* **145**, 940 (1907)
Crawford, Watanabe., *J. Biol. Chem.,* **24**, 169 (1916)

ALKALOID VH-A

$C_{22}H_{24}O_2N_2$

M.p. 174–7°C

A minor constituent of *Vinca herbacea* grown in Azerbaidzhan, this base has $[\alpha]_D^{23} + 595°$ (c 0.48, pyridine) and the same specific rotation in $CHCl_3$. The ultraviolet spectrum is stated to resemble that of α-methyleneindoline or 2-acylindole derivatives.

Aliev, Babaev., *Farmatsiya* (Moscow), **17**, 23 (1968)

ALKALOID VH-A₁

M.p. 175–7°C

The Et_2O-soluble fraction of the alkaloidal residue from *Vinca herbacea* grown in Georgia, SSR contains four alkaloids which have been isolated by Vachnadze and his colleagues. The solutions of this base show a marked green fluorescence and the ultraviolet spectrum has absorption maxima at 245, 302 and 365.5 mμ. The alkaloid has been classed among the akuammicine group.

Vachnadze *et al., Soobshch. Akad. Nauk. Gruz. SSR*, **53**, 117 (1969)

ALKALOID VH-A₂

M.p. 210–2°C

A mitraphylline type alkaloid present in *Vinca herbacea*, this base has $[\alpha]_D^{22} -$ 105° ($CHCl_3$). The ultraviolet spectrum is stated to be typical of alkaloids with the oxyindole structure.

Vachnadze *et al., Soobshch. Akad. Nauk. Gruz. SSR*, **53**, 117 (1969)

ALKALOID VH-A₅

M.p. 189–191°C

Also present in *Vinca herbacea* grown in Georgia SSR, this alkaloid has $[\alpha]_D^{22} -$ 105° ($CHCl_3$) and an ultraviolet spectrum similar to that of the preceding base. The infrared spectrum shows the presence of a benzene ring, a methoxycarbonyl group, an amidocarbonyl group and an imino group. The base is a stereoisomer of Alkaloid VH-A₂.

Vachnadze *et al., Soobshch. Akad. Nauk. Gruz. SSR*, **53**, 117 (1969)

ALKALOID VH-A₇

M.p. 278–280°C

The fourth alkaloid isolated from the Et_2O-soluble extract of *Vinca herbacea* shows a blue fluorescence in solution and gives an ultraviolet spectrum with absorption maxima at 243 and 315 mμ. It belongs to the indole group of sarpagine and amaline alkaloids.

Vachnadze *et al.*, *Soobshch. Akad. Nauk. Gruz. SSR*, **53**, 117 (1969)

ALKALOID VM-A

$C_{20}H_{24}O_2N_2$

M.p. 169–170°C

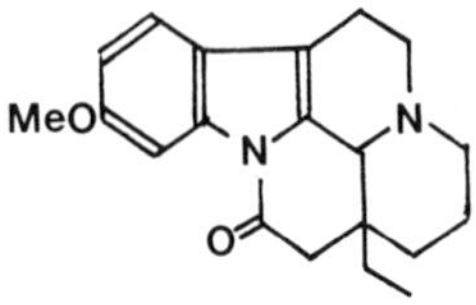

This carboline alkaloid has been isolated from the weakly basic fraction of *Vinca minor*. It is laevorotatory with $[\alpha]_D^{22} - 107°$ (CHCl$_3$) and has assigned the above 11-methoxyeburnamonine structure on the basis of spectroscopic evidence. The alkaloid may also be obtained by the reduction of Vincine (q.v.) with LiAlH$_4$ in tetrahydrofuran.

Döpke *et al.*, *Tetrahedron Lett.*, 1803 (1968)

ALKALOID VM-1

$C_{21}H_{26}O_3N_2$

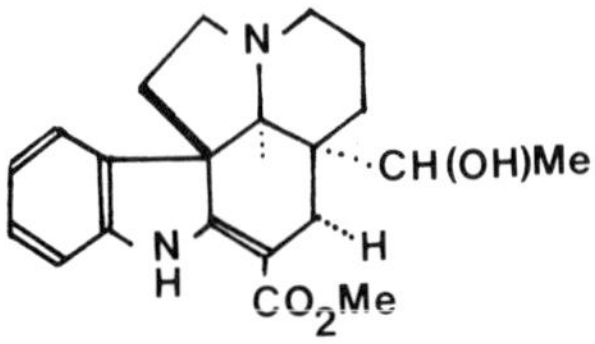

This imidazolidinocarbazole alkaloid has recently been isolated from *Vinca minor*. It is strongly laevorotatory with $[\alpha]_D - 580°$ (c 0.2, EtOH) and its spectra closely resemble those of Minovincinine (q.v.). The above structure has been assigned on the basis of chemical evidence.

Döpke., *Tetrahedron Lett.*, 749 (1970)

ALKALOID VN-1

M.p. 100°C

A minor constituent of *Verbascum nobile*, this alkaloid has not yet been isolated in sufficient quantity for further chemical or physical identification.

Ninova *et al.*, *Khim. Prir. Soedin.*, **7**, 540 (1971)

120

ALKALOID VO-A

M.p. 208–210°C (*dec.*).

This alkaloid from *Vincetoxicum officinale* forms colourless crystals from CHCl$_3$. It has been suggested that it is identical with Antofine (q.v.).

Pailer, Streicher., *Monatsh.*, **96**, 1094 (1965)

ALKALOID VP-A

C$_{21}$H$_{26}$O$_3$N$_2$

M.p. 269°C (*dec.*).

This new alkaloid from *Vinca pusilla* has a yohimbine structure according to the infrared, ultraviolet, NMR and mass spectral data. The hydrogen atom at C-3 has been shown to be α and possess equatorial configuration.

Chatterjee, Biswas, Kundu., *Ind. J. Chem.*, **11**, 7 (1973)

ALKALOID VS-1

M.p. 195–6°C

The buds and leaves of *Verbascum songaricum* yield this minor alkaloid which forms colourless crystals from EtOH. No salts or derivatives have been reported.

Ziyaev *et al.*, *Khim. Prir. Soedin.*, **7**, 853 (1971)

ALKALOID WP-A

M.p. 153–160°C and 175°C

A minor constituent of *Wurmbea purpurea*, this base is crystalline having the double melting point given above.

Pijewska *et al.*, *Collect. Czech. Chem. Commun.*, **32**, 158 (1967)

ALKALOID WP-B

M.p. 175–7°C

A second minor base obtained from *Wurmbea purpurea*, this alkaloid yields colourless prisms from AcOEt. No salts or derivatives have been reported.

Pijewska *et al.*, *Collect. Czech. Chem. Commun.*, **32**, 158 (1967)

ALKALOID WS-A

M.p. Indefinite

An amorphous alkaloid from *Withania somnifera* Dunal, this base furnishes an aurichloride as yellow needles, m.p. 185°C. When boiled with alcoholic KOH, the alkaloid gives a crystalline base, $C_{12}H_{16}N_2$, as colourless leaflets, M.p. 116°C.

Power, Salway., *J. Chem. Soc.*, **99**, 490 (1911)

ALKALOID WS-1

M.p. 113–5°C

A further alkaloid of *Wurmbea* species, this base occurs in *W. spicata* and is laevorotatory with $[\alpha]_D^{22} - 6.2°$ (c 0.650, CHCl$_3$).

Pijewska *et al.*, *Collect. Czech. Chem. Commun.*, **32**, 158 (1967)

ALKALOID ZN-1

$C_{21}H_{17}O_5N$

M.p. 274°C (*dec.*).

One of two closely related alkaloids present in the root bark of *Zanthoxylum nitidum*, this base contains two methoxyl groups and one methylenedioxy group. Treatment with PCl$_5$ followed by reduction with Zn and HCl yields the following base. The alkaloid is stated to resemble those of the chelidonine group.

Arthus., *Proc. Pacif. Sci. Congr., Pacif. Sci. Assoc., Bangkok,* **5**, 61 (1957), Publ. 1963

ALKALOID ZN-2

$C_{21}H_{19}O_4N$

M.p. 211–3°C

This second alkaloid of *Zanthoxylum nitidum* also resembles Chelidonine (q.v.) and contains two methoxyl groups and one methylenedioxy group. No salts have yet been described.

Arthur., *Proc. Pacif. Sci. Congr., Pacif. Sci. Assoc., Bangkok,* **5**, 61 (1957), Publ. 1963

ALKALOID 13

$C_{16}H_{17}O_4N$

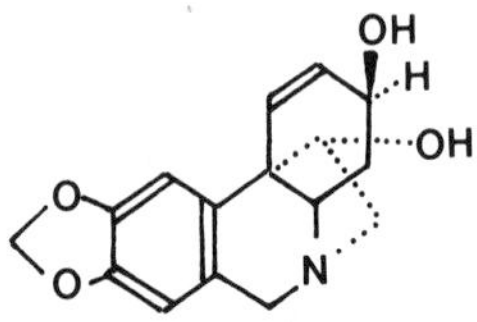

This Amaryllidaceous alkaloid has been described by de Angelis and Wildman. The base is of the *iso*quinoline type and contains one methylenedioxy group and two non-phenolic hydroxyl groups in the molecule.

De Angelis, Wildman., *Tetrahedron Lett.*, 729 (1969)

ALKAMINE G2

$C_{27}H_{43}O_3N$

M.p. 248–250°C

This alkaloid has been isolated from the mother liquors of the alkaloidal extract from *Amianthum muscaetoxicum*. Structurally, the base is isomeric with Cevine (q.v.) and Germine (q.v.).

Smith, Miller, Smith., *Chem. & Ind.*, **30**, 1362 (1964)

ALLOANODENDRINE

$C_{13}H_{21}O_2N$

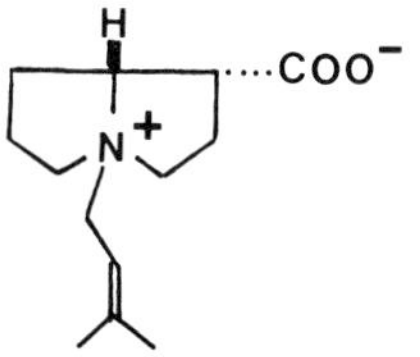

One of the bases obtained from *Anodendron affine* Druce., the alkaloid is slightly dextrorotatory with $[\alpha]_D^{25} + 18°$ (c 1.0, EtOH). In MeOH, the ultraviolet spectrum exhibits a single absorption maximum at 212 mμ. The base is best characterized as the *p*-bromophenacyl ester hydrobromide, m.p. 82–4°C. On hydrogenation, it forms 8 H-pyrrolizidine-1β-carboxylic acid.

Sasaki, Hirata., *Tetrahedron Lett.*, 4065 (1969)

ALLOFERINE

$C_{44}H_{50}O_2N_4^{++}$

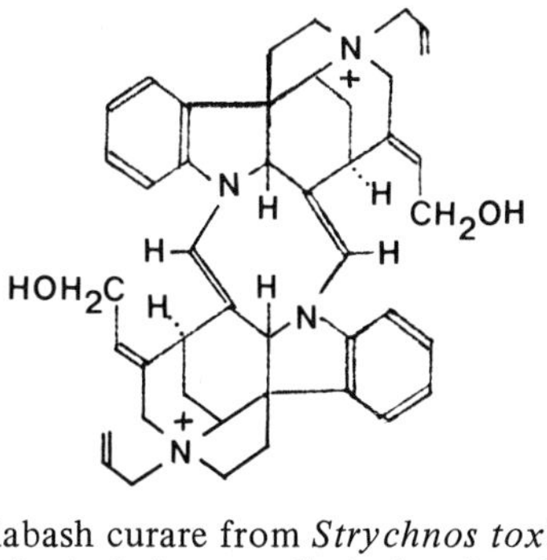

A minor alkaloid of calabash curare from *Strychnos toxifera*, the structure has been confirmed by synthesis. It is normally isolated as the dichloride.

Schmid., *Bull. Schweiz. Akad. Med. Wiss.*, **22**, 415 (1967)

α-ALLOCRYPTOPINE (β-Homochelidonine)

$C_{21}H_{23}O_5N$

M.p. 159–160°C

This alkaloid, which is stereoisomeric with β-allocryptopine, has been recorded in a number of plant genera belonging to the order Rhoeadales (Fumariaceae and Papavericeae), e.g. *Adlumia cirrhosa* Rap., *Bocconia arborea* Wats., *B. cordata* Willd., *B. frutescens* L., *Chelidonum majus* L., *Corydalis aurea* Willd., *C. caseana* A. Grey, *C. cheilantheifolia* Hemsl., *C. ophiocarpa* Hook, *C. scouleri* HK., *C. ternata* Nakai, *Dactylicapnos macrocapnos*, *Dicentra oregana* Eastwood, *Eschscholtzia californica* Cham, *Glaucium fimbrilligerum* and *Sanguinaria canadenses* L. The alkaloid crystallizes from AcOEt in monoclinic prisms and is freely soluble in $CHCl_3$ or AcOEt but less so in EtOH. Several crystalline salts are known: the hydrochloride sesquihydrate, colourless needles soluble in H_2O; platinichloride, an amorphous powder and the aurichloride, blood-red crystals, m.p. 187°C. The base contains two methoxyl groups and yields two methiodides, m.p. 185°C and 211°C indicating the tertiary nature of the base. In concentrated H_2SO_4, the alkaloid forms a yellow solution changing through violet to carmine-red. With $POCl_3$ it gives dihydroberberine methochloride as colourless needles, m.p. 200–1°C. On reduction with sodium amalgam it forms the dihydro derivative, m.p. 167–8°C which, with $POCl_3$, goes to tetrahydroanhydroberberine methochloride, m.p. 249–251°C. The alkaloid has been synthesized from berberine, establishing the structure given above.

Schlotterbeck., *Amer. Chem. J.*, **24**, 249 (1900)
Schlotterbeck, Watkins., *Pharm. Archiv.*, **6**, 17 (1903)
Howarth, Perkin., *J. Chem. Soc.*, 445 (1926)
Manske., *Can. J. Res.*, **9**, 436 (1933)
Manske., *ibid*, **15**, 159 (1937)
Manske., *ibid*, **16**, 81 (1938)
Manske, Miller., *ibid*, **16B**, 153 (1938)
Manske, Miller., *ibid*, **17B**, 94 (1939)
Manske, Miller., *ibid*, **18B**, 288 (1940)

β-ALLOCRYPTOPINE

$C_{21}H_{23}O_5N$

M.p. 170–1°C

This alkaloid does not appear to occur as widely as the preceding base, having been found in *Bocconia frutescens* L., *Chelidonium majus* L., *Eschscholtzia californica* Cham. and *Sanguinaria canadensis* L. An exceptional occurrence of the alkaloid is that reported from *Zanthoxylum brachyacanthum* Mull. (Rutaceae). The alkaloid crystallizes from EtOH in colourless needles as the solvate and is optically inactive. The hydrochloride sesquihydrate is obtained as small, colourless needles, m.p. 175°C (*dec.*); the aurichloride, deep-red crystals, m.p. 192° (*dec.*); stated to be identical with that of α-allocryptopine and the methiodide which crystallizes with 2.5 H_2O occurs in the form of yellow prisms.

Schmidt, Selle., *Arch. Pharm.*, **239**, 409, 421 (1901)
Jowett, Pyman., *J. Chem. Soc.*, **103**, 291 (1913)

ALLOTHIOBINUPHARIDINE

$C_{30}H_{42}O_2N_2S$

The rhizomes of *Nuphar luteum* contain a number of sulphur-containing alkaloids of which this is one. The base is characterized as the perchlorate which forms colourless plates, m.p. 320–5°C.

Achmatowicz, Bellen., *Tetrahedron Lett.*, 1121 (1962)

ALLOYOHIMBINE

$C_{21}H_{26}O_3N_2$

M.p. 135–140°C (*capillary*);
    165–170°C (*block*)

This base occurs in the bark of *Corynanthe yohimbe* and forms colourless crystals from EtOH of the trihydrate. The specific rotation of the hydrate is reported as $[\alpha]_D^{19} - 71.6°$ (pyridine) while that of the anhydrous alkaloid in the same solvent is − 84°. The hydrochloride has m.p. 279–280°C (*dec.*); $[\alpha]_D^{19} + 33°$ (H_2O) and the O-acetate, colourless needles from MeOH, m.p. 136°C; $[\alpha]_D^{20} - 25°$ (pyridine). Alkaline hydrolysis yields acetic acid and alloyohimbic acid, m.p. 248–250°C; $[\alpha]_D - 79.5°$ (pyridine). Both the free base and alloyohimbic acid yield alloyohimbone, $C_{19}H_{22}ON_2$, m.p. 230°C (*dec.*); $[\alpha]_D^{18} + 144.6°$ (pyridine) when subjected to the Oppenauer process, i.e. dehydrogenation by means of aluminium phenoxide and cyclohexane in xylene. Alloyohimbone gives a crystalline 2:4-dinitrophenylhydrazone hydrochloride, m.p. 264°C (*dec.*).

Warnat., *Ber.*, **59**, 2388 (1926)
Warnat., *ibid*, **60**, 1118 (1927)
Le Hir, Janot, Goutarel., *Bull. Soc. Chim. Fr.*, 1023 (1953)
Janot *et al.*, *Helv. Chim. Acta*, **38**, 1073 (1955)

ALOLYCOPINE

$C_{16}H_{21}O_2N$

M.p. 53–6°C

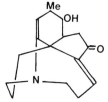

One of the *Lycopodium* alkaloids isolated from *L. alopecuroides,* the base crystallizes from Et$_2$O. In MeOH solution, the alkaloid exhibits an absorption maximum in the ultraviolet region at 237 mμ. The crystalline O-acetate has m.p. 180–2°C.

Ayer *et al., Can. J. Chem.,* **47,** 2449 (1967)
Structure:
Ayer, Altenkirk., *Can. J. Chem.,* **47,** 2457 (1969)

ALOPECURINE

$C_{23}H_{29}O_3N$

M.p. 244–5°C

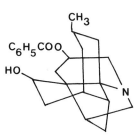

A further *Lycopodium* alkaloid from *L. alopecuroides,* this base is obtained in the crystalline form from Me$_2$CO. The ultraviolet spectrum has absorption maxima at 230, 272 and 280 mμ.

Ayer *et al., Can. J. Chem.,* **46,** 15 (1968)
Structure:
Ayer *et al., Can. J. Chem.,* **47,** 2449 (1969)

ALOPERINE

$C_{15}H_{24}N_2$

M.p. 73–5°C

A minor constituent of *Sophora alopecuroides,* this low-melting base has $[\alpha]_D$ + 85.7°. It yields a crystalline hydrochloride, m.p. 261–3°C; $[\alpha]_D$ + 92.4° (H$_2$O); an aurichloride, m.p. 204–6°C and a picrate, m.p. 235°C (*dec.*). The N-benzoyl derivative has m.p. 161–2°C. The alkaloid contains one imino group and with methyl iodide gives N-methylaloperine methiodide, m.p. 247–9°C.

Orekhov *et al., Ber.,* **66,** 948 (1933)
Orekhov *et al., ibid,* **68,** 431 (1935)
Orekhov *et al., Arch. Pharm.,* **272.** 673 (1934)

ALPINIGENINE

$C_{22}H_{27}O_6N$

M.p. 193.5°C

Alpinigenine and its 14-O-methyl ether, Alpinine (q.v.), occur in *Papaver alpinum* and the dried latex of *P. bracteatum* Lindl. The former crystallizes from AcOEt as colourless prisms, $[\alpha]_D^{22} + 286°$ (c 0.63, MeOH). A re-examination of this alkaloid by Giggisberg *et al* gives m.p. 186.5–187.5°C; $[\alpha]_D^{20} + 306°$ (c 1.084, MeOH). The ultraviolet spectrum shows two main absorption maxima at 230 and 284 mμ. The hydrochloride has been obtained as colourless crystals, m.p. 161–3°C (*dec.*); $[\alpha]_D^{20} + 210°$ (c 0.796, MeOH) but the acetate is amorphous and all attempts to obtain it crystalline have so far failed. The structure has been determined mainly by spectroscopic methods, notably by mass spectrometry.

Neubauer, Mothes., *Planta Med.*, **11**, 387 (1963)
Maturova, Pavlaskova, Santavy., *ibid*, **14**, 22 (1966)
Maturova *et al.*, *Collect. Czech. Chem. Commun.*, **32**, 419 (1967)
Guggisberg *et al.*, *Helv. Chim. Acta*, **50**, 621 (1967)

Mass spectra:
Dolejs, Hanus., *Tetrahedron*, **23**, 2997 (1967)

Stereochemistry:
Santavy *et al.*, *Collect. Czech. Chem. Commun.*, **32**, 4452 (1967)
Shamma *et al.*, *Chem. Commun.*, 212 (1968)
Lalazari, Shafiee, Nasseri-Nouri., *J. Pharm. Sci.*, **62**, 1718 (1973)

ALPININE (*O-methylalpinigenine*)

$C_{23}H_{29}O_6N$

M.p. Indefinite

This base is present in *Papaver alpinum* and is obtained as an amorphous powder with $[\alpha]_D^{22} + 288°$ (c 0.82, CHCl$_3$). The ultraviolet spectrum is virtually identical with that of the preceding base with absorption maxima at 231 and 286 mμ. It yields alpinigenine on hydrolysis.

Maturova *et al.*, *Collect. Czech. Chem. Commun.*, **32**, 419 (1967)

Mass spectra:
Dolejs, Hanus., *Tetrahedron*, **23**, 2997 (1967)

Stereochemistry:
Shamma *et al.*, *Chem. Commun.*, 212 (1968)

ALSTONAMINE

This crystalline alkaloid has been reported from *Alstonia spectabilis* R. Br. but its composition has not yet been determined, nor does it appear to have been examined further since its isolation.

Hesse., *Ber.*, **11**, 1546 (1878)
Hesse., *Annalen*, **203**, 170 (1880)

ALSTONERINE

$C_{21}H_{24}O_2N_2$

M.p. 172–3°C

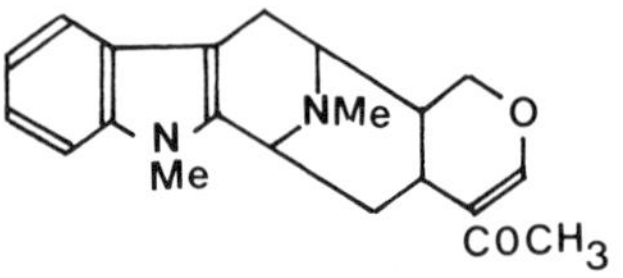

An indolchromotropane alkaloid from *Alstonia muelleriana*, the base has $[\alpha]_D^{25} - 195°$ (EtOH). The mass spectral fragmentation patterns are almost identical with those found for certain ajmaline derivatives while the NMR spectrum is similar to that of Alstophylline (q.v.).

Cook, LeQuesne, Elderfield., *J. Chem. Soc., D,* 1306 (1969)
Elderfield, Gilman., *Phytochem.*, **11**, 339 (1972)

ALSTONIDINE

$C_{22}H_{24}O_4N_2$

M.p. 188–190°C

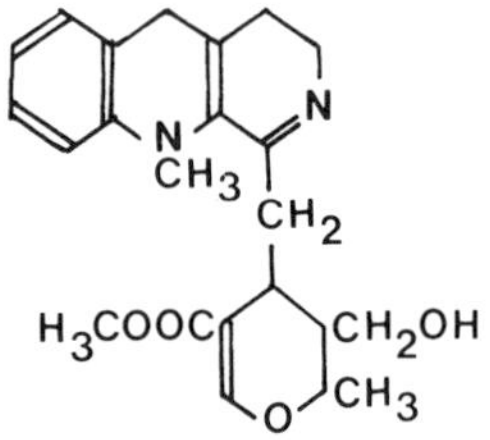

This alkaloid is a carboline type base and has been isolated from the root bark of *Alstonia constricta* F. Muell. When recrystallized from aqueous MeOH it is obtained as colourless, needle-shaped crystals. Treatment with Ac_2O gives the acetate which crystallizes as the trihydrate from aqueous Me_2CO with m.p. 92–6°C. The structure has been determined from chemical analysis and spectroscopic evidence.

Hesse., *Annalen*, **205**, 260 (1880)
Svoboda., *J. Amer. Pharm. Assoc.*, **46**, 508 (1957)
Boaz, Elderfield, Schenker., *ibid*, **46**, 510 (1957)

Stereochemistry:
Crow, Hancox, Johns, Lamberton., *Austral. J. Chem.*, **23**, 2489 (1970)

ALSTONILIDINE

$C_{23}H_{18}O_6N_2$

M.p. 244–5°C

The root bark of *Alstonia constricta* F. Muell yields several crystalline alkaloids. This minor constituent forms colourless needles when purified by recrystallization from EtOH. There are four absorption maxima in the ultraviolet spectrum occurring at 215, 255, 289 and 335 mμ, in solution in EtOH. The structure given above has been deduced from chemical degradative experiments and confirmed by the infrared, ultraviolet, NMR and mass spectra.

One methoxyl group and two methoxycarbonyl groups have been shown to be present in the molecule, the latter being substituted in a benzoyl moiety. An imino group is present although no salts or derivatives have yet been described. The structure as 1-(2:6-dimethoxycarbonylbenzoyl)-7-methoxy-β-carboline, has been confirmed by synthesis.

Crow, Hancox, Johns, Lamberton., *Austral. J. Chem.*, **23**, 2489 (1970)

ALSTONILINE

$C_{22}H_{18}O_3N_2$

M.p. 372°C (*dec.*).

This alkaloid was first obtained by Hawkins and Elderfield during the working up of *Alstonia constricta* F. Muell bark by a special process for the preparation of Alstonine. Like the latter, it has a protoberberine and not a carboline structure. The base exists as the monohydrate, yellow-brown needles, decomposing at 356°C and also in the anhydrous form which decomposes sharply at 372°C. Both of these forms give their own series of salts although it is clear from the close similarity of their ultraviolet spectra that hydration does not bring about any fundamental change in the molecule. There is now evidence that the hydrochloride (H_2O) exists naturally.

The anhydrous form gives the following salts: sulphate, m.p. 260–4°C (*dec.*); methiodide decomposing over a wide range and the picrate which explodes above 350°C.

The monohydrate yields: the hydrochloride, fine red needles, again decomposing over a wide range; picrate, m.p. 294°C (*dec.*). Attempts have been made to produce the methiodide, but these produced a new hydrate of the alkaloid, m.p. 189–190°C, as fine yellow needles.

The alkaloid is susceptible to oxidation yielding the oxide, $C_{22}H_{18}O_4N_2.H_2O$, m.p. 212–3°C or 219–221.5°C (*dry*). The sulphate and hydrochloride are stated to absorb 8 and 4 moles of hydrogen respectively over PtO_2 giving stable products with m.p. 233–4°C (*dec.*) and 231–2°C.

Alstoniline has been synthesized by ring closure of 2-2-(6-methoxy indol-3-yl) ethyl-5-(methoxycarbonyl)isoquinolinium bromide without reduction of the ester group to give tetrahydroalstoniline. The hydrochloride of the tetrahydro derivative in 0.1 N EtOH/KOAc, when added to hot iodine/KOAc/EtOH gave alstonilidine.

Hawkins, Elderfield., *J. Org. Chem.*, **7**, 573 (1942)
Elderfield, Wythe., *ibid*, **19**, 683 (1954)
Ban, Seo., *ibid*, **27**, 3380 (1962)

Synthesis:
Beisler., *Chem. Ber.*, **103**, 3360 (1970)

ALSTONINE

$C_{21}H_{20}O_3N_2$

M.p. 205–210°C (*dec.*).

Among the *Alstonia* species, this alkaloid has, so far, been found only in *Alstonia constricta* F. Muell although it occurs in certain *Rauwolfia* species. The free base is unstable and cannot be recrystallized without loss although it may be prepared in the form of a microcrystalline, yellow powder by precipitation followed by trituration with H_2O. This form is stated to be the tetrahydrate, sintering at 77° and decomposing at 130°C. Several well-crystallized salts have been prepared: hydrochloride, yellow, pentagonal plates, m.p. 278–9°C (*dec.*); nitrate, m.p. 252–4°C (*dec.*); hydriodide, m.p. 270°C (*dec.*); platinichloride (H_2O), m.p. 220–1°C (*dec.*); perchlorate, m.p. 239–240°C, sulphate (anhydrous), m.p. 243–4°C (*dec.*), with 2 H_2O, m.p. 195–6°C, frothing at 209°C, with 4 H_2O, m.p. 203–4°C and with 5 H_2O, pale orange rods, m.p. 209°C (*dec.*); acid sulphate, m.p. 244°C; picrate, rosettes of orange-red needles from EtOH, m.p. 194–5°C. In dilute solution, the salts are yellow with a marked blue fluorescence.

Catalytic reduction yields the tetrahydro-derivative, $C_{21}H_{24}O_3N_2$, as colour-less rods with m.p. 230–1°C; $[\alpha]_D - 107°$ (CHCl$_3$) or $- 88°$ (pyridine). Hydrolysis of this compound furnishes MeOH and tetrahydroalstoninic acid (hydrochloride, hygroscopic needles, m.p. 296° (*dec.*)). Dehydrogenation with Se yields the oxygen-free base, alstyrine, $C_{18}H_{20}N_2$ or $C_{19}H_{22}N$, as pale yellow plates, m.p. 113°C.

Hesse., *Annalen,* **205**, 360 (1880)
Sharp., *J. Chem. Soc.,* 287 (1934)
Leonard, Elderfield., *J. Org. Chem.,* **7**, 573 (1942)
Raymond-Hamet., *Compt. rend.,* **227**, 344 (1948)
Elderfield, Gray., *J. Org. Chem.,* **16**, 506 (1951)
Bader., *Helv. Chim. Acta,* **36**, 215 (1953)

ALSTONISIDINE

$C_{42}H_{48}O_4N_4$

M.p. 325°C (*dec.*).

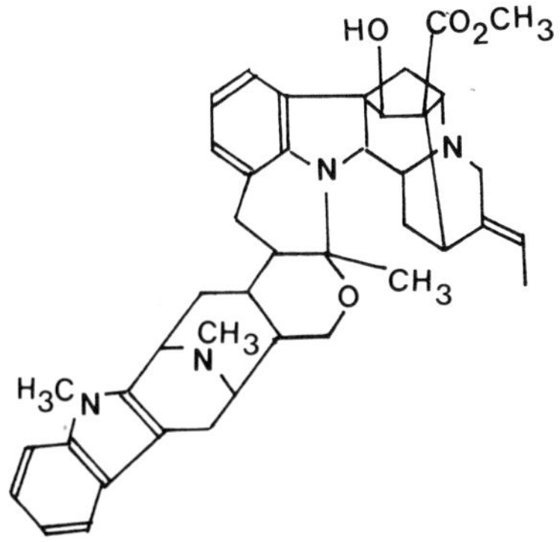

This complex *Alstonia* alkaloid occurs in the aerial bark of *Alstonia* muelleriana and forms colourless crystals from MeOH. It has $[\alpha]_D - 234°$ (EtOH) and shows three absorption maxima in the ultraviolet spectrum at 230, 286 and 294 mμ. The base contains four methyl, one hydroxyl and a methoxycarbonyl group. The structure given has recently been confirmed by synthesis.

Elderfield., *Amer. Scientist*, **48**, 193 (1960)

Cook, LeQuesne., *J. Org. Chem.*, **36**, 582 (1971)

Burke, Cook, LeQuesne., *J. Chem. Soc., Chem. Commun.*, 697 (1972)

ALSTONISINE

$C_{20}H_{22}O_3N_2$

M.p. 168–9°C

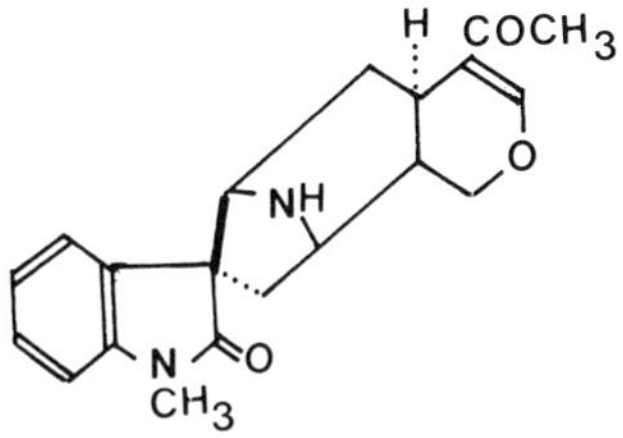

The aerial bark of *Alstonia muelleriana* also yields this alkaloid which has $[\alpha]_D^{25} + 200°$ (c 1.0, EtOH). The base is characterized as the hydrochloride, m.p. 250–260°C (*dec.*); $[\alpha]_D^{25} + 155°$ (c 1.0, H$_2$O).

Elderfield., *Amer. Scientist*, **48**, 193 (1960)

Nordman, Nakatsu., *J. Amer. Chem. Soc.*, **85**, 353 (1963)

Elderfield, Gilman., *Phytochem.*, **11**, 339 (1972)

ALSTOPHYLLINE

$C_{22}H_{26}O_3N_2$

M.p. 155–8°C

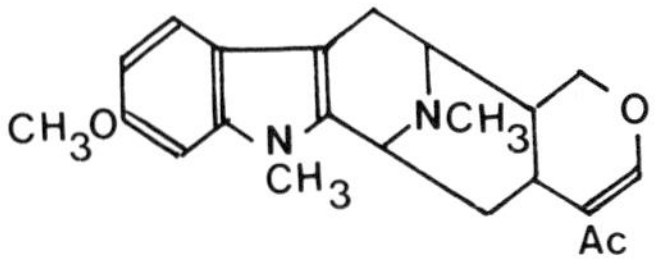

An alkaloid found in the rind of *Alstonia macrophylla,* this base is laevorotatory with $[\alpha]_D^{26} - 151° \pm 7°$ (c 0.326, CH_2Cl_2). With $NaBH_4$ it gives alstophyllinol, m.p. 170–4°C.

Kishi *et al., Helv. Chim. Acta,* **48**, 1349 (1965)

ALSTOVENINE

$C_{22}H_{28}O_4N_2$

M.p. 172°C

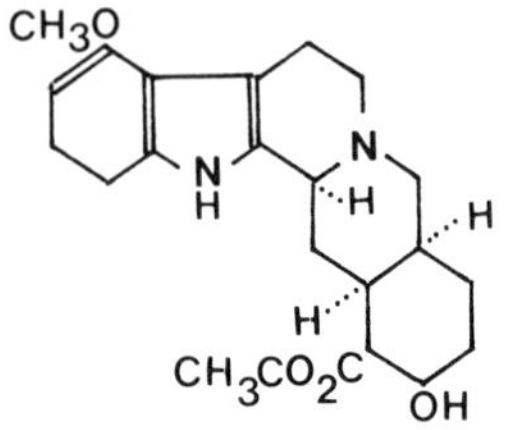

This protoberberine type alkaloid is present in *Alstonia venenata.* It contains one methoxyl, one hydroxyl and one methoxycarbonyl group in the molecule.

Chatterjee, Ray., *J. Ind. Chem. Soc.,* **41**, 638 (1964)

ALTERAMINE

$C_{15}H_{20}ON_2$

M.p. 112°C

From *Thermopsis alterniflora,* Shairmardanov *et al* have isolated this base with $[\alpha]_D - 43°$. It forms crystalline salts, e.g. the hydrochloride, m.p. 185–6°C; hydriodide, m.p. 212–3°C; perchlorate, m.p. 234–5°C and picrate, m.p. 215–6°C. The methiodide has also been prepared, m.p. 225–6°C.

Shaimardanov, Iskandarov, Yunusov., *Khim. Prir. Soedin.,* **6**, 276 (1970)

ALVANIDINE

$C_{20}H_{33}O_2N$

M.p. 235–6°C

The tubers of *Fritillaria raddeana* yield two alkaloids, this base being characterized as the crystalline hydrochloride, m.p. 174–5°C.

Aslanov, Sadykov., *J. Gen. Chem., USSR,* **26**, 579 (1956)

ALVANINE

$C_{26}H_{43}O_3N$

M.p. 185–7°C

The second base from *Fritillaria raddeana* tubers gives a crystalline hydrochloride, m.p. 163–5°C.

Aslanov, Sadykov., *J. Gen. Chem., USSR*, **26**, 579 (1956)

AMABILINE

$C_{16}H_{27}O_4N$

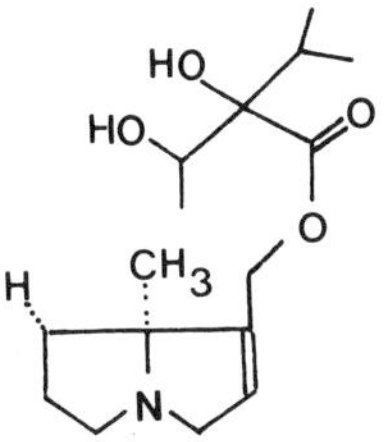

A pyrrolizidine alkaloid found in *Cynoglossum australe,* the structure of this base has been investigated by Culvenor and Smith.

Culvenor, Smith., *Austral. J. Chem.*, **20**, 2499 (1967)

AMARYLLISINE

$C_{18}H_{23}O_4N$

M.p. 255–8°C

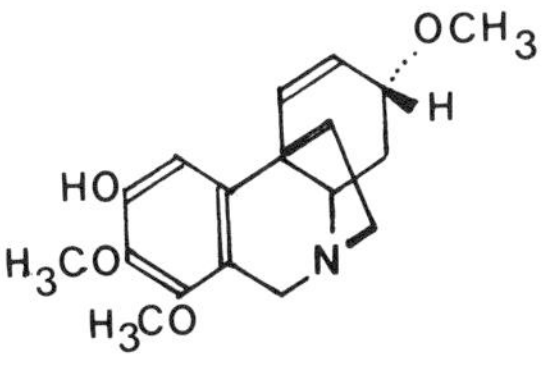

This benz*iso*quinoline base is found in *Brunsvigia rosea* (Syn. *Amaryllis belladona*). It forms colourless prisms from MeOH; $[\alpha]_D^{24} + 2.4°$ and $[\alpha]_{436}^{24} -$ 6.6° (c 0.27, CHCl$_3$). The ultraviolet spectrum shows one absorption maximum at 283 mμ. With Ac$_2$O, the alkaloid yields the O-acetyl derivative, m.p. 181–2°C The O-methyl ether is obtained as prisms from cyclohexane, m.p. 99–100°C; $[\alpha]_D^{24} - 16.4°$; $[\alpha]_{436}^{24} - 41.3°$ (c 1.6, CHCl$_3$). The latter may be characterized by the perchlorate, m.p. 236–7°C; $[\alpha]_D^{24} - 4.2°$ (c 1.5, CHCl$_3$).

Burlingame, Fales, Highte., *J. Amer. Chem. Soc.*, **86**, 4976 (1964)

AMATAINE

$C_{43}H_{48}O_6N_4$

M.p. 216–221°C

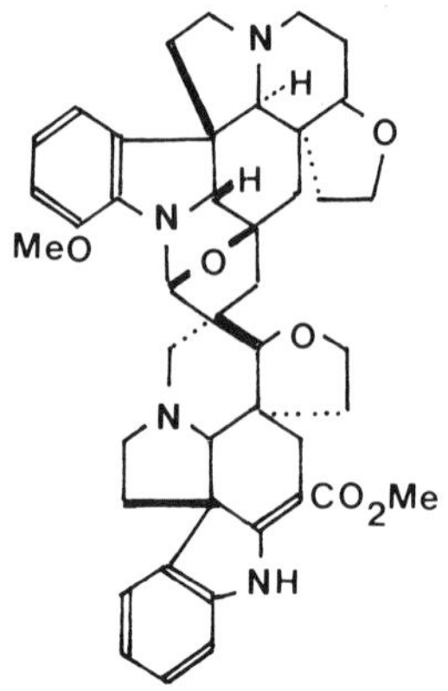

This complex imidazolinocarbazole alkaloid occurs in the root bark of *Hedranthera barteri* Pichon. It has $[\alpha]_D^{26} - 262°$ (c 0.7, $CHCl_3$).

Agwada, Patel, Hesse, Schmid., *Helv. Chim. Acta,* **53,** 1567 (1970)

AMBALINE

$C_{38}H_{42}O_{10}N_2$

M.p. 123°C

Isolated from *Pycnarrhena manillensis* Vidal, this base has $[\alpha]_D^{26} + 143.2°$ ($CHCl_3$). It forms a crystalline dihydrochloride, m.p. 265°C; an aurichloride, m.p. 185°C (*dec.*); and an oxime, m.p. 197°C (*dec.*). The structure has not yet been determined. Chemical evidence indicates the presence of three methoxyl, a carbonyl, a methylenedioxy and a methylimino group. The possibility that the second nitrogen is also present as a methylimino group appears likely.

Quibilan, Santos., *Univ. Philipp. Nat. Appl. Sci. Bull.,* **3,** 353 (1933)

AMBALININE

$C_{18}H_{21}O_3N$

M.p. 203–4°C

A second alkaloid isolated from *Pycnarrhena manillensis* Vidal, the base two methoxyl groups and one methylimino group in the molecule. It forms well-crystallized salts, e.g. the aurichloride, m.p. 170°C (*dec.*); the platinichloride, m.p. 240°C (*dec.*) and the picrate, m.p. 238°C (*dec.*). Like the preceding base, the structure of this alkaloid has not yet been elucidated.

Villanos, Santos., *Univ. Philipp. Nat. Appl. Sci. Bull.,* **3,** 353 (1933)

AMBELLINE

$C_{18}H_{21}O_5N$

M.p. 261°C (*dec.*).

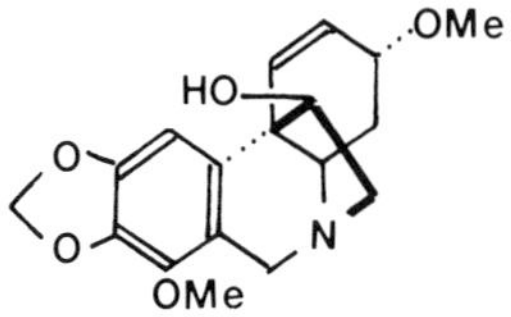

From *Brunswigia rosea,* this alkaloid has been obtained as colourless crystals from MeOH-Et$_2$O. It yields several crystalline salts and derivatives: the hydrochloride, m.p. 230°C (*dec.*); perchlorate, m.p. 200°C (*dec.*) and the methiodide, m.p. 298°C. Degradative evidence shows that it possesses the stereo structure given above.

Naegelli, Warnhoff, Fales, Lyle, Wildman., *J. Org. Chem.,* **28**, 206 (1963)

Mass spectrum:
Duffield, Aplin, Budzikiewicz, Djerassi, Murphy, Wildman., *J. Amer. Chem. Soc.,* **87**, 4902 (1965)

AMERICINE

$C_{31}H_{39}O_4N_5$

M.p. 135.5−137°C (142−182°C)

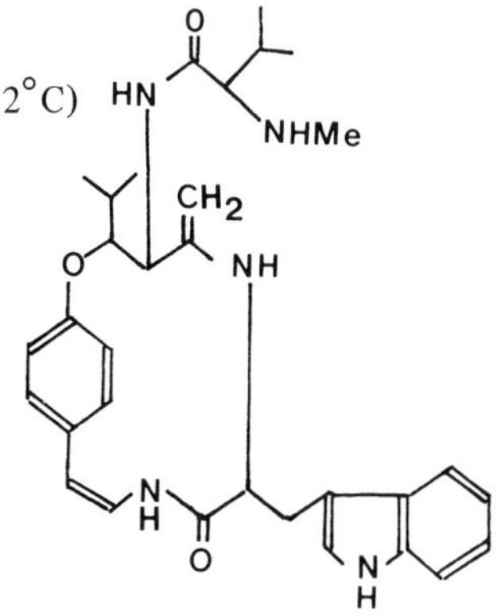

From the root bark of *Ceanothus americanus* L., Klein and Rapoport have isolated this peptide alkaloid which forms dimorphous crystals from EtOH-C$_6$H$_6$ having the above melting points. The base has $[\alpha]_D^{20} - 198°$ (c 0.51, MeOH). The ultraviolet spectrum of the alkaloid in MeOH shows absorption maxima at 221, 273, 280 and 290 mμ.

Klein, Rapoport., *J. Amer. Chem. Soc.,* **90**, 2398 (1968)

AMIANTHINE

M.p. 251−3°C

This alkaloid occurs in the roots and leaves of *Amianthium muscaetoxicum* Gray and yields colourless crystals from CHCl$_3$. It is laevorotatory having $[\alpha]_D^{20} - 87°$ (c 0.1728, CHCl$_3$) and gives a crystalline O-acetate, m.p. 206−7°C.

Neuss., *J. Amer. Chem. Soc.,* **75**, 2772 (1933)

(22R,25S)-3β-AMINO-5α-SPIROSTANE (*Jurubidine*)

$C_{27}H_{45}O_2N$

M.p. 182–6°C

This steroidal base occurs in the root of *Solanum paniculatum* L. It has $[\alpha]_D^{20}$ – 48.9° (pyridine). The alkaloid yields a crystalline hydrochloride from EtOH, m.p. 280–5°C. The N-acetyl derivative has m.p. 266°C; $[\alpha]_D^{20}$ – 74.3° ($CHCl_3$) and the N-salicylidene derivative, m.p. 203–5°C; $[\alpha]_D^{20}$ – 42.4° ($CHCl_3$).
For the 26-O-β-D-Glucopyranosyl derivative see Jurubine.

Schreiber, Ripperger, Budzikiewicz., *Tetrahedron Lett.,* 3999 (1965)
Ripperger, Budzikiewicz, Schreiber., *Chem. Ber.,* **100**, 1725 (1967)

AMMOCALLINE

$C_{19}H_{22}N_2$

M.p. > 335°C (*dec.*).

One of a number of alkaloids which occur in the roots of *Vinca rosea* L., this base shows two absorption maxima in the ultraviolet spectrum at 218 and 288 mμ. The complete structure has not yet been determined.

Svoboda, Oliver, Bedwell., *Lloydia,* **26**, 141 (1963)

AMMODENDRINE

$C_{12}H_{20}ON_2$

M.p. 50–60°C (*anhydrous*)

One of the Papilionaceous alkaloids, this base has been obtained from *Ammodendron Conollyi* Bge. It is isolated as the monohydrate, m.p. 73–4°C which becomes anhydrous at 70–80°C and then has the melting point given above. All of the salts are amorphous with the exception of the hydriodide which forms colourless crystals from EtOH, m.p. 218–220°C and the perchlorate which can be crystallized from Me_2CO, m.p. 199–200°C (208–9°C). The N-benzoyl derivative has been prepared as an amorphous powder. With CH_3I, the alkaloid behaves as a secondary base, giving first N-methylammodendrine hydriodide as a crystalline precipitate from EtOH-Me_2CO, m.p. 183–5°C and then N-methylammodendrine methiodide, m.p. 163–5°C. The N-methyl derivative itself has m.p. 65–6°C when crystallized from petroleum ether.

On hydrogenation, the alkaloid furnishes the dihydro-derivative which can be hydrolyzed into acetic acid and 2:3'-dipiperidyl and consequently, the dihydro form is dl-N-acetyl-3-α-piperidylpiperidine. Ammodendrine is therefore acetyl-tetrahydroanabasine. Biologically, the base is of interest in being the first recorded occurrence of this type of alkaloid in the Leguminosae.

Orekhov, Proskurnina, Lazurevskii., *Ber.*, **68**, 1807 (1935)
Orekhov, Proskurnina., *Bull. soc. chim.*, **5**, 29 (1938)
Schöpf, Braun., *Naturwiss.*, **36**, 377 (1949)
Schöpf, Braun, Kreibich., *Annalen*, **674**, 87 (1954)

AMMOROSINE

M.p. 221–5°C

This alkaloid has been reported as occurring in the roots of *Vinca rosea* L. The ultraviolet spectrum has absorption maxima at 227, 280, 295 and 305 mμ.

Svoboda, Oliver, Bedwell., *Lloydia*, **26**, 141 (1963)

AMMOTHAMNINE

$C_{15}H_{24}O_3N_2$

M.p. 199–201°C

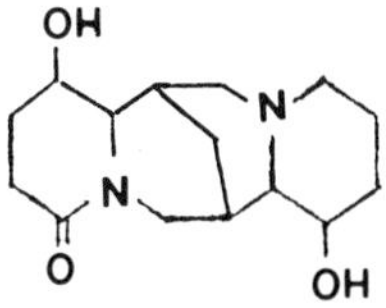

A base found in *Ammothamnus lehmannii* Bge., the alkaloid has $[\alpha]_D \pm 0°$. It forms a crystalline picrate, m.p. 212–4°C (*dec.*).

Sadykov, Proskurnina., *J. Gen. Chem., USSR*, **13**, 314 (1943)

AMPHIBIN A

$C_{33}H_{43}O_4N_5$

M.p. 237–9°C (*dec.*).

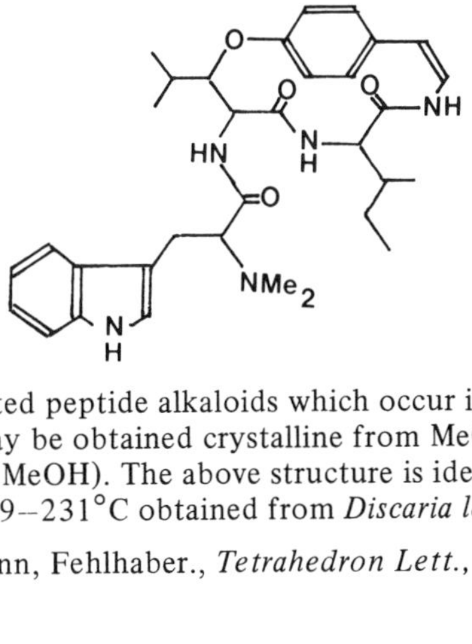

One of five closely-related peptide alkaloids which occur in *Ziziphus amphibia* A. Cheval. This base may be obtained crystalline from MeOH-CH$_2$Cl$_2$ with $[\alpha]_D^{20} - 310°$ (c 0.021, MeOH). The above structure is identical with that given to Discarine A, m.p. 229–231°C obtained from *Discaria longispina* (q.v.).

Tschesche, Kauffmann, Fehlhaber., *Tetrahedron Lett.*, 865 (1972)

AMPHIBIN B

C$_{39}$H$_{47}$O$_5$N$_5$

M.p. Indefinite

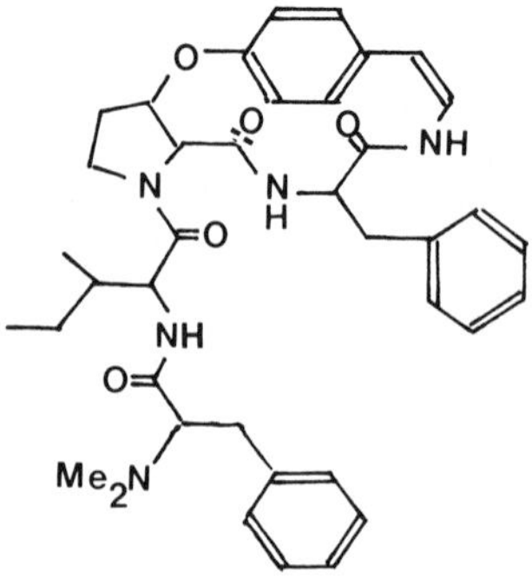

This base, and the remaining three alkaloids, have not been obtained in the crystalline form. Amphibin B is found in the bark of *Ziziphus amphibia* A. Cheval and has $[\alpha]_D^{20} - 181°$ (c 0.08, MeOH).

Teschesche, Kauffmann, Fehlhaber., *Chem. Ber.,* **105**, 3094 (1972)

AMPHIBIN C

C$_{36}$H$_{49}$O$_5$N$_5$

M.p. Indefinite

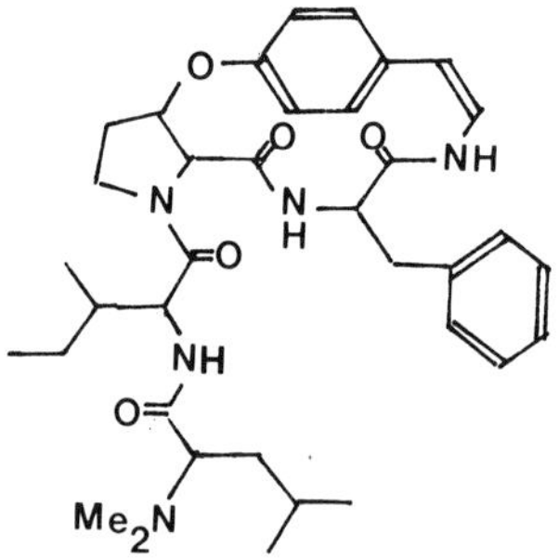

An amorphous alkaloid from *Ziziphus amphibia* A. Cheval, the base has $[\alpha]_D^{20} - 244°$ (c 0.075, MeOH).

Tschesche, Kauffmann, Fehlhaber., *Chem. Ber.,* **105**, 3094 (1972)

AMPHIBIN D

C$_{36}$H$_{49}$O$_5$N$_5$

M.p. Indefinite

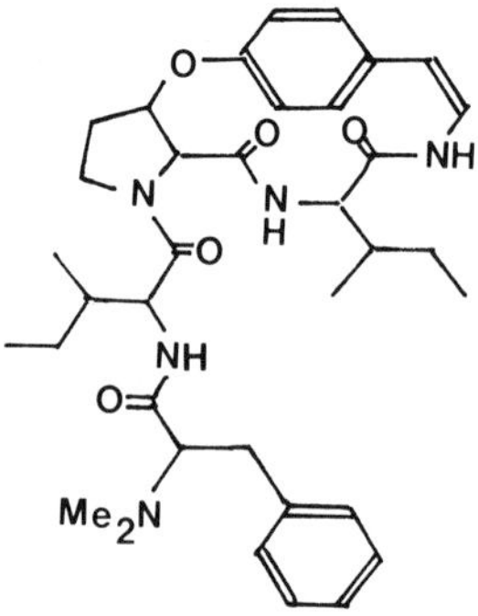

Also amorphous, this alkaloid of *Ziziphus amphibia* A. Cheval is isomeric with the preceding base. It has $[\alpha]_D^{20} - 203°$ (c 0.09, MeOH).

Tschesche, Kauffmann, Fehlhaber., *Chem. Ber.,* **105**, 3094 (1972)

AMPHIBIN E

$C_{38}H_{50}O_6N_5$

M.p. Indefinite

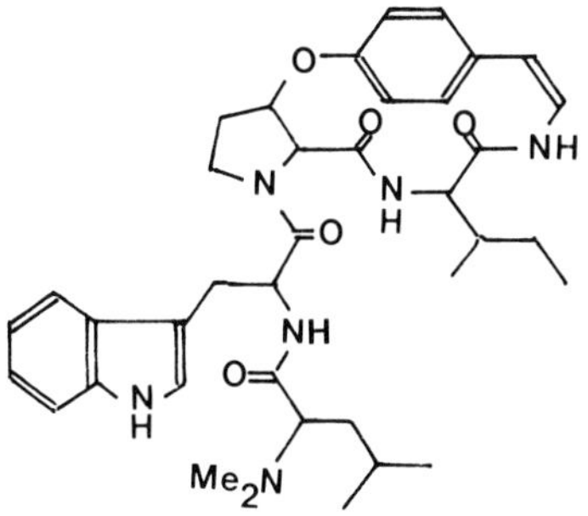

The fifth alkaloid occurring in the bark of *Ziziphus amphibia* A. Cheval is also amorphous with $[\alpha]_D^{20} - 175°$ (c 0.14, MeOH). Like Amphibin A, it possesses an indolyl group.

Tschesche, Kauffmann, Fehlhaber., *Chem. Ber.,* **105**, 3094 (1972)

AMPHIBINE F

$C_{29}H_{36}O_4N_4$

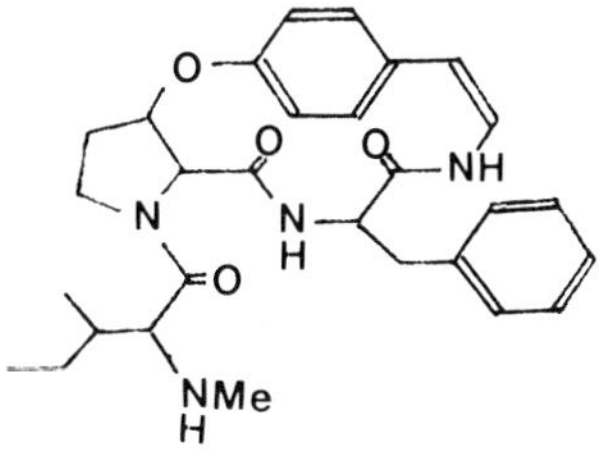

A further minor alkaloid found in *Zizyphus amphibia,* the structure of this peptide base has been determined by spectroscopic methods.

Tschesche, Spilles, Eckhardt., *Chem. Ber.,* **107**, 686 (1974)

AMPHIBINE G

$C_{32}H_{39}O_4N_5$

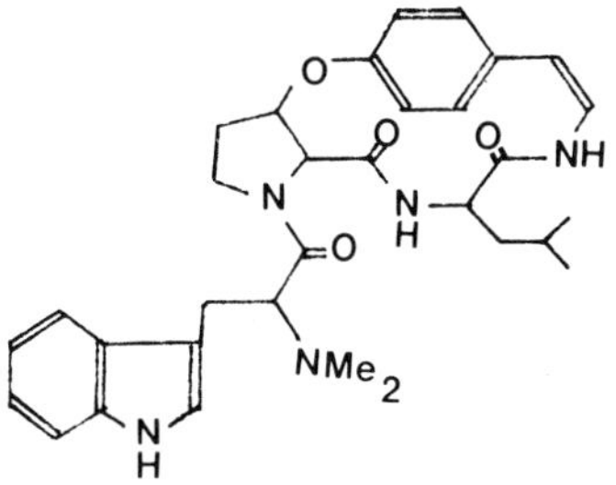

This peptide alkaloid has also been discovered recently in *Zizyphus amphibia*. The additional nitrogen atom is present in an indole nucleus.

Tschesche, Spilles, Eckhardt., *Chem. Ber.*, **107**, 686 (1974)

AMPHIBINE H

$C_{33}H_{43}O_5N_5$

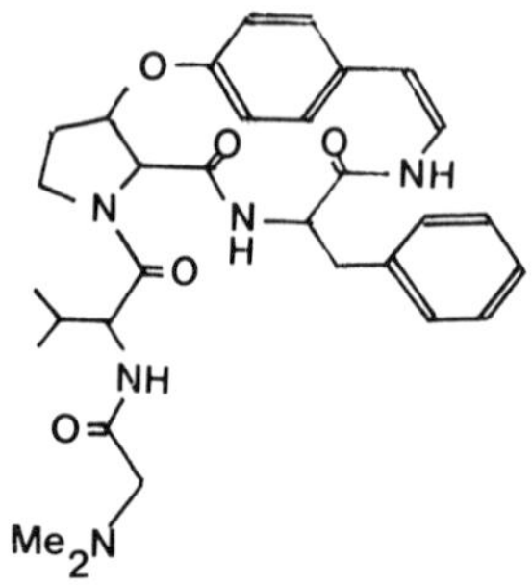

The third of the peptide alkaloids to be discovered recently in *Zizyphus amphibia*. The structure has been established from chemical analysis and the infrared, NMR and mass spectra.

Tschesche, Spilles, Eckhardt., *Chem. Ber.*, **107**, 686 (1974)

AMPHIPORINE

This base has been obtained only in minute quantities from the marine worm, *Amphiporus lactifloreus*. It has not been examined in detail but it is stated to closely resemble nicotine in its pharmacological action.

King., *J. Chem. Soc.*, 1365 (1939)

AMSONINE

$C_{21}H_{28}O_4N_2$

M.p. 234–5°C (*dec.*).

This alkaloid, of unknown structure, occurs in *Amsonia elliptica* and crystallizes as colourless needles from AcOEt. It has $[\alpha]_D^{22} - 19.8°$. Alkaline hydrolysis yields an aminoacid which may be decarboxylated to form yohimbol. The latter was originally considered to be a secondary alcohol but Witkop has demonstrated that it is a ketone and is more correctly termed yohimbone, $C_{19}H_{22}ON_2$, m.p. 307°C (*dec.*).

Witkop, *Annalen.*, **554**, 83 (1943)
Kimoto, Inoue., *J. Pharm. Soc. Japan,* **62**, 95 (1942)
Kimoto, Honjo., *ibid,* **63**, 159 (1943)

AMURENSINE (*Xanthopetalin*)

$C_{19}H_{19}O_4N$

M.p. 213°C

From several *Papaver* species, particularly *Papaver alpinum* and *P. nudicaule* var. *amurense*, two closely related alkaloids have been obtained namely amurensine and amurensinine. The former crystallizes from Me_2CO in colourless prisms with $[\alpha]_D^{23} - 194°$ (c 0.25, $CHCl_3$). The hydriodide, m.p. 255°C (*dec.*) and the picrate, m.p. 132°C are both crystalline. The infrared spectrum of the alkaloid bears a strong resemblance to known *iso*pavine bases but not to the pavine alkaloids. Oxidation of the base with alkaline $KMnO_4$ gives hydrastic acid while a two-step Hofmann degradation furnishes an optically inactive nitrogen-free compound, $C_{19}H_{16}O_4$, m.p. 179–181°C.

The 100 MHz NMR spectrum shows the presence of one hydroxyl and one methoxyl, two aromatic protons in the ortho-position and two in the para-position as well as the methimino group and a methylenedioxy group. The relative positions of the hydroxyl and methoxyl groups in the aromatic ring has been proved by synthesis.

Boit, Flentje., *Naturwiss.*, **46**, 514 (1959)
Boit, Flentje., *ibid*, **47**, 180 (1960)
Maturova, Moza, Sitar, Santavy., *Planta Medica.*, **10**, 345 (1962)
Maturova, Pavlaskova, Santavy., *ibid*, **14**, 22 (1966)

Structure:
Santavy, Maturova, Hruban., *Chem. Commun.*, **26**, 144 (1966)

Synthesis:
Dyke, Ellis., *Tetrahedron*, **28**, 3999 (1972)

AMURENSININE

$C_{20}H_{21}O_4N$

M.p. 164°C

Isolated together with the foregoing alkaloid, the base has $[\alpha]_D - 175°$ (MeOH). Chemical and spectroscopic evidence show that the alkaloid is the O-methyl ether of amurensine.

Boit, Flentje., *Naturwiss.*, **46**, 514 (1959)
Boit, Flentje., *ibid*, **47**, 180 (1960)
Maturova, Moza, Sitar, Santavy., *Planta Medica.*, **10**, 345 (1962)
Maturova, Pavlaskova, Santavy., *ibid*, **14**, 22 (1966)

Structure:
Santavy, Maturova, Hruban., *Chem. Commun.*, **26**, 144 (1966)

141

AMURINE

$C_{19}H_{19}O_4N$

M.p. 213–5°C

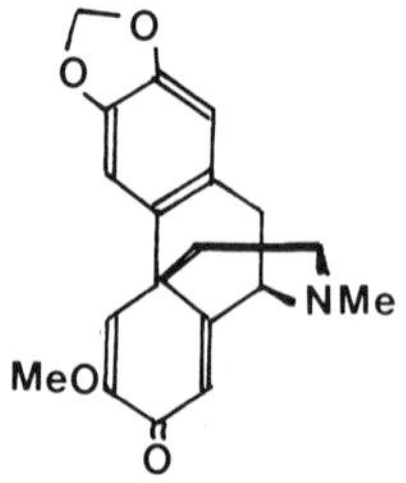

Isolated from *Papaver auranticum* and *P. nudicaule* var. *amurense,* this base forms colourless crystals from Me_2CO; $[\alpha]_D^{26} + 10°$ (c 1.0, $CHCl_3$). It yields crystalline salts, e.g. the hydriodide, m.p. 216–8°C; perchlorate, m.p. 215–7°C and the picrate, m.p. 226–7°C. The (±)-form gives a crystalline methiodide, m.p. 222–4°C and has been synthesized from 1-(2-amino-4:5-methylenedioxy-benzyl-)-7:8-dimethoxyisoquinoline which, on diazotization and coupling at 70° gives *dl*-dicentrine and dl-amurine.

Boit, Flentje., *Naturwiss.,* **46**, 514 (1959)
Boit, Flentje., *ibid,* **47**, 180 (1960)
Maturova, Moza, Sitar, Santavy., *Planta Medica,* **10**, 345 (1962)
Döpke, Flentje, Jeffs., *Tetrahedron,* **24**, 4459 (1968)

Synthesis:
Kametani, Fukumoto, Sugahara., *Tetrahedron Lett.,* 5459 (1968)
Kametani, Fukumoto, Sugahara., *J. Chem. Soc., C,* 801 (1969)

Circular Dichroism:
Snatzke, Wollenberg., *J. Chem. Soc., C,* 1681 (1966)

AMUROLINE

$C_{19}H_{25}O_3N$

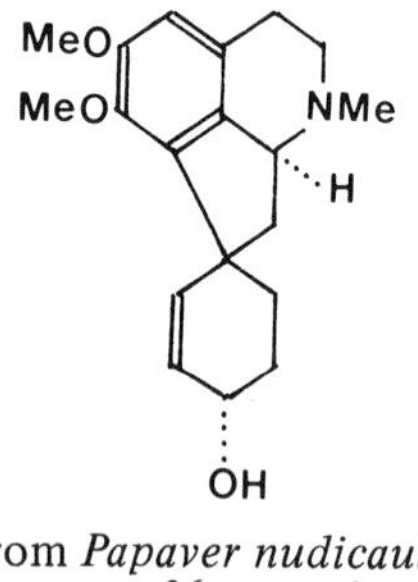

A further alkaloid isolated from *Papaver nudicaule* var. amurense, this base forms crystals from Me_2CO with $[\alpha]_D^{26} + 106°$ (c 0.3, $CHCl_3$). The perchlorate is crystalline with m.p. 151–3°C while the O-acetate forms yellow prisms from Me_2CO with m.p. 152–4°C and $[\alpha]_D^{24} + 147°$ (c 0.85, $CHCl_3$).

Boit, Flentje., *Naturwiss.,* **46**, 514 (1959)
Dopke, Flentje, Jeffs., *Tetrahedron,* **24**, 2297 (1968)

Circular Dichroism:
Snatzke, Wollenberg., *J. Chem. Soc., C,* 1681 (1966)

AMURONINE

$C_{19}H_{23}O_3N$

M.p. 119–120°C and 132–3°C

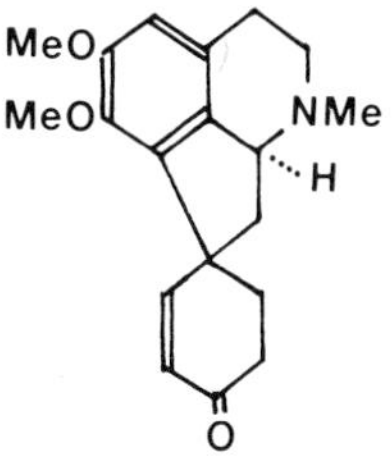

This base from *Papaver nudicaule* var. *amurense,* when crystallized from light petroleum exhibits a double melting point as shown above. It has $[\alpha]_D^{26} + 140°$ (c 0.3, $CHCl_3$). The salts are crystalline, e.g. hydriodide, m.p. 249–250°C; perchlorate, m.p. 252–4°C and methiodide, m.p. 234–7°C (*dec.*); $[\alpha]_D^{22} + 71°$ (c 0.5, $CHCl_3$).

Boit, Flentje., *Naturwiss.,* **46**, 514 (1959)

Circular Dichroism:
Snatzke, Wollenberg., *J. Chem. Soc., C,* 1681 (1966)

Structure:
Flentje, Döpke, Jeffs., *Pharmazie,* **21**, 379 (1966)
Döpke, Flentje, Jeffs., *Tetrahedron,* **24**, 2297 (1968)

ANABASAMINE

$C_{16}H_{19}N_3$

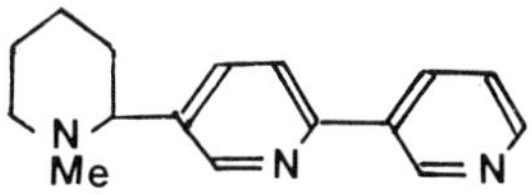

A pyridine-type base isolated from *Anabasis aphylla,* this alkaloid was previously assigned the formula $C_{17}H_{21}N_3$, later revised to that given above. The structure has been determined mainly from spectroscopic evidence, in particular the ultraviolet spectrum which is similar to that of 2:3'-bipyridyl and the infrared spectrum (KBr disc) which shows the presence of an aromatic iminogroup, a CH_3 to a tertiary nitrogen and 1:3 substitution in the A ring and 1:2:4 substitution in the B ring. Oxidation of the alkaloid with $KMnO_4$ gives 2:3'-bipyryl-5-carboxylic acid.

Sadykov, Mukhamedzhanov, Aslanov., *Dokl. Akad. Nauk, Uzb. SSR.,* **24**, 34 (1967)
Mukhamedzhanov, Aslanov, Sadykov, Leont'ev, Kiryakhin., *Khim. Prir. Soedin.,* **4**, 158 (1968)

ANABASINE

$C_{10}H_{14}N_2$

B.p. 276°C

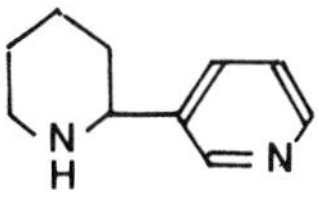

A liquid alkaloid obtained from *Anabasis aphylla* and *Nicotiana glauca,* the base has $[\alpha]_D^{20} - 82.2°$. It is readily soluble in H_2O and most organic solvents. The imino hydrogen is readily substituted with the formation of crystalline derivatives: N-benzoylanabasine, colourless needles, m.p. 82–3°C, b.p. 222°C/2 mm. 2 mm.

The N-methyl derivative is an oil, b.p. 127–8°C/12 mm; $[\alpha]_D^{15} - 136.9°$, which is also present in small quantities in tobacco. The nitroso compound has b.p. 176°C/4 mm; $[\alpha]_D^{20} - 155°$, the dipicrate has m.p. 198–199.5°C (dec.) and the dinitrophenate, m.p. 265°C (in vacuo).

(+)-anabasine also forms a dipicrate, m.p. 198–9°C (dec.) and a dinitrophenate, m.p. 264–5°C. The (±)-form has b.p. 280–2°C/775 mm and forms a crystalline dipicrate, m.p. 213–4°C. This base has been named Neonicotine.

Hydrogenation of the alkaloid with PtO_2 gives a mixture of bases including 1-2:3-dipiperidyl, m.p. 66–8°C, b.p. 113–4°C/5 mm; $[\alpha]_D^{20} - 5°$ (EtOH). With $NaNH_2$ in the presence of dimethylaniline, it yields 2-(2'-amino-3'-pyridyl) piperidine, m.p. 89.5–90°C and 2-(6'-amino-3'-pyridyl)piperidine, m.p. 109°C. The alkaloid has been synthesized by condensing 1-benzoylpiperidone with ethyl nicotinate at 130°C with HCl to give anabaseine, $C_{10}H_{12}N_2$, b.p. 110–120°C/1 mm which gives dl-anabasine on reduction.

Orekhov., Compt. rend., 189, 945 (1929)
Orekhov, Menschikoff., Ber., 64, 266 (1931)
Orekhov, Menschikoff., ibid, 65, 232 (1932)
Orekhov, Norkina., ibid, 65, 742, 1126 (1932)
Smith., J. Amer. Chem. Soc., 54, 397 (1932)
Späth, Mamoli., Ber., 69, 1082 (1936)
Späth, Kesztler., ibid, 70, 72 (1937)
Goshaev, Otroshchenko, Sadykov., Izv. Akad. Nauk. Turkm. SSR, Ser Fiz-Tekh., Khim. Geol. Nauk., 4, 105 (1970)

ANACROTINE

$C_{18}H_{25}O_6N$

M.p. 191–2°C (195°C)

This alkaloid occurs in several Crotalaria species, mainly in C. anagyroides and C. incana. It has $[\alpha]_D^{20} + 30°$ (EtOH) and + 37.4° (MeOH). From EtOH, the base forms slender, colourless needles. The picrate is obtained as leaflet from EtOH, m.p. 224°C (dec.) and the methiodide, also as colourless leaflets from EtOH-AcOEt, m.p. 222°C (dec.). Hydrolysis with aqueous alkalies yields crotanecine and senecic acid, $CH_3CH:C(COOH).CH_2.CH(CH_3).C(OH)(COOH).CH_3$.

Atal, Kapur, Culvenor, Smith., Tetrahedron Lett., 537 (1966)
Mattocks., J. Chem. Soc., C, 235 (1968)

ANADOLINE

$C_{20}H_{29}O_6N$

M.p. $186°C$ (dec.).

The roots of *Symphytum orientale* contain this alkaloid: $[\alpha]_D^{22} + 9.2°$ (c 0.7, $CHCl_3$). The ultraviolet spectrum shows one absorption maximum at 226 mμ. The NMR spectrum reveals the presence of five methyl groups while the infrared spectrum shows a hydroxyl group, two ester carbonyls, a double bond and an *iso*propyl group in the molecule. Hydrolysis with 10 per cent aqueous NaOH gives an acid, white crystals, m.p. $64°C$, $C_5H_8O_2$, while thin layer chromatography reveals the presence of a second acid component, $C_7H_{14}O_4$, m.p. $90°C$. From their mixed melting points, these have been found to be tiglic and trachelantic acids respectively. The alkamine produced by the hydrolysis is shown by hydrogenation to have two double bonds, giving the tetrahydro derivative as an oil (picrate, m.p. $199-201°C$). The picrate has been identified with that of 7-(2-methylbutyryl)retronecanol.

Ulubelen, Doganca., *Tetrahedron Lett.*, **30**, 2583 (1970)

ANAFERINE

$C_{13}H_{24}ON_2$

B.p. $55°C/0.01$ mm

This oily base is obtained from the root of *Uithania somnifera*. It is somewhat unstable and rapidly darkens on exposure to air. The alkaloid behaves as a diacidic base forming the dihydrochloride, m.p. $222.5-223.5°C$; $[\alpha]_D^{22}$ $0°$. The distyphnate has m.p. $229-231°C$ and the dipicrate, m.p. $184-5°C$ (*dec.*). The structure of the base has been proved by synthesis.

Rother, Bobbitt, Schwarting., *Chem. & Ind.*, 654 (1962)

Synthesis:
Schöpf, Benz, Braun, Hinkel, Krüger, Rokohl, Hutzler., *Annalen,* 737, 1 (1970)

ANAGYRINE (*Monolupine, Rhombinine*)

$C_{15}H_{20}ON_2$

B.p. $165-8°C/0.3$ mm;
$\quad 210-215°C/4$ mm

This alkaloid occurs in *Anagyris foetida* and *Lupinus laxiflorus* var. *silvicola* and is also identical with ulexine obtained from *Ulex europaeus*. The base is best

145

isolated as the crystalline perchlorate which forms colourless needles from H_2O, decomposing between 270°C and 298.5°C without melting. The free base is soluble in most organic solvents except ligroin and is more soluble in cold H_2O than in hot. It has $[\alpha]_D^{20} - 165.3°$ (EtOH) and gives an intense red colour with aqueous $FeCl_3$. As usually obtained, it forms a pale yellow glassy solid which is deliquescent. Crystalline salts and derivatives include: the hydrochloride (3 H_2O), m.p. 235–6°C or 295–7°C (*dry*); platinichloride, ruby-red crystals (1.5 H_2O), m.p. 250–1°C and 278°C (*dec. dry*); aurichloride, yellow needles from aqueous HCl, m.p. 167–8°C; picrate, m.p. 242–4°C according to most workers but Couch has recorded 169.5°C; methiodide, m.p. 263–4°C (*dec.*). The mercuri-chloride exists in three modifications although that normally obtained has m.p. 221–4°C. With $Ba(MnO_4)_2$, the base gives anagyramide, $C_{15}H_{18}O_2N_2$, colourless needles, m.p. 201–2°C. Catalytic hydrogenation at 80°C furnishes a tetrahydro-derivative, b.p. 186–190°C/1 mm; $[\alpha]_D - 61.45$ (Me$_2$CO).

Gerrard., *Pharm. J.*, **17**, 109, 227 (1886)
Clemo, Raper., *J. Chem. Soc.*, 10 (1935)
Ing., *ibid*, 504 (1933)
Couch., *J. Amer. Chem. Soc.*, **61**, 3327 (1939)
Marion, Quellet., *ibid*, **70**, 2076 (1940)
van Tamelen, Baran., *ibid*, **78**, 2913 (1956)

ANAHYGRINE

$C_{13}H_{24}ON_2$

B.p. 106°C/0.2 mm

From the root extract of *Withania somnifera* Dunal, this base is obtained as a pale yellow oil. It forms a crystalline dihydrochloride, m.p. 216.5–217.5°C and a dipicrate, m.p. 173–174.5°C.

Leary *et al.*, *Chem. & Ind.*, 283 (1964)

ANANTINE

$C_{15}H_{15}ON_3$

This imidazole alkaloid occurs in the leaves of *Cynometra ananta*, together with Cynodine and Cynometrine (q.v.). The structure has been deduced by chemical and spectroscopic means.

Khuong Huu Laine *et al.*, *Tetrahedron Lett.*, 1757 (1973)

146

(−)-ANATABINE

$C_{10}H_{12}N_2$

B.p. 145−6°C/10 mm

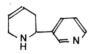

In an investigation of the subsidiary bases of *Nicotiana tabacum*, Späth and Kesztler obtained a crude base with $[\alpha]_D - 141°$ which, after purification via the (−)-6:6'-dinitro-2:2'-diphenate yielded this alkaloid having $[\alpha]_D^{17} - 177.8°$. It yields a monohydrochloride, $[\alpha]_D^{17} - 61.9°$ (H_2O); a dihydrochloride, $[\alpha]_D^{17} - 65.4°$ (H_2O); a dipicrate, m.p. 191−3°C (*vac. dec.*); dipicrolonate, m.p. 234−5°C (*dec.*); dinitrophenate, m.p. 238−238.5°C; N-benzoyl derivative, b.p. 160−170°C/0.01 mm; $[\alpha]_D^{15} - 15.4°$ (MeOH) and the N-*p*-nitrobenzoyl derivative, m.p. 101−2°C, followed by solidification and remelting at 130−1°C; $[\alpha]_D^{15} - 174.5°$ (MeOH). The N-methyl compound has $[\alpha]_D^{15} - 167°$, yields a dipicrate, m.p. 207−8°C, and is also present in minute quantities in *N. tabacum*.

Späth, Kesztler., *Ber.*, **70**, 239, 704 (1937)

Synthesis:
Quan, Karns, Quin., *Chem. & Ind.*, 1553 (1964)

(±)-ANATABINE

$C_{10}H_{12}N_2$

This base is also present in *Nicotiana tabacum* and yields crystalline derivatives including the diperchlorate, m.p. 129−130°C; picrolonate, m.p. 233−5°C and the dipicrate, m.p. 201−201.5°C. The (+)-alkaloid does not occur naturally in any quantity and has been obtained as the N-*p*-nitrobenzoyl derivative, m.p. 101−2°C, solidifying and remelting at 129−130°C; $[\alpha]_D + 168.7°$ (MeOH).

Spath, Kesztler., *Ber.*, **70**, 239, 704 (1937)

Synthesis:
Quin, Karns, Quin., *Chem. & Ind.*, 1553 (1964)

ANATALLINE

$C_{15}H_{17}N_3$

B.p. 225°C/3 mm

From a 70 per cent MeOH extract of the roots of *Nicotiana tabacum*, this base is separated by chromatography on an alumina column and obtained as the perchlorate, m.p. 244−252°C. The alkaloid also forms a crystalline picrate, m.p. 258.5°C and a benzoate, b.p. 274°C/3 mm. Its identification as 2:4-di (pyridyl)piperidine is shown by elemental analysis and spectroscopic methods together with its dehydrogenation to nicotelline.

Kisaki, Mizusaki, Tamaki., *Phytochem.*, 7, 323 (1968)

ANCISTROCLADINE

$C_{25}H_{29}O_4N$

M.p. 265–7°C (dec.).

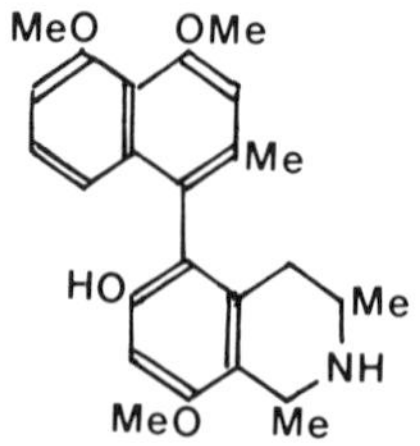

This *iso*quinoline alkaloid occurs in *Ancistrocladus heyneanus* Wall. Both the hydrochloride, m.p. 220–4°C (dec.); $[\alpha]_D^{25} - 25.5°$ (c 2.3, MeOH) and the hydrobromide, m.p. 229–231°C (dec.) have been obtained in the crystalline form. The structure has been determined from spectroscopic evidence and the synthesis of the various degradation products. The position of the *iso*quinoline methoxyl group has been located at C-8.

Govindachari, Parthasarathy., *Ind. J. Chem.*, **8**, 567 (1970)
Govindachari, Parthasarathy., *Tetrahedron*, **27**, 1013 (1971)

ANCISTROCLADININE

$C_{25}H_{27}O_4N$

M.p. 235–8°C (dec.).

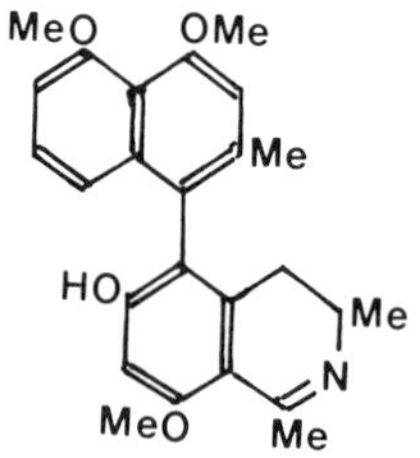

This alkaloid is present as a minor constituent of *Ancistrocladus heyneana* Wall and has $[\alpha]_D^{25} - 321.8°$ (c 1.06, pyridine). The ultraviolet spectrum shows absorption maxima at 217, 295, 306, 320 and 334 mμ. The base differs in structure from the preceding alkaloid only in having a double bond in the *iso*quinoline nucleus at the 1:2-position.

Govindachari, Parthasarathy, Desai., *Ind. J. Chem.*, **9**, 1421 (1971)
Govindachari, Parthasarathy, Desai., *ibid*, **11**, 1180 (1973)

ANCISTROCLADISINE

$C_{26}H_{29}O_4N$

M.p. 178–180°C

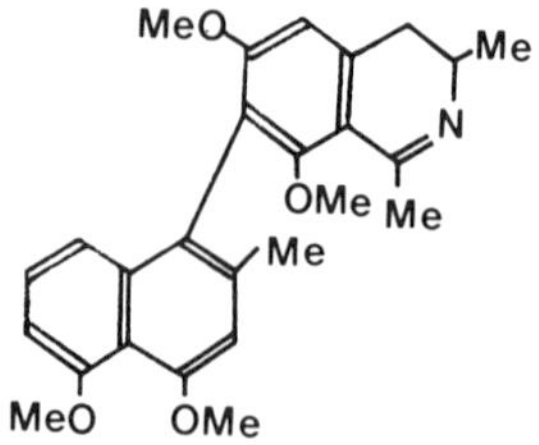

Found in the roots of *Ancistrocladus heyneanus* Wall, this alkaloid is laevorotatory with $[\alpha]_D - 16.13°$. The structure has been deduced from spectroscopic data and the results of Hofmann degradation.

Govindachari, Parthasarathy, Desai., *Ind. J. Chem.*, **10**, 1117 (1972)

ANDRACHNINE

$C_{11}H_{17}O_2N$

M.p. 97–9°C (*vac.*).

An alkaloid isolated from *Andrachne rotundifolia,* the base gives an ultraviolet spectrum with two absorption maxima occurring at 235 and 335 mμ. The perchlorate forms colourless crystals, m.p. 139–140°C whereas the diacetyl derivative is a non-crystallizable solid. The alkaloid contains one methoxyl group, an alcoholic hydroxyl, an imino group and an aromatic ring according to the infrared spectrum.

Vil'yams *et al., Khim. Prir. Soedin.*, **2**, 257 (1966)

ANDROCYMBINE

$C_{21}H_{25}O_5N$

M.p. 199–201°C

From *Androcymbium melanthoides* var. *strictia* Baker, this base is obtained in the form of colourless prisms from either Me_2CO or AcOEt. It is laevorotatory with $[\alpha]_D^{22} - 260°$ (c 0.5, $CHCl_3$). In concentrated H_2SO_4 it gives a vivid red colour.

Hrbek, Santavy., *Collect. Czech. Chem. Commun.*, **27**, 255 (1962)
Battersby *et al., Chem. Commun.*, 228 (1965)

Synthesis:
Kametani, Koizumi, Fukumoto., *J. Org. Chem.*, **36**, 3729 (1971)
Kametani *et al., ibid*, **36**, 3733 (1971)
Kametani, Satoh, Fukumoto., *J. Chem. Soc., Perkin I*, 2160 (1972)

O[7]-ANGELOYLHELIOTRIDINE

$C_{13}H_{19}O_3N$

M.p. 116–7°C

A pyrrolizidine alkaloid found in *Senecio rivularis,* the base forms colourless needles from AcOEt and has the following specific rotations, $[\alpha]_D^{24} - 18° \pm 2°$

(c 0.783, CHCl$_3$) and + 19° (c 0.658, EtOH). Alkaline hydrolysis of the alkaloid furnishes angelic acid, m.p. 45–6°C and heliotridine, m.p. 116–8°C; $[\alpha]_D^{24}$ + 35.2° (c 0.483, MeOH), the latter being characterized as the hydrochloride, m.p. 122–4°C.

Klasek, Vrublovsky, Santavy., *Collect. Czech. Chem. Commun.*, **32**, 2512 (1967)

ANGELOYLZYGADENINE

C$_{32}$H$_{49}$O$_8$N

M.p. 234°C (*dec.*).

This steroidal alkaloid occurs in *Veratrum album* and is obtained as colourless columnar crystals from Me$_2$CO. Catalytic hydrogenation with Pd-C gives the dihydro derivative as colourless plates from aqueous EtOH, m.p. 203.5–205°C. Ac$_2$O in pyridine yields the diacetate, m.p. 167–9°C which, on saponification, provides the monoacetate as crystals from C$_6$H$_6$, m.p. 243.5°C. Hydrolysis with EtONa furnishes tiglic acid and pseudozygadenine, m.p. 168°C. Among the other crystalline derivatives that have been prepared to characterize the base are: the 16-propionate, m.p. 224–6°C; $[\alpha]_D^{21}$ + 34°; the 15:16-dipropionate, m.p. 210–3°C and the 14:15-acetonide-16-priopionate, m.p. 228–230°C.

Suzuku *et al.*, *J. Pharm. Soc., Japan*, **79**, 619 (1959)
Shimizu., *ibid*, **80**, 32 (1960)

ANGOLINE

C$_{22}$H$_{22}$O$_5$N

M.p. 209°C

Occurring in both *Fagara angolensis* Engl. and *F. lepieurii* Engl., this alkaloid forms colourless prisms when crystallized from MeOH. The ultraviolet spectrum of this naphthylphenanthridine base has absorption maxima at 230, 289 and 325 mμ. The salts are normally crystalline: hydrochloride, colourless needles, m.p. 267–8°C; picrate, orange needles, m.p. 238–9°C. The structure has been determined primarily from spectroscopic evidence.

Palmer, Paris., *Ann. Pharm. Fr.*, **13**, 657 (1955)
Calderwood, Fish., *J. Pharm. Pharmacol.*, **18**, 119S (1966)

Structure:
Fonzes, Winternitz., *Phytochem.*, **7**, 1889 (1968)

ANGULARINE

$C_{18}H_{15}O_6N$

This pyrrolizidine alkaloid, isolated from *Senecio angulatus,* has been shown to be the seneciphyllic ester of rosmarinecine.

Porter, Geissman., *J. Org. Chem.,* 27, 4132 (1962)

ANGUSTIDINE

$C_{19}H_{15}ON_3$

M.p. 309—311°C

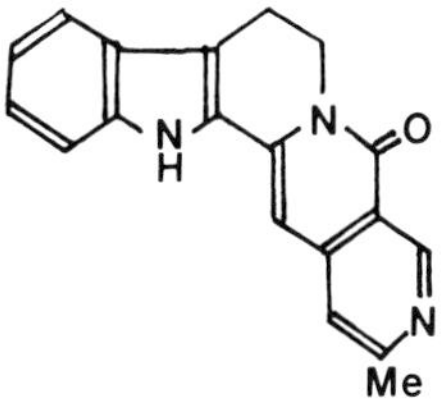

The leaves of *Strychnos angustiflora* Benth. which is indigenous to Southern China, yields three closely related carboline type alkaloids, all of which have high melting points. This particular base yields yellow needles when crystallized from $CHCl_3$. Two of the nitrogen atoms are tertiary, the third being present as an imino group. One methyl group is also present as a substituent.

Au, Cheung, Sternhell., *J. Chem. Soc., Perkin I,* 13 (1973)

ANGUSTIFOLINE

$C_{14}H_{22}ON_2$

M.p. 79—80°C

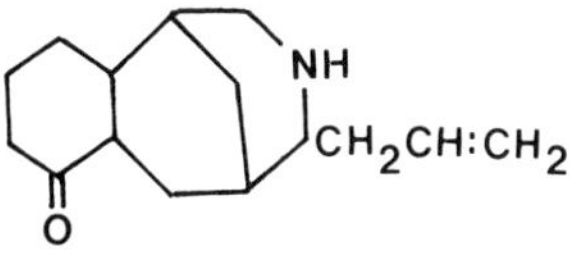

This base occurs in several species of *Ormosia* and also in *Lupinus angustifolius* and *L. perennis.* From petroleum ether, it crystallizes in colourless needles, $[\alpha]_D^{20} - 1.66°$ ($CHCl_3$) or $- 7.5°$ (EtOH). A figure of $+ 5.2°$ (EtOH) has also been recorded. The hydrochloride monohydrate has m.p. 134—5°C or 96—7°C (*dry*); the picrate forms colourless crystals from EtOH, m.p. 186°C and the N-acetyl derivative has m.p. 151—2°C.

Bohlmann, Winterfeldt., *Ber.,* 93, 1956 (1956)
Wiewiorowski, Galinovsky, Bratek., *Monatsh.,* 88, 663 (1957)

ANGUSTINE

$C_{20}H_{15}ON_3$

M.p. 340°C

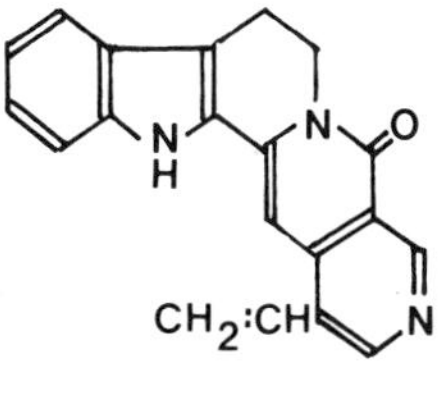

This alkaloid occurs in the leaves of *Strychnos angustiflora* Benth and forms yellow plates from a mixture of MeOH and $CHCl_3$. A vinyl group is present and reduction over PtO_2 yields the dihydro derivative which forms crystals from MeOH, m.p. 290–4°C.

Au, Cheung, Sternhell., *J. Chem. Soc., Perkin I*, 13 (1973)

ANGUSTOLINE

$C_{20}H_{17}O_2N_3$

M.p. 310–4°C

CH₃(OH)CH

The third alkaloid found in the leaves of *Strychnos angustiflora* Benth, this base has $[\alpha]_D - 34°$ ($CHCl_3$) and forms yellow needles from MeOH-$CHCl_3$. Treatment with Ac_2O in pyridine gives the O-acetate as yellow needles from $CHCl_3$, m.p. 148–152°C. Concentrated H_2SO_4 in MeOH furnishes Angustine (q.v.).

Au, Cheung, Sternhell., *J. Chem. Soc., Perkin I*, 13 (1973)

ANHALAMINE

$C_{11}H_{15}O_3N$

M.p. 187–8°C

The presence of alkaloids has been recorded in a number of cacti (Cactaceae) although only those of the *Anhalonium* species have been investigated in detail. This particular base occurs in *A. Lewinii* Hennings and forms microscopic needles from EtOH. It is readily soluble in H_2O, hot EtOH and aqueous alkalies but only sparingly so in C_6H_6, $CHCl_3$, Et_2O or petroleum ether. The hydrochloride dihydrate forms lustrous leaflets, m.p. 256–8°C; the sulphate, colourless prisms, and the picrate has m.p. 234–6°C. The N-benzoyl derivative has m.p. 167–8°C and the O,N-dibenzoyl compound, m.p. 128–9°C. The former is soluble in alkalies whereas the latter is not. The N-*m*-nitrobenzoyl derivative has m.p. 174–5°C. The O-methyl ether is Anhalinine (q.v.) and the N-methyl compound is Anhalidine (q.v.).

Heffter., *Ber.*, 3004 (1901)
Späth, Becke., *ibid*, **67**, 2100 (1934)
Späth, Becke., *ibid*, **68**, 501, 944 (1935)
Späth, Becke., *Monatsh.*, **66**, 327 (1935)
Späth, Roder., *ibid*, **43**, 93 (1922)

ANHALIDINE

$C_{12}H_{17}O_3N$

M.p. 131–3°C

A second alkaloid present in *Anhalonium Lewinii* Hennings, the base is purified by sublimation. The infrared spectrum shows the presence of a methylimino group in the molecule indicating that the alkaloid is N-methylanhalamine.

Späth, Becke., *Ber.*, **68**, 944 (1935)
Späth, Becke., *Monatsh.*, **66**, 335 (1935)

ANHALINE

$C_{10}H_{15}ON$

This alkaloid, isolated from *Anhalonium fissuratum* by Heffter has subsequently been shown to be identical with Hordenine (q.v.).

Heffter., *Ber.*, **34**, 3004 (1901)
Späth., *ibid*, **75**, 1558 (1942)

ANHALININE

$C_{12}H_{17}O_3N$

M.p. 61–3°C;
B.p. 144–5°C/0.1 mm

One of the Cactaceous alkaloids from *Anhalonium Lewinii* Hennings, the base is normally purified by sublimation when it forms colourless crystals with the above constant.

Späth, Becke., *Ber.*, **68**, 501 (1935)
Späth, Becke., *Monatsh.*, **66**, 327 (1935)

ANHALONIDINE

$C_{12}H_{17}O_3N$

M.p. 160°C

Also obtained from *Anhalonium Lewinii* Hennings, this base crystallizes in small, colourless octahedra, soluble in H_2O, $CHCl_3$ and EtOH, only moderately so in Et_2O and insoluble in petroleum ether. The hydrochloride forms colourless prisms but both the aurichloride and platinichloride are amorphous. The picrate has m.p. 201–8°C. Among other crystalline derivatives that have been prepared are the N-benzoyl, m.p. 189°C; N-*m*-nitrobenzoyl, m.p. 207–8°C and the O,N-dibenzoyl, m.p. 125–6°C. With methyl iodide, the alkaloid gives pellotine hydriodide as yellow prisms, m.p. 125–130°C.

Heffter., *Ber.*, **29**, 216 (1896)
Späth., *Monatsh.*, **43**, 477 (1922)
Späth, Passl., *Ber.*, **65**, 1778 (1932)
Späth, Boschan., *Monatsh.*, **63**, 141 (1933)
Kapadia, Fales., *Chem. Commun.*, 1688 (1968)
Biosynthesis:
Leete., *J. Amer. Chem. Soc.*, **88**, 4218 (1966)

ANHALONINE

$C_{12}H_{15}O_3N$

M.p. 85°C

This alkaloid has been obtained from *Anhalonium Lewinii* Hennings and *A. Jourdanianum* Lem. and crystallizes from light petroleum in colourless needles; $[\alpha]_D - 56.3°$ (CHCl$_3$). It is freely soluble in H$_2$O, CHCl$_3$, EtOH and Et$_2$O. The hydrochloride forms colourless prisms with $[\alpha]_D^{17} - 41.9°$ (H$_2$O); the platini-chloride is obtained as golden-yellow needles. With methyl iodide, it gives the N-methyl derivative identical with Lophophorine methiodide, m.p. 223°C.

Späth, Gangl., *Monatsh.*, **44**, 103 (1923)
Kapadia, Fales., *J. Pharm. Sci.*, **57**, 2017 (1968)
Kapadia, Fales., *Chem. Commun.*, 1688 (1968)

ANHYDREUOXINE

$C_{18}H_{19}O_5N$

M.p. 141–4°C

This furoquinoline alkaloid is present in *Evodia zanthoxyloides* F. Muell and crystallizes in colourless plates from a mixture of hexane and AcOEt. It is slightly dextrorotatory with $[\alpha]_D + 13°$ (CHCl$_3$) and gives an ultraviolet spectrum with absorption maxima at 248, 310, 320, 332 and 342 mμ.

Dreyer., *J. Org. Chem.*, **35**, 2420 (1970)

ANHYDROIGNAVINOL

$C_{20}H_{28}O_4N$

The methiodide of this base has been examined by X-ray techniques. It forms orthorhombic crystals with space group P2$_1$2$_1$2$_1$, a = 13.28, b = 13.87, c = 10.58 Å and Z = 4.

Pelletier, Page, Newton., *Tetrahedron Lett.*, **55**, 4825 (1970)

ANHYDROLYCOCERNUINE

An uncharacterized alkaloid present in *Lycopodium carolinianum* var. *affine*. The structure is unknown and no salts or derivatives have been recorded.

Miller *et al.*, *Bull. Soc. Chim. Belg.*, **80**, 629 (1971)

ANHYDRONUPHARAMINE

$C_{15}H_{23}ON$

B.p. $108-9°C/4$ mm

This alkaloid has been isolated from the rhizomes of *Nuphar japonicum* and forms a crystalline picrolonate, m.p. 203.5°C. Catalytic hydrogenation over Pd-C, followed by treatment with NaOH gives (−)-deoxynupharamine, b.p. $130-4°C/3$ mm, yielding a hydrochloride, m.p. 233°C. When dissolved in 5 per cent HCl for 7 days and then made alkaline with KOH, the alkaloid yields (−)-nupharamine, b.p. $145-150°C/3.5$ mm, forming a crystalline picrolonate, m.p. $171-171.5°C$.

Arata, Ohashi, Yomemitsu, Yasuda., *J. Pharm. Soc., Japan,* **87**, 1094 (1967)

ANHYDROVOBASINEDIOL

$C_{20}H_{24}ON_2$

M.p. $200-4°C$

First isolated from the trunk bark of *Conopharyngia durissima* Stapf., this alkaloid has recently been discovered in the bark of *Tabernaemontana brachyantha*. It is best crystallized from a mixture of MeOH and Et$_2$O. It is laevorotatory with $[\alpha]_D - 284°$ (c 0.873, CHCl$_3$) and gives an ultraviolet spectrum with absorption maxima at 224, 285 and 293 mμ.

Dugan *et al., Helv. Chim. Acta,* **52**, 701 (1969)
Patel *et al., Phytochem.,* **12**, 451 (1973)

ANIBINE

$C_{11}H_9O_3N$

M.p. $179-180°C$

This alkaloid occurs in certain species of *Aniba* but mainly in *A. coco* and may be obtained as colourless crystals from both EtOH and by sublimation. In EtOH solution, the ultraviolet spectrum shows absorption maxima at 228.5, 254 and 315 mμ. The hydrochloride has m.p. $179-209°C$ (*dec.*) although a higher melting point of $205-230°C$ (*dec.*) is obtained in a sealed capillary tube. The picrate yields pale yellow crystals with m.p. $199-201°C$.

155

Mors, Gottleib, Djerassi., *J. Amer. Chem. Soc.*, **79**, 4507 (1957)
Ziegler, Nolken., *Monatsh.*, **89**, 391, 716 (1958)
Mors, Gottlieb., *Anais. Assoc. Brasil. Quim.*, **18**, 185 (1959)
Mors, Magdalhaes, Gottlieb., *ibid*, **19**, 193 (1960)

ANIFLORINE

$C_{20}H_{21}O_3N_3$

M.p. 195–7°C

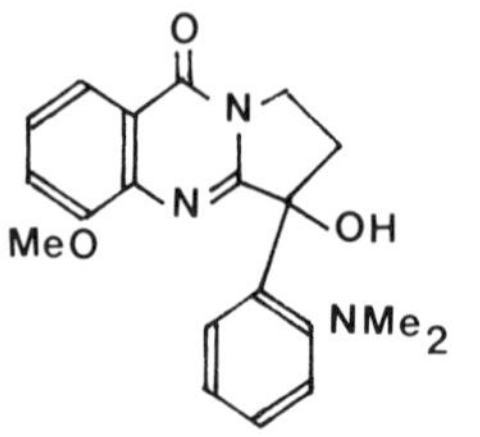

An alkaloid from *Anisotes sessiliflorus* C.B. Cl, the base crystallizes from MeOH as colourless needles. In neutral ethanol solution, the ultraviolet spectrum shows absorption maxima at 207, 235, 286, 312 and 324 mμ. In acidified EtOH (HCl) the absorption maxima are found at 207, 236, 291, 312 and 324 mμ.

Arndt, Eggers, Jordaan., *Tetrahedron*, **23**, 3521 (1967)

ANISESSINE

$C_{20}H_{19}O_3N_3$

M.p. 170–1°C

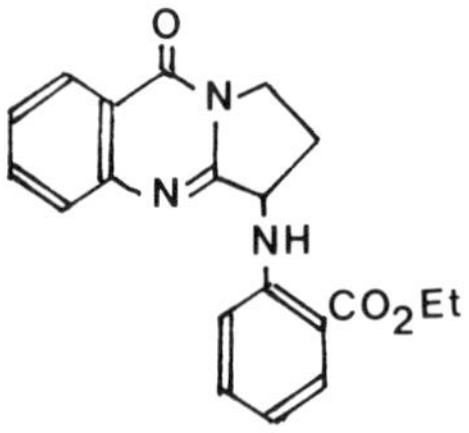

A second base found in *Anisotes sessiliflorus* C.B. Cl, this alkaloid also forms colourless crystals from MeOH. The ultraviolet spectrum has absorption maxima at 207, 225, 253, 300, 311 and 340 mμ.

Arndt, Eggers, Jordaan., *Tetrahedron*, **23**, 3521 (1967)

ANISOTINE

$C_{20}H_{19}O_3N_3$

M.p. 189–190°C

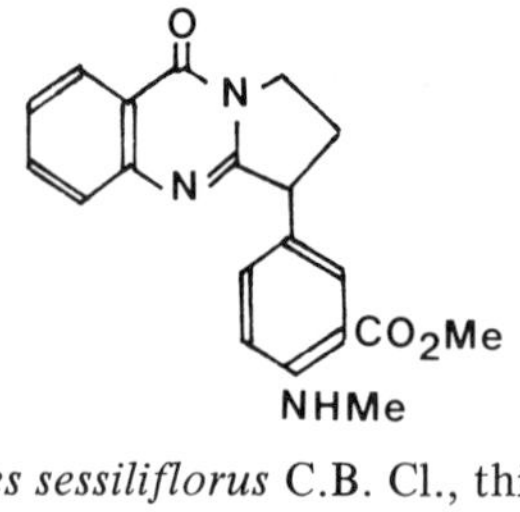

Also isolated from *Anisotes sessiliflorus* C.B. Cl., this alkaloid crystallizes from Me$_2$CO-hexane. The ultraviolet spectrum is similar to that of aniflorine with absorption maxima at 212, 226, 259, 301, 312 and 356 mμ.

Arndt, Eggers, Jordaan., *Tetrahedron*, **23**, 3521 (1967)

ANKORINE

$C_{19}H_{29}O_4N$

M.p. 174–6°C

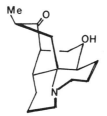

This alkaloid occurs in *Alangium lamarckii* Thw. and forms lustrous plates from Me$_2$CO. It has $[\alpha]_D^{26}$ – 62° (CHCl$_3$). The ultraviolet spectrum has absorption maxima at 272 mμ in EtOH and 287 mμ in 0.1 N/NaOH. Several crystalline salts are known: the hydrochloride, m.p. 233–4°C; hydrobromide, colourless needles, m.p. 220–2°C (*dec.*); oxalate, m.p. 190–1°C (*dec.*) and sulphate, m.p. 286°C (*dec.*).

Dasgupta., *J. Pharm. Sci.*, **54**, 481 (1965)

Battersby, Kapil, Bhakuni, Popli, Merchant, Salgar., *Tetrahedron Lett.*, 4965 (1966)

ANNOFOLINE

$C_{16}H_{25}O_2N$

M.p. 156–7°C

One of the Lycopodium alkaloids, this base occurs in *L. annotinum* and forms colourless crystals from Et$_2$O-MeOH. It has $[\alpha]_D$ – 131° (c 2.0, EtOH). The perchlorate has m.p. 234–6°C and the methiodide, m.p. 308–9°C.

Anet, Khan., *Can. J. Chem.*, **37**, 1589 (1959)

Burnell, Taylor., *Tetrahedron*, **15**, 173 (1961)

ANNOPODINE

$C_{17}H_{25}O_3N$

M.p. 211–2°C

A minor constituent of *Lycopodium annotinum* L. this alkaloid is obtained from the mother liquor after removal of -obscurine, lycodoline and annotoxine. It forms a crystalline hydrobromide, m.p. 230–2°C; hydroperchlorate, m.p. 210–2°C and a methiodide, m.p. 240–2°C. The base also forms the O-acetate as an oil (perchlorate, m.p. 250–2°C). Dehydration with POCl$_3$ in pyridine at 20°C yields an oily anhydrocompound while dehydrogenation furnishes basic products which appear to be C_{15} and C_{16} alkylquinolines. The structure of the alkaloid has been examined by X-ray analysis of the crystalline hydrobromide which forms orthorhombic crystals, space group $P2_12_12_1$ with four molecules in each unit, $a = 13.4$, $b = 14.0$ and $c = 9.0$ Å.

Ayer, Iverach, Jenkins, Masaki., *Tetrahedron Lett.*, 4597 (1968)

ANNOTINE (*Alkaloid L-11*)

$C_{16}H_{21}O_3N$

M.p. 173–4°C

Several species of *Lycopodium* have been examined for alkaloids by Manske and Marion who distinguished the bases provisionally by the letter L followed by a number, a trivial name being assigned once the individuality of the alkaloid had been established. This alkaloid occurs in *L. annotinum* L. and was first isolated as the perchlorate, m.p. 239°C. It also forms a crystalline nitrate as large prisms, m.p. > 380°C and a methiodide, m.p. 236–7°C (*dec.*). The free base is soluble in most organic solvents but only sparingly so in H_2O. It has $[\alpha]_D^{21} - 114°$ (c 1.0, CHCl$_3$). LiAlH$_4$ yields a compound, $C_{16}H_{23}O_3N$, m.p. 162–3°C.

Manske, Marion., *Can. J. Res.*, **21B**, 92 (1943)
Manske, Marion., *ibid*, **22B**, 53 (1944)
Bentho, Stoll., *Ber.*, **85**, 663 (1952)
Structure:
Szarek, Adams, Curcumelli-Rodostamo, MacLean., *Can. J. Chem.*, **42**, 2584 (1964)

Mass spectra:
MacLean, Curcumelli-Rodostamo., *ibid*, **44**, 611 (1966)

ANNOTININE (*Alkaloid L-7*)

$C_{16}H_{21}O_3N$

M.p. 232°C

A further base obtained from *Lycopodium annotinum* L, the alkaloid crystallizes from MeOH-CHCl$_3$ as colourless prisms. It forms several crystalline salts: perchlorate, m.p. 267°C; hydrochloride (0.5 H_2O), m.p. 210–1°C (*dec.*); hydrobromide, m.p. 260°C (*dec.*) and hydriodide, m.p. 237–9°C (*dec.*). Manske and Marion have discussed the results of the action of alkali and halogen acids on this base, and of the oxidation products and shown that two of the oxygen atoms are present as a lactone group and the third as an ether bridge.

Manske, Marion., *Can. J. Res.,* **21B**, 92 (1943)
Wiesner *et al., Chem. & Ind.,* 564 (1957)
Przybylska, Marion., *Can. J. Chem.,* 35, 1075 (1957)
Martin-Smith, Greenhalgh, Marion., *ibid,* **35**, 409 (1957)
Wiesner *et al., Tetrahedron,* 4, 87 (1958)

Mass spectra:
MacLean., *Can. J. Chem.,* **41**, 2654 (1963)

Crystal structure:
Przybylska, Ahmed., *Acta Cryst.,* **11**, 718 (1958)

Total Synthesis:
Wiesner, Poon., *Tetrahedron Lett.,* 4937 (1967)

ANNOTOXINE

$C_{31}H_{42}O_5N_2$

M.p. 197°C

Also present in *Lycopodium annotinum* L. this alkaloid crystallizes from Me_2CO
or MeOH as plates or rhombic crystals; $[\alpha]_D^{20} - 179°$ (c 1.0, $CHCl_3$). It is
readily soluble in most organic solvents. The perchlorate forms colourless
needles, monohydrate, m.p. 277–8°C (*dec.*) and the dinitrate, m.p. 215–7°C.

Bertho, Stoll., *Ber.,* **85**, 663 (1952)

ANNULOLINE

$C_{20}H_{19}O_4N$

M.p. 114°C

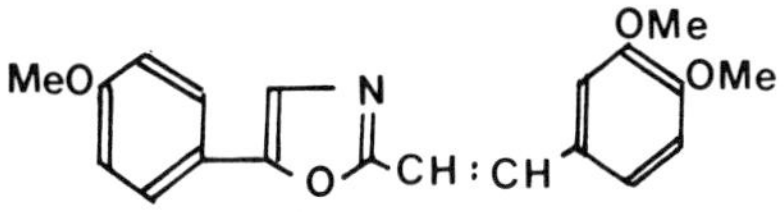

This alkaloid occurs in *Lolium multiflorum* and crystallizes from benzene-light
petroleum as colourless needles or plates. Some workers have reported a lower
melting point of 105–6°C for this base. The ultraviolet spectrum shows an
absorption maximum at 354 mμ. The hydrochloride is crystalline m.p. 174–7°C
and the picrate, from aqueous EtOH has m.p. 216–8°C.

Axelrod, Belzile., *J. Org. Chem.,* **23**, 919 (1958)
Karimoto *et al., Tetrahedron Lett.,* 83 (1962)

ANODENDRINE

$C_{13}H_{21}O_2N$

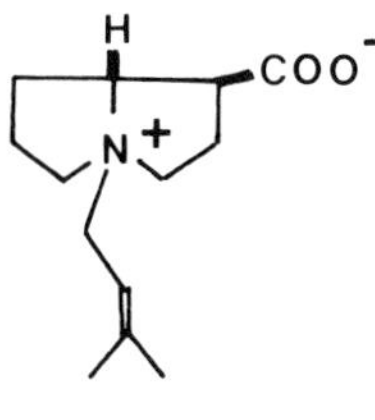

Obtained from *Anodendron affine* Druce, this alkaloid had $[\alpha]_D^{25} + 9.5°$ (EtOH) and shows one absorption maximum in the ultraviolet spectrum in methanol solution at 212 mμ. The picrate forms yellow needles, m.p. 123–4°C. Hydrogenation with 10 per cent Pd-C in MeOH gives laburninic acid, $C_8H_{13}O_2N$, $[\alpha]_D^{25} + 44.2°$ (H_2O), forming a picrate, m.p. 175–6°C. The structure is shown to be N-*iso*propyllaburninic acid both by physical and chemical techniques and by synthesis.

Isolation and synthesis:
Sasaki, Hirata., *Tetrahedron Lett.*, **46**, 4065 (1969)

ANODMINE

This base occurs only in a minute quantity in tobacco smoke and is present in .the fraction which is not volatile in steam. The picrolonate is stated to have m.p. 310°C.

Spath, Wenuschand, Zajic., *Ber.*, **69**, 393 (1936)

ANOLOBINE

$C_{17}H_{15}O_3N$

M.p. 262°C (*dec.*).

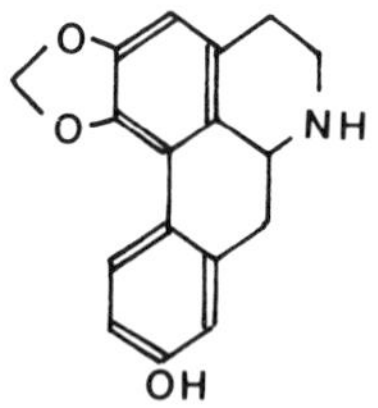

One of the aporphine alkaloids found in *Asimina triloba,* the base has $[\alpha]_D^{27} - 22.5°$ (MeOH-CHCl$_3$). The *dl*-O,N-dimethyl derivative has been synthesized by Marion. It yields a hydrochloride, m.p. 266°C (*dec.*); methiodide, colourless prisms from MeOH, m.p. 241°C and a picrate, m.p. 226°C, all identical with those prepared by methylation of analobine. The O-methyl ether of the alkaloid is Xylopine (q.v.).

Manske., *Can. J. Res.*, **16B**, 76 (1938)
Govindachari., *Chem. Abstr.*, **35**, 6963 (1941)
Marion., *J. Amer. Chem. Soc.*, **66**, 1125 (1944)
Tomita, Kozuka., *J. Pharm. Soc.*, (*Japan*), **85**, 77 (1965)

(−)-ANONAINE

$C_{17}H_{15}O_2N$

M.p. 122–3°C

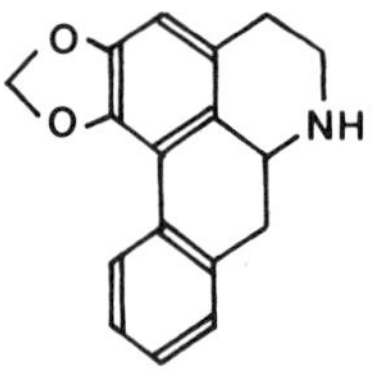

This aporphine base occurs in *Anona reticulata* and has $[\alpha]_D^{20} - 52°$ (CHCl$_3$). The crystalline hydrochloride has m.p. 277.5°C (*dec.*). The nitrogen is secondary and the alkaloid gives a monoacetyl derivative, m.p. 229–230°C and a neutral nitroso-compound, m.p. 229–230°C. With CH$_3$I it furnishes the quaternary iodide, $C_{19}H_{20}O_2NI$, m.p. 217°C which is decomposed by alkali into the methine base, m.p. 87–90°C. The methiodide of the latter, m.p. 270.5°C (*dec.*) yields a methylenedioxy vinyl phenanthrene, $C_{17}H_{12}O_2$, m.p. 87°C.

The *dl*-form, small prisms from Et$_2$O, m.p. 116.5°C has been synthesized from O-nitrophenylacetyl chloride and *homo*piperonylamine. It forms a hydrochloride, m.p. 295°C and an N-benzoyl derivative with a double melting point at 129°C and 146°C.

Formaldehyde and formic acid react with the free base to give the N-methyl derivative, identical with *dl*-roermerine (q.v.).

Santos., *Philipp. J. Sci.*, **43**, 561 (1930)
Gopinath *et al.*, *Chem. Ber.*, **92**, 776 (1959)

Synthesis:
Marion, Lemay, Ayotte., *Can. J. Res.*, **28B**, 21 (1950)
Cava, Dalton., *J. Org. Chem.*, **31**, 1281 (1966)

Biosynthesis:
Barton, Bhakuni, Chapman, Kirby., *Chem. Commun.*, 259 (1966)
Barton, Bhakuni, Chapman, Kirby., *J. Chem. Soc., C.*, 2134 (1967)

ANTHEROSPERMIDINE

$C_{18}H_{11}O_4N$

M.p. 275–6°C (*dec.*).

From *Anthosperma moschatum* Labill. this alkaloid is obtained in the crystalline form from CHCl$_3$. The ultraviol spectrum in ethanol solution exhibits absorption maxima at 247, 281 and 312 mμ. In acid solution (0.1 N/HCl) the absorption maxima occur at 262.2 and 283 mμ.

Bick, Clezy, Crow., *Austral. J. Chem.*, **9**, 111 (1956)
Bick, Douglas., *Tetrahedron Lett.*, 1629 (1964)

ANTHRANILOYLLYCOCTONINE

$C_{31}H_{46}O_8N_2$

M.p. 132–5°C (block);
160–165.5°C (capillary)

One of the aconite alkaloids obtained from the roots of *Delphinium barkeyi,* this base crystallizes as the hemihydrate.It has $[\alpha]_D^{20.5} + 50.6°$ (CHCl$_3$). The alkaloid forms numerous crystalline salts and derivatives: hydrochloride, colourless needles from Et$_2$O-MeOH, m.p. 182°C (*dec.*); hydrobromide, m.p. 185°C (*dec.*); hydriodide, pale yellow needles, *dec.* at 183°C; perchlorate, colourless plates from Et$_2$O-MeOH, m.p. 202.5–203°C; aurichloride, brown amorphous powder, *dec.* at 159°C; methiodide, light yellow needles from Et$_2$O-MeOH, m.p. 177°C (*dec.*) and picrate, m.p. 159–160°C. It has also been stated to form a crystalline diperchlorate, m.p. > 235°C. The N-acetyl derivative is Ajacine (q.v.). Hydrolysis with alkalies furnishes anthranilic acid and lycoctonine.

Goodson., *J. Chem. Soc.,* 139 (1943)
Marion, Manske., *Can. J. Res.,* **24B**, 1 (1946)
Cook, Beath., *J. Amer. Chem. Soc.,* **74**, 1411 (1952)

ANTIRHINE

$C_{19}H_{21}ON_2$

M.p. 112–4°C

A carboline-type alkaloid present in *Antirhea putaminosa* (F. Muell.) Bail, the base forms an adduct with CHCl$_3$ which has the melting point given above. It has $[\alpha]_D - 2°$ (CHCl$_3$). The ultraviolet spectrum shows absorption maxima at 225, 282 and 289 (infl.) mμ. Hydrogenation yields the dihydro-derivative (1 H$_2$O), m.p. 105–8°C; $[\alpha]_D + 23°$.

Johns, Lamberton, Occolowicz., *Austral. J. Chem.,* **20**, 1463 (1967)
Johns, Lamberton, Occolowicz., *Chem. Commun.,* 229 (1967)

ANTIRHINE METHOCHLORIDE

$C_{20}H_{24}ON_2Cl$

This alkaloid has recently been discovered as a minor constituent of the roots of *Amsonia elliptica.*

Sakai *et al., J. Pharm. Soc., Japan,* **93**, 483 (1973)

ANTOFINE

$C_{23}H_{25}O_3N$

M.p. 213–5°C

A phenanthroindolizidine alkaloid present in *Antitoxicum funebre,* the base forms colourless crystals from Me$_2$CO. It has been shown to contain three methoxyl groups but no hydroxyl groups. The structure has recently been confirmed by the synthesis of the optically inactive form of the base.

Platonova, Kuzovkov, Massagetov., *J. Gen. Chem., USSR,* **28**, 3131 (1958)
Synthesis:
Chauncy, Gellert., *Austral. J. Chem.,* **23**, 2503 (1970)

(+)-APHYLLIDINE

C$_{15}$H$_{22}$ON$_2$

M.p. 112–3°C

This alkaloid occurs in the high-boiling fraction obtained from *Anabasis aphylla* and crystallizes in colourless plates from petroleum ether. It has $[\alpha]_D^{18} + 5.57°$ (MeOH). It is readily soluble in EtOH or Et$_2$O, moderately so in light petroleum and only slightly soluble in H$_2$O. It forms crystalline salts and derivatives: the hydrochloride, m.p. 235–7°C; $[\alpha]_D + 30°$ (H$_2$O); picrolonate, yellow prisms, m.p. 235–6°C and methiodide, m.p. 223–5°C; $[\alpha]_D + 9.8°$ (H$_2$O). With bromine in CHCl$_3$, it forms an unstable dibromide which readily reverts to bromoaphyllidine hydrobromide, colourless needles, m.p. 210–1°C. From the latter, bromoaphyllidine, m.p. 150–2°C may easily be obtained.

Orekhov, Men'schikov., *Ber.,* **65**, 234 (1932)
Orekhov, Norkina., *ibid,* **67**, 1845 (1934)
Orekhov, Men'schikov, Norkina, Maximova., *ibid,* **67**, 1976 (1934)
Orekhov., *Chem. Zentr.,* **I**, 2365 (1938)
Spath *et al., Ber.,* **75**, 805 (1942)

(−)-APHYLLINE

C$_{15}$H$_{22}$ON$_2$

M.p. 101–6°C

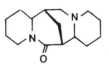

The laevorotatory form of this alkaloid is present in *Argyolobium megorhizum* Bol. and forms colourless prisms from Et$_2$O-hexane with $[\alpha]_D - 9.1°$ (c 2.2, EtOH). It forms a hydrochloride as prisms from Et$_2$O-MeOH-Me$_2$CO, m.p. 228–230°C (*dec.*); picrolonate, yellow needles, m.p. 241–3°C (*dec.*).

Tsuda, Marion., *Can. J. Chem.,* **42**, 764 (1964)

APHYLLINE

C$_{15}$H$_{24}$ON$_2$

B.p. 200°C/4 mm

Also present in the high boiling fraction from *Anabasis aphylla,* this alkaloid has been obtained crystalline by rubbing the oil, m.p. 52–3°C; $[\alpha]_D^{20} + 10.3°$ (aqueous MeOH). It is readily soluble in all organic solvents. The hydrochloride has m.p. 207–9°C; $[\alpha]_D^{20} + 13.6°$ (H_2O); the methiodide, large colourless crystals, m.p. 212–3° (*dec.*) and the picrolonate, small yellow prisms, m.p. 230–1°C. On exhaustive methylation, the alkaloid loses one nitrogen atom to give hemiaphylline, $C_{15}H_{21}ON$, a viscous yellow oil, b.p. 217–220°C which is not markedly basic.

Orekhov, Men'schikov., *Ber.,* **64**, 266 (1931)
Orekhov, Men'schikov., *ibid,* **65**, 234 (1932)
Orekhov., *Chem. Zentr.,* **I**, 2365 (1938)
Spath *et al., Ber.,* **75**, 805 (1942)
Edwards, Clarke, Douglas., *Can. J. Chem.,* **32**, 235 (1954)
Galinovsky, Knoth, Fischer., *Monatsh.,* **86**, 1014 (1955)

APOATROPINE (*Atropamine*)

$C_{17}H_{21}O_2N$

M.p. 60–2°C

The anhydride of atropine, this alkaloid was first obtained synthetically by Pesci and subsequently by Merck and Hesse. It was found naturally under the name of Atropamine in the roots of *Atropa belladonna* by Hesse, the identity of the two being established by Mercke. The base crystallizes in colourless prisms from Et_2O or $CHCl_3$. It is very soluble in most organic solvents although only moderately so in *iso*amyl alcohol and ligroin and sparingly soluble in H_2O. The hydrochloride forms colourless leaflets, m.p. 237–9°C; the hydrobromide, m.p. 248°C, the aurichloride, yellow needles, m.p. 112°C and the picrate, yellow needles, m.p. 166–8°C.

When heated alone, the base passes partly into belladonnine (q.v.) and partially decomposes into tropine and atropic acid. $Ba(OH)_2$ at 100°C also yields tropine and atropic acid while concentrated HCl at 130°C gives tropine and *iso*tropic acid, together with atropic acid.

Pesci., *Gazzetta,* **11**, 538 (1881)
Merck., *Arch. Pharm.,* **229**, 134 (1891)
Hesse., *Annalen,* **361**, 87 (1891)
Hesse., *ibid,* **271**, 124 (1892)
Hesse., *ibid,* **277**, 292 (1893)

Synthesis:
Ladenberg., *Annalen,* **217**, 102 (1883)

APOCINCHENE

$C_{19}H_{19}ON$

M.p. 209–210°C

One of the Cinchona alkaloids, the base is obtained from cinchene by reaction with HBr. It forms colourless crystals from EtOH and is freely soluble in both alkalies and acids. The hydrobromide forms colourless needles, m.p. 256°C. Methylation yields the O-methyl ether as an oil, forming a crystalline picrate, m.p. 200°C (*dec.*).

Comstock, Koenigs., *Ber.*, **20**, 2517 (1887)

(+)-APOGLAZIOVINE

This minor base has recently been discovered in *Ocotea variabilis*. It is still under investigation.

Cava *et al.*, *Tetrahedron Lett.*, 4647 (1972)

APOHYOSCINE

$C_{17}H_{19}O_3N$

M.p. 97°C

This tropane alkaloid occurs in both *Datura innoxia* Miller and *D. meteloides* D.C. It is obtained in the form of colourless needles from Et_2O and gives a series of crystalline salts, e.g. the nitrate, colourless plates from H_2O, m.p. 157°C; aurichloride, m.p. 186°C; methiodide, m.p. 238°C.

Willstätter, Hug., *Z. physiol. Chem.*, **79**, 146 (1912)
Evans, Woolley., *J. Chem. Soc.*, 4936 (1965)

APOREIDINE

M.p. 176–8°C

Isolated from *Papaver dubium* L., this alkaloid forms glistening rhombic plates from EtOH. It is possible that it does not occur naturally in the plant but is produced by the action of light and air on Aporeine (q.v.).

Pavesi., *Chem. Soc. Abstr.*, i, 368 (1905)
Pavesi., *ibid*, i, 870 (1907)

APOREINE

$C_{18}H_{16}O_2N$

M.p. 88–9°C

A major alkaloid of *Papaver dubium* L., the base forms greenish-yellow prisms and can be distilled unchanged in H_2 or CO_2. It is readily soluble in most organic solvents except hot light petroleum from which it is best crystallized. It has $[\alpha]_D^{15} + 75.19°$. The alkaloid is only slightly basic but gives well crystallized salts: hydrochloride, glistening plates from H_2O or EtOH, m.p. 230°C (*dec.*);

hydrobromide, yellow-green scales that discolour at 190°C and decompose at 210°C; acid oxalate, plates from EtOH, m.p. 89–90°C. The free base can be sublimed at 220–230°C in CO_2 but on exposure to sunlight it passes to aporegenine and Aporeidine (q.v.). The alkaloid is stated to be a tetanizing poison similar to thebaine.

Pavesi., *Chem. Soc. Abstr.*, i, 368 (1905)
Pavesi., *ibid*, i, 870 (1907)

(+)-APOVINCAMINE

$C_{21}H_{24}O_3N_2$

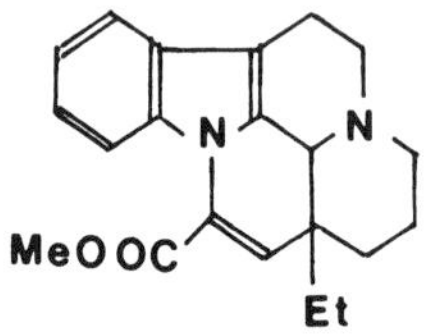

This imidazolidinocarbazole alkaloid occurs in two Amazonian species of *Tabernaemontana,* namely *T. riedelii* and *T. rigida,* although it occurs only in minute traces in the former. The structure has been determined from the infrared, ultraviolet, NMR and mass spectra.

Cava *et al., J. Org. Chem.*, **33**, 1055 (1968)

(+)-APPARICINE

$C_{18}H_{20}N_2$

M.p. 178°C

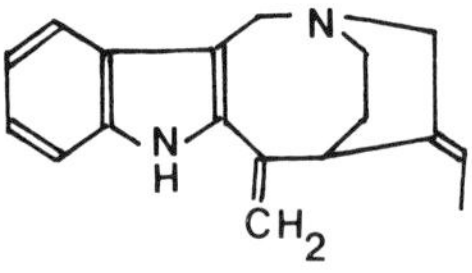

This form of the alkaloid occurs in *Aspidosperma dasycarpon* A. DC and is dextrorotatory with $[\alpha]_D^{27} + 177°$ (c 2.16, $CHCl_3$).

Gilbert *et al., Tetrahedron,* **21**, 1141 (1965)

(−)-APPARICINE

$C_{18}H_{20}N_2$

M.p. 192–4°C

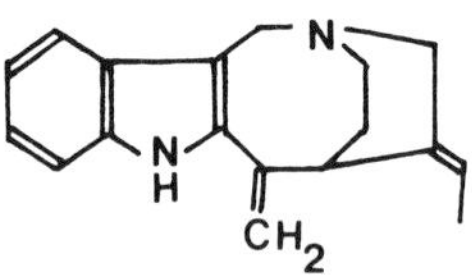

This alkaloid has been obtained from several *Aspidosperma* species, e.g. *A. eburneum* Fr. All., *A. dasycarpon* A. DC., *A. gomezianum* A. DC., *A. multiflorum* A. DC. and *A. olivaceum* Mull-Arg. It forms colourless crystals from Me_2CO and undergoes a phase transition to fine needles at about 160°C. It is laevorotatory with $[\alpha]_D^{27} - 177°$ (c 2.16, $CHCl_3$). The ultraviolet spectrum exhibits absorption maxima at 203, 230, 303 and 312 mμ. The methiodide forms an amorphous powder.

166

Gilbert *et al.*, *Tetrahedron*, **21**, 1141 (1965)

Structure:

Joule *et al.*, *J. Chem. Soc.*, 4773 (1965)

ARACHINE

$C_5H_{14}ON_2$

This base occurs along with choline and betaine in *Arachis hypogoea* L., forming a yellow-green syrup. The platinichloride is crystalline, m.p. 216°C and the alkaloid is stated to also form a crystalline aurichloride. It produces transient narcosis in frogs and rabbits with partial paralysis.

Mooser., *Landw. Versuchs-stat.*, **60**, 321 (1904)

Mooser., *Chem. Soc. Abstr.*, **i**, 79 (1905)

ARALIONINE

$C_{34}H_{38}O_5N_4$

M.p. 165−7°C

A peptide alkaloid present in *Araliorhamnus vaginatus* Perrier, the base is isolated as colourless crystals having $[\alpha]_D^{20} + 82°$ (c 0.2, MeOH). The ultraviolet spectrum in MeOH has a single absorption maximum at 246 mμ. When hydrogenated catalytically over PtO_2, the alkaloid gives an amorphous tetrahydro derivative. Hydrolysis with 6N HCl furnishes β-phenylnaphthalene, N,N-dimethyl-*iso*leucine and ω-aminoacetophenone, m.p. 85.5−86.5°C.

Tschesche, Behrendt, Fehlhaber., *Chem. Ber.*, **102**, 50 (1969)

ARBORINE

$C_{16}H_{14}ON_2$

M.p. 155−6°C

From the leaves of *Glycosmis arborea correa*, this alkaloid is obtained as colourless plates containing $EtOH-C_6H_6$ of solvation. It is soluble in C_6H_6, EtOH, $CHCl_3$, AcOH and dioxan, sparingly so in Et_2O or hot H_2O and insoluble in petroleum ether. Hydrolysis with alcoholic KOH yields NH_3, N-methylanthranilic acid and benzylic acid. When heated with soda line, it gives NH_3, toluene and N-methylaniline. The hydrochloride crystallizes from H_2O as the dihydrate, m.p. 106−8°C which solidifies and subsequently remelts at 215°C; hydrobromide, m.p. 75−6°C; hydriodide, m.p. 95−6°C; nitrate, m.p. 116−7°C;

picrate, m.p. $172-3°C$ and the styphnate, m.p. $194-5°C$. The base also forms a methiodide, m.p. $126-7°C$ and a picrolonate, m.p. $171°C$.

Chakravarti, Chakravarti., *J. Proc. Inst. Chem.* (India), 24, 96 (1952)
Chakravarti, Chakravarti, Chakravarti., *J. Chem. Soc.*, 3337 (1953)
Chakravarti *et al., Tetrahedron*, 16, 224 (1961)

ARBORININE

$C_{16}H_{15}O_4N$

M.p. $175-6°C$

An acridone alkaloid first isolated from *Evodia alata* and *Glycosmis arborea correa*, the base has subsequently been found in *Teclea natalensis*. From the leaf extract it may be crystallizes from EtOH and gives a deep green colour with alcoholic $FeCl_3$. It is soluble in dioxan or $CHCl_3$, only moderately so in petroleum ether or Et_2O and insoluble in H_2O. The O-benzoate crystallizes as fine, colourless needles from a mixture of EtOH and $CHCl_3$, m.p. $257-8°C$; the O-acetate, also colourless needles, has m.p. $215-6°C$. The O-methyl ether is a constituent of *Evodia alata* (q.v.).

Hughes *et al., Austral. J. Sci. Res.*, 3A, 500 (1950)
Hughes *et al., ibid*, 4A, 430 (1951)
Chakravarti, Chakravarti., *J. Proc. Inst. Chem.* (India), 24, 96 (1952)
Chakravarti, Chakravarti, Chakravarti., *J. Chem. Soc.*, 3337 (1953)
Sell, Hughes, Ritchie., *Austral. J. Chem.*, 8, 114 (1955)
Banerjee *et al., Tetrahedron*, 16, 251 (1961)
Pakrashi *et al., Chem. & Ind.*, 464 (1961)
Pegel, Wright., *J. Chem. Soc.*, C, 2327 (1969)

ARECAIDINE (*Arecaine*)

$C_7H_{11}O_2N$

M.p. $232°C$

One of several alkaloids obtained from the seeds of *Areca catechu*, the base crystallizes from aqueous EtOH with 1 H_2O in the form of colourless tetragonal or hexagonal tablets. The melting point has been recorded as $223-4°C$ by Jahns as well as that given above. The hydrochloride forms slender colourless needles, m.p. $262-3°C$ (rapid heating); the hydrobromide crystallizes from MeOH, m.p. $248-9°C$ with decomposition beginning around $190°C$; aurichloride, prisms from dilute HCl, m.p. $200°C$ (*dec.*); platinichloride, yellow octahedra, m.p. $234-5°C$ (*dec.*); methopicrate, m.p. $224-5°C$; methochloride, m.p. $256-8°C$ and amide, m.p. $161°C$ although $152°C$ has been reported for this last compound.

Various esters of the acid have been prepared. The methyl ester is the naturally-occurring Arecoline (q.v.); the ethyl ester forms a crystalline hydrochloride, m.p. $104-7°C$; propyl ester hydrochloride, m.p. $132-5°C$ and the butyl ester hydrochloride, m.p. $126-8°C$.

On a commercial scale the alkaloid may be prepared by loss of H_2O from 1-methyl-4-hydroxypiperidine-3-carboxylic acid, a process patented by Merck and Maeder. The alkaloid is not markedly toxic.

Freudenberg., *Ber.*, **51**, 976 (1918)
Hess, Liebbrandt., *ibid*, **51**, 806 (1918)
Merck, Maeder., D.R.P. 485,139
Ugryumov., *Chem. Abstr.*, **35**, 3644 (1941)
Dankova *et al.*, *ibid*, **37**, 381 (1943)
Sapara., *Chem. Listy.*, **45**, 454 (1951)
Panouse., *Compt. rend.*, **233**, 1200 (1951)
Tsukamoto, Komori., *J. Pharm. Soc. Japan*, **73**, 779 (1953)

ARECOLIDINE

$C_8H_{13}O_2N$

M.p. 105°C

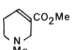

A weak base isolated from *Areca catechu,* the alkaloid crystallizes from dry Et_2O as glassy needles and after sublimation it has m.p. 110°C and is hygroscopic. It forms several crystalline salts: hydrochloride (monohydrate), m.p. 95–8°C; hydrobromide, m.p. 268–271°C (*dec.*); aurichloride, yellow leaflets, m.p. 219–220°C (*dec.*); platinichloride, thick orange needles, m.p. 222–3°C (*dec.*) and methiodide, colourless prisms, m.p. 264°C (*dec.*). The structure given is that proposed by Emde.

Emde., *Apoth. Zeit.*, **30**, 240 (1915)

ARECOLINE

$C_8H_{13}O_2N$

B.p. 209°C

This is the most important alkaloidal constituent of *Areca catechu* and is a colourless, alkaline oil which is volatile in steam and soluble in most organic solvents and H_2O although it may be extracted from the latter by Et_2O in the presence of dissolved salts. The salts of the base are normally crystalline but deliquescent: hydrochloride, colourless needles, m.p. 157–8°C; hydrobromide, prisms from EtOH, m.p. 170–2°C; platinichloride, orange-red crystals, m.p. 176°C and methiodide, m.p. 173–4°C. The aurichloride is, like the free base, an oil.

Arecoline exhibits markedly toxic properties, showing a profound parasympathetic stimulant action. With large doses central paralysis may occur. The hydrobromide has been employed in small doses as a diaphoretic, anthelmintic and sialogogue.

Hess, Liebbrandt., *Ber.*, **51**, 806 (1918)
Freudenberg., *ibid*, **51**, 976 (1918)
Chemnitius., *J. pr. Chem.*, **117**, 147 (1927)

Ugryumov., *Chem. Abstr.*, **35**, 3644 (1941)
Mannich., *Ber.*, **75**, 1480 (1942)
Dankova *et al.*, *Chem. Abstr.*, **37**, 381 (1943)
Panouse., *Compt. rend.*, **233**, 1200 (1951)
Dobrowsky., *Monatsh.*, **83**, 443 (1952)

(−)-ARGEMONINE

$C_{21}H_{25}O_4N$

M.p. 155.5−156.5°C

Several *Argemone* species contain this alkaloid, in particular *A. mexicana* L. The base forms colourless prisms with $[\alpha]_D^{20} - 226°$ (c 0.1, CHCl$_3$). The ultraviolet spectrum has an absorption maximum at 287 mμ. The hydrochloride has been assigned various melting points of 65−81°C; 80−2°C and 72−5°C. The methiodide exists in two modifications as the tetrahydrate, m.p. 118−120°C (*dec.*) and the dihydrate, m.p. 270−280°C (*dec.*). The picrate has m.p. 119−121°C although 219°C has also been reported.

Schlotterbeck., *J. Amer. Chem. Soc.*, **24**, 238 (1902)
Santos, Adkillen., *ibid*, **54**, 2923 (1932)
Soine, Gisvold., *J. Amer. Pharm. Assoc.*, **33**, 185 (1944)
Martell, Soine, Kier., *J. Amer. Chem. Soc.*, **85**, 1022 (1963)

(−)-ARGEMONINE METHOHYDROXIDE

$C_{22}H_{29}O_5N$

M.p. Indefinite

This minor alkaloid of *Argemone gracilenta* Greene is an amorphous powder which cannot be crystallized. It occurs only in small quantities in the plant.

Sternetz, McMurtry., *J. Org. Chem.*, **34**, 555 (1969)

(−)-ARGEMONINE N-OXIDE

$C_{21}H_{25}O_5N$

M.p. 140−168°C
(effervescence)

From *Argemone gracilenta* Greene, this alkaloid has been isolated as a transparent glass. It is laevorotatory with $[\alpha]_D^{25} - 185°$ (c 2.81, CHCl$_3$). Treatment with methyl iodide yields (−)-Argemonine.

Sternetz, McMurtry., *J. Org. Chem.*, **34**, 555 (1969)

ARGENTAMINE

$C_{15}H_{20}O_2N_2$

M.p. 203°C

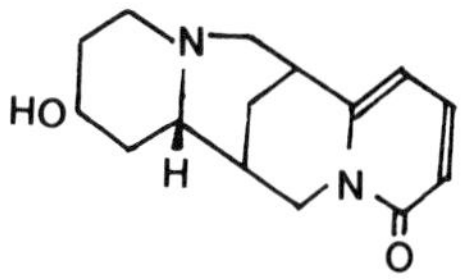

An alkaloid of *Ammodendron argentum*, the base crystallizes from C_6H_6. It forms a crystalline hydrochloride, m.p. 298°C and a picrate, m.p. 230°C. Raney Ni yields the tetrahydro derivative, m.p. 210°C, while hydrogenation with Pt gives the deoxyhexahydro compound, m.p. 147°C which yields α-*iso*sparteine with P_2O_5 in xylene. The structure has been determined from the above chemical reactions and from infrared and mass spectrometry.

Ngok *et al., Khim. Prir. Soedin.*, **6**, 111 (1970)

ARGENTINE

$C_{23}H_{26}O_3N_4$

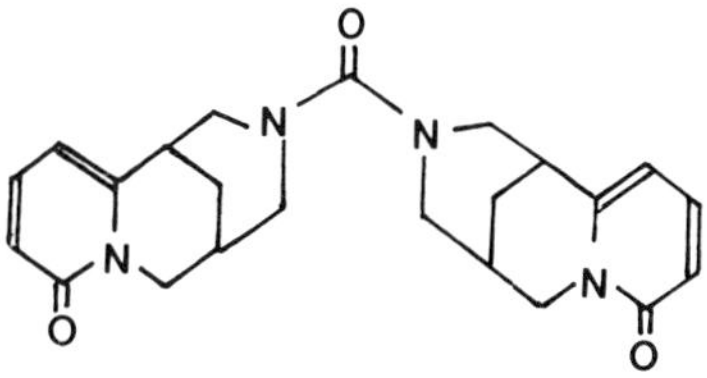

A second alkaloid from *Ammodendron argentum*, this base has been shown to possess the above structure from infrared and mass spectrometry.

Ngok, Kushmuradov, Aslanov, Sadykov, Ziyavitdinov, Zaiken, Vul'fson., *Khim. Prir. Soedin.*, **6**, 111 (1970)

ARGYROLOBINE

$C_{15}H_{22}O_2N_2$

M.p. 168–9°C

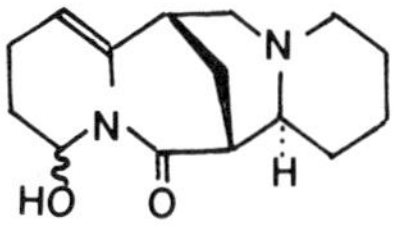

Isolated from *Argyrolobium megarhizum*, this alkaloid forms colourless prisms from Me_2CO with $[\alpha]_D$ + 13.3° (c 1.4, $CHCl_3$). The ultraviolet spectrum exhibits an absorption maximum at 239 mμ. Of the salts and derivatives that have been prepared to characterize the alkaloid, the hydrochloride has m.p. 170–2°C; the methiodide, m.p. 180–3°C (*dec.*) and the acetate, m.p. 61°C.

Tsuda, Marion., *Can. J. Chem.*, **42**, 764 (1964)

ARIBINE

$C_{23}H_{20}N_4$

This alkaloid, isolated from the bark of *Arariba rubra*, has been shown to be identical with Harman (q.v.).

Rieth, Wohler., *Annalen.*, **120**, 247 (1861)
Späth., *Monatsh.*, **40**, 351 (1919)
Späth., *ibid*, **41**, 401 (1920)

ARICINE (*Cusconine, heterophylline*)

$C_{22}H_{26}O_4N_2$

M.p. 188–9°C

One of the alkaloids found in the bark of *Cinchona Pelletierana* Wedd. the base crystallizes from aqueous EtOH as colourless prisms, $[\alpha]_D - 58.18°$ (EtOH), $- 63°$ (pyridine), $- 91°$ ($CHCl_3$) and $- 92.5°$ (Et_2O). It is readily soluble in Et_2O but insoluble in H_2O. The hydrochloride has m.p. 254°C; $[\alpha]_D - 14.5°$ (EtOH); hydrobromide, m.p. 262–3°C; succinate, m.p. 208–9°C (*dec.*) and the oxalate, m.p. 235°C (*dec.*).

Pelletier, Corriol., *J. Pharm.*, **15**, 565 (1829)
Howard., *J. Chem. Soc.*, **28**, 309 (1875)
Moissan, Landrin., *Bull. soc. chim.*, **4**, 258 (1890)
Moissan, Landrin., *Compt. rend.*, **110**, 469 (1890)
Hamet., *ibid*, **221**, 307 (1945)
Stoll, Hofmann, Brunner., *Helv. Chim. Acta*, **38**, 270 (1955)
Prelog *et al.*, *ibid*, **37**, 1805 (1954)
Shamma, Moss., *J. Amer. Chem. Soc.*, **83**, 5038 (1961)

Stereochemistry:
Shamma, Richey., *J. Amer. Chem. Soc.*, **85**, 2507 (1963)
Finch, Taylor, Emerson, Klyne, Swan., *Tetrahedron*, **22**, 1327 (1966)

ARISTOLOCHINE

$C_{17}H_{19}O_3N$

M.p. 215°C (*dec.*).

This alkaloid from *Aristolchia clematis* is obtained as a microcrystalline powder with $[\alpha]_D - 268.6°$. It dissolves readily in alkaline solutions but is only sparingly soluble in organic solvents. The hydrochloride has m.p. 268°C (*dec.*); $[\alpha]_D^{25} - 236.2°$ and the picrate, m.p. 222°C (*dec.*). The base contains one replaceable hydrogen, one methoxyl group and the nitrogen atom carries two methyl groups.

A great deal of confusion has arisen concerning this alkaloid. Three bases of the same name have been isolated from *Aristolchia* species. One was isolated by Pohl from *A. clematis* and *A. rotunda* L, originally assigned the formula $C_{32}H_{22}O_{13}N$, later reduced to $C_{17}H_{11}O_7N$, and subsequently obtained from *A. Sipho* and *A. debili*. The second, found in *A. argentina* Griseb. by Hesse is amorphous but yielding crystalline salts, while the third, found in various *Aristolchia* species by Krishnaswamy *et al,* is that described above and now generally accepted as aristolochine.

Castille., *J. Pharm. Belg.,* **4**, 569 (1922)

Ryo., *Folio Pharmacol. Japan,* **4**, 123 (1927)

Rosenmund, Reichstein., *Pharm. Acta Helv.,* **18**, 243 (1943)

ARMEPAVINE

$C_{19}H_{23}O_3N$

M.p. 148–9°C

A benzylisoquinoline alkaloid from *Papaver armeniacum* and *P. floribundum,* the base forms colourless needles from Et_2O-Me_2CO with $[\alpha]_D^{18} - 109.1°$ ($CHCl_3$). It is soluble in $CHCl_3$ or EtOH, moderately so in Et_2O and insoluble in H_2O. The alkaloid gives a crystalline hydrochloride, m.p. 151–2°C; methiodide, m.p. 199–200°C and an oxalate, m.p. 211–2°C. CH_2N_2 converts it into the O-methyl derivative, m.p. 63–4°C; $[\alpha]_D - 84.48°$ ($CHCl_3$), oxidized by HNO_3 to anisic acid. With CH_3I and MeONa it furnishes O-methylarmepavine methiodide, m.p. 135–6°C. Oxidation with $KMnO_4$ yields *p*-hydroxybenzoic acid and 1-keto-6:7-dimethoxy-2-methyl-1:2:3:4-tetrahydro*iso*quinoline. The alkaloid has been resolved via the O-benzoyl derivatives into its enantiomorphs: *S*(+)-armepavine, m.p. 149–150°C; $[\alpha]_D^{23} + 112°$ and *R*(−)-armepavine with $[\alpha]_D^{23} - 103.2°$.

Yunusov, Konovalova, Orekhov., *J. Gen. Chem. USSR,* **10**, 641 (1940)

Konovalova, Yunusov, Orekhov., *Ber.,* **68**, 2161 (1935)

Tomita, Fujita, Murai., *J. Pharm. Soc., Japan,* **71**, 226 (1951)

Inubushi., *Pharm. Bull. Japan,* **3**, 384 (1955)

Farber, Giacomazi., *Chem. & Ind.,* 57 (1968)

AROMOLINE

$C_{36}H_{38}O_6N_2$

This alkaloid of *Daphnandra aromatica* has been characterized as the crystalline compound with $CHCl_3$, m.p. 174–5°C. It is strongly dextrorotatory with $[\alpha]_D^{17} + 327°$ ($CHCl_3$). The structure has been determined by spectroscopic methods.

Bick, Whalley., *Univ. Queensland Papers; Dept. Chem.,* **1**, No. 33 (1948)

ARTABOTRINE

$C_{20}H_{23}O_4N$

M.p. 185–6°C

This aporphine alkaloid occurs in *Artabotyris suaveolens* Blume and forms large, tabular, orthorhombic crystals with $[\alpha]_D^{15} + 194.8°$ (c 1.86, CHCl$_3$). The hydrochloride has m.p. 226–7°C and the acetate, crystals of the dihydrate, m.p. 97–9°C or 118–9°C (*dry*). The O-methyl ether is a syrup, $[\alpha]_D^{16} + 182.2°$ (c 2.9, CHCl$_3$) but forms a crystalline methiodide, m.p. 254–5°C. Artabotrine methiodide, m.p. 224–5°C furnishes the methine base when boiled with alcoholic KOH, m.p. 122–3°C; $[\alpha]_D^{18} - 183°$ (c 1.65, EtOH). Oxidation with KMnO$_4$ gives a monocarboxylic lactone acid, $C_{11}H_{10}O_6$, m.p. 203–4°C which contains two methoxyl groups and gives the fluorescein reaction.

Maranon., *Philipp. J. Sci.*, **38**, 259 (1928)
Santos, Reyes., *Univ. Philipp. Nat. Appl. Sci. Bull.*, **2**, 407 (1932)
Barger, Sargent., *J. Chem. Soc.*, 991 (1939)

ARTABOTRININE

$C_{18}H_{17}O_3N$

M.p. Indefinite

OMe

An amorphous aporphine alkaloid from *Artabotyris suaveolens* Blume, this base has $[\alpha]_D^{18} - 18.9°$ (c 2.69, CHCl$_3$) and forms a crystalline hydrochloride, m.p. 273–4°C. It also gives a nitroso-derivative as hexagonal plates, m.p. 203–4°C and an N-methyl derivative, m.p. 132–3°C; $[\alpha]_D^{16} - 53.8°$ (c 0.424, EtOH) yielding a methiodide, m.p. 223–4°C.

Maranon., *Philipp. J. Sci.*, **38**, 259 (1928)

ARTARINE

$C_{21}H_{23}O_4N$

M.p. Indefinite

This alkaloid obtained from *Zanthoxylum senegalense* DC (syn. *Fagara xanthoxyloides*) is amorphous but yields crystalline salts: hydrochloride (4 H$_2$O), yellow crystals, m.p. 194°C and platinichloride, yellow needles, m.p. 290°C.

Giacosa, Monari., *Gazzetta*, **17**, 362 (1887)
Giacosa, Soave., *ibid*, **19**, 303 (1889)

ASARINE

This uncharacterized alkaloid is stated to be present in the roots of *Asarum europeum* L to the extent of 1.7 per cent. It is said to produce nausea, emesis and acceleration of respiration in rabbits, frogs and dogs.

Abdul'menev., *Farmatsiya*, 8, 39 (1945)

ASIMILOBINE

$C_{17}H_{17}O_2N$

M.p. 177–9°C

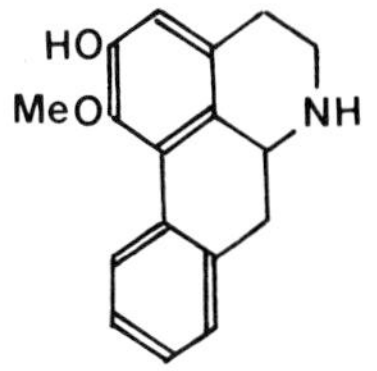

Isolated from *Asimina triloba* Dunal and certain species of *Popowia*, the alkaloid crystallizes from Me_2CO with $[\alpha]_D^{14} - 213°$ (c 0.64, $CHCl_3$). The O,N-diacetyl derivative forms crystals from Et_2O-$CHCl_3$, m.p. 146°C.

Tomita, Kozuka., *J. Pharm. Soc. Japan*, 85, 77 (1965)
Johns, Lamberton, Li, Sioumis., *Austral. J. Chem.*, 23, 363 (1970)

ASIMININE

An uncharacterized alkaloid present in *Anona triloba* Dunal, this base is amorphous but is said to yield crystalline salts.

Lloyd., *Arch. Pharm.*, 25, 503 (1887)
Fletcher., *Amer. J. Pharm.*, 476 (1891)

ASPERUMINE

$C_{18}H_{25}O_4N$

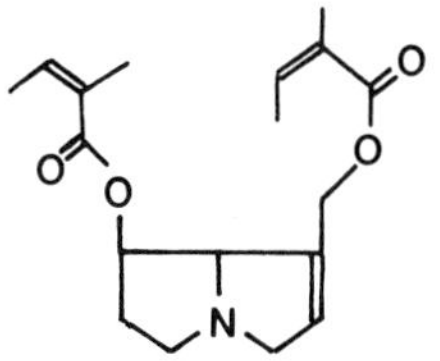

This pyrrolizidine alkaloid occurs in *Symphytum asperum* and forms a crystalline picrate, m.p. 135–7°C and picrolonate, m.p. 169–171°C.

Man'ko, Kotovskii., *J. Gen. Chem. USSR*, 40, 2519 (1970)

ASPIDOALBIDINE

$C_{19}H_{24}ON_2$

M.p. 180°C

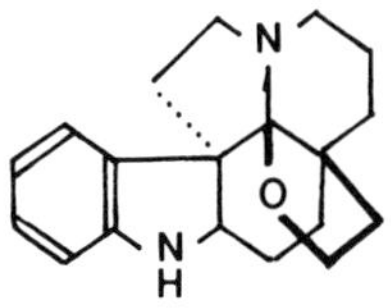

This base does not occur naturally, but it is of importance in being the parent structure of a large group of alkaloids. It is difficult to obtain in a crystalline form.

Brown, Budzikiewicz, Djerassi., *Tetrahedron Lett.*, 1731 (1963)

ASPIDOALBINE

$C_{24}H_{32}O_5N_2$

M.p. 174–7°C

The stem bark of both *Aspidosperma album* (Vahl) R. Bent. and *A. spruceanum* Benth yields this alkaloid which forms colourless prisms; $[\alpha]_D^{25} + 164°$ (c 2.12, CHCl$_3$). In the ultraviolet spectrum, the absorption maxima appear at 227 and 267 mμ. The O-methyl ether has m.p. 128–131°C; $[\alpha]_D^{25} + 9.2°$ (c 1.84, MeOH).

Djerassi, Antonaccio, Budzikiewicz, Wilson, Gilbert., *Tetrahedron Lett.*, 1001 (1962)
Ferrari, MacLean, Marion, Palmer., *Can. J. Chem.*, **41**, 1531 (1963)
Gilbert, Duarte, Nakagawa, Joule, Flores, Brissolese, Campello, Carrazzoni, Owellen, Blossey, Brown, Djerassi., *Tetrahedron*, **21**, 1141 (1965)

ASPIDOCARPINE

$C_{22}H_{30}O_3N_2$

M.p. 168.5–169.5°C

This *Aspidosperma* alkaloid occurs in the root bark of *A. megalacarpon* Muell Arg. It crystallizes as colourless prisms from MeOH and has $[\alpha]_D^{25} + 140°$ (c 2.3, CHCl$_3$). It forms several salts: the hydrochloride, m.p. 224–230°C (*dec.*); hydrobromide (0.5 H$_2$O), m.p. 288–290°C; hydriodide, m.p. 272–4°C (*dec.*); perchlorate, m.p. 280–2°C (*dec.*); the O-acetyl derivative, m.p. 165–7°C; $[\alpha]_D^{25} - 8.4°$ (c 0.81, CHCl$_3$) and the O-methyl ether, m.p. 152–4°C; $[\alpha]_D^{25} - 94°$ (c 1.5, CHCl$_3$).

MacLean, Palmer, Marion., *Can. J. Chem.*, **38**, 1547 (1960)

ASPIDODASYCARPINE

$C_{21}H_{26}O_4N_2$

M.p. 207–9°C

This alkaloid was originally isolated from *Aspidosperma dasycarpon* A. DC. and subsequently from *A. cuspa*. It forms colourless crystals from Me_2CO with $[\alpha]_D - 101°$ (c 1.42, $CHCl_3$). The ultraviolet spectrum exhibits two absorption maxima at 240 and 297 mμ. A crystalline diacetate has been prepared, m.p. 111–4°C; $[\alpha]_D - 35°$ (c 1.42, $CHCl_3$). The structure has been determined primarily from mass spectroscopic evidence.

Ohashi, Joule, Djerassi., *Tetrahedron Lett.*, 3899 (1964)
Burnell, Medina., *Phytochem.*, 7, 2045 (1968)

Mass spectra:
Joule, Ohashi, Gilbert, Djerassi., *Tetrahedron,* 21, 1717 (1965)

16-epi-ASPIDODASYCARPINE (*Lonicerine*)

$C_{21}H_{26}O_4N_2$

M.p. 105–7°C

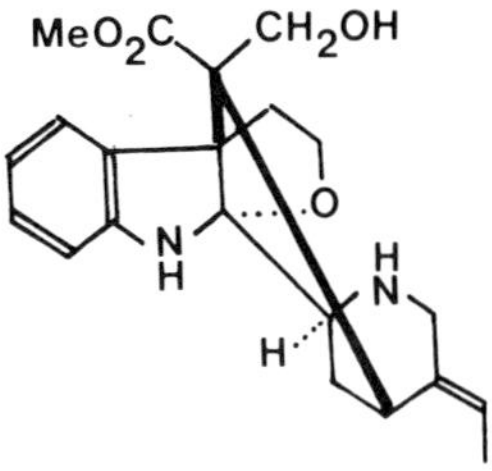

The epimer of Aspidodasycarpine occurs in *Callichilia barteri* and forms colourless plates from hexane-Me_2CO. It has $[\alpha]_D^{24} - 127°$ (c 0.98, $CHCl_3$). The ultraviolet spectrum in ethanol solution has absorption maxima at 244 and 295 mμ.

Naranjo, Hesse, Schmid., *Helv. Chim. Acta,* 53, 749 (1970)

ASPIDODISPERMINE

$C_{19}H_{24}O_3N_2$

M.p. Indefinite

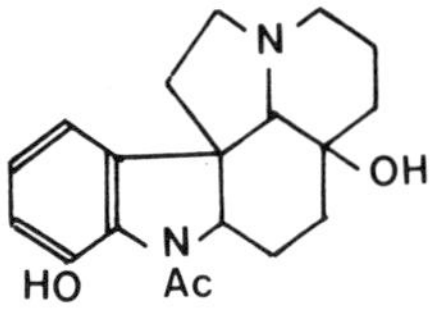

An amorphous base obtained from *Aspidosperma dispermum*, this alkaloid has $[\alpha]_D + 119°$ (MeOH). The ultraviolet spectrum shows absorption maxima at 219, 260 and 290 mμ in MeOH. In NaOH-MeOH solution, there is a peak at 302 mμ. The O-methyl ether has m.p. 189–190°C; $[\alpha]_D - 43°$ (MeOH) and the 17-acetate is amorphous.

Ikeda, Djerassi., *Tetrahedron Lett.*, 5837 (1968)

ASPIDOFILINE

$C_{20}H_{26}O_2N_2$

M.p. 186–7°C ·

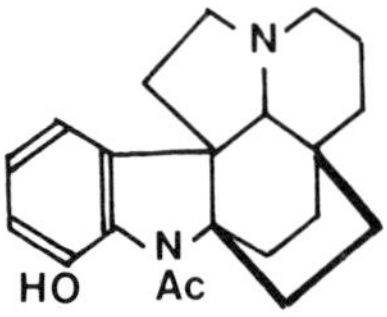

From *Aspidosperma pyrifolium* Mart. this alkaloid is obtained as colourless needles, $[\alpha]_D^{20} - 174°$ (CHCl₃). The ultraviolet spectrum shows absorption maxima at 231 and 308 mμ in alcoholic KOH solution. The picrate crystallizes from Me₂CO with m.p. 146°C; the O-acetyl derivative has m.p. 179–181°C; $[\alpha]_D^{30} + 53°$ (CHCl₃) and the methyl ether is an oil, b.p. 175°C/7 X 10⁻⁶ mm.

Antonaccio., *J. Org. Chem.*, **25**, 1262 (1960)
Djerassi *et al.*, *Experientia*, **18**, 397 (1962)

ASPIDOFRACTINE (*N-Formylkopsine*)

$C_{22}H_{26}O_3N$

M.p. 193–193.5°C

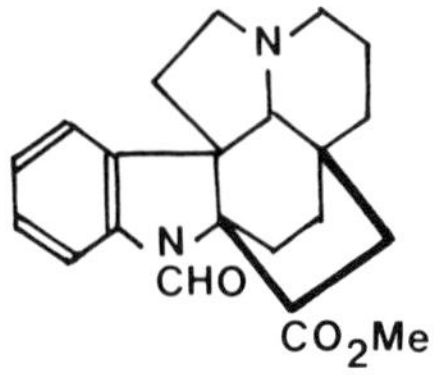

This alkaloid is a constituent of *Aspidosperma refractum* Mart. It has $[\alpha]_D - 142°$ (CHCl₃).

Djerassi *et al.*, *J. Amer. Chem. Soc.*, **84**, 1499 (1962)

ASPIDOFRACTININE

$C_{19}H_{24}N_2$

M.p. 101–2°C;
B.p. 110°C/0.001 mm

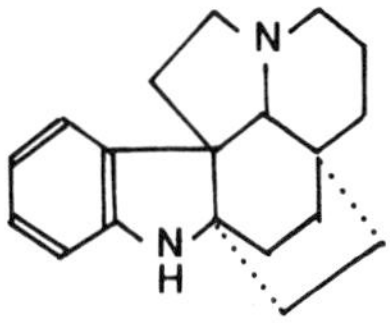

This base is present in *Aspidosperma refractum* Mart. and also in *Pleiocarpa tubicina* Stapf. The crude alkaloid is an oil which can be crystallized from pentane. In the ultraviolet spectrum the absorption maxima occur at 241 and 391 mμ. The N-acetyl derivative has b.p. 125°C/0.001 mm but may be crystallized from Me₂CO with m.p. 127–130°C.

Djerassi, Budzikiewicz, Owellen, Wilson, Kump, Le Court, Battersby, Schmid., *Helv. Chim. Acta,* **46**, 742 (1963)
Bycroft, Schumann, Patel, Schmid., *ibid*, **47**, 1147 (1964)

ASPIDOLIMIDINE

$C_{22}H_{28}O_4N_2$

M.p. 196–9°C

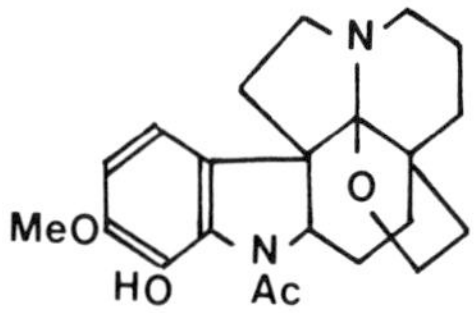

Found in *Aspidosperma limae* Woodson, this base has $[\alpha]_D + 239°$ (CHCl₃).

Gilbert *et al.*, *Chem. & Ind.*, 1949 (1962)

ASPIDOLIMINE

$C_{23}H_{32}O_3N_2$

M.p. 150–1°C

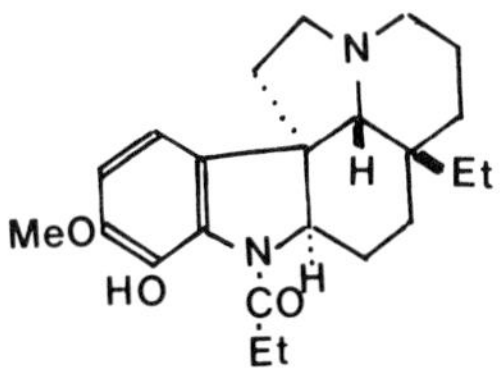

A second alkaloid found in *Aspidosperma limae* Woodson, this base has $[\alpha]_D^{21}$ + 133° ± 3° (c 1.156, CHCl$_3$). It forms a crystalline hydrochloride from Et$_2$O-AcOEt, m.p. 200–5°C (*dec.*); a picrate, m.p. 189–192°C and the O-acetate which is an oil but yields a crystalline picrate, m.p. 193–193.5°C (*dec.*).

Pinar, Schmid., *Helv. Chim. Acta*, 45, 1283 (1962)
Gilbert *et al.*, *Chem. & Ind.*, 1949 (1962)

ASPIDOSAMINE

$C_{20}H_{28}O_2N_2$

One of the Quebracho alkaloids, this base is said to occur in *Aspidosperma quirandy* Hassler according to Floriani and also in A. *quebracho blanco* Schlecht f. *pendulae* Speg. The above formula was assigned to the alkaloid by Floriani.

Floriani., *Rev. Cent. Estud. Farm. Bioquim.*, 25, 373, 423 (1935)

ASPIDOSPERMATINE

$C_{21}H_{26}O_2N_2$

M.p. 162°C

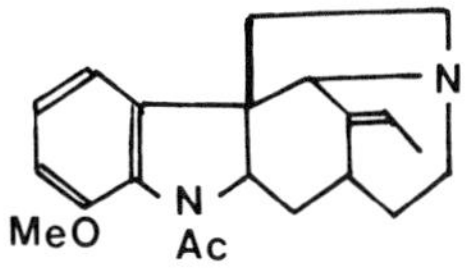

This alkaloid was first isolated by Hesse from *Aspidosperma quebracho blanco* and has $[\alpha]_D$ − 72.3° (EtOH). The platinichloride (4 H$_2$O) is amorphous.

Hesse., *Annalen*, 211, 249 (1882)
Biemann, Spiteller-Friedmann, Spiteller., *J. Amer. Chem. Soc.*, 85, 631 (1963)

ASPIDOSPERMICINE

$C_{17}H_{24}ON$

This base occurs along with aspidosamine in *Aspidosperma quebracho blanco*. It crystallizes with 1.5 H$_2$O. The structure has not yet been elucidated.

Floriani., *Rev. Farm.* (Buenos Aires), 80, 47, 135 (1938)

ASPIDOSPERMIDINE

$C_{19}H_{26}N_2$

M.p. 110–2°C

One of the alkaloids isolated from *Aspidosperma quebracho blanco* Schlecht f. *pendulae* Speg. The (±)-form has been synthesized using 4-ethyl-4-formylkept-6-enoate as the starting material. This synthesis appears to be entirely stereospecific, the skeletal rearrangement being considered to be initiated by the formation of a carbonium ion at C-16 of the tetracyclic lactam formed as an intermediate.

Synthesis:
Harley-Mason, Kaplan., *Chem. Commun.*, 915 (1967)
Kutney, Abdurahman, Gletsos, LeQuesne, Piers, Vlattas., *J. Amer. Chem. Soc.*, **92**, 1727 (1970)

Mass spectra:
Biemann, Spiteller-Friedmann, Spiteller., *Tetrahedron Lett.*, 485 (1961)
Biemann, Spiteller-Friedmann, Spiteller., *J. Amer. Chem. Soc.*, **85**, 631 (1963)

ASPIDOSPERMINE

$C_{22}H_{30}O_2N_2$

M.p. 208°C

This alkaloid is widely distributed among the *Aspidosperma* and *Vallesia* species, being found in *A. quebracho blanco* Schlecht, *A. quirandy*, *V. dichotoma* and *V. glabra*. The base forms colourless needles from EtOH with the above melting point and boiling at 220°C/1–2 mm. It has $[\alpha]_D^{18}$ – 99° (EtOH) or – 93° (CHCl$_3$), and is readily soluble in C_6H_6, CHCl$_3$, moderately so in EtOH and only sparingly soluble in H_2O. The solution in concentrated H_2SO_4 is colourless. The alkaloid is only feebly basic and does not form crystalline salts.

On boiling with dilute HCl, the alkaloid yields acetic acid and deacetylaspidospermine, $C_{20}H_{28}ON_2$, colourless needles, m.p. 110–1°C, b.p. 210°C/1–2 mm. $[\alpha]_D$ + 2.8° (EtOH). This compound forms crystalline salts, e.g. the hydriodide, m.p. 235–243°C; a benzoyl derivative, m.p. 186–7°C; dimethiodide, m.p. 176–7°C. Oxidation of aspidospermine with chromic acid furnishes a base, $C_{15}H_{24}O_2N_2$, stout prisms from AcOEt, m.p. 192–3°C.

Ewins., *J. Chem. Soc.*, **105**, 2738 (1914)
Field., *ibid*, **125**, 1444 (1924)
Deulofeu *et al.*, *Chem. Abstr.*, **32**, 2135 (1938)
Witkop., *J. Amer. Chem. Soc.*, **70**, 3712 (1948)
Openshaw, Smith., *Experientia*, **4**, 428 (1948)
Conroy *et al.*, *J. Amer. Chem. Soc.*, **79**, 1763 (1957)

Chalmers, Openshaw, Smith., *J. Chem. Soc.,* 1115 (1957)
Everett, Openshaw, Smith., *ibid,* 1120 (1957)
Mill, Nyburg., *ibid,* 1458 (1960)
Smith, Wrobel., *ibid,* 1463 (1960)
Ling, Djerassi., *Tetrahedron Lett.,* 3015 (1970)

ASTROCASINE

$C_{20}H_{26}ON_2$

M.p. 171–2°C

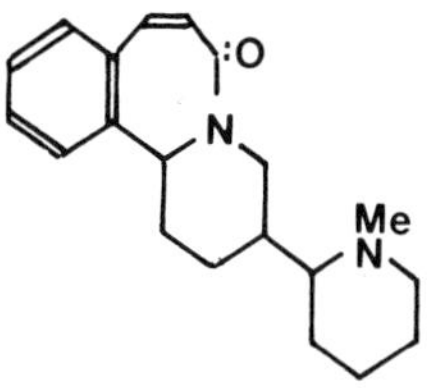

This alkaloid has been isolated from *Astrocasia phyllantoides* and has $[\alpha]_D^{24}$ – 270° (EtOH). The ultraviolet spectrum exhibits one absorption maximum at 263 mμ. It forms crystalline salts and derivatives, e.g. the perchlorate, colourless needles, m.p. 149–151°C and the methiodide, m.p. 227–8°C. The structure has been determined mainly on the basis of infrared, NMR and mass spectrometry.

Lloyf., *Tetrahedron Lett.,* 1761 (1965)

ASTROPHYLLINE

$C_{19}H_{26}ON_2$

B.p. 115°C/0.001 mm

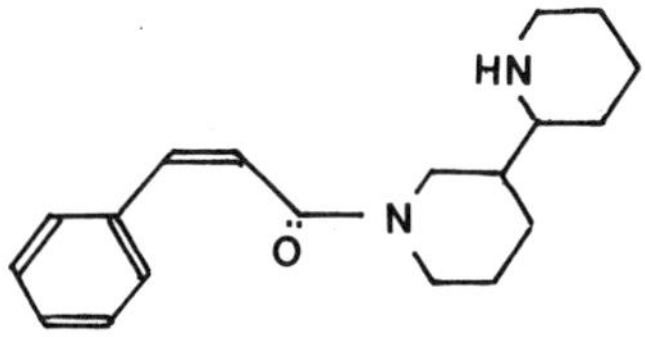

Obtained as a viscous oil from *Astrocasia phyllantoides,* this base has an ultra-violet spectrum similar to that of the preceding alkaloid with an absorption maximum at 254 mμ. It also forms crystalline salts and derivatives, e.g. the perchlorate, m.p. 172–4°C; picrate, m.p. 146–8°C (*dec.*). The N-methyl derivative is also an oil with $[\alpha]_D$ + 92° (EtOH) which yields a crystalline perchlorate with m.p. 152–4°C.

Lloyd., *Tetrahedron Lett.,* 4537 (1965)

ATALANTINE

$C_{34}H_{30}O_9N_2$

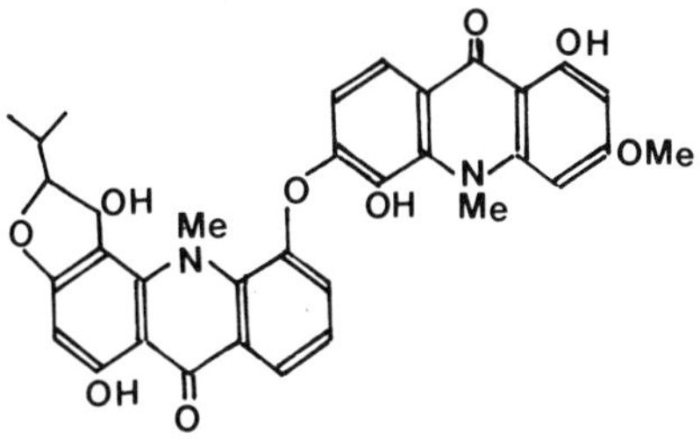

This complex diacridone alkaloid has recently been isolated from *Atalantia ceylanica*. The structure has been determined on the basis of spectroscopic evidence, particularly the mass spectral fragmentation patterns.

Fraser, Lewis., *J. Chem. Soc., Chem. Commun.*, 615 (1973)

ATALINE

$C_{38}H_{35}O_9N_2$

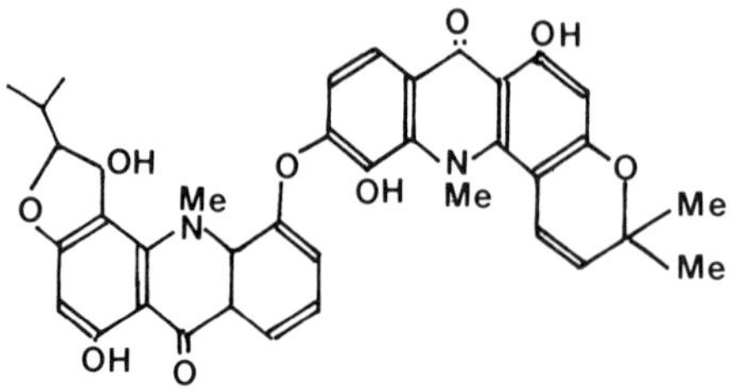

An alkaloid similar in structure to the preceding base, also present in *Atalantia ceylanica*. The structure has been determined in a similar manner from the mass spectra.

Fraser, Lewis., *J. Chem. Soc., Chem. Commun.*, 615 (1973)

ATALAPHYLLINE

$C_{23}H_{25}O_4N$

M.p. 246°C

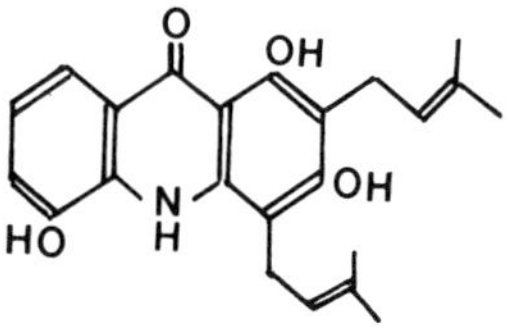

An acridone alkaloid from the root bark of *Atalantia monophylla* Correa, the base crystallizes from AcOEt-C_6H_6 as yellow needles. The solution in EtOH gives an ultraviolet spectrum with absorption maxima at 255, 265, 285, 312 and 402 mμ. The 3:5-di-O-methyl ether also forms yellow needles from Et$_2$O-hexane with m.p. 145–7°C. The structure has been assigned on the basis of chemical degradations and spectroscopic investigation. The N-methyl derivative also occurs naturally in *Atalantia monophylla*.

Govindachari *et al.*, *Tetrahedron*, **26**, 2906 (1970)

ATANINE

$C_{15}H_{19}O_2N$

M.p. 134°C

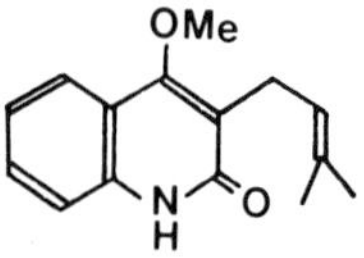

A quinolone alkaloid present in *Ravenia spectabilis*, the structure has been established from spectroscopic data. Treatment with HBr in AcOH gives dihydroflindersine.

Paul, Bose., *J. Ind. Chem. Soc.*, **45**, 552 (1968)

ATHEROLINE

$C_{19}H_{15}O_5N$

M.p. 250–260°C (*dec.*).

This oxodibenzoquinoline alkaloid was first isolated from the phenolic extract of *Atherosperma moschatum* Labill. It has also been found as a constituent of the bark of the New Caledonian monimiaceous plant *Nemuaron vieillardii* together with Laurotetanine, N-methyllaurotetanine and Norisocorydine. The alkaloid is purified by column chromatography followed by recrystallization from Et_2O-MeOH when it yields irregularly-shaped yellow crystals. In EtOH solution, the ultraviolet spectrum exhibits absorption maxima at 244, 273, 292 (shoulder), 355, 380 (shoulder), and 435 mμ. In 0.05 N/NaOH, the absorption maxima are found at 252, 294, 320, 390 and 535 mμ while in 0.5 N/HCl, they occur at 257, 282, 385 and 500 mμ. With Ac_2O in pyridine, the base yields the O-acetyl derivative, $C_{21}H_{17}O_6N$, as yellow needles, m.p. 190–5°C.

Bick, Douglas., *Tetrahedron Lett.*, 28, 2399 (1965)
Bick, Bowie, Douglas., *Austral. J. Chem.*, 20, 1403 (1967)

ATHEROSPERMIDINE (*Psilopine*)

$C_{18}H_{13}O_4N$

M.p. 276–8°C (*dec.*).

This aporphine base also occurs both in *Atherosperma moschatum* Labill. and *Guatteria psilopus*. It crystallizes as yellow needles from pyridine or $CHCl_3$. The hydrochloride forms deep-red needles, m.p. 256–8°C (*dec.*). The structure given has been confirmed by synthesis.

Bick, Clezy, Crow., *Austral. J. Chem.*, 9, 111 (1956)
Bick, Douglas., *Tetrahedron Lett.*, 1629 (1964)
Bick, Douglas., *Austral. J. Chem.*, 18, 1997 (1965)

Mass spectra:
Bick, Bowie, Douglas., *Austral. J. Chem.*, 20, 1403 (1967)

Synthesis:
Pai, Shanmugasundram., *Tetrahedron*, 21, 2579 (1965)

ATHEROSPERMINE

$C_{30}H_{40}O_5N_2$

This alkaloid was isolated from *Atherosperma moschatum* Labill and assigned the above formula by Zeyer. It is stated to be an amorphous powder which could not be crystallized.

Zeyer., *Vjschr. prakt. Pharm.*, **10**, 504 (1861)

ATHEROSPERMOLINE

$C_{35}H_{36}O_6N_2$

M.p. 183–8°C

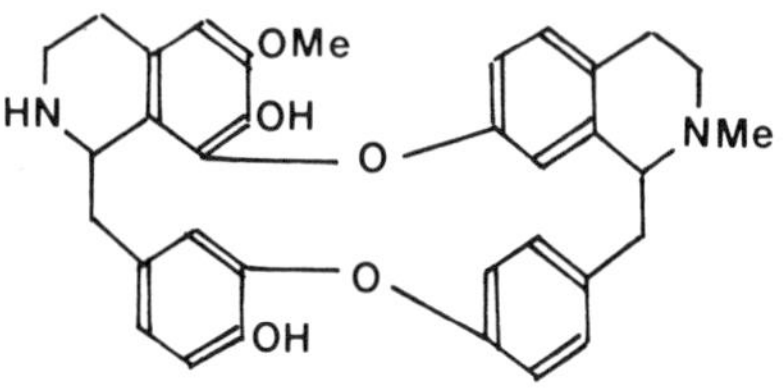

A bisbenzyl*iso*quinoline alkaloid, also from *Atherosperma moschatum* Labill. this base crystallizes from $CHCl_3$ as colourless prisms which contain solvate of crystallization. It has $[\alpha]_D^{18} + 202°$ (c 0.15, $CHCl_3$). The ultraviolet spectrum shows one absorption maximum at 284 mμ.

Bick, Douglas., *Chem. & Ind.*, 695 (1965)

ATIDINE

$C_{22}H_{33}O_3N$

M.p. 182.5–183.5°C

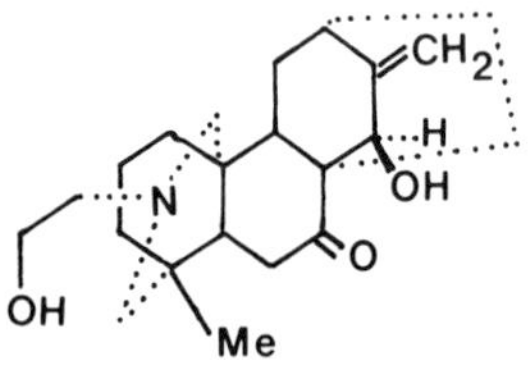

One of the aconite alkaloids found in the roots of *Aconitum heterophyllum*, this base has $[\alpha]_D^{29} - 47°$. It forms a crystalline hydrochloride, m.p. 204–215°C and a diacetyl derivative, colourless crystals from Me_2CO, m.p. 182–190°C. On reduction, the base furnishes dihydroatidine, m.p. 156–9°C; $[\alpha]_D^{27} - 44°$ ($CHCl_3$); diacetate, m.p. 122.5–123.5°C; $[\alpha]_D^{27} - 82°$ ($CHCl_3$).

Pelletier., *Chem. & Ind.*, 1016 (1956)
Pelletier., *ibid*, 1670 (1957)
Solo, Pelletier., *ibid*, 1108 (1960)
Vorbrüggen, Djerassi., *J. Amer. Chem. Soc.*, **84**, 2999 (1962)

Stereochemistry:
Pelletier., *J. Amer. Chem. Soc.*, **87**, 799 (1965)

184

ATISINE (*Anthorine*)

$C_{22}H_{33}O_2N$

M.p. 57–60°C

The major constituent of *Aconitum heterophyllum*, this base also occurs in
other *Aconitum* species. Atisine forms a colourless varnish that can be sublimed
in a molecular still to form an opaque film with the above melting point. It is
unstable in solution, especially in alkalies. The salts crystallize well: hydrochloride, m.p. 311–2°C (*dec.*); $[\alpha]_D^{25} + 28°$ (H_2O); hydrobromide, m.p. 273°C;
$[\alpha]_D + 24.3°$ (H_2O) and hydriodide, m.p. 279°C (*dec.*); $[\alpha]_D + 27.4°$ (H_2O).
The aurichloride is amorphous while the platinichloride forms a microcrystalline
powder. The Diacetate gives a crystalline hydrochloride, m.p. 241–3°C (*dec.*).

Mild hydrolysis with MeOH/KOH gives *iso*atisine, m.p. 150–1°C forming a
hydrochloride, m.p. 295–9°C (*dec.*) while more drastic treatment with the same
reagent yields a mixture of dihydro derivatives, one of which has been isolated
as $C_{22}H_{35}O_2N$, m.p. 171–4°C. Dehydrogenation with Se furnishes a mixture of
1-methylphenanthrene and 1-methyl-6-ethyl-phenanthrene. With Br_2, the
alkaloid forms a bromo-derivative, m.p. 172–5°C; $[\alpha]_D^{30} - 38°$ ($CHCl_3$).
Hydrogenation with PtO_2 gives the tetrahydro compound. Compared with the
aconitines, atisine is relatively non-toxic.

Broughton., 'Cinchona Cultivation in East India', 133 (1877)
Wasowicz., *Arch. Pharm.*, **214**, 193 (1879)
Lawson, Toffs., *J. Chem. Soc.*, 1640 (1937)
Goris., *Compt. rend.*, **205**, 1007 (1937)
Jacobs, Craig., *J. Biol. Chem.*, **143**, 589 (1942)
Jacobs., *J. Org. Chem.*, **16**, 1593 (1951)
Edwards, Singh., *Can. J. Chem.*, **32**, 465 (1954)
Edwards, Singh., *ibid*, **33**, 448 (1955)
Pelletier., *J. Amer. Chem. Soc.*, **82**, 2398 (1960)
Vorbrüggen, Djerassi., *J. Amer. Chem. Soc.*, **84**, 2990 (1962)
Apsimon, Edwards, Howe., *Can. J. Chem.*, **40**, 630, 896 (1962)

Total synthesis:
Nagata *et al.*, *J. Amer. Chem. Soc.*, **85**, 2342 (1963)
Masamune., *ibid*, **86**, 291 (1964)

Stereochemistry:
Dvornik, Edwards., *Can. J. Chem.*, **42**, 137 (1964)

ATROPINE

$C_{17}H_{23}O_3N$

M.p. 118°C

This alkaloid normally occurs only in minute quantities in solanaceous plants,
e.g. *Atropa belladonna* and *Datura stramonium* and it is considered possible that

185

it is formed by racemisation of (−)-hyoscyamine during the extraction process. It is soluble to varying degrees in organic solvents, sparingly soluble in H_2O and insoluble in petroleum ether. It is optically inactive and a strong base forming crystalline salts. The hydrobromide forms slender needles, m.p. 163−4°; the oxalate, minute prisms, m.p. 198°C; platinichloride, monoclinic crystals, m.p. 207−8°C; aurichloride, an oil which solidifies on standing, m.p. 137−9°C; picrate, m.p. 175−6°C; sulphate (1 H_2O), m.p. 194°C (*dry*); methobromide, m.p. 223−5°C and methonitrate, m.p. 166−8°C. The last three compounds are those normally used in medicine.

Atropine is very readily hydrolyzed with alkalies, dilute acids and even H_2O. With $Ba(OH)_2$ or concentrated HCl in a sealed tube, it is completely resolved into tropine, $C_8H_{15}ON$, and tropic acid, $C_9H_{10}O_3$. Several syntheses of atropine have been reported. These include more recent syntheses with isotopically-labelled carbon in the molecule.

When administered internally in toxic doses, atropine first stimulates and then eventually depresses the central nervous system, giving rise to hallucinations, delirium and convulsions, followed by coma. The alkaloid is employed principally in medicine as a mydriatic to cause dilatation of the pupil of the eye. It may also be used where paralysis of parasympathetic nervouc activity is desired as in bronchial or intestinal spasms.

Mein., *Annalen,* **6**, 67 (1833)
Geiger, Hesse., *ibid,* **5**, 33 (1833)
von Planta., *Arch. Pharm.,* **74**, 245 (1850)
Gadamer., *ibid,* **239**, 294 (1901)
Schmidt, Eling., *U.S. Clearinghouse Fed. Sci. Tech. Inform.,* AD 657787 (1967)
Eling, McOwen, Schmidt., *J. Pharm. Sci.,* **57**, 1357 (1968)

AUREINE

$C_{18}H_{25}O_5N$

M.p. 232°C

This alkaloid, isolated from *Senecio aureus,* has been shown to be identical with senecionine (q.v.).

Manske., *Can. J. Res.,* **14**, 6 (1936)
Barger, Blackie., *J. Chem. Soc.,* 584 (1937)

AURICULARINE

$C_{42}H_{55}ON_5$

M.p. 201°C (*dec.*).

Isolated in small quantity from *Hedyotis auricularia* Linn., the alkaloid crystallizes from aqueous EtOH with 1 H_2O. It is said to form an oxalate, m.p. > 230°C (*dec.*) and a picrate, m.p. 217−8°C (*dec.*). The structure has not yet been elucidated.

Ratnagiriswaran, Venkatachalam., *J. Ind. Chem. Soc.,* **19**, 389 (1942)

AURICULINE

$C_{31}H_{45}O_8N$

M.p. Indefinite

A base obtained from *Liparis auriculata* Blume, this alkaloid forms an amorphous powder which cannot be crystallized. It has $[\alpha]_D^{20} - 19.9°$ (MeOH). The ultraviolet spectrum in MeOH solution shows one absorption maximum at 246 mμ. Alkaline hydrolysis yields glucose and 1β-hydroxymethyl-8Hβ-pyrrolizidine. The alkaloid forms a crystalline picrate, m.p. 97–100°C. Methylation yields the N-methyl ion identical with Kumokirine (q.v.).

Nishikawa, Hirata., *Tetrahedron Lett.*, 6289 (1968)

AUROTENSINE

M.p. 128°C

From the following Papaveraceous plants, Manske isolated this alkaloid which forms rhombic crystals with $[\alpha]_D - 69.9°$; *Corydalis aureus, C. ochotensis* Turez, *C. platycarpa* Makino, *Fumaria officinalis* L., *Glaucium flavum* Crantz, *G. serpieri* Heldr. According to Manske, the alkaloid appears to be an addition compound of l- and dl-scoulerine. Its identity with isoboldine has been suggested although this alkaloid gives a green-blue colour with concentrated H_2SO_4 whereas authentic aurotensince gives a purple colour with this reagent.

Manske., *Can. J. Res.,* **9**, 436 (1933)
Manske., *ibid,* **15**, 459 (1937)
Manske., *ibid,* **16**, 81 (1938)
Knörck., *Inaug. Diss. Marburg*, 1926
Slavik., *Collect. Czech. Chem. Commun.,* **33**, 323 (1968)

AUSTAMIDE

$C_{21}H_{21}O_3N_3$

This dioxopiperazine base occurs in *Aspergillus ustus*. Although possibly not an alkaloid in the strict sense of the definition it is included here for completeness. The structure has been determined from spectroscopic analysis and chemical data. It has been suggested that this base is formed from Alkaloid AU-III (q.v.).

Steyn., *Tetrahedron,* **29**, 107 (1973)

AUTUMNALINE

$C_{21}H_{27}O_5N$

M.p. 166–8°C

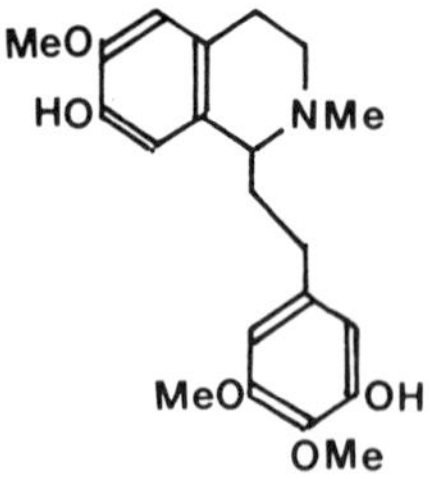

An isoquinoline alkaloid occurring in *Colchicum cornigerum* Tackh. et Drar., this base forms colourless crystals from AcOEt. The structure has been determined primarily from spectroscopic evidence.

Battersby *et al.*, *J. Chem. Soc., C*, 3514 (1971)

AVICINE

$C_{20}H_{14}O_4N^+$

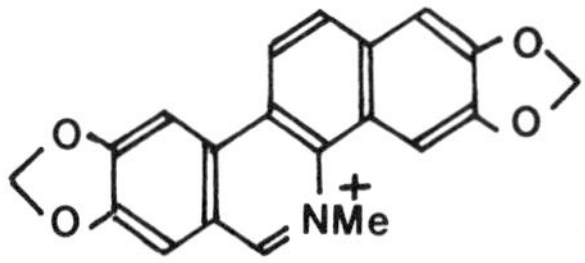

This quaternary alkaloid belongs to the naphthylphenanthridine type and is found in the root bark of *Zanthoxylum avicennae* (Lam.) DC. In the presence of alkali it disproportionates into oxyavicine and dihydroavicine, m.p. 211–212.5°C. It forms an acetate as yellow needles from EtOH, m.p. 160°C (*vac. dec.*). The pseudocyanide crystallizes as needles from EtOH with m.p. > 340°C.

Arthur, Hui, Ng., *J. Chem. Soc.*, 4007 (1959)

AXILLARIDINE

$C_{18}H_{27}O_6N$

M.p. 148–152°C (*dec.*).

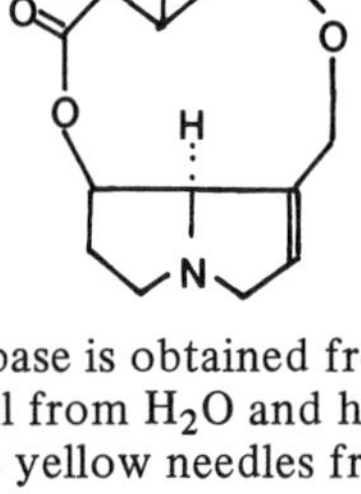

A pyrrolizidine alkaloid, this base is obtained from the seeds of *Crotalaria axillaris* Ait. It crystallizes well from H_2O and has $[\alpha]_{400}^{21}$ + 241° (c 0.12, MeOH). The picrate crystallizes as pale yellow needles from EtOH with m.p. 235°C (*dec.*).

Crout., *J. Chem. Soc., C*, 1379 (1969)

AXILLARINE

$C_{18}H_{27}O_7N$

M.p. 205°C (dec.).

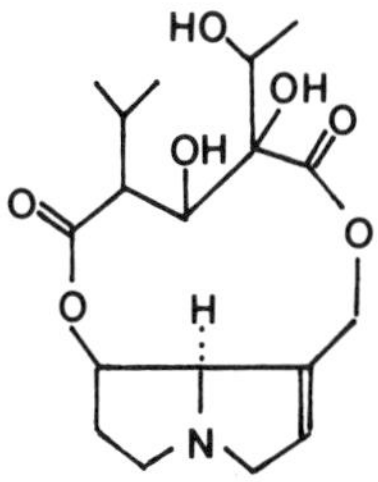

The major component of the seeds of *Crotalaria axillaris* Ait., this alkaloid crystallizes from $CHCl_3$-MeOH and has $[\alpha]_D^{20} + 65.1°$ (c 0.82, pyridine). The hydrochloride forms colourless needles from MeOH, m.p. 228°C. The picrate is also crystalline, m.p. 214–6°C (dec.). Hydrogenation of the base followed by hydrolysis gives retronecanol. The structure of the necic acid component represents a fifth member of the class of C_{10} necic acids and it has been suggested that it arises *in vivo* from *iso*leucine and valine, accompanied by the loss of the carboxyl group of the former. The structure of the alkaloid has been elucidated from infrared, NMR and mass spectral data.

Crout., *Chem. Commun.*, 429 (1968)
Crout., *J. Chem. Soc., C,* 1379 (1969)

(+)-AZA-1-METHYLBICYCLO 3,3,1-NONAN-3-ONE

$C_9H_{16}ON$

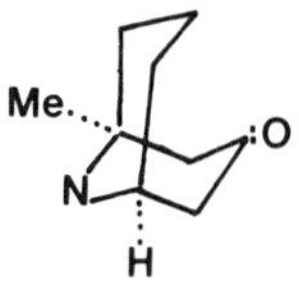

An alkaloid from *Euphorbia atoto,* the structure and absolute configuration have been assigned on the basis of spectroscopic and circular dichroism determinations. The C.D. spectrum shows a weak negative peak in the carbonyl absorption region indicating that the perturbing methyl substituent is separated from the chromophore.

Beecham, Johns, Lamberton., *Austral. J. Chem.*, **20**, 2291 (1967)

AZARIDINE

The fruit of *Melia azadirachta* L. is said to be toxic and to contain this alkaloid. So far, the base has not been characterized.

Carratala., *Rev. Assoc. med. Argentina,* **53**, 338 (1939)

AZCARPINE

$C_{26}H_{46}O_4N_2$

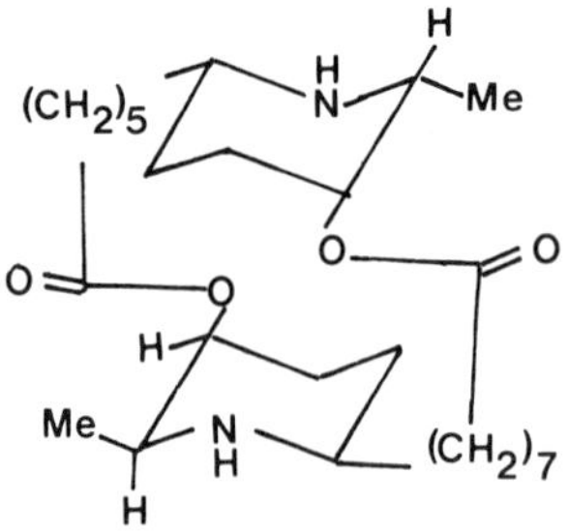

This alkaloid has been isolated from the leaf extract of *Azima tetracantha* Lam. One of the macrocyclic bases, it closely resembles Azimine (q.v.) in structure. The alkaloid itself cannot be crystallized.

Configuration:
Smalberger *et al.*, *Tetrahedron*, **24**, 6417 (1968)

Mass spectra:
Rall *et al.*, *Tetrahedron Lett.*, 3465 (1967)
Rall *et al.*, *ibid*, 896 (1968)

AZIMINE

$C_{24}H_{42}O_4N_2$

M.p. 112–3°C

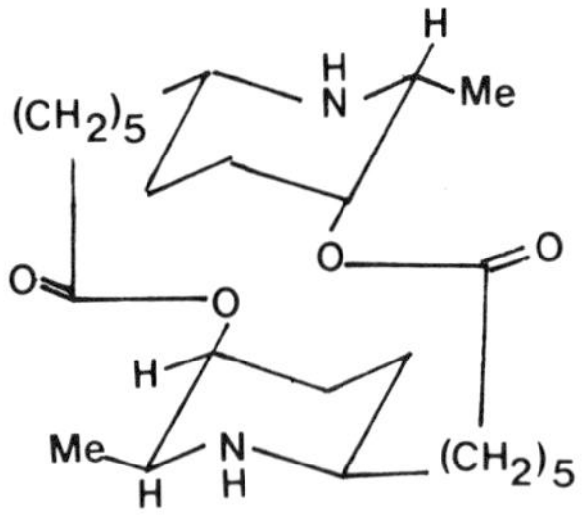

A second alkaloid obtained from the leaves of *Azima tetracantha* Lam., this base forms colourless crystals. A crystalline hydrochloride has been prepared, m.p. 284–7°C. The bis-N-methyl derivative is also crystalline with m.p. 92–3°C.

Configuration:
Smalberger, Rall, de Waal, Arndt., *Tetrahedron,* **24**, 6417 (1968)

Mass spectra:
Rall, Smalberger, de Waal, Arndt., *Tetrahedron Lett.*, 3465 (1967)
Rall, Smalberger, de Waal, Arndt., *ibid*, 896 (1968)

AZTEQUINE

$C_{36}H_{40}O_7N_2$

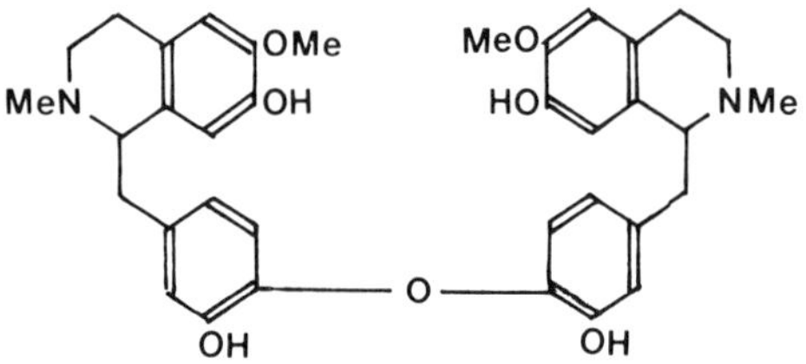

The leaves of *Talauma mexicana* Don. have been stated to have a nicotine-like action and to contain this alkaloid together with talaumine (q.v.). From the series of degradation products which have been obtained it is suggested that the alkaloid belongs to the bisbenzyl*iso*quinoline group.

Pallares, Garza., *Arch. Inst. Cardiol. Mex.,* **17**, 883 (1947)
Pallares, Garza., *Archiv. Biochem.,* **16**, 275 (1948)

B

BACANCOSINE

$C_{16}H_{23}O_8N.H_2O$

M.p. 157°C and 211°C

This glucosidic alkaloid is found in *Strychnos vacacoua* Baillon. Although discovered many years ago it has only comparatively recently been investigated in any detail. It forms colourless crystals from EtOH, melts at 157°C and then resolidifies, melting again at 211°C. It has $[\alpha]_D - 205.2°$. With dilute acids, it is hydrolyzed to *d*-glucose and an aglycone, $C_{10}H_{13}O_3N$. It is said to be non-toxic.

Bourquelot, Herissey., *Compt. rend.,* **144**, 575 (1907)
Bourquelot, Herissey., *ibid,* **147**, 750 (1908)
Bourquelot, Herissey., *J. Pharm. Chim.,* **25**, 417 (1907)
Bourquelot, Herissey., *ibid,* **28**, 433 (1908)
Bourquelot, Herissey., *Arch. Pharm.,* **247**, 857 (1909)
Balencovic *et al., Helv. Chim. Acta,* **35**, 2519 (1952)

BAIKEIDINE (*Baikeine 3-acetate*)

$C_{29}H_{47}O_4N$

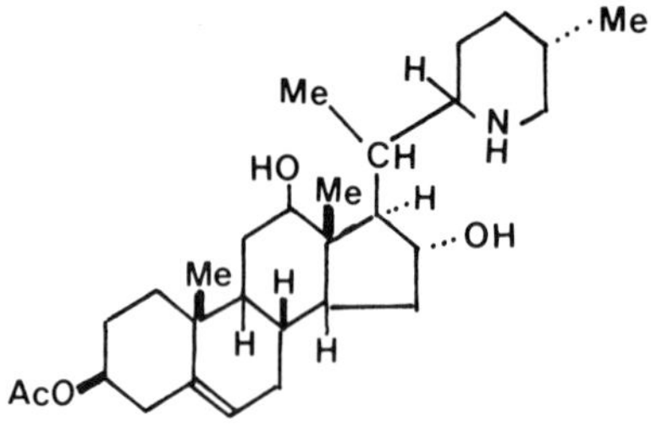

A minor constituent of *Veratrum grandiflorum,* this steroidal base has been shown to have the above structure on the basis of spectroscopic evidence.

Ito, Miyashita, Fukuzawa, Mori, Iwai, Yoshimura., *Tetrahedron Lett.,* 2961 (1972)

BAIKEINE

$C_{27}H_{45}O_3N$

M.p. 153–153.5°C

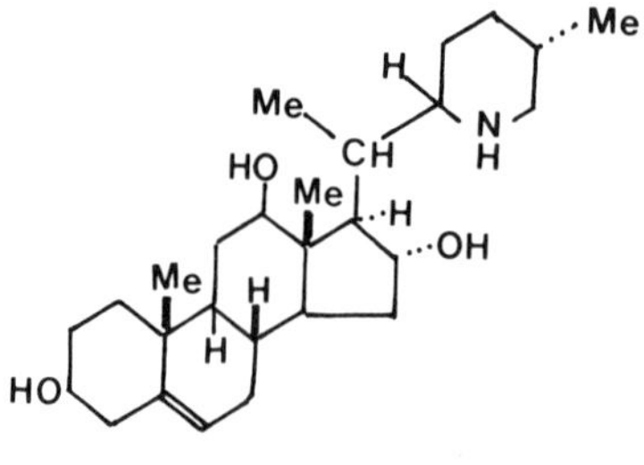

Isolated from *Veratrum grandiflorum*, this steroidal alkaloid has $[\alpha]_D$ $- 97.9°$. It forms a crystalline hydrochloride, m.p. 285°C; a picrate, m.p. 177.5–178°C; the N-acetyl derivative, m.p. 141–3°C and the tetraacetate, m.p. 230–4°C. The structure has been determined by spectroscopic techniques to be (22R,25S)-epiminocholest-5-ene-3β, 12α, 16-triol.

Ito, Miyashita, Fukuzawa, Mori, Iwai, Yoshimura., *Tetrahedron Lett.*, 2961 (1972)

BALEABUXINE (*N-Isobutyrylbaleabuxine F*)

$C_{30}H_{50}O_2N_2$

M.p. 258–9°C

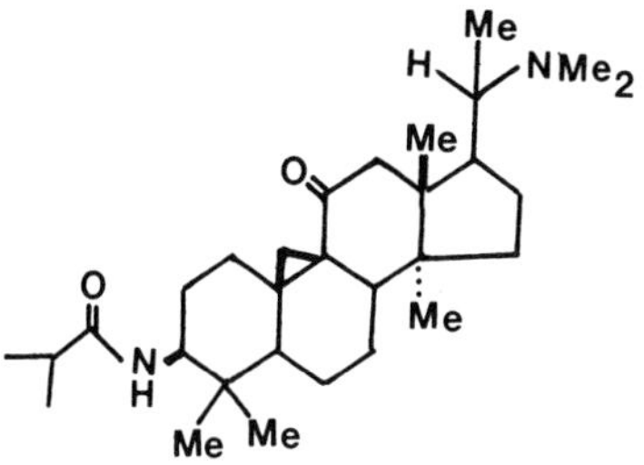

The various *Buxus* species yield a large number of closely-related alkaloids whose structures have been determined only in the last two decades. This alkaloid from *Buxus balearica* Willd. crystallizes from AcOEt as colourless needles with $[\alpha]_D$ $+ 115°$ (c 0.6, CHCl$_3$). The ultraviolet spectrum in dioxan shows an absorption maximum at 219 mμ. The structure had been determined from degradation and spectroscopic studies.

Herlem-Gaulier, Khuong-Huu-Laine, Stanislas, Goutarel., *Bull. soc. chim. Fr.*, 657 (1965)

BALEABUXOXAZINE C

$C_{27}H_{41}O_3N_2$

M.p. 292°C

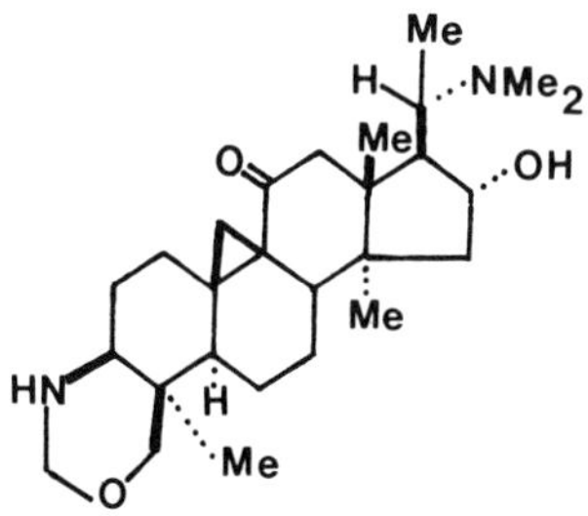

This base is also a constituent of *Buxus balearica* Willd., occurring mainly in the leaves of the plant. It has $[\alpha]_D$ $+ 116°$ (CHCl$_3$) and gives an ultraviolet spectrum virtually identical with that of the preceding alkaloid with the absorption maximum occurring at 219 mμ.

Khuong-Huu-Laine, Herlem-Gaulier, Khuong-Huu, Stanislas, Goutarel., *Tetrahedron*, 22, 3321 (1966)

BALFOURODINE

$C_{16}H_{19}O_4N$

M.p. 188–9°C

Obtained from *Balfourodendron riedelianum,* this furoquinolone alkaloid forms colourless crystals from C_6H_6-$CHCl_3$ with $[\alpha]_D + 49°$ (c 1.0, EtOH). The ultraviolet spectrum in MeOH shows several absorption maxima at 219, 241, 299, 312 and 325 mμ. That in 0.1 N/HCl-MeOH has absorption maxima at 214, 257, 299, 315 (shoulder) mμ. The (±)-form has m.p. 189–191°C and forms colourless prisms from AcOEt. It gives a crystalline perchlorate, crystallizing from Et_2O-MeOH with m.p. 212–3°C.

Rapoport, Holden., *J. Amer. Chem. Soc.,* **81**, 3738 (1959)
Rapoport, Holden., *ibid,* **82**, 4395 (1960)
Clarke, Grundon., *J. Chem. Soc.,* 4196 (1964)

BALOXINE

$C_{21}H_{24}O_4N_2$

M.p. Indefinite

Melodinus balansae Baill. yields this amorphous imidolizinocarbazole base. Infrared spectroscopy shows the presence of an imino and a secondary hydroxyl group in the molecule.

Mehri, Koch, Plat, Potier., *Bull. Soc. Chim. Fr.,* 3291 (1972)

BAPTIFOLINE

$C_{15}H_{20}O_2N_2$

M.p. 210°C

The Papilionaceae form a subgroup of the Leguminosae and yield a large number of alkaloids. This sparteine-type base is found in *Baptisia minor* Lehm. and also in *B. perfoliata* Linn., R. Br. It is readily soluble in EtOH and has $[\alpha]_D^{18} - 147.7°$ (c 0.325, EtOH). The diperchlorate is crystalline with m.p. 289.5°; $[\alpha]_D^{16} - 89.05°$ (c 1.415, H_2O); the picrate forms colourless crystals from MeOH with 1 mole of solvent, m.p. 145°C and 256°C (*dry*).

Marion, Turcotte., *J. Amer. Chem. Soc.,* **70**, 3253 (1948)
Bohlmann *et al., Chem. Ber.,* **95**, 944 (1962)

194

BAPTITOXINE

See Cytisine

BATRACHOTOXIN

$C_{31}H_{42}O_6N_2$

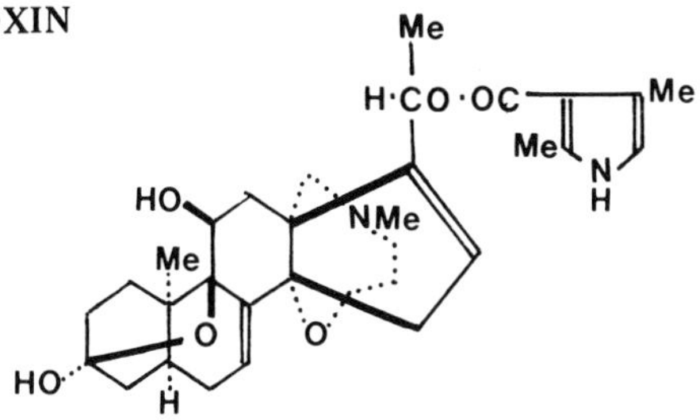

From the skin of *Phyllobates aurotaenia* (the Columbian arrow poison frog), this toxic alkaloid may be isolated as colourless crystals with $[\alpha]_D + 5°$ to $- 10°$; $[\alpha]_{300} - 260°$ (c 0.23, MeOH). The earlier formula of $C_{24}H_{33}O_4N$ has recently been revised to that given above. The ultraviolet spectrum in HCl-MeOH solution has two absorption maxima at 234 and 262 mμ. Hydrogenation with Pd-C gives the dihydro derivative. This alkaloid is said to be the most potent venom known at the present time.

Marki, Witkop., *Experientia*, **19**, 329 (1963)

Daly, Witkop, Bommer, Biemann., *J. Amer. Chem. Soc.*, **87**, 124 (1965)

Structure:

Tokuyama, Daly, Witkop., *J. Amer. Chem. Soc.*, **91**, 3931 (1969)

BATRACHOTOXININ A

$C_{24}H_{35}O_5N$

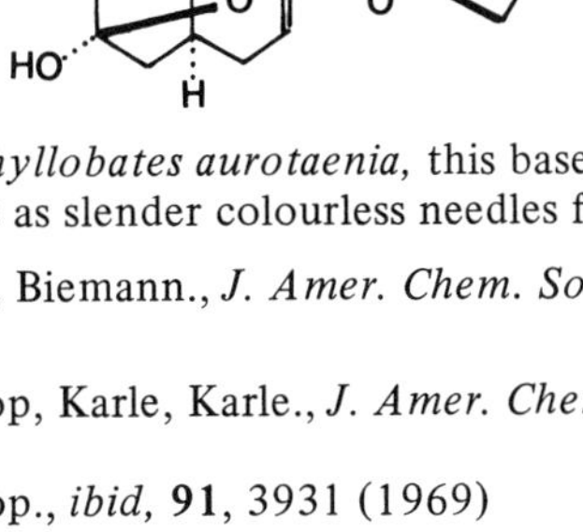

A second constituent of *Phyllobates aurotaenia,* this base forms a crystalline *p*-bromobenzoyl derivative as slender colourless needles from Me$_2$CO, m.p. 213°C.

Daly, Witkop, Bommer, Biemann., *J. Amer. Chem. Soc.*, **87**, 124 (1965)

Crystal structure:

Tokuyama, Daly, Witkop, Karle, Karle., *J. Amer. Chem. Soc.*, **90**, 1917 (1968)

Tokuyama, Daly, Witkop., *ibid*, **91**, 3931 (1969)

BEBEERINE B

$C_{22}H_{23}O_5N$

M.p. 220°C (*dec.*).

This name has been given to an alkaloid isolated from *Chondrodendron* platy-phyllum (St. Hill.) Miers. It is described as a yellow, amorphous powder with $[\alpha]_D + 56.7°$ and containing two hydroxyl, one methoxyl and one methylimino groups in the molecule. Fusion with KOH is said to give protocatechuic acid. The available data concerning this base almost certainly requires revision.

Scholtz., *Ber.*, **29**, 2054 (1896)
Scholtz., *Arch. Pharm.*, **236**, 530 (1898)
Scholtz, Koch., *Arch. Pharm.*, **252**, 513 (1914)
Faltis., *Monatsh.*, **33**, 873 (1912)
Faltis, Neumann., *ibid*, **42**, 311 (1921)

α-BEBEERINE

$C_{21}H_{23}O_4N$

M.p. 124–150°C

An amorphous base occurring in *Chondrodendron platyphyllum* (St. Hill.) Miers., this alkaloid has $[\alpha]_D^{21} + 28.6°$ (EtOH) or $- 24.7°$ (pyridine). It yields amorphous salts and is stated to contain one methoxyl, one hydroxyl and one methylimino group. According to Scholtz (1913) it has the formula $C_{18}H_{21}O_3N$ and furnishes a crystalline methiodide, m.p. 80°C (1 H_2O) or 258–9°C (*dry*). It has been suggested that this alkaloid may be a diastereoisomeride of curine (q.v.). As in the case of the preceding alkaloid, the data concerning this base is extremely confusing.

Scholtz., *Ber.*, **29**, 2054 (1896)
Scholtz., *Arch. Pharm.*, **251**, 136 (1913)
Faltis, Kadiera, Doblhammer., *Ber.*, **69**, 1271 (1936)

BELARINE

$C_{37}H_{40}O_6N_2$

M.p. 158–160°C

This bisbenzyl*iso*quinoline alkaloid has been isolated from the root bark of *Berberis laurina* Billb. It has $[\alpha]_D - 222°$ (c 0.2, $CHCl_3$).

Falco, de Vries, Maccio, Bick., *Chem. Commun.*, 1056 (1971)

196

BELLADINE

$C_{19}H_{25}O_3N$

MeO⟨⟩ ⟨⟩OMe
MeO⟨⟩CH$_2$·N·(CH$_2$)$_2$⟨⟩
       |
       Me

This amine base is present in several *Amaryllidaceae* species. It forms
crystalline salts and derivatives including the perchlorate, m.p. 128–129.5°C;
methiodide, m.p. 224–225.5°C and the picrate, m.p. 138.5–139.5°C.

Surrey *et al.*, *J. Amer. Chem. Soc.*, **71**, 2421 (1949)
Warnhoff., *Chem. & Ind.*, 1385 (1957)

BELLADONNINE

$C_{34}H_{42}O_4N_2$

M.p. 129°C

Hübschmann first isolated this base from the berries of *Hyoscyamus* species. A
subsequent examination by Kraut and Merling suggested that it was an isomer of
*apo*atropine, $C_{17}H_{21}O_2N$. Molecular weight determinations, however, show it to
be a dimeride. It forms a crystalline hydrochloride, m.p. 195–6°C (*dry*). The
base may be prepared synthetically by heating hyoscyamine at 120–130°C or by
heating *apo*atropine at 110°C for 48 hours. It is readily soluble in most organic
solvents but only sparingly so in light petroleum or H_2O. With alcoholic NaOH
in a sealed tube at 100°C it is hydrolyzed to give tropine and -isatropic acid.

Hübschmann., *Jahresb.*, 376 (1858)
Kraut., *Ber.*, **13**, 165 (1880)
Merling., *ibid*, **17**, 381 (1884)
Küssner., *Arch. Pharm.*, **276**, 617 (1938)

BELLARIDINE

$C_7H_{13}ON$

A minor constituent of *Atropa Belladonna* Linn, this base is an oil which yields
crystalline salts. The hydrochloride is hygroscopic, m.p. about 159°C; aurichloride (unstable), m.p. 189°C; picrate, m.p. 224–5°C; methiodide, m.p. 253°C
and methopicrate, orange needles from H_2O, m.p. 228°C.

King, Ware., *J. Chem. Soc.*, 331 (1941)

BELLATROPINE

Considered by Hesse to be an individual alkaloid, this compound has been shown
to be a mixture of bases, the main component being chlorotropane.

Hesse., *Annalen*, **261**, 87 (1891)
Polonovski, Polonovski., *Bull. Soc. Chim.*, **45**, 304 (1929)

197

BENININE

$C_{20}H_{26}O_2N_2$

M.p. 225–7°C

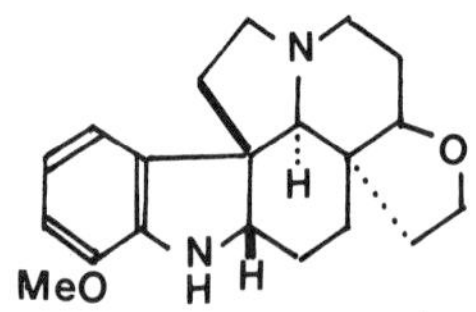

An alkaloid occurring in *Callichilia barteri* Hook, the base may be crystallized either by sublimation or from AcOEt. The ultraviolet spectra have been examined in detail. In EtOH solution, the absorption maxima occur at 246 and 291 mμ; in concentrated H_2SO_4 at 270 and 277 mμ and in 0.05 N/HCl-EtOH at 248, 270 and 277 mμ. The N(a)-acetyl derivative forms a transparent glass which may be crystallized by sublimation, m.p. 220°C. The structure has been determined mainly from mass spectral data.

Gorman *et al., Helv. Chim. Acta,* **49**, 2072 (1966)

N-BENZOYL-O-ACETYLBUXODIENINE E

$C_{35}H_{49}O_2N_2$

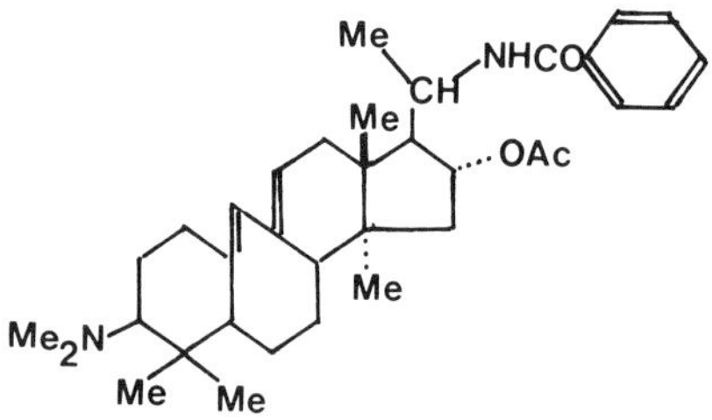

A recently discovered alkaloid of *Buxus sempervirens,* the structure of the base has been determined on the basis of infrared, ultraviolet, NMR and mass spectrometry.

Dopke, Haertel., *Z. Chem.,* **13**, 135 (1973)

N-BENZOYLBALEABUXIDIENE F

$C_{33}H_{48}O_3N_2$

M.p. 291°C

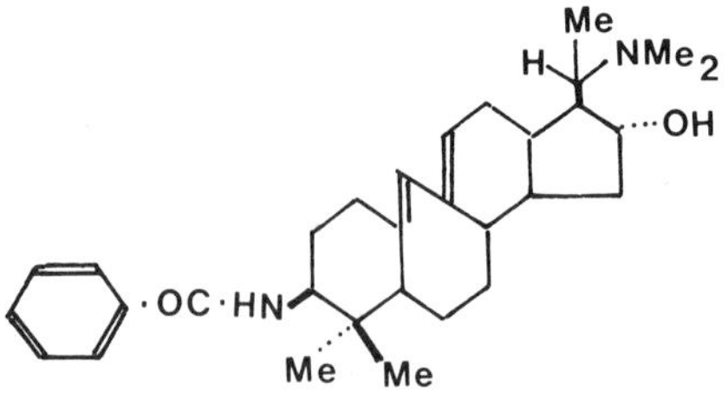

This alkaloid has been isolated from the leaves of *Buxus balearica* Willd. It is laevorotatory with $[\alpha]_D - 29°$ (CHCl$_3$). It contains both a primary and a secondary hydroxyl group in the molecule.

Khuong Huu Laine *et al., Tetrahedron,* **22**, 3321 (1966)

N-BENZOYLBALEABUXIDINE F

$C_{33}H_{48}O_4N_2$

M.p. 277°C

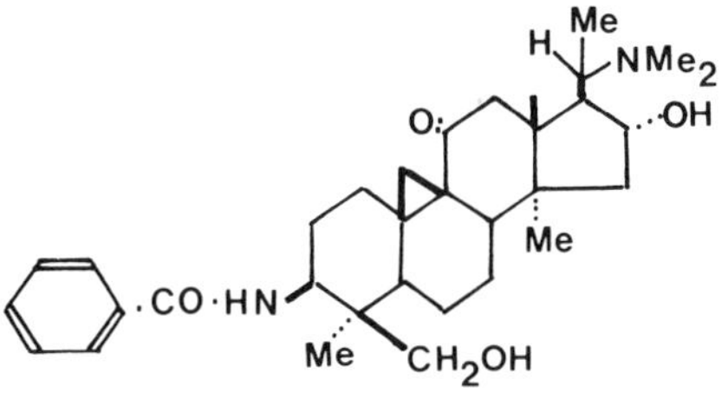

Also present in the leaves of *Buxus balearica* Willd., this alkaloid has $[\alpha]_D + 52°$ (CHCl$_3$). The structure is very similar to that of the preceding base.

Khuong Huu Laine *et al.*, *Tetrahedron*, **22**, 3321 (1966)

N-BENZOYLBUXODIENINE E

$C_{33}H_{49}ON_2$

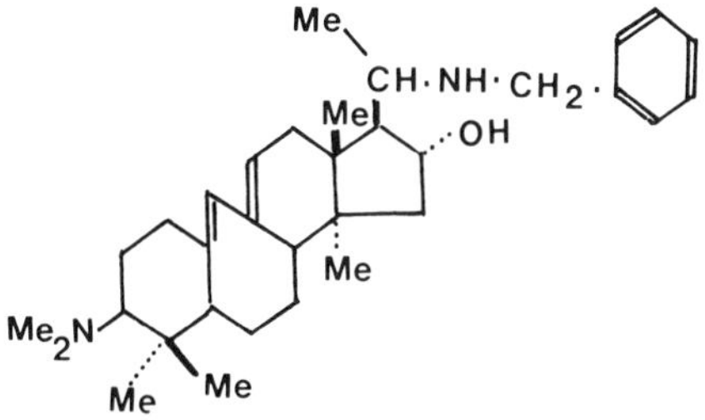

Buxus sempervirens has recently been found to contain this alkaloid, the structure of which has been assigned on the basis of spectroscopic data and comparison with similar *Buxus* alkaloids.

Döpke, Haertel., *Z. Chem.*, **13**, 135 (1973)

N-3-BENZOYLCYCLOBUXIDINE F

$C_{30}H_{50}O_4N_2$

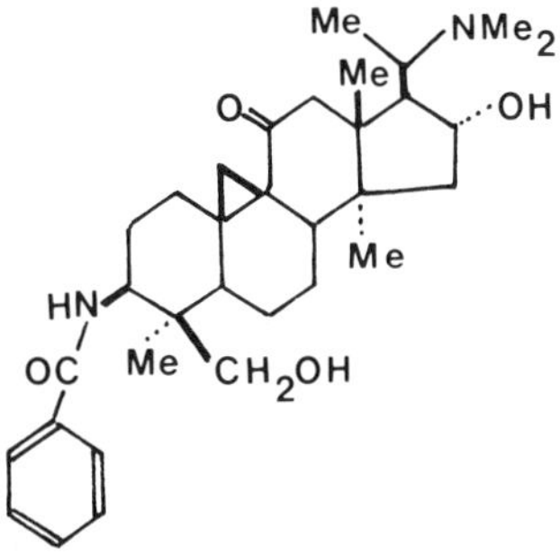

A steroidal alkaloid of *Buxus balearica* Willd. Based upon the infrared, ultraviolet, NMR and mass spectra, the structure given above has been assigned to this alkaloid.

Herlem-Gaulier, Khuong Huu Laine, Goutarel., *Bull. Soc. Chim. Fr.*, 763 (1968)

N-BENZOYL-17-DEMETHYL-20-OXOCYLINDROCARINE

$C_{27}H_{28}O_5N_2$

M.p. 84–5°C

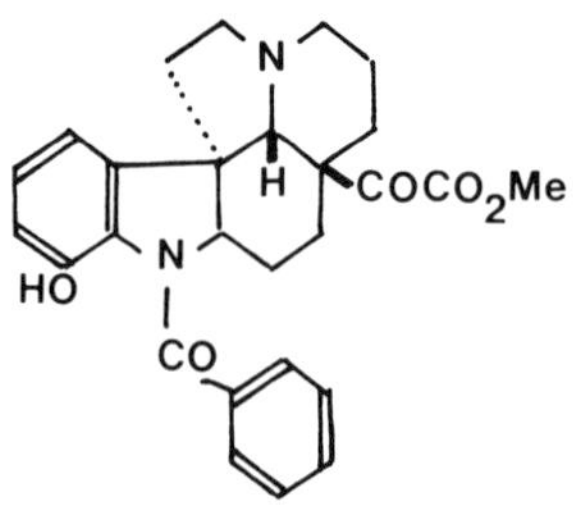

One of the *Aspidosperma* alkaloids, this base is found in *A. cylindrocarpon*. The structure follows from infrared, ultraviolet, NMR and mass spectrometry.

Milborrow, Djerassi., *J. Chem. Soc., C*, 417 (1969)

1β-BENZOYLMETHYL-8Hβ-PYRROLIZIDINE

$C_{15}H_{19}O_2N$

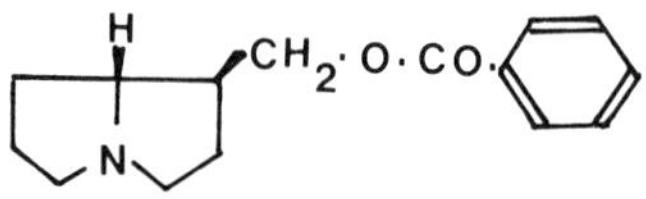

A hepatotoxic alkaloid present in *Planchonella anteridifera* (White & Francis) H. J. Lam, the base is a colourless oil which yields a hydrochloride as colourless needles, m.p. 202–4°C.

Hart, Lamberton., *Austral. J. Chem.*, **19**, 1259 (1966)

O-BENZOYLVINCAMAJINE

$C_{29}H_{30}O_4N_2$

M.p. 267–9°C

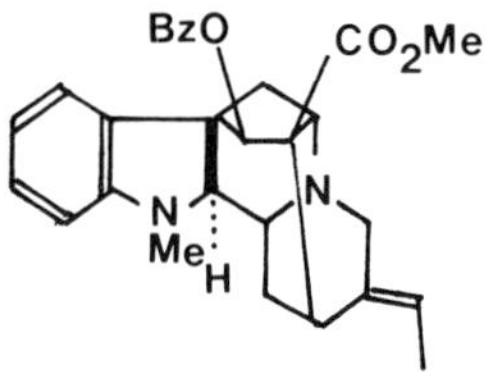

The leaves of *Alstonia macrophylla* contain this alkaloid which is laevorotatory having $[\alpha]_D^{30} - 147°$ (CHCl$_3$). Hydrolysis with 6N H_2SO_4 followed by methylation with CH_2N_2 gives Vincamajine (q.v.). The mass spectrum of the alkaloid shows a relationship with that of quebrachidine.

Mukherjee *et al.*, *Chem. Ind.*, **39**, 1387 (1969)

200

BERBAMINE

$C_{37}H_{40}O_6N_2$

M.p. 156°C

(197–210°C)

This alkaloid of the bisbenzyl*iso*quinoline group is present in *Atherosperma moschatum* Labill, *Berberis thunbergii* and *B. vulgaris*. The recorded melting points vary according to the solvent used for crystallization, e.g. from EtOH, the base forms colourless leaflets of the dihydrate, m.p. 156°C (*dry*); from C_6H_6, it crystallizes with one mole of solvent, m.p. 129–134°C (*dec.*) and from petroleum ether it forms colourless crystals, m.p. 197–210°C; $[\alpha]_D$ + 108.6° (CHCl$_3$). The dihydrochloride yields colourless needles of the heptahydrate, m.p. 257–8°C (*dec.*); the dimethiodide, colourless needles from Me$_2$CO-MeOH; m.p. 287–9°C (*dec.*). The ethyl ether has m.p. 188°C; $[\alpha]_D^{20}$ + 129° (c 0.5, CHCl$_3$). The methyl ether is the alkaloid isoTetrandine (q.v.).

Hesse., *Ber.*, **19**, 3190 (1886)
Rüdel., *Arch. Pharm.*, **229**, 631 (1891)
Santos., *Chem. Abstr.*, **24**, 1647 (1930)
Bruchhausen, Gericke., *Arch. Pharm.*, **269**, 119 (1931)
Tomita, Fujita, Murai., *J. Pharm. Soc., Japan*, **71**, 226, 301 (1951)
Tomita, Kugo., *ibid*, **75**, 753 (1955)
Bick, Clezy, Crow., *Austral. J. Chem.*, **9**, 111 (1956)
Craig *et al.*, *Tetrahedron*, **22**, 1335 (1966)

BERBAMUNINE

$C_{36}H_{40}O_6N_2$

M.p. 190–1°C

From *Berberis amurensis* Rupr. var. *japonica* (Regel) Rehd., this bisbenzyl*iso*quinoline alkaloid is obtained as colourless needles from MeOH or Me$_2$CO with $[\alpha]_D^9$ + 90.9° (c 0.44, MeOH) or + 53.3° (c 0.57, Me$_2$CO). The trimethyl ether has m.p. 179–180°C (*dec.*); $[\alpha]_D^{10}$ + 60.7° and the tribenzoyl derivative has m.p. 113–7°C.

Kametani, Sakurai, Iida., *J. Pharm. Soc., Japan*, **88**, 1163 (1968)

BERBENINE

$C_{19}H_{21}O_3N$

M.p. 152–3°C

This alkaloid from the roots of *Berberis lycium* has been shown to be identical with Berbamine (q.v.).

Ikram, Huq, Warsi., *Pakistan J. Sci. Ind. Res.*, **9**, 343 (1966)
Miana *et al., ibid,* **12**, 159 (1969)

BERBERASTINE

$C_{20}H_{18}O_5N^+$

A quaternary protoberberine alkaloid from *Hydrastis canadensis* L., this base is present in only small amounts in the plant. It has $[\alpha]_D + 107°$ (c 0.06, 90% EtOH) as the iodide. The ultraviolet spectrum of this salt has absorption maxima at 228, 265, 344 and 424 mμ. The biosynthesis of this alkaloid has been discussed by Monkovic and Spenser.

Nijland., *Pharm. Weekbl.*, **96**, 640 (1961)
Nijland., *ibid,* **98**, 301 (1963)

Biosynthesis:
Monkovic, Spenser., *J. Amer. Chem. Soc.*, **87**, 1137 (1965)

BERBERICINE

$C_{20}H_{17}O_4N$

M.p. 162–3°C (*dec.*).

Obtained from *Berberis lycium,* this alkaloid forms yellow crystals and is optically inactive. Several crystalline salts and derivatives have been prepared including the hydrochloride, m.p. 199–200°C (*dec.*); hydriodide, m.p. 269–270°C (*dec.*); nitrate, m.p. 263–4°C (*dec.*); sulphate, m.p. 274–5°C (*dec.*); picrate, m.p. 227–8°C (*dec.*) and the N-nitroso derivative, m.p. 239–240°C (*dec.*).

Ikram, Huq, Warsi., *Pakistan J. Sci. Ind. Res.*, **9**, 343 (1966)

BERBERICININE HYDRIODIDE

$C_{21}H_{22}O_4NI$

M.p. 205–6°C (*dec.*).

Also present in the roots of *Berberis lycium,* this alkaloid is optically inactive. The empirical formula has been obtained from combustion analysis.

Ikram, Huq, Warsi., *Pakistan J. Sci. Ind. Res.*, **9**, 343 (1966)

BERBERINE

$C_{20}H_{18}O_4N$

M.p. 145°C

This protoberberine alkaloid was first isolated from *Xanthoxylum Clava Herculis* under the name of 'Xanthopicrit' and obtained independently from *Berberis vulgaris*. The base occurs in several plants including those of the Ranunculaceae (*Coptis japonica, C. trifolia, C. occidentalis* and *Thalictrum foliosum*), the Berberidaceae (*Berberis buxifolia* Lam., *B. Darwinii* Hook, *B. glauca* DC., *B. nervosa, Mahonia aquifolium* Nutt., *M. trifoliata* Fedde, and *Nandina domestica* Thunb.), the Anonaceae (*Coelocline polycarpa* DC), the Menispermaceae *Archangelisia flava* L., *Cocsinium blumeanum* Miers, *C. fenestratum* Colebr.), the Papaveraceae (*Argemone mexicana* L., *Chelidonium majus* L., *Corydalis cheilantheifolia* Hemsl., *C. ophiocarpa* Hook.) and the Rutaceae (*Evodia meliifolia* Benth, *Phellodendron amurense* Rupr., *Toddalia aculeata* Pers. and *Zanthoxylum caribaeum* Lam.).

The alkaloid crystallizes from H_2O or aqueous EtOH as the hexahydrate or from $CHCl_3$ with one mole of solvent as yellow needles. The base is readily purified via the acetone compound, B, Me_2CO, which forms reddish-yellow tablets. The salts are mostly yellow in colour and crystallize well: the hydrochloride dihydrate as small yellow needles; the hydriodide also as yellow needles; nitrate as green-yellow needles and the sulphate as slender yellow needles. The phosphate sesquihydrate is a bright yellow and also crystalline.

Berberine is moderately toxic to larger animals causing cardiac damage, dyspnoea, lowered blood pressure and paresis in rabbits. In man large amounts are present in the urine after oral administration. Its main use in Western medicine is as a bitter tonic and stomachic. It has some trypanocidal action and had been used as an adjunct to quinine in the treatment of malaria. The sulphate, in concentrations of 1–3 mg. per ml. decreases the anticoagulant action of heparin in dog and human blood *in vitro*.

Chevalier, Pelletan., *J. chim. med.*, 2, 314 (1826)
Buchner, Herberger., *Annalen, Suppl.*, 24, 228 (1837)
Perrins., *J. Chem. Soc.*, 15, 339 (1862)
Haworth, Perkin, Rankin., *ibid*, 125, 1686 (1924)
Perkin, Ray, Robinson., *ibid*, 127, 740 (1925)
Mizuno, Yoshida., *Japanese Patent*, 99, 230
Awe., *Arch. Pharm.*, 284, 352 (1951)

Biosynthesis:
Barton, Hesse, Kirby., *Proc. Chem. Soc.*, 267 (1963)
Barton, Hesse, Kirby., *J. Chem. Soc.*, 6379 (1965)
Monkovic, Spenser., *Proc. Chem. Soc.*, 223 (1964)
Monkovic, Spenser., *Can. J. Chem.*, 43, 2017 (1965)
Gupta, Spenser., *ibid*, 43, 133 (1965)

Pharmacology:
Chopra, Dikshit, Chowhan., *Ind. J. Med. Res.*, 19, 1193 (1932)
Seery, Bieter., *J. Pharmacol. exp. Ther.*, 69, 64 (1940)
Brahmachari., *Ind. Med. Gaz.*, 79, 259 (1944)

BERLAMBINE

$C_{20}H_{17}O_5N$

M.p. 199–200°C

This alkaloid has been isolated from *Berberis lambertii*. Very little further investigation has been carried out on it since its isolation.

Chatterjee, Banerjee., *J. Ind. Chem. Soc.*, **30**, 705 (1953)

BERVULCINE

$C_{18}H_{19}O_3N$

M.p. 125–6°C (*dec.*).

Isolated from *Berberis vulgaris* L., this base has $[\alpha]_D^{24} - 185°$ (c 0.2, $CHCl_3$). It forms crystalline salts and derivatives: hydriodide, colourless prisms from H_2O, m.p. 236°C (*dec.*); perchlorate, m.p. 258–260°C (*dec.*); methiodide, m.p. 269°C (*dec.*) and picrate, needles from MeOH, m.p. 188–190°C (*dec.*).

Döpke., *Naturwiss.*, **50**, 595 (1963)

BETONICINE

$C_7H_{13}O_3N$

M.p. 252°C (*dec.*).

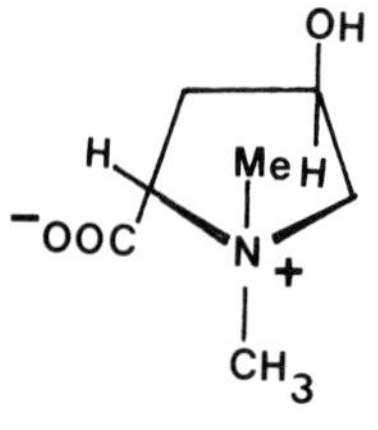

This simple pyrrolidine base occurs in *Betonica officinalis, Marrubium vulgare* L. and *Stachys silvatica*. It is stereoisomeric with turicine and forms colourless prisms from EtOH with $[\alpha]_D^{15} - 36.6°$ (H_2O). The base is only sparingly soluble in cold EtOH. It readily forms crystalline salts: hydrochloride, needles from EtOH, m.p. 232°C (*dec.*); platinichloride (dihydrate), m.p. 225–6°C (*dec.*) and the aurichloride, *dec.* at 230–2°C.

Küng., *Z. physiol. Chem.*, **85**, 217 (1913)
Goodson, Clewer., *J. Chem. Soc.*, **115**, 923 (1919)
Paudler, Wagner., *Chem. & Ind.*, 1693 (1963)

BICUCINE

$C_{20}H_{19}O_7N$

M.p. 222°C (dec.).

A constituent of *Corydalis aurea* Willd., this alkaloid $[\alpha]_D^{52} - 115.4°$ (0.1 N/KOH). In N/HCl, however, it shows mutarotation $- 145°$ to $- 100°$ due to the formation of an equilibrium mixture of bicucine and bicuculline (q.v.). Oxidation with alkaline $KMnO_4$ gives 3:4-methylene dioxy-phthalic acid, characterized as the ethylimide. The preferred structure is that given above, representing it as the hydroxyacid corresponding to bicuculline as the lactone.

Manske., *Can. J. Res.,* **9**, 436 (1933)
Manske., *ibid,* **15**, 159 (1937)
Manske., *ibid,* **16**, 81 (1938)

BICUCULLINE (*Adlumidine, capnoidine*)

$C_{20}H_{17}O_6N$

M.p. 215°C (177°C, 196°C)

This alkaloid is widespread among the species of the genera Rhoeadales, being found in *Adlumia fungosa* Greene (*A. cirrhosa* Rap.), *Corydalis aurea* Willd., *C. caseana* A. Gray, *C. crystallina* Engelm., *C. nobilis* Pers., *C. ochroleuca* Koch, *C. platycarpa* Makino, *C. scouleri* HK., *C. sempervirens* (L) Pers., *C. sibirica* Pers., *Dicentra chrysantha* Walp., *D. cucullaria* (Ker) Torr. and *D. ochroleuca* Engelm.

The base forms colourless plates from $CHCl_3$-MeOH and is soluble in $CHCl_3$, but only moderately so in EtOH or MeOH. It contains no methoxyl groups and shows behaviour characteristic of a lactone being converted by alkalies into bicucine. On oxidation it yields hydrastinine and 2-carboxy-3:4-methylenedioxy-benzaldehyde, m.p. 155°C. The alkaloid has been synthesized by Groenewoud and Robinson.

Manske., *Can. J. Res.,* **7**, 265 (1932)
Manske., *ibid,* **8**, 210, 407 (1933)
Manske., *ibid,* **9**, 436 (1933)
Manske., *ibid,* **18**, 288 (1940)
Groenewoud, Robinson., *J. Chem. Soc.,* 199 (1936)

Manske., *J. Amer. Chem. Soc.,* **72**, 3207 (1950)

Edwards, Handa., *Can. J. Chem.,* **39**, 1801 (1961)

Stereochemistry:

Safe, Moir., *Can. J. Chem.,* **42**, 160 (1964)

BICYCLOMAHANIMBICINE

$C_{23}H_{25}ON$

M.p. 218°C (*dec.*).

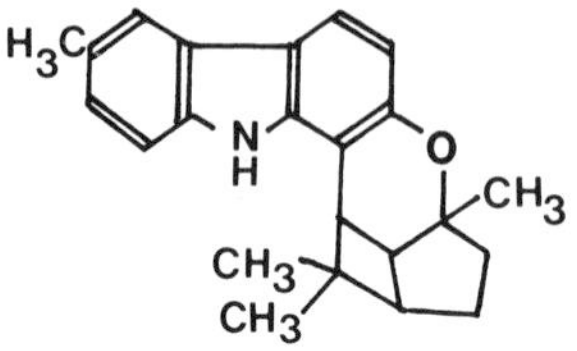

A constituent of the leaves of *Murraya koenigii* Spreng., this base has an ultra-violet spectrum in which the absorption maxima occur at 243, 257, 263 and 305 mμ. The earlier structure has recently been revised to that given above.

Kureel, Kapil, Popli., *Chem. & Ind.,* 958 (1970)

Structure revision:
Begley, Clarke, Crombie, Whiting., *Chem. Commun.,* 1547 (1970)

BICYCLOMAHANIMBIN

$C_{23}H_{25}ON$

M.p. 145°C

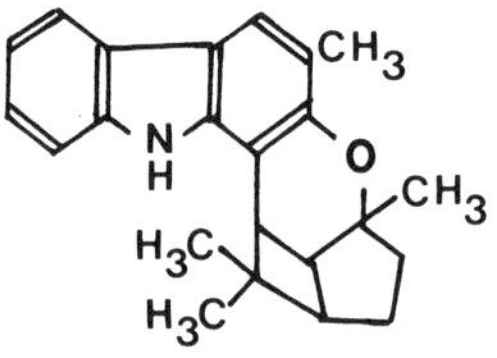

The leaves of *Murraya koenigii* Spreng. also yield this alkaloid which is closely related to the preceding base. It has $[\alpha]_D^{23} - 1.23°$ (CHCl$_3$). The ultraviolet spectrum exhibits absorption maxima at 242, 255, 260, 305 and 331 mμ, in EtOH solution. The N-methyl derivative, m.p. 156°C has been prepared.

Kureel, Kapil, Popli., *Tetrahedron Lett.,* 3857 (1969)
Kureel, Kapil, Popli., *Chem. Commun.,* 1120 (1969)

Structure revision:
Begley, Clarke, Crombie, Whiting., *Chem. Commun.,* 1547 (1970)

BIFLORINE

$C_{17}H_{17}O_4N$

M.p. 206°C

This alkaloid occurs in *Oldenlandia biflora* and forms colourless needles from EtOH. It has $[\alpha]_D - 135.4°$ and is readily soluble in Me$_2$CO or CHCl$_3$ but only sparingly so in Et$_2$O, EtOH or C$_6$H$_6$. It yields several crystalline salts, e.g. the hydrochloride, m.p. 259°C; platinichloride, m.p. 231°C; nitrate, m.p. 278°C and

206

methiodide, m.p. 124°C. This alkaloid must not be confused with the antibiotic of the same name obtained from Capraria biflora, $C_{20}H_{20}O_3$, m.p. 97°C.

Chauhan, Tiwari., *J. Ind. Chem. Soc.*, **29**, 386 (1952)

BIKHACONITINE

$C_{36}H_{51}O_{11}N$

M.p. 163.5−164°C

This aconite alkaloid was first isolated from the roots of *Aconitum spicatum* Stapf. From Et_2O, the base crystallizes in button-shaped masses, m.p. 118−123°C and from EtOH, on addition of H_2O, as the monohydrate in colourless granules, m.p. 113−6°C (dry); $[\alpha]_D + 16°$ (c 1.6, EtOH). The salts all crystallize well: hydrochloride (pentahydrate), m.p. 159−161°C (*dry*); hydrobromide (penta-hydrate), m.p. 173−5°C (*dry*); perchlorate, needles from EtOH, m.p. 240−2°C; aurichloride, m.p. 232−3°C; acetate, prisms from MeOH, m.p. 197−9°C; $[\alpha]_D + 21.6°$ (c 1.5, $CHCl_3$). The alkaloid contains six methoxyl groups of which two are present in the veratroyl radical. Hydrolysis of the base in H_2O at 130°C in a sealed tube yields acetic acid and veratroylbikhaconine, $C_{34}H_{49}O_{10}N$, m.p. 120−5°C. Alkaline hydrolysis gives acetic and veratric acids and bikhaconine, $C_{25}H_{41}O_7N$, which is amorphous; $[\alpha]_D^{22} + 33.85°$ but yields readily crystallizable salts, e.g. hydrobromide, m.p. 145−150°C; nitrate, m.p. 125−8°C and the aurichloride trihydrate, m.p. 129−132°C or 187−8°C (*dry*). When heated alone at 180°C, the alkaloid furnishes acetic acid and pyrobikhaconitine, $C_{34}H_{47}O_9N$, a colourless glassy solid giving amorphous salts, e.g. the aurichloride, m.p. 115−123°C. Like all of the aconitines, the base is highly toxic producing respiratory paralysis and a direct toxic action upon the heart which normally terminates in ventricular fibrillation. Prickling in the throat and of the skin are characteristic symptoms of poisoning by this alkaloid.

Dunstan, Andrews., *J. Chem. Soc.*, **87**, 1636 (1905)
Tsuda, Marion., *Can. J. Chem.*, **41**, 3055 (1963)

2:5-BISDIACETYLEVONINE

$C_{32}H_{35}O_{15}N$

A minor alkaloid recently isolated from the seeds of *Euonymus europea*. The structure has been determined from spectroscopic and chemical data.

Crombie, Whiting., *Phytochem.*, **12**, 703 (1973)

18:18'-BIS(O-DEMETHYLASPIDOCARPINE)

$C_{42}H_{54}O_6N_4$

M.p. 174–5°C

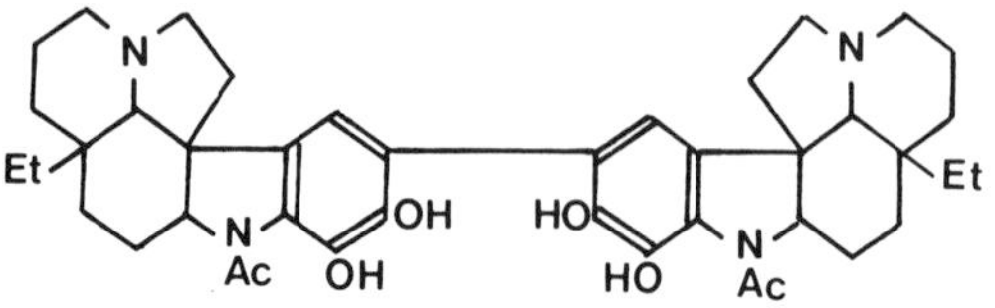

A dimeric alkaloid from the bark of *Aspidosperma melanocalyx* Muell-Arg., this base forms colourless crystals from hexane. It has $[\alpha]_D^{25} + 108°$ (c 1.01, pyridine). The ultraviolet spectrum in EtOH has absorption maxima at 236 and 297 mμ. That in NaOH-EtOH has maxima at 243, 302 and 335 mμ.

Miranda, Gilbert., *Experientia*, **25**, 575 (1969)

BISDIHYDRODEOXOHOMALINE

$C_{30}H_{46}N_4$

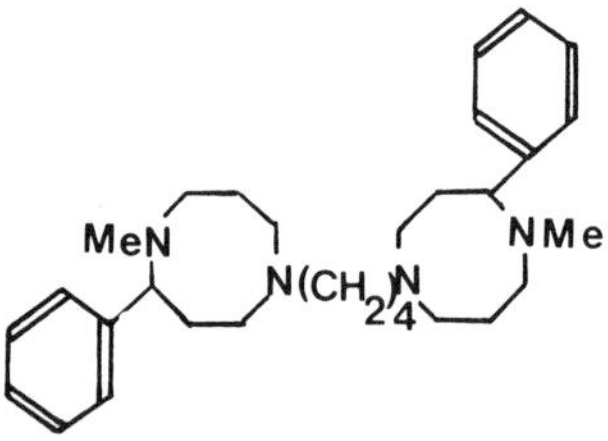

A minor alkaloid obtained from *Homalium* species. The structure of the base has been confirmed by synthesis, the dimerization of diazacyclooctane with succinyl chloride, followed by reduction of the oxo groups with LiAlH$_4$ giving 5:5'-butylenedi(1-methyl-2-phenyl-1:5-diazacyclooctane) which proves to be identical with the natural alkaloid.

Pais, Sarfati, Jarreau., *Bull. Soc. Chim. Fr.*, **1**, 331 (1973)

1:3-BIS(11-HYDROCHELERYTHRINYL)ACETONE

$C_{45}H_{40}O_9N_2$

M.p. 304°C

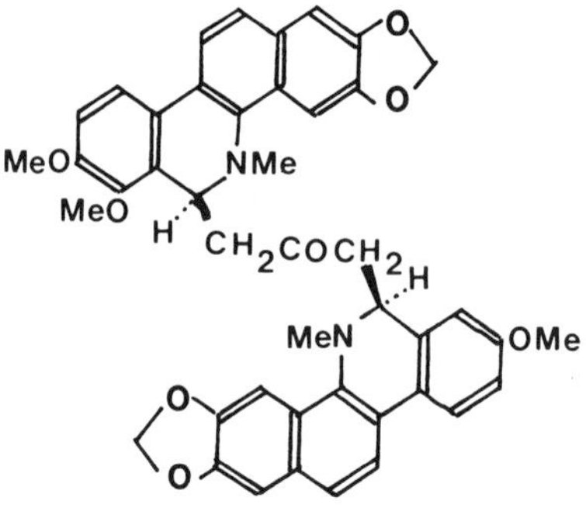

This dimeric naphthylphenanthridine alkaloid occurs in *Bocconia arborea*. The structure has been determined primarily from degradation, infrared, NMR and mass spectrometry studies.

MacLean *et al., Can. J. Chem.*, **47**, 1951 (1969)

3:3'-BIS(INDOLYLMETHYL)-DIMETHYL-AMMONIUM HYDROXIDE

$C_{20}H_{20}ON_3$

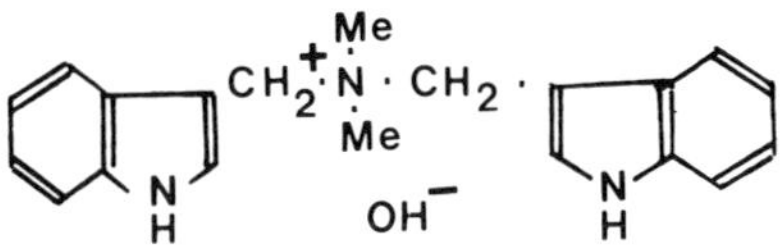

A quaternary alkaloid recently discovered in the flowers of *Arundo donax*. The structure given above follows from chemical and spectroscopic data.

Ghosal, Chaudhuri, Dutta., *Phytochem.*, **10**, 2852 (1971)

BISJATRORRHIZINE

$C_{40}H_{38}O_8N_2^{++}$

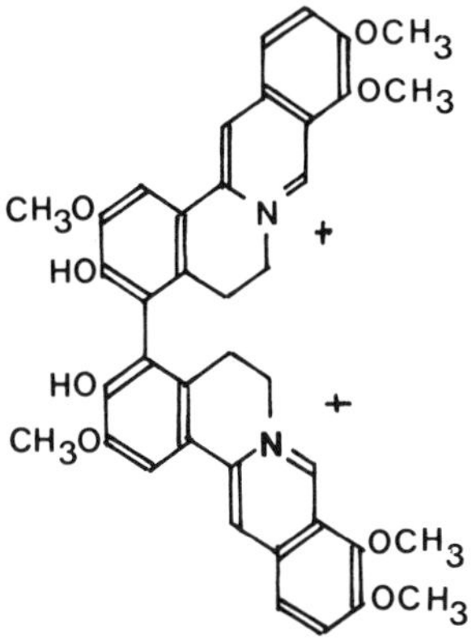

A dimeric quaternary base obtained from the roots of *Jatrorrhiza palmata* Miers, the alkaloid is normally isolated as the dichloride which forms orange-yellow crystals from MeOH. The crystals do not show a sharp melting point but darken above about 270°C. In the ultraviolet spectrum in H_2O, the absorption maxima occur at 228, 263, 345 and 420 mμ with a shoulder at 275 mμ. The structure has been determined from molecular weight studies and comparison with Jatrorrhizine (q.v.).

Carvalhas., *J. Chem. Soc., Perkin I*, 327 (1972)

BIS-6:7β-OXIDODEOXYNUPHARIDINE

$C_{30}H_{42}O_4N_2$

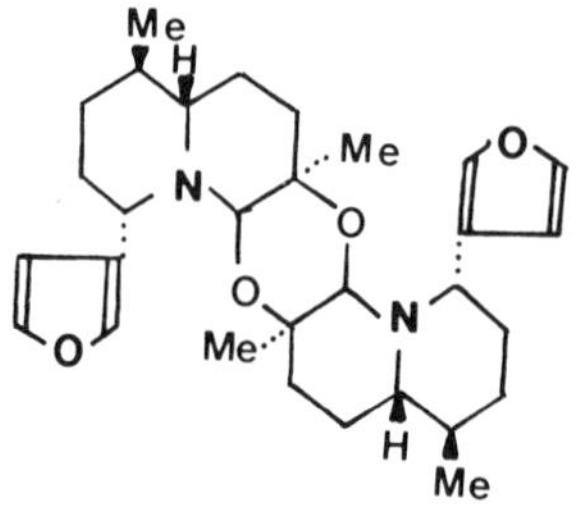

One of the more recently discovered alkaloids of *Nuphar luteum* subsp. *macrophyllum*, this base is dimeric about two ether bridges. The structure has been established by chemical and spectroscopic methods.

LaLonde, Wong, Das., *J. Amer. Chem. Soc.*, **94**, 8522 (1972)

BLEEKERINE

$C_{23}H_{24}O_5N_2$

M.p. 276–7°C

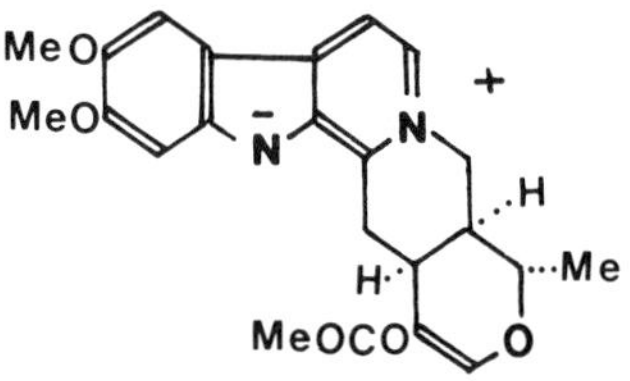

The stem bark of *Bleekeria vitiensis* yields this alkaloid which is obtained as yellow prisms when recrystallized from EtOH. It is dextrorotatory with $[\alpha]_{546}^{22.5} + 612°$ (MeOH). The ultraviolet spectrum contains several absorption maxima at 208, 242, 276, 336 and 394 mμ.

Sainsbury, Webb., *Phytochem.*, **11**, 2337 (1972)

BOCCONINE

$C_{21}H_{17}O_6N$

M.p. 201°C

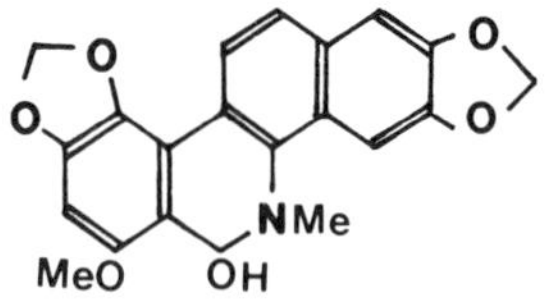

This naphthylphenanthridine alkaloid is present in *Bocconia cordata* Willd. The structure has been determined both by chemical and spectroscopic methods.

Onda, Takiguchi, Hirakura, Fukushima, Akagawa, Naoi., *Nippon Nogeikagaku Kaishi.*, **39**, 168 (1965)

Structure:
Onda, Abe, Yonezawa, Esumi, Suzuki., *Chem. Pharm. Bull.* (Tokyo), **18**, 1435 (1970)

BOCCONOLINE

$C_{22}H_{21}O_5N$

M.p. 232–3°C

A second naphthylphenanthridine base isolated from *Bocconia cordata* Willd., the alkaloid crystallizes as colourless rods. It contains a primary hydroxyl group and forms a crystalline acetate, m.p. 188.5–189.5°C.

Tani, Takao., *J. Pharm. Soc., Japan,* 82, 755 (1962)
Ishii, Hosoya, Takao., *Tetrahedron Lett.,* 2429 (1971)

BOKITAMINE

$C_{21}H_{35}O_2N$

M.p. 191°C

A steroidal alkaloid, this base occurs in the leaves of various *Holarrhena* species. It crystallizes well from AcOEt. The N-acetyl derivative forms colourless crystals, m.p. 247–8°C.

Nelle, Charles, Cave, Goutarel., *Compt. rend.,* 271C, 153 (1970)

BOLDINE

$C_{19}H_{21}O_4N$

M.p. 161–3°C

An aporphine alkaloid isolated from *Boldea fragrans* Gray (*B. chilensis* Juss., *Pneumus Boldus* Molina), this is an amorphous, light-sensitive compound which crystallizes from $CHCl_3$ or CS_2 with one mole of solvent. It has $[\alpha]_D + 72.7°$ ($CHCl_3$-EtOH) and does not form crystalline salts. With HNO_3 it gives a deep red colour. Reaction with C_6H_5COCl gives mainly the tribenzoyl derivative, m.p. 171°C in which one acyl radical is attached to nitrogen due to scission of a reduced pyridine ring in which the nitrogen atom is tertiary. A small amount of the dibenzoyl derivative, m.p. 124–7°C is also formed. The dimethyl ether has m.p. 117–8°C and is identical with glaucine (q.v.). The location of the two hydroxyl groups in boldine has been determined by exhaustive methylation of the diethyl ether to give trimethylamine and 3:5-dimethoxy-2:6-diethoxy-8-

vinylphenanthrene, m.p. 112–3°C which is oxidized by $KMnO_4$ to 3:5-dimethoxy-2:6-diethoxyphenanthrene-8-carboxylic acid. The latter, on decarb-oxylation, yields 3:5-dimethoxy-2:6-diethoxyphenanthrene, m.p. 133–4°C, identified by comparison with a synthesized specimen. Boldine is therefore 3:5-dimethoxy-2:6-dihydroxyaporphine.

Bourgoin, Verne., *J. Pharm. Chim.*, **16**, 191 (1872)
Merck., *Jahresb.*, **36**, 110 (1922)
Warnat., *Ber.*, **58**, 2768 (1925)
Warnat., *ibid*, **59**, 85 (1926)
Späth, Tharrer., *ibid*, **66**, 904 (1933)
Schlittler., *ibid*, **66**, 988 (1933)

BOSCHNIAKINE

$C_{10}H_{11}ON$

B.p. 80–90°C/3 mm

This pyridine derivative is not generally considered to be an alkaloid although it possesses a marked physiological action on the cat. It is found in *Boschniakia rossica* Hult. and is obtained as a pleasant-smelling liquid, $[\alpha]_D^{20} + 21.02°$ (c 0.98, $CHCl_3$). It forms a semicarbazone, m.p. 277–8°C (*dec.*).

BRACTEOLIN

$C_{19}H_{21}O_4N$

M.p. 218–221°C

Papaver bracteatum also yields this alkaloid, shown to be 1:10-dihydroxy-2:9-dimethoxyaporphine. It is dextrorotatory with $[\alpha]_D^{20} + 35° \pm 8°$ (c 0.16, $CHCl_3$). In MeOH solution, the ultraviolet spectrum shows absorption maxima at 218, 278 and 304 mμ with a shoulder at 268 mμ. The structure has been confirmed by synthesis.

Heydenreich, Pfeifer., *Pharmazie*, **22**, 124 (1967)
Synthesis:
Kerekes, Heydenreich, Pfeifer., *Tetrahedron Lett.*, 2483 (1970)

BRASILINECINE

M.p. 169–171°C (*dec.*).

This hepatotoxic alkaloid has been reported from *Senecio brasiliensis*. It is laevo-rotatory with $[\alpha]_D^{20} - 68.2°$ ($CHCl_3$). The salts and derivatives crystallize well, e.g. the aurichloride, m.p. 146–8°C; picrate, m.p. 191–2°C; picrolonate, m.p. 67–9°C and the methiodide, m.p. 235–7°C (*dec.*). The alkaloid gives a red colour with HCl or HNO$_3$ and a yellow colour with H$_2$SO$_4$.

De Camargo Fonseca., *Anais faculdade farm. e odontol., Univ. Sao Paulo*, **9**, 85 (1951)

BREVICARINE

C$_{16}$H$_{19}$N$_3$

M.p. 112°C

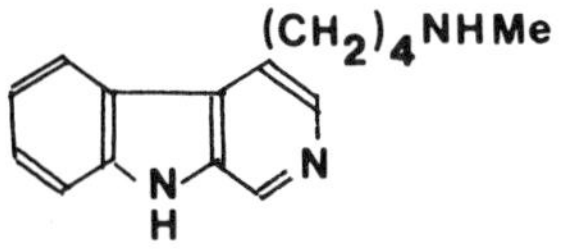

This carboline alkaloid occurs in *Carex brevicollis*. It forms a crystalline dihydrochloride, m.p. 195–6°C.

Terent'eva, Lazur'evskii, Shirshova., *Khim. Prir. Soedin.*, **5**, 397 (1969)

BREVICOLLINE

C$_{17}$H$_{19}$N$_3$

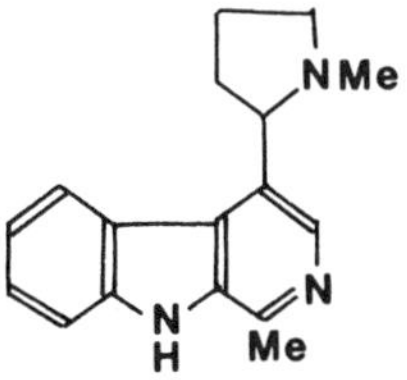

The major constituent of *Carex brevicollis*, this carboline alkaloid yields harman-4-carboxylic acid on oxidation. The methyl ester of this acid has been unambiguously synthesized to afford proof of the structure of the alkaloid. Spectroscopic data also confirms the above structure.

Vember, Terent'eva, Ul'yanova., *Khim. Prir. Soedin.*, **4**, 98 (1968)
Terent'eva, Lazur'evskii, Vember., *Brevikollin-Alkaloid Osoki Parvskoi*, 5 (1969)

4-BROMOPHAKELLIN

C$_{11}$H$_{16}$N$_5$Br

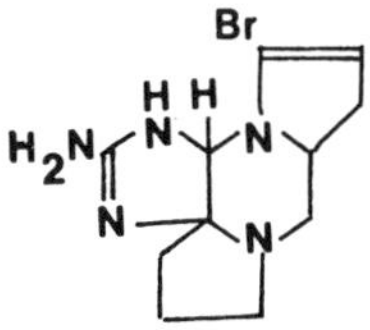

This unique alkaloid has recently been isolated from the marine sponge *Phakellia flabellata*. The structure given has been determined from chemical and spectroscopic evidence.

Sharma, Burkholder., *J. Chem. Soc., C*, **3**, 151 (1971)

BROWNIINE

$C_{25}H_{41}O_7N$

M.p. Indefinite

This aconite alkaloid is found in *Delphinium brownii* Rybd., forming an amorphous powder. The salts, however, are crystalline: hydriodide, colourless crystals from Me CO-AcOEt, m.p. 193–6°C and the perchlorate, m.p. 212°C; $[\alpha]_D + 25°$ (EtOH). Not being as ester alkaloid, the base is relatively non-toxic.

Benn, Cameron, Edwards., *Can. J. Chem.*, **41**, 477 (1963)

BRUCINE

$C_{23}H_{26}O_4N_2$

M.p. 178°C

The seeds of several plants yield this alkaloid, e.g. *Ignatia amara* L., *Strychnos aculeata* Solered, *S. ligustrina* Blume, *S. Nux-vomica* (bark and seeds) and *S. Rheedei* Clarke. The base crystallizes from H_2O or aqueous EtOH in monoclinic prisms of the tetrahydrate, m.p. 105°C or 178°C (*dry*). It has $[\alpha]_D^{20} - 80.1°$ (EtOH) or $- 119°$ to $- 127°$ (CHCl$_3$). It is only slightly soluble in cold H_2O, more so in hot H_2O or Et$_2O$ and very soluble in CHCl$_3$, EtOH or amyl alcohol. Brucine acts as a monoacidic base yielding salts that crystallize well. The hydrochloride forms colourless needles from H_2O; hydriodide, leaflets that are only sparingly soluble in H_2O; sulphate, long needles of the heptahydrate. The nitrate is obtained as the crystalline dihydrate, m.p. 230°C (*dec.*). The alkaloid may be readily distinguished from Strychnine (q.v.) by not giving the series of colours with chromic acid in H_2SO_4. With HNO_3 it affords an intense red colour, distinguished from that given by morphine by adding $SnCl_2$ when the colour changes to violet.

Pharmacologically, brucine resembles strychnine in its action but it is much less toxic. It also has a more marked curare-like action on the nerve endings in voluntary muscle.

Regnault., *Annalen,* **26**, 17 (1838)
Saunders., *J. Amer. Chem. Soc.,* **50**, 1231 (1928)
Menon, Perkin, Robinson., *J. Chem. Soc.,* 833 (1930)
Späth, Bretschneider., *Ber.,* **63**, 3005 (1930)
Leuchs, Kröhnke., *ibid,* **64**, 455 (1931)
Leuchs., *ibid,* **65**, 1230 (1932)
Woodward., *J. Amer. Chem. Soc.,* **70**, 2107 (1948)
Kaeser., *J. Chem. Soc.,* 2098 (1950)
Robinson., *Progress in Organic Chemistry,* **1**, 1 (1952)

ψ-BRUCINE

$C_{23}H_{26}O_4N_2$

This alkaloid is a minor constituent of the leaves of *Strychnos wallichiana*. The base has only recently been discovered and is still under chemical investigation.

Bisset, Choudhury., *Phytochem.*, **13**, 259 (1974)

BRUCINE N-OXIDE

$C_{23}H_{26}O_5N_2$

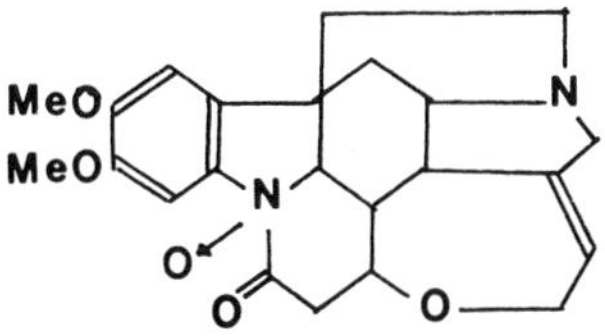

A second recently discovered alkaloid present as a minor constituent of the leaves of *Strychnos wallichiana*, the structure of the base has been determined by chemical and spectroscopic means.

Bisset, Choudhury., *Phytochem.*, **13**, 259 (1974)

BRUGINE

$C_{12}H_{19}O_2NS_2$

M.p. Indefinite

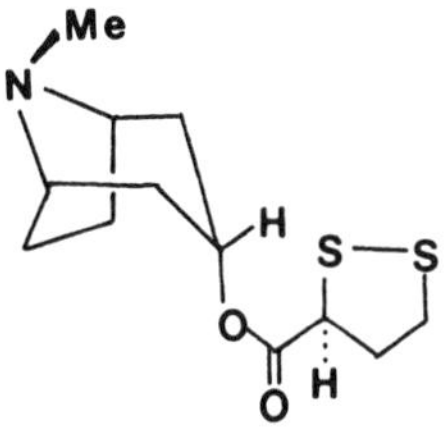

The bark of the mangrove tree, *Bruguiera sexangula* (Lour.) Poir. yields this sulphur-containing alkaloid which is obtained in the form of a pale yellow, glassy solid with no definite melting point. On standing, the alkaloid slowly darkens and polymerizes. The ultraviolet spectrum in EtOH has absorption maxima at 277 and 320 (shoulder) mμ. Brugine may be hydrolyzed by dilute acids or alkalies to give tropine and 1,2-thiolane-3-carboxylic acid.

Loder, Russell., *Tetrahedron Lett.*, 6327 (1966)
Beecham, Loder, Russell., *ibid*, 1785 (1968)

BUCHARAINE

$C_{19}H_{25}O_4N$

M.p. 151–2°C

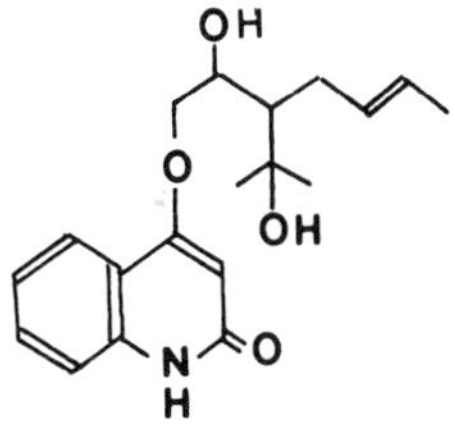

215

This quinolone alkaloid has been isolated from *Haplophyllum* bucharicum. It contains one secondary and one tertiary hydroxyl group and a double bond in the side chain. The structure has been determined mainly from degradative and spectroscopic evidence. Oxidation with KIO_4 in MeOH furnishes an aldehyde, bucharainal, m.p. $121-2°C$, giving an oxime, m.p. $181-2°C$ and a 2:4-dinitro-phenylhydrazone, m.p. $202-3°C$. When the alkaloid is refluxed for 8 hours in tetralin it yields Bucharidine (q.v.).

Sharafutdinova, Yunusov., *Khim. Prir. Soedin.*, 5, 394 (1969)
Faizutdinova, Bessonova, Rashkes, Yunusov., *ibid*, 6, 239 (1970)

BUCHARAMINE

$C_{21}H_{29}O_3N$

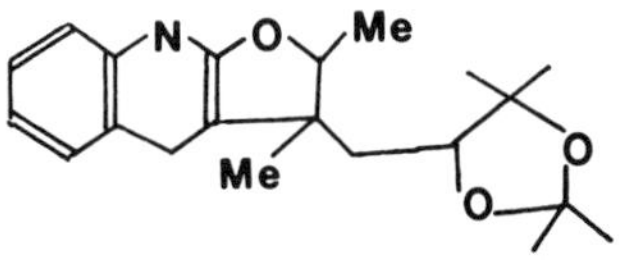

A further alkaloid occurring in *Haplophyllum bucharicum,* this base has the possible structure given above based upon chemical and spectroscopic data, particularly the NMR and mass spectra.

Ubaidullaev, Bessonova, Yunusov., *Khim. Prir. Soedin.*, 8, 343 (1972)

BUCHARIDINE

$C_{19}H_{25}O_4N$

M.p. $250-1°C$

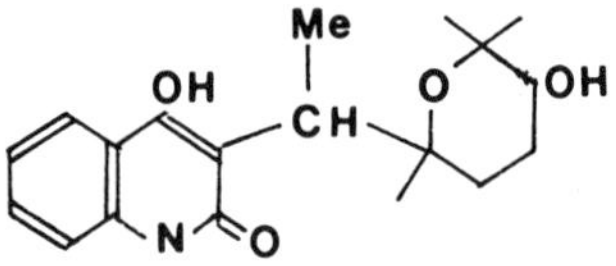

This alkaloid from *Haplophyllum bucharicum* is isomeric with Bucharaine (q.v.). The earlier structure due to Faizutdinova *et al* has been shown to be incorrect. The ultraviolet spectrum of the alkaloid has absorption maxima at 228, 274, 282, 314 and 328 mμ. Oxidation of the base with chromic acid in H_2SO_4 yields acetone, characterized as the 2:4-dinitrophenylhydrazone. The above structure has been confirmed by determination of the functional groups as well as by infrared, NMR and mass spectral data. Bucharidine may be prepared from bucharaine using a Claisen rearrangement.

Faizutdinova, Bessonova, Yunusov., *Khim. Prir. Soedin.*, 5, 455 (1969)
Structure revision:
Faizutdinova *et al., ibid*, 6, 239 (1970)

BUDRUGAINE

From the bark of *Zanthoxylum budrunga,* Khastagir has isolated two alkaloids which have, as yet, not been fully characterized. This particular base chars above 180°C but does not melt.

Khastagir., *Curr. Sci.,* 16, 185 (1947)
Khastagir., *Chem. Abstr.,* 42, 326 (1948)

BUDRUGAININE

M.p. 155°C

The second alkaloid to be obtained from the bark of *Zanthoxylum budrunga*, this base has the melting point given above. So far, its formula and structure have not been determined.

Khastagir., *Curr. Sci.*, **16**, 185 (1947)
Khastagir., *Chem. Abstr.*, **42**, 326 (1948)

BUFOTENIDINE

$C_{13}H_{18}ON_2$

M.p. Indefinite

This amorphous base is present in various toad toxins. It forms crystalline salts: the hydriodide, m.p. 209°C; flavianate, orange-red prisms, decomposing above 198°C; picrate as red needles, m.p. 198°C and the picrolonate, yellow crystals, m.p. 120–1°C.

Wieland, Konz, Mittasch., *Annalen*, **513**, 1 (1934)
Jensen., *J. Biol. Chem.*, **116**, 87 (1936)

BUFOTENINE (*Mappine*)

$C_{12}H_{16}ON_2$

M.p. 146–7°C;
B.p. 320°C/0.1 mm

This base occurs in both the plant and animal kingdom, being found in the toxic secretion of toads, *Bufo vulgaris,* in the fungus *Amanita mappa* and in the seeds of *Piptadenia peregrina.* It forms colourless prisms from Et_2O-Me_2CO and is freely soluble in EtOH or MeOH, moderately soluble in Me_2CO, slightly soluble in Et_2O and insoluble in H_2O. The oxalate forms colourless needles of the monohydrate from Et_2O, m.p. 96.5°C; monopicrate, m.p. 179–180°C; dipicrate, red crystals from MeOH, m.p. 177–8°C; methiodide, m.p. 213–4°C; picrolonate, yellow crystals, m.p. 120–1°C.

The methyl ether has m.p. 66–7°C, b.p. 208–210°C/4 mm. It forms a crystalline picrate, m.p. 176–7°C. The ethyl ether is an oil, b.p. 230–2°C/5 mm, also forming a picrate, yellow prisms, m.p. 144–5°C; dipicrate, red needles from MeOH, m.p. 124–5°C.

Wieland, Konz, Mittasch., *Annalen*, **513**, 10 (1934)
Hoshino, Shimodaira., *ibid*, **520**, 28 (1935)
Hoshino, Shimodaira., *Bull. Chem. Soc. Japan,* **11**, 221 (1936)
Wieland, Motzel, Merz., *Annalen*, **581**, 10 (1953)
Stromberg., *J. Amer. Chem. Soc.,* **76**, 1707 (1954)
Harley-Mason, Jackson., *J. Chem. Soc.*, 1167 (1954)

BUFOTOXIN

$C_{40}H_{60}O_{10}N_4$

M.p. 204–5°C (*dec.*).

OC·(CH$_2$)$_6$·CO·O
HN
HC·COOH
(CH$_2$)$_3$
NH·C·NH$_2$
NH

Like the two preceding bases, this compound is found mainly in the poisonous secretion of *Bufo vulgaris*. It crystallizes in colourless needles from aqueous EtOH and is soluble in pyridine and MeOH, only slightly so in EtOH or H_2O and insoluble in most other organic solvents. It has $[\alpha]_D^{19} + 3.6°$ or $[\alpha]_D^{24} + 3.9°$ (MeOH). Hydrolysis with dilute acids furnishes acetic and suberic acids, arginine and bufotalein. The earlier structure has recently been revised.

Wieland, Alles., *Ber.*, **55**, 1793 (1922)
Wieland *et al.*, *Annalen*, **549**, 209 (1941)

Structure revision:
Kamano, Yamamoto, Tanaka, Komatsu., *Tetrahedron Lett.*, 5673 (1968)

BULBOCAPNINE

$C_{19}H_{19}O_4N$

M.p. 199°C

This alkaloid occurs in the tubers of *Bulbocapnus cavus* Bernh., *Corydalis decumbens* Pers., *C. solida* Sm., *C. tuberosa* DC., and *Dicentra canadensis* Walp. The base crystallizes from EtOH in rhombic needles, $[\alpha]_D + 237.1°$ (CHCl$_3$). It is soluble in alkalies developing a green colouration, being reprecipitated by CO$_2$. The alkaloid dissolves in H_2SO_4 with an orange-red colour changing slowly to violet. It forms crystalline salts, e.g. the hydrochloride, colourless needles, m.p. 270°C (*dec.*); the platinichloride, m.p. 200°C and 230°C (*dec.*) and the methiodide, needles, m.p. 257°C. The *dl*-methyl ether has m.p. 135°C and forms the hydriodide, m.p. 250°C (*dec.*); picrate, m.p. 213–4°C (*dec.*) and the methiodide, m.p. 243°C while the *d*-methyl ether has m.p. 128–9°C.

Exhaustive methylation yields trimethylamine and 3:4-dimethoxy-5:6-methylenedioxy-8-vinylphenanthrene. Mild oxidation of the ethyl ether with KMnO$_4$ furnishes 4-methoxy-3-ethoxybenzene-1:2-dicarboxylic acid, thereby establishing the relative positions of the hydroxyl and methoxyl groups in the molecule.

Bulbocapnine produces a cataleptic condition in warm-blooded animals, expecially in cats, and also stimulates the secretion of tears and saliva. In non-toxic doses it accelerates respiration but with lethal doses respiratory failure occurs shortly before heart failure. In small doses, the alkaloid induces a moderate hyperglycaemia in rabbits and lowers the glutathione content of the blood and liver while increasing it in the spleen. The phosphate is sometimes used in medicine in the treatment of Paralysis agitans and St. Vitus' dance.

Freund, Josephi., *Annalen,* **277,** 10 (1893)
Gadamer, Kuntz., *Arch. Pharm.,* **249,** 503, 598 (1911)
Gulland, Haworth., *J. Chem. Soc.,* 1132 (1928)
Späth, Hromatka., *Ber.,* **61,** 1334 (1928)
Kikkawa., *J. Pharm. Soc., Japan,* **79,** 1244 (1959)

Crystal structure:
Ashida, Pepinsky, Okaya., *Acta Cryst.,* **16,** A.48 (1963)

Mass spectra:
Jackson, Martin., *J. Chem. Soc., C,* 2181 (1966)

BULBOCODINE

$C_{19}H_{23}O_3N$

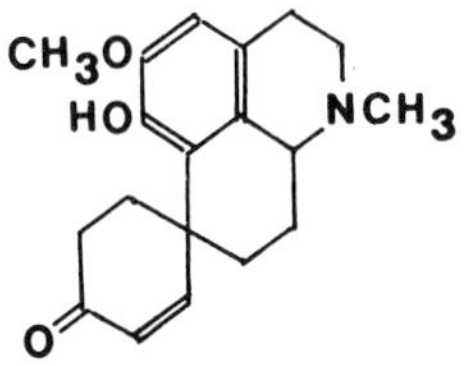

An alkaloid found in *Bulbocodium vernum,* the above structure has been assigned to this base on spectroscopic and circular dichroism determinations.

Reichstein, Snatzke, Santavy., *Planta Med.,* **16,** 357 (1968)

BULLATINE A

An uncharacterized alkaloid present in *Aconitum bullatifolium* var. *homostrichum.* The base is obtained by column chromatography of the alkaloidal extract and is present only in trace quantities.

Chu, Fang., *Hua Hsueh Hsueh Pao.,* **31,** 222 (1965)

BULLATINE B

A further minor constituent of *Aconitum bullatifolium* var. *homostrichum,* this base has not yet been obtained in sufficient quantity for a chemical analysis to be carried out.

Chu, Fang., *Hua Hseuh Hseuh Pao.,* **31,** 222 (1965)

BULLATINE C

Column chromatography of the alkaloid extract of *Aconitum bullatifolium* var. *homostrichum* affords this minor alkaloid which has not yet been characterized.

Chu, Fang., *Hua Hseuh Hseuh Pao.*, **31**, 222 (1965)

BULLATINE D

A fourth uncharacterized alkaloid from *Aconitum bullatifolium* var. *homostrichum*, this base is also present only in trace amounts.

Chu, Fang., *Hua Hseuh Hseuh Pao.*, **31**, 222 (1965)

BULLATINE E

$C_{24}H_{39}O_6N$

M.p. 182–3°C

This alkaloid from *Aconitum bullatifolium* var. *homostrichum* forms colourless crystals. It is dextrorotatory with $[\alpha]_D^{24} + 79.6°$ (Me_2CO) and contains three methoxyl groups, three hydroxyl groups and an ethylimino group in the molecule.

Chu, Fang., *Hua Hseuh Hseuh Pao.*, **31**, 222 (1965)

BULLATINE F

$C_{24}H_{39}O_7N$

M.p. 186°C

A major constituent of *Aconitum bullatifolium* var. *homostrichum*, this alkaloid also yields colourless needles. It is dextrorotatory with $[\alpha]_D^{14} + 23°$ ($CHCl_3$). There are three methoxyl groups, four hydroxyl groups and an ethylimino group present.

Chu, Fang., *Hua Hseuh Hseuh Pao.*, **31**, 222 (1965)

BULLATINE G

$C_{21}H_{31}O_3N$

M.p. 200–1°C

Also present in *Aconitum bullatifolium* var. *homostrichum*, this alkaloid is strongly laevorotatory having $[\alpha]_D^{20} - 168°$ ($CHCl_3$). It contains two hydroxyl groups, a keto group and an ethylimino group.

Chu, Fang., *Hua Hseuh Hseuh Pao.*, **31**, 222 (1965)

BUPHANAMINE

$C_{17}H_{19}O_4N$

M.p. 184–6°C

An alkaloid found in *Boöphone disticha* Herb. and *B. fischerii* Baker, the base forms colourless crystals from Me_2CO. It has $[\alpha]_D^{20} - 205°$ (c 1.0, 90% EtOH) and $[\alpha]_{436}^{24} - 408°$ (c 0.97, $CHCl_3$). The ultraviolet spectrum shows one absorption maximum at 287 mμ. The salts are crystalline, the hydrochloride, m.p. 180°C; nitrate, m.p. 136–140°C and the perchlorate, m.p. 232–4°C having been prepared.

Humbold, Taylor., *Can. J. Chem.,* 33, 1268 (1955)
Renz, Stauffacher, Seebeck., *Helv. Chim. Acta,* 38, 1209 (1955)
Fales, Wildman., *J. Org. Chem.,* 26, 881 (1961)

BUPHANIDRINE

$C_{18}H_{21}O_4N$

M.p. 90–2°C;
B.p. 150–170°C/0.04 mm

Like the preceding base, this alkaloid is present in *Boöphone disticha* Herb. and *B. fischerii* Baker. It yields colourless prisms from Et_2O with the above melting and boiling points. From aqueous MeOH it crystallizes in needles of the sesquihydrate, m.p. 144°C. This material still contains 0.5 mole of H_2O after sublimation. It is slightly dextrorotatory with $[\alpha]_D^{20} + 1.8°$ (90% EtOH). Its solution in concentrated H_2SO_4 is violet in colour. Several crystalline salts have been prepared including the hydrobromide, m.p. 195–7°C; the perchlorate, m.p. 240–2°C; the platinichloride, orange-yellow crystals, m.p. 223°C; the thiocyanate, m.p. 200–2°C (*dec.*); the picrate as yellow needles, m.p. 235°C; the styphnate, m.p. 239–241°C and the methiodide, m.p. 271°C.

Renz, Stauffacher, Seebeck., *Helv. Chim. Acta,* 38, 1209 (1955)
Bates *et al., J. Chem. Soc.,* 2537 (1957)
Goosen, Warren., *ibid,* 1094 (1960)
Wildman., *J. Amer. Chem. Soc.,* 80, 2567 (1958)
Haugwitz, Jeffs, Wenkert., *J. Chem. Soc.,* 2001 (1965)

BUPHANINE

From *Boöphane disticha* Herb. (Syn. *Haemanthus toxicarius* Herb.), Tutin isolated this amorphous alkaloid which has not yet been characterized. It is converted by KOH into Buphanitine (q.v.) which is also present in very small amounts in *B. disticha* Herb.

Tutin., *J. Chem. Soc.,* 99, 1240 (1911)

BUPHANISINE

$C_{17}H_{19}O_3N$

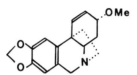

A further alkaloid from *Boöphane disticha* Herb. and *B. fischerii* Baker, this base yields colourless prisms when recrystallized from EtOH. It is laevorotatory with $[\alpha]_D^{20} - 26°$ (90% EtOH). The structure has been determined from spectroscopic evidence.

Renz, Stauffacher, Seebeck., *Helv. Chim. Acta*, **38**, 1209 (1955)
Fales, Wildman., *J. Amer. Chem. Soc.*, **82**, 3368 (1960)
Mass spectra:
Duffield *et al.*, *J. Amer. Chem. Soc.*, **87**, 4902 (1965)

(+)-epi-BUPHANISINE

$C_{17}H_{19}O_3N$

M.p. 123–5°C

This epimer of buphanisine occurs in *Ammocharis coranica* (Ker. Gaul) Herb. It has $[\alpha]_D^{21} + 133°$ (c 0.22, 95% EtOH) and $+ 141°$ (c 0.27, $CHCl_3$). The base is characterized as the crystalline perchlorate which forms colourless prisms with m.p. 244–6°C (*dec.*). The (–)-form of the alkaloid has m.p. 124–6°C; $[\alpha]_D^{22} - 139°$ (c 0.168, $CHCl_3$).

Hauth, Stauffacher., *Helv. Chim. Acta*, **45**, 1307 (1962)

BUPHANITINE

$C_{17}H_{21}O_5N$

M.p. 234°C

The alkaloid of this name obtained by Tutin from *Boöphane disticha* Herb., $C_{23}H_{24}O_6N_2$, m.p. 240°C (*dec.*) has since been resolved into two components, Buphanamine (q.v.) and this alkaloid which has the empirical formula given above. The base crystallizes from $CHCl_3$-Et_2O as slender needles which show a change in crystal form at 210°C into colourless prisms, m.p. 232°C. This latter form, with the same melting point, is also obtained when Me_2CO is employed as the crystallizing solvent. The alkaloid is laevorotatory with $[\alpha]_D^{20} - 102°$ (c 1.0, $CHCl_3$). It forms a crystalline nitrate, m.p. 222–4°C and a hydrochloride, m.p. 265°C. In the literature, this alkaloid is sometimes termed 'crystalline' haemanthine; buphanamine being referred to as 'oily' haemanthine.

Tutin., *J. Chem. Soc.*, **99**, 1240 (1911)
Lewin., *Arch. expt. Path. Pharm.*, **68**, 333 (1912)
Goosen, Warren., *J. Chem. Soc.*, 1094 (1960)

BURASAINE

$C_{21}H_{23}O_4N$

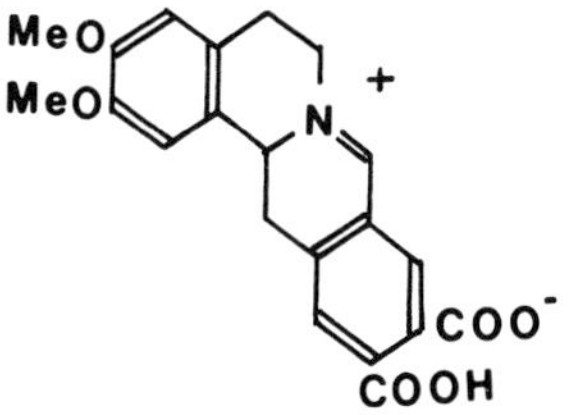

From one of the fractions obtained by column chromatography of the alkaloidal extract of *Burasia madagascariensis,* this alkaloid was obtained as the crystalline nitrate. The base differs from the accompanying Palmatine (q.v.) only by the absence of a double bond. The protoberberine structure of the base is confirmed by hydrogenation which yields optically inactive tetrahydropalmatine.

Resplandy., *Mem. Inst. Sci. Madagascar.,* **10D**, 37 (1961)

BURMANNALINE

$C_{21}H_{23}O_4N$

M.p. 165°C

This alkaloid occurs in *Cyclea burmanni* but apart from the formula and melting point, the base does not appear to have been examined in any further detail.

Saradamma., *Bull. Cent. Res. Inst. Univ. Travancore, Trivandrum.,* Ser. A, 3, 55 (1954)

BURMANNINE

$C_{18}H_{21}O_3N$

M.p. 218°C

A second alkaloid found in *Cyclea burmanni,* this base yields a crystàlline acetate, m.p. 140°C; hydrochloride, m.p. 304°C; picrate, m.p. 246°C (*dec.*) and a methiodide, m.p. 292°C.

Saradamma., *Bull. Cent. Res. Inst. Univ. Travancore, Trivandrum.,* Ser. A, 3, 55 (1954)

BURNAMICINE

$C_{20}H_{26}O_2N_2$

M.p. 198–200°C

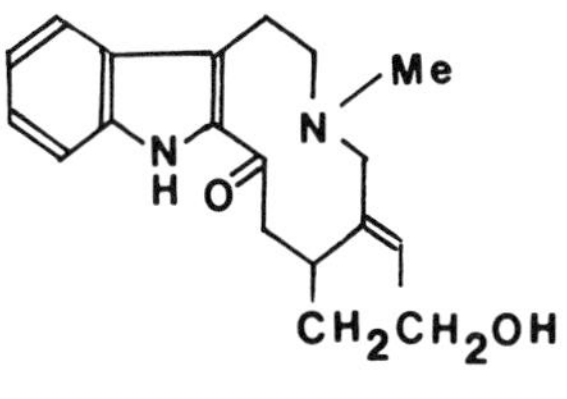

This indole alkaloid is a minor constituent of *Hunteria eburnea* and has $[\alpha]_D$ − 281°. The ultraviolet spectrum shows a broad absorption maximum at 309−312 mμ.

Bartlett, Taylor., *J. Amer. Chem. Soc.*, **85**, 1203 (1963)

BURNAMINE

$C_{21}H_{24}O_4N_2$

M.p. 197−8°C

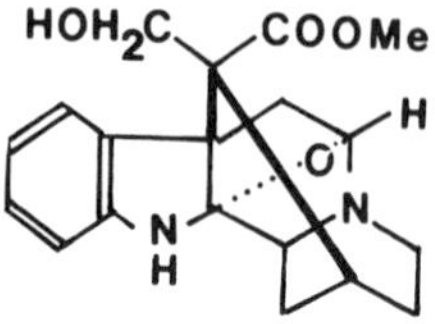

A carboline base which occurs in *Aspidosperma cuspa*, *Hunteria eburnea* and *Picralima nitida*, the alkaloid is laevorotatory with $[\alpha]_D$ − 131° (− 119°) (CHCl$_3$). The ultraviolet spectrum exhibits two absorption maxima at 234 and 288 mμ. The base may be characterized as the picrate which crystallizes as colourless needles from MeOH with m.p. 147−9°C.

Bartlett *et al.*, *J. Org. Chem.*, **28**, 2197 (1963)
Britten, Smith., *J. Chem. Soc.*, 3850 (1963)
Taylor *et al.*, *Bull. Soc. Chim. Fr.*, 392 (1964)

BUTROPINE

$C_{12}H_{21}O_2N$

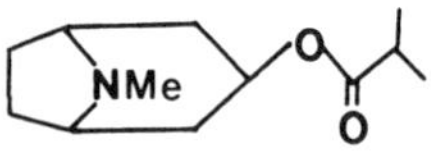

A liquid alkaloid, this base is obtained by steam distillation of the leaves of *Duboisia leuchhardtii*. It is strongly basic and optically inactive. The hydrobromide forms colourless prisms, m.p. 242°C; the aurichloride, golden-yellow needles, m.p. 149°C and the picrate has m.p. 224−5°C. On alkaline hydrolysis, the alkaloid furnishes tropine and *iso*butyric acid.

Rosenblum, Taylor., *J. Pharm. Pharmacol.*, **6**, 410 (1954)

BUXALTINE

$C_{35}H_{50}O_2N_2$

M.p. 188−191°C

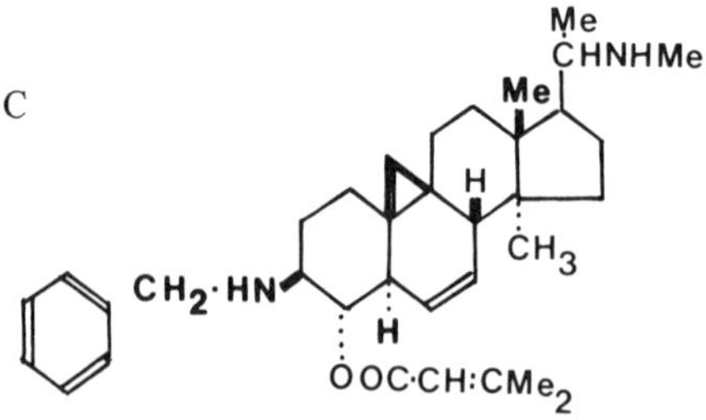

One of the numerous alkaloids isolated from *Buxus* species, this base occurs in

B. sempervirens. It forms colourless crystals when purified by recrystallization from Me_2CO. The structure has been assigned on the basis of spectroscopic data.

Döpke, Mueller., *Pharmazie,* **24**, 649 (1969)
Döpke *et al., Tetrahedron Lett.,* 4247 (1967)

BUXAMINE

See Buxamine E

BUXAMINE A

$C_{28}H_{48}N_2$

M.p. 134°C

This crystalline steroidal alkaloid is obtained from the roots of *Buxus madagascarica* and has $[\alpha]_D + 40°$. The ultraviolet spectrum shows three main absorption maxima at 238, 246 and 254 mμ. The base is the 20-N-methyl derivative of Buxamine E (q.v.).

Khuong Huu Laine *et al., Compt. rend.,* **273C**, 558 (1971)

BUXAMINE E

$C_{26}H_{44}N_2$

M.p. Indefinite

This alkaloid was formerly known simply as Buxamine. It occurs in the leaves of *Buxus balearica* Willd. and also in *B. sempervirens.* It is dextrorotatory with $[\alpha]_D^{20} + 32°$ (c 0.57, $CHCl_3$) and has an ultraviolet spectrum virtually identical with that of the preceding alkaloid with absorption maxima also at 238, 246 and 254 mμ. Of the crystalline salts and derivatives that have been prepared, the oxalate has m.p. 263–7°C; $[\alpha]_D^{20} + 18°$ (c 0.5, aqueous MeOH); bis hydrogen tartrate, colourless needles from EtOH, m.p. 210°C (*dec.*); $[\alpha]_D^{20} + 26°$ (c 0.52, aqueous EtOH); the N-*iso*propylidene derivative, m.p. 187°C; $[\alpha]_D^{20} + 48°$ (c 0.5, $CHCl_3$) and the 20-N-acetyl derivative, m.p. 237°C; $[\alpha]_D^{20} + 5°$ (c 0.5, $CHCl_3$).

Stauffacher., *Helv. Chim. Acta,* **47**, 968 (1964)
Khuong Huu Laine *et al., Tetrahedron,* **22**, 3321 (1966)

BUXAMINOL E

$C_{26}H_{44}ON_2$

M.p. 199–200°C

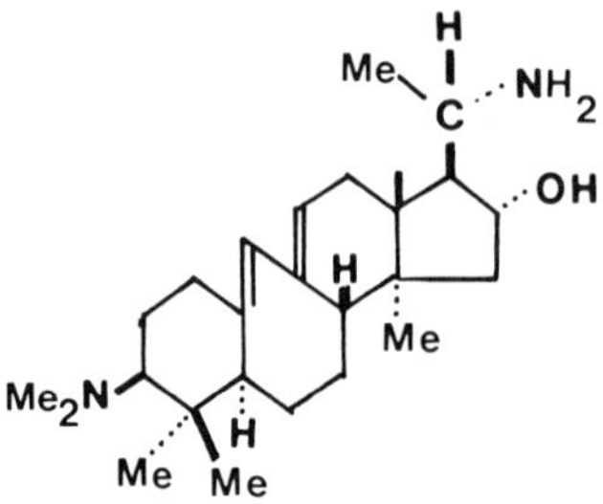

In order to standardize the names of the various *Buxus* alkaloids, the base originally known as Buxaminol has now been renamed Buxaminol E. It occurs in *B. sempervirens* and in the leaves of *B. balearica* Willd. When crystallized from aqueous MeOH, it forms short, colourless needles. It may also be crystallized from C_6H_6-hexane. It sublimes at 200°C and has $[\alpha]_D^{20} + 38°$ (c 0.5, CHCl$_3$). The ultraviolet spectrum has absorption maxima at 238, 245, 254, 277 and 287 mμ. The N-*iso*propylidene derivative has m.p. 206–9°C; $[\alpha]_D^{20} + 95°$ (c 0.5, CHCl$_3$) and the bis-hydrogen tartrate, m.p. 210°C; $[\alpha]_D^{20} + 14°$ (c 0.5, CHCl$_3$).

Stauffacher., *Helv. Chim. Acta,* **47**, 968 (1964)

Khuong-Huu-Laine, Herlem-Gaulier, Khuong-Huu, Stanislas, Goutarel., *Tetrahedron,* **22**, 3321 (1966)

BUXANDRINE

$C_{35}H_{52}O_4N_2$

M.p. 289–290°C (*dec.*).

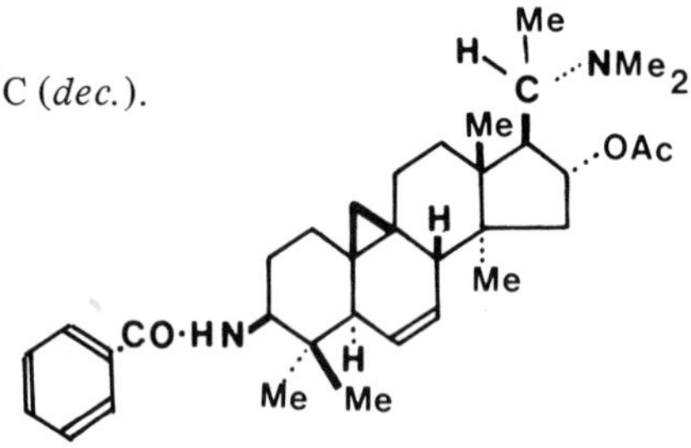

A further minor alkaloid present in *Buxus sempervirens,* this base forms colourless needles when crystallized from Me$_2$CO.

Döpke, Mueller, Spiteller, Spiteller-Friedmann., *Tetrahedron Lett.,* 4247 (1967)

226

BUXANINE

$C_{32}H_{43}O_2N$

M.p. 196–9°C

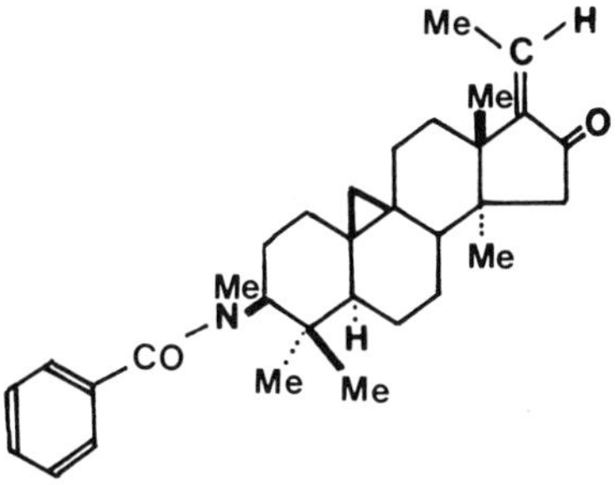

This steroidal alkaloid also occurs in *Buxus sempervirens* and forms colourless prisms from Me_2CO with $[\alpha]_D - 38°$ (c 0.2, $CHCl_3$).

Döpke, Mueller., *Pharmazie*, **21**, 769 (1966)

BUXARINE

$C_{33}H_{48}O_3N_2$

M.p. 210–2°C

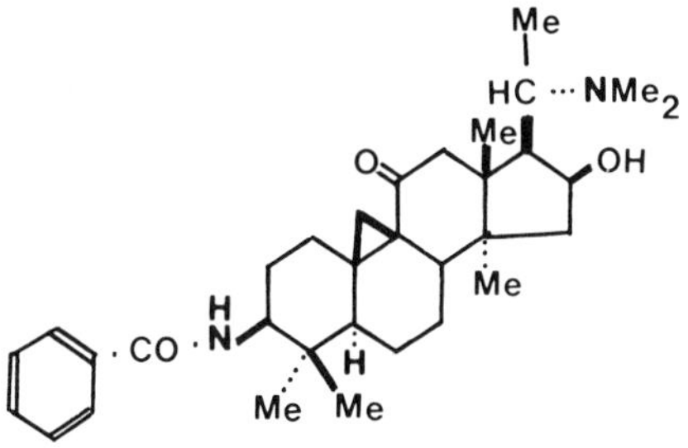

A minor constituent of *Buxus sempervirens*, this base crystallizes from Me_2CO in colourless prisms. It forms a dihydrochloride, m.p. 257–260°C. The N-methyl derivative has m.p. 175°C.

Döpke, Mueller, Jeffs., *Pharmazie*, **21**, 643 (1966)

BUXATINE

$C_{33}H_{48}O_2N_2$

M.p. 214–7°C (*dec.*).

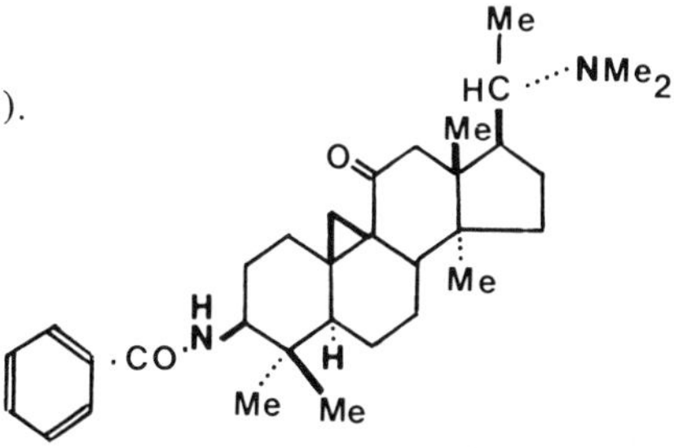

This alkaloid is closely related to Buxarine and also occurs in *Buxus sempervirens* from which it may be obtained as colourless needles from Me_2CO. It has $[\alpha]_D^{24} + 112°$ (c 0.2, $CHCl_3$).

Döpke, Mueller, Jeffs., *Naturwiss.*, **54**, 249 (1967)

BUXAZIDINE B

$C_{27}H_{46}O_2N_2$

M.p. 234–6°C

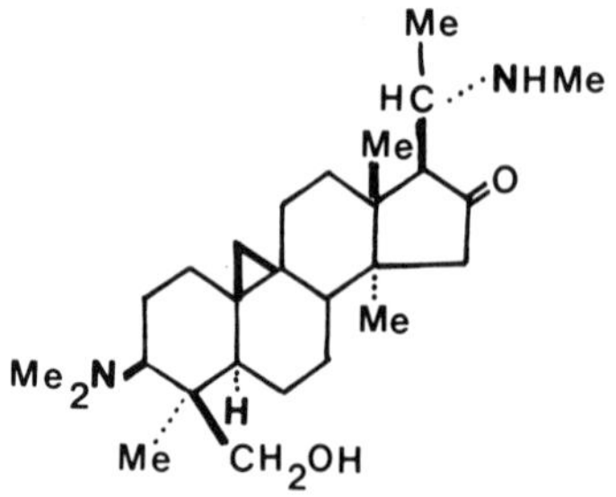

Also present in *Buxus sempervirens,* this base crystallizes in colourless needles from Me_2CO. It has $[\alpha]_D^{21} - 31°$ (c 0.1, $CHCl_3$).

Döpke, Mueller, Spiteller, Spiteller-Friedmann., *Naturwiss.,* 54, 200 (1967)

BUXAZINE

$C_{28}H_{48}O_2N_2$

M.p. 238–9°C (*dec.*).

A minor alkaloid from *Buxus sempervirens* obtained as colourless prisms from MeOH. This base has $[\alpha]_D^{24} + 93°$ (c 0.2, $CHCl_3$). The oxalate is amorphous with m.p. 257–260°C (*dec.*) but the acetyl derivative is crystalline, m.p. 238°C. The alkaloid may be reduced to the dihydroderivative, m.p. 262°C (*dec.*).

Döpke, Mueller., *Naturwiss.,* 52, 61 (1965)

BUXENE

$C_{27}H_{41}O_3N$

M.p. 202–4°C

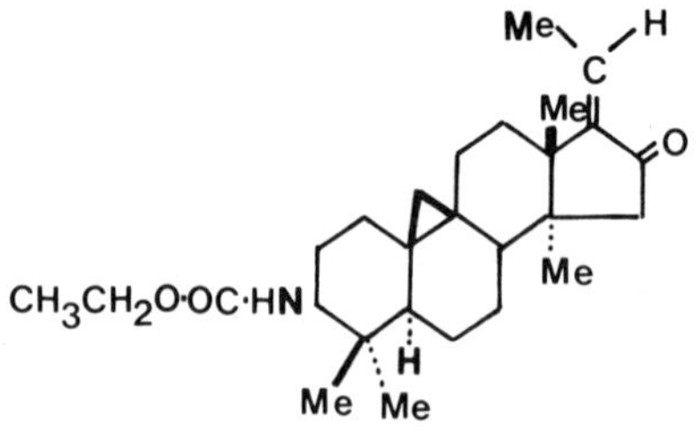

A further constituent of *Buxus sempervirens,* this base crystallizes from MeOH in colourless prisms. The ultraviolet spectrum in MeOH shows a single absorption maximum at 243 mμ. The N-methyl derivative (q.v.) is also present in this plant.

Döpke, Hartel, Fehlhaber., *Tetrahedron Lett.,* 4423 (1969)

BUXENINE G

$C_{25}H_{42}N_2$

M.p. Indefinite

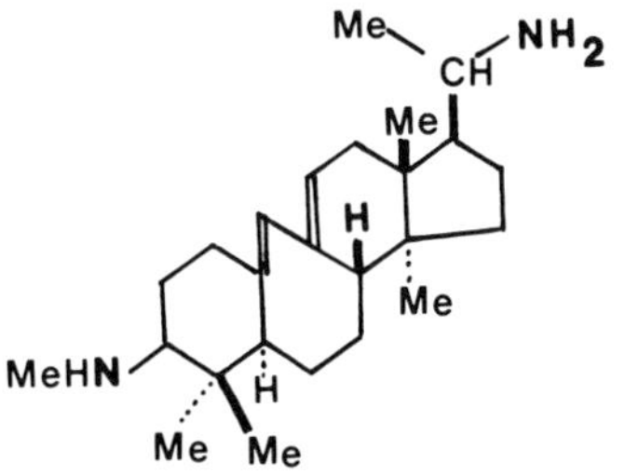

Buxus sempervirens also yields this cytotoxic alkaloid which is present in the Me_2CO-soluble portion of the strong bases. The base is isolated as the isopropylideneimine, $C_{28}H_{46}N_2$, m.p. 186–8°C (m.p. 194–6°C after vacuum sublimation); $[\alpha]_D^{22} + 51°$ (c 0.72, $CHCl_3$) or as the dihydriodide which forms orthorhombic crystals from EtOH-AcOEt, m.p. 298–300°C (*dec.*). The ultraviolet spectrum of the alkaloid in EtOH shows absorption maxima at 238, 247, and 255 mμ with shoulders at 215, 230 and 290 mμ. On catalytic hydrogen with Pt in AcOH the base yields the tetrahydro derivative, characterized as the *iso*propylideneimine, m.p. 140–3°C; $[\alpha]_D^{20} + 3°$ (c 0.6, $CHCl_3$). The salicylaldimine has also been prepared as colourless crystals, m.p. 216–220°C; $[\alpha]_D^{24} + 130°$ (c 1.1, $CHCl_3$).

Kupchan, Asbun., *Tetrahedron Lett.*, **42**, 3145 (1964)
Puckett *et al., ibid,* 3815 (1966)

BUXENONE

$C_{25}H_{39}ON$

M.p. 174°C

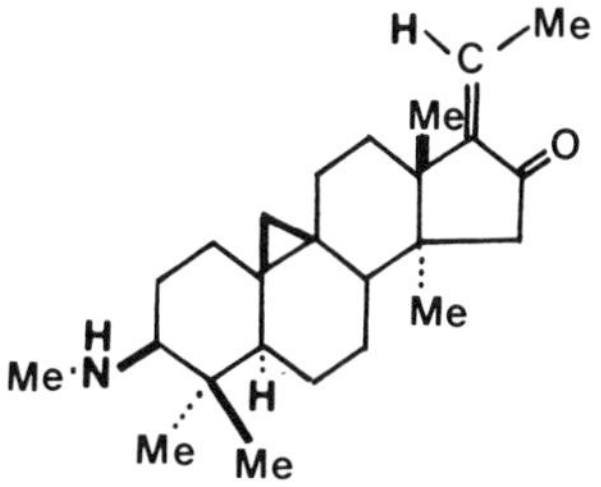

Also present in *Buxus sempervirens*, this minor alkaloid crystallizes as colourless prisms from Me_2CO. It is laevorotatory with $[\alpha]_D - 48°$ (c 0.28, $CHCl_3$). The hydrochloride is also crystalline, m.p. 290°C (*dec.*). The N-methyl derivative has m.p. 201–3°C.

Döpke, Mueller, Jeffs., *Pharmazie,* **21**, 643 (1966)

BUXERIDINE

$C_{34}H_{50}ON_2$

M.p. 208–211°C

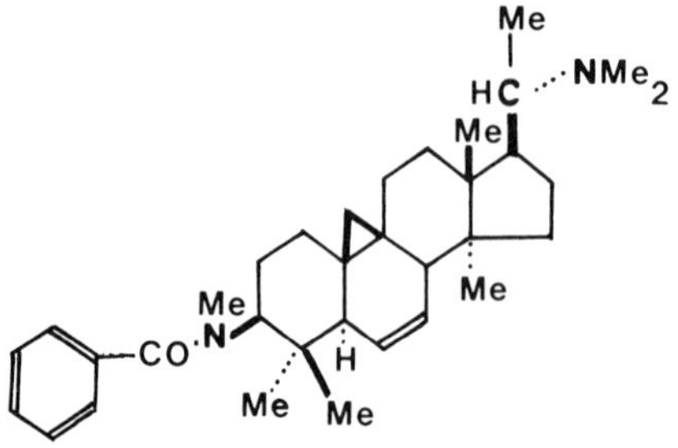

A further minor constituent of *Buxus sempervirens*, this alkaloid crystallizes from Me_2CO in colourless prisms. It is slightly dextrorotatory with $[\alpha]_D^{21} + 14°$ (c 0.18, $CHCl_3$).

Döpke *et al.*, *Naturwiss.*, **54**, 200 (1967)

BUXIDINE

$C_{33}H_{48}O_3N_2$

M.p. 154–7°C

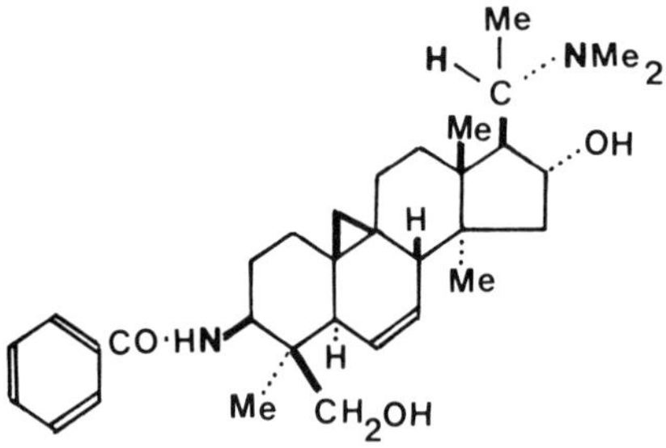

A minor alkaloid of *Buxus sempervirens*, this base is obtained in the form of slender, colourless needles from Me_2CO. It has $[\alpha]_D^{24} + 67.5°$ (c 0.2, $CHCl_3$). The N-methyl derivative is the alkaloid Cyclomicrosine (q.v.) and the 15-O-acetate is Buxandrine (q.v.).

Döpke *et al.*, *Tetrahedron Lett.*, 4247 (1967)

BUXIRAMINE

$C_{25}H_{42}ON_2$

M.p. 213–5°C

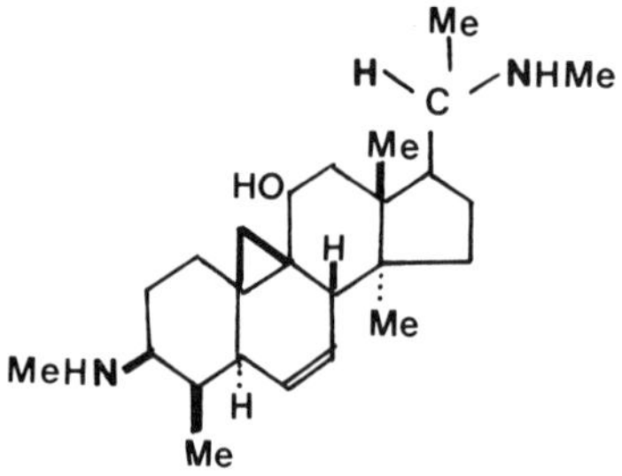

A further steroidal alkaloid from *Buxus sempervirens,* the base crystallizes from Me_2CO as colourless prisms.

Döpke, Mueller., *Pharmazie,* **24,** 649 (1969)

BUXITRIENINE C

$C_{27}H_{44}ON_2$

M.p. 192°C

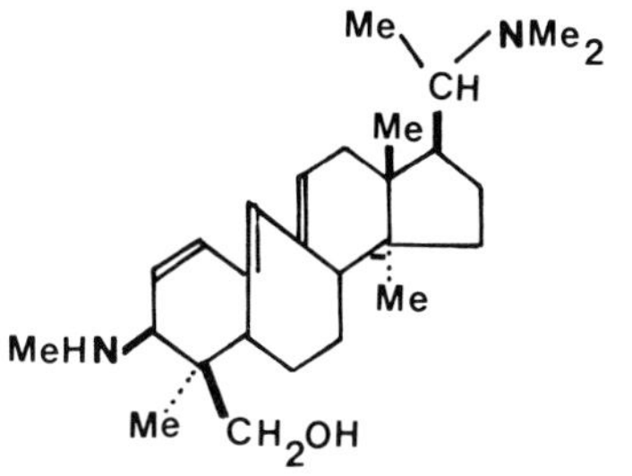

This alkaloid occurs in the roots of *Buxus madascarica* and forms colourless crystals from C_6H_6-hexane. It has $[\alpha]_D + 57°$ and the ultraviolet spectrum exhibits absorption maxima at 270, 278 and 289 mμ.

Khuong-Huu-Laine, Paris, Razafindrambao, Cave, Goutarel., *Compt. rend.,* **273C,** 558 (1971)

BUXOCYALAMINE A

$C_{27}H_{48}N_2$

M.p. 187–8°C

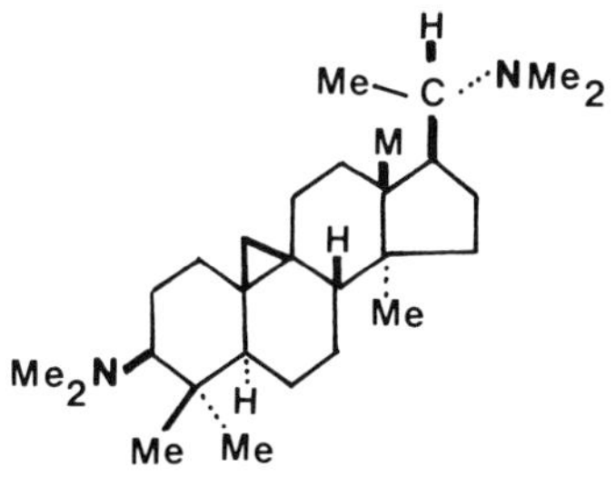

This base has been isolated by chromatographic purification of the extract from *Buxus sempervirens.* It forms colourless needles when crystallized from Me_2CO and has $[\alpha]_D^{24} + 87°$ (c 0.15, $CHCl_3$). The infrared spectrum shows strong bands at 1455 and 3030 cm^{-1} while the mass spectra exhibit intense peaks at m/e 400 (M$^+$), 84 and 72.

Döpke, Mueller, Jeffs., *Pharmazie,* **23,** 37 (1968)

BUXPSIINE (*Buxamideine K*)

$C_{26}H_{39}ON$

M.p. 176–8°C

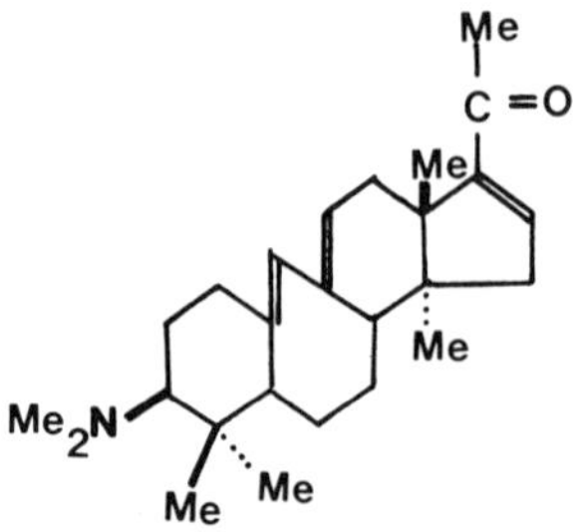

A norhomopregnane type alkaloid from *Buxus sempervirens,* this base forms crystals from Me_2CO and has $[\alpha]_D^{24}$ + 105° (c 0.18, $CHCl_3$). The ultraviolet spectrum shows absorption maxima at 240, 247 and 255 (shoulder) mμ.

Tomko, Bauerova, Voticky, Goutarel, Longevialle., *Tetrahedron Lett.,* 915 (1966)

C

CAAVERINE

$C_{17}H_{17}O_2N_2$

M.p. 208–210°C (*dec.*).

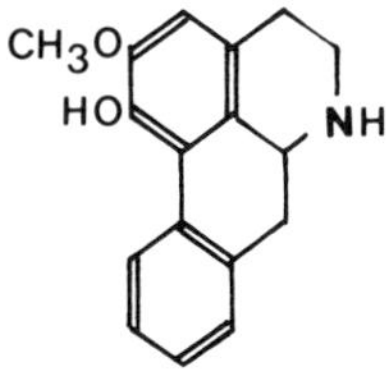

A noraporphine alkaloid isolated from the bark of *Symplocos celastrinea* Mart. The base is obtained as colourless crystals from C_6H_6 and has $[\alpha]_D^{25} - 89°$ (c 1.0, MeOH). The O,N-diacetyl derivative forms slender, colourless needles when recrystallized from MeOH, m.p. 236–8°C. The structure has been shown to be 5-hydroxy-6-methoxynoraporphine by degradative and spectroscopic studies.

Tschesche *et al., Tetrahedron*, **20**, 1435 (1964)

CABUCINE (*10-Methoxyajmaline*)

$C_{23}H_{26}O_4N_2$

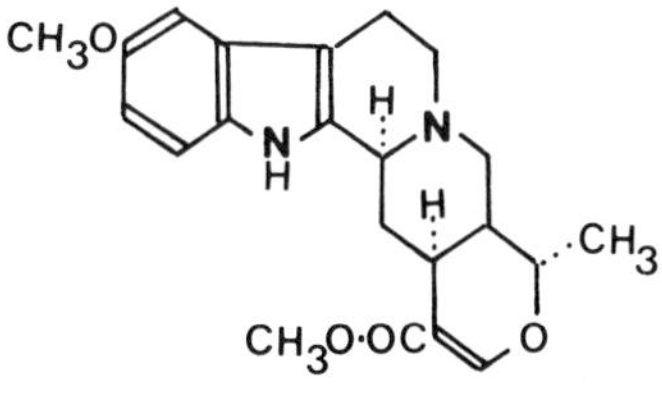

Obtained from *Cabucala madagascariensis* Pichon, this alkaloid is laevorotatory with $[\alpha]_D - 60°$ (CHCl$_3$). The structure has been assigned on the basis of chemical and spectroscopic investigation and comparison with Ajmaline (q.v.).

Douzoua *et al., Ann. Pharm.*, **30**, 199 (1972)

CABUCININE

$C_{22}H_{28}O_5N_2$

M.p. 170°C

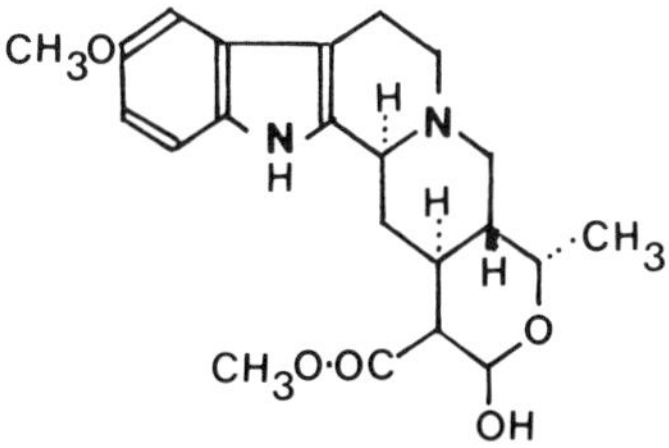

A second base found in *Cabucala madagascariensis* Pichon., this alkaloid is structurally very similar to the preceding base. It is optically inactive in CHCl$_3$.

Douzoua *et al., Ann. Pharm.*, **30**, 199 (1972)

CADAINE

$C_{23}H_{30}O_4N_2$

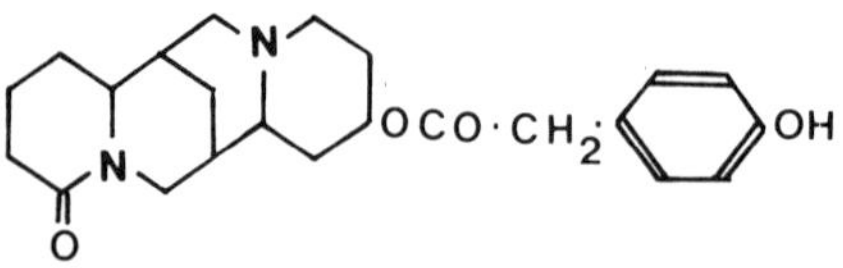

A sparteine type alkaloid recently isolated from *Cadia purpurea*, the structure of this base has been established from spectroscopic data.

Van Eijk, Radena., *Pharm. Weekbl.*, **107**, 13 (1972)

CAFFAEOSCHIZIN

$C_{20}H_{20}O_4N_2$

M.p. 208–212°C

Found in *Schizozygia caffaeoides* (Boj.) Baill., this base has the tentative structure and formula given above. It is dextrorotatory with $[\alpha]_D^{24} + 25.6°$ (c 1.0, $CHCl_3$) and the ultraviolet spectrum shows absorption maxima at 264 and 307 mμ. The structure is not yet known with certainty.

Renner, Kernweisz., *Experientia*, **19**, 244 (1963)

CAFFEINE (*Theine*)

$C_8H_{10}O_2N_4$

Subl. 178°C

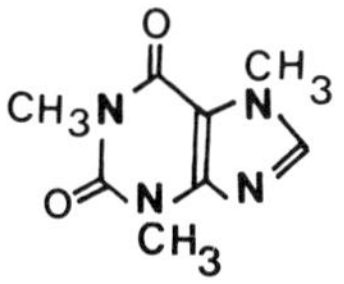

This purine alkaloid occurs in tea, coffee and cocoa and forms colourless crystals of the monohydrate from H_2O. It is almost insoluble in Et_2O, somewhat more so in H_2O or EtOH and dissolves to the extent of 12.5 per cent in $CHCl_3$. The crystals do not melt but sublime at 178°C. Caffeine is only a weak base and the salts formed are unstable, e.g. the aurichloride, m.p. 248°C; perchlorate, m.p. 89°C; styphnate, m.p. 199°C and the (±)-α-camphorsulphonate, m.p. 151°C; $[\alpha]_D^{15} + 2°$. The base is decomposed when heated with alkalies to form caffeidine. Pharmacologically, caffeine acts as a mild stimulant.

Rodionov., *Bull. soc. chim.*, **39**, 305 (1926)
Biltz, Beck., *J. prakt. Chem.*, **118**, 198 (1928)
Poggi., *Chem. Abstr.*, **44**, 1069 (1950)
Pirrone, Riparbelli., *ibid*, **45**, 1069 (1951)
Bredereck, Hennig, Muller., *Ber.*, **86**, 850 (1953)

CALABACIN

$C_{17}H_{25}O_3N_3$

M.p. 138°C

This minor alkaloid of *Physostigma venenosum* Balf., has $[\alpha]_D^{27} - 198°$ (c 0.2, $CHCl_3$). As yet the complete structure has not been determined. It forms a crystalline picrate as prisms from MeOH, m.p. 215°C and the salicylate, also crystalline, m.p. 138°C.

Döpke., *Naturwiss.*, **50**, 713 (1963)

CALABATIN

$C_{17}H_{25}O_2N$

M.p. 119°C

A further minor constituent of *Physostigma venenosum* Balf. seeds, this base has $[\alpha]_D^{24} - 98°$ (c 0.2, $CHCl_3$). It too, forms a crystalline picrate, m.p. 128°C and salicylate, m.p. 211°C.

Döpke., *Naturwiss.*, **50**, 713 (1963)

CALEBASSINE (*C-Toxiferine II, C-Strychnotoxine I*)

$C_{40}H_{48}O_2N_4^{++}$

Several alkaloids have been isolated and characterized from gourd or calabash curare whose botanical source has been shown to be the bark of *Strychnos toxifera* Schomb. This particular alkaloid is one of the major constituents of calabash curare and is also formed from C-dihydrotoxiferine I by photo-oxidation. The dichloride is obtained as needles of the hexahydrate from H_2O; $[\alpha]_D^{24} + 72.1°$ (H_2O). In high vacuum it slowly forms the dihydrate on warming. It gives characteristic colour reactions with various reagents, e.g. with $Ce(SO_4)_2$ it gives a deep blue-violet colour gradually changing to carmine. In concentrated HNO_3 the colour is deep crimson. The picrate crystallizes from Me_2CO with m.p. 216–8°C (*dec.*).

Wieland, Bähr, Witkop., *Annalen*, **547**, 156 (1941)
Karrer, Schmid., *Helv. Chim. Acta*, **29**, 1853 (1946)

Karrer, Schmid., *ibid*, **30**, 2081 (1947)
Wieland, Merz., *Chem. Ber.*, **85**, 731 (1952)
Meyer, Schmid, Karrer., *Helv. Chim. Acta*, **39**, 1208 (1956)
Hesse *et al.*, *ibid*, **44**, 2211 (1961)

CALEBASSINE A

$C_{20}H_{23}O_2N_2$

A minor alkaloid of *Strychnos toxifera* Schomb., this base forms a crystalline picrate, m.p. 228°C.

Kebrle *et al.*, *Helv. Chim. Acta.*, **36**, 102 (1953)

CALEBASSINE F

$C_{20}H_{25}O_2N_2$

Also present in calabash curare from *Strychnos toxifera* Schomb., the picrate of this base has m.p. 209−210°C.

Kebrle *et al.*, *Helv. Chim. Acta*, **36**, 102 (1953)

CALEBASSINE I

$C_{19-20}H_{23-25}N_2$

Calabash curare also contains this base in very small amounts. As yet it has not been fully characterized. It yields a crystalline picrate with m.p. 194°C.

Kebrle *et al.*, *Helv. Chim. Acta*, **36**, 102 (1953)

CALEBASSININE

$C_{19}H_{23}O_2N_2$

This alkaloid is normally isolated as the picrate from calabash curare, crystallizing in small yellow needles, m.p. 260°C and giving an intense carmine colour with $Ce(SO_4)_2$ although the colour test is negative in 50 per cent H_2SO_4. The chloride hemihydrate is amorphous and has $[\alpha]_D + 63°$ (H_2O). The iodide, however, is crystalline, forming minute, hygroscopic needles. The base is stated to contain no methoxyl groups.

Schmid, Karrer., *Helv. Chim. Acta*, **29**, 1853 (1946)
Schmid, Karrer., *ibid*, **30**, 1162, 2081 (1947)

CALIFORNIDINE

A quaternary alkaloid found in *Eschscholtzia californica* and also in *E. douglasi* appears to be an aporphine derivative although the structure is still unknown.

Slavik, Dolejs, Sedmera., *Collect. Czech. Chem. Commun.*, **35**, 2597 (1970)

C-ALKALOID A

$C_{40}H_{48}O_4N_4^{++}$

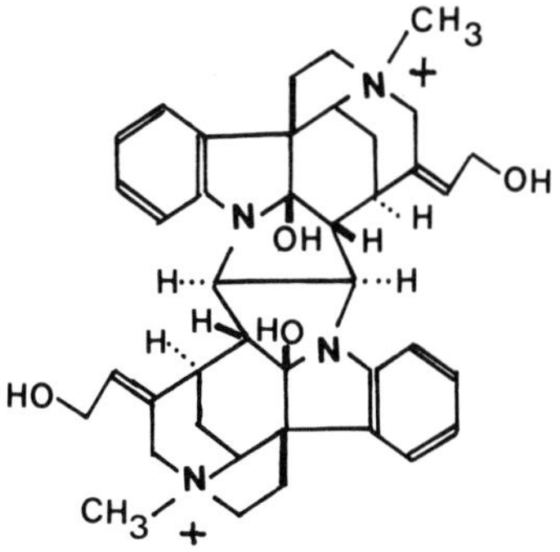

A dimeric alkaloid obtained from the bark of *Strychnos toxifera* Schomb and calabash curare, this base is also formed by photo-oxidation of C-toxiferine. Like most of these alkaloids it gives characteristic colour reactions with certain reagents. $Ce(SO_4)_2$ in H_2SO_4 produces a blue-violet colour changing to carmine red. The dichloride is obtained in the form of colourless needles from MeOH-di-*iso*propyl ether and the picrate from 80 per cent aqueous Me_2CO, m.p. 269°C (*dec.*). Pharmacologically, the base is a strong curarizing poison.

Karrer, Schmid., *Helv. Chim. Acta,* **29**, 1853 (1946)
King., *J. Chem. Soc.,* 3263 (1949)
Schmid, Kebrle, Karrer., *Helv. Chim. Acta,* **35**, 1864 (1952)
Kebrle *et al., ibid,* **36**, 102 (1953)
Hesse *et al., ibid,* **44**, 2211 (1961)

C-ALKALOID B

$(C_{20}H_{23}ON_2)_n$

Isolated from calabash curare, this polymeric alkaloid forms a chloride, colourless needles from MeOH-Et$_2$O and a crystalline picrate, m.p. > 280°C. The value of n in the above formula is probably 2.

Karrer, Schmid., *Helv. Chim. Acta,* **29**, 1853 (1946)
Kebrle *et al., ibid,* **36**, 102 (1953)

C-ALKALOID D

$C_{40}H_{48}O_2N_4^{++}$

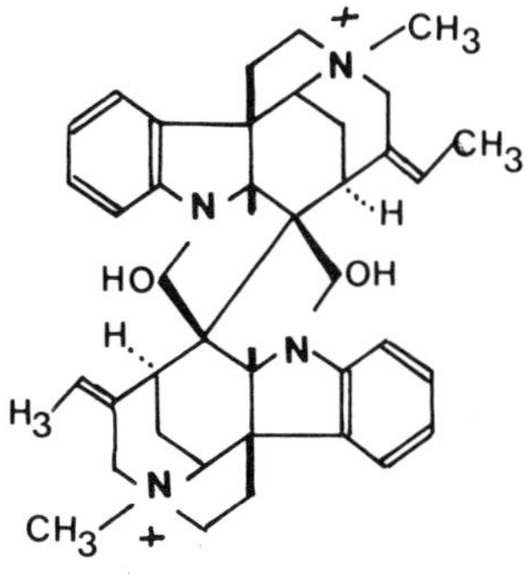

Occurring in calabash curare, this alkaloid is also formed by the action of acids on C-dihydrotoxiferine I. With $Ce(SO_4)_2$ in H_2SO_4 it gives a reddish-violet colour that slowly changes to yellow. The picrate is crystalline and has m.p. $> 270°C$.

Schmid, Kebrle, Karrer., *Helv. Chim. Acta,* **35**, 1864 (1952)
Kebrle *et al., ibid,* **36**, 102 (1953)
Battersby, Hodson., *Proc. Chem. Soc.,* 287 (1958)
Battersby *et al., ibid,* 412, 413 (1961)
McPhail, Sim., *ibid,* 416 (1961)
Hesse *et al., Helv. Chim. Acta,* **44**, 2211 (1961)

C-ALKALOID E

$C_{40}H_{46}O_2N_4^{++}$

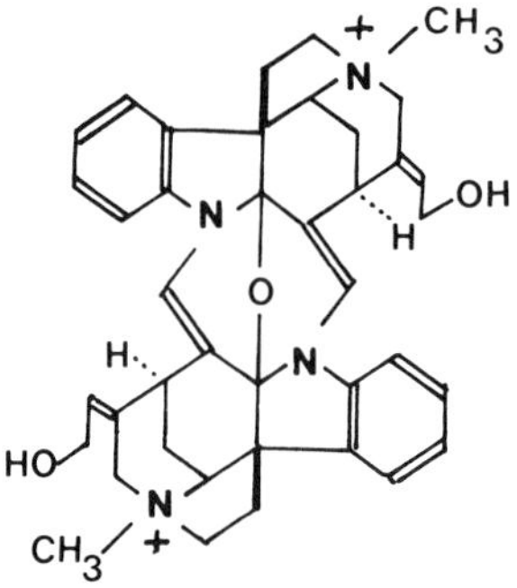

A further alkaloid found in calabash curare, this quaternary base is also obtained by photo-oxidation of C-toxiferine I. With $Ce(SO_4)_2$ in H_2SO_4 it produces a blue colour turning to green. The chloride is formed as colourless needles from $MeOH-Et_2O$ and the picrate, needles from aqueous Me_2CO has m.p. 272°C.

Kebrle *et al., Helv. Chim. Acta,* **36**, 102 (1953)
Schmid, Kebrle, Karrer., *ibid,* **35**, 1864 (1952)
Battersby, Hodson., *Quart. Rev.,* **14**, 77 (1960)
Nagyvary *et al., Tetrahedron,* **14**, 138 (1961)
Grdinic, Nelson, Boekelheide., *J. Amer. Chem. Soc.,* **86**, 3357 (1964)

C-ALKALOID F (*18-Hydroxy-C-calebassine*)

$C_{40}H_{48}O_3N_4^{++}$

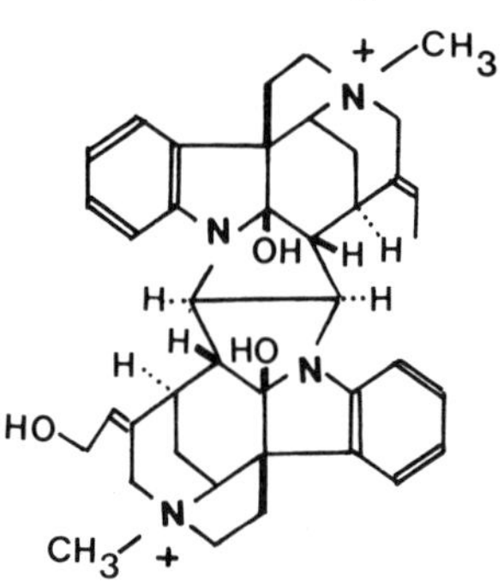

This alkaloid is also present in calabash curare and is also formed by oxidation of C-Alkaloid H (q.v.). It produces a carmine red colour with $Ce(SO_4)_2$ in H_2SO_4. The crystalline picrate has m.p. 209–210°C.

Schmid, Kebrle, Karrer., *Helv. Chim. Acta*, **35**, 1864 (1952)
Kebrle *et al.*, *ibid*, **36**, 102 (1953)
Berlage *et al.*, *ibid*, **42**, 2650 (1959)

C-ALKALOID G (*18-Hydroxy-C-curarine I*)

$C_{40}H_{44}O_2N_4^{++}$

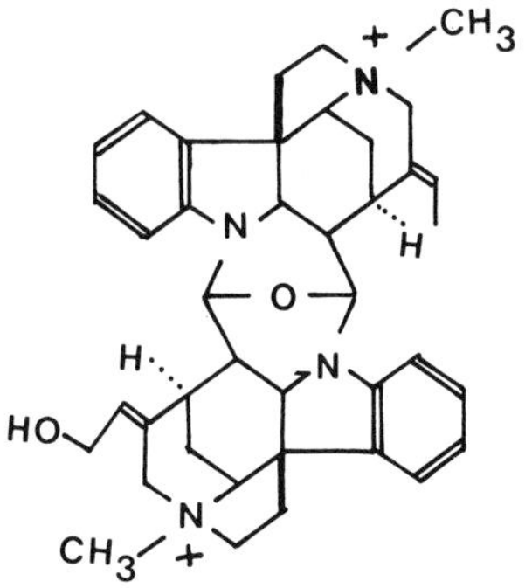

A minor alkaloid found in calabash curare, this quaternary base forms a picrate as slender needles from aqueous Me_2CO, m.p. 285–6°C. With $Ce(SO_4)_2$ in H_2SO_4 it produces a blue colour going to green on standing.

Schmid, Kebrle, Karrer., *Helv. Chim. Acta*, **35**, 1864 (1952)
Kebrle *et al.*, *ibid*, **36**, 102 (1953)
Berlage *et al.*, *ibid*, **42**, 2650 (1959)

C-ALKALOID H

$C_{40}H_{46}ON_4^{++}$

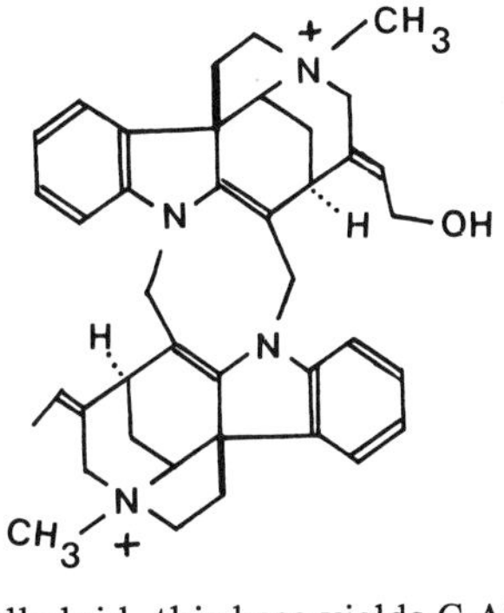

A further calabash curare alkaloid, this base yields C-Alkaloid F when oxidized. It gives a reddish-violet colour with $Ce(SO_4)_2$ in H_2SO_4 which becomes colourless on standing. The picrate crystallizes from aqueous Me_2CO with m.p. 189–192°C. The dichloride has $[\alpha]_D^{24} - 544.9°$ (c 0.3307, H_2O).

Schmid, Kebrle, Karrer., *Helv. Chim. Acta*, **35**, 1864 (1952)
Kebrle *et al.*, *ibid*, **36**, 102 (1953)
Berlage *et al.*, *ibid*, **42**, 2650 (1959)

C-ALKALOID I

$C_{19-20}H_{23-25}N_2$

This alkaloid of calabash curare has been characterized as the picrate, m.p. 194°C. It does not appear to have been examined further since its discovery.

Kebrle *et al., Helv. Chim. Acta,* **36**, 102 (1953)

C-ALKALOID J

$(C_{19}H_{21}N_2^+)_n$

Present in calabash curare, this alkaloid forms a crystalline picrate with m.p. > 260°C. In the formula given above it is probable that n = 2.

Kebrle *et al., Helv. Chim. Acta,* **36**, 102 (1953)

C-ALKALOID L

This alkaloid from calabash curare has been characterized only by the picrate which forms prisms from aqueous Me_2CO with m.p. 171°C.

Kebrle *et al., Helv. Chim. Acta,* **36**, 102 (1953)

C-ALKALOID M

Like the preceding alkaloid, this base is found in calabash curare but so far has not been characterized. The chloride is crystalline.

Asmis *et al., Helv. Chim. Acta,* **37**, 1968 (1954)

C-ALKALOID O

$C_{20}H_{27}ON_2^+$

Obtained from calabash curare, this base forms a crystalline chloride from EtOH with $[\alpha]_D^{20} - 124°$ (c 0.864, MeOH). The picrate crystallizes as needles from aqueous Me_2CO with m.p. 237–8°C.

Asmis *et al., Helv. Chim. Acta,* **37**, 1968 (1954)
Giesbrecht *et al., ibid,* **37**, 1974 (1954)

C-ALKALOID P

$C_{20}H_{23}ON_2^+$

This base has been isolated from calabash curare as the picrate which crystallizes from aqueous Me_2CO with m.p. 224–232°C (*dec.*).

Asmis *et al., Helv. Chim. Acta,* **37**, 1968 (1954)
Giesbrecht *et al., ibid,* **37**, 1974 (1954)

C-ALKALOID Q

$(C_{22}H_{27}O_3N_3)_n$

One of the minor calabash curare alkaloids, this base is said to crystallize from aqueous MeOH with m.p. 276–283°C (*dec.*). It has not been characterized further.

Meyer, Schmid, Karrer., *Helv. Chim. Acta*, **39**, 1208 (1956)

C-ALKALOID R

$(C_{21}H_{27}O_2N_2^+)_n$

A further minor constituent of calabash curare, the chloride may be obtained in the crystalline form from PrOH, m.p. 312°C (*dec.*). The crystalline perchlorate has m.p. 317°C.

Meyer, Schmid, Karrer., *Helv. Chim. Acta*, **39**, 1208 (1956)

C-ALKALOID S

$C_{19-20}H_{22-24}N_2$

Also present in calabash curare, the picrate of this alkaloid has m.p. 250°C.

Meyer, Schmid, Karrer., *Helv. Chim. Acta*, **39**, 1208 (1956)

C-ALKALOID X

This alkaloid has been obtained in minute quantity from calabash curare as the crystalline chloride which gives a deep, although unstable, carmine colour and violet fluorescence with HNO_3. With $Ce(SO_4)_2$ the colour is orange, slowly turning to red.

Karrer, Schmid., *Helv. Chim. Acta*, **29**, 1853 (1946)
Karrer, Schmid., *ibid*, **30**, 1162, 2081 (1947)

C-ALKALOID Y (*C-Profluorocurine*)

$C_{20}H_{27}O_3N_2^+$

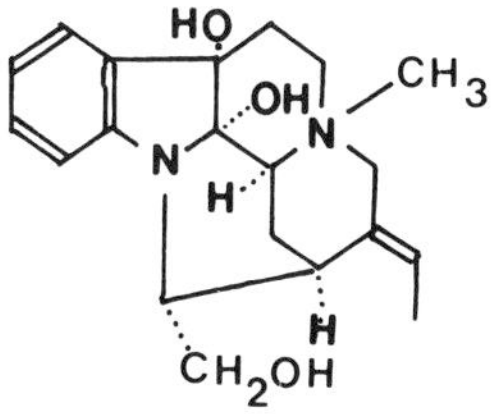

As well as occurring in the bark of *Strychnos toxifera* Schomb, this alkaloid is formed by oxidation of C-Mavacurine (q.v.). With acids, the alkaloid gives C-fluorocurine. With $Ce(SO_4)_2$ the alkaloid furnishes a reddish-violet colour and with HNO_3 the colour is a deep carmine. The chloride is obtained as colourless crystals from aqueous Me_2CO. The earlier structure of this base has now been revised to that given above.

Asmis *et al., Helv. Chim. Acta,* **37**, 1968 (1954)
Fritz, Wieland, Besch., *Annalen,* **611**, 268 (1958)
Structure revision:
Hesse, von Phillipsborn, Schumann, Spiteller, Spiteller-Friedmann, Taylor, Schmid, Karrer., *Helv. Chim. Acta,* **47**, 878 (1964)

C-ALKALOID UB

$C_{19}H_{23}O_3N_2$

The picrate of this calabash curare alkaloid, m.p. 238–240°C gives an intense carmine colour with $Ce(SO_4)_2$ in H_2SO_4 which is unstable and soon fades. The crystalline iodide is obtained from the picrate.

Kebrle *et al., Helv. Chim. Acta,* **36**, 102 (1953)
Asmis *et al., ibid,* **37**, 1968 (1954)

CALLICHILINE

$C_{42}H_{48}O_5N_4$

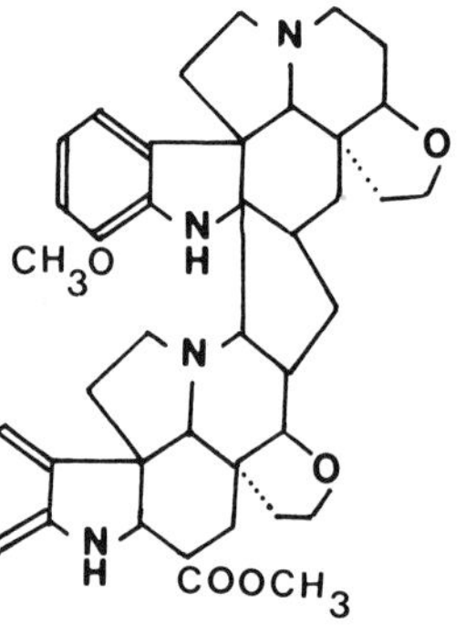

This dimeric indole alkaloid is present in *Callichilia barteri* together with beninine and vobtusine. The probable structure given has been determined on the basis of chemical reactions and spectroscopic evidence, particularly from the mass spectra.

Agwada, Gorman, Hesse, Schmid., *Helv. Chim. Acta,* **50**, 1939 (1967)

CALLIGONINE

$C_{12}H_{14}N_2$

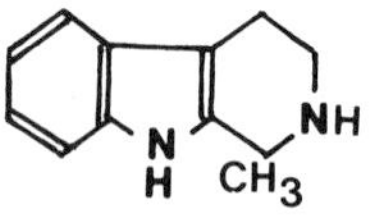

This tetrahydroharman base is the major alkaloid of *Calligonum minimum.* It forms colourless crystals from Me_2CO and a number of derivatives, some of which possess marked pharmacological properties, have been prepared, particu-

242

larly by Abdusalamov and Sadykov. These include the 3:4:5-trimethoxy-benzoyloxy acetyl derivative, m.p. 200–2°C; the diethylaminoacetyl compound, m.p. 177–9°C; the 3-aminopropyl derivative which is isolated as the hydrochloride, m.p. 117–9°C; the α-hydroxylethyl compound obtained as the oxalate, m.p. 177–8°C and the 3-(3:4:5-trimethoxybenzamido)propyl compound, m.p. 169–170°C, yielding a picrate, m.p. 138–9°C (*dec.*). The latter causes a powerful and lasting depression of blood pressure which is very like that produced by Reserpine (q.v.).

Abdusalamov, Sadykov., *Nauch. Tr., Tashkent. Gos. Univ.*, No. 286, 76 (1966)

CALPURNINE

$C_{20}H_{27}O_3N_3$

M.p. 152–4°C

This alkaloid has been isolated from *Calpurnia subdecandra* and *Virgilia oroboides*. It forms colourless prisms when crystallized from AcOEt with $[\alpha]_D^{22} + 59°$ (c 1.0, $CHCl_3$). It may be characterized by the perchlorate, m.p. 255–260°C and the methiodide, colourless rods from Me_2CO, m.p. 230–3°C. On hydrolysis, the base yields pyrrole-2-carboxylic acid and 13-hydroxylupanine.

Goosen., *J. Chem. Soc.*, 3067 (1963)

CALYCANTHIDINE

$C_{23}H_{28}N_4$

M.p. 142°C

In 1938, Berger *et al.* isolated this base from the seeds of *Calycanthus floridus* L. and assigned to it the formula $C_{13}H_{16}N_2$. This has since been revised to that given above. The base has $[\alpha]_D^{20} - 285.1°$ (MeOH) and − 317° (EtOH). It yields the following salts: hydriodide, m.p. 182°C; perchlorate, m.p. 158°C; chromate, m.p. > 300°C; platinichloride, m.p. 198–200°C and picrate, m.p. 192°C. With MeI it furnishes a compound with m.p. 180–215°C which, on further treatment with MeI and KOH gives a salt, m.p. 221°C, the latter also being obtained directly from the alkaloid itself by similar treatment.

Barger, Jacob, Madinaveitia., *Rev. trav. chim.*, 57, 548 (1938)
Saxton, Bardsley, Smith., *Proc. Chem. Soc.*, 148 (1962)

CALYCANTHINE

$C_{22}H_{26}N_4$

M.p. 245°C

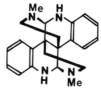

First obtained from the seeds of *Calycanthus glaucus* Willd., this alkaloid has subsequently been discovered in other species of *Calycanthus,* including *C. floridus* L., *C. occidentalis,* Hook and Arn. and *Meratia praecox* Rehd. and Wils. The original formula of $C_{11}H_{14}N_2$ due to Gordin was doubled by Späth and Stroh and finally altered to that given above by Barger *et al.*

Calycanthine crystallizes from aqueous Me_2CO in colourless octahedra, m.p. 219—220°C, which lose H_2O under vacuum to form the anhydrous base. It has $[\alpha]_D^{18} + 684.3°$ (EtOH). The dihydrobromide forms colourless prisms of the dihydrate from aqueous MeOH, m.p. 213—4°C. The nitrosamine has m.p. 175—6°C (*dec.*) and the phenylcarbamoyl derivative, m.p. 252°C. According to Späth and Stroh, the action of MeI yields the dimethiodide, m.p. 261—2°C but later workers obtained a mixture of compounds; the hydriodide, m.p. 260°C, the dihydriodide (H_2O), m.p. 226—7°C; a quaternary salt, $C_{22}H_{26}ON_3I$, m.p. 240—2°C and an oxygen-free quaternary salt, $C_{21}H_{22}N_3I$, m.p. 317—8°C. When heated in a sealed tube with soda lime, the alkaloid furnishes N-methyltryptamine, m.p. 86°C. With phosphorus and hydriodic acid, the base gives quinoline.

Pharmacologically, calycanthine produces similar symptoms to those due to strychnine acting as a stimulant to the spinal cord and as a cardiac depressant. The hydrochloride is toxic to rats at a dosage of 17.2 mgm per kilo. It also reduces blood pressure and cardiac contraction in anaesthetized cats.

Eccles., *Proc. Amer. Pharm. Assoc.,* **84**, 382 (1888)
Gordin., *J. Amer. Chem. Soc.,* **27**, 144, 1418 (1905)
Späth, Stroh., *Ber.,* **58**, 2131 (1925)
Manske., *J. Amer. Chem. Soc.,* **51**, 1836 (1929)
Manske., *Chem. Zentr.,* **I**, 3689 (1931)
Barger, Madinaveitia, Streuli., *J. Chem. Soc.,* 510 (1939)
Mason., *Proc. Chem. Soc.,* 362 (1962)
Hamor, Robertson., *J. Chem. Soc.,* 194 (1962)
Takamizawa, Takahashi, Sakakibara, Kobayashi., *Tetrahedron,* **23**, 2959 (1967)

Synthesis:
Hall, McCapra, Scott., *Tetrahedron,* **23**, 4131 (1967)

Absolute configuration:
Mason, Vane., *J. Chem. Soc., B,* 370 (1966)

CALYCOTAMINE

$C_{11}H_{15-17}O_3N$

The seeds of *Calycotome spinosa* Link. are said to contain trace amounts of this alkaloid isolated as the hydrochloride, m.p. 206°C; $[\alpha]_D + 20°$ (H_2O). The picrate is an oil while the mercurichloride crystallizes as slender needles. Two methoxyl groups are present in the molecule.

White., *New Zealand J. Sci. Tech.,* B, **25**, 93 (1943)

CALYCOTOMINE

$C_{12}H_{17}O_3N$

M.p. 139–141°C

The major base of *Calycotome spinosa* Link. where it occurs in the seeds as the *d*-form, together with traces of the *dl*-form, this alkaloid is also found as the main constituent of *Cytisus nigricans* var. *elongatus* Willd. and in the seeds of *C. proliferus*. The base has $[\alpha]_D^{20} + 21°$ (H_2O). The hydrochloride has m.p. 193°C; $[\alpha]_D^{20} + 15°$ (H_2O); the perchlorate, m.p. 176–7°C; the picrate (1 H_2O), m.p. 163–6°C after melting at 99–100°C and then resolidifying; and the mercurichloride, m.p. 118–9°C. The dibenzoyl derivative has m.p. 120–2°C. With MeI, the alkaloid yields N-methylcalycotomine hydriodide, m.p. 228–9°C. The nitrosamine is amorphous.

White., *New Zealand J. Sci. Tech.*, B, **25**, 93 (1943)
White., *ibid, B,* **25**, 152 (1944)

CAMMACONINE

$C_{23}H_{37}O_5N$

M.p. 135–7°C

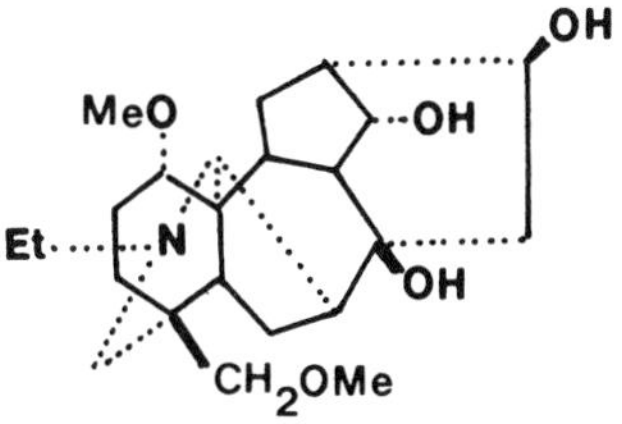

An atisine-type alkaloid found in *Aconitum variegatum,* this base contains three hydroxyl, two methoxyl and an ethylimino group. The trimethyl ether has m.p. 103.5–105°C. The 16-methyl ether is Talatisamine (q.v.).

Khaimova, Palamareva, Mollov, Krestev., *Tetrahedron,* **27**, 819 (1971)

CAMPESTRINE

$C_{13}H_{19}O_3N$

M.p. 93°C

One of the less clearly defined 'hepatotoxic' alkaloids, this base has been obtained from *Senecio camprestris* var. *maritima*.

Blackie., *Pharm. J.,* **138**, 102 (1937)

CAMPTOTHECIN

$C_{20}H_{16}O_4N_2$

M.p. 264–7°C (*dec.*).

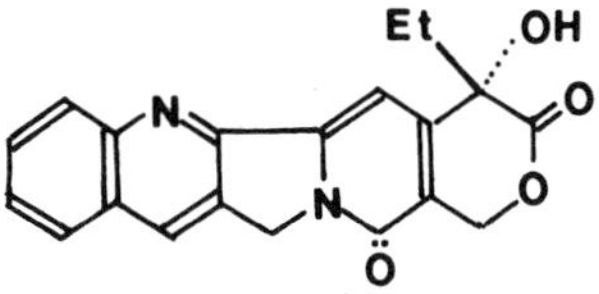

This important alkaloid has been isolated from *Camptotheca acuminata*. It forms light yellow needles from MeOH-MeCN with $[\alpha]_D^{25} + 31.3°$ (8:2 $CHCl_3$-MeOH). The ultraviolet spectrum shows absorption maxima at 220, 254, 290 and 370 mμ. The acetate has m.p. 271–4°C (*dec.*); the chloroacetyl derivative, m.p. 245–8°C (*dec.*) and the iodoacetyl derivative, m.p. 238–240°C (*dec.*). The alkaloid does not form stable salts with inorganic acids.

The importance of camptothecin lies in its pronounced antitumour and antileukaemia activity. When treated against leukaemia L1210 in mice on a daily dosage of 0.25–1.0 mg/kg, it gave life prolongation as high as 100 per cent. Similarly, a significant growth inhibition occurred when Walker 256 rat tumours were treated with the alkaloid. The sodium salt has been subjected to preliminary and phase II clinical studies with gastrointestinal cancer but unfortunately, the alkaloid has an extremely high toxicity in both animals and man. Structural modifications of the alkaloid, however, may hold future promise in clinical screening.

Wall *et al.*, *J. Amer. Chem. Soc.*, **88**, 3888 (1966)
McPhail, Sim., *J. Chem. Soc., B*, 923 (1968)
Shamma., *Experientia*, **24**, 107 (1968)

Synthesis:
Stork, Schultz., *J. Amer. Chem. Soc.*, **93**, 4074 (1971)
Winterfeldt, Korth, Pike, Boch., *Angew. Chem.*, **84**, 265 (1972)
Kende *et al.*, *Tetrahedron Lett.*, **16**, 1307 (1973)

Chemotherapeutic studies:
Gottlieb *et al.*, *Cancer Chemother. Rep.*, **54**, 461 (1970)
Moertel *et al.*, *Proc. Amer. Ass. Cancer Res.*, **12**, 18 (1971)
Muggia., *ibid*, **12**, 41 (1971)

Toxicity:
Schaeppi, Cooney, Davis., *U.S. Clearinghouse Fed. Sci. Tech. Inform.*, PB Rep 1967, PB-180549
Schaeppi *et al.*, *ibid*, PB Rep 1968, PB-179993

(+)-CANADINE

$C_{20}H_{21}O_4N$

M.p. 132°C

This form of the alkaloid has, so far, been isolated from *Corydalis tuberosa*, D.C. It has $[\alpha]_D^{15} + 299°$ ($CHCl_3$).

Gadamer, Knörck., *Apoth. Zeit.*, **41**, 928 (1926)

(−)-CANADINE

$C_{20}H_{21}O_4N$

M.p. 133–4°C

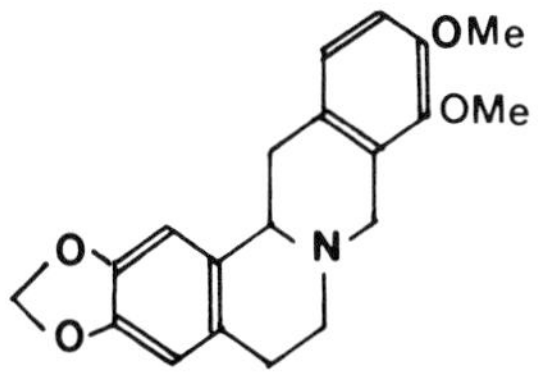

The (−)-form of canadine has been obtained from several species, e.g. *Corydalis cheilantheifolia* Hemsl., *Fagara rhoifolia* Lam., *Hydrastis canadensis* L., *Zanthoxylum brachyacanthum* F. Muell. and *Z. veneficum* F.M. Bail. The alkaloid forms silky needles with $[\alpha]_D - 299°$ (CHCl$_3$) or $- 432°$ (CS$_2$). It is insoluble in H$_2$O but readily soluble in Et$_2$O or CHCl$_3$. Both the hydrochloride and nitrate are crystalline, laevorotatory and only slightly soluble in H$_2$O. When the alkaloid is treated with mercuric acetate, it yields berberine.

Schmidt, Wilhelm., *Arch. Pharm.*, **226**, 329 (1888)
Go., *Chem. Abstr.*, **24**, 620 (1930)
Späth, Julian., *Ber.*, **64**, 1131 (1931)
Manske., *Can. J. Res.*, **20B**, 53 (1942)

CANCENTRINE

$C_{36}H_{32}O_7N_2$

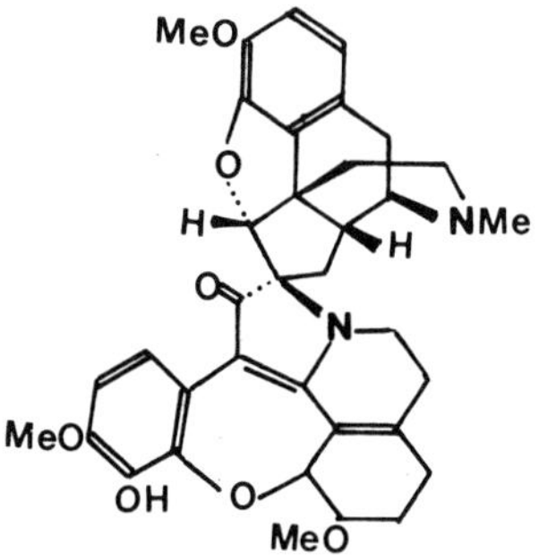

This dimeric benzylisoquinoline alkaloid is found in *Dicentra canadensis*. The structure has been elucidated by comparison of its NMR spectrum with that of codeine.

Clark, Manske, Palenik, Rodrigo, MacLean, Baczynski, Gracey, Saunders., *J. Amer. Chem. Soc.*, **92**, 4998 (1970)

CANDICINE

$C_{11}H_{18}ON$

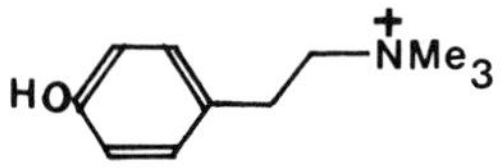

First isolated from the cactus *Trichocereus candicans*, this quaternary base has also been obtained from certain *Fagara* species, *Hordeum vulgare* and *Magnolia grandiflora*. In the plant itself, it appears to be present as the hydroxide. The chloride forms colourless crystals which are hygroscopic, m.p. 285°C (*dec.*); the iodide, m.p. 229–230°C; platinichloride, m.p. 208–9°C; picrate, m.p. 165°C and the picrolonate, m.p. 218–9°C. The pharmacological action of the alkaloid has been studied, among others, by Luduena.

Luduena., *Compt. rend. soc. biol.,* **114**, 809, 950, 951, 953 (1933)
Reit., *ibid,* 811 (1933)
Rabtzsch., *Planta Medica.,* **6**, 103 (1958)
Erspamer., *Arch. Biochem. Biophys.,* **82**, 431 (1959)

CANDIMINE

$C_{18}H_{19}O_6N$

M.p. 218–220°C

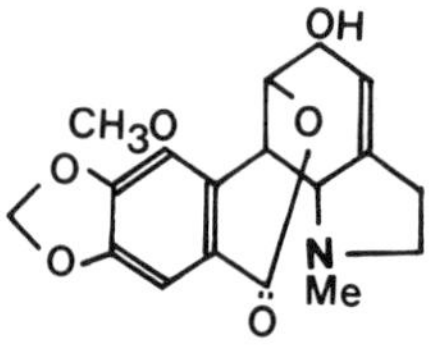

Isolated from *Hippeastrum candidum.*, this alkaloid forms colourless crystals from MeOH; $[\alpha]_D^{24}$ + 220° (c 0.2, CHCl$_3$). The crystalline perchlorate has m.p. 177–9°C and the picrate, m.p. 220°C. With Ac$_2$O it yields an acetyl derivative, m.p. 239–241°C (*dec.*), the perchlorate of which is also crystalline with m.p. 262°C (*dec.*).

Döpke., *Arch. Pharm.,* **295**, 920 (1962)

CANNAGUNINE

$C_{20}H_{22}O_2N_2$

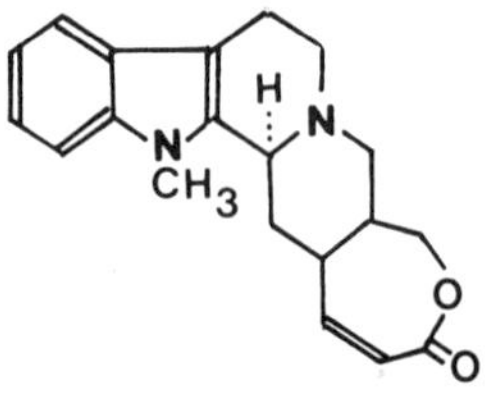

This base has recently been obtained from *Vaccinium oxycoccus.* The structure is noteworthy for the seven-membered lactone ring present in the molecule.

Jankowski, Boudreau, Jankowska., *Experientia,* **27**, 1141 (1971)

CANTHIN-6-ONE

$C_{14}H_8ON_2$

M.p. 162.5–163.5°C

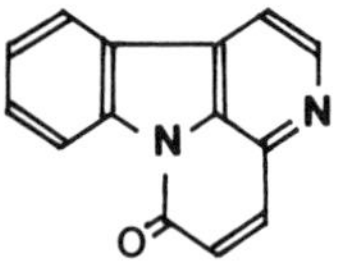

An alkaloid present in *Pentaceras australis* Hook., the base forms colourless needles when crystallized from MeOH. The ultraviolet spectrum exhibits absorption maxima at 251, 259, 269, 293, 299, 347, 362 and 381 mμ. The following salts and derivatives have been prepared: hydrochloride, yellow needles, m.p. 244–6°C (*dec.*); picrate, yellow rods, m.p. 262–4°C and the methiodide, orange-red crystals, m.p. 271–3°C.

Haynes, Nelson, Price., *Austral. J. Sci. Res.,* **5A**, 387 (1952)

Synthesis:
Rosenkranz, Botyos, Schmid., *Annalen,* **691**, 159 (1966)

CANTHIUMINE

$C_{33}H_{36}O_4N_4$

M.p. 232–3°C

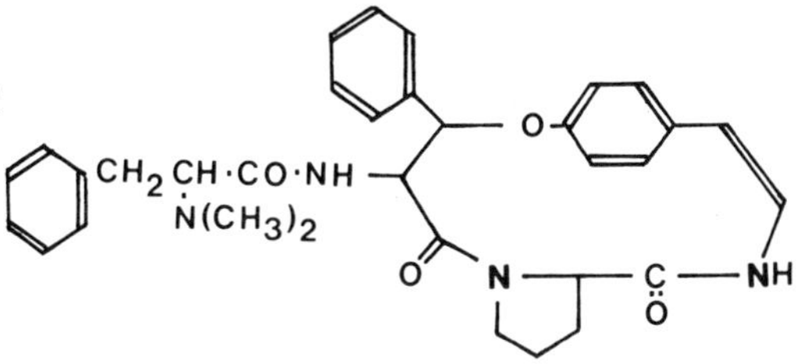

A macrocyclic alkaloid from *Canthium euryoides,* this compound has $[\alpha]_D$ – 254° (c 1.0, CHCl$_3$).

Boulvin, Ottinger, Pais, Chiuroglu., *Bull. Soc. Chim. Belg.,* **78**, 583 (1969)

CANTLEYINE

$C_{10}H_{11}O_2N$

M.p. 130°C

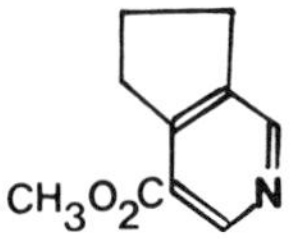

This monoterpene alkaloid occurs in the trunk bark of *Cantleya corniculata* and has $[\alpha]_D^{20}$ – 40 ± 2° (CHCl$_3$). The above biogenetically-favoured structure was assigned to the alkaloid from spectroscopic data and subsequently confirmed by conversion of loganoside, of previously known structure, into cantleyine. It has been suggested that the alkaloid is, in reality, an artifact of the ammoniacal extraction.

Sevenet, Das, Parello, Potier., *Bull. Soc. Chim. Fr.,* **8**, 3120 (1970)

CAPAURIDINE (*dl-Capaurine*)

$C_{21}H_{25}O_5N$

M.p. 208°C

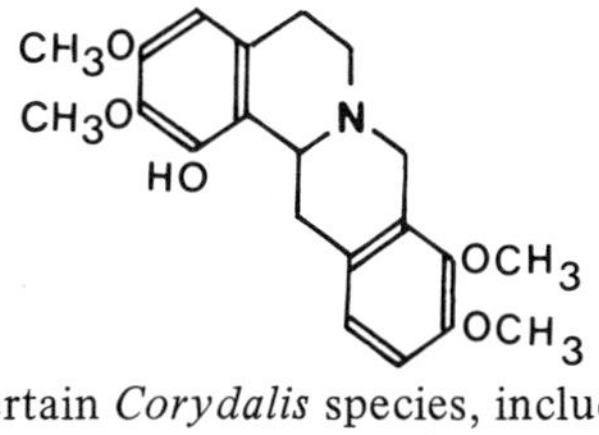

This alkaloid is found in certain *Corydalis* species, including *C. aurea* Willd., *C. micrantha* (Engelm) Gray, *C. montana* (Engelm) Britton and *C. pallida* Pers. The alkaloid has $[\alpha]_D$ ± 0°. On methylation with CH_2N_2 it furnishes *dl*-capaurine O-methyl ether, m.p. 142°C.

Manske., *Can. J. Res.*, **9**, 436 (1933)
Manske., *ibid*, **15**, 159 (1937)
Manske., *ibid*, **16**, 81 (1938)

CAPAURIMINE

$C_{20}H_{23}O_5N$

M.p. 212°C

A protoberbering type alkaloid, this base occurs in *Corydalis montana* (Engelm)
Britton and *C. pallida* Pers. It has $[\alpha]_D^{24} - 287°$ (c 0.4, $CHCl_3$). The 10-methyl
ether is Capaurine (q.v.). The 1:10-dimethyl ether crystallizes from MeOH as
colourless needles, m.p. 150°C. The original structure in which the two hydroxyl
groups were located at C-1 and C-9 has been shown, by synthesis, to be incorrect,
the revised structure with the hydroxyls at C-1 and C-10 being given above.

Manske., *Can. J. Res.*, **18B**, 80 (1940)
Manske., *ibid*, **20B**, 49 (1942)
Manske., *J. Amer. Chem. Soc.*, **69**, 1800 (1947)
Kametani, Ihara, Fukumoto, Yagi, Shinmanouchi, Sasada., *Tetrahedron,
Lett.*, 4251 (1968)
Kametani, Fukumoto, Yagi, Iida, Kikuchi., *J. Chem. Soc., C*, 1178 (1968)

Structure revision:
Kametani, Ihara, Honda., *J. Chem. Soc., C*, 2342 (1970)

Crystal structure:
Kametani, Ihara, Kitahara, Kabuto, Shimanouchi, Sasada., *Chem. Commun.*,
1241 (1970)

CAPAURINE (*Capaurimine 10-methyl ether*)

$C_{21}H_{25}O_5N$

M.p. 164°C

Several species of *Corydalis* yield this particular alkaloid, e.g. *C. aurea* Willd.,
C. micrantha (Engelm) Gray, *C. montana* (Engelm) Britton and *C. pallida* Pers.
The hydrobromide has been prepared as light yellow crystals from MeOH, m.p.
198–9°C; $[\alpha]_D - 423°$. The O-methyl ether forms prisms when crystallized
from MeOH, m.p. 152°C and the corresponding ethyl ether is obtained as
colourless prisms from Et_2O, m.p. 134°C. The latter, an oxidation with $KMnO_4$,
yields 3-ethoxy-4:5-dimethoxyphthalic acid. The alkaloid itself, on oxidation,
gives hemipinic acid.

Manske., *Can. J. Res.*, **9**, 436 (1933)

Manske., *ibid*, **15**, 159 (1937)

Manske., *ibid*, **16**, 81 (1938)

Crystal structure:

Shimanouchi, Sasada, Ihara, Kametani., *Acta Cryst.*, **25B**, 1310 (1969)

Synthesis:

Kametani, Iida, Kikuchi, Honda, Ihara., *J. Heterocyclic Chem.*, **7**, 491 (1970)

CAPNOIDINE

$C_{20}H_{17}O_6N$

M.p. 238°C

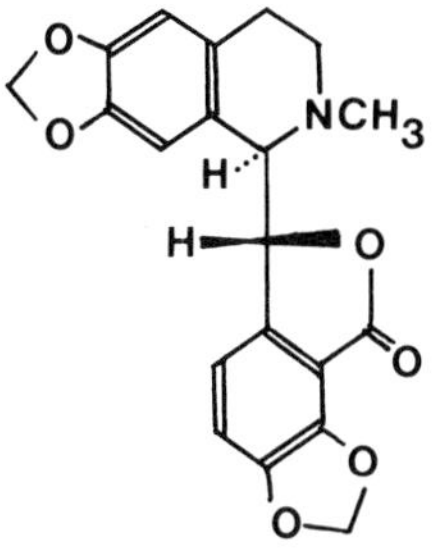

This alkaloid has been isolated from *Corydalis scouleri* HK. and *C. sempervirens* (L) Pers. It forms colourless crystals from MeOH or Me$_2$CO and gives a crystalline hydrochloride, m.p. 244°C. It is isomeric with Adlumine (q.v.) and contains no methoxyl groups. The pharmacological action of capnoidine has been investigated by Anderson and Chen. It stimulates isolated guinea-pig or rabbit uterus and also inhibits isolated rabbit intestine. The alkaloid is exceptional in resembling *l-iso*corypalmine in inducing catalepsy in young monkeys.

Manske., *Can. J. Res.*, **8**, 407 (1933)

Manske., *ibid*, **14**, 347 (1936)

Anderson, Chen., *Fed. Proc.*, **5**, 163 (1946)

CARACURINE I

A minor constituent of *Strychnos toxifera* bark, this base has, so far, been obtained only in the form of the picrate, orange crystals, m.p. > 300°C.

Asmis, Schmid, Karrer., *Helv. Chim. Acta*, **37**, 1983, 1993 (1954)

CARACURINE II

$C_{38}H_{38}O_2N_4$

M.p. 248–9°C

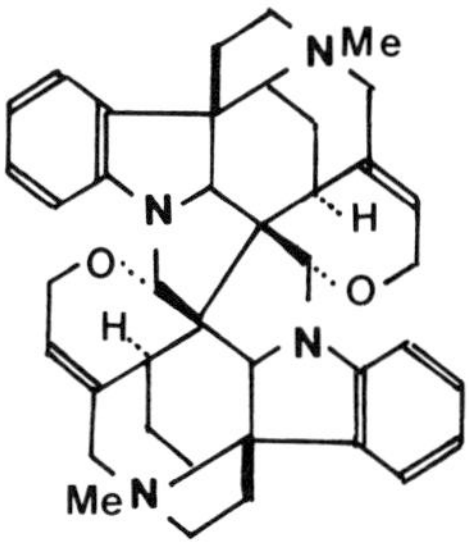

This dimeric alkaloid occurs in the bark of *Strychnos toxifera*. It yields a crystalline picrate, m.p. > 300°C and the methochloride which is identical with Toxiferine IX (q.v.).

Asmis, Schmid, Karrer., *Helv. Chim. Acta,* **37**, 1983, 1993 (1954)
Battersby *et al., Proc. Chem. Soc.,* 412, 413 (1961)
McPhail, Sim., *ibid,* 416 (1961)
Mason, Vane., *J. Chem. Soc., B,* 370 (1966)
Crystal structure:
McPhail, Sim., *Proc. Chem. Soc.,* 1663 (1965)

CARACURINE III

The bark of *Strychnos toxifera* yields minute amounts of this alkaloid which has only been obtained as the picrate, orange crystals, m.p. > 300°C.

Asmis, Schmid, Karrer., *Helv. Chim. Acta,* **37**, 1983, 1993 (1954)

CARACURINE IV

$C_{21}H_{24}O_2N_2$

A further component of the bark of *Strychnos toxifera,* this base yields a crystalline hydrochloride and picrate, the latter having m.p. > 300°C.

Asmis, Schmid, Karrer., *Helv. Chim. Acta,* **37**, 1983, 1993 (1954)

CARACURINE V

$C_{38}H_{40}O_2N_4$

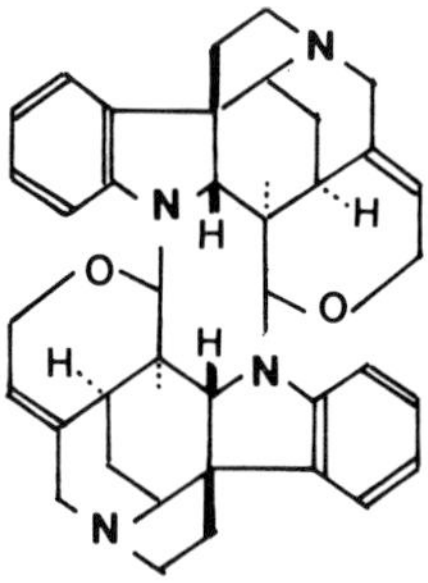

Present in *Strychnos toxifera* bark, this alkaloid forms a crystalline hydrochloride and picrate, both having m.p. > 300°C. With HCl the alkaloid gives Caracurine Va (nortoxiferine I), $C_{20}H_{22}O_2N_2$, amorphous, giving a crystalline picrate, m.p. > 310°C. Reaction with NH_2SO_4 furnishes a mixture of caracurines II and VII.

Asmis, Schmid, Karrer., *Helv. Chim. Acta,* **37**, 1983, 1993 (1954)
Bernauer *et al., ibid,* **41**, 1405 (1958)

CARACURINE VI

$C_{38}H_{40}ON_4$

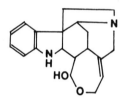

This alkaloid, also obtained from the bark of *Strychnos toxifera*, has only been isolated as the picrate, m.p. > 300°C.

Asmis, Schmid, Karrer., *Helv. Chim. Acta*, **37**, 1983, 1993 (1954)
Berlage *et al.*, *ibid*, **42**, 2650 (1959)

CARACURINE VII (*Wieland-Gumlich aldehyde*)

$C_{19}H_{22}O_2N_2$

M.p. 211–3°C (*dec.*).

Isolated from the bark of *Strychnos toxifera*, this alkaloid has $[\alpha]_D^{22} - 133.8°$ (c 0.5194, MeOH). The hydrochloride forms colourless crystals from MeOH, m.p. > 300°C and the picrate is obtained as orange-red needles from aqueous Me_2CO, m.p. 230–231.5°C. The N(a)-acetyl derivative is Diaboline (q.v.).

Asmis, Schmid, Karrer., *Helv. Chim. Acta*, **37**, 1983, 1993 (1954)
Bernauer *et al.*, *ibid*, **41**, 1405 (1958)
Deyrup, Schmid, Karrer., *ibid*, **45**, 2266 (1962)

CARANINE

$C_{16}H_{17}O_3N$

M.p. 178–180°C

Several *Amaryllidaceous* species contain this alkaloid which crystallizes as colourless prisms from AcOEt with $[\alpha]_D^{27} - 196.6°$ (c 2.0, $CHCl_3$). The hydrochloride is crystalline as is also the perchlorate, m.p. 260–270°C (*dec.*). The methiodide is obtained in the forms of light-brown crystals from MeOH, m.p. 316–8°C (*dec.*). The acetate also occurs in *Amaryllidaceae* species.

Mason, Puschett, Wildman., *J. Amer. Chem. Soc.*, **77**, 1253 (1955)
Warnhoff, Wildmann., *ibid*, **79**, 2192 (1957)
Takeda, Kotera, Mizukami., *ibid*, **80**, 2562 (1958)

Mass spectra:
Kinstle, Wildman, Brown., *Tetrahedron Lett.*, 4659 (1966)
Ibuka, Irie, Uyeo, Kotera, Nagawa., *ibid,* 4745 (1966)

Stereochemistry:
Kotera, Hamada, Tori, Aono, Kuriyama., *Tetrahedron Lett.*, 2009 (1966)

CARAPANAUBINE

$C_{23}H_{28}O_6N_2$

M.p. 221–3°C

This alkaloid occurs in *Aspidosperma carapanauba* M. Pichon. It forms colourless crystals from AcOEt-hexane and has $[\alpha]_D^{20} - 101°$ (c 1.0, $CHCl_3$). The ultra-violet spectrum shows absorption maxima at 215, 244, 278 and 300 (inflexion) mμ. The absolute configuration has been determined as (7R, 3S, 4R, 15S, 19S, 20S)-.

Gilbert *et al., J. Amer. Chem. Soc.*, **85**, 1523 (1963)
Finch *et al., ibid,* **85**, 1520 (1963)

Absolute configuration:
Poisson, Pousset., *Tetrahedron Lett.*, 1919 (1967)

CARATAGINE

This uncharacterized alkaloid has been isolated from *Rindera oblongifolia.* The amount obtained so far has proved insufficient for a chemical analysis to be carried out and no salts or derivatives have been described.

Akramov, Kiyamitdinova, Yunusov., *Dokl. Akad. Nauk. Uzbek SSR.*, **22**, 35 (1965)

N(a)-CARBOMETHOXY-10:22-DIOXOKOPSANE

$C_{22}H_{22}O_4N_2$

M.p. 264–5°C

The stem bark of *Pleiocarpa mutica* Benth yields this alkaloid which forms opaque white needles when recrystallized from $CHCl_3$-light petroleum. It is dextrorotatory with $[\alpha]_D^{30} + 110°$ (c 1.31, $CHCl_3$). The ultraviolet spectrum exhibits absorption maxima at 240, 279 and an inflexion at 285 mμ. The structure is based mainly upon the mass spectra fragmentation patterns.

Achenbach, Biemann., *J. Amer. Chem. Soc.*, **87**, 4944 (1965)

5α-CARBOXYSTRICTOSIDINE

$C_{28}H_{34}O_{11}N_2$

M.p. 232°C

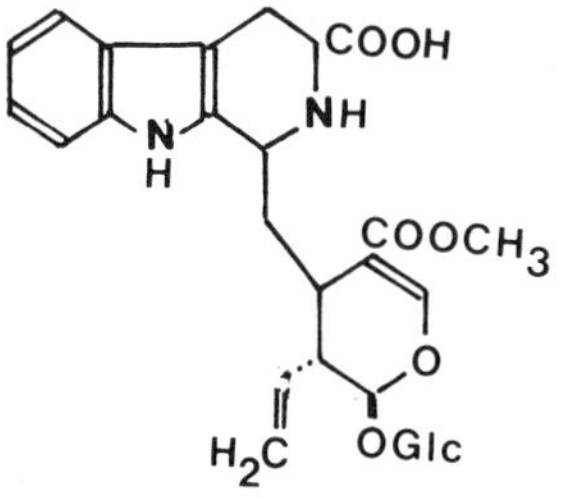

A glucosidic alkaloid from the roots of *Rhazya stricta* and *R.* orientalis, this base is strongly laevorotatory having $[\alpha]_D - 280°$ (MeOH).

De Silva, King, Smith., *Chem. Commun.*, 908 (1971)

CARMICHAELINE

M.p. 185–6°C

This novel alkaloid has been obtained from the column chromatographic fractionation of the alkaloidal bases of *Aconitum carmichaeli*. It has $[\alpha]_D^{25} - 16.7°$ (c 0.59, MeOH) and yields a hydrobromide, m.p. 214–6°C and a diacetate, m.p. 121–4°C. The structure is still unknown.

Iwasa, Naruto., *J. Pharm. Soc., Japan,* **86**, 585 (1966)

CARNAVALINE

$C_{18}H_{37}O_2N$

M.p. 60.7–61.2°C

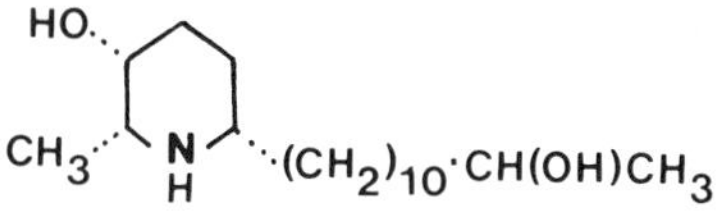

This piperidine alkaloid occurs in *Cassia carnaval* Speg. It contains two secondary hydroxyl groups, one of which is present in the long, saturated side chain and the other in the piperidine ring.

Lythgoe, Vernengo., *Tetrahedron Lett.,* 1133 (1967)

CARNEGINE (*Pectenine*)

$C_{13}H_{19}O_2N$

M.p. 262–3°C;
B.p. 170°C/1 mm

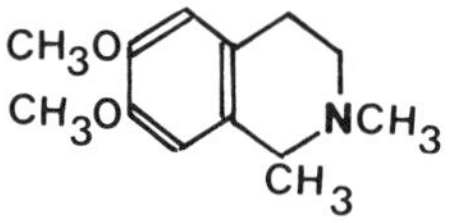

First isolated from the cactus *Cereus pecten aboriginum* under the name Pectenine, this was subsequently shown to be identical with carnegine obtained from *Carnegia gigantea* (Engelm.). Britton. and Rose. The base is a highly alkaline oil which can be crystallized and yields crystalline salts: the hydrochloride, m.p. 210–1°C; picrate, m.p. 212–3°C (*dec.*) and the methiodide, m.p. 210–1°C (*dec.*).

Heyl., *Arch. Pharm.*, **239**, 451 (1901)
Heyl., *ibid*, **266**, 668 (1928)
Späth, Kuffner., *Ber.*, **62**, 2242 (1929)
Späth, Dengel., *ibid*, **71**, 113 (1938)

CAROLINIANINE

$C_{16}H_{24}O_2N_2$

A minor alkaloid of *Lycopodium carolinianum* var. *affine*, this base is found in the petroleum ether extract of the plant. The structure has not yet been elucidated.

Miller *et al.*, *Bull. Soc. Chim. Belg.*, **80**, 629 (1971)

CAROSIDINE

M.p. 283°C (*dec.*).

This alkaloid occurs in *Vinca rosea* L. and forms colourless crystals from $CHCl_3$-Me_2CO which begin to darken at 263°C before melting. It is laevorotatory with $[\alpha]_D^{26} - 89.8°$ (c 1.0, $CHCl_3$). The ultraviolet spectrum in EtOH exhibits three absorption maxima occurring at 212, 254 and 303 mμ.

Svoboda *et al.*, *J. Pharm. Sci.*, **51**, 518 (1962)

CAROSINE

$C_{46}H_{56}O_{10}N_4$

M.p. 214–8°C

Like the preceding base, this alkaloid is present in *Vinca rosea* L. and forms colourless needles when recrystallized from a mixture of CH_2Cl_2 and Et_2O. It is slightly dextrorotatory with $[\alpha]_D^{26} + 6.0°$ (c 1.0, $CHCl_3$) and the ultraviolet spectrum in EtOH shows absorption maxima at 255 and 294 mμ.

Svoboda *et al.*, *J. Pharm. Sci.*, **51**, 518 (1962)

CARPAINE

$C_{28}H_{50}O_4N_2$

M.p. 121°C;
B.p. 215–235°C (*vac.*)

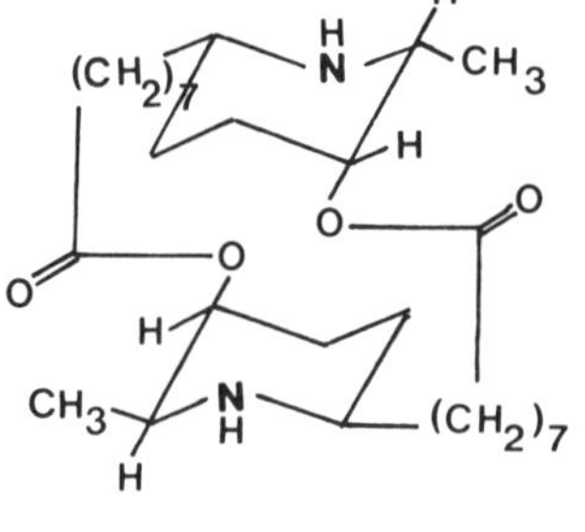

Greshoff isolated this alkaloid from the fruit, seeds and leaves of *Carica papaya* L. and it has subsequently been found in *Vascanella hastata*. The base crystallizes in monoclinic prisms from EtOH or Me_2CO. It has $[\alpha]_D + 21.9°$ (EtOH) and is insoluble in H_2O but soluble in most organic solvents. The hydrochloride forms colourless needles and the aurichloride, yellow needles of the pentahydrate, m.p. 205°C (*dry*). The methyl derivative forms colourless prisms, m.p. 71°C; the N-acetyl derivative has m.p. 114°C and the nitroso compound, small prisms, has m.p. 144–5°C.

Hofmann degradation of the alkaloid yields myristic acid. With 10 per cent HCl at 130–140°C, or EtONa, the base behaves as a lactone and is converted into carpamic acid, long colourless needles, m.p. 224°C. Distillation with Se *in vacuo* gives carpyrine, $C_{14}H_{21}O_2N$, b.p. 210°C/5 mm, but at 360°C and atmospheric pressure, *apo*carpyrine is formed, b.p. 145–150°C/21 mm.

The original formula, $C_{14}H_{25}O_2N$ has been doubled on mass spectral evidence.

The pharmacological action of carpaine has been investigated by several workers. Essentially it is a heart poison although not of the cardiac glucoside type. It lowers pulse frequency and depresses the central nervous system. According to To and Kyu it is also a potent amoebicide.

Greshoff., *Meded. uit's Lands. Plant.*, No. 7, 5, (1890)
van Rijn., *Arch. Pharm.*, **231**, 184 (1893)
Webster., *Ber. Deut. Pharm. Ges.*, **24**, 123 (1914)
Rapoport, Baldridge., *J. Amer. Chem. Soc.*, **73**, 343 (1951)
Rapoport, Baldridge., *ibid*, **74**, 5365 (1952)
Govindachari, Narasimhan., *J. Chem. Soc.*, 2635 (1953)
Rapoport, Baldridge, Volcheck., *J. Amer. Chem. Soc.*, **75**, 5290 (1953)

Structure revision:
Spiteller-Friedmann, Spiteller., *Monatsh.*, **95**, 1234 (1964)
Govindachari, Nagarajan, Viswanathan., *Tetrahedron Lett.*, 1907 (1965)

Pharmacology:
Alcock, Meyer., *Arch. Physiol.*, 225 (1903)
Kakowski., *Arch. inst. Pharmacodyn*, **15**, 84 (1905)
Kyu., *Folia Pharmacol. Japan*, **10**, 333 (1930)
To, Kyu., *Jap. J. Med. Sci.*, **8**, 52 (1934)

ψ-CARPAINE

$C_{28}H_{50}O_4N_2$

M.p. 65–8°C

The stereoisomer of carpaine has been obtained from the leaves of *Carica papaya* L. It crystallizes from light petroleum and has $[\alpha]_D^{28} + 4.95°$ (c 1.62, EtOH). The crystalline hydrochloride has m.p. 295°C. Hydrolysis with hot HCl gives a mixture of carpamic acid, m.p. 224°C and ψ-carpamic acid (ethyl ester hydrochloride, m.p. 122–4°C). The earlier formula for this alkaloid has also been doubled on the basis of mass spectral data.

Govindachari, Pai, Narasimhan., *J. Chem. Soc.*, 1847 (1954)

Govindachari, Nagarajan, Viswanathan., *Tetrahedron Lett.*, 1907 (1965)

CARTHAMOIDINE

This base is stated to be present in *Senecio carthamoides* although it has not yet been characterized chemically. Pharmacologically, it is said to resemble pterophine (q.v.) in that it produces predominantly periportal necrosis of the liver.

Adams, Carmack, Rogers., *J. Amer. Chem. Soc.*, **64**, 571 (1942)

(–)-CARYACHINE

$C_{19}H_{19}O_4N$

M.p. 174–5°C

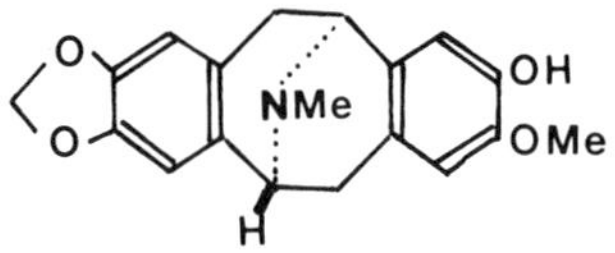

The leaves of *Cryptocarya chinensis* contain this alkaloid which may be crystallized from Me_2CO and has $[\alpha]_D^{21} - 269.6°$ (c 1.0, EtOH). The hydrobromide is crystalline with m.p. 295–6°C (*dec.*).

Lu, Lan., *J. Pharm. Soc. Japan*, **83**, 177 (1966)

Absolute configuration:
Barker, Battersby., *J. Chem. Soc.*, C, 1317 (1967)

(±)-CARYACHINE

$C_{19}H_{19}O_4N$

M.p. 241–2°C

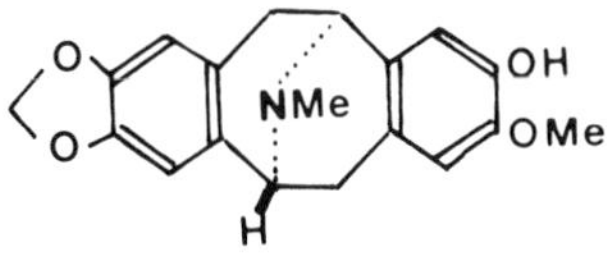

The racemate of caryachine is also present in the leaves of *Cryptocarya chinensis*. It forms colourless crystals from MeOH or EtOH.

Lu, Lan., *J. Pharm. Soc. Japan*, **83**, 177 (1966)

CASEADINE (*Alkaloid F-35*)

$C_{20}H_{23}O_4N$

M.p. 145°C

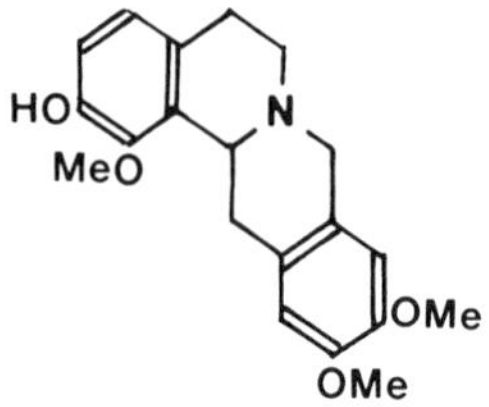

A tetrahydroprotoberberine alkaloid isolated from *Corydalis caseana* A. Gray. This base has $[\alpha]_D - 393°$ (c 1.12, $CHCl_3$). The ultraviolet spectrum shows absorption maxima at 206, 228 and 286 mμ in EtOH. CH_2N_2 yields the O-methyl ether, m.p. 186°C; $[\alpha]_D - 360°$ (c 0.4, $CHCl_3$). The structure has been determined mainly by infrared and NMR spectral data. The present of Bohlmann bands in the infrared spectrum indicates a trans quinolizidine nucleus in the molecule.

Manske, Miller., *Can. J. Res.,* **16B**, 153 (1938)
Chen, MacLean, Manske., *Tetrahedron Lett.,* 349 (1968)

Structure revision:
Kametani, Nakano, Shishido, Fukumoto., *J. Chem. Soc., C,* 3350 (1971)

CASEAMINE (*Alkaloid F-33*)

$C_{19}H_{21}O_4N$

M.p. 257°C

Also present in *Corydalis caseana* A. Gray., this tetrahydroprotoberberine alkaloid has $[\alpha]_D - 406°$ (c 0.12, $CHCl_3$). The ultraviolet spectrum of the ethanol solution shows absorption maxima at 206, 228 and 286 mμ. Methylation with CH_2N_2 gives the same tetramethoxy derivative as caseadine, m.p. 186°C; $[\alpha]_D - 360°$ (c 0.4, $CHCl_3$).

Manske, Miller., *Can. J. Res.,* **16B**, 153 (1938)
Chen, MacLean, Manske., *Tetrahedron Lett.,* 349 (1968)

CASEANADINE

$C_{20}H_{23}O_4N$

M.p. 170°C

A further tetrahydroprotoberberine alkaloid found in *Corydalis caseana* A. Gray. This base has $[\alpha]_D - 212°$ ($CHCl_3$). The ultraviolet spectrum in methanol solution shows one absorption maximum at 282 mμ. The O-acetate is an oil which has not yet been obtained in a crystalline form.

Yu, MacLean, Rodrigo, Manske., *Can. J. Chem.,* **49**, 124 (1971)

259

CASIMIROEDINE

$C_{21}H_{27}O_6N_3$

M.p. 223–4°C

The seeds of *Casimiroa edulis* Le Llave et Lejarza contain this glucosidic alkaloid which crystallizes in colourless needles from EtOH with $[\alpha]_D - 36.5°$ (CHCl$_3$) or $- 27°$ (1% HCl). The ultraviolet spectrum shows absorption maxima at 219 and 280 mμ. The aurichloride has m.p. 90°C or 145–8°C (*dry, dec.*), the picrate, yellow needles, m.p. 110–2°C; tetraacetate, colourless crystals, m.p. 80°C and the tetrabenzoyl derivative, m.p. 97–105°C.

Hydrogenation over PtO$_2$ yields the dihydro derivative, m.p. 176–7°C; $[\alpha]_D + 12°$ (EtOH).

Bickern., *Arch. Pharm.*, **241**, 166 (1903)
Power, Callan., *J. Chem. Soc.*, 1993 (1911)
de Lille., *An. Inst. Biol. Univ. Mex.*, **5**, 45 (1934)
Aebi., *Helv. Chim. Acta*, **39**, 1495 (1956)
Djerassi, Bankiewicz, Kapuor, Riniker., *J. Org. Chem.*, **21**, 1510 (1956)
Djerassi, Bankiewicz, Kapuor, Riniker., *Tetrahedron*, **2**, 168a (1958)
Raman, Riddy, Lipscomb., *Tetrahedron Lett.*, 357 (1962)

CASIMIROINE

$C_{12}H_{11}O_4N$

M.p. 202–3°C

This simple quinolone alkaloid is also present in the seeds and bark of *Casimiroa edulis* Llave et Lejarza. The base crystallizes from Me$_2$CO-hexane in rosettes of colourless needles. The ultraviolet spectrum exhibits absorption maxima at 227, 237, 252, 260 and 301 mμ. The earlier formula of $C_{24}H_{30}O_8N_2$ has been shown to be incorrect.

Bickern., *Arch. Pharm.*, **241**, 166 (1903)
Power, Callan., *J. Chem. Soc.*, **99**, 1993 (1911)
Kincl *et al.*, *ibid*, 4163, 4170 (1956)
Weinstein, Hylton., *Tetrahedron*, **20**, 1725 (1964)

CASSAIDE

$C_{22}H_{35}O_4N$

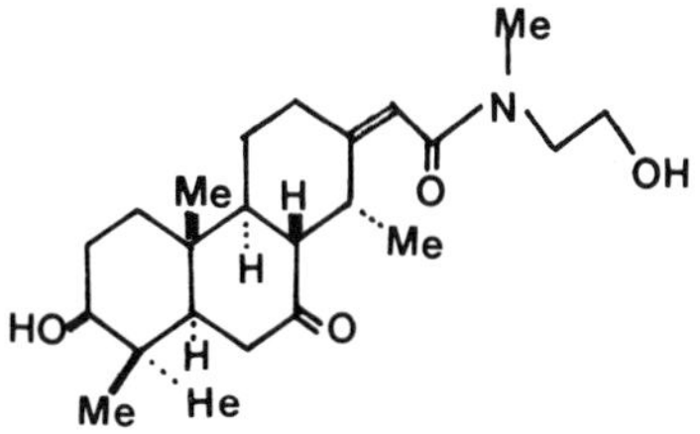

This reduced phenanthrene alkaloid has recently been discovered in *Erythrophleum ivorense*. The structure has been assigned mainly on the basis of spectroscopic data, particularly the NMR and mass spectra.

Cronlund, Sandberg., *Acta Pharm. Suecica.*, 8, 351 (1971)

CASSAIDINE

$C_{24}H_{41}O_4N$

M.p. 139.5°C

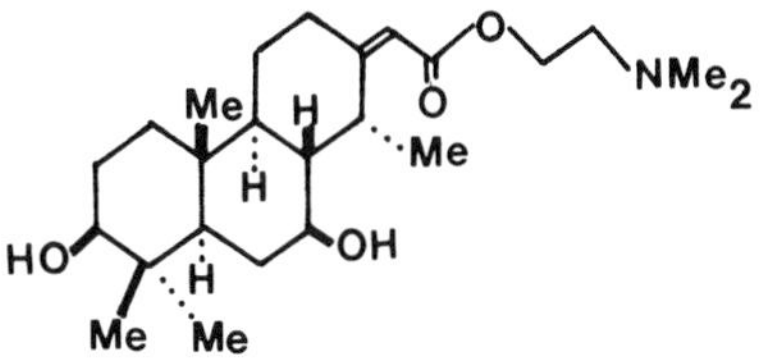

First isolated by Dalma in 1935, this alkaloid is obtained from the mother liquors containing the Et_2O-soluble bases of *Erythrophleum* guineense G. Don. bark after removal of Cassaine (q.v.), as the acid sulphate. Cassaidine crystallizes from $Me_2CO\text{-}Et_2O$ and has $[\alpha]_D^{20} - 98°$ (EtOH). It forms a crystalline hydrochloride, m.p. 251°C; $[\alpha]_D^{17} - 84°$ (H_2O) and amorphous acetyl and benzoyl derivatives. Hydrolysis with boiling 2N HCl gives dimethylaminoethanol (aurichloride, m.p. 194°C) and cassaidic acid, $C_{22}H_{32}O_4$, decomposing at 275–7°C; $[\alpha]_D^{20} - 100°$ (EtOH), giving a methyl ester, m.p. 162–3°C. Hydrogenation with PtO_2 as the catalyst yields a mixture of bases including dihydrocassaidine, m.p. 96–7°C; $[\alpha]_D^{20} \pm 0°$ (EtOH), yielding a hydrochloride, m.p. 247°C.

Dalma., *Ann. Chim. Appl.*, **25**, 569 (1935)
Dalma., *Helv. Chim. Acta*, **22**, 1497 (1939)
Ruzicka, Dalma., *ibid*, **23**, 753 (1940)
Engel, Tondeur., *ibid*, **32**, 2364 (1949)

Synthesis:
Engel., *Helv. Chim. Acta*, **42**, 1127 (1959)
Turner *et al.*, *J. Amer. Chem. Soc.*, **88**, 1766 (1966)

Stereochemistry:
Clarke *et al.*, *J. Amer. Chem. Soc.*, **88**, 5865 (1966)

CASSAINE

$C_{24}H_{39}O_4N$

M.p. 142.5°C;
B.p. 405°C

This alkaloid from the bark of *Erythrophleum guineense* G. Don. was first isolated by Dalma and subsequently examined in detail by Faltis and Holzinger. The base is virtually insoluble in H_2O or petroleum ether but soluble in most other organic solvents. It forms white leaflets when crystallized from hot H_2O and has $[\alpha]_D^{20} - 103°$ (EtOH) or $- 117°$ (0.1 N/HCl). Cassaine forms several crystalline salts and derivative, e.g. the hydrochloride monohydrate, m.p. 212–3°C; hydrobromide, m.p. 221–5°C; $[\alpha]_D^{25} - 93°$ (H_2O); perchlorate, m.p. 202–4°C (*dec.*); acid sulphate dihydrate, m.p. 290°C (*dec.*); oxalate hemihydrate, m.p. 210–2°C; $[\alpha]_D^{27} - 97°$ (H_2O) and the oxime, m.p. 123–5°C. The O-acetate forms colourless crystals, m.p. 123–4°C and gives a perchlorate, m.p. 160–3°C. The alkaloid is hydrolyzed with boiling HCl to yield dimethylaminoethanol and cassaic acid, $C_{20}H_{30}O_4$, m.p. 203°C; $[\alpha]_D^{20} - 126.3°$ (EtOH). If hydrolysis is carried out with alkali, *allo*cassaic acid, m.p. 222–4°C; $[\alpha]_D^{20} + 81.8°$ (EtOH) is produced in place of cassaic acid.

Pharmacologically, the alkaloid is a heart stimulant and is distinguished from the other *Erythrophleum* alkaloids by producing intense excitation. It is only a moderate local anaesthetic. Acetylation reduces the cardiac activity but raises slightly the emetic action of the alkaloid.

Dalma., *Ann. Chim. Appl.*, **25**, 569 (1935)
Dalma., *Helv. Chim. Acta*, **22**, 1497 (1939)
Faltis, Holzinger., *Ber.*, **72**, 1443 (1939)
Engel, Tondeur., *Helv. Chim. Acta*, **32**, 2364 (1949)

Synthesis:
Turner *et al.*, *J. Amer. Chem. Soc.*, **88**, 1766 (1966)

Pharmacology:
Santi, Zweifel., *Boll. Soc. ital. Biol. sper.*, **11**, 758, 760 (1936)
Trabucci., *Arch. Farm. sperim.*, **64**, 97 (1937)

CASSAMEDINE

$C_{19}H_{11}O_6N$

M.p. 278°C

Isolated from *Cassytha americana* (Syn. *C. filliformis* L.), this alkaloid forms an orange microcrystalline powder from $CHCl_3$-Et_2O. The ultraviolet spectrum of the solution in EtOH shows absorption maxima at 252, 281, 324, 364 and 460 mµ. That in EtOH-HCl solution exhibits absorption maxima at 272, 286, 408 and 534 mµ.

Cava *et al., J. Org. Chem.*, **33**, 2443 (1968)

CASSAMERIDINE

$C_{18}H_9O_5N$

M.p. 300°C

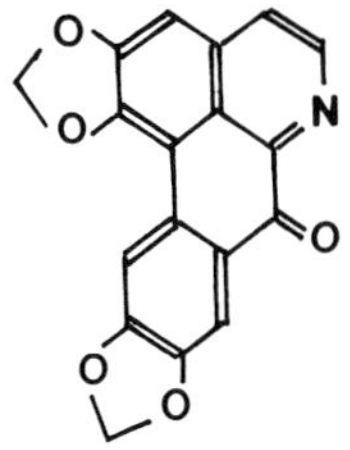

Also present in *Cassytha americana,* this base is obtained as a yellow micro-crystalline powder. With dilute mineral acids, the alkaloid yields a red solution while its solution in $CHCl_3$ exhibits a green fluorescence. The ultraviolet spectrum in EtOH shows absorption maxima at 251, 274, 323, 353, 388 and 440 mµ. The above structure for the base has been confirmed by synthesis.

Cava *et al., J. Org. Chem.*, **33**, 2443 (1968)
Synthesis:
Lahey, Mak., *Tetrahedron Lett.*, 4511 (1970)

CASSAMIDE

$C_{23}H_{35}O_6N$

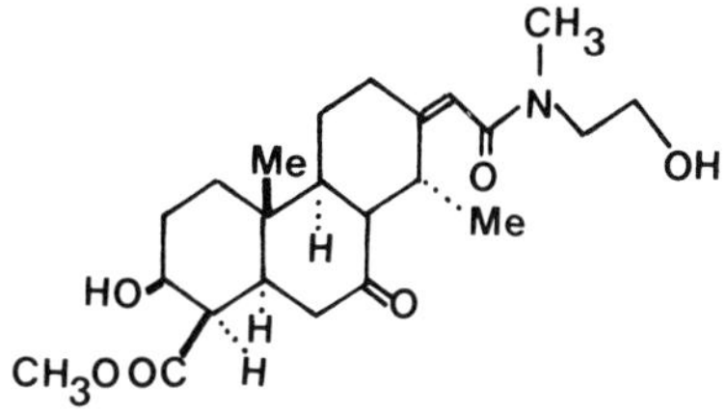

A second phenanthrene type alkaloid isolated from the bark of *Erythrophleum ivorense* (*See Cassaide*). The base resembles the latter alkaloid in structure, containing an acetoxy group in place of a methyl group.

Cronlund, Sandberg., *Acta Pharm. Suecica,* **8**, 351 (1971)

CASSAMINE

$C_{25}H_{39}O_5N$

M.p. 76–80°C

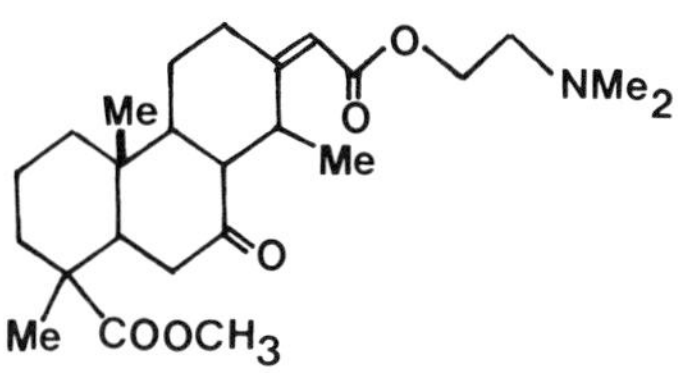

The bark and twigs of *Erythrophleum quincense* G. Dom. contain this alkaloid which has $[\alpha]_D^{19} - 56°$ (c 0.84, 95% EtOH). The ultraviolet spectrum shows only one main absorption maximum at 225 mμ. The alkaloid forms crystalline salts, e.g. the hydrochloride, m.p. 214–7°C (*dec.*); perchlorate, m.p. 200–210°C (*dec.*); $[\alpha]_D^{20} - 50°$ (c 0.59, 50% EtOH) and the sulphate, m.p. 191–4°C.

Engel, Tondeur., *Helv. Chim. Acta*, **32**, 2364 (1949)
Engel, Tondeur, Ruzicka., *Rec. trav. chim.*, **69**, 396 (1950)
Mathieson *et al.*, *Experientia*, **16**, 404 (1960)

CASSINE

$C_{18}H_{35}O_2N$

M.p. 57–58.5°C;
B.p. 90°C/0.001 mm

This alkaloid has been obtained from the leaves and twigs of *Cassia excelsa* Shrad. and is also present in *C. carnaval* Speg. The base has $[\alpha]_D^{25} - 0.6°$, a value which, although small, is consistent and appears to be real and not due to any impurity. The hydrochloride forms clusters of colourless needles from EtOH, m.p. 173–5°C; the nitrate crystallizes from dilute HNO_3 with m.p. 116–7°C. Ac_2O yields the O,N-diacetyl derivative as a neutral oil, b.p. 110°C/0.002 mm. Reduction with $NaBH_4$ furnishes the dihydro compound, m.p. 57–61°C, shown to be identical with Carnavaline (q.v.). When heated alone over Pd-C at 220°C in a stream of nitrogen, the alkaloid gives the dehydro derivative, m.p. 104–5°C. The N-methyl compound is an oil which forms a hydrochloride, m.p. 110–111.5°C; $[\alpha]_D^{26} + 6.5°$ and a methiodide, m.p. 91–3°C; $[\alpha]_D^{26} + 15.8°$.

Highet., *J. Org. Chem.*, **29**, 471 (1964)
Lythgoe, Vernengo., *Tetrahedron Lett.*, 1133 (1967)

Structure:
Rice, Coke., *J. Org. Chem.*, **31**, 1010 (1966)
Highet, Highet., *ibid*, 1275 (1966)

CASSIPOURINE

$C_{14}H_{22}N_2S_4$

M.p. 212°C

This dimeric pyrrolizidine sulphur-containing alkaloid is a constituent of *Cassipourea gummiflua* Tul. var. *verticellata* Lewis. It forms colourless needles when recrystallized from Me_2CO and has $[\alpha]_D^{20} - 11.8°$ (c 1.0, $CHCl_3$). The di-salts are all crystalline, e.g. the dihydrobromide, m.p. 185–190°C; dipicrate, yellow granules, m.p. 211–220°C (*dec.*) and the dimethiodide, m.p. 258–260°C.

Wright, Warren., *J. Chem. Soc.*, C, 283 (1967)
Cooks, Warren, Williams., *ibid*, 286 (1967)

CASSYFILINE

$C_{19}H_{19}O_5N$

M.p. 217°C (dec.).

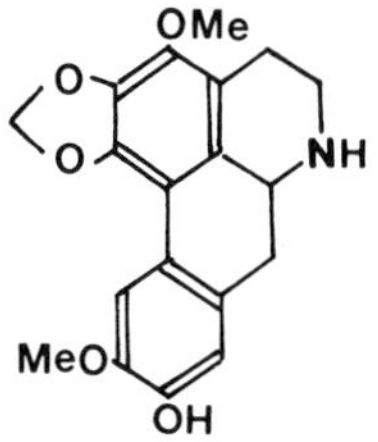

The stems of *Cassytha filiformis* grown in Formosa yield this alkaloid which forms pale orange-brown granules. It is laevorotatory having $[\alpha]_D^{15} - 89.6°$ (c 1.0, CHCl$_3$). The O-methyl ether forms needles with m.p. 150–1°C, giving a crystalline hydrochloride, m.p. 260–1°C while the N-methyl derivative crystallizes from MeOH as colourless needles, m.p. 210–1°C. The O,N-dimethyl compound is obtained as columnar crystals, m.p. 139–140°C.

Tomita *et al., J. Pharm. Soc., Japan,* **85**, 827 (1965)

CASSYTHICINE

$C_{19}H_{19}O_4N$

M.p. 210–2°C

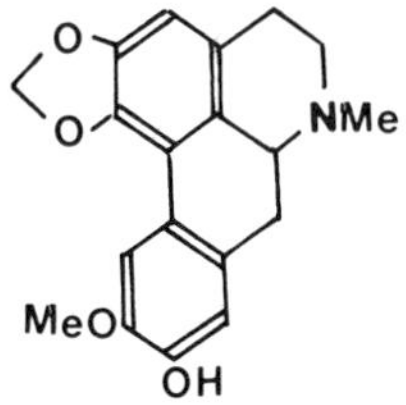

An alkaloid from *Cassytha melantha* R. Br. and *C. glabella* R. Br., this base crystallizes from CHCl$_3$ with one mole of solvent. It is dextrorotatory with $[\alpha]_D + 62°$ (c 0.43, CHCl$_3$) and the ultraviolet spectrum in EtOH has absorption maxima at 219, 283 and 305 mμ with an inflexion at 272 mμ. The structure as 9-hydroxy-10-methoxy-1:2-methylenedioxyaporphine has been confirmed by the synthesis of the optically inactive form, m.p. 111–3°C. The O-methyl ether is identical with (+)-Dicentrine (q.v.).

Tomita, Kikkawa., *J. Pharm. Soc., Japan,* **52**, 3833 (1958)

CASSYTHIDINE

$C_{19}H_{17}O_5N$

M.p. 206–7°C

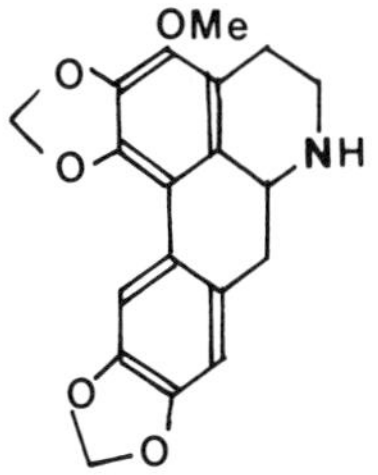

Obtained from the leaves of *Cassytha filiformis* L., this alkaloid forms colourless prisms when recrystallized from $CHCl_3$-MeOH and has $[\alpha]_D + 15°$ (c 0.64, $CHCl_3$). The ultraviolet spectrum shows absorption maxima at 217, 286 and 309 mμ.

Johns, Lamberton., *Austral. J. Chem.*, **19**, 297 (1966)

CASTORAMINE

$C_{15}H_{23}O_2N$

An alkaloid isolated from the glands of the beaver, the base is obtained as the crystalline hydrochloride, m.p. 215−235°C. Ac_2O yields the acetyl derivative which can be crystallized as colourless needles. The deoxy derivative forms a hydrochloride, m.p. 207−215°C (*dec.*).

Khaleque., *Sci. Res.*, (Dacca), **6**, 29 (1969)

CATALAUDESMINE

$C_{25}H_{34}O_7N_2$

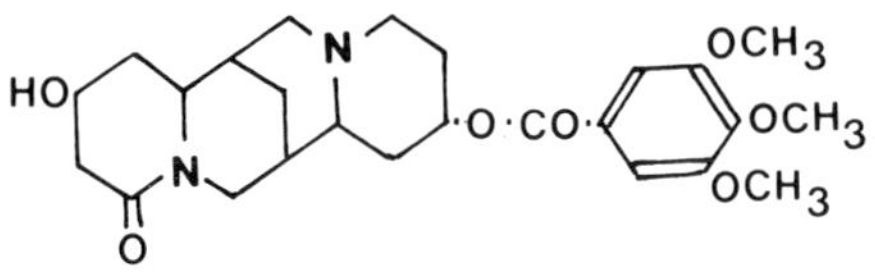

This sparteine type alkaloid is present in *Sarothamnus catalaunicus* Webb. Few further details have been recorded for this base.

Faugeras, Paris., *Plant. Med. Phytother.*, **5**, 134 (1971)

CATALAUVERINE

$C_{24}H_{32}O_6N_2$

M.p. 152−3°C

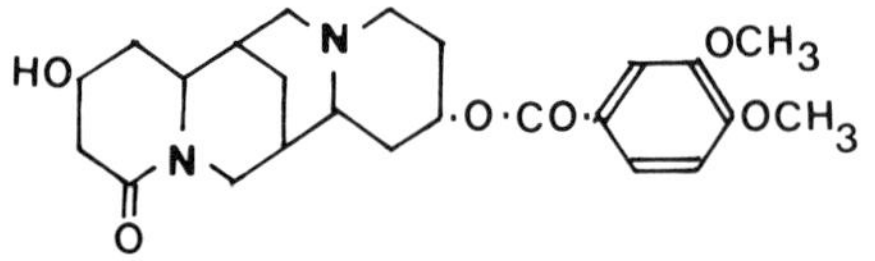

A second sparteine type alkaloid occurring in *Sarothamnus catalaunicus* Webb, this alkaloid differs from the preceding base only in the lesser degree of substitution in the aromatic ring.

Faugeras, Paris., *Plant. Med. Phytother.*, **5**, 134 (1971)

CATALINE

$C_{21}H_{25}O_5N$

M.p. 183°C

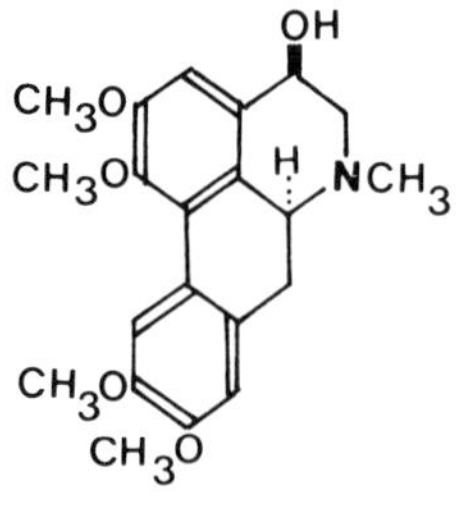

This aporphine alkaloid is present in *Glaucium flavum* Cr. and is obtained as colourless crystals with $[\alpha]_D + 166°$ (CHCl$_3$). The ultraviolet spectrum shows absorption maxima at 282 and 303 mμ in EtOH solution. The alkaloid contains four methoxyl groups, one hydroxyl and a methylimino group. It forms a crystalline O-acetate, m.p. 91–2°C.

Ribas, Sueiras, Castedo., *Tetrahedron Lett.,* 2033 (1972)

CATALPIFOLINE (*2:10-Dimethylhernovine*)

C$_{20}$H$_{23}$O$_4$N

M.p. 174–5°C

A noraporphine base occurring in *Hernandia catalpifolia,* this alkaloid is obtained as colourless crystals from EtOH. It has $[\alpha]_D^{22} + 220°$ (c 0.10, EtOH). The alkaloid contains four methoxyl groups and one imino group in the molecule. The structure has been determined mainly from spectroscopic data and comparison with hernovine (q.v.).

Cava, Bessho, Douglas, Markey, Weisbach., *Tetrahedron Lett.,* 4279 (1966)

CATHALANCEINE

M.p. 188–190°C (*dec.*).

Occurring in the roots of *Catharanthus lanceus,* this alkaloid crystallizes from Me$_2$CO. The ultraviolet spectrum exhibits absorption maxima at 226, 296 and 323 mμ.

Blomster, Martello, Farnsworth, Draus., *Lloydia,* **27**, 480 (1964)

CATHANNEINE

C$_{24}$H$_{30}$O$_5$N$_2$

M.p. 76–7°C

A further base from the roots of *Catharanthus lanceus,* this alkaloid has $[\alpha]_D^{25} - 73°$ (MeOH). The ultraviolet spectrum shows absorption maxima at 208, 255 and 308 mμ.

Aynilian, Tin-Wa, Farnsworth, Gorman., *Tetrahedron Lett.,* 89 (1972)
Aynilian, Farnsworth, Lyon, Fong., *J. Pharm. Sci.,* **61**, 298 (1972)
Absolute configuration:
Aynilian, Robinson, Farnsworth., *Tetrahedron Lett.,* 391 (1972)

CATHARANTHINE

$C_{21}H_{24}O_2N_2$

M.p. 126–8°C

A constituent of *Vinca rosea* Linn. this alkaloid forms colourless crystals from MeOH and has $[\alpha]_D^{27} + 29.8°$ (CHCl$_3$). The ultraviolet spectrum has absorption maxima at 226, 284 and 292 mμ. The base forms crystalline salts which crystallize from MeOH or EtOH, e.g. the sulphate, m.p. 164–7°C (*dec.*); the hemitartrate, m.p. 148–150°C (*dec.*) and the methiodide, m.p. 232–4°C (*dec.*). In a biogenetic-type synthesis of this alkaloid, Qureshi and Scott have shown that either geissoschizine or corynantheine aldehyde when refluxed in HOAc for 72 hours under N$_2$ give a mixture of pseudocatharanthine and catharanthine. Under the reaction conditions, these two products are in equilibrium.

Gorman *et al., J. Amer. Pharm. Assoc. Sci. Ed.,* **48**, 256, 659 (1959)
Neuss, Gorman., *Tetrahedron Lett.,* 206 (1961)
Kutney *et al., Chem. & Ind.,* 648 (1963)

Synthesis:
Qureshi, Scott., *Chem. Commun.,* 945, 947 (1968)

NMR spectra:
Gorman, Neuss, Cone., *J. Amer. Chem. Soc.,* **87**, 93 (1965)

Biosynthesis:
Battersby, Brown, Kapil, Plunkett, Taylor., *Chem. Commun.,* 46 (1966)
Battersby, Brown, Knight, Martin, Plunkett., *ibid,* 346 (1966)
Battersby, Brown, Kapil, Knight, Martin, Plunkett., *ibid,* 810, 888 (1966)
Leete, Ueda., *Tetrahedron Lett.,* 4915 (1966)

CATHARICINE

$C_{46}H_{52}O_{10}N_4$

M.p. 231–4°C

A dimeric alkaloid present in *Vinca rosea* L. the base forms colourless crystals from Me$_2$CO. It has $[\alpha]_D^{26} + 34.8°$ (c 1.0, CHCl$_3$). The ultraviolet spectrum exhibits absorption maxima at 214, 268, 283 (shoulder), 293 and 315 mμ.

Svoboda, Gorman, Barnes, Oliver., *J. Pharm. Sci.,* **51**, 518 (1962)

CATHARINE

$C_{46}H_{52}O_9N_4$

M.p. 271–5°C (*dec.*).

This closely-allied alkaloid also occurs in *Vinca rosea* L. and crystallizes from MeOH with one mole of solvent. It has $[\alpha]_D - 54.2°$ (CHCl$_3$). There are three absorption maxima present in the ultraviolet spectrum at 222, 265 and 292 mμ.

Svoboda, Gorman, Neuss, Barnes., *J. Pharm. Sci.,* **50**, 409 (1961)

268

CATHAROSINE

$C_{22}H_{28}O_4N_2$

M.p. 141–3°C

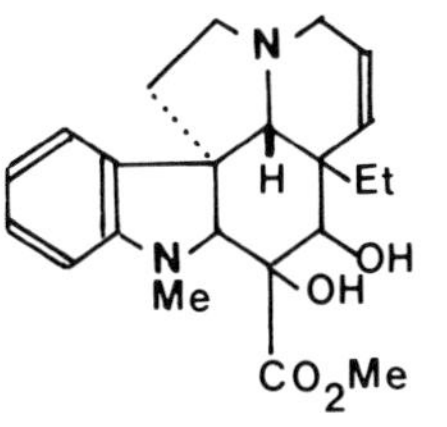

Found in *Vinca rosea* L. (*Catharanthus roseus* G. Don), this alkaloid crystallizes as colourless, slender needles from C_6H_6-light petroleum and has $[\alpha]_D$ 0°. The ultraviolet spectrum shows absorption maxima at 252 and 306 mμ. The 4-O-acetate is Vindolidine (q.v.).

Moza, Trojanek, Hanus, Dolejs., *Collect. Czech. Chem. Commun.*, **29**, 1913 (1964)
Moza, Trojanek., *Chem. Ind.*, 1260 (1965)

CATHINDINE

This uncharacterized alkaloid from the roots of *Vinca rosea* L. has been isolated as the crystalline sulphate, m.p. 239–245°C (*dec.*). In MeOH solution, the ultraviolet spectrum of the alkaloid has absorption maxima at 224, 282 and 289 mμ.

Svoboda, Oliver, Bedwell., *Lloydia*, **26**, 141 (1963)

CATHOVALINE

$C_{24}H_{30}O_5N_2$

M.p. 88–90°C

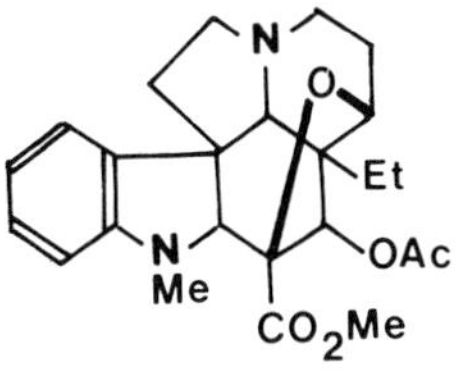

A crystalline alkaloid obtained from *Catharanthus ovalis* Markgraf. the base crystallizes from cyclohexane and has $[\alpha]_D$ − 73° (c 0.5, CHCl₃).

Langlois, Potier., *Compt. Rend.*, **273C**, 994 (1971)

CAULOPHYLLINE (*N-Methylcytisine*)

$C_{12}H_{16}ON_2$

M.p. 137°C

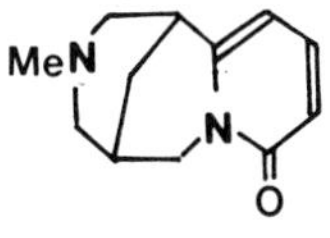

This base occurs together with cytisine in several species of *Gerista* and in *Caulophyllum thalictroides* Michx. It forms glancing prisms when crystallized from EtOH and has $[\alpha]_D$ − 221.6°. The salts and derivatives are generally well crystalline, e.g. the perchlorate, m.p. 282°C; picrate, m.p. 230–1°C and the tartrate, m.p. 158–9°C; $[\alpha]_D^{24} + 94.5°$.

Power, Salway., *J. Chem. Soc.*, **103**, 191 (1913)
Orekhov, Norkina, Gurevitsch., *Ber.*, **67**, 1394 (1934)

CAVINCIDINE

A further minor constituent of *Vinca rosea* L, this alkaloid has been characterized as the crystalline sulphate, m.p. 236–9°C (*dec.*).

Svoboda, Oliver, Bedwell., *Lloydia,* **26**, 141 (1963)

CAVINCINE

$C_{20}H_{24}O_2N_2$

M.p. Indefinite

This alkaloid is also a constituent of *Vinca rosea* L. It is obtained as a glassy solid which is not crystallizable. The sulphate forms colourless plates of the monohydrate from EtOH, m.p. 275–7°C (*dec.*).

Svoboda, Oliver, Bedwell., *Lloydia,* **26**, 141 (1963)

CEANOTHAMINE A

See Frangulanine

CEANOTHAMINE B

See Adouetin X

CEANOTHINE A

$C_{30}H_{40}O_4N_4$

M.p. 256–9°C

From the root bark of *Ceanothus americanus,* this alkaloid is obtained as slender, colourless needles from CH_2Cl_2-Et_2O. It has $[\alpha]_D - 256°$ (c 0.5, $CHCl_3$).

Warnhoff, Pradham, Ma., *Can. J. Chem.*, **43**, 2594 (1965)

CEANOTHINE B

$C_{29}H_{36}O_4N_4$

M.p. 238.5–240.5°C

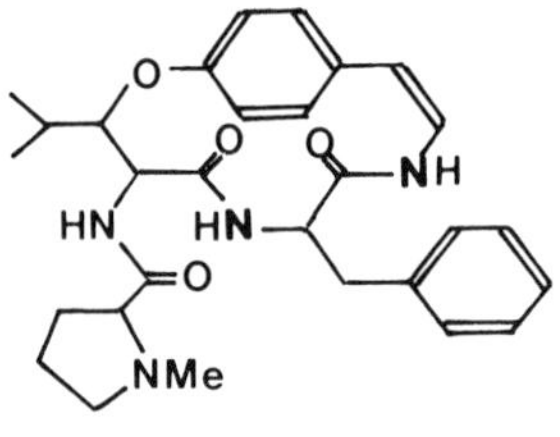

This alkaloid is the major constituent of the root bark of *Ceanothus americanus* and forms colourless needles when crystallized from $CHCl_3$-Et_2O. It has $[\alpha]_D^{25}$ − 293° (c 0.68, $CHCl_3$). The hydriodide is crystalline, forming lustrous plates, m.p. 195−200°C.

Hydrogenation of the alkaloid yields the dihydro derivative, m.p. 263−273°C; $[\alpha]_D^{25}$ − 91° (c 0.38, $CHCl_3$).

Warnhoff, Pradhan, Ma., *Can. J. Chem.*, **43**, 2594 (1965)
Warnhoff, Ma, Reynolds-Warnhoff., *J. Amer. Chem. Soc.*, **87**, 4198 (1965)

Structure revision:
Klein, Rapoport., *J. Amer. Chem. Soc.*, **90**, 3576 (1968)
Servis, Kosak., *ibid*, **90**, 4179, 6895 (1968)

CEANOTHINE C

$C_{26}H_{38}O_4N_4$

M.p. 223−9°C

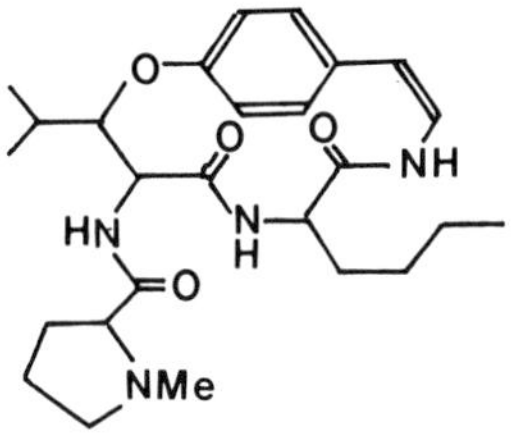

A minor peptide alkaloid from the root bark of *Ceanothus americanus*, this base also forms colourless needles from $CHCl_3$-Et_2O. It has $[\alpha]_D^{25}$ − 368° (c 1.01, $CHCl_3$).

Warnhoff, Pradhan, Ma., *Can. J. Chem.*, **43**, 2594 (1965)
Fehlhaber., *Z. Anal. Chem.*, **91**, 235 (1968)
Servis *et al.*, *J. Amer. Chem. Soc.*, **91**, 5619 (1969)

CEANOTHINE D

$C_{26}H_{38}O_4N_4$

M.p. 227−9°C

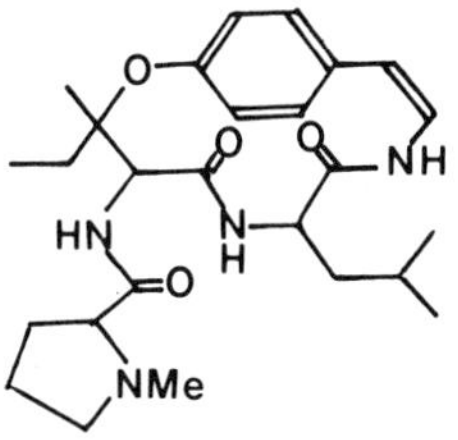

A further peptide alkaloid found in the root bark of *Ceanothus americanus*, this base also crystallizes well from $CHCl_3$-Et_2O and has $[\alpha]_D$ − 347° ($CHCl_3$).

Servis *et al.*, *J. Amer. Chem. Soc.*, **91**, 5619 (1969)

CEANOTHINE E

$C_{34}H_{40}O_4N_4$

M.p. 238–9°C

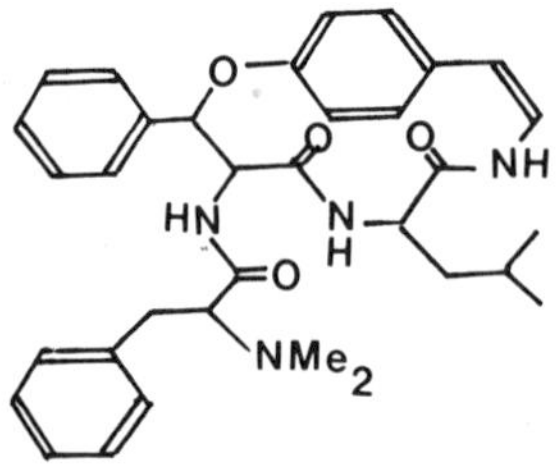

This peptide base also occurs in the root bark of *Ceanothus americanus* and forms colourless crystals from CH_2Cl_2-Et_2O. It is laevorotatory with $[\alpha]_D$ − 285° ($CHCl_3$).

Servis *et al., J. Amer. Chem. Soc.*, **91**, 5619 (1969)

CELEPANIGINE

$C_{33}H_{31}O_9N$

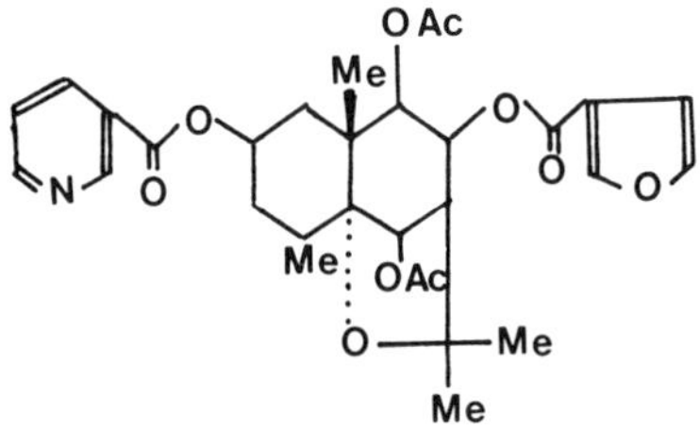

A recently discovered sesquiterpene alkaloid present in *Celastrus paniculatus*. Spectroscopic data shows that the base is a diacetyl benzoylnicotinoyl ester.

Wagner, Heckel, Sonnenbichler., *Tetrahedron Lett.*, 213 (1974)

CELAPANINE

$C_{30}H_{29}O_{10}N$

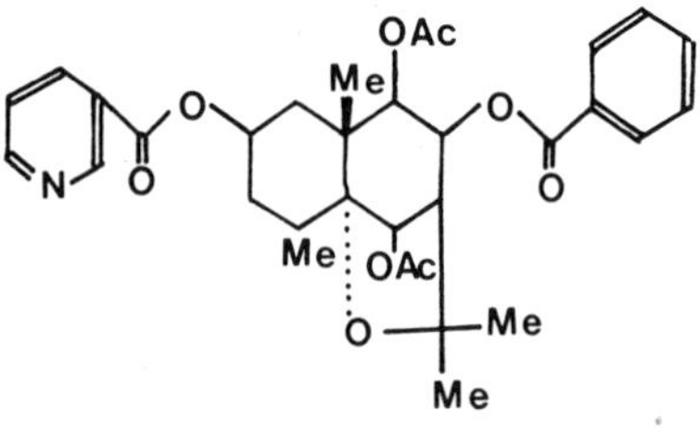

This sesquiterpene alkaloid also occurs in *Celastrus paniculatus*. The structure, determined spectroscopically, is similar to that of the preceding base, being a diacetylfuranoylnicotinoyl tetraester.

Wagner, Heckel, Sonnenbichler., *Tetrahedron Lett.*, 213 (1974)

272

CEPHAELINE

$C_{28}H_{38}O_4N_2$

M.p. 120–130°C

One of the alkaloids obtained from ipecacuanha (*Cephaelis Ipecacuanha* (Brot.) A. Rich), Cephaeline is most readily purified by regenerating the base from the hydrochloride or hydrobromide and crystallizing the alkaloid from Et_2O. It forms colourless needles and has $[\alpha]_D - 43.4°$ ($CHCl_3$) or $- 21.2°$ (EtOH). The hydrochloride crystallizes as stout prisms of the heptahydrate, m.p. 245–270°C; $[\alpha]_D + 25°$ to 29.5° (c 1.7 to 6.7, H_2O). An acid hydrochloride is also known, B, 5HCl, m.p. 84–6°C, which separates from concentrated acid solutions. The hydrobromide, like the chloride, forms crystals of the heptahydrate, m.p. 266–293°C. The hydriodide, nitrate and sulphate are all amorphous solids with no definite melting points. The dimethiodide is crystalline with m.p. 225–8°C; the diacetyl derivative, m.p. 116°C and the dibenzoyl compound, m.p. 128°C, are also known. The O-methyl ether is Emetine (q.v.). The free alkaloid couples with p-nitroazobenzene to form a dye which gives a deep purple colour in aqueous NaOH.

Brindley, Pyman., *J. Chem. Soc.*, 1067 (1927)

Späth, Leithe., *Ber.*, **60**, 688 (1927)

Späth, Pailer., *Monatsh.*, **78**, 348 (1948)

Pailer., *ibid*, **79**, 127 (1949)

Battersby, Openshaw., *J. Chem. Soc., Suppl.*, 59 (1949)

Janot., *Bull. Soc. Chim. Fr.*, 185 (1949)

CEPHALOTAXINE

$C_{18}H_{21}O_4N$

M.p. 131–2°C

This base occurs in both *Cephalotaxus drupacea* and *C. fortuni* and is obtained as colourless crystals from C_6H_6. It has $[\alpha]_D^{25} - 204°$ (c 1.8, $CHCl_3$) and the ultraviolet spectrum in EtOH shows absorption maxima at 238 and 290 mμ. The salts are crystalline, e.g. the hydrochloride with a double melting point at 174–7°C and 188°C (*dec.*); the perchlorate, m.p. 213–6°C (*dec.*) and the acetyl derivative which crystallizes from Et_2O, m.p. 140–2°C; $[\alpha]_D^{27} - 97°$ (c 2.2, $CHCl_3$).

Paundler, Kerley, McKay., *J. Org. Chem.*, **28**, 2194 (1963)

CEPHALOTAXINONE

$C_{18}H_{19}O_4N$

M.p. 198–200°C (dec.).

A minor alkaloid of *Cephalotaxus fortuni,* this base is laevorotatory with $[\alpha]_D^{24} - 146°$ (c 0.63, $CHCl_3$) and $- 155°$ (c 0.35, $CHCl_3$). The structure has been established by comparison with Cephalotaxine (q.v.).

Paundler, McKay., *J. Org. Chem.,* **38,** 2110 (1973)

CEPHARAMINE

$C_{19}H_{23}O_4N$

M.p. 186–7°C

This alkaloid is one of the major constituents of *Stephania cepharantha* Hayata, occurring mainly in the tubers of the plant. The alkaloidal extract may be separated into phenolic and non-phenolic components with cepharamine being found in the former after removal of Berbamine (q.v.). The alkaloid has $[\alpha]_D^{40} - 248°$ ($CHCl_3$) and the ultraviolet spectrum in EtOH shows a single absorption maximum at 259 mμ. The hydrobromide is crystalline with m.p. 241–3°C. With $NaBH_4$, the base yields an oily dihydro derivative. The structure has been confirmed by total synthesis.

Tomita, Kosuka., *Tetrahedron Lett.,* 6229 (1966)
Tomita, Kosuka., *J. Pharm. Soc., Japan,* **87,** 1203 (1967)
Synthesis:
Keely, Martinez, Takh., *Tetrahedron,* 4729 (1970)
Inubushi, Kitano, Ibuka., *Chem. Pharm. Bull.,* (Tokyo), **19,** 1820 (1971)
Kametani *et al., Chem. Ind.,* 538 (1972)

CEPHAROLINE

$C_{36}H_{36}O_6N_2$

M.p. 270°C (dec.).

A bisbenzyl*iso*quinoline alkaloid occurring in the roots of Stephania cephalantha, this base is strongly dextrorotatory with $[\alpha]_D^{35} + 319°$ ($CHCl_3$). It forms a crystalline O-methyl ether with m.p. 103°C.

Tomita *et al., J. Pharm. Soc., Japan,* **89,** 1678 (1969)

CEPHARANTHINE

$C_{37}H_{38}O_6N_2$

M.p. 145–155°C

A further constituent of *Stephania cepharantha* tubers, this bisbenzyl*iso*quinoline alkaloid crystallizes from C_6H_6-Me_2CO with C_6H_6 of crystallization, m.p. 103°C (*dec.*); removal of solvent under vacuum gives the anhydrous base as a yellow powder which is soluble in most organic solvents and mineral acids but only sparingly so in petroleum ether. The alkaloid has $[\alpha]_D^{20} + 277°$ (CHCl$_3$). All of the salts and the methiodide are amorphous solids with indefinite melting points. The first stage of the Hofmann degradation yields two methine bases; the α-methine, $C_{39}H_{42}O_6N_2$, as the trihydrate, m.p. 98–100°C which is optically inactive, forming a methiodide, m.p. 305–6°C. The isomeric β-methine has m.p. 183–4°C and $[\alpha]_D^{27} + 58°$ (CHCl$_3$).

According to work done in Japan during the last war, this alkaloid appears to show some promise in the treatment of leprosy and tuberculosis although it has now been superseded by other drugs.

Kondo *et al., J. Pharm. Soc., Japan,* **58**, 276 (1938)
Kondo, Keimatsu., *Ber.,* **71**, 2553 (1938)
Kondo, Kataoka, Nakagawa., *Chem. Abstr.,* **47**, 7519 (1953)
Tomita, Sasaki., *Chem. Pharm. Bull.,* (Tokyo), **1**, 105 (1953)
Tomita, Sasaki., *ibid,* **2**, 89, 375 (1954)
Tomita, Sasaki., *ibid,* **3**, 178, 250 (1955)

Absolute configuration:
Kunimoto., *J. Pharm. Soc., Japan,* **83**, 981 (1962)

Synthesis:
Tomita, Fujitani, Aoyagi., *Tetrahedron Lett.,* 1201 (1967)

Pharmacology:
Buchi., *Schweiz. Apoth. Zeit.,* **83**, 198 (1945)

CERNUINE (*Alkaloid L-32*)

$C_{16}H_{26}ON_2$

M.p. 106°C

This tetracyclic alkaloid is present in *Lycopodium cernuum* L. and forms colourless crystals from MeOH. The perchlorate is also crystalline, forming the sesquihydrate, m.p. 110°C. Some confusion has arisen in the literature due to the above name also having been assigned to an aurone, the latter now being renamed Aureusidin.

Marion, Manske., *Can. J. Res.,* **26B**, 1 (1948)
Ayer *et al., Tetrahedron Lett.,* 2201 (1964)

CEVACINE

$C_{27}H_{45}O_2N$

M.p. 178–183°C

A steroidal alkaloid found in the corms of *Fritillaria imperialis.* The base is laevorotatory with $[\alpha]_D - 21°$. No salts of this alkaloid have been reported.

Suri, Ram., *Ind. J. Chem.*, **7**, 1057 (1969)

CEVADILLINE (*Sabadilline*)

$C_{34}H_{52}O_8N$

M.p. Indefinite

This amorphous base is obtained during the purification of Cevadine (q.v.). It is insoluble in Et_2O and may be hydrolyzed with warm alkali to give tiglic acid and cevilline, $C_{29}H_{47}O_7N$.

Wright, Luff., *J. Chem. Soc.*, **33**, 338 (1878)

CEVADINE (*Veratrine*)

$C_{32}H_{49}O_9N$

M.p. 205°C (*dec.*).

This complex steroidal alkaloid was first obtained in a crystalline form by Merck from the seeds of *Schoenocaulon officinale,* A. Gray (sabadilla or cevadilla) and subsequently from *Veratrum viride.* In the literature it is sometimes termed 'crystallized' veratrine. The base crystallizes from EtOH with two moles of solvent which are lost at 130–140°C. It has $[\alpha]_D^{17} + 12.5°$ (EtOH), $+ 6.4°$ (pyridine) or $+ 1.25°$ (Me$_2$CO). While it dissolves readily in hot EtOH, the alkaloid is insoluble in H_2O. The hydrochloride forms colourless needles; the aurichloride, yellow needles, m.p. 182°C (*dec.*); the picrate darkens at 225°C and the mercurichloride forms lustrous, silvery scales, m.p. 172°C (*dec.*). The base also forms a monoacetate, m.p. 225–8°C (*dec.*); $[\alpha]_D^{20} + 11.3°$ (EtOH); a diacetate, m.p. 254–7°C (*dec.*); a benzoyl derivative, m.p. 255°C and an *o*-nitro-benzoyl compound, m.p. 236°C; $[\alpha]_D^{17} - 37.5°$ (EtOH). Cevadine gives no colour with HCl but with H_2SO_4 it produces a yellow colour with a green fluorescence, gradually turning orange and then crimson. With alcoholic NaOH it is hydrolyzed to form tiglic and angelic acids and cevine (q.v.), while gaseous HCl in EtOH furnishes ethyl tiglate and cevine.

Merck., *Annalen*, **95**, 200 (1855)
Wright, Luff., *J. Chem. Soc.*, **33**, 338 (1878)
McBeth, Robinson., *ibid*, **121**, 1571 (1922)
Blount., *ibid*, 124 (1935)
Stoll, Seebeck., *Helv. Chim. Acta*, **35**, 1942 (1952)

CEVAGENINE

$C_{27}H_{43}O_8N$

M.p. 246–8°C

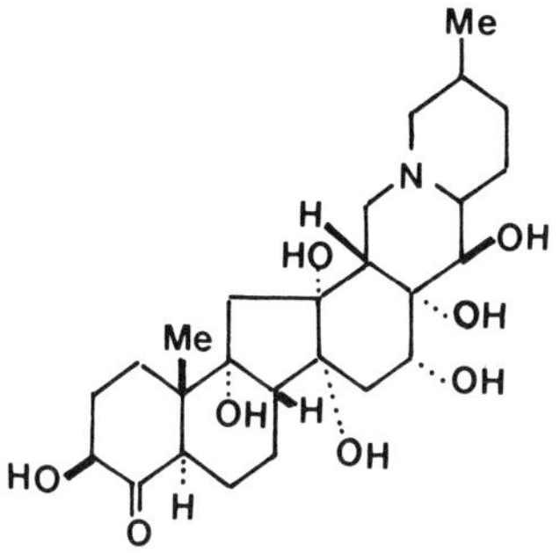

A steroidal alkaloid present in various *Veratrum* species, this base is laevorotatory having $[\alpha]_D^{20} - 52°$ (CHCl$_3$) and $- 47.5°$ (EtOH).

Vejdelek, Macek, Katac., *Chem. Listy.*, **49**, 1538 (1955)

CEVANINE

$C_{27}H_{44}O_2N_2$

M.p. 272–3°C

The corms of *Fritillaria imperialis* contain this steroidal alkaloid which is dextrorotatory with $[\alpha]_D + 49°$. No salts have yet been reported.

Suri, Ram., *Ind. J. Chem.*, **7**, 1057 (1969)

CEVINE

$C_{27}H_{43}O_8N$

M.p. 165–172°C (*dec.*).

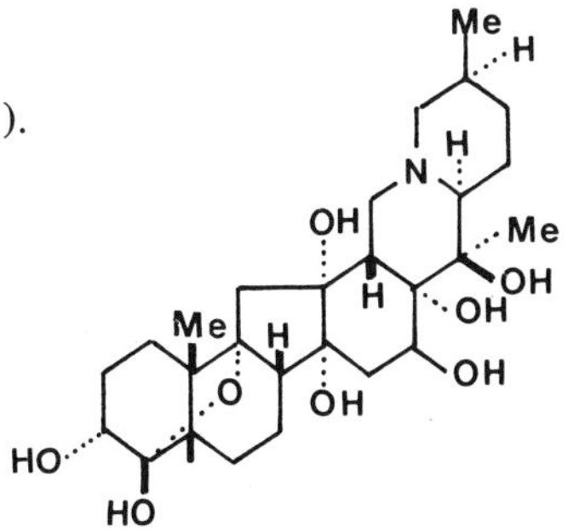

Although first obtained as a hydrolysis product of cevadine, this base also occurs naturally in the seeds of *Veratrum sabadilla*. It crystallizes from aqueous EtOH with 3.5 H_2O, m.p. 110°C in triclinic prisms. It has $[\alpha]_D^{17} - 17.52°$ (EtOH). The hydrochloride crystallizes as colourless needles, m.p. 247°C; the aurichloride, m.p. 162°C (*dec.*); the methiodide, m.p. 257°C (*dec.*); the monobenzoyl derivative, m.p. 195°C; the dibenzoyl compound, m.p. 195–6°C; the diacetyl derivative, m.p. 190°C and the di-*o*-nitrobenzoyl compound, m.p. 175°C. With alcoholic KOH, the alkaloid forms a characteristic crystalline potassium derivative.

Oxidation with H_2O_2 yields cevine oxide, $C_{27}H_{43}O_9N$, while dehydrogenation with Se gives, as the main products cevanthrol, $C_{17}H_{16}O$, colourless plates from C_6H_6, m.p. 197–8°C and cevanthridine, $C_{25}H_{27}N$, m.p. 211–2°C. The latter forms crystalline salts and derivatives, e.g. the hydrochloride, m.p. 245°C; methiodide, m.p. 268–270°C (*dec.*); picrate, m.p. 230–240°C (*dec.*) and an acetyl derivative, m.p. 206–7°C.

Wright, Luff., *J. Chem. Soc.,* **33**, 338 (1878)
Freund, Schwartz., *Ber.,* **32**, 800 (1899)
Hess, Mohr., *ibid*, **52**, 1984 (1919)
MacBeth, Robinson., *J. Chem. Soc.,* 1571 (1922)
Ikawa *et al.,* *J. Biol. Chem.,* **159**, 517 (1945)
Heubner, Jacobs., *ibid*, **170**, 181 (1947)
Jacobs, Pelletier., *J. Org. Chem.,* **18**, 765 (1953)
Barton *et al., Experientia,* **10**, 81 (1954)
Kupchan, Johnson, Rajacopalan., *Tetrahedron,* **7**, 47 (1959)
Eeles., *Tetrahedron Lett.,* **24**, (1960)

CHAENORHINE

$C_{31}H_{40}O_5N_4$

M.p. 263–8°C (*dec.*).

A macrocyclic spermine alkaloid, this base has been isolated from *Chaenorhinium organifolium* (Family Scrophilariaceae). The base has $[\alpha]_D^{25} + 46.7°$ (c 1.5008, $CHCl_3$-MeOH) and the ultraviolet spectrum shows an absorption maximum at 264 mμ and an inflexion at 280 mμ. Ac_2O in pyridine gives the N(2)-acetyl derivative which is amorphous as is also the N(2)-methyl compound. Catalytic hydrogenation with PtO_2 yields the 13:14-dihydro derivative, m.p. 230–6°C; $[\alpha]_D^{25} - 10° \pm 4°$ (c 0.111, MeOH).

Hesse, Schmid., *Izv. Otd. Khim. Nauk., Bulg. Akad. Nauk.,* **5**, 279 (1972)
Bernhard *et al., Helv. Chim. Acta,* **56**, 1266 (1973)

CHAIRAMIDINE

$C_{22}H_{26}O_4N_2$

M.p. 126–8°C

This amorphous alkaloid is obtained from the bark of *Remija Purdieana*, being present as a minor constituent. It has $[\alpha]_D^{15} + 7.3°$ (EtOH) and gives a green colour with H_2SO_4.

Hesse., *Annalen*, **185**, 296, 323 (1877)
Hesse., *ibid*, **225**, 211 (1884)

CHAIRAMINE

$C_{22}H_{26}O_4N_2$

M.p. 233°C

A minor constituent of the bark of *Remija Purdieana,* this alkaloid is stated to form colourless needles or prisms from EtOH. It has $[\alpha]_D + 100°$ (EtOH). The solution in AcOH gives a dark green colour with HNO_3.

Hesse., *Annalen*, **185**, 296, 323 (1877)
Hesse., *ibid*, **225**, 211 (1884)

CHAKSINE

$C_{11}H_{21}O_3N_3$

This alkaloid from *Cassia absus* has only been prepared as the free base in the impure form. It has $[\alpha]_D + 32°$ (EtOH). It behaves as a quaternary base forming salts with mineral acids by loss of water. The chloride has m.p. 178°C; bromide, m.p. 186°C; iodide, m.p. 168°C (*dec.*); the nitrate, m.p. 220–1°C (*dec.*); the sulphate, m.p. 316°C (*dec.*); the hydrogen carbonate, m.p. 117–9°C; the platinichloride, m.p. 232°C (*dec.*) and the picrate, m.p. 239–240°C (*dec.*). Treatment of the sulphate with Ba(OH)$_2$ yields *iso*chaksine, forming a carbonate, m.p. 128°C (*dec.*); platinichloride, m.p. 172°C (*dec.*) and a picrate, m.p. 184°C. It has been reported that *iso*chaksine also occurs naturally in the seeds of *Cassia absus* although it seems possible that this base is produced as a rearrangement product during the isolation of chaksine.

Siddiqui, Ahmen., *Proc. Ind. Acad. Sci.,* **2**, 421 (1935)
Kapur *et al., J. Ind. Chem. Soc.,* **17**, 281 (1940)
Aggarwal, Ray, Sen., *Sci. & Cult.,* **12**, 201 (1946)
Lala, Gupta., *Res. Bull. East Punjab Univ.,* No. 21, 95 (1952)
Gupta, Mahajan., *J. Sci. Ind. Res.,* **14B**, 602 (1955)
Guka, Ray., *J. Ind. Chem. Soc.,* **33**, 225 (1956)
Wiesner *et al., J. Amer. Chem. Soc.,* **80**, 1521 (1958)
Fowler, Valenta, Wiesner., *Chem. & Ind.,* 95 (1962)

CHALCHUPINE A

M.p. 168°C

This alkaloid is stated to occur in *Rauwolfia heterophylla* Roem. and Sch. It forms a hydriodide, m.p. 240°C; platinichloride, m.p. 261–2°C and a picrate, m.p. 150–2°C. The formula has not yet been rigorously established.

Deger., *Arch. Pharm.,* **275**, 496 (1937)
Paris, Daza., *Bull. Sci. Pharmacol.,* **48**, 46 (1941)

CHALCHUPINE B

M.p. 240°C

A second alkaloid found in *Rauwolfia heterophylla* Roem. and Sch., this base yields a hydriodide, m.p. 258–260°C; a tartrate, m.p. 250–6°C and a picrate, m.p. 154–6°C. Like the preceding base, the formula has not yet been established.

Deger., *Arch. Pharm.,* **275**, 496 (1937)
Paris, Daza., *Bull. Sci. Pharmacol.,* **48**, 46 (1941)

CHANDRINE

$C_{25}H_{30}O_8N_2$

M.p. 230–1°C

A minor constituent of the roots of *Rauwolfia serpentina,* this alkaloid forms crystalline salts, e.g. the hydrochloride, m.p. 185°C; the nitrate, m.p. 220–1°C; the chromate, m.p. 280–5°C; oxalate, m.p. 255–6°C; tartrate, m.p. 270–1°C and picrate, m.p. 180°C.

Rakshit., *Indian Pharmacist,* **9**, 226 (1954)
Rakshit., *ibid,* **10**, 84 (1954)

CHANOCLAVINE I

$C_{16}H_{20}ON_2$

M.p. 220–2°C (*dec.*).

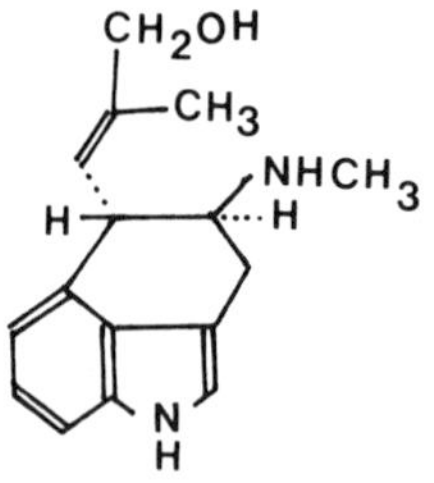

This alkaloid, originally designated chanoclavine or secaclavine, is produced by *Claviceps purpurea* (Fries) Tul. and forms colourless crystals from MeOH. It has $[\alpha]_D^{20} - 240°$ (pyridine) and the ultraviolet spectrum exhibits absorption maxima at 222, 275 (shoulder), 281 and 291 mμ in MeOH. Hydrogenation at 1 atmosphere over Pd-C yields festuclavine (q.v.), pyroclavine (q.v.) and, as the major product, a mixture of dihydrochanoclavine I and *iso*dihydrochanoclavine I.

Hofmann *et al., Helv. Chim. Acta,* **40**, 1358 (1957)
Abe *et al., Bull. Agr. Chem. Soc.* (Japan), **23**, 246 (1959)
Voigt, Zier., *Pharmazie,* 272 (1970)
Stereochemistry:
Acklin, Fehr, Arigoni., *Chem. Commun.,* 799 (1966)

(−)-CHANOCLAVINE II

$C_{16}H_{20}ON_2$

M.p. 174°C

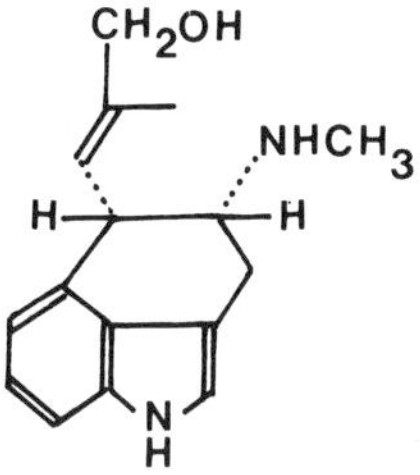

Also produces by *Claviceps purpurea* (Fries) Tul. this base has $[\alpha]_D^{20} - 332°$ (c 0.5, pyridine). The hydrochloride forms colourless needles from EtOH, m.p. 247°C; $[\alpha]_D^{20} - 271°$ (c 0.5, EtOH). The N-acetyl derivative has m.p. 203°C; $[\alpha]_D^{20} - 455°$ (c 0.54, pyridine) and the O,N-diacetyl compound, which cannot be crystallized, has $[\alpha]_D^{20} - 377°$ (c 0.5, pyridine).

Spectra:
Stauffacher, Tscherter., *Helv. Chim. Acta,* **47**, 2186 (1964)

(±)-CHANOCLAVINE II

$C_{16}H_{20}ON_2$

M.p. 179°C

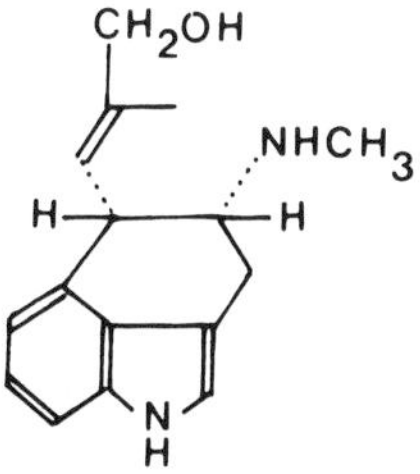

This alkaloid has been obtained from *Claviceps purpurea* (Fries) Tul. and forms colourless crystals from Me_2CO or $CHCl_3$.

Stauffacher, Tscherter., *Helv. Chim. Acta,* **47**, 2186 (1964)

CHASMACONITINE

$C_{34}H_{47}O_9N$

M.p. 165–7°C
or 181–2°C (dec.).

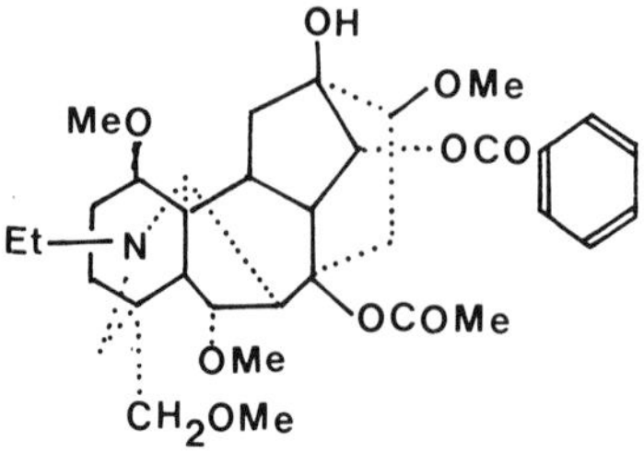

One of the aconite alkaloids, this base occurs in the roots of *Aconitum chasmanthum* Stapf and exists in two crystalline forms. From Et_2O it is obtained as clusters of slender needles, m.p. 165–7°C; $[\alpha]_D^{25}$ + 10.3° (c 1.26, EtOH). When crystallized from hexane, however, it forms colourless prisms, m.p. 181–2°C (*dec.*). The alkaloid contains four methoxyl groups, one tertiary hydroxyl and an ethylimino group. Acid hydrolysis furnishes acetic acid and benzoylchasmaconine while alkaline hydrolysis produces acetic and benzoic acids and chasmaconine.

Achmatowicz, Marion., *Can. J. Chem.,* **42**, 154 (1964)

CHASMANINE (*Toroko-base II*)

$C_{25}H_{41}O_6N$

M.p. 90–1°C;
B.p. 150°C/0.00005 mm

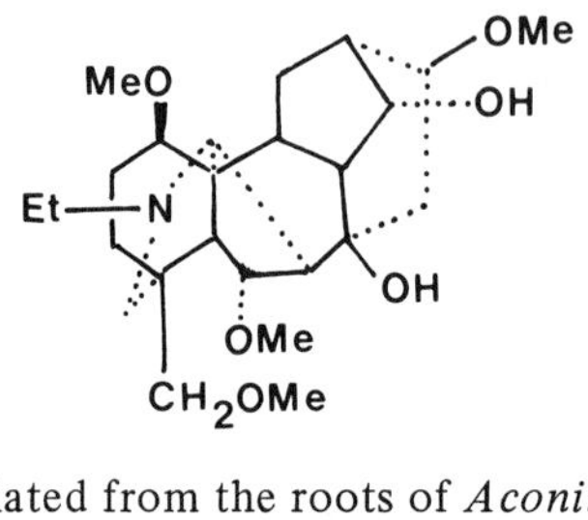

This alkaloid has been isolated from the roots of *Aconitum chasmanthum* Stapf, *A. subcuneatum* Nakai and *A. yesoensis* Nakai. It forms clusters of fine needles from hexane and has $[\alpha]_D^{25}$ + 23.6° (c 2.5, EtOH). The 8:10-diacetate has m.p. 139–141°C and the 10-benzoyl derivative which is non-crystallizable has b.p. 145°C/0.00005 mm. The latter forms a crystalline hydrochloride, m.p. 248–9°C and an O-acetate, m.p. 148–156°C.

Ochiai, Okamoto, Sakai., *J. Pharm. Soc. Japan,* **75**, 550 (1955)
Achmatowicz, Marion., *Can. J. Chem.,* **42**, 154 (1964)
Achmatowicz, Tsuda, Marion, Okamoto, Natsume, Chang, Kajima., *ibid,* **43**, 825 (1965)

CHASMANTHININE

$C_{36}H_{49}O_9N$

M.p. 160–1°C

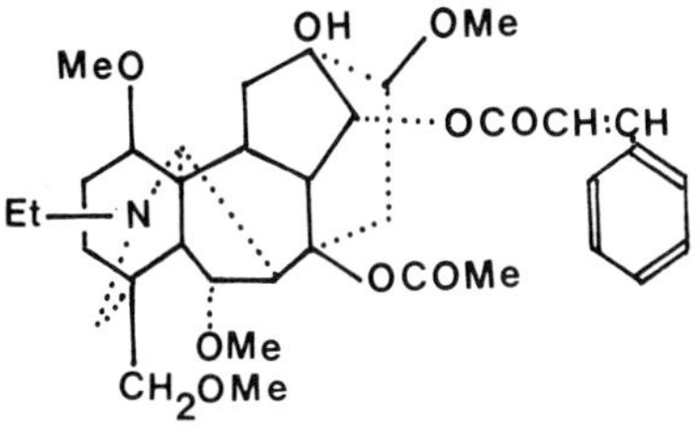

This base from the roots of *Aconitum chasmanthum* Stapf forms colourless needles from Et_2O or hexane. It has $[\alpha]_D^{25} + 9.6°$ (c 1.09, EtOH). It contains four methoxyl groups, one hydroxyl, a cinnamic acid moiety and an ethylimino group in the molecule.

Achmatowicz, Marion., *Can. J. Chem.*, **42**, 154 (1964)

CHATININE

This alkaloid has been obtained from the fresh roots of *Valeriana officinalis* and characterized as the hydrochloride, m.p. 115°C and the picrate, m.p. 97–8°C.

Chevalier., *Compt. rend.*, **144**, 154 (1907)

CHAVICINE

$C_{17}H_{19}O_3N$

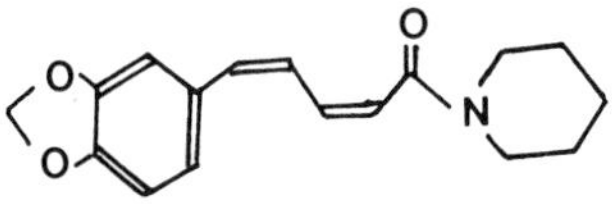

This weak base occurs in *Piper nigrum, P. longum* and *P. officinarum* along with piperine (q.v.). Chemically, it is the geometrical isomeride of piperine being the cis-cis form of the former. Like piperine, it possesses very little pharmacological action being merely a local irritant.

Ott *et al., Annalen*, **425**, 314 (1921)
Ott *et al., Ber.*, **55**, 2653 (1922)
Ott *et al., ibid*, **57**, 214 (1924)

CHEILANTHIFOLINE

$C_{19}H_{19}O_4N$

M.p. 184°C

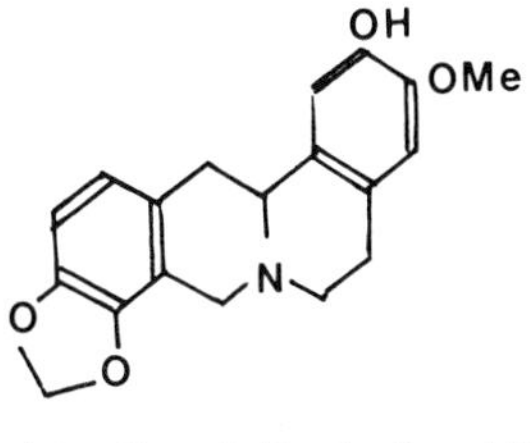

A berberine type alkaloid found in *Corydalis cheilanthifolia, C. scouleri* and *C. siberica*, this base has $[\alpha]_D^{20} - 311°$ (MeOH). The O-methyl ether is identical with sinactine (q.v.) and the O-ethyl ether has m.p. 144°C and on oxidation with $KMnO_4$ furnishes 6-methoxy-7-ethoxy-1-keto-1:2:3:4-tetrahydro*iso*quinoline, m.p. 195°C. From the latter observation it may be deduced that the hydroxyl group in the alkaloid is located at C-2, proving its constitution as 2-O-demethyltetrahydro*epi*berberine.

Manske., *Can. J. Res.,* **14B**, 347, 354 (1936)
Manske., *ibid,* **16B**, 438 (1938)
Manske., *ibid,* **18B**, 100 (1940)
Manske., *ibid,* **20B**, 57 (1942)

CHEIRANTHIN

This uncharacterized compound, obtained from the leaves and seeds of certain *Cheiranthus* species, has been described as a glucoside with a digitalis-like action.

Reeb., *Arch. exp. Path. Pharm.,* **41**, 302 (1898)
Reeb., *ibid,* **43**, 130 (1899)

CHEIRININE

$C_{18}H_{35}O_{17}N_3$

This base has also been reported as occurring in the leaves and seeds of *Cheiranthus* species. It is said to possess a pharmacological action rather like that of quinine.

Reeb., *Arch. exp. Path. Pharm.,* **41**, 302 (1898)
Reeb., *ibid,* **43**, 130 (1899)

CHEIROLINE

$C_5H_9O_2NS_2$

M.p. 47–8°C

Wagner obtained this compound from the seeds of *Cheiranthus* species and supposed it to be an alkaloid. It forms colourless prisms which, when heated with mercuric oxide and H_2O, yield cheirole as colourless needles, m.p. 172.5°C. Schneider subsequently proved that the compound is methyl-γ-thiocarbimino-propylsulphone, $CH_3.SO_2.(CH_2)_3.NCS$. In the plant, cheiroline appears to exist as a glucoside. Cheiroline has also been obtained from the seeds of *Erysimum aureum* and *E. arkansanum*.

Wagner., *Chem. Zeit.,* **32**, 76 (1908)
Schneider., *Ber.,* **41**, 4466 (1908)
Schlagdenhauffen, Reeb., *Compt. rend.,* **131**, 753 (1900)

CHELAMIDINE

M.p. 225–6°C

A minor alkaloid of *Chelidonium majus,* this base crystallizes as colourless needles from $CHCl_3$-EtOH. It is dextrorotatory with $[\alpha]_D^{21} + 123° \pm 2°$ (c 0.5, $CHCl_3$).

Slavik, Slavikova, Brabenec., *Collect. Czech. Chem. Commun.,* **30**, 3697 (1965)

CHELAMINE

M.p. 203–4°C

A further minor constituent of *Chelidonium majus,* this base may be recrystallized from EtOH when it yields clusters of colourless crystals. It has $[\alpha]_D^{20} + 107° \pm 2°$ ($CHCl_3$).

Slavik, Slavikova, Brabenec., *Collect. Czech. Chem. Commun.,* **30**, 3697 (1965)

CHELERYTHRINE

$C_{21}H_{19}O_5N$

M.p. 207°C

This quaternary alkaloid is quite widespread in occurrence being found in *Bocconia frutescens* Linn, *B. arborea, Chelidonium majus, Eschscholtzia californica* Cham., *Fagara seniarticulata* and *Toddalia aculeata.* The alkaloid crystallizes from EtOH with one mole of solvent. It is somewhat unstable, absorbing CO_2 from the air and very readily forming an oxidation product. When the latter impurity is present, the solutions show a marked blue fluorescence. The salts, which are quaternary, are all a bright yellow: the hydrochloride, m.p. 210°C (*dec.*); nitrate, m.p. 240°C; aurichloride, m.p. 233°C (*dec.*) and the picrate, m.p. 238°C. The base also forms a pseudocyanide, m.p. 261°C and the 9-ethyl ether, m.p. 239–242°C. On reduction with Zn and HCl it yields the dihydro derivative, m.p. 162–3°C, which is non-basic. The contradictory observations which have been recorded regarding chelerythrine and sanguinarine were due, in part, to the difficulty in separating these alkaloids.

Probst., *Annalen,* **29**, 120 (1839)
König, Tietz., *Arch. Pharm.,* **231**, 145 (1893)
Schmidt, Selle., *ibid,* **239**, 405 (1901)
Bauer, Hedinger., *ibid,* **258**, 167 (1920)
Späth, Kuffner., *Ber.,* **64**, 1123, 2034 (1931)
Manske., *Can. J. Res.,* **21B**, 140 (1943)
Schuer, Chang, Suanholm., *J. Org. Chem.,* **27**, 1472 (1962)

CHELIDAMINE

$C_{19}H_{19}O_4N$

M.p. 204–5°C

A further minor alkaloid of *Chelidonium majus*, this base is strongly laevo-rotatory with $[\alpha]_D - 316.9°$. It yields a crystalline hydrochloride, m.p. 254–6°C and a methiodide, m.p. 275°C.

Platonova *et al., J. Gen. Chem., USSR*, **26**, 181 (1956)

CHELIDIMERINE

$C_{43}H_{32}O_9N_2$

M.p. 258–260°C

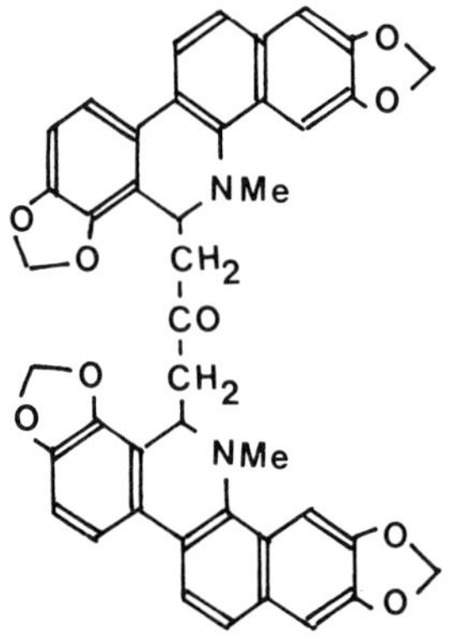

This dimeric alkaloid has recently been isolated from *Chelidonium majus*. It has been shown to possess the structure given above from chemical and spectroscopic evidence. This has also been confirmed by synthesis.

Kim *et al., J. Pharm. Sci.*, **58**, 372 (1969)

Synthesis:
Tin-Wa *et al., Lloydia*, **35**, 87 (1972)

CHELIDONINE

$C_{20}H_{19}O_5N$

M.p. 135–6°C

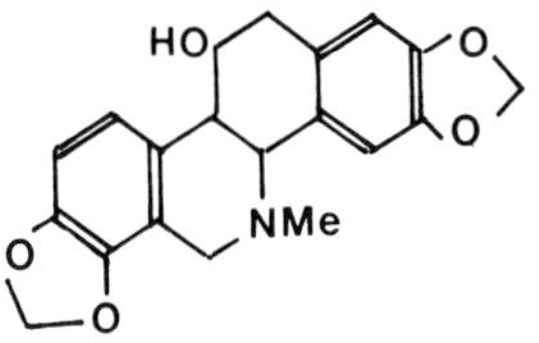

A major constituent of several Fumariaceous plants including *Chelidonium majus, Dicranostigma franchetianum* (Prain) Fedde. and *Stylophorum diphyllum* Nutt. The alkaloid separates with Protopine (q.v.) and is isolated by means of its greater solubility in Et_2O and the low solubility of the hydrochloride in HCl. Chelidonine crystallizes from aqueous HCl or MeOH as the monohydrate but is best purified by recrystallization from AcOH. It forms monoclinic tablets with

$[\alpha]_D$ + 115.4° (EtOH). The hydrochloride and nitrate are crystalline and insoluble in H_2O. With H_2SO_4 and guaiacol it gives an intense crimson colour. The aurichloride has m.p. 155°C, the benzoyl derivative, m.p. 217°C and the acetate, m.p. 165–6°C; $[\alpha]_D$ + 110°. The latter forms a crystalline platini-chloride, m.p. 200°C. With boiling Ac_2O, N-acetylanhydrochelidonine, $C_{22}H_{19}O_5N$, m.p. 152°C is formed.

Späth, Kuffner., *Ber.*, **64**, 370 (1931)

Manske., *Can. J. Res.*, **20B**, 53 (1942)

Chen, MacLean., *Can. J. Chem.*, **45**, 3001 (1967)

(–)-CHELIDONINE

$C_{20}H_{19}O_5N$

M.p. 136°C

This alkaloid occurs in *Glacium corniculatum* Curt. It is laevorotatory with $[\alpha]_D^{22} - 112°$ (EtOH) and has been identified by dehydrogenation and dehydration to Sanguinarine (q.v.).

Slavik, Slavikova., *Chem. Listy.*, **50**, 969 (1956)

CHELILUTINE

An uncharacterized alkaloid present in *Chelidonium majus* L. and also in *Eschscholtzia californica* Cham. The base is stated to yield a series of orange salts.

Slavik, Slavikova., *Collect. Czech. Chem. Commun.*, **20**, 2127 (1954)

Slavik, Slavikova., *Chem. Listy.*, **48**, 1382, 1387 (1954)

CHELIRUBINE

A second uncharacterized alkaloid isolated from *Chelidonium majus* L. and *Eschscholtzia californica* Cham, this base forms purple salts and is normally obtained as the crystalline pseudocyanide.

Slavik, Slavikova., *Collect. Czech. Chem. Commun.*, **20**, 2127 (1954)

Slavik, Slavikova., *Chem. Listy.*, **48**, 1382, 1387 (1954)

CHERYLLINE (*Crinine*)

$C_{17}H_{19}O_3N$

M.p. 217–8°C

The bulbs of *Crinum powellii* contain this alkaloid which forms colourless crystals from Me_2CO. The base is laevorotatory with $[\alpha]_D^{26} - 69°$ (c 0.2, MeOH). The ultraviolet spectrum exhibits absorption maxima at 225, 280 and 285 mμ with a shoulder at 294 mμ. The hydrochloride is crystalline with m.p. 238–9°C.

Boit., *Chem. Ber.*, **87**, 1704 (1954)
Brossi *et al.*, *J. Org. Chem.*, **35**, 1100 (1970)

Synthesis:
Brossi, Teitel., *J. Org. Chem.*, **35**, 3559 (1970)
Brossi, Teitel., *Tetrahedron Lett.*, 417 (1970)

(−)-CHIMONANTHINE

$C_{22}H_{26}N_4$

M.p. 188–9°C

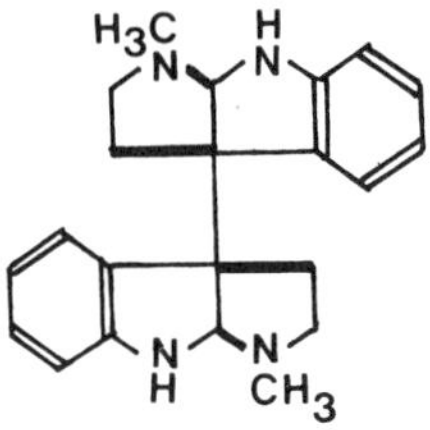

This dimeric alkaloid is found in the leaves of *Chimonanthus fragrans* Lindle (Syn. *Meratia praecox* Rehd. and Wils.). It has $[\alpha]_D - 329°$ and forms a crystalline dihydrobromide, m.p. 188–9°C; a dimethiodide, m.p. 235–6°C and a mono-N-methyl derivative which is identical with Calycanthidine (q.v.). The optically inactive form of the base has been prepared and has m.p. 185–6°C.

Hodson, Robinson., *Proc. Chem. Soc.*, 465 (1961)
Grant *et al.*, *ibid*, 383 (1962)
Hendrickson *et al.*, *ibid*, 383 (1962)
Grant *et al.*, *J. Chem. Soc.*, 5678 (1965)

Meso-CHIMONANTHINE

$C_{22}H_{26}N_4$

M.p. 199–202°C

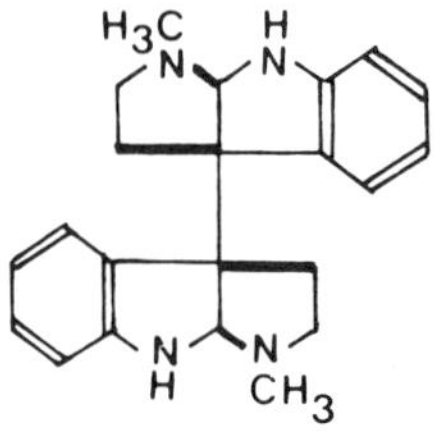

This alkaloid, which forms colourless prisms from C_6H_6, has been isolated from *Calycanthus floridus*. The structure has been confirmed by independent syntheses.

Hendrickson *et al.*, *Tetrahedron*, **20**, 565 (1964)
Scott, McCapra, Hall., *J. Amer. Chem. Soc.*, **86**, 302 (1964)
Hall, McCapra, Scott., *Tetrahedron*, **23**, 4131 (1967)

CHLIDANTHINE

$C_{17}H_{21}O_3N$

M.p. 238–9°C

From *Chlidanthus fragrans* and *Hippeastrum caubium* var. *robustum,* this alkaloid is obtained as colourless plates when crystallized from MeOH. It has $[\alpha]_D - 140°$ (EtOH). The base has been characterized as the methiodide which has m.p. 263–4°C (*dec.*) and the methoperchlorate, m.p. 255–6°C (*dec.*). The location of the double bond and the methoxyl group have been determined by Döpke and Dalmer.

Boit., *Chem. Ber.,* **89**, 1129 (1956)
Ehmke., *ibid,* **90**, 57 (1957)
Böit, Dopke., *Naturwiss.,* **47**, 109 (1960)
Döpke, Dalmer., *ibid,* **52**, 60 (1965)

CHLOROXYLONINE

$C_{22}H_{23}O_7N$

M.p. 182–3°C

The timber of *Chloroxylon swietania* D.C. contains this alkaloid which has $[\alpha]_D^{18} - 9.3°$. It forms crystalline salts: hydrochloride, m.p. 95°C; hydrobromide, m.p. 125°C and the aurichloride, m.p. 70°C. The alkaloid contains four methoxyl groups but no hydroxyl. It is stated to be a local irritant causing dermatitis when applied to the skin. Mukherjee and Bose have identified this alkaloid with Skimmianine (q.v.), isolated from the bark of this tree.

Auld., *J. Chem. Soc.,* **95**, 964 (1909)
Cash., *Brit. Med. J.,* ii, 784 (1911)
Mukherjee, Bose., *J. Ind. Chem. Soc.,* **23**, 1 (1946)

CHONDROCURARINE CHLORIDE

$C_{38}H_{44}O_6N_2Cl_2$

M.p. Indefinite

This salt of the quaternary base is an amorphous power which occurs naturally in *Chondrodendron tomentosum* along with (+)-tubocurarine chloride (q.v.). The base has $[\alpha]_D^{23} + 188°$ (H_2O) or $+ 195°$ (MeOH). The corresponding iodide forms prisms from MeOH-$CHCl_3$ containing 1 mole of $CHCl_3$. The unsolvated compound has m.p. 277–280°C (*dec.*) and $[\alpha]_D^{23} + 150°$ (H$_2$O) or $+ 128°$ (MeOH). The positions of the adjacent methoxyl and hydroxyl groups have recently been reversed in the revised structure.

Dutcher., *J. Amer. Chem. Soc.*, **74**, 2221 (1952)

Structure revision:
Everett, Lowe, Wilkinson., *Chem. Commun.*, 1020 (1970)

(+)-CHONDROCURINE (*Tubocurine*)

C$_{36}$H$_{38}$O$_6$N$_2$

M.p. 232–4°C

A further alkaloid present in *Chondrodendron tomentosum*, this base has $[\alpha]_D^{24} + 105°$ (pyridine) or $+ 200°$ (0.1 N/HCl). It gives a hydrochloride, m.p. 280–2°C, a sulphate (tetrahydrate), m.p. 263–5°C (*dec.*); $[\alpha]_D^{24} + 193°$ (H$_2$O) and a methochloride, m.p. 259–261°C (*dec.*); $[\alpha]_D^{12} + 198°$ (MeOH). Complete methylation by CH$_3$I in the presence of KOH gives *d*-O-dimethylchondrocurine dimethiodide, m.p. 266°C; $[\alpha]_D^{24} + 160°$ (H$_2$O) which is identical with *d*-O-dimethyltubocurarine iodide. Like the preceding alkaloid, the structure has recently been revised with the positions of the adjacent methoxyl and hydroxyl groups being reversed.

Dutcher., *J. Amer. Chem. Soc.*, **74**, 2221 (1952)
Kondo, Satomi, Odera., *Ann. Rept. ITSUU Lab.*, **4**, 45 (1953)
Bick, Clezy., *J. Chem. Soc.*, 3893 (1953)

Structure revision:
Everett, Lowe, Wilkinson., *Chem. Commun.*, 1020 (1970)

CHONDRODINE

C$_{18}$H$_{21}$O$_4$N

M.p. 218–220°C

This amorphous alkaloid has been reported as present in *Nectandra* Rodioei, Hook being present in the bark with bebeerine. It has $[\alpha]_D - 75°$ (EtOH). The hydrochloride has m.p. 274–5°C; the picrate is a yellow crystalline powder, m.p. 193–4°C and the picrolonate, greenish-yellow crystals, has m.p. 185–6°C. The alkaloid also yields a crystalline benzoyl derivative, m.p. 295°C and the diethyl ether hydrochloride, m.p. 258°C forms yellow needles. In spite of the above evidence, it still appears likely that much of this data requires some revision.

Scholtz., *Ber.*, **29**, 2054 (1896)
Scholtz, Koch., *Arch. Pharm.*, **252**, 513 (1914)
Faltis., *Monatsh.*, **33**, 873 (1912)
Faltis, Neumann., *ibid*, **42**, 311 (1921)
Faltis, Kadiera, Doblhammer., *Ber.*, **69**, 1271 (1936)

CHONDROFOLINE

$C_{37}H_{40}O_6N_2$

M.p. about 135°C

A bisbenzylisoquinoline alkaloid obtained from *Chondrodendron platyphyllum*, this base crystallizes from MeOH as triangular plates with 2 H_2O. It has $[\alpha]_{5461}^{20}$ − 280.6° (0.1 N/HCl) and is a phenolic base, giving no Millon reaction but forming a faint pink-purple colour with $FeCl_3$. The alkaloid forms a crystalline dinitrate, m.p. 225°C (*dec.*). When boiled with 20 per cent NaOH it produces a mixture of methine bases which can be separated as the methiodides into O-methylbebeerine methine methiodide, m.p. 237°C and the *l*-enantiomorph of d-O-methylbebeering methine methiodide, m.p. 190°C. The structure has recently been revised to (*S,S*)-7-O-methylcurine on the basis of NMR and mass spectroscopy.

King., *J. Chem. Soc.*, 737 (1940)

Baldas, Bick, Porter, Vernengo., *Chem. Commun.*, 132 (1971)

CHONEMORPHINE

$C_{23}H_{42}N_2$

M.p. 144−6°C

This steroidal alkaloid is the main constituent of the root bark of *Chonemorpha macrophylla* and *C. penangensis*. It forms crystalline salts, e.g. the dihydrochloride as colourless needles of the dihydrate, m.p. 418−420°C; the dihydriodide, also the dihydrate, m.p. 312−4°C; the platinichloride, m.p. 365°C (with charring); the aurichloride as yellow needles, m.p. 216°C; the N-acetyl derivative, m.p. 270°C and the benzylidene compound, m.p. 184°C.

With $NaNO_2$ in HOAc, the base is deaminated to form deaminooxychonemorphine, $C_{23}H_{39}ON_3$, m.p. 190°C.

Das, Pillay., *J. Sci. Ind. Res.*, **13B**, 602, 701 (1954)

Chatterjee, Das., *Chem. & Ind.*, 1445 (1959)

Chatterjee, Das., *ibid*, 290, 1247 (1960)

CHRYCENTRINE

$C_{18}H_{15}O_5N$

M.p. 216°C

Various *Corydalis* species yield this alkaloid, particularly *Dicentra chrysantha* Walp. It is stated to contain a methylenedioxy group but no methoxyl groups.

Manske., *Can. J. Res.*, **15B**, 274 (1937)

CHRYSANTHEMINE

This base, isolated from *Chrysanthemum cinerariaefolium* Bocc. has now been shown to be a mixture of choline and stachydrine.

Marino-Zuco., *Chem. Soc. Abstr.*, **60**, 333 (1891)
Marino-Zuco., *ibid*, **62**, 84 (1892)
Yoshimura, Trier., *Zeit. Physiol. Chem.*, **77**, 290 (1912)

CHUAN-WU BASE A

$C_{23}H_{37}O_6N$

M.p. 111°C

One of two minor alkaloids isolated from *Aconitum carmichaeli*, this base is optically inactive in $CHCl_3$. At present, insufficient material has been obtained for any salts or derivatives to be prepared.

Chen, Chu, Chu., *Yao Hseuh Hseuh Pao.*, **12**, 435 (1965)

CHUAN-WU BASE B

$C_{32}H_{35}O_4N$

M.p. 185°C

The second minor constituent of *Aconitum carmichaeli*, this alkaloid is also optically inactive in $CHCl_3$. Only small quantities of the base have so far been isolated.

Chen, Chu, Chu., *Yao Hseuh Hseuh Pao.*, **12**, 435 (1965)

CHYSINE A

$C_9H_{15}O_2N$

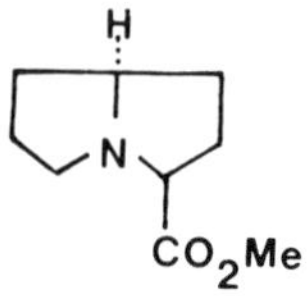

This pyrrolizidine alkaloid is found in *Chysis bractescens* and has $[\alpha]_D$ + 63.6°. The structure has been determined from chemical and spectroscopic studies.

Lüning, Tränkner., *Tetrahedron Lett.*, **14**, 921 (1965)

CHYSINE B

$C_{10}H_{17}O_2N$

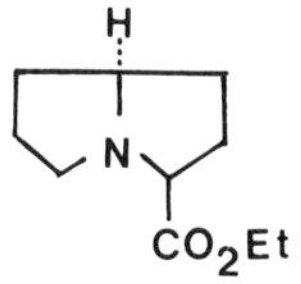

A second base isolated from *Chysis bractescens,* this alkaloid is closely related to the preceding base.

Lüning, Tränkner., *Tetrahedron Lett.*, **14**, 921 (1965)

CILIAPHYLLINE

$C_{23}H_{30}O_5N_2$

M.p. 222–3°C

An alkaloid of *Mitragyna ciliata,* the base is purified via the picrate, m.p. 130–1°C. It is laevorotatory with $[\alpha]_D^{25.5}$ − 89.5° (c 0.65, $CHCl_3$). The alkaloid is an orally effective analgetic and antitussive agent.

Beckett., *British Patent,* 1,056,537, 25 January 1967

CIMICIDINE

$C_{23}H_{28}O_5N_2$

M.p. 268–270°C (*dec.*).

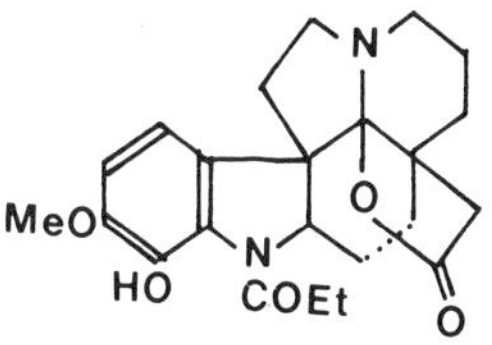

The Mexican shrub *Haplophyton cimicidum* A.D.C. contains this alkaloid which crystallizes as colourless prisms from a mixture of Me_2CO and EtOH. It has $[\alpha]_D^{25}$ + 23° (c 1–3, $CHCl_3$). The ultraviolet spectrum shows absorption maxima at 227.5 and 260 mμ. The salts crystallize well, e.g. the hydrochloride, m.p. 247–9°C (*dec.*); platinichloride, m.p. 208–215°C (*dec.*) and the picrate, m.p. 136–8°C. The alkaloid is a potent insecticide.

Rogers, Snyder, Fischer., *J. Amer. Chem. Soc.,* **74**, 1987 (1952)
Snyder *et al., ibid,* **76**, 2819, 4601 (1954)
Cava *et al., Chem. & Ind.,* 1875 (1963)

CIMICINE

$C_{22}H_{26}O_4N_2$

M.p. 229–231°C

Also present in *Haplophyton cimicidum* A.D.C., this alkaloid is dextrorotatory with $[\alpha]_D + 113°$ (CHCl$_3$).

Cava *et al., Chem. & Ind.*, 1875 (1963)

CINCHONAMINE

$C_{19}H_{24}ON_2$

M.p. 186°C

First isolated by Arnaud, this alkaloid occurs in the bark of *Remija Purdieana* and crystallizes in triboluminescent, orthorhombic needles. The base has $[\alpha]_D + 121.1°$ (EtOH) and forms a series of crystalline double chlorides with cadmium, copper and zinc. It does not give the thalleioquin reaction nor are solutions of the sulphate fluorescent. It is a diacidic base and forms two series of salts. The nitrate forms minute prisms, m.p. 227°C (*dec.*) and the methiodide has m.p. 208°C. With strong HNO$_3$, the alkaloid furnishes dinitrocinchonamine. The monoacetyl derivative is amorphous.

Arnaud., *Compt. rend.*, **93**, 593 (1881)
Arnaud., *ibid*, **97**, 174 (1883)
Tschugaeff., *Ber.*, **34**, 1824 (1901)
Goutarel *et al., Helv. Chim. Acta*, **33**, 150 (1950)
Culvenor *et al. J. Chem. Soc.*, 1485 (1950)

CINCHONIDINE

$C_{19}H_{22}ON_2$

M.p. 210.5°C

This alkaloid occurs in several *Cinchona* species and forms the major constituent of *C. succirubra*, Pav. The base crystallizes in large trimetric prisms and has $[\alpha]_D^{15} - 107.48°$ (EtOH) or $- 178°$ (0.1 N/H$_2$SO$_4$). It is only sparingly soluble in H$_2$O, more so in EtOH and Et$_2$O. As a diacidic base it yields two series of salts: the hydrochloride forms a dihydrate, m.p. 242°C (*dec.*); $[\alpha]_D^{20} - 117.6°$ (H$_2$O); the acid hydrochloride forms large monoclinic crystals of the hydrate; the

neutral sulphate forms prisms of the hexahydrate from H_2O and has m.p. 205°C
(*dry, dec.*). The dihydrobromide has $[\alpha]_D^{15} - 114.3°$ (H_2O) and the tartrate
forms a crystalline precipitate, insoluble in sodium potassium tartrate solution
and is the form in which the alkaloid is normally estimated. In addition to the
above, the acetyl derivative has m.p. 47–9°C; the benzoyl derivative, m.p.
183°C; the benzenesulphonyl compound, m.p. 166°C and the picrate, m.p.
208–9°C.

Hesse., *Annalen*, **205**, 196 (1880)
Heidelberger, Jacobs., *J. Amer. Chem. Soc.*, **41**, 819 (1919)
Rabe., *Ber.*, **55**, 522 (1922)

CINCHONINE

$C_{19}H_{22}ON_2$

M.p. 255°C (264°C)

Normally present in cinchona and cuprea barks, this alkaloid is best obtained
from *Cinchona micrantha*. It occurs in the crude mother liquors from the
preparation of quinine sulphate. The base crystallizes from EtOH in rhombic
prisms which sublime at 220°C. It has $[\alpha]_D + 229°$ (EtOH) or $+ 234.5°$
(EtOH-CHCl$_3$). It is sparingly soluble in H_2O, more so in EtOH, Et_2O and amyl
alcohol. Like most of the cinchona alkaloids it is a diacidic base forming normal
and acid salts: the normal sulphate forms rhombic crystals of the dihydrate,
m.p. 200°C (*dry, dec.*); the acid sulphate occurs as octahedral crystals of the
tetrahydrate; the normal hydrochloride has m.p. 166°C; $[\alpha]_D^{20} + 45.5°$ (CHCl$_3$)
and the hydrobromide has $[\alpha]_D^{15} + 143.6°$ (H_2O). Other derivatives that have
been prepared in a crystalline forms are the picrate, m.p. 193–4°C; styphnate,
m.p. 106°C; O-benzoyl compound, m.p. 105–6°C; $[\alpha]_D^{15} + 114.1°$ (EtOH);
O-benzenesulphonyl derivative, m.p. 89–93°C; $[\alpha]_D^{20} + 62.2°$ (CHCl$_3$) and the
O-*p*-toluenesulphonyl derivative, m.p. 173°C; $[\alpha]_D^{20} + 51°$ (CHCl$_3$).

Pharmacologically, cinchonine shows the usual activity against *Plasmodium
lophurae* being equal in potency to quinine. It is, however, more potent against
Plasmodium gallinaceum in chicks.

Martinotti., *Industria chimica*, **6**, 395 (1931)
Rabe, Buchholz., *Ber.*, **41**, 62 (1908)
Rabe., *ibid*, **55**, 522 (1922)

Pharmacological activity:
Dusenbery, Malanga., *J. Pharm. exp. Ther.*, **78**, 159 (1943)
Marshall., *ibid*, **85**, 299 (1945)

CINCHOPHYLLAMINE

$C_{31}H_{37}ON_4$

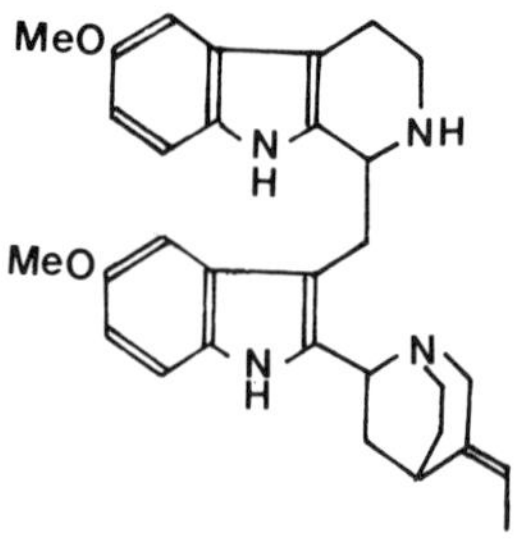

A dimeric alkaloid present in *Cinchona ledgeriana* leaves, this base occurs with Isocinchophyllamine (q.v.). The alkaloid shows a typical 5-methoxyindole ultraviolet spectrum and on treatment with Pd-C at 200°C under nitrogen is degraded to 7-methoxyharman. Catalytic hydrogenation gives the dihydro derivative, m.p. 238°C; $[\alpha]_D + 17°$ (CHCl$_3$) yielding the N-acetyl compound, m.p. 197°C; $[\alpha]_D + 145°$ (CHCl$_3$). With cold Ac$_2$O, the alkaloid furnishes the N-acetyl derivative, m.p. 204°C; $[\alpha]_D + 147°$ (CHCl$_3$) whereas hot Ac$_2$O gives a mixture of complex products. The dihydrochloride crystallizes as the mono-hydrate, m.p. 274°C; $[\alpha]_D + 98°$ (CHCl$_3$). The structure of the alkaloid has been deduced from chemical and spectroscopic data.

Potier *et al.*, *Bull. Soc. Chim. Fr.*, **7**, 2309 (1966)

CINEGALLEINE (*3'-O-Methylcinegalline*)

$C_{24}H_{32}O_6N_2$

M.p. 182°C

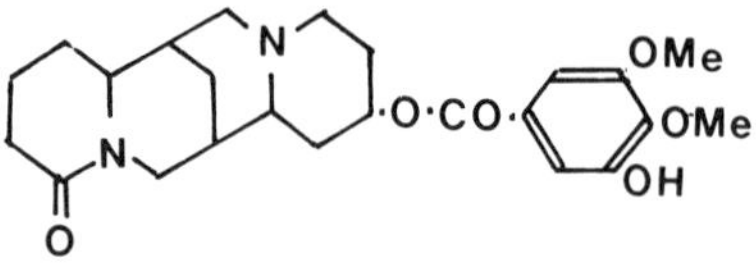

A lupanine alkaloid occurring in *Genista cinerea* D.C., the base forms colourless needles when recrystallized from MeOH. It has $[\alpha]_D^{20} + 48°$ (c 0.25, MeOH).

Faugeras, Paris., *Compt. Rend.*, **270D**, 203 (1970)

CINEGALLINE

$C_{23}H_{30}O_6N_2$

M.p. 223–6°C

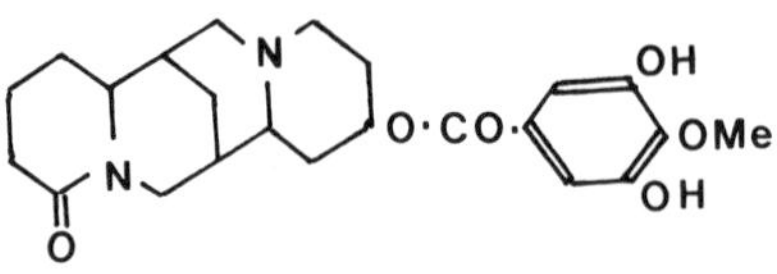

A further lupinine alkaloid found in *Genista cinerea* D.C. The base is dextro-rotatory with $[\alpha]_D + 46.7°$ (MeOH).

Faugeras, Paris., *Compt. Rend.*, **267D**, 538 (1968)
Faugeras, Paris., *Plant. Med. Phytother.*, **5**, 134 (1971)

CINEVANINE

$C_{23}H_{30}O_5N_2$

M.p. 207–8°C

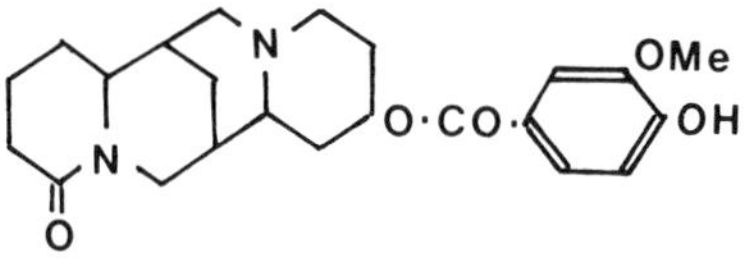

This alkaloid also occurs in *Genista cinerea* D.C. and has $[\alpha]_D + 69°$ (MeOH). Like the previous alkaloids, it possesses the lupinine skeleton and differs from them only in the nature of the acid substituent.

Faugeras, Paris., *Plant. Med. Phytother.*, **5**, 134 (1971)

CINEVERINE

$C_{24}H_{32}O_5N_2$

M.p. 155–7°C

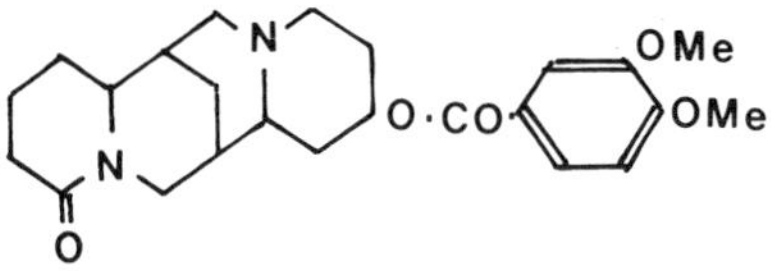

A fourth alkaloid which has been isolated from *Genista cinerea* D.C., this base has $[\alpha]_D + 71°$ (MeOH) and has been shown to be the O-methyl ether of Cinevanine.

Faugeras, Paris., *Compt. Rend.*, **263D**, 435 (1966)
Faugeras, Paris., *Plant. Med. Phytother.*, **5**, 134 (1971)

CINNAMOLAURINE

$C_{18}H_{19}O_3N$

M.p. 212–3°C (*dec.*).

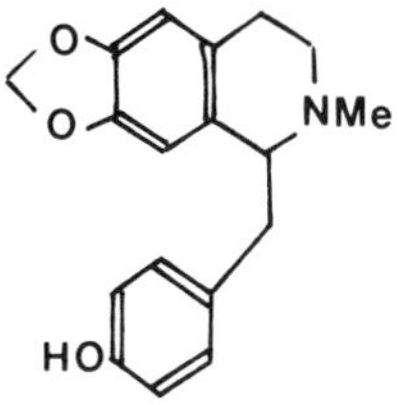

A benzyl*iso*quinoline alkaloid, this base occurs in various species of *Cinnamomum*. It is laevorotatory with $[\alpha]_D^{25} - 100°$ (EtOH) and the ultraviolet spectrum in EtOH has a single absorption maximum at 287 mμ. The alkaloid may be characterized as the hydrochloride, m.p. 230–3°C (*dec.*). The optically inactive form has been synthesized and has m.p. 212°C (*dec.*).

Gellert, Summons., *Tetrahedron Lett.*, 5055 (1969)

CINNAMOYLCOCAINE

$C_{19}H_{23}O_4N$

M.p. 121°C

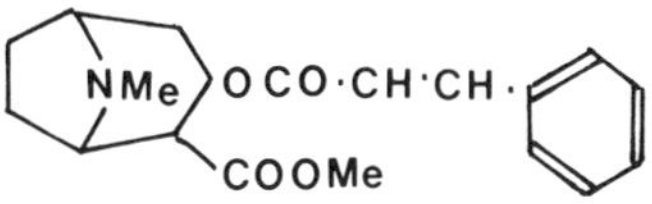

First prepared synthetically, this alkaloid was isolated by Giesel from the young leaves of *Erythroxylon truxillense* Rusby grown in Java where it is the major alkaloid. The base is almost insoluble in H_2O but is readily soluble in most organic solvents and crystallizes from C_6H_6 or light petroleum in rosettes of needles. It has $[\alpha]_D - 4.7°$ ($CHCl_3$). The hydrochloride forms flattened needles of the dihydrate, m.p. 176°C (*dec.*); the aurichloride, yellow needles, m.p. 156°C and the platinichloride, m.p. 217°C is amorphous when first precipitated but crystallizes on standing. When warmed with alkali, the base is hydrolyzed to MeOH, cinnamic acid and (−)-ecgonine. The isomeric (+)-alkaloid forms colourless prisms, m.p. 68°C; $[\alpha]_D + 2°$ (EtOH). It also forms crystalline salts including the hydrochloride as needles, m.p. 186°C; platinichloride, m.p. 208°C and the aurichloride, orange needles, m.p. 164°C.

Liebermann., *Ber.*, **21**, 3372 (1888)
Giesel., *Pharm. Zeit.*, **34**, 516 (1889)
Deckers, Einhorn., *Ber.*, **24**, 7 (1891)

CINNAMOYLHISTAMINE

$C_{14}H_{15}O_2N_3$

M.p. 179–180°C

This histamine derivative occurs in the leaves of *Acacia argentea* and in the bark of *A. polystacha* and *Glochida philippicum*. The crystalline picrate has m.p. 96–7°C when crystallized from H_2O and 165–6°C when obtained from EtOH. The structure has been confirmed by synthesis from histamine and cinnamoyl chloride which yields the optically inactive form of the base.

FitzGerald., *Austral. J. Chem.*, **17**, 375 (1964)
Johns, Lamberton., *ibid*, **20**, 555 (1967)

(+)-13-trans-CINNAMYLHYDROXYLUPANINE

$C_{24}H_{30}O_3N_2$

M.p. 165–6°C

This alkaloid is separated from the other lupine bases of *Lupinus angustifolius* by extraction of the acid solution with $CHCl_3$. It forms colourless crystals from hexane and has $[\alpha]_D^{20} + 41.4°$ ($CHCl_3$). The hydrochloride crystallizes from Me_2CO as colourless needles, m.p. 271–2°C; $[\alpha]_D^{20} + 24.1°$ (MeOH). Hydrolysis of the base furnishes *trans*-cinnamic acid and (+)-13-hydroxylupanine, the alkaloid being synthesized by esterification of these two products.

Wiewiorowski, Bratek., *Bull. Acad. Polon. Sci., Ser. Biol.*, **10**, 349 (1962)

CISSAMINE

This alkaloid, found in the roots of *Cissampelos pareira* has been shown to be identical with Cyclanoline (q.v.) by spectroscopic examination of the chlorides.

Anwer *et al., Experientia,* **24**, 999 (1968)

CISSAMPAREINE

$C_{37}H_{38}O_6N_2$

M.p. 239–240°C (*dec.*).

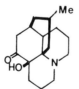

This cytotoxic bisbenzyl*iso*quinoline alkaloid is present in the bark of *Cissampelos pareira* and forms colourless columns from Me_2CO. The ultraviolet spectrum shows absorption maxima at 282 and 320 (shoulder) mμ and the base itself has $[\alpha]_D^{26} - 111°$ (c 1.05, $CHCl_3$). The alkaloid contains one hydroxyl group and forms an O-methyl ether as colourless crystals, m.p. 192–4°C; $[\alpha]_D^{26} - 121°$ (c 1.36, $CHCl_3$) and an O-ethyl ether, m.p. 152–3°C; $[\alpha]_D^{27} - 157°$ (c 1.02, $CHCl_3$). Hydrogenation over Pd-C affords the dihydro derivative, m.p. 208–212°C; $[\alpha]_D^{27} - 157°$ (c 0.7, $CHCl_3$).

Kupchan, Patel, Fujita., *J. Pharm. Sci.,* **54**, 580 (1965)

Structure:
Kupchan *et al., J. Amer. Chem. Soc.,* **88**, 4212 (1966)

CLAVATINE

$C_{16}H_{25}O_2N$

M.p. 212–3°C

This alkaloid has been isolated from the European species of *Lycopodium clavatum* L. Since neither it, nor clavatoxine (q.v.) have been found in American specimens of this plant, it has been suggested that these are either different varieties of the one species, or distinct species. This alkaloid crystallizes as colourless plates from petroleum ether. It forms a methiodide, m.p. 317–8°C.

Achmatowicz, Uzieblo., *Rocz. Chem.,* **18**, 88 (1938)
Marion, Manske., *Can. J. Res.,* **22B**, 137 (1944)

CLAVATOXINE

$C_{17}H_{27}O_2N$

M.p. 185–6°C

A second base from the European species of *Lycopodium clavatum* L., this alkaloid forms colourless needles from petroleum ether. Both methoxyl and methylimino groups are absent. Rodewald and Grynkiewicz have produced evidence to indicate that clavatoxine is, in reality, a 1:1 molar cimplex of clavatine and lycodoline.

Achmatowicz, Uzieblo., *Rocz. Chem.*, **18**, 88 (1938)
Rodewald, Grynkiewicz., *Bull. Acad. Pol. Sci., Ser. Chim.*, **15**, 579 (1967)

CLAVOLONINE

$C_{16}H_{25}O_2N$

M.p. 238°C

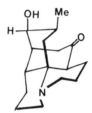

Also present in *Lycopodium clavatum* L., this alkaloid is characterized as the crystalline methiodide, m.p. 325–8°C (*dec.*).

Burnell, Mootoo., *Can. J. Chem.*, **39**, 1090 (1961)
Burnell, Taylor., *Tetrahedron*, **15**, 173 (1961)

CLIVATIN

$C_{21}H_{25}O_7N$

M.p. 166–9°C

This alkaloid occurs in *Clivia miniata* Regel and forms colourless crystals from Et_2O. It has $[\alpha]_D^{25} + 52°$ (c 0.2, $CHCl_3$). The structure has not yet been fully determined.

Boit, Mehlis., *Naturwiss.*, **48**, 603 (1961)

CLIVIASINE

$C_{17}H_{19}O_5N$

M.p. 195–7°C

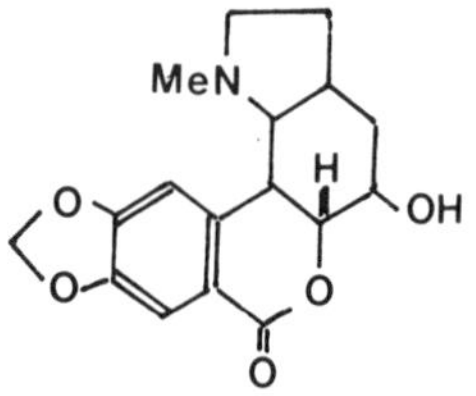

Isolated from *Clivia miniata* Regel., this alkaloid forms a crystalline perchlorate, m.p. 273–6°C. It has the structure of dihydrohippeastrine. With LiAlH$_4$ it is reduced to a tetrahydro derivative. For the 5α- and 5-β epimers, see clivonine and clividine.

Döpke, Bienert., *Pharmazie*, **25**, 700 (1970)

CLIVIDINE

C$_{17}$H$_{19}$O$_5$N

M.p. 195–7°C

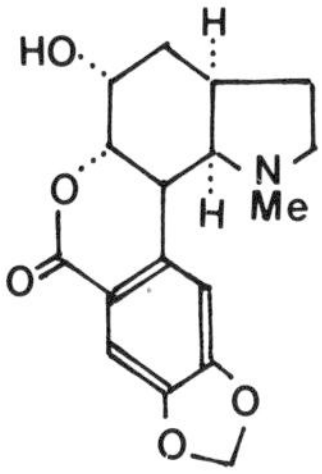

This epimer of cliviasine (q.v.) is also present in Clivia miniata Regel. It has [α]$_D^{22}$ − 75° (c 0.2, CHCl$_3$) and the ultraviolet spectrum in MeOH solution shows absorption maxima at 225, 267 and 308 mμ. The alkaloid has the structure of dihydro-5-epihippeastrine.

Döpke, Bienert., *Tetrahedron Lett.*, 3245 (1970)
Döpke, Bienart., *Pharmazie*, **25**, 700 (1970)

CLIVIMINE

C$_{43}$H$_{43}$O$_{12}$N$_3$

M.p. 264–6°C (*dec.*).

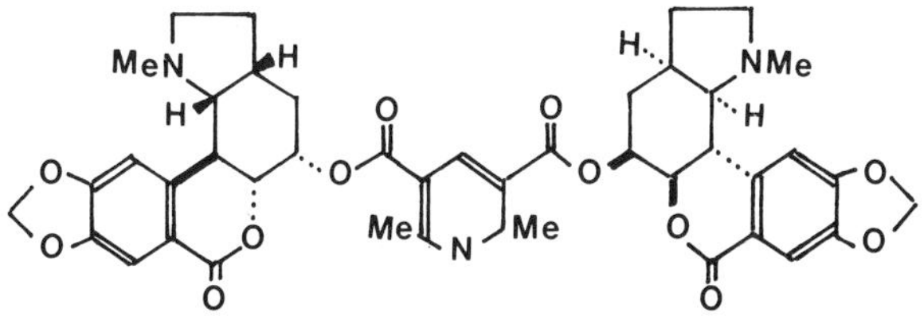

Also isolated from *Clivia miniata* Regel, this alkaloid forms colourless crystals from C$_6$H$_6$. It has [α]$_D^{28}$ + 32° (c 0.25, CHCl$_3$).

Boit, Mehlis., *Naturwiss.*, **48**, 603 (1961)
Döpke *et al.*, *Tetrahedron Lett.*, 451 (1967)

CLIVONINE

C$_{17}$H$_{19}$O$_5$N

M.p. 199–200°C

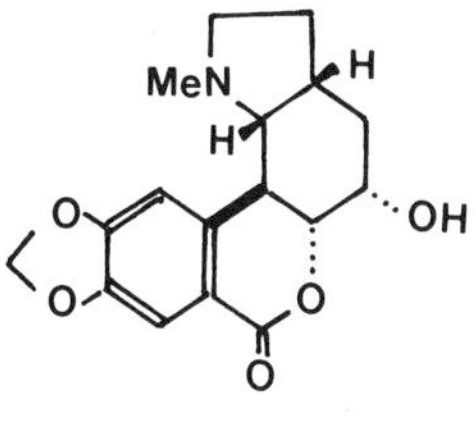

A further base to be isolated from *Clivia miniata* Regel. this alkaloid is present to the extent of 0.07 per cent in the rhizomes of this plant. It forms colourless crystals from EtOAc with $[\alpha]_{589}^{23} + 41.24°$ (CHCl$_3$), $[\alpha]_{436}^{23} + 103.44°$ (CHCl$_3$). The hydrochloride has m.p. 282–7°C; picrate, m.p. 250–4°C (*dec.*); metho-picrate, m.p. 285°C (*dec.*) and the O-acetyl derivative, m.p. 194–6°C. With LiAlH$_4$ the alkaloid yields a tetrahydro derivative as an oil which is not crystal-lizable. The structure is that of dihydro-5-epihippeastrine.

Briggs *et al., J. Amer. Chem. Soc.*, **78**, 2899 (1956)
Döpke *et al., Tetrahedron Lett.*, 451 (1967)
Döpke, Bienert., *Pharmazie*, **25**, 700 (1970)

CLIVORINE

$C_{21}H_{27}O_7N$

M.p. 148–150°C

A pyrrolizidine alkaloid found in *Ligularia clivorum* Maxim. The base forms colourless crystals from EtOAc. The structure has been determined from chemical and spectroscopic evidence.

Klasek, Vrublovsky, Santavy., *Collect. Czech. Chem. Commun.*, **32**, 2512 (1967)
Klasek, Sedmera, Santavy., *ibid*, **35**, 956 (1970)
Structure revision:
Birnbaum *et al., Tetrahedron Lett.*, 3421 (1971)

β-COCAINE

$C_{17}H_{21}O_4N$

M.p. 98°C

This is, by far, the most important of the alkaloids of *Erythroxylon* species. It occurs mainly in *Erythroxylon coca* Lam. and *E. truxillense* Rusby although small quantities are also found in the leaves of *E. areolatum, E. laurifolium, E. monogynum, E. montanum, E. ovatum, E. pulchrum* and *E. retusum*. In general, cocaine is found in the older leaves, the youngest leaves containing mainly cinnamoylcocaine.

The alkaloid crystallizes from EtOH in monoclinic four- or six-sided prisms and becomes volatile above 90°C, boiling at 187–8°C/0.1 mm. It is laevorotatory, having $[\alpha]_D^{20} - 15.83°$ (CHCl$_3$). It is only slightly soluble in H$_2$O (with an alkaline reaction to litmus) but readily soluble in most organic solvents. The hydrochloride crystallizes as short prisms, m.p. 197°C; $[\alpha]_D - 71.95°$ (H$_2$O); the platinichloride is microcrystalline and almost insoluble in H$_2$O; the chromate forms orange-yellow leaflets of the monohydrate, m.p. 127°C; the stypnate, m.p. 187°C; methiodide, m.p. 169°C; methochloride, m.p. 152.5°C and the mercurichloride, m.p. 123°C.

With mineral acids or Ba(OH)$_2$, the alkaloid is hydrolyzed to MeOH, benzoic acid and *l*-ecgonine. When boiled with H$_2$O, hydrolysis gives MeOH and benzoyl-l-ecgonine.

Commercially, the base is prepared either from the crude alkaloid obtained from South America or synthetically from ecgonine (obtained by hydrolysis of the total alkaloids from Java coca leaves) by methylation and benzoylation. The alkaloid is a potent anaesthetic, mydriatic and sedative.

The (±)-form has m.p. 79–80°C and forms a crystalline hydrochloride, m.p. 187°C.

Willstätter, Wolfes, Mäder., *Annalen*, **434**, 266 (1923)
Merck., B.P. 214,917
Chemnitius., *J. prakt. Chem.*, **116**, 285 (1927)
Elgazin., *Chem. Abstr.*, **26**, 3331 (1932)
Perrot., *Bull. sci. pharmacol.*, **42**, 266 (1935)
Kovacs, Fodor, Weisz., *Helv. Chim. Acta*, **37**, 892 (1954)

(+)-ψ-COCAINE (*d-Cocaine*)

$C_{17}H_{21}O_4N$

M.p. 46°C

This stereoisomer of β-cocaine has been isolated from the leaves of *Erythroxylon truxillense* Rusby but it appears likely that it is produced during the process of extraction by the action of alkali. The base differs considerably from β-cocaine. It has $[\alpha]_D^{20} + 42.2°$ (CHCl$_3$) and forms a hydrochloride, m.p. 208°C; $[\alpha]_D^{20} + 49.8°$ (H$_2$O); an aurichloride, m.p. 148°C and a methiodide, m.p. 172°C. The optically inactive form has m.p. 81.5°C and also yields crystalline salts, e.g. the hydrochloride, m.p. 205–6°C; aurichloride, m.p. 164–5°C and the methiodide, m.p. 213°C.

Liebermann, Giesel., *Ber.*, **23**, 508, 925 (1890)
Einhorn, Marquardt., *ibid*, **23**, 468, 981 (1890)
Willstätter, Bode., *Annalen,* **326**, 42 (1903)
Willstätter, Bommer., *ibid*, **422**, 34 (1921)
Willstätter, Wolfes, Mäder., *ibid*, **434**, 138 (1923)
Willstätter *et al.*, *Münch. med. Woch.*, **71**, 849 (1924)

COCCINELLIN

$C_{13}H_{23}ON$

Decomposes $235°C$

This alkaloid is obtained as colourless crystals from the whole-body homogenate of the European ladybird (*Coccinella septempunctata*). It has been shown to be the N-oxide of an amorphous substance named Precoccinellin, $C_{13}H_{23}N$.

Tursch *et al.*, *Experientia*, **27**, 1380 (1971)

COCCININE

$C_{17}H_{19}O_4N$

M.p. $162-3°C$

This anthracene type alkaloid is present in *Haemanthus trigrinus* and is obtained as colourless crystals from EtOH. It has $[\alpha]_D^{27} - 188.8°$ (c 1.89, EtOH). The base contains one hydroxyl group and forms a perchlorate, m.p. $254-5°C$ (*dec.*); picrate, m.p. $155-160°C$ (*dec.*) and a methiodide, m.p. $223-4°C$; $[\alpha]_D^{26} - 60.5°$ (c 1.41, H_2O). It also yields an O-methyl ether, m.p. $122-6°C$; $[\alpha]_{5890}^{25} - 131°$ (c 0.36, $CHCl_3$).

Wildman, Kaufman., *J. Amer. Chem. Soc.*, **77**, 1248 (1955)
Fales, Warnhoff, Wildman., *J. Org. Chem.*, **25**, 2153 (1960)

COCCULIDINE

$C_{18}H_{23}O_2N$

M.p. $86-7°C$

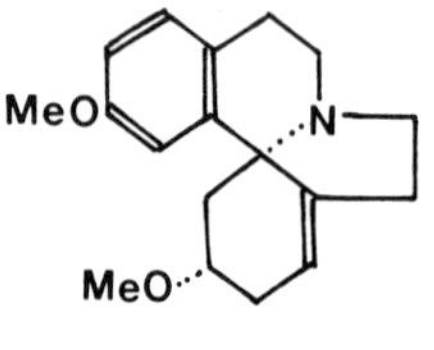

Obtained from *Cocculus laurifolius,* this alkaloid crystallizes as colourless crystals from petroleum ether and has $[\alpha]_D + 250.9°$ ($CHCl_3$). It forms crystalline salts, e.g. the nitrate, m.p. $131.5-132.5°C$; the hydriodide, m.p. $174-5°C$ and the methiodide, m.p. $238-9°C$. The structure has recently been revised to include a seven-membered ring as shown above.

Yunusov., *J. Gen. Chem., USSR*, **20**, 368 (1950)
Yunusov., *Trudy Akad. Nauk. Uzbek SSR*, **3**, 3 (1952)

Structure revision:
Vul'fson, Bochkarev., *Izv. Akad. Nauk SSSR, Ser. Khim.*, 500 (1972)

COCCULINE

$C_{17}H_{21}O_2N$

M.p. 217–8°C

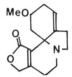

A further alkaloid of *Cocculus laurifolium*, the base forms colourless prisms from Me_2CO. It has $[\alpha]_D$ + 271.1° (MeOH) and yields a crystalline hydrochloride, m.p. 222–3°C and a nitrate, m.p. 196–7°C. With CH_2N_2 it furnishes Cocculidine (q.v.) while with methyl iodide it gives cocculidine methiodide.

Yunusov., *J. Gen. Chem., USSR,* **20**, 368 (1950)
Yunusov., *Trudy Akad. Nauk SSSR, Ser. Khim.,* **3**, 3 (1952)
Rozakov *et al., Izv. Akad. Nauk SSSR, Ser. Khim.,* **1**, 218 (1974)

Structure revision:
Vul'fson, Bochkarev., *Izv. Akad. Nauk SSSR, Ser. Khim.,* 500 (1972)

COCCULOLIDINE

$C_{15}H_{19}O_3N$

M.p. 144–6°C

The leaves of *Cocculus trilobus* yield this insecticidal alkaloid which is dextrorotatory with $[\alpha]_D^{25}$ + 273° (c 1.0, $CHCl_3$). The ultraviolet spectrum has one absorption maximum at 215 mμ. Chemical analysis and the infrared spectrum confirm the structure given above. The base yields a hydrochloride, m.p. 247–251°C (*dec.*) and a methiodide, m.p. 261–4°C. Reduction with $NaBH_4$ gives the dihydro derivative, m.p. 121–121.5°C which forms colourless crystals from CCl_4–Et_2O. Hydrogenation at room temperature over Pt in AcOH, on the other hand, gives the tetrahydro derivative, m.p. 187–9°C. Cocculolidine is demethylated by treatment with HBr in AcOH at 100°C to give the demethyl compound, m.p. 220–2°C (*dec.*) and hydrogenation of this derivative over PtO_2 yields dihydrodemethylcocculolidine, m.p. 171–3°C in which intramolecular hydrogen bonding occurs between the nitrogen atom and the hydroxyl group indicating that these are *cis* to each other and thereby establishing the stereochemistry of the alkaloid.

Wada, Marumo, Munakata., *Tetrahedron Lett.,* 5179 (1966)
Wada, Marumo, Munakata., *Agr. Biol. Chem.* (Tokyo), **31**, 452 (1967)
Wada, Marumo, Munakata., *ibid,* **32**, 1187 (1968)

COCHLEARINE

$C_{15}H_{19}O_3N$

M.p. 235–6°C

This alkaloid occurs in *Cochlearia arctica* and has been characterized as the hydrochloride, m.p. 307°C (*dec.*); perchlorate, m.p. 202–5°C (*dec.*) and picrate, m.p. 276°C. On hydrolysis it furnishes tropine and *m*-hydroxybenzoic acid.

Platonova, Kuzovkov., *Med. Prom. SSSR*, **17**, 19 (1963)

COCLANDINE

$C_{19}H_{23}O_4N$

MeO
HO
NMe
OMe
OH

A bisbenzyl*iso*quinoline alkaloid isolated from *Cocculus laurifolius*, the probable structure is that given above although this has still to be verified by synthesis. The base yields an oxalate, m.p. 120–1°C and a dimethyl ether, forming a methiodide, m.p. 200°C.

Kusuda., *Pharm. Bull.* (Japan), **1**, 189 (1953)

COCLANOLINE

This alkaloid is identical with Coclandine (q.v.)

(±)-COCLAURINE

$C_{17}H_{19}O_3N$

M.p. 220–1°C

MeO
HO
NH
OH

This alkaloid is found in *Cocculus laurifolius* and crystallizes in colourless plates. The hydrochloride forms crystals of the monohydrate, m.p. 258–9°C (*dec.*) although a higher melting point of 264°C (*dec.*) has been recorded. The fact that the alkaloid is soluble in alkali indicates the presence of a phenolic hydroxyl group and the formation of a non-basic O,O,N-triacetyl derivative, m.p. 174°C and a tribenzoyl compound, m.p. 207°C shows the presence of two such groups. The O,O,-dimethyl ether has m.p. 200–3°C while the N-methyl compound has m.p. 162–3°C, forming a methosulphate, m.p. 174.5°C. Coclaurine also forms a crystalline methiodide, m.p. 200–2°C and a methopicrate, m.p. 177–8°C. This alkaloid is of special interest since *nor*coclaurine may be regarded as the parent compound from which this series of bisbenzyl*iso*quinoline bases may be formed by ether formation.

Kondo, Kondo., *J. Pharm. Soc., Japan*, **45**, 876 (1925)
Kondo, Kondo., *ibid*, **46**, 104 (1926)
Kondo, Kondo., *J. prakt. Chem.*, **126**, 24 (1930)
Finkelstein., *J. Amer. Chem. Soc.*, **73**, 550 (1951)
Kratzl, Billek., *Monatsh.*, **82**, 568 (1951)
Kratzl, Billek., *ibid*, **83**, 1045 (1952)
Tomita, Kusuda., *J. Pharm. Soc., Japan*, **72**, 280, 793 (1952)
Tomita, Yamaguchi., *Pharm. Bull.* (Japan), **1**, 10 (1953)
Kidd *et al.*, *Chem. & Ind.*, 748 (1955)
Arndt., *J. Chem. Soc.*, 2547 (1963)

(+)-COCLAURINE

$C_{17}H_{19}O_3N$

M.p. 217–8°C

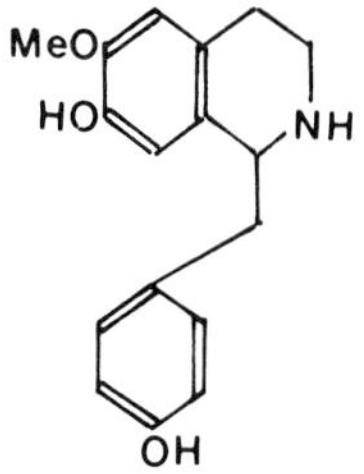

Isolated from *Xylopia papuana* Diels., this alkaloid forms colourless prisms when recrystallized from EtOH. It has $[\alpha]_D + 47°$ (EtOH). The O,O,N-triacetyl derivative melts at 199°C; $[\alpha]_D - 76°$ (EtOH) and the N-methyl compound has m.p. 182–3°C; $[\alpha]_D - 62°$ (c 0.13, CHCl$_3$), $- 115°$ (c 0.19, MeOH) and $- 80°$ (c 0.17, EtOH).

Kidd *et al.*, *Chem. & Ind.*, 748 (1955)
Arndt., *J. Chem. Soc.*, 2547 (1963)

COCLOBINE

$C_{37}H_{38}O_6N_2$

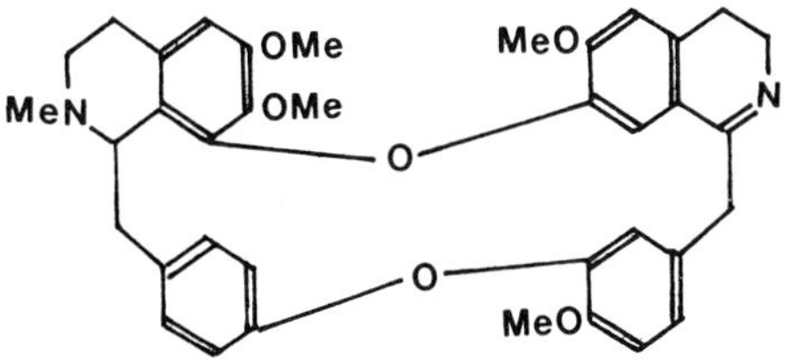

This biscoclaurine alkaloid has been isolated from *Cocculus trilobus* and the above structure determined by chemical degradation and spectroscopic investigation. Four methoxyl groups and one methylimino group are present in the molecule.

Ito, Furukawa, Sato, Takahashi., *J. Pharm. Soc., Japan*, **89**, 1163 (1969)

COCSARMINE

$C_{21}H_{26}O_4N^+$

The roots of *Cocculus sarmentosus* yield this quaternary alkaloid which has been characterized as the iodide trihydrate, m.p. 205–7°C after sintering at 185°C; $[\alpha]_D^{22} + 27.9°$ (EtOH). The base also yields a crystalline picrate, m.p. 226–7°C (*dec.*).

Tomita, Furukawa., *J. Pharm. Soc., Japan,* **83**, 190 (1963)

L(+)-CODAMINE

$C_{20}H_{25}O_4N$

M.p. 126–7°C

A minor constituent of the latex of *Papaver somniferum* L., this alkaloid crystallizes in hexagonal prisms from light petroleum and has $[\alpha]_D^{23.5} + 75.7°$ (c 0.5, EtOH). Most of the salts are amorphous but the hydriodide sesquihydrate is crystalline and sparingly soluble in H_2O and the acid tartrate may be obtained in the form of colourless needles. The methiodide may be crystallized from 2-propanol, m.p. 200.5–201°C as may be the picrate, m.p. 146–9°C. On oxidation with $KMnO_4$ the ethyl ether yields veratric acid showing that the hydroxyl group is present in the *iso*quinoline nucleus. The alkaloid dissolves in HNO_3 to give a deep green solution. The solution in H_2SO_4 is colourless but changes through green to red-violet on warming.

The D(−)-form of the alkaloid has m.p. 127–8°C; $[\alpha]_D^{17} - 68.8°$ (c 1.0, EtOH), forming a picrate, m.p. 147–9°C; $[\alpha]_D^{24} - 84.4°$ (c 1.0, $CHCl_3$). The optically inactive form yields colourless needles from light petroleum, m.p. 106–8°C, giving a picrate with m.p. 187–187.5°C.

Hesse., *Annalen.,* **153**, 47 (1870)
Späth, Epstein., *Ber.,* **59**, 2791 (1926)
Späth, Epstein., *ibid,* **61**, 334 (1928)
Brochmann-Hanssen, Nielsen, Utzinger., *J. Pharm. Sci.,* **54**, 1531 (1965)
Cassels, Deulofeu., *Tetrahedron,* 485 (1966)

308

CODAPHNIPHYLLINE

$C_{30}H_{47}O_3N$

This complex alkaloid occurs in the leaves and bark of *Daphniphyllum macro-podum* Miq., and has been characterized as the hydrochloride, m.p. 266–7°C (sealed tube); $[\alpha]_D + 4.2°$ (c 1.4, $CHCl_3$).

Irikawa *et al.*, *Tetrahedron Lett.*, 5363 (1966)
Irikawa *et al.*, *ibid*, 553 (1967)
Irikawa *et al.*, *Tetrahedron*, 24, 5691 (1968)

CODEINE

$C_{18}H_{21}O_3N$

M.p. 155°C

First isolated from opium by Robiquet, this alkaloid is obtained therefrom, along with morphine, as the hydrochloride. Commercially, the base is prepared by methylation of morphine. Codeine crystallizes from H_2O as large, ortho-rhombic prisms of the monohydrate although from Et_2O it separates as small, anhydrous prisms. It is slightly soluble in H_2O, more so in Et_2O and readily in EtOH or $CHCl_3$. The aqueous solution is strongly alkaline to litmus.

The hydrochloride dihydrate forms short, colourless needles; $[\alpha]_D^{22} - 108.2°$ (H_2O); the sulphate, obtained as the pentahydrate, m.p. 278°C (*dec.*); $[\alpha]_D^{15} - 101.2°$ (H_2O), readily loses 2 H_2O on exposure to air, is completely dehydrated at 100°C and then absorbs 3 H_2O on exposure to air. The phosphate forms three hydrates with 1, 1.5 and 2 H_2O and has m.p. 235°C (*dec.*) when anhydrous. The alkaloid also forms a crystalline picrate, m.p. 196–7°C; a styphnate, m.p. 115°C (195–7°C) and an acetate, m.p. 133.5°C. With sulphoacetic acid, the alkaloid is converted into 6-acetyl-1-acetodeine which occurs in two forms with m.p. 146–7°C and 125–126.5°C, both forms having $[\alpha]_D^{20} - 207°C$ ($CHCl_3$). When treated with $SOCl_2$, PCl_3 or PBr_3, codeine forms α-chlorocodide, m.p. 152–3°C; β-chlorocodide, m.p. 156–7°C and bromocodide, m.p. 162°C respectively. In this series of compounds, which are analogous to those formed by morphine with the same reagents, the alcoholic hydroxyl is replaced by halogen.

Pharmacologically, codeine resembles morphine but is less toxic and its depressant action is less marked and prolonged while its stimulating action involves not only the spinal cord but also the lower parts of the brain. In small doses it induces sleep but in large doses it causes restlessness and increased reflex excitability. The respiration is slowed less than in the case of morphine. Cases of addiction can occur but they are far less common than those due to morphine.

Robiquet., *Annalen,* **5**, 106 (1833)
Grimaux., *Compt. rend.,* **92**, 1140 (1881)
Freund, Melber, Schlesinger., *J. prakt. Chem.,* **101**, 1 (1921)
Speyer, Krauss., *Annalen,* **432**, 233 (1923)
Gulland, Robinson., *Chem. Abstr.,* **20**, 765 (1926)
Schöpf., *Annalen,* **452**, 211 (1927)
Rodionov., *Bull. Soc. Chim. Fr.,* **45**, 119 (1929)

Crystal structure:
Kartha, Ahmed, Barnes., *Acta Cryst.,* **15**, 326 (1962)

Mass spectra:
Wheeler, Kinstle, Rinehart., *J. Amer. Chem. Soc.,* **89**, 4494 (1967)

NMR spectrum:
Batterham, Bell, Weiss., *Austral. J. Chem.,* **18**, 1799 (1965)

Addiction:
Wolff., *Bull. Health Org. League of Nations,* VII, 546 (1938)

CODONOCARPINE

$C_{26}H_{31}O_5N_3$

M.p. 187°C (*dec.*).

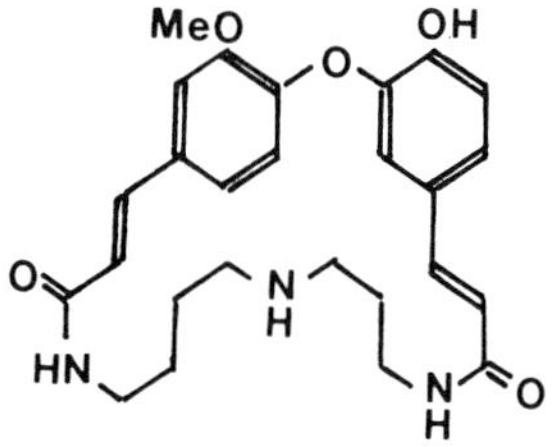

A macrocyclic alkaloid found in the bark of *Codoncarpus australis* A. Cunn, the base forms yellow needles when crystallized from MeOH. It contains one methoxyl, one hydroxyl and three imino groups in the molecule, the structure of which has been determined by chemical analysis and spectroscopic methods.

Doskotch, Ray, Beal., *Chem. Commun.,* 300 (1971)

CODONOPSINE

$C_{14}H_{21}O_4N$

M.p. 150–1°C

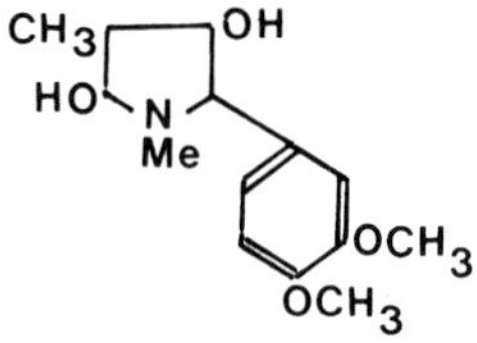

The aerial parts of *Codonopsis clematidea* contain this alkaloid which is laevo-rotatory with $[\alpha]_D^{20} - 16°$ (MeOH). An earlier structure has recently been revised, based upon NMR spectra and Hofmann degradation.

Matkhalikova, Malikov, Yunusov., *Khim. Prir. Soedin.,* **5**, 30 (1969)
Matkhalikova, Malikov, Yunusov., *ibid,* **5**, 606 (1969)

CODONOPSININE

$C_{13}H_{19}O_3N$

M.p. 169–170°C

A second alkaloid present in the aerial portions of *Codonopsis clematidea,* this base occurs in the mother liquors after the removal of the preceding base. It is also paevorotatory having $[\alpha]_D^{20} - 31°$ (MeOH). The structure differs from Codonopsine only in the lesser degree of substitution in the phenyl ring.

Matkhalikova, Malikov, Yunusov., *Khim. Prir. Soedin.,* **5,** 607 (1969)

COLCHAMINE (*Alkaloid F*)

$C_{21}H_{25}O_5N$

M.p. 181–2°C

This colchicine alkaloid occurs in the roots of *Colchicum speciosum* and forms colourless plates from AcOEt. It has $[\alpha]_D^{20} + 117.6°$ (CHCl$_3$) and gives yellow solutions with mineral acids, turning green on warming. The salts and derivatives are crystalline: hydrochloride, m.p. 216–7°C (*dec.*); perchlorate, m.p. 264°C (*dec.*) and the benzoate, m.p. 209–210°C. The N-methyl derivative crystallizes from AcOEt with m.p. 201–2°C; $[\alpha]_D - 127.8°$ (EtOH). The N-acetyl compound is identical with N-methylcolchicine.

Kiselev, Men'shikov, Beer., *Dokl. Akad. Nauk. SSSR,* **87,** 227 (1952)
Kiselev, Men'shikov., *ibid,* **88,** 825 (1953)

COLCHICERINE

$C_{22}H_{25}O_6N$

M.p. 187–187.5°C

An alkaloid of *Colchicum speciosum,* this base forms colourless crystals from Me$_2$CO. It has the following specific rotations; $[\alpha]_D - 390°$ (H$_2$O), $- 155°$ (CHCl$_3$), $- 180°$ (EtOH) and $- 166°$ (AcOH). The alkaloid is very soluble in CHCl$_3$ and yields an aurichloride, m.p. 170–171.5°C. It gives a red colour with FeCl$_3$. The toxicity is very similar to that of Colchicine (q.v.).

Beer., *Dokl. Akad. Nauk. SSSR,* **69,** 369 (1949)

311

COLCHICINE

$C_{22}H_{25}O_6N$

M.p. 155–7°C

This important alkaloid was first isolated from the seeds and corms of *Colchicum autumnale* L. and has subsequently been obtained from other *Colchicum* species and numerous members of the Liliaceae. According to Niemann, the flowers of *C. autumnale* L. also contain 0.8 per cent of this alkaloid.

Colchicine forms yellow flakes or crystals containing $CHCl_3$ or C_6H_6 of crystallization. From H_2O, it forms the trihydrate. It has $[\alpha]_D^{16.5}$ – 120.8° ($CHCl_3$) or – 429° (H_2O). In concentrated H_2SO_4, the colour is yellow, turning blue-green and then red on addition of a drop of HNO_3. The aurichloride is crystalline, m.p. 209°C and the base also forms a series of amide derivatives including the methylamide, m.p. 173–4°C; dimethylamide, m.p. 204–6°C; ethylamide, m.p. 160–2°C and allylamide, m.p. 152°C. On heating with dilute HCl or H_2SO_4, the alkaloid forms colchiceine, $C_{21}H_{23}O_6N$, m.p. 172°C; $[\alpha]_D$ – 253° ($CHCl_3$). With CH_2N_2, this base yields colchicine and *iso*colchicine, m.p. 225°C; $[\alpha]_D$ – 307° ($CHCl_3$).

The constitution of colchicine has been drastically revised since the original phenanthrene structure was put forward and it has now been shown that both rings B and C are seven-membered.

Colchicine has no direct action upon the heart but is, among other things, a capillary poison. Large doses cause an ascending paralysis of the central nervous system accompanied by vasomotor and respiratory paralysis. The fact that the base induces regression of tumours in mice and effectively treats spontaneous tumours in dogs has led to investigation of its effect on cell-division in normal and malignant cells. Unfortunately the inhibition of cell division is not specific for tumour cells and the dosage necessary to arrest the growth of a transplanted tumour approaches the lethal dose for the host. All colchicine derivatives which has so far been examined have proved to be less potent than the parent alkaloid.

Pelletier, Caventou., *Ann. Chim. Phys.,* **14**, 82 (1820)
Albo., *Arch. Sci. phys. nat.,* **12**, 227 (1901)
Perrot., *Compt. rend.,* **202**, 1088 (1936)
Cohen, Cook, Roe., *J. Chem. Soc.,* 194 (1940)
Santavy., *Compt. rend. soc. biol.,* **140**, 932 (1946)
Tarbell, Frank, Fanta., *J. Amer. Chem. Soc.,* **68**, 502 (1946)
Dewar., *Nature,* **155**, 141 (1945)
Cook, Loudon., *Quart. Rev.,* **5**, 104 (1951)
Eigsti, Pierre., *Colchicine.* Ames: Iowa State College Press, 1955
van Tamelen *et al., Tetrahedron,* **14**, 8 (1961)
Schreiber *et al., Helv. Chim. Acta,* **44**, 540 (1961)
Pharmacology:
Dixon, Malden., *J. Physiol.,* **37**, 50 (1908)
Fühner., *Arch. exp. Path. Pharm.,* **63**, 357 (1910)
Lipps, Beck, Jacobson., *ibid,* **85**, 235 (1920)
Amoroso., *Nature,* **135**, 266 (1935)
Brues, Cohen., *Biochem. J.,* **30**, 1363 (1936)
Lettre, Fernholz., *Zeit. Physiol. Chem.,* **278**, 175 (1943)

COLLETINE

$C_{20}H_{26}O_3N$

M.p. 130–2°C (chloride)

A quaternary alkaloid which occurs in *Colletia spinosissima* Gmel. this base is usually isolated as the chloride, crystallizing from AcOEt-EtOH. This salt has $[\alpha]_D^{20} - 132.8°$ (c 1.07, EtOH). The ultraviolet spectrum has absorption maxima at 227 and 284 mμ in EtOH and at 253 and 303 mμ in NaOH-EtOH. The corresponding iodide forms crystals from MeOH-isopropanol, m.p. 169–173°C.

Sanchez, Comin., *Tetrahedron*, 23, 1139 (1963)
Albonico *et al.*, *J. Chem. Soc., C*, 1340 (1966)

α-COLUBRIN

$C_{22}H_{24}O_3N_2$

M.p. 184°C

One of the strychnine alkaloids, this base occurs in *Strychnos Nux-vomica* L. and crystallizes from aqueous EtOH as crystals of the tetrahydrate. It has $[\alpha]_D^{19} - 76.5°$ (EtOH). The hydrochloride forms long colourless leaflets of the trihydrate from H_2O; $[\alpha]_D^{18} - 3.1°$ (EtOH) and the sulphate forms glancing leaflets of the decahydrate. On oxidation with alkaline $KMnO_4$, the alkaloid yields N-oxalyl-4-methoxyanthranilic acid (dimethyl ester, m.p. 163°C). The structure has confirmed by the synthesis of the base from strychnine.

Warnat., *Helv. Chim. Acta*, 14, 997 (1931)
Synthesis:
Rosenmund, Franke., *Chem. Ber.*, 97, 1677 (1964)

β-COLUBRINE

$C_{22}H_{24}O_3N_2$

M.p. 222°C

This isomeric alkaloid also forms colourless leaflets from aqueous EtOH and has $[\alpha]_D^{19} - 107.7°$ (EtOH). It yields a crystalline hydrochloride, $[\alpha]_D^{18} - 32.7°$ (H_2O); a sulphate crystallizing in long, narrow prisms of the nonahydrate and a methiodide, m.p. 318°C (*dec.*). The alkaloid is soluble in C_6H_6, EtOH or $CHCl_3$.

Warnat., *Helv. Chim. Acta*, 14, 997 (1931)
Rosenmund., *Chem. Ber.*, 95, 2639 (1962)

COLUMBAMINE

$C_{20}H_{21}O_5N$

A quaternary alkaloid which has been isolated from the root bark of various species including *Archangelisia flava* L. (Merr.); *Berberis heteropoda* Schrenk., *B. lambertii, B. japonica* Mak., *B. Thunbergii* DC var *Maximowiczii, B. vulgaris* L., *Coptis japonica* and *Jatrorrhiza palmata* Lam. (Meirs.). The iodide has m.p. 223–4°C and is the form in which the alkaloid is normally isolated. When reduced wtih Zn in $AcOH-H_2SO_4$, the base yields the tetrahydro derivative, m.p. 223°C which furnishes tetrahydropalmatine with CH_2N_2.

Späth, Bohm., *Ber.,* **55**, 2985 (1922)
Späth, Duschinsky., *ibid,* **58**, 1939 (1925)
Späth, Burger., *ibid,* **59**, 1486 (1926)
Murayama, Shinozaki., *J. Pharm. Soc. Japan,* **32**, 530 (1926)
Späth, Polgar., *Monatsh.,* **52**, 118, 120, 127 (1929)
Kondo, Tomita., *Arch. Pharm.,* **268**, 549 (1930)
Orekhov., *ibid,* **271**, 323 (1933)
Santos., *Univ. Philipp. Nat. Appl. Sci. Bull.,* **1**, 153 (1931)
Chatterjee, Banerjee., *J. Ind. Chem. Soc.,* **30**, 705 (1953)
Cava, Reed, Beal., *Lloydia,* **28**, 73 (1965)

COMBRETINE

From the leaves of the West African tree *Combretum micranthum,* this non-volatile alkaloid has been obtained by Lahmann. So far, the base has not been chemically characterized.

Lahmann., *Heil u. Gewurz-Pflanzen,* **22**, 1 (1943)

COMPACTINERVINE

$C_{20}H_{24}O_4N_2$

M.p. 111–120°C

(*dec.* 235–245°C)

The bark of *Aspidosperma compactinervium* Kuhlmann yields this alkaloid which crystallizes from aqueous EtOH with ethanol of solvation. The base has $[\alpha]_D^{25} - 515°$ (c 0.55, EtOH) or $- 680°$ (c 0.15, pyridine). The ultraviolet spectrum exhibits absorption maxima at 237, 297 and 331 mμ. The salts are

314

crystalline, e.g. the hydrochloride, m.p. 191–2°C (*dec.*); hydrobromide, hygroscopic prisms, m.p. 199–200°C; methiodide, m.p. 254–260°C (*dec.*) and the picrate, m.p. 219–220°C (*dec.*). The alkaloid forms an O-acetate, m.p. 223–5°C and an O,O-diacetate, m.p. 198°C (*dec.*); $[\alpha]_D^{23} - 623°$ (c 0.43, $CHCl_3$).

Djerassi *et al.*, *Experientia*, **19**, 467 (1963)
Gilbert *et al.*, *Tetrahedron*, **21**, 1141 (1965)

COMPLANATINE

$C_{18}H_{31}ON$

M.p. 169°C

This alkaloid has been obtained from *Lycopodium flabelliforme* Fernald now re-named *L. complanatum* L. The base is characterized as the diperchlorate which forms crystals of the monohydrate, m.p. 190°C. It is stated to have a marked pressor action in cats. Intravenous injection into anaesthetised cats, however, does not affect the respiration.

Manske, Marion., *Can. J. Res.*, **20B**, 87 (1942)
Pharmacology:
Lee, Chen., *J. Amer. Pharm. Assoc.*, **34**, 197 (1945)

CONAMINE

$C_{22}H_{36}N_2$

M.p. 130°C

This alkaloid is said to occur in the bark of *Holarrhena antidysenterica* Wall. It has $[\alpha]_D^{28} - 19°$ (EtOH) and contains an amino and a methylimino group.

Siddiqui., *J. Ind. Chem. Soc.*, **11**, 283 (1934)
Siddiqui., *Proc. Ind. Acad. Sci.*, **3A**, 249, 257 (1936)
Siddiqui, Pillay., *J. Ind. Chem. Soc.*, **9**, 553 (1932)

CONARRHIMINE

$C_{21}H_{34}N_2$

M.p. 160°C and 175°C

This base, from the bark of *Holarrhena antidysenterica* Wall. has not been obtained in the pure state since it forms eutectic mixtures with holarrhimine having the melting points given above. However, its presence is established by the isolation of nitrosohydroxyapoconarrhimine, $C_{21}H_{32}O_2N_2$, m.p. 160–3°C, from these mixtures.

Siddiqui., *J. Ind. Chem. Soc.*, **11**, 283 (1934)
Siddiqui., *Proc. Ind. Acad. Sci.*, **3A**, 249, 257 (1936)

CONCHAIRAMIDINE

$C_{22}H_{26}O_4N_2$

M.p. 114°C

A minor constituent of the bark of *Cinchona Pelletierana*, Wedd., this alkaloid crystallizes as the monohydrate. It has $[\alpha]_D^{15} - 60°$ (EtOH) and gives a deep green colour with concentrated H_2SO_4.

Hesse., *Annalen*, **185**, 296, 323 (1877)

CONCHAIRAMINE

$C_{22}H_{26}O_4N_2$

M.p. 120°C

A further minor constituent of the bark of *Cinchona Pelletierana* Wedd and also found in *Rejima Purdieana,* this base forms colourless prisms of the monohydrate and has $[\alpha]_D^{15} + 68.4°$ (EtOH). In H_2SO_4 it gives a brown colour, changing to green while the solution in AcOH-HNO$_3$ is dark green.

Hesse., *Annalen*, **185**, 296, 323 (1877)

CONCURCHINE (*Conkurchine*)

$C_{21}H_{32}N_2$

M.p. 153°C

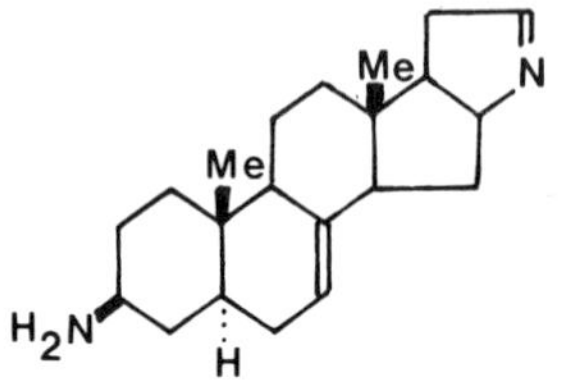

This alkaloid is found in *Holarrhena* species and has $[\alpha]_D^{21} - 67.4°$ (EtOH). It forms a number of crystalline salts and derivatives: hydriodide, m.p. 278°C (*dec.*); oxalate, m.p. 325°C (*dec.*); sulphate, m.p. 342°C; carbonate, m.p. 149–150°C; azide., m.p. 204.5°C (*dec.*); N,N-dibenzoate, m.p. 267°C; benzylidene derivative, m.p. 205.5–206°C and salicylidene compound, m.p. 244.5–245°C. The alkaloid contains two methyl and one amino group.

Bertho *et al., Ber.,* **66B**, 786 (1933)
Bertho., *ibid,* **80**, 316 (1947)
Tschesche, Roy., *Chem. Ber.,* **89**, 1288 (1956)

Identity with Irehline:
Janot *et al., Compt. Rend.,* **258**, 2089 (1964)

CONCURCHININE (*Conkurchinine*)

$C_{25}H_{36}N_2$

M.p. 161°C

A ditertiary alkaloid obtained from *Holarrhena* species, this base has $[\alpha]_D^{23}$ – 47.0° (EtOH). It forms a diperchlorate as the dihydrate which darkens at 260°C and a dimethiodide, m.p. 255–6°C (*dec.*). With dilute HNO_3 it yields concurchine nitrate by hydrolysis. The second product is believed to be a hydroxybutyraldehyde.

Bertho., *Arch. Pharm.*, **277**, 237 (1939)

CONDELPHINE

$C_{25}H_{39}O_6N$

M.p. 158–9°C

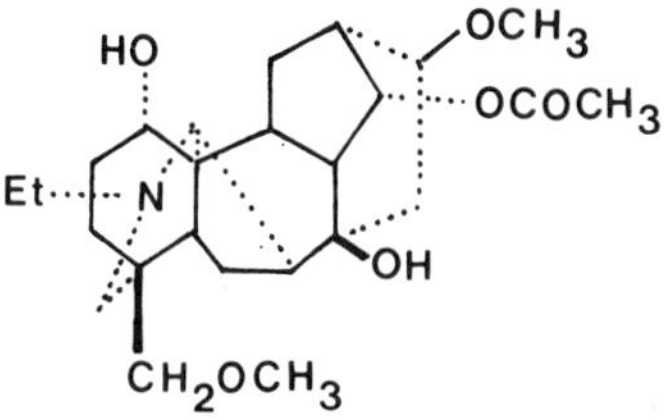

This aconite alkaloid occurs in *Delphinium confusum* Pop. and *D. denudatum*. It has $[\alpha]_D$ + 26.8° and forms a perchlorate, m.p. 209–210°C; an oxalate, m.p. 160–2°C (*dec.*); a methiodide, m.p. 203–5°C (*dec.*) and a diacetate, m.p. 130–4°C. Alkaline hydrolysis furnishes acetic acid and *iso*talatisidine (q.v.). Selenium dehydrogenation of the alkaloid gives 1:3-dimethylphenanthrene.

Rabinovitch, Konovalova., *J. Gen. Chem., USSR*, **12**, 329 (1942)
Kuzuvkov, Platonova., *ibid*, 1286 (1961)
Pelletier, Keith, Parthasarathy., *Tetrahedron Lett.*, 4217 (1966)
Pelletier, Keith, Parthasarathy., *J. Amer. Chem. Soc.*, **89**, 4146 (1967)
Tandon, Tiwari., *Proc. Nat. Acad. Sci., India*, **39A**, 233 (1969)

CONDENSAMINE

$C_{24}H_{28}O_5N_2$

M.p. 264–5°C

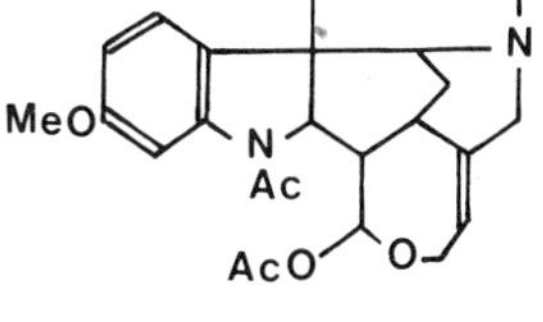

A strychnine alkaloid obtained from *Strychnos holstii*, this base contains one methoxyl, one O-acetyl and one N-acetyl group in the molecule. The structure has been determined from chemical analysis and spectroscopic data.

Denöel *et al., Arch. intern. physiol.*, **59**, 341 (1951)

CONDYFOLINE

$C_{18}H_{22}N_2$

M.p. 76–80°C

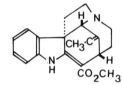

This alkaloid is a minor component of *Diplorrhynchus condylocarpon*. It has $[\alpha]_D^{21} + 348°$ (c 0.668, AcOEt). The ultraviolet spectrum has a single absorption maximum at 250 mμ in EtOH solution. The structure has been confirmed by the synthesis of the (±)-form.

Schumann, Schmid., *Helv. Chim. Acta*, **46**, 1996 (1963)
Synthesis:
Dadson, Harley-Mason, Foster., *Chem. Commun.*, 1233 (1968)

CONDYLOCARPINE

$C_{20}H_{22}O_2N_2$

M.p. 167–8°C

A further constituent of *Diplorrhynchus condylocarpon*, this alkaloid has $[\alpha]_D + 876°$ (AcOEt). On hydrogenation with Pd-C it yields tubotaiwin (q.v.).

Stauffacher., *Helv. Chim. Acta*, **44**, 2006 (1961)
Sandoval *et al.*, *Tetrahedron Lett.*, 409 (1962)
Schumann, Schmid., *Helv. Chim. Acta*, **46**, 1996 (1963)

CONESSIDINE

$C_{22}H_{34}N_2$

M.p. 123°C

This alkaloid occurs in *Holarrhena antidysenterica* Wall. It forms a stable dihydrate, m.p. 291–2°C (*dec.*) and yields crystalline salts, e.g. the dihydrochloride, darkening at 200°C; dihydriodide, m.p. 259°C (*dec.*); diperchlorate, m.p. 243°C (*dec.*) and a dimethiodide, m.p. 269°C (*dec.*). It has $[\alpha]_D^{21} - 63.5°$ (CHCl$_3$).

von Schuckmann, Bertho, Schönberger., *Ber.*, **66**, 786 (1933)
Bertho., *Arch. Pharm.*, **277**, 237 (1939)
Bertho., *Annalen.*, **555**, 214 (1944)
Tschesche, Petersen., *Chem. Ber.*, **87**, 1719 (1954)
Tschesche, Roy., *ibid*, **89**, 1288 (1956)

CONESSIMINE

$C_{23}H_{38}N_2$

M.p. 100°C;
B.p. 230°C/1.8 mm

Also present in *Holarrhena antidysenterica* Wall., this base forms colourless needles from petroleum ether or AcOEt and has $[\alpha]_D^{35}$ − 22.25° (CHCl₃) or $[\alpha]_D^{26}$ − 24.1° (H₂O). The salts which have been prepared include the hydrochloride, m.p. 342−4°C; $[\alpha]_D^{26}$ − 15.1° (H₂O); hydriodide, m.p. 318−9°C (*dec.*); platinichloride, m.p. 301°C (*dec.*); carbonate, m.p. 105°C; aurichloride, m.p. 165°C (*dec.*) and picrate, m.p. 172−4°C. The alkaloid also forms a nitroso derivative, m.p. 240°C (*dec.*) and on methylation with H.COOH and H.CHO it yields conessine (q.v.).

Siddiqui, Pillay., *J. Ind. Chem. Soc.,* **9**, 553 (1932)
Siddiqui., *ibid,* **11**, 283 (1934)
Tschesche, Petersen., *Chem. Ber.,* **87**, 1719 (1954)

CONESSINE (*Wrightine*)

$C_{24}H_{40}N_2$

M.p. 123−4°C

This steroidal alkaloid occurs in several *Holarrhena* species. It was first isolated from the bark of *Holarrhena antidysenterica* Wall., and has since been found in *H. africana* D.C., *H. congolensis* Stapf., *H. febrifuga* Klotsch. and *H. Wulfsbergii*. The base crystallizes from boiling Me₂CO in large colourless plates and has $[\alpha]_D^{20}$ + 21.6° (EtOH) or − 1.9° (CHCl₃). In its reactions it behaves as a ditertiary base giving a hydrochloride (monohydrate) as masses of silky needles, m.p. > 340°C; $[\alpha]_D^{20}$ + 9.3° (H₂O); hydrobromide with $[\alpha]_D$ + 7.4° (H₂O); acid oxalate, m.p. 280°C (*dec.*); platinichloride as a microcrystalline powder and the picrate, m.p. 222−4°C. The dimethiodide forms as the trihydrate, m.p. 285°C and the dimethosulphate has m.p. 240−2°C. On reduction, the alkaloid gives the dihydro derivative, m.p. 97.5°C; $[\alpha]_D^{19}$ + 37.3° (EtOH). Oxidation with KIO₄ in dilute H₂SO₄ furnishes dioxyconessine, $C_{24}H_{42}O_2N_2$, m.p. 294−5°C; $[\alpha]_D$ + 11.79° (EtOH). More vigorous oxidation with chromic acid yields dimethylamine and a lactone acid, $C_{22}H_{33}O_4N$. With H₂SO₄ in AcOH the alkaloid is isomerized to *neo*conessine, m.p. 128−9°C; $[\alpha]_D^{37}$ + 96.8° (EtOH) which, on further reaction gives *iso*conessine, b.p. 239−241°C/3 mm; $[\alpha]_D^{35}$ + 97° (EtOH).

Although conessine induces narcosis in frogs, this effect is minimal in mammals. The alkaloid produces local anaesthesia but causes local necrosis on subcutaneous injection. An interesting observation by Meissner and Hesse is that conessine inhibits the growth of *Mycobacterium tuberculosis in vitro*. The major use of this alkaloid, in common with other *Holarrhena* bases is as a remedy for amoebic dysentery, although the major alkaloid for this is emetine or its salts.

Siddiqui, Pillay., *J. Ind. Chem. Soc.,* **9**, 553 (1932)
Siddiqui., *ibid,* **11**, 283 (1934)
Späth, Hromatka., *Ber.,* **63**, 127 (1930)
Haworth, McKenna., *Chem. & Ind.,* 312 (1951)
Haworth *et al., ibid,* 215 (1952)
Haworth., *Chem. Soc. Spec. Publ.,* **3**, 1 (1955)
Barton, Morgan., *J. Chem. Soc.,* 622 (1962)
Marshall, Johnson., *J. Amer. Chem. Soc.,* **84**, 1485 (1962)
Stork *et al., ibid,* **84**, 2018 (1962)

Pharmacology:
Burns., *J. Pharm. exp. Ther.,* **6**, 305 (1915)
Meissner, Hesse., *Arch. exp. Path. Pharm.,* **147**, 339 (1930)

CONHYDRINE

$C_8H_{17}ON$

M.p. 121°C;
B.p. 226°C

A piperidine alkaloid found in *Conium maculatum* (hemlock), this base was first isolated by Wertheim. It forms colourless leaflets and has an odour similar to that of coniine (q.v.). It is strongly basic and can be readily sublimed. The alkaloid has $[\alpha]_D + 10°$ and is soluble in EtOH or $CHCl_3$, moderately so in H_2O or Et_2O from which it is readily crystallized. The salts are also crystalline: aurichloride, m.p. 133°C and the hydrazone, m.p. 124–5°C. The base forms a benzoyl derivative, m.p. 132°C and an N-acetyl compound, b.p. 133–5°C/3 mm. On oxidation with chromic acid, conhydrine yields *l*-piperidyl-2-carboxylic acid. By reaction with hydriodic acid and phosphorus at 180°C, the alkaloid is converted into iodoconiin, $C_8H_{16}NI$, which may then be reduced to give coniine.

Although all of the hemlock alkaloids are highly poisonous, the substitution of a hydroxyl group as in conhydrine, reduces the toxicity. Nevertheless, the alkaloid produces paralysis of the motor nerve terminations and stimulation followed by depression of the central nervous system. Large doses slow the action of the heart. Nausea and vomiting are produced at an early stage of its action.

Wertheim., *Annalen,* **100**, 1329 (1856)
Willstätter., *Ber.,* **34**, 3166 (1901)
Chemnitius., *J. prakt. Chem.,* **118**, 25 (1928)
Späth, Adler., *Monatsh.,* **63**, 127 (1933)
Galinovsky, Nulley., *ibid,* **79**, 426 (1948)

α-CONHYDRINE

$C_8H_{17}ON$

M.p. 105–6°C;
B.p. 236.5°C

320

This isomer of conhydrine was obtained from *Conium maculatum* by Merck and examined by Ladenburg and Adam. It may be separated from conhydrine by crystallization of the mixed hydrochlorides, that of the latter being hygroscopic while the α-conhydrine salt crystallizes well from EtOH. The alkaloid forms slender needles from Et_2O and has $[\alpha]_D^{15} + 11°$ (EtOH). The hydrochloride has m.p. 212–3°C; the aurichloride, m.p. 133–4°C; the platinichloride as golden-yellow needles, m.p. 185–6°C and the N-benzoyl derivative has m.p. 132–3°C; $[\alpha]_D^{17} + 23.4°$. The last compound can be oxidized with alkaline $KMnO_4$ to give the benzoyl derivative of two aminoacids (a) $C_7H_{15}O_2N$ which has been shown to be α-aminoheptoic acid, isolated as the lactam, m.p. 45–7°C and (b) α-amino-*n*-hexoic acid, m.p. 205–7°C. This confirms that the hydroxyl group is present in the piperidyl nucleus.

In its pharmacological action, this alkaloid closely resembles conhydrine.

Ladenburg, Adam., *Annalen, 24,* 1071 (1891)
Loeffler., *Ber., 42,* 116 (1909)
Spath, Kuffner, Ensfellner., *ibid, 66,* 591 (1933)

γ-CONICEINE

$C_8H_{15}N$

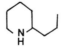

B.p. 171–2°C/746 mm

This is the only one of the six coniceines known which occurs naturally in *Conium maculatum.* It is a coniine-like oil, optically inactive and strongly alkaline. The salts crystallize well: the hydrochloride, m.p. 143°C is hygroscopic; the hydrobromide has m.p. 139°C; the hydriodide, m.p. 102°C; the aurichloride, m.p. 69–70°C; picrate, m.p. 79°C, picrolonate, m.p. 140°C and the N-acetyl derivative, b.p. 252–5°C. The cadmium iodide salt crystallizes from H_2O in long needles, m.p. 146–7°C.

The alkaloid is a secondary base and on reduction yields *dl*-coniine. It has been synthesized by hydrolysis of γ-phthaliminobutyl propyl ketone.

Gabriel., *Ber., 42,* 4059 (1909)
Loeffler, Tschunke., *ibid, 42,* 945 (1909)
Lukes, Sorm, Arnold., *Collect. Czech. Chem. Commun., 12,* 641 (1947)
Beyerman *et al., Rec. trav. chim., 80,* 513 (1961)

(+)-CONIINE

$C_8H_{17}N$

M.p. – 2°C;
B.p. 166–7°C

This alkaloid, obtained from *Conium maculatum,* is a colourless, alkaline liquid having a burning taste and a characteristic, penetrating odour. It is volatile in steam and has $[\alpha]_D^{19} + 15.7°$ (+ 13.79°). The refractive index is $n_D^{23°}$ 1.4505. It is miscible in all proportions with EtOH and readily soluble in Et_2O and most organic solvents. When allowed to stand in air for some time it forms a resin. The hydrochloride forms colourless rhombs from H_2O, m.p. 220°C; $[\alpha]_D^{20} + 10.1°$

(liquid NH_3); the hydrobromide, needles, m.p. 211°C; the d-acid tartrate, m.p. 54°C as the dihydrate; the aurichloride, m.p. 77°C; the platinichloride which separates as an oil, crystallizes on standing with m.p. 175°C; the picrate, m.p. 75°C; the 2:4-dinitrobenzoyl derivative, m.p. 139–139.5°C and the 3:5-dinitrobenzoyl compound, m.p. 108–9°C. The precipitate formed with potassium cadmium iodide is also crystalline, m.p. 118°C.

When distilled with Zn dust or heated with silver acetate, the alkaloid yields conyrine, $C_8H_{11}N$, which an oxidation furnishes pyridine-2-carboxylic acid. Heated with hydriodic acid at 300°C, the base yields n-octane. These reactions confirm the structure of the alkaloid as α-propylpiperidine.

The alkaloid is highly toxic, inducing nausea and vomiting at an early stage with paralysis of the motor nerve endings followed by depression of the central nervous system. Respiration is usually accelerated and deepened at first but then becomes slow and laboured and finally ceases while the heart still beats and consciousness has just disappeared. Both (+)- and (−)-coniine are identical in their action.

(−)-Coniine has b.p. 166.5°C and $[\alpha]_D$ − 15.6° but in other respects it closely resembles the (+)-isomeride. The salts, however, have slightly different characteristics. The hydrochloride has m.p. 220–1°C; the hydrobromide, m.p. 205°C; hydriodide, m.p. 145–6°C; aurichloride, m.p. 59°C; nitrate, m.p. 82–3°C and platinichloride, m.p. 160°C.

The (±)-form has b.p. 166°C and forms a crystalline hydrochloride, m.p. 216–7°C and platinichloride, m.p. 160°C.

Giesecke., *Arch. Pharm.,* **20**, 97 (1827)

Blyth., *Annalen,* **70**, 73 (1849)

Hofmann., *Ber.,* **14**, 705 (1881)

Hofmann., *ibid,* **17**, 825 (1884)

Tafel., *ibid,* **25**, 1619 (1892)

Chemnitius., *J. prakt. Chem.,* **118**, 25 (1928)

CONIMINE

$C_{22}H_{36}N_2$

M.p. 130°C

This alkaloid has been isolated by Siddiqui from *Holarrhena* species. The base has $[\alpha]_D^{28}$ − 30° (EtOH) and forms a hydrochloride, m.p. 318–320°C (*dec.*); platinichloride, m.p. 296–8°C (*dec.*) and a picrate, m.p. 140–1°C. It contains two reactive hydrogens and one methylimino group. Methylation furnishes conessine and it may be produced by the demethylation of the latter with cyanogen bromide. With H_2SO_4 it isomerizes to *iso*conimine which has $[\alpha]_D^{35}$ + 89° (EtOH) and forms a hydriodide, m.p. 332°C (*dec.*) and a picrate, m.p. 135°C.

Siddiqui, Siddiqui., *J. Ind. Chem. Soc.,* **11**, 787 (1934)

CONODURAMINE

$C_{41}H_{50}O_6N_4$

M.p. 215–8°C

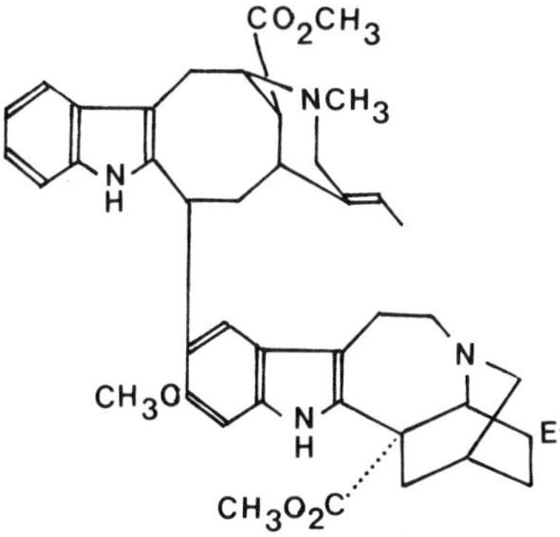

A dimeric alkaloid from the root bark of *Conopharyngia durissima* Stapf. The alkaloid is obtained as colourless needles from MeOH-Me$_2$CO and has $[\alpha]_D^{23}$ – 77.5° (c 1.0, CHCl$_3$). The ultraviolet spectrum has absorption maxima at 228, 287 and 294.5 mμ.

Renner, Prins, Stoll., *Helv. Chim. Acta*, **42**, 1572 (1959)
Renner, Fritz., *Tetrahedron Lett.*, 283 (1964)

CONODURINE

$C_{41}H_{50}O_5N_4$

M.p. 222–5°C (*dec.*).

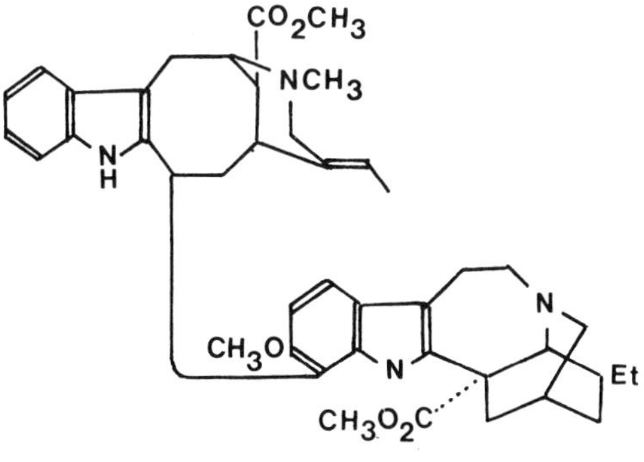

A second dimeric alkaloid found in the root bark of *Conopharyngia durissima* Stapf., the base has $[\alpha]_D^{22}$ – 101°C (c 1.0, CHCl$_3$). The ultraviolet spectrum exhibits absorption maxima at 225, 285 and 292.5 m.

Renner, Prins, Stoll., *Helv. Chim. Acta*, **42**, 1572 (1959)
Renner, Fritz., *Tetrahedron Lett.*, 283 (1964)

CONOFLORINE

$C_{19}H_{24}ON_2$

M.p. 166–8°C

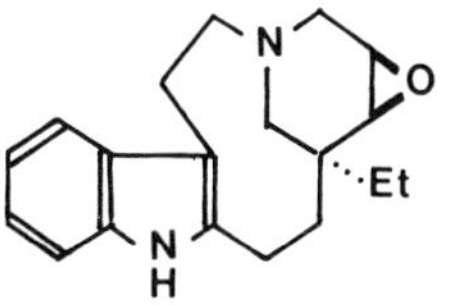

The leaves of *Conopharyngia longiflora* Stapf. contain this alkaloid which forms colourless crystals from MeOH. It has $[\alpha]_D^{24}$ + 24.4° (c 1.04, CHCl$_3$). The ultraviolet spectrum of the solution in EtOH has absorption maxima at 230, 286 and 292 mμ. The base contains an imino and an epoxy group in the molecule.

Dugan *et al.*, *Helv. Chim. Acta*, **50**, 60 (1967)

CONOLLINE

C$_{13}$H$_{20}$ON$_2$

M.p. 192.5–193.5°C

An alkaloid occurring in *Ammodendron conollyi* Bge. the base forms a series of crystalline salts including the hydrochloride, m.p. 180–2°C; hydriodide, m.p. 195–6°C and the platinichloride, m.p. 136–8°C (*dec.*). A crystalline perchlorate, m.p. 197–8°C has also been prepared.

Proskurnina, Merlis., *J. Gen. Chem. USSR*, **19**, 1396 (1949)

CONOPHARYNGINE

C$_{23}$H$_{30}$O$_4$N$_2$

M.p. 141–3°C

Both the stem and root bark of *Conopharyngia durissima* Stapf. yield this alkaloid which has $[\alpha]_D^{25}$ – 40.5° (c 1.0, CHCl$_3$). Alcoholic KOH furnishes the decarboxy derivative which, with HCl gives decarbomethoxyconopharyngine, C$_{21}$H$_{28}$O$_2$N$_2$, m.p. 136–7°C; $[\alpha]_D^{22}$ – 42.6° (c 0.82, CHCl$_3$).

Renner, Prins, Stoll., *Helv. Chim. Acta*, **42**, 1572 (1959)

CONQUINAMINE

C$_{19}$H$_{24}$O$_2$N$_2$

M.p. 121°C

A minor constituent of *Cinchona Ledgeriana* and *C. succirubra*, this alkaloid forms triclinic crystals from EtOH and has $[\alpha]_D$ + 204.6° (EtOH).

Hesse., *Ber.*, **10**, 2158 (1877)
Hesse., *Annalen*, **209**, 62 (1881)
Oudemans., *ibid*, **209**, 38 (1881)

CONQUININE

See Quinidine

CONSOLICINE

This alkaloid is stated to be present in *Anchusa officinalis* L., *Cynoglossum officinale* L. and *Echium vulgare* L. It is also formed by the hydrolysis of the gluco-alkaloid consolidine (q.v.).

Greiner., *Arch. Pharm.*, **238**, 505 (1900)

CONSOLIDINE

This name has been given to two alkaloids.

A gluco-alkaloid found in *Anchusa officinalis* L. and also present in *Cynoglossum officinale* L. and *Echium vulgare* L. This alkaloid has not been characterized. On alkaline hydrolysis it furnishes glucose and consolicine (q.v.). It is stated to paralyze the central nervous system.

Greiner., *Arch. Pharm.*, **238**, 505 (1900)

$C_{33}H_{49}O_9N$

M.p. 153–7°C

One of the aconite alkaloids isolated from *Delphinium consolida Linn.* this base has $[\alpha]_D$ + 64° (MeOH). It forms a crystalline perchlorate, m.p. 252°C; $[\alpha]_D^{28}$ + 33° (EtOH). Hydrolysis with alcoholic KOH furnishes benzoic acid and an alkamine, consoline, which has not been obtained crystalline.

Marion, Edwards., *J. Amer. Chem. Soc.*, **69**, 2010 (1947)

CONVOLVAMINE (*Veratroyltropine*)

$C_{17}H_{23}O_4N$

M.p. 114–5°C

The seeds of *Convolvulus pseudocantabricus* Schrenk contain about 0.5 per cent of alkaloids from which this base and the three succeeding alkaloids have been isolated by fractional crystallization of the crude mixed hydrochlorides. Convolvamine also occurs in *C. subhirsutus*. It crystallizes as colourless prisms from petroleum ether and is soluble in most organic solvents although only sparingly so in Et_2O and hot H_2O. When hydrolyzed with hot alcoholic KOH it yields veratric acid and tropine.
 The salts are crystalline, e.g. the hydrochloride, m.p. 237–9°C; aurichloride, m.p. 201–2°C; platinichloride, m.p. 216–7°C; methiodide, m.p. 257–9°C and the picrate, m.p. 263–4°C (*dec.*).

Orekhov, Konovalova., *Arch. Pharm.*, **271**, 145 (1933)
Orekhov, Konovalova., *Ber.*, **67**, 1153 (1934)
Orekhov, Konovalova., *ibid*, **68**, 814 (1935)
Orekhov., *Arch. Pharm.*, **272**, 673 (1934)
Yunusov, Shakirov, Plekhanova., *Dokl. Akad. Nauk. Uzbek. SSR*, 17 (1958)

CONVOLVICINE

$C_{10}H_{16}N_2$

B.p. 250–260°C

This liquid alkaloid is found in *Convolvulus pseudocantabricus* Schrenk and *C. subhirsutus* and yields a crystalline picrate, m.p. 260–2°C.

Orekhov, Konovalova., *Arch. Pharm.*, **271**, 145 (1933)
Orekhov, Konovalova., *Ber.*, **67**, 1153 (1934)
Orekhov, Konovalova., *Ber.*, **68**, 814 (1935)
Orekhov., *Arch. Pharm.*, **272**, 673 (1934)
Yunusov, Shakirov, Plekhanova., *Dokl. Akad. Nauk, Uzbek SSR*, 17 (1958)

CONVOLVIDINE

$C_{32-33}H_{42-44}O_8N_2$

M.p. 192–3°C

This alkaloid from *Convolvulus pseudocantabricus* Shrenk. is also a veratroyl ester but the alkamine has not yet been identified. The latter has m.p. 274–6°C; picrate, m.p. 229–231°C.

Orekhov, Konovalova., *Arch. Pharm.*, **271**, 145 (1933)
Orekhov, Konovalova., *Ber.*, **67**, 1153 (1934)
Orekhov, Konovalova., *ibid*, **68**, 814 (1935)

CONVOLVINE (*Veratroylnortropine*)

$C_{16}H_{21}O_4N$

M.p. 114–5°C

Present in *Convolvulus pseudocantabricus* Shrenk and *C. subhirsutus*, this alkaloid is soluble in $CHCl_3$, Me_2CO or EtOH, sparingly so in Et_2O, petroleum ether or H_2O. It forms crystalline salts, e.g. hydrochloride, m.p. 260–1°C; oxalate, m.p. 265–6°C (*dec.*); nitrate, m.p. 212–3°C; aurichloride, m.p. 217°C and picrate, m.p. 261–3°C. The methiodide has also been prepared, m.p. 230–1°C. The alkaloid is stated to possess local anaesthetic properties.

Orekhov, Konovalova., *Arch. Pharm.*, **271**, 145 (1933)
Orekhov, Konovalova., *Ber.*, **67**, 1153 (1934)
Orekhov, Konovalova., *ibid*, **68**, 814 (1935)
Orekhov., *Arch. Pharm.*, **272**, 673 (1934)
Yunusov, Shakirov, Plekhanova., *Dokl. Akad. Nauk. Uzbek, SSR*, 17 (1958)

Pharmacology:
Nolle., *Khim. Farm. Prom.*, 39 (1934)
Awrutowa., *Chem. Zentr.*, 496 (1938)

COPTINE

This uncharacterized yellow alkaloid has been reported as occurring in *Coptis Teeta* Wall. It does not appear to have been investigated further since its isolation.

Gross., *Amer. J. Pharm.*, **14**, 193 (1873)

COPTISINE

$C_{19}H_{15}O_5N$

M.p. 216–8°C

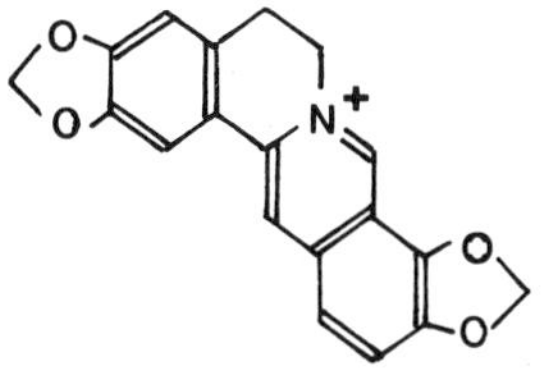

This alkaloid was first isolated as the tetrahydro derivative by reduction of the mixture of bases remaining after removal of berberine as the sulphate from the total alkaloids of *Coptis japonica* Mak. The free base forms yellow needles from EtOH. The chloride is obtained as thin orange prisms, m.p. 280–300°C and the iodide forms yellow crystals, m.p. > 280°C. $KMnO_4$ oxidizes the base to hydrastic acid.

Kitasato., *J. Pharm. Soc. Japan*, **542**, 48 (1927)
Kitasato., *Proc. Imp. Acad. Tokyo.*, **2**, 124 (1926)
Späth, Posega., *Ber.*, **62**, 1029 (1929)
Huang-Minlon., *ibid*, **69**, 1737 (1936)

CORANICINE

$C_{16}H_{17}O_4N$

M.p. Indefinite

An amorphous alkaloid found in *Ammocharis coranica* (Ker.-Gawl) Herb. this base has $[\alpha]_D^{21} + 156°$ (c 0.198, $CHCl_3$). The perchlorate forms colourless crystals from Me_2CO, m.p. 192–4°C (*dec.*); the methiodide, m.p. > 300°C (*dec.*) and the Diacetyl derivative, m.p. 118–9°C; $[\alpha]_D^{21} + 90°$ (c 0.21 EtOH) or + 80° (c 0.21, $CHCl_3$).

Hauth, Stauffacher., *Helv. Chim. Acta*, **45**, 1305 (1962)

CORDIFOLINE

$C_{30}H_{32}O_{13}N_2$

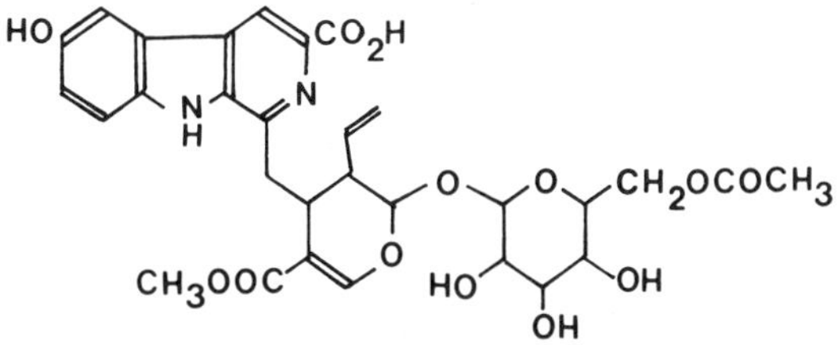

This complex β-carboline alkaloid is present in *Adina cordifolia* and is characterized as the pentaacetate, m.p. 142–4°C. The ultraviolet spectrum of the acetate has absorption maxima at 239, 271, 305 (infl.), 338 and 350 mμ. There is a pronounced bathochromic shift in acid solution. The alkaloid contains four hydroxyl and one carboxylic acid group.

Brown, Row., *Chem. Commun.*, 453 (1967)

CORDRASTINE

$C_{22}H_{25}O_6N$

M.p. 196°C

This phthalide*iso*quinoline alkaloid has been isolated from *Corydalis aurea* Willd. by Manske. It forms colourless needles from EtOH. The structure has been determined by chemical and spectroscopic investigation.

Manske., *Can. J. Res.*, **9**, 436 (1933)
Manske., *ibid*, **15**, 159 (1937)
Manske., *ibid*, **16**, 81 (1938)

COREXIMINE (*Alkaloid F29*)

$C_{19}H_{21}O_4N$

M.p. 262°C

A protoberberine alkaloid present in *Dicentra eximia* (Ker) Torr. The base is obtained as colourless prisms from CHCl$_3$ or a mixture of EtOH and dioxan. On heating, it begins to darken at 250–5°C. The O,O-dimethyl ether has m.p. 177°C forming a hydrochloride, m.p. 236–7°C. Both the dimethyl ether and its hydrochloride have been synthesized and have [α]$_D$ − 277° (c 1.0, CHCl$_3$) and − 277 (c 1.0, EtOH) respectively. The O,O-diethyl ether has m.p. 170°C and forms a picrate, m.p. 131°C. The (±)-form of the alkaloid has m.p. 233–4°C, forming a diethyl ether, m.p. 170°C and a picrate, m.p. 131°C.

Manske., *Can. J. Res.*, **16B**, 81 (1938)
Manske., *J. Amer. Chem. Soc.*, **72**, 4796 (1950)
Manske, Ashford., *ibid*, **73**, 5144 (1951)
Corrodi, Hardegger., *Helv. Chim. Acta*, **39**, 889 (1956)
Battersby *et al.*, *Tetrahedron*, **14**, 46 (1961)

CORGOINE

$C_{17}H_{19}O_3N$

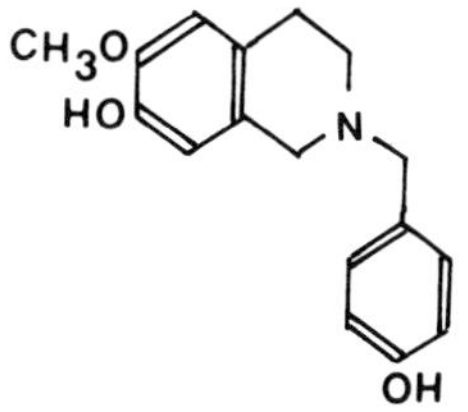

This alkaloid occurs in *Corydalis gortschakovii*. The structure has been shown to be that given above by chemical analysis and spectroscopic data, particularly an investigation of the NMR spectrum and mass spectrometry.

Ibragimova, Yunusov, Yunusov., *Khim. Prir. Soedin.*, **6**, 638 (1970)

CORLUMIDINE

$C_{20}H_{19}O_6N$

M.p. 236°C

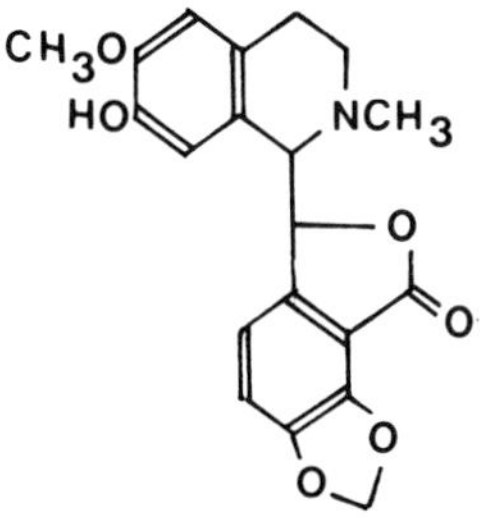

A phthalide*iso*quinoline alkaloid found in *Corydalis scouleri* HK, the base crystallizes in colourless prisms with $[\alpha]_D^{23} + 80°$. It contains one hydroxyl group and on methylation yields corlumine (q.v.).

Manske., *Can. J. Res.*, **14B**, 347 (1936)
Manske., *ibid*, **18B**, 100 (1940)

CORLUMINE

$C_{21}H_{21}O_6N$

M.p. 158–160°C (*dec.*).

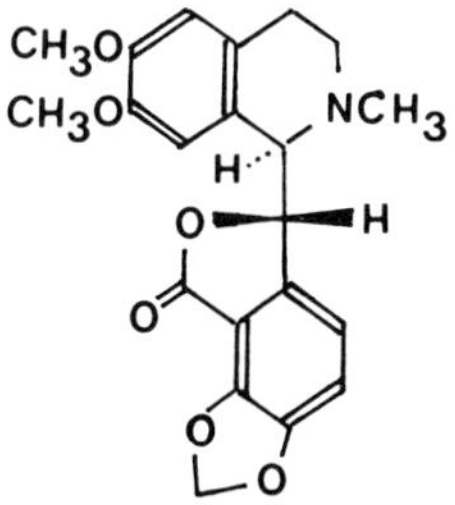

This alkaloid occurs in *Corydalis nobilis* Pers., *C. scouleri* HK, *C. sibirica* Pers. and *Dicentra cucullaria* (L) Bernh. The base has $[\alpha]_D^{25} + 77.6°$ (c 1.13, CHCl$_3$) and ± 0° (EtOH). It is laevorotatory in acid solution. Oxidation with HNO$_3$ furnishes 2-carboxy-3:4-methylenedioxybenzaldehyde and 4:5-dimethoxy-2β-methylaminoethylbenzaldehyde. It has been shown to be stereoisomeric, but

329

not enantiomorphic with adlumine (q.v.). The (+)-hydrogen tartrate has m.p. 127–140°C.

The (−)-form of the alkaloid has m.p. 158–160°C (*dec.*); $[\alpha]_D^{26-} - 73°$ (c 1.32, $CHCl_3$). It also forms a (+)-hydrogen tartrate, m.p. 208–208.5°C (*dec.*).

Manske., *Can. J. Res.*, **14B**, 325, 347 (1936)
Manske., *ibid*, **16B**, 81 (1938)
Manske., *ibid*, **18B**, 288 (1940)
Whaley, Meadow., *J. Chem. Soc.*, 1067 (1953)

Stereochemistry:
Edwards *et al.*, *Can. J. Chem.*, **39**, 1801 (1961)
Safe, Moir., *ibid*, **42**, 160 (1964)

CORNIGERINE

$C_{21}H_{21}O_6N$

M.p. 268–270°C

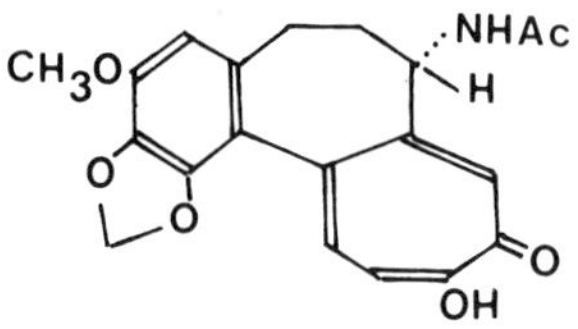

A colchicine alkaloid isolated from the corms of *Colchicum cornigerum* (Schweinf.) Täckh et Drar., this base crystallizes from AcOEt–Et_2O and has $[\alpha]_D^{20} - 150°$ (c 0.63, $CHCl_3$), − 233° (c 0.73, MeOH). On acid or alkaline hydrolysis it yields cornigereine, $C_{20}H_{19}O_6N$, m.p. 168–170°C; $[\alpha]_D^{22} - 222°$ (c 0.758, $CHCl_3$).

El-Hamidi, Santavy., *Collect. Czech. Chem. Commun.*, **27**, 2111 (1962)
Cross *et al.*, *ibid*, **29**, 1187 (1964)

CORNUCERVINE

$C_{17}H_{29}O_5N$

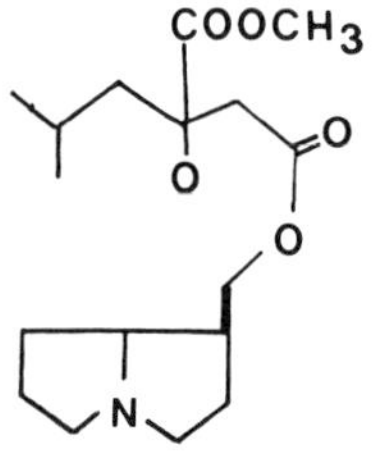

A pyrrolizidine alkaloid isolated from *Phalaenopsis cornu-cervi* Rchb. this base is an oil which cannot be crystallized. It has $[\alpha]_D^{22} - 4.3°$ (c 1.6, EtOH). The structure has been determined from its mass spectrum and the products of acid methanolysis.

Brandange *et al.*, *Acta Chem. Scand.*, **25**, 349 (1971)

CORNUTINE

See Ergotoxine

CORONARIDINE

$C_{21}H_{26}O_2N_2$

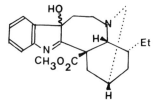

This ibogamine alkaloid occurs in *Tabernaemontana coronaria* (Syn. *Ervatamia coronaria*) and also in *T. oppositifolia*. It forms a crystalline hydrochloride, m.p. 235°C (*dec.*); $[\alpha]_D^{25} - 8.5°$ (c 1.0, MeOH). When treated with KOH followed by HCl, the alkaloid is converted into Ibogamine (q.v.).

Gorman *et al., J. Amer. Chem. Soc.*, **82**, 1142 (1960)
Neuss, Gorman., *Tetrahedron Lett.*, 206 (1961)

CORONARIDINE HYDROXYINDOLENINE

$C_{21}H_{26}O_3N_2$

M.p. 113–7°C

The ligroine extract of the seeds of *Conopharyngia durissima* contains this alkaloid together with Coronaridine and Tabersonine (q.v.). It has been separated from the accompanying bases by column chromatography on alkaline Kieselgel G. The mass spectrum is very like that of Voacangine hydroxyindolenine (q.v.).

Das, Fellion, Plat., *Compt. Rend.*, **264C**, 1765 (1967)

CORONARINE

$C_{44}H_{56}O_6N_4$

M.p. 196–8°C (*dec.*).

This complex alkaloid has been obtained, together with Tabernaemontanine (q.v.) from *Tabernaemontana coronaria*. Its structure has not yet been determined, nor have any salts been reported.

Ratnagiriswaran, Ventatachalan., *Quart. J. Pharm.*, **12**, 174 (1939)

CORPAVERINE

This supposed alkaloid has been shown to be a 1:1-molecular complex of sandaverine and (−)-capaurine. It has m.p. 138°C and $[\alpha]_D - 154.2°$ (CHCl$_3$).

Kametani *et al., Tetrahedron Lett.*, 3345 (1965)
Kametani *et al., ibid*, 985 (1966)

CORUNNINE

$C_{20}H_{17}O_5N$

M.p. 255–7°C

This alkaloid from *Glaucium flavum* Cr. var. *vestitum* forms violet needles on crystallization from EtOH. In EtOH solution, the ultraviolet spectrum shows absorption maxima at 258, 325, 400, 440 and 630 mμ. The perchlorate also yields violet needles, m.p. 293–5°C.

Ribas, Sueiras, Castedo., *Tetrahedron Lett.*, 3093 (1971)

CORUSCINE

$C_{18}H_{23}O_5N$

M.p. 170°C

Isolated from *Nerine corusca* and subsequently from *Brunsdonna tubergenii*, this alkaloid forms colourless crystals from Me$_2$CO and has $[\alpha]_D$ + 70° (CHCl$_3$). The hydriodide is crystalline, m.p. 179–180°C (*dec.*), as are the methiodide, m.p. 311°C (*dec.*) and the methoperchlorate, m.p. 278–280°C (*dec.*).

Boit, Ehmke., *Chem. Ber.*, **90**, 369 (1957)
Boit, Döpke., *Naturwiss.*, **47**, 159 (1960)

CORYBULBINE (*Corydalis-G*)

$C_{21}H_{25}O_4N$

M.p. 235°C; 244°C
(evacuated tube)

This berberine alkaloid is present in the roots of *Corydalis ambigua* Cham. and Sch., *C. platycarpa* Makino and *C. tuberosa* DC (Syn. *C. cava* Schwg.). It crystallizes from boiling EtOH in small, colourless needles, $[\alpha]_D$ + 303.3° (CHCl$_3$) and is readily soluble in CHCl$_3$, Me$_2$CO or C$_6$H$_6$ but only sparingly so in MeOH or Et$_2$O. The hydrochloride forms pale yellow prisms from H$_2$O, m.p. 245–250°C (*dec.*). Both the aurichloride and the platinichloride are amorphous. The O-ethyl ether has m.p. 129–130°C; $[\alpha]_D^{20}$ + 299° (EtOH) and forms a hydrochloride m.p. 245–250°C and a methiodide which exists in two forms with m.p. 223–4°C and 240–1°C.

The optically inactive form has m.p. 220–2°C and yields a crystalline nitrate, m.p. 207–8°C and a platinichloride which is also crystalline, m.p. 223°C.

When treated with iodine, the alkaloid is oxidized to dehydrocorybulbine hydriodide, m.p. 175–8°C.

Freund, Joseph i., *Ber.*, **25**, 2411 (1892)
Freund, Joseph i., *Annalen*, **277**, 1 (1893)
Makoshi., *Arch. Pharm.*, **246**, 381 (1908)
Späth *et al.*, *Ber.*, **56**, 876 (1923)
Späth, Dobrowsky., *ibid*, **58**, 1274 (1925)
Späth, Holter., *ibid*, **59**, 2800 (1926)
Huang-Minlon., *ibid*, **69**, 1742 (1936)

CORYCAVAMINE

$C_{21}H_{21}O_5N$

M.p. 148–9°C

Isolated from the root nodules of *Corydalis tuberosa* D.C., this alkaloid is desmotropic with corycavine (q.v.), changing to the latter when melted. When crystallized from Et_2O it forms colourless prisms and has $[\alpha]_D^{20} + 166.6°$ ($CHCl_3$). The hydrochloride and hydriodide crystallize in needles but the platinichloride is amorphous. Like corycavine it dissolves in H_2SO_4 giving a dirty green solution which gradually changes to reddish-violet. In HNO_3 the colour is greenish-yellow becoming orange-red.

Gadamer, Ziegenbein, Wagner., *Arch. Pharm.*, **234**, 528 (1896)
Gadamer., *ibid*, **240**, 21, 83 (1902)
Gadamer, Bruchhausen., *ibid*, **260**, 101, 113 (1922)
Bruchhausen., *ibid*, **263**, 584 (1925)
Späth, Holter., *Ber.*, **60**, 1892 (1927)

CORYCAVIDINE

$C_{22}H_{25}O_5N$

M.p. 212–3°C

A further constituent of the root nodules of *Corydalis tuberosa* D.C., this alkaloid crystallizes from MeOH and has $[\alpha]_D^{20} + 210–218°$ ($CHCl_3$). At its melting point, it is converted into the (±)-form. The alkaloid is insoluble in Et_2O or EtOH and is also unstable to light. The nitrate and hydrochloride are crystalline but the red aurichloride is amorphous, m.p. 170°C (*dec.*). The methiodide is obtained as the trihydrate, m.p. 207–210°C (*dec.*) and is optically inactive.

The alkaloid is not converted by AcOCl or $POCl_3$ into the quaternary chloride but the dihydro derivative, m.p. $147-8°C$; $[\alpha]_D^{20} - 44.3°$ ($CHCl_3$), is so converted into *iso*dihydrocorycavidine chloride isolated as the crystalline mercurichloride. Corycavidine methosulphate is reduced with sodium amalgam in dilute H_2SO_4 to tetrahydromethylcorycavidine, an oil with $[\alpha]_D^{20} + 39.9°$ ($CHCl_3$), hydrochloride, m.p. $190°C$. On evaporation in dilute HCl the latter yields the corresponding anhydro base, $C_{23}H_{29}O_4N$, as an oil giving a crystalline hydrochloride, m.p. $233-5°C$ which may be oxidized by $KMnO_4$ in Me_2CO to 2-methyl-3:4-dimethoxyacetophenone and N-methylhydrastinine. These reactions provide confirmation for the above structure.

Gadamer., *Arch. Pharm.*, **249**, 30 (1911)
Gadamer, Lederlotz., *ibid*, **256**, 162 (1918)
Bruchhausen., *ibid*, **263**, 583, 600 (1925)

CORYCAVINE

$C_{21}H_{21}O_5N$

M.p. $218-9°C$

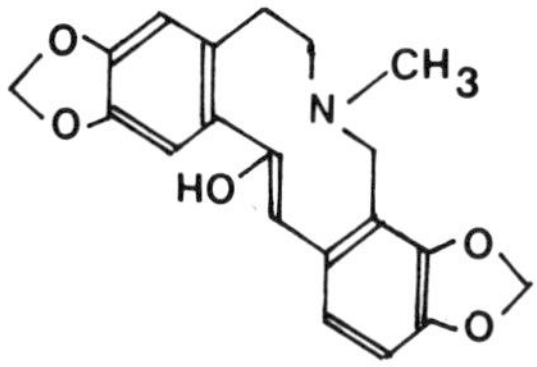

Also present in *Corydalis tuberosa* D.C., this base forms colourless plates from EtOH. It is optically inactive, insoluble in H_2O, alkalies or cold EtOH. The melting points is raised to $221-2°C$ in an evacuated tube. The salts are all crystalline: hydrochloride, m.p. $219°C$; hydriodide, small yellow crystals, m.p. $236°C$ of the monohydrate; aurichloride, m.p. $178-9°C$ (*dec.*); platinichloride as yellow crystals, m.p. $214°C$ (*dec.*) and the methiodide as rhombic tablets, m.p. $218°C$. The alkaloid gives a dirty green colour with H_2SO_4 changing to reddish-violet, and a green-yellow colour with HNO_3, gradually becoming orange.

Freund, Josephi., *Annalen,* **277**, 1 (1893)
Gadamer, Ziegenbein, Wagner., *Arch. Pharm.,* **234**, 528 (1896)
Gadamer, Ziegenbein, Wagner., *ibid,* **240**, 19 (1902)
Gaebel., *ibid,* **248**, 247 (1910)
Legerlotz., *ibid,* **256**, 161 (1918)
Gadamer, Bruchhausen., *ibid,* **259**, 247 (1921)
Gadamer, Bruchhausen., *ibid,* **260**, 97 (1922)
Späth, Holter., *Ber.,* **60**, 1891 (1927)

CORYCIDINE

m.p. $290-1°C$

An alkaloid of *Corydalis stewartii,* this base yields crystalline salts and derivatives, e.g. the hydriodide, m.p. $265-270°C$ (*dec.*); aurichloride, m.p. $148-150°C$ (*dec.*); platinichloride, m.p. $233-5°C$ (*dec.*) and the picrate, m.p. $158-160°C$ (*dec.*).

Ikram, Huq, Warsi., *Pakistan J. Sci. Ind. Res.,* **9**, 34 (1966)

CORYDALIC ACID METHYL ESTER

$C_{22}H_{23}O_6N$

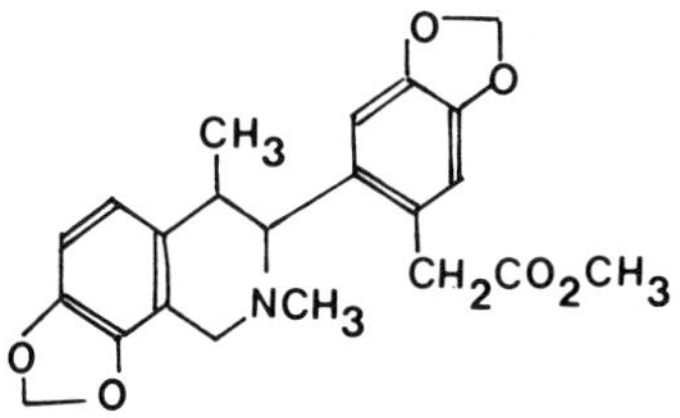

This alkaloid is present in *Corydalis incisa* only when the plant is in the vegetative stage. The structure has been established by spectroscopic studies and correlation with mesotetrahydrocorysamine. On the basis of the stereochemical investigation of this latter base, the stereostructure of the alkaloid has been determined.

Nonaka, Kodera, Fukuoka., *Chem. Pharm. Bull.*, **21**, 1020 (1973)

CORYDALIDZINE

$C_{20}H_{23}O_4N$

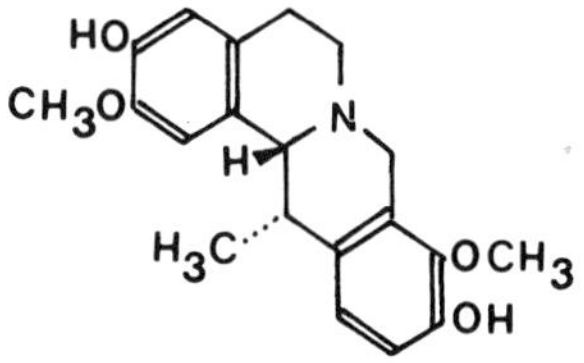

This alkaloid has recently been isolated from *Corydalis koidzumiana* and assigned the above structure on the basis of spectroscopic data. The alkaloid has been synthesized in nine stages from 3-benzyloxy-4-methoxy-phenethylamine and 4-benzyloxy-3-hydroxyphenylacetic acid.

Tani, Nagakura, Hattori., *Tetrahedron Lett.*, **11**, 803 (1973)

CORYDALINE

$C_{22}H_{27}O_4N$

M.p. 135°C

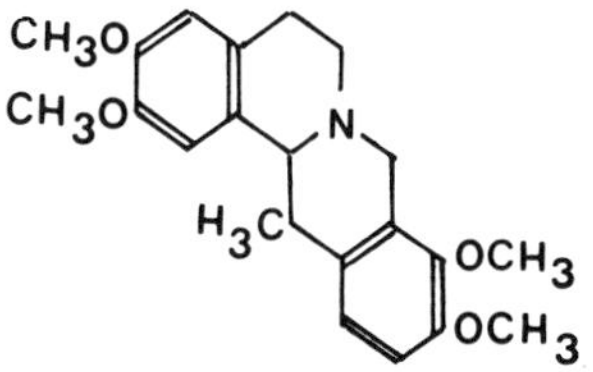

Present in *Corydalis ambigua* Chem. and Sch., *C. aurea* Willd. and *C. tuberosa* D.C. The original formula of $C_{18}H_{19}O_4N$ due to Wicke has been modified several times before that given above was finally adopted. The alkaloid crystallized from EtOH in short, six-sided prisms and has $[\alpha]_D^{20} + 300°$ (CHCl$_3$) or + 295° (EtOH). It is sparingly soluble in cold EtOH but dissolves on warming, is readily soluble in Et$_2$O or CHCl$_3$ and insoluble in H$_2$O. When exposed to air it slowly oxidizes to the yellow dehydrocorydaline. It forms well crystallized salts: the hydrochloride as the dihydrate, m.p. 214°C; nitrate, m.p. 197°C; aurichloride, m.p. 207°C; platinichloride, m.p. 227°C; methiodide, m.p. 228°C (crystalline form) and 64–8°C (amorphous form) and the ethyl sulphate as large prisms of the monohydrate, m.p. 152.5°C. Oxidation with $KMnO_4$ yields m-hemipinic acid and corydaldine, $C_{11}H_{13}O_3N$, as prismatic crystals, m.p. 175°C. HNO_3, on the other hand, gives dehydrocorydaline, $C_{22}H_{23}O_4N$, oxidized further by the same reagent to corydic acid, $C_{18}H_{17}O_6N$, which crystallizes as the dihydrate in yellow leaflets, m.p. 218°C and behaves as a dibasic acid. On further oxidation with $KMnO_4$, the latter furnishes cirydilic acid, $C_{17}H_{15}O_8N$, a tribasic acid, m.p. 228°C.

The (±)-form of the alkaloid has m.p. 135°C while the *meso* form melts at 158–9°C and forms crystalline salts, e.g. the hydrochloride, m.p. 247–8°C (*dry*); nitrate, m.p. 207–8°C (*dec.*) and the aurichloride, m.p. 191–2°C (*dec.*).

Weckenroder., *Berz. Jahrb.*, 7, 220 (1826)
Wicke., *Annalen*, 137, 274 (1866)
Freund, Josephi., *ibid*, 277, 1 (1893)
Gadamer, Bruchhausen., *J. Chem. Soc.*, 122, 675 (1922)
Späth, Mosettig., *Annalen*, 433, 138 (1923)
Bruchhausen., *Chem. Abstr.*, 18, 2900 (1924)
Bruchhausen, Stippler., *ibid*, 21, 1963 (1927)
Chou., *ibid*, 22, 2359 (1928)
Späth, Kruta., *Ber.*, 62, 1024 (1929)
Huang-Minlon., *ibid*, 69, 1744 (1936)

CORYDALIS I

M.p. 104°C

This alkaloid is present in the tubers of *Corydalis ambigua* and is dextrorotatory with $[\alpha]_D^{25}$ + 112.5°. It gives a crystalline hydrochloride, m.p. 236°C; hydrobromide, m.p. 241°C and a hydrogen oxalate, m.p. 185°C. Pharmacologically, the alkaloid is a depressor of the central nervous system.

Chou., *Chin. J. Physiol.*, 3, 301 (1929)

CORYDAMINE

$C_{20}H_{18}O_4N_2$

This alkaloid of *Corydalis incisa* has recently been isolated as the crystalline hydrochloride. The structure has been determined by chemical analysis and spectroscopic examination.

Nonaka, Nishioka., *Chem. Pharm. Bull.*, 21, 1410 (1973)

CORYDICINE

M.p. 181–4°C

An alkaloid of *Corydalis stewartii*, this base yields crystalline salts including the hydrochloride, m.p. 244–5°C (*dec.*); platinichloride, m.p. 212–3°C (*dec.*) and the picrate, m.p. 268–270°C (*dec.*).

Ikram, Huq, Warsi., *Pakistan J. Sci. Ind. Res.*, **9**, 34 (1966)

(–)-CORYDINE

$C_{20}H_{23}O_4N$

M.p. 149°C

This alkaloid occurs in several species of the order Rhoeadales, e.g. *Corydalis ternata*, Nakai., *C. tuberosa* D.C., *Dicentra canadensis* Walp., *D. eximia* (Ker) Torr., *D. formosa* Walp., *D. oregana* Eastwood and *Glaucium fimbrilligerum*. The alkaloid crystallizes from EtOH with 0.5 mole of solvent, m.p. 124–5°C or from moist Et$_2$O as the hemihydrate, m.p. 129–130°C. The melting point given above is that of the anhydrous base. The alkaloid is readily soluble in CHCl$_3$, EtOH or AcOEt. It is laevorotatory with $[\alpha]_D^{26} - 206°$ (EtOH). The optically inactive form has m.p. 165–7°C and is somewhat less soluble in solvents than either of the two optically active forms.

Späth, Haworth., *Ber.*, **61**, 1692 (1928)
Gulland, Haworth., *J. Chem. Soc.*, 1834 (1928)
Go., *Chem. Abstr.*, **24**, 620 (1930)
Späth, Berger., *Ber.*, **64**, 2038 (1931)
Hey, Palluel., *J. Chem. Soc.*, 2926 (1957)
Arumugam *et al.*, *Chem. Ber.*, **91**, 40 (1958)

(+)-CORYDINE

$C_{20}H_{23}O_4N$

M.p. 149°C

This form of the alkaloid is present in *Corydalis tuberosa* DC, *Dicentra eximia* (Ker) Torr. and *Stephania venosa*. It has $[\alpha]_D^{26} + 209°$ and yields a hydrochloride, m.p. 258°C (*dec.*) and a methiodide, m.p. 228–230°C (*dec.*).

Manske., *Can. J. Res.*, **8**, 592 (1933)
Tomita, Furukawa, Ikeda., *J. Pharm. Soc., Japan*, **87**, 880 (1967)

CORYDININE

This alkaloid, isolated from *Corydalis stewartii* has been shown to be identical with Protopine (q.v.).

Ikran, Huq, Warsi., *Pakistan J. Sci. Ind. Res.,* **9**, 34 (1966)
Miana, Ikram, Warsi., *ibid,* **11**, 337 (1968)

CORYMINE

$C_{22}H_{26}O_4N_2$

M.p. 189–192°C

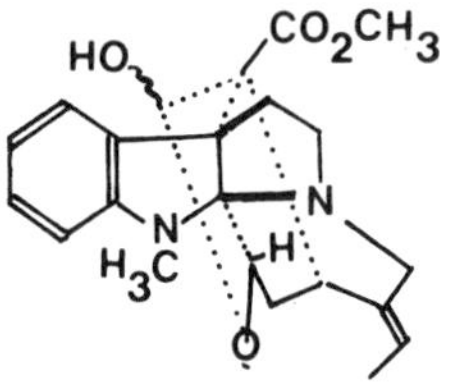

Isolated from *Hunteria corymbosa*, this alkaloid is dextrorotatory with $[\alpha]_D^{18}$ + 27.3° (CHCl$_3$). It furnishes a crystalline nitrate, m.p. 204–5°C; a picrate, m.p. 136–7°C; methiodide, m.p. 188–190°C and the O-acetyl derivative, m.p. 159–161°C. Heating with KOH decomposes the alkaloid to the deformyl derivative, m.p. 170–2°C.

Kiang, Smith., *Proc. Chem. Soc.,* 298 (1962)

(−)-CORYNANTHEIDINE

$C_{22}H_{28}O_3N_2$

M.p. 117°C

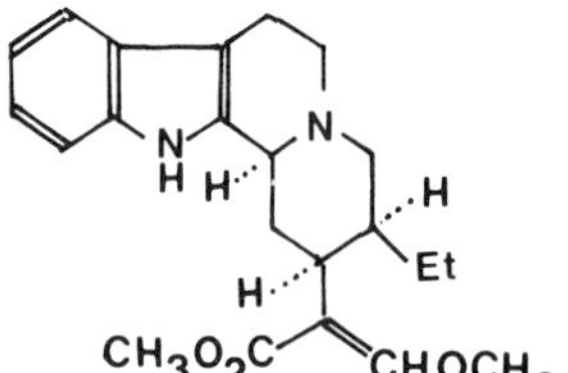

This isomeride of Corynantheine (q.v.) was isolated by Janot and Goutarel from the C_6H_6-soluble alkaloids of *Pseudocinchona africana*. It crystallizes with one mole of solvent from Me$_2$CO and has $[\alpha]_D^{15}$ − 142° (MeOH) or − 165° (MeOH) when freed of solvent. The alkaloid yields a hydrochloride as the dihydrate, m.p. 213°C; $[\alpha]_D^{15}$ − 128° (MeOH); a styphnate, m.p. 246°C; $[\alpha]_D^{14}$ − 138° (Me$_2$CO) and a picrate, m.p. 252°C; $[\alpha]_D^{15}$ − 152° (Me$_2$CO).

Janot, Goutarel., *Compt. rend.,* **218**, 852 (1944)
Tamelen, Aldrich, Katz., *J. Amer. Chem. Soc.,* **79**, 6426 (1957)
Bartlett *et al., ibid,* **84**, 622 (1962)

Synthesis:
Szantay, Barczai-Beke., *Tetrahedron Lett.,* **11**, 1405 (1968)
Weisbach *et al., ibid,* 3457 (1965)
Wenkert *et al., J. Amer. Chem. Soc.,* **89**, 6741 (1967)

CORYNANTHEINE

$C_{22}H_{28}O_3N_2$

M.p. Indefinite

An amorphous base found in the bark of *Pseudocinchona africana*, this alkaloid has $[\alpha]_D^{20} + 28.8°$ (MeOH) and yields a crystalline hydrochloride, m.p. 205°C; $[\alpha]_D^{20} + 43.8°$ (MeOH) or $+ 12.15°$ (H_2O), which is soluble in $CHCl_3$. Alkaline hydrolysis gives corynantheic acid, $C_{21}H_{26}O_3N_2$, which crystallizes from MeOH and has $[\alpha]_D^{21} + 7.53°$ (MeOH).

Karrer, Salomon., *Helv. Chim. Acta*, **9**, 1059 (1926)
Janot, Goutarel., *Bull. Soc. Chim.*, **8**, 625 (1941)
Karrer *et al.*, *Helv. Chim. Acta*, **34**, 933 (1951)
Janot *et al.*, *ibid*, **34**, 1207 (1951)
Karrer *et al.*, *ibid*, **35**, 851 (1952)

Synthesis:
Tamelen, Wright., *Tetrahedron Lett.*, 295 (1964)

CORYNANTHIDINE

$C_{21}H_{26}O_3N_2$

M.p. 243–4°C

Another crystalline alkaloid isolated from the bark of *Pseudocinchona africana*, this alkaloid is an isomeride of yohimbine (q.v.) and has $[\alpha]_D^{12} - 11.5°$ (MeOH) or $- 18.3°$ (pyridine). It forms a hydrochloride, m.p. 288°C; $[\alpha]_D^{12} + 57.4°$ (H_2O); a picrate, m.p. 231–2°C; $[\alpha]_D^{12} + 6°$ (Me_2CO) and a monoacetyl derivative, m.p. 231–2°C. On alkaline hydrolysis it furnishes corynanthidic acid, m.p. 322–3°C; $[\alpha]_D^{12} + 48.3°$ (pyridine) and on Se dehydrogenation it yields yobyrine, tetrahydroyobyrine and ketoyobyrine.

Janot, Goutarel., *Compt. rend.*, **206**, 1183 (1938)
Janot, Goutarel., *ibid*, **218**, 852 (1944)
Janot, Goutarel., *ibid*, **220**, 617 (1945)
Janot, Goutarel., *Bull. Soc. Chim.*, **10**, 383 (1943)

CORYNANTHINE

$C_{21}H_{26}O_3N_2$

M.p. 242°C

A fourth crystalline alkaloid isolated from the bark of *Pseudocinchona africana,* this base is the *cis*-isomer of Yohimbine (q.v.) and has $[\alpha]_D - 125°$ (EtOH) or $- 73°$ (pyridine). It forms a hydrochloride, m.p. 285–290°C; $[\alpha]_D - 63°$ (H_2O); a monoacetyl derivative, m.p. 147°C; $[\alpha]_D - 60.4°$ (pyridine) and a diacetyl compound, m.p. 194–5°C; $[\alpha]_D - 105°$ (pyridine). Hydrolysis with dilute mineral acids yields corynanthic acid.

Fourneau, Fiore., *Bull. Soc. Chim. Fr.,* **9**, 1037 (1911)
Janot, Goutarel., *ibid,* **10**, 383 (1943)
Janot *et al., ibid,* 1085 (1952)

CORYNOLINE

$C_{21}H_{24}O_5N$

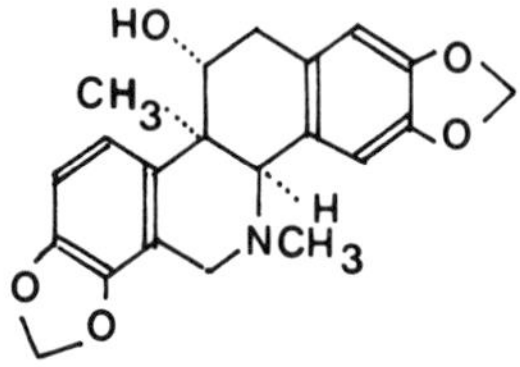

This alkaloid has been reported from *Corydalis incisa* Pers. The crystal structure of the *p*-bromobenzoyl derivative has recently been determined by X-ray analysis and it has also been demonstrated that the B and C rings are fused in the *cis* position. The hydroxyl group is axial. The Emde degradation of the acetate gives a product which, on Hofmann degradation, yields Corynoxoline (q.v.).

Takao., *Chem. Pharm. Bull.,* **11**, 1306, 1312 (1963)
Naruto, Arakawa, Kanedo., *Tetrahedron Lett.,* 1705 (1968)
Takao, Bersch, Takao., *Chem. Pharm. Bull.,* **19**, 259 (1971)

Crystal structure:
Kametani *et al., Tetrahedron Lett.,* 3729 (1972)

(+)-14-*epi*-CORYNOLINE

$C_{21}H_{24}O_5N$

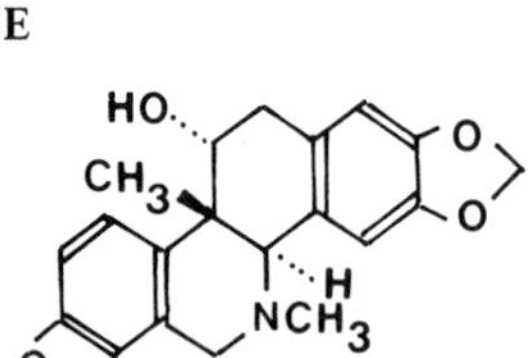

A further minor alkaloid of *Corydalis incisa,* the structure of the base has been determined from spectroscopic and chemical data.

Takao, Bersch, Takao., *Chem. Pharm. Bull.,* **21**, 1096 (1973)

340

CORYNOLOXINE

$C_{21}H_{19}O_5N$

M.p. 209–210°C

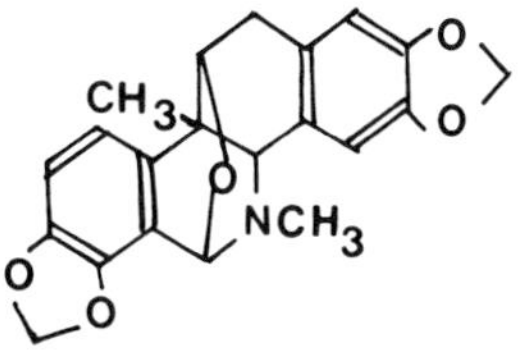

A minor constituent of *Corydalis incisa,* this alkaloid crystallizes as colourless needles from either MeOH or CHCl₃. Like the preceding alkaloids, the B and C rings have been shown to be *cis* fused. Reduction with LiAlH₄ yields Corynoline (q.v.).

Takao., *Chem. Pharm. Bull.,* **19**, 247 (1971)
Takao, Bersch, Takao., *ibid,* **19**, 259 (1971)

CORYNOXEINE

$C_{22}H_{26}O_4N_2$

M.p. 210°C

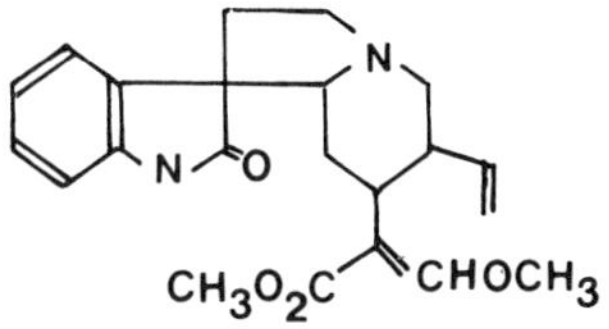

An alkaloid found in the bark of *Pseudocinchona africana,* this base forms colourless, prismatic needles from CHCl₃. It has $[\alpha]_D + 23°$ (c 1.0, pyridine) or $- 21.5°$ (c 1.0, CHCl₃). The alkaloid may be reduced to the dihydro derivative which is identical with Rhyncophylline (q.v.).

Cu, Goutarel, Janot., *Bull. Soc. Chim. Fr.,* 1292 (1957)
Finch, Taylor., *J. Amer. Chem. Soc.,* **84**, 3871 (1962)

CORYNOXINE

$C_{22}H_{28}O_4N_2$

M.p. 166–8°C

A further base present in *Pseudocinchona africana,* this alkaloid is also obtained in the form of colourless, prismatic needles. It has $[\alpha]_D - 14°$ (c 1.0, pyridine).

Cu, Goutarel, Janot., *Bull. Soc. Chim. Fr.,* 1292 (1957)

CORYPALLINE

$C_{11}H_{15}O_2N$

M.p. 168°C

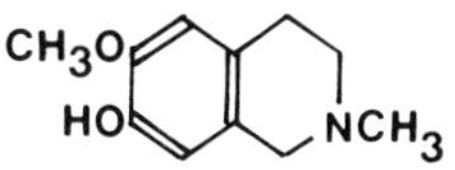

This alkaloid has been obtained from the seeds of *Corydalis aurea* Willd. and *C. pallida* Pers. The alkaloid is a phenolic base and yields a crystalline picrate,

341

m.p. 178°C and a methyl ether, m.p. 82°C. On ethylation it gives 2-methyl-6-methoxy-7-ethoxytetrahydro*iso*quinoline, m.p. 65°C indicating that the free hydroxyl is present at C-7. This has been confirmed by synthesis of the alkaloid.

Manske., *Can. J. Res.*, **15B**, 159 (1937)

(+)-CORYPALMINE

$C_{20}H_{23}O_4N$

M.p. 235–6°C

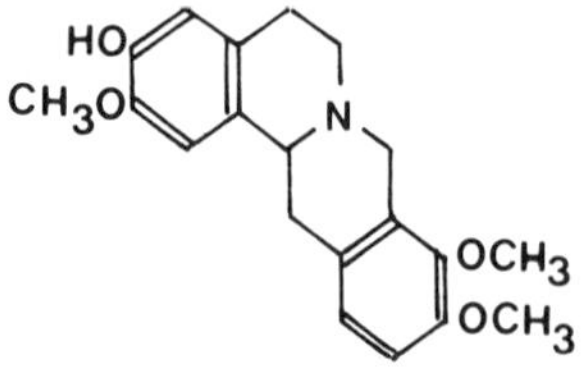

This alkaloid has, so far, only been obtained from *Corydalis tuberosa* DC. It has $[\alpha]_D^{16} + 280°$ (CHCl$_3$). With CH$_2$N$_2$ it is methylated to (+)-tetrahydropalmatine. The position of the hydroxyl group was determined by Späth and Mosettig by oxidizing the ethyl ether with KMnO$_4$ to 7-methoxy-6-ethoxy-1-keto-1:2:3:4-tetrahydro*iso*quinoline.

Späth, Mosettig, Trothandl., *Ber.*, **56**, 877 (1923)
Späth, Mosettig., *Arch. Pharm.*, **58**, 2133 (1925)

(−)-CORYPALMINE

$C_{20}H_{23}O_4N$

M.p. 230°C

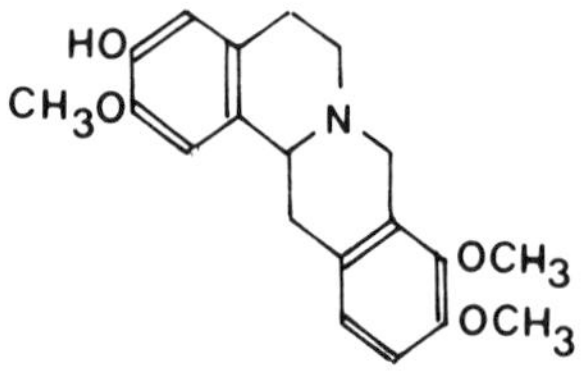

This alkaloid is of more widespread occurrence than the preceding base, being found in *Berberis floribunda*, *B. himaloica*, *Coptis Teeta*, *Corydalis cheilanthei-folia* Hemsl., *C. incisa*, *C. ochroleuca* Koch., *C. ophiocarpa* Hook, *C. thalictrifolia* Franch and *Dicentra oregana* Eastwood.

Gadamer, Knörck., *Apoth. Zeit.*, **41**, 928 (1926)
Manske., *Can. J. Res.*, **17B**, 51, 95 (1939)
Manske., *ibid*, **20B**, 57 (1942)
Chatterjee, Juha, Gupta., *J. Ind. Chem. Soc.*, **29**, 921 (1952)

(±)-CORYPALMINE

$C_{20}H_{23}O_4N$

M.p. 215–7°C

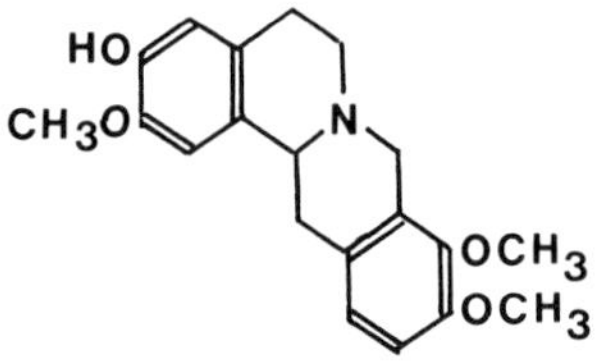

The optically inactive form of this alkaloid is present only in *Corydalis caseana* A. Gray. It may also be prepared by mixing equimolar amounts of the two active forms and crystallizing the mixture.

Manske., *Can. J. Res.,* **16B**, 153 (1935)
Manske., *ibid,* **18B**, 288 (1940)
Corrodi, Hardegger., *Helv. Chim. Acta,* **39**, 889 (1956)
Govindachari, Rajadurai, Ramada., *Chem. Ber.,* **92**, 1654 (1959)

CORYSAMINE

This alkaloid exists as the chloride in *Chelidonium majus.* Reduction with Zn and HCl yields tetrahydrocorysamine m.p. $201-2°C$, obtained as colourless crystals from $CHCl_3$-MeOH.

Slavik, Slavikova, Brabenec., *Collect. Czech. Chem. Commun.,* **30**, 3697 (1965)

CORYTUBERINE

$C_{19}H_{21}O_4N$

M.p. 240°C

Obtained from *Corydalis nobilis* Pers., *C. tuberosa* D.C., *Dicentra formosa* Walp. and *Glaucium vitellum,* this alkaloid forms colourless needles from EtOH. It has $[\alpha]_D^{20} + 282.65°$ (EtOH) and is insoluble in most organic solvents, but soluble in hot H_2O. The solution in EtOH exhibits a violet fluorescence. When dissolved in alkalies, the solution darkens rapidly on exposure to air. The salts are crystalline but unstable. On methylation it yields a mixture of corydine and *iso*corydine. The O,O-dimethyl ether has b.p. $200-240°C/0.06$ mm and forms a methiodide, m.p. 248°C. The corresponding diethyl ether is amorphous and is oxidized with $KMnO_4$ to 4-methoxy-3-ethoxyphthalic acid, characterized by the ethylimide, m.p. 85°C.

Corytuberine does not induce narcosis in frogs but induces increased reflex irritability. In warm-blooded animals it gives rise to tonic convulsions and stimulates the secretion of saliva and tears. It also slows the pulse rate by vagus action, increasing the blood pressure during convulsions.

The (±)-form crystallizes as leaflets from MeOH, m.p. 242°C. It forms a crystalline hydrochloride, m.p. 250°C (*dec.*).

Dobbie, Lauder., *J. Chem. Soc.,* **63**, 485 (1893)
Gadamer., *Arch. Pharm.,* **249**, 641 (1911)
Shinoda., *Chem. Abstr.,* **21**, 2272 (1927)
Gulland, Haworth., *J. Chem. Soc.,* 1834 (1928)
Späth, Berger., *Ber.,* **64**, 2038 (1931)
Manske., *Can. J. Res.,* **10**, 521 (1934)
Tomita, Kikkawa., *J. Pharm. Soc. Japan,* **77**, 195 (1957)
Slavik., *Collect. Czech. Chem. Commun.,* **24**, 3999 (1959)

COSTACLAVINE

$C_{16}H_{20}N_2$

M.p. 182–4°C

One of the ergot alkaloids produced by *Claviceps purpurea* (Fries) Tul. and by *Penicillium chermesinum*. The base has $[\alpha]_D^{20} + 44°$ (c 0.2, pyridine) and the ultraviolet spectrum shows absorption maxima at 275, 282 and 293 mμ.

Abe *et al., Bull. Agric. Chem. Soc. Japan,* **20**, 59 (1956)
Agurell., *Experientia,* **20**, 25 (1964)

COULTEROPINE

$C_{21}H_{21}O_6N$

M.p. 168–170°C

An alkaloid found in the roots of *Romneya coulteri* var. *trichocalyx* (Eastwood) Jepson, the base is obtained as white crystals from C_6H_6. The ultraviolet spectrum shows a single absorption maximum at 286 mμ. The salts are crystalline, the hydrochloride, m.p. 149–150°C; hydrobromide, rhomboidal prisms, m.p. 231–2°C and the methiodide, m.p. 198–200°C.

The infrared evidence shows clearly that the acid salts cannot be represented as the N-protonated structure but involve closure of the 10-membered ring, although NMR studies indicate that, under carefully controlled conditions, such salts can be prepared where no ring closure occurs. These studies also show that whereas the freshly formed salts have the trans configuration, on standing a proportion of the cis compound is also formed.

Stermitz, Chen, White., *Tetrahedron,* **22**, 1095 (1966)
Stermitz, Coomes, Harris., *Tetrahedron Lett.,* 3915 (1968)

COUMINGIDINE

$C_{28}H_{45}O_6N$

M.p. 160–1°C

This alkaloid from the bark of *Erythrophleum couminga* is best isolated as the nitroso compound, m.p. 174°C from which the free base is obtained by the action of cuprous chloride. The base forms a hydrochloride, m.p. 217–9°C; an acetyl derivative, m.p. 155°C and a phenylthiocarbamate, m.p. 146°C. Catalytic hydrogenation yields the dihydro derivative, isolated as the perchlorate, m.p. 166–8°C, and forming an acetyl derivative, m.p. 115–116.5°C. Alkaline hydrolysis gives, among other products, cassaic acid.

Schlittler., *Helv. Chim. Acta,* **24,** 319E (1941)
Jones, Kenner., *J. Chem. Soc.,* 713 (1932)

COUMINGINE

$C_{29}H_{47}O_6N$

M.p. 142°C

This alkaloid was isolated from the bark of *Erythrophleum couminga* by Dalma, the original formula of $C_{28}H_{45}O_6N$ being changed to that now given. The base has $[\alpha]_D^{20} - 70°$ (EtOH) and forms a hydrochloride, m.p. 195°C and an oxime, m.p. 165°C. The crude alkaloid, but not the purified form, reacts with Ac_2O in pyridine to form the acetyl derivative, m.p. 154–5°C. The alkaloid may be hydrogenated using PtO_2 as catalyst to give the dihydro derivative, m.p. 95–6°C; $[\alpha]_D^{20} + 8°$ (EtOH), yielding a hydrochloride, m.p. 160–2°C and converted by KOH in EtOH to ketohydroxycassanic acid, $C_{20}H_{32}O_4$. On acid hydrolysis, the base furnishes dimethylaminoethanol and coumingic acid, $C_{25}H_{38}O_6$, m.p. 200°C; $[\alpha]_D^{20} - 81°$ (EtOH), methyl ester, m.p. 217–8°C; $[\alpha]_D^{20} - 83°$ (EtOH), oxime, m.p. 124–5°C. Alkaline hydrolysis yields cassaic acid, $C_{20}H_{30}O_4$, m.p. 223–4°C; $[\alpha]_D^{20} - 123°$ (EtOH), methyl ester, m.p. 188–9°C; $[\alpha]_D^{20} - 124°$ (EtOH). From the above results, it is concluded that the alkaloid is the α-hydroxy*iso*valerate of cassaine.

Ruzicka, Dalma, Scott., *Helv. Chim. Acta,* **24,** 63, 1449 (1941)

CRASSANINE

$C_{23}H_{30}O_5N_2$

Isolated from *Tabernaemontana crassa,* this alkaloid is isomeric with 20-hydroxy-conopharyngine (q.v.). It has been assigned the oxindole conopharyngine structure mainly on the basis of NMR data.

Cava, Watanabe, Bessho., *J. Org. Chem.,* **33,** 3350 (1968)

CREBANINE

$C_{20}H_{21}O_4N$

M.p. 126°C

This aporphine alkaloid occurs in *Stephania capitata* and *S. sasakii,* forming colourless needles with $[\alpha]_D^{20} - 57.5°$ (CHCl$_3$). It contains two methoxyl, one methylenedioxy and one methylimino group in the molecule.

Tomita, Shirai., *J. Pharm. Soc., Japan,* **62**, 381 (1942)

Tomita, Shirai., *ibid,* **63**, 233, 517, 532 (1943)

Tomita, Shirai., *ibid,* **78**, 733 (1958)

Tomita, Kishikita., *ibid,* **64**, 240 (1944)

Govindachari, Nagarajan, Ramadas., *J. Chem. Soc.,* 983 (1958)

CRENATIDINE

$C_{15}H_{16}O_2N_2$

M.p. 157–8°C

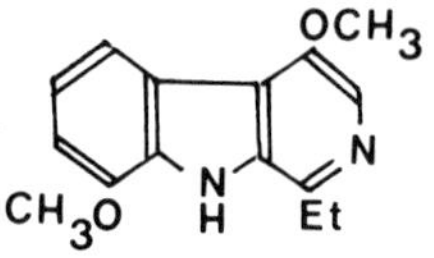

A β-carboline alkaloid occurring in the bark of *Aeschrion crenata* Vell. The ultraviolet spectrum shows absorption maxima in EtOH at 243, 267, 283, 334 and 346 mμ. The structure has been shown, by chemical and spectroscopic evidence, to be 1-ethyl-4:8-dimethoxy-β-carboline.

Sanchez, Comin., *Phytochem.,* **10**, 2155 (1971)

CRENATINE

$C_{14}H_{14}ON_2$

M.p. 177–9°C

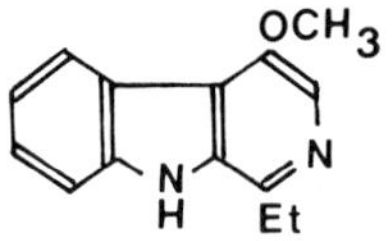

A further constituent of the bark of *Aeschrion crenata* Vell. The ultraviolet spectrum of this alkaloid in EtOH is very similar to that of the preceding base, having absorption maxima at 243, 265, 274, 284, 331 and 348 mμ. The structure is that of 1-ethyl-4-methoxy-β-carboline.

Sanchez, Comin., *Phytochem.,* **10**, 2155 (1971)

CREPIDAMINE

$C_{18}H_{25}O_2N$

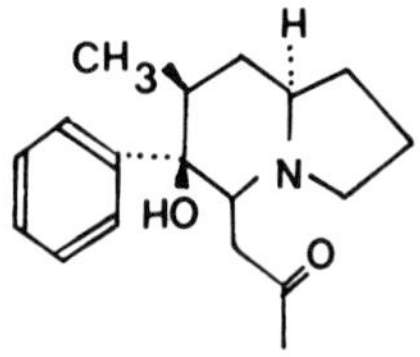

This alkaloid from *Dendrobium crepidatum* is epimeric with the following base. The structure has been established by spectropic methods, particularly X-ray and NMR spectra.

Elander *et al., Acta Chem. Scand.,* **27**, 1907 (1973)

CREPIDINE

$C_{18}H_{25}O_2N$

M.p. 221–2°C

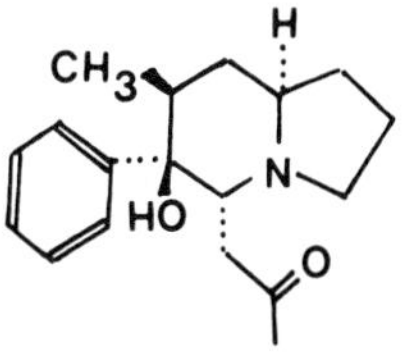

Isolated from *Dendrobium crepidatum*, this alkaloid forms colourless needles when recrystallized from EtOH. It has $[\alpha]_D^{24} - 78°$ (c 0.5, CHCl$_3$) and forms a crystalline methiodide, m.p. 240–2°C (*dec.*). The crystal structure has been determined by X-ray analysis.

Kierkegaard, Pilotti, Leander., *Acta Chem. Scand.*, 24, 3757 (1970)
Elander *et al.*, *ibid*, 27, 1907 (1973)

CINALBINE

$C_{17}H_{19}O_5N$

M.p. 235–6°C

One of the alkaloids isolated from *Crinium powellii*, this base has $[\alpha]_D^{25} - 23°$ (c 0.2, CHCl$_3$). It has been shown to be the optical antipode of Crinamidine (q.v.).

Boit, Döpke., *Naturwiss.*, 47, 498 (1960)

CRINAMIDINE

$C_{17}H_{19}O_5N$

M.p. 235–6°C

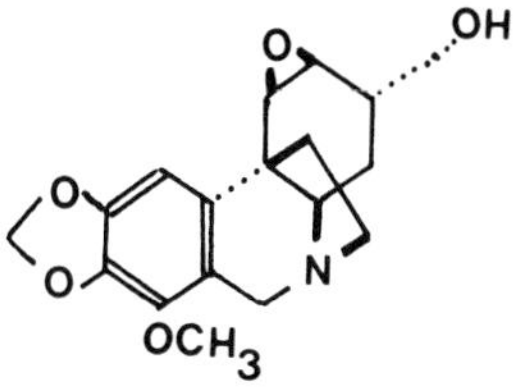

This alkaloid is present in *Crinium moorei* Hook F. and is also found in certain *Nerine* species. It forms colourless needles from Me$_2$CO and has $[\alpha]_D^{23} - 24°$ (c 0.6, CHCl$_3$). It yields a crystalline methiodide, m.p. 263–6°C (*dec.*) and a picrate, m.p. 131–2°C. With concentrated H$_2$SO$_4$ it gives a deep red colour.

Boit, Ehmke., *Chem. Ber.*, 87, 1704 (1954)
Boit, Ehmke., *ibid*, 89, 2093 (1956)
Boit, Ehmke., *ibid*, 90, 369 (1957)
Lyle *et al.*, *J. Amer. Chem. Soc.*, 82, 2620 (1960)
Fales, Wildman., *J. Org. Chem.*, 26, 181 (1961)

CRINAMINE

$C_{17}H_{19}O_4N$

M.p. 198–9°C

One of the minor Amaryllidaceous alkaloids, this base occurs mainly in *Crinium asiaticum* L. It has $[\alpha]_D^{28} + 156.6°$ (c 1.65, $CHCl_3$) and the ultraviolet spectrum exhibits absorption maxima at 234–240 and 297 mμ. The perchlorate is crystalline with m.p. 201–201.5° (*dec.*), as is the picrate, m.p. 273–4°C (*dec.*) and the O-acetate, m.p. 161.5–163°C; $[\alpha]_D^{24} + 18.2°$ (c 0.55, $CHCl_3$).

Kutani, Matsumoto., *J. Pharm. Soc., Japan,* **64**, 239 (1944)
Mason, Puschett, Wildman., *J. Amer. Chem. Soc.,* **77**, 1253 (1955)
Jeffs, Warren, Wright., *J. Chem. Soc.,* 1090 (1960)

Mass spectra:
Duffield *et al., J. Amer. Chem. Soc.,* **87**, 4902 (1965)

Stereochemistry:
Fales, Wildman., *Chem. & Ind.,* 561 (1958)
Wildman, Fales., *J. Amer. Chem. Soc.,* **80**, 6465 (1958)

CRININE (*Crinidine*)

$C_{16}H_{17}O_3N$

M.p. 208–210°C

This alkaloid occurs in several species including *Buphane Fischeri* Baker, *Calostemma purpureum, Crinium moorei* Hook., *Nerine bowdenii* and *Zephyranthus* species. Boit and Ehmke give $[\alpha]_D^{22} - 44°$ (c 0.48, $CHCl_3$), $- 25°$ (c 1.02, $CHCl_3$) and $- 11°$ (c 2.04, $CHCl_3$) but other workers have found the following specific rotations: $[\alpha]_D^{20} - 23°$ (c 0.5, $CHCl_3$), $- 19°$ (c 1.0, $CHCl_3$), $- 9.6°$ (c 2.0, $CHCl_3$) and $- 21°$ (EtOH). With strong H_2SO_4 the alkaloid gives a yellow colour. Crystalline salts and derivatives have been prepared including the perchlorate, m.p. 135–7°C; methiodide, m.p. 198°C; picrate, m.p. 237–9°C and the O-acetate with m.p. 145–6°C; $[\alpha]_D^{20} + 68°$ (c 1.11, 95% EtOH). On reduction with Pt in HCl, the base yields the dihydro derivative, m.p. 212–3°C.

Boit, Ehmke., *Chem. Ber.,* **87**, 1704 (1954)
Renz, Stauffacher, Seebeck., *Helv. Chim. Acta,* **38**, 1209 (1955)
Mason, Puschett, Wildman., *J. Amer. Chem. Soc.,* **77**, 1253 (1955)
Wildman., *ibid,* **78**, 4180 (1956)
Boit, Ehmke., *Chem. Ber.,* **89**, 2093 (1956)
Boit, Döpke., *ibid,* **90**, 369, 2203 (1957)
Fales, Wildman., *J. Amer. Chem. Soc.,* **82**, 197 (1960)
Jeffs, Warren, Wright., *J. Chem. Soc.,* 1090 (1960)
Lyle *et al., J. Amer. Chem. Soc.,* **82**, 2620 (1960)
Boit, Döpke., *Naturwiss.,* **48**, 406 (1961)

Synthesis:
Muxfeldt, Schneider, Mooberry., *J. Amer. Chem. Soc.,* **88**, 3670 (1966)
Whitlock, Smith., *ibid,* **89**, 3600 (1967)

Mass spectra:
Duffield *et al., ibid,* **87**, 4902 (1965)

(+)-*epi*-CRININE

$C_{16}H_{17}O_3N$

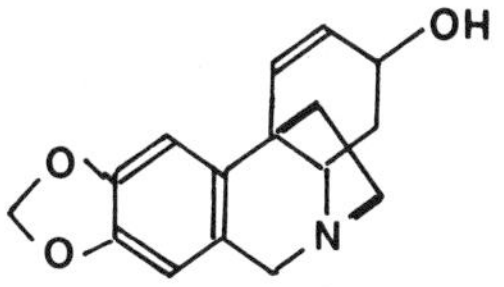

This alkaloid is a minor constituent of the bulbs of *Nerine bowdenii.* The stereochemistry has been elucidated from the NMR spectra.

Lyle *et al., J. Amer. Chem. Soc.,* **82**, 2620 (1960)

CRINOSINE

$C_{17}H_{21}O_4N$

M.p. 195°C

An alkaloid isolated from *Crinium powellii,* the base forms colourless prisms and is dextrorotatory with $[\alpha]_D^{21} + 210°$ (c 0.2, EtOH).

Döpke, Fritsch., *Pharmazie,* **20**, 586 (1965)

CRIOPHYLLINE

$C_{40}H_{46}O_4N_4$

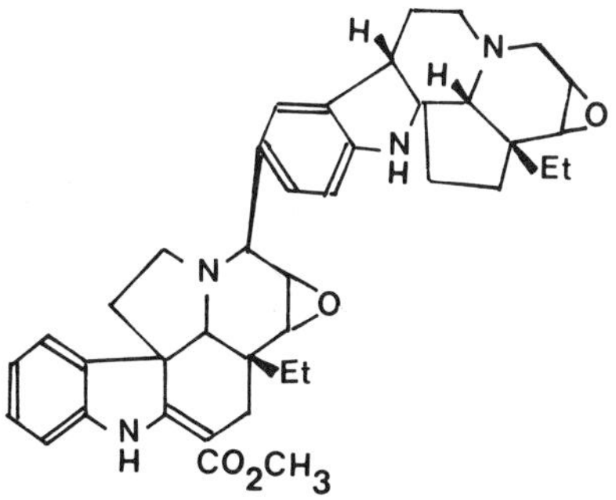

A dimeric imidazolidinocarbazole alkaloid, the above structure has been determined on the basis of carbon-13 NMR spectra.

Cave *et al., Tetrahedron Lett.,* 5081 (1973)

CRIPALINE

$C_{16}H_{17}O_3N$

M.p. 198–9°C

This alkaloid occurs in *Crinium powellii* var. *harlemense* and is obtained from the alkaloidal extract by countercurrent distribution methods. It crystallizes as colourless needles from Me_2CO and is dextrorotatory with $[\alpha]_D^{24} + 50°$ (c 0.2, $CHCl_3$). The alkaloid is characterized as the perchlorate, m.p. 257–8°C and the picrate, m.p. 185–6°C. With MnO_2 in $CHCl_3$, the base yields an unsaturated ketone, m.p. 166°C. The base has been shown to be the optical isomer of Powellamine (q.v.).

Döpke., *Arch. Pharm.*, **295**, 868 (1962)

CRISPANINE

$C_{18}H_{21}O_5N$

M.p. 139–141°C

Isolated from *Nerine crispa* Hort., this base has $[\alpha]_D^{24} + 78°$ (c 0.2, $CHCl_3$). It forms a crystalline perchlorate, m.p. 221°C (*dec.*) and a picrate, m.p. 201°C (*dec.*). With concentrated H_2SO_4 it gives an intense blue colour.

Döpke., *Naturwiss.*, **49**, 469 (1962)

CRISPATINE

$C_{16}H_{23}O_5N$

M.p. 137–8°C

A pyrrolizidine alkaloid isolated from *Crotalaria crispata* F. Muell., the base forms colourless needles when recrystallized from light petroleum and has $[\alpha]_D^{20} + 40.7°$ (c 1.94, EtOH). Alkaline hydrolysis furnishes retronecine and crispatic acid, the latter shown to be 3-hydroxy-2:3:4-trimethylglutaric acid.

Culvenor, Smith., *Austral. J. Chem.*, **16**, 239 (1963)

CRISPINE

$C_{18}H_{23}O_6N$

M.p. 275°C (*dec.*).

This alkaloid occurs in *Nerine undulata* and crystallizes from Me_2CO as colourless rods with $[\alpha]_D - 96°$ (c 0.25, $CHCl_3$). It forms crystalline salts, e.g. the perchlorate, m.p. 268–9° (*dec.*), methoperchlorate, m.p. 282–3°C (*dec.*) and the picrate, m.p. 258°C (*dec.*).

Boit., *Chem. Ber.,* **89**, 1129 (1956)

CRIWELLINE (*Criucelline*)

$C_{18}H_{21}O_5N$

M.p. 205–6°C

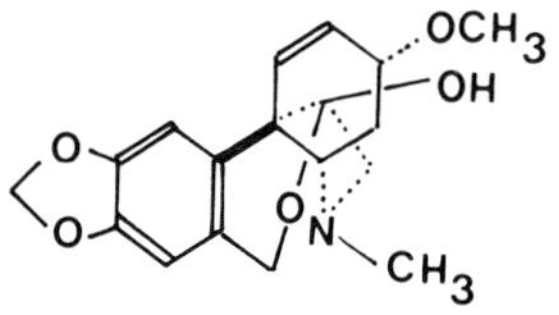

One of the alkaloids isolated from *Nerine powellii,* the base crystallizes as colourless columnar rods from Me$_2$CO. It has $[\alpha]_D^{25} + 220°$ (c 0.15, CHCl$_3$). The perchlorate forms colourless prisms from H$_2$O, m.p. 217–8°C; the hydriodide has m.p. 228–9°C and the picrate, m.p. 233°C. The structure has been determined from both chemical and spectroscopic data.

Boit, Ehmke., *Chem. Ber.,* **89**, 2093 (1956)
Fales, Horn, Wildman., *Chem. & Ind.,* 1415 (1959)
Jeffs, Warren, Wright., *J. Chem. Soc.,* 1090 (1960)

Mass spectra:
Duffield *et al., J. Amer. Chem. Soc.,* **87**, 4902 (1965)

NMR spectra:
Haugwitz, Jeffs, Wenkert., *J. Chem. Soc.,* 2001 (1965)

CROALBIDINE

$C_{18}H_{29}O_7N$

M.p. 208–9°C

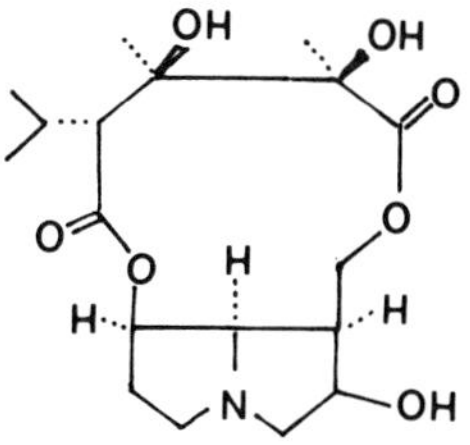

A pyrrolizidine alkaloid present in *Crotalaria albida,* the base has been shown by spectroscopy and chemical evidence to be the diester of croalbinecine and trichodesmic acid.

Sawhney, Atal., *Ind. J. Chem.,* **11**, 88 (1973)

CROBARBATINE

$C_{14}H_{21}O_5N$

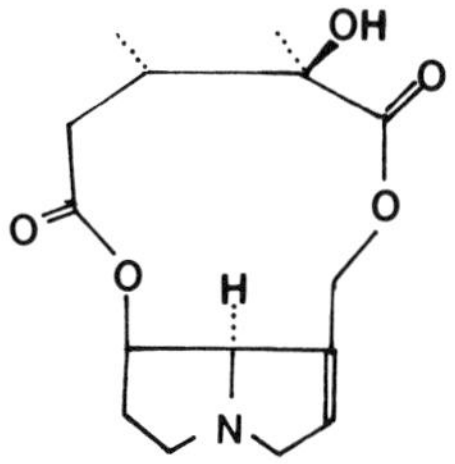

The seeds of *Crotalaria barbata* have recently been shown to contain this pyrrolizidine alkaloid, the structure of which has been elucidated from chemical and spectroscopic data.

Puri, Sawhney, Atal., *Experientia*, **29**, 390 (1973)

CROSEMPERINE

$C_{19}H_{29}O_6N$

M.p. 117–8°C

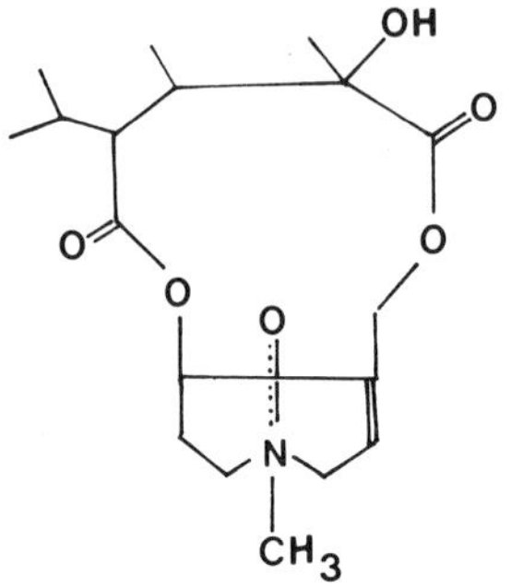

A pyrrolizidine alkaloid obtained from *Crotalaria semperflorens* Vent. The base is dextrorotatory with $[\alpha]_D^{29} + 45°$ (CHCl$_3$) or $[\alpha]_D^{20} + 2.2°$ (c 1.5, EtOH). The hydrochloride is crystalline and has m.p. 180°C (*dec.*); the methiodide crystallizes from EtOH-CHCl$_3$ with m.p. 208–9°C (*dec.*) and the reineckate has m.p. 151–2°C. The structure follows from the acid hydrolysis to otonecine and incanic acid, m.p. 163–4°C, the formation of dihydrodeoxyotonecine on hydrogenolysis and the infrared, NMR and mass spectra.

Atal *et al.*, *Austral. J. Chem.*, **20**, 805 (1967)

CROSSOPTINE

$C_{22}H_{28}O_4N_2$

M.p. 218–9°C

This alkaloid was isolated from *Crossopteryx kotschyana* Fenzl. by Blaise and has subsequently been re-examined by Raymond-Hamet who found $[\alpha]_D - 24°$ (CHCl$_3$). The latter has suggested that it is identical with mitrinermine, now renamed Rhyncophylline (q.v.). Raymond-Hamet also considered that the bark used in the original isolation was derived from a *Mitragyna* species.

Blaise., *Les Crossopteryx africains. Etude botanique. Thesis,* Paris, (1932)
Raymond-Hamet., *Bull. Sci. Pharmacol.*, **47**, 194 (1940)

CROTAFOLINE

$C_{18}H_{25}O_6N$

M.p. 176–182°C (dec.).

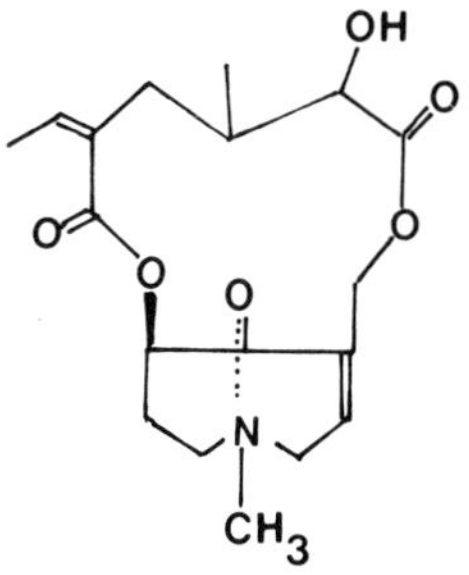

A pyrrolizidine alkaloid occurring in *Crotalaria laburnifolia* L. subsp. eldomae. The base forms colourless crystals from Me₂CO.

Crout., *J. Chem. Soc., Perkin I,* 1602 (1972)

CROTALABURNINE

M.p. 185–6°C (dec.); (194–5°C)

This alkaloid was first isolated from the seeds of *Crotalaria laburnifolia* of Indian origin by Emmanuel and Ghosh and examined by Snehelata and his colleagues who found a m.p. of 185–6°C (dec.). The higher melting point was found by Subramanian and Nagarajan for the base obtained from the seeds of *C. verrucosa.* There is now some evidence that the alkaloid is identical with Anacrotine (q.v.).

Emmanuel, Ghosh., *Ind. J. Pharm.,* **26**, 322 (1964)
Snehelata *et al., ibid,* **28**, 277 (1966)
Subramanian, Nagarajan., *ibid,* **29**, 311 (1967)

CROTASTRIATINE

$C_{19}H_{25}O_6N$

M.p. 133°C

This pyrrolizidine alkaloid has been obtained from the seeds of *Crotalaria striata.* It has $[\alpha]_D^{26} + 9.6°$ (c 1.04, CHCl₃) and + 32.2° (c 1.24, EtOH). Hydrolysis with Ba(OH)₂ yields retronecine and striatic acid, m.p. 138°C; $[\alpha]_D^{25} - 14.0°$ (c 1.0, EtOH) with the formula $C_9H_{14}O_5$. The manner in which the two fragments are linked is still undecided.

Gandi, Rajagopalan, Seshadri., *Curr. Sci.,* **37**, 285 (1968)

CROTONOSINE

$C_{17}H_{17}O_3N$

M.p. 300°C

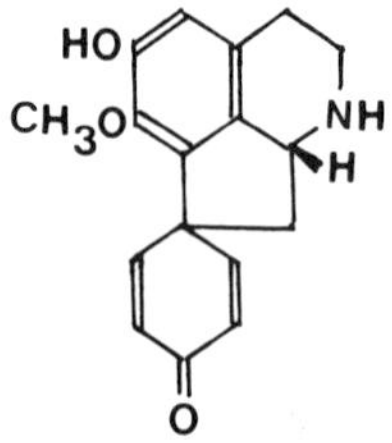

Isolated from *Croton linearis*, this alkaloid darkens at 165°C and softens around 197°C. It has $[\alpha]_D^{28} + 180°$ (c 0.83, MeOH) and the ultraviolet spectrum exhibits absorption maxima at 226, 235, 282 and 290 mμ. The methiodide crystallizes as colourless rods from MeOH and melts above 250°C. The O,N-diacetyl derivative has m.p. 203–5°C. The O-methyl ether is Stepharine (q.v.) and the O,N-dimethyl derivative is Pronuciferine (q.v.).

Hayes, Stuart., *J. Chem. Soc.*, 1784, 1789 (1963)
Hayes *et al.*, *Proc. Chem. Soc.*, 280 (1963)
Hayes *et al.*, *ibid*, 261 (1964)

Mass spectra:
Baldwin *et al.*, *J. Chem. Soc.*, C, 154 (1967)

Biosynthesis:
Haynes *et al.*, *Chem. Commun.*, 141 (1965)
Barton *et al.*, *J. Chem. Soc.*, C. 1295 (1967)

CROTSPARINE

$C_{17}H_{17}O_3N$

M.p. 193–5°C

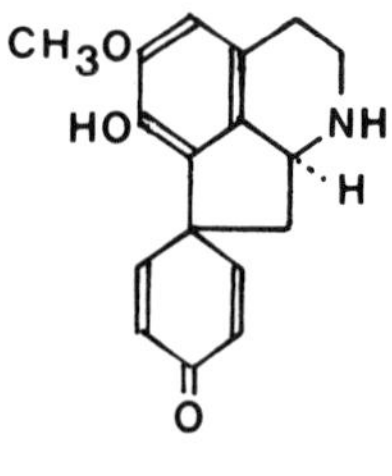

This alkaloid is present in *Croton sparsiflorus* Morong. It has $[\alpha]_D - 30°$ (c 1.22, CHCl$_3$), the ultraviolet spectrum showing a single absorption maximum at 235 mμ. The hydrochloride is crystalline, m.p. 278°C (*dec.*); the O,N-diacetyl derivative, m.p. 185–6°C and the N-methyl compound, m.p. 233–5°C; $[\alpha]_D - 113°$ (c 1.52, CHCl$_3$) are also crystalline. It is interesting to note that the base isolated from plants grown in Calcutta is laevorotatory while that obtained from similar plants grown in Lucknow is dextrorotatory.

Bhakuni, Dhar., *Experientia*, **24**, 10 (1968)

CROTSPARININE

$C_{17}H_{19}O_3N$

M.p. 184–5°C

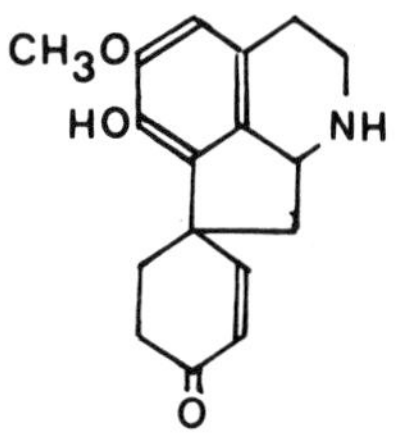

A second alkaloid occurring in *Croton sparsiflorus* Morong., this base has $[\alpha]_D$ + 215° (c 2.37, CHCl$_3$). The ultraviolet spectrum shows absorption maxima at 228 and 285 mμ. The N-methyl derivative is crystalline with m.p. 160–1°C; $[\alpha]_D$ + 244° (c 0.92, CHCl$_3$), identical with an isomer of Linearisine (q.v.).

Bhakuni, Dhar., *Experientia*, **25**, 354 (1969)

CRYCHINE

This alkaloid occurs in the phenolic portion of the alkaloidal extract from *Cryptocarya chinensis*. It is laevorotatory with $[\alpha]_D^{15}$ − 220.2° (c 1.0, EtOH) and forms a crystalline picrate, m.p. 177°C and methiodide, m.p. 286°C (*dec.*).

Lu, Lan., *J. Pharm. Soc., Japan*, **86**, 177 (1966)

CRYKONISINE

$C_{18}H_{17}O_3N$

M.p. 235–6°C (*dec.*).

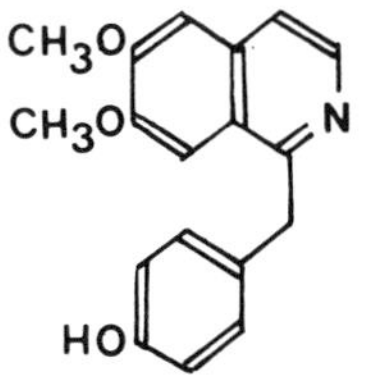

An alkaloid of the benzyl*iso*quinoline group, this base occurs in *Cryptocarya konishii* and forms colourless needles when recrystallized from MeOH. When reduced with Zn and HCl it yields optically inactive N-norarmepavine.

Lu., *J. Pharm. Soc., Japan*, **87**, 1278 (1967)

CRYPTAUSTOLINE

$C_{20}H_{24}O_4N^+$

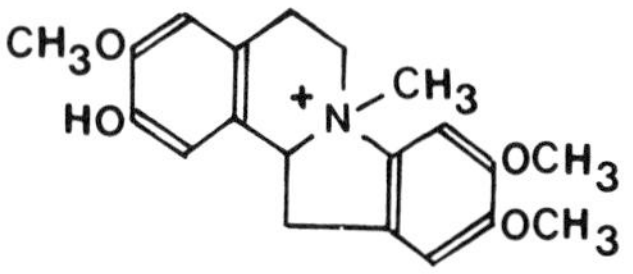

A quaternary alkaloid occurring in *Cryptocarya bowiei*, this base is normally isolated as the iodide, m.p. 214°C (*dec.*); $[\alpha]_D^{20}$ − 151° (EtOH). The O-ethyl derivative has m.p. 90–5°C. When the alkaloid is refluxed with methyl iodide and KOH it yields O-methylcryptaustoline iodide, m.p. 80–90°C as the dihydrate and 153–4°C (*dry*). This salt, on refluxing with NaOH, gives O-methyl-cryptaustoline methine iodide, m.p. 101°C; $[\alpha]_D^{20} - 221°$ (CHCl$_3$), furnishing a crystalline methiodide, m.p. 195°C. The structure given has been confirmed by synthesis.

Ewing *et al., Austral. J. Chem.*, **6**, 78 (1953)

Synthesis:
Kametani *et al., Chem. Pharm. Bull.*, **21**, 766 (1973)

CRYPTOCAVINE

C$_{21}$H$_{23}$O$_5$N

M.p. 233°C

This alkaloid is present in *Corydalis ochotensis* Turez., *C. ophiocarpa* Hook, *Dicentra crysantha* Walp and *Fumaria officinalis* L. It is optically inactive in CHCl$_3$ and gives the protopine colour reaction, being isomeric with Cryptopine (q.v.). Both the perchlorate, m.p. 226–8°C and the methosulphate, m.p. 210–1°C are crystalline. The latter may be degraded by a series of reactions to 4:5-dimethoxy-2-β-dimethylaminoethyl benzaldehyde and 5:6-methylenedioxy-*o*-toluic aldehyde. In this degradation the keto group is reduced to a secondary hydroxyl which is then lost as H$_2$O. The anhydrotetrahydromethylcryptocavine has m.p. 111°C and forms a hydrochloride, m.p. 258–264°C. Theoretically, this should be identical with the corresponding cryptopine base but they are not quite identical. As pointed out by Manske, this is possibly due to *cis-trans* isomerism.

Manske, Marion., *J. Amer. Chem. Soc.*, **62**, 2042 (1940)

CRYPTOCURINE

C$_{20}$H$_{28-30}$O$_2$N$_2$

This alkaloid, isolated from calabash curare (*Strychnos toxifera*), has been obtained as the tetraphenylborate derivative, m.p. 127°C.

Meyer *et al., Helv. Chim. Acta*, **39**, 1214 (1956)

CRYPTODORINE

C$_{18}$H$_{21}$O$_4$N

An alkaloid occurring in the bark of *Cryptocarya odorata,* the base has been characterized as the sulphate, m.p. 219–221°C.

Bick, Preston, Potier., *Bull. Soc. Chim., Fr.,* **12**, 4596 (1972)

CRYPTOLEPINE

$C_{17}H_{16}ON_2$

M.p. 193–4°C

This alkaloid from *Cryptolepis sanguinolenta* Sch. has been described as forming golden-yellow needles. It yields a crystalline hydrochloride as the trihydrate, also yellow needles. The alkaloid is stated to produce a lowering of the body temperature and has marked vasodilator properties.

Clinquart., *Bull. Acad. Med. Belg.,* **9**, 627 (1929)
Delvaux., *J. Pharm. Belg.,* **13**, 955, 973 (1931)
Raymond-Hamet., *Compt. rend.,* **207**, 1016 (1938)
Raymond-Hamet., *C.R. Soc. Biol.,* **126**, 768 (1937)

CRYPTOPALMATINE

$C_{22}H_{27}O_5N$

M.p. 148–150°C

This base has not yet been found to occur naturally but is formed from tetra-hydropalmatine by the action of perbenzoic acid on the anhydromethyl derivative. It crystallizes from Et_2O as colourless prisms and, like Cryptopine (q.v.), gives a reddish-violet colour with H_2SO_4.

Haworth, Koepfli, Perkin., *J. Chem. Soc.,* 2261 (1927)

CRYPTOPINE

$C_{21}H_{23}O_5N$

M.p. 221–3°C

Several species of the order Rhoeadales contain this alkaloid, e.g. *Corydalis nobilis* Pers., *C. scouleri* HK, *C. sempervirens* (L.) Pers., *C. sibirica* Pers., *Dicentra chrysantha* Walp., *D. cucullaria* (L.) Bernh., *D. ochroleuca* Engelm, *Fumaria officinalis* L. and *Papaver somniferum* L. The alkaloid is optically inactive and forms colourless crystals from MeOH-CHCl₃. The salts normally separate as gels but may usually be crystallized by warming. The hydrochloride forms gelatinous masses of crystals of the pentahydrate, soluble in H_2O or CHCl₃; the oxalate forms a tetrahydrate; the platinichloride crystallizes as concentrically-shaped needles, m.p. 204°C (*dec.*); the perchlorate has m.p. 226–8°C; the aurichloride, brown-yellow needles, m.p. 205°C (*dec.*) and the picrate, m.p. 163°C. With H_2SO_4, the alkaloid gives a violet colour changing to green when warmed to 150°C. The methosulphate may be reduced in acid solution with sodium amalgam to tetrahydromethylcryptopine, m.p. 107°C from which AcOCl eliminates H_2O forming the anhydro derivative, also melting at 107°C. This substance, on oxidation with $KMnO_4$ in Me_2CO gives 5:6-methylenedioxy-*o*-toluic acid, 5:6-methylenedioxytoluic aldehyde, N-formyl-4:5-dimethoxy-2 -methylamino-ethylbenzoic acid and 4:5-dimethoxy-2- -dimethylaminoethylbenzaldehyde.

Perkin., *J. Chem. Soc.*, **109**, 815 (1916)
Perkin., *ibid*, **115**, 713 (1919)
Manske., *Can. J. Res.*, **7**, 265 (1932)
Manske., *ibid*, **8**, 407 (1933)
Manske., *ibid*, **14B**, 347, 354 (1936)
Manske., *ibid*, **16B**, 438 (1938)
Manske., *ibid*, **17B**, 51 (1939)
Manske., *ibid*, **18B**, 75, 288 (1940)

Synthesis:
Haworth, Perkin., *J. Chem. Soc.*, 1769 (1926)

CRYPTOPLEURIDINE

$C_{23}H_{23}O_4N$

M.p. 196–7°C

The bark of *Cryptocarya pleurosperma* White and Francis yields this alkaloid which crystallizes as colourless needles from C_6H_6. The base has $[\alpha]_D + 90°$ (c 1.13, $CHCl_3$) and the ultraviolet spectrum exhibits absorption maxima at 257, 290, 325 and 344 mμ. With inflexions at 220, 252, 272, 283, 302 and 312 mμ. The alkaloid contains one methoxyl and one methylenedioxy group and yields a crystalline acetyl derivative, m.p. 268–9°C.

Johns *et al.*, *Austral. J. Chem.*, **23**, 353 (1970)

CRYPTOPLEURINE

$C_{24}H_{29}O_3N$

M.p. 197–8°C

An alkaloid isolated from *Cryptocarya pleurosperma*, the base forms long,

colourless prisms from several organic solvents. It has $[\alpha]_D^{18} - 106°$ (CHCl$_3$).
Several crystalline salts and derivatives have been prepared, e.g. the hydrochloride,
m.p. 262°C (*dec.*); hydrobromide, m.p. 258–260°C (*dec.*); hydriodide, m.p.
256–8°C (*dec.*); perchlorate, m.p. 177–8°C and remelting at 253–5°C;
methiodide, m.p. 215–7°C; $[\alpha]_D^{15} - 74°$; methopicrate, m.p. 240–2°C (*dec.*)
and the picrate, m.p. 220–1°C. The optically inactive form has m.p. 199–200°C
and yields a crystalline methiodide, m.p. 272–4°C.

Lande., *Austral. J. exp. Biol. Med. Sci.,* **26**, 181 (1948)
Fridrichsons, Mathieson., *Nature,* **173**, 732 (1954)
Gellert., *ibid,* **9**, 489 (1956)
Bradsher, Berger., *J. Amer. Chem. Soc.,* **79**, 3287 (1957)
Bradsher, Berger., *ibid,* **80**, 930 (1958)
Marchini, Belleau., *Can. J. Chem.,* **36**, 581 (1958)

Isolation from *Boehmeria* species:
Hart, Johns, Lamberton., *Austral. J. Chem.,* **21**, 2579 (1968)
Farnsworth *et al., ibid,* **22**, 1805 (1969)

CRYPTOSTYLINE I

$C_{19}H_{21}O_4N$

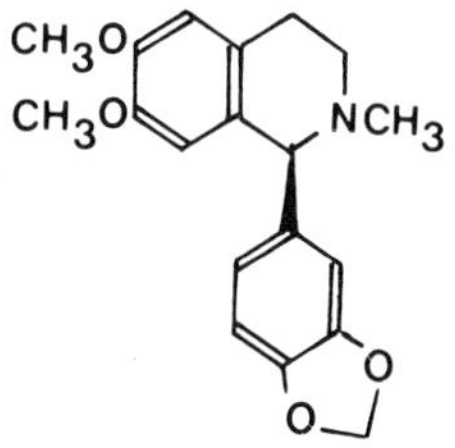

Isolated from *Cryptostylis fulva*, this alkaloid has been shown to possess the
above structure from circular dichroism and X-ray crystallographic studies.

Leander, Luning, Ruusa., *Acta Chem. Scand.,* **23**, 244 (1969)
Leander, Luning, Westin., *ibid,* **27**, 710 (1973)
Blount *et al., Tetrahedron,* **29**, 31 (1973)

CRYPTOSTYLINE II

$C_{20}H_{25}O_4N$

M.p. 117–8°C

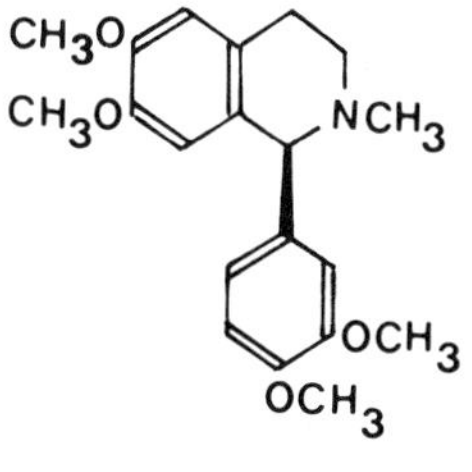

This closely related alkaloid from *Cryptostylis fulva* has $[\alpha]_D^{25} + 58°$ (c 0.28,
CHCl$_3$). The ultraviolet spectrum has absorption maxima at 228 and 281 mμ.

Leander, Luning, Ruusa., *Acta Chem. Scand.,* **23**, 244 (1969)
Leander, Luning, Westin., *ibid,* **27**, 710 (1973)
Blount *et al., Tetrahedron,* **29**, 31 (1973)

CRYPTOSTYLINE III

$C_{21}H_{27}O_5N$

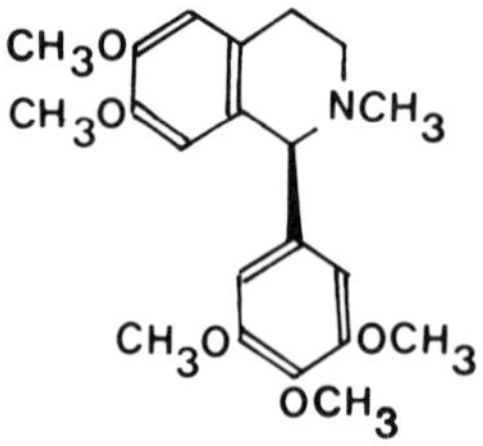

A third alkaloid found in *Cryptostylis fulva*, this base has been shown to be methoxycryptostyline II from circular dichroism and X-ray crystallographic studies.

Leander, Luning, Westin., *Acta Chem. Scand.*, **27**, 710 (1973)
Blount *et al.*, *Tetrahedron*, **29**, 31 (1973)

CRYPTOWOLINE

$C_{19}H_{20}O_4NI$

M.p. 245–6°C (*dec.*).

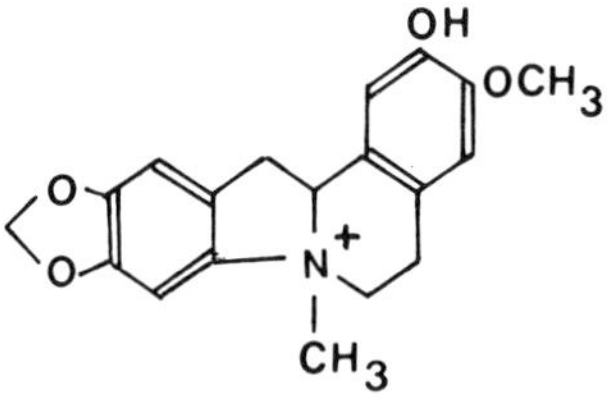

A quaternary alkaloid found in *Cryptocarya bawri* and isolated as the iodide with $[\alpha]_D^{20}$ − 186° (EtOH). The crystalline methyl ether has m.p. 227°C; $[\alpha]_D^{20}$ − 179° (EtOH) and the ethyl ether, m.p. 215°C.

Ewing *et al.*, *Nature*, **169**, 618 (1952)
Ewing *et al.*, *Austral. J. Chem.*, **6**, 78 (1953)
Hughes, Ritchie, Taylor., *ibid*, **6**, 315 (1953)

Synthesis:
Kametani, Ogasawara., *J. Chem. Soc., C*, 2208 (1967)

CUAUCHICHICINE

$C_{22}H_{33}O_2N$

M.p. 152–5°C

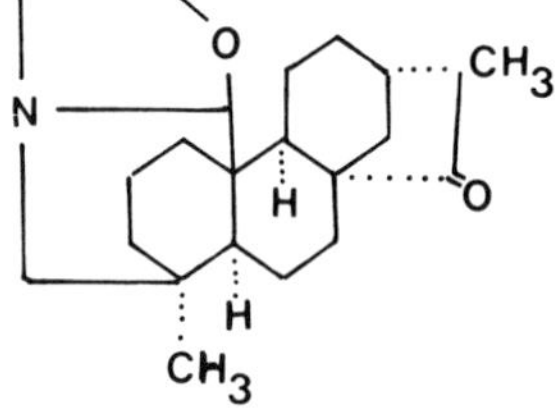

A garrya alkaloid isolated from the bark of *Garrya laurifolia* Hartw. this base forms colourless crystals from Et_2O and has $[\alpha]_D$ − 71.4°. When heated in MeOH the base isomerizes to isocuauchichicine, m.p. 134–6°C; $[\alpha]_D$ − 84°

forming a crystalline oxime, m.p. 192–4°C. Cuauchichicine hydrochloride is also crystalline with m.p. 259–262°C.

Djerassi et al., J. Amer. Chem. Soc., 77, 4801, 6633 (1955)

CUCULLARINE

This alkaloid was reported as occurring in Dicentra cucullaria (L) Bernh. by Black et al but later work by Manske was unable to confirm the presence of this base.

Black et al., J. Agr. Res., 23, 55 (1923)
Manske., Can. J. Res., 7, 265 (1932)

CULARICINE

$C_{18}H_{17}O_4N$

M.p. 185°C

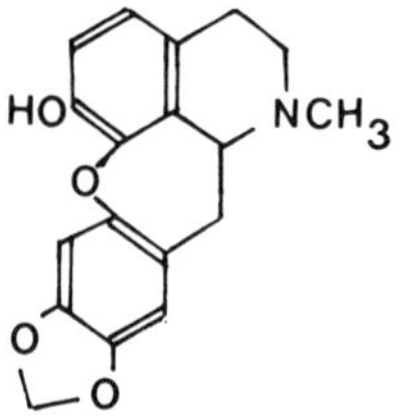

Manske has obtained this alkaloid from Corydalis claviculata (L) DC as colourless prisms having $[\alpha]_D^{22} + 295°$ (c 0.96, CHCl$_3$). The O-methyl ether forms a non-crystallizable resin which may, however, be characterized as the crystalline hydrochloride, m.p. 267°C. The O-ethyl ether is crystalline, m.p. 114°C and forming a hydrochloride, m.p. 275°C.

Manske., Can. J. Res., 18B, 97 (1940)
Manske., Can. J. Chem., 43, 989 (1965)

CULARIDINE

$C_{19}H_{21}O_4N$

M.p. 156°C

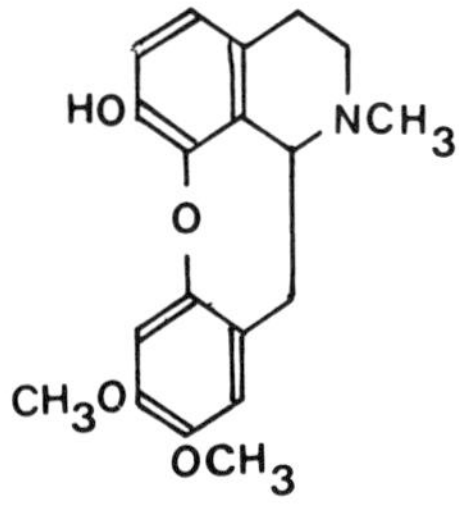

A minor Corydalis alkaloid isolated from Corydalis claviculata (L) DC and Dicentra cucullaria (L) Bernh., the base crystallizes as colourless prisms from MeOH and has $[\alpha]_D^{22} + 295°$ (c 0.99, CHCl$_3$). It forms a perchlorate, m.p. 297°C and on methylation with CH_2N_2 yields cularine (q.v.).

Manske., Can. J. Res., 16B, 81 (1938)
Manske., Can. J. Chem., 43, 989 (1965)

Structure:
Kametani *et al.*, *Tetrahedron Lett.*, 3215 (1966)
Manske., *Can. J. Chem.*, **44**, 561 (1966)

CULARIMINE (*Alkaloid F 30*)

$C_{20}H_{23}O_4N$

M.p. 102°C

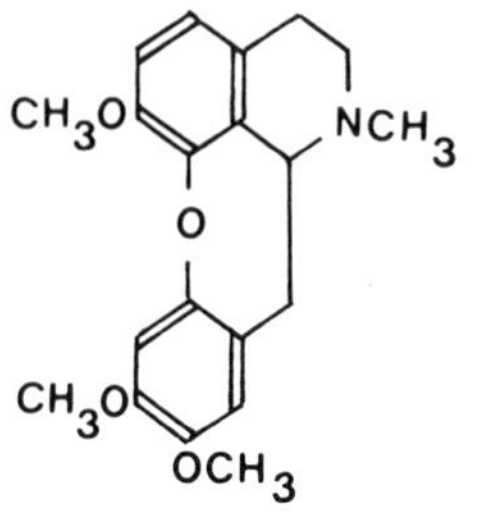

A minor constituent of *Dicentra eximinia*, this non-phenolic base yields a crystalline N-benzoyl derivative, m.p. 102°C. The (+)-form of the alkaloid has m.p. 100–1°C; $[\alpha]_D$ + 259.5° (c 0.94, MeOH) and yields a (+)-tartrate, m.p. 205–6°C. The (−)-form also has m.p. 100–1°C; $[\alpha]_D$ − 262.9° (c 2.13, MeOH).

Manske., *Can. J. Res.*, **16B**, 81 (1938)
Manske., *J. Amer. Chem. Soc.*, **72**, 55 (1950)

Synthesis:
Kametani *et al.*, *Tetrahedron Lett.*, 25 (1954)
Kametani *et al.*, *J. Chem. Soc.*, 4146 (1964)
Kametani, Shibuya., *J. Chem. Soc.*, 5565 (1965)

CULARINE

$C_{20}H_{23}O_4N$

M.p. 115°C

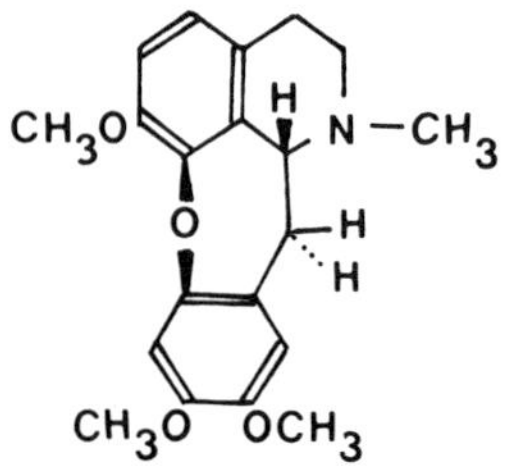

This *iso*lquinoline base is present in a number of Fulariaceae species including *Corydalis claviculata* (L) DC, *Dicentra cucullaria* (L) Bernh., *D. eximia* (Ker) Torr., *D. formosa* Walp. and *D. oregana* Eastwood. It has $[\alpha]_D$ + 285° (c 0.8, MeOH) and the ultraviolet spectrum exhibits absorption maxima at 274, and 283 mμ with shoulders occurring at 229 and 295 mμ. The acid oxalate is sparingly soluble in H_2O and has m.p. 245°C (*dec.*) while the methiodide has m.p. 205°C. In *Corydalis claviculata* it is accompanied by cularidine (q.v.) while in *Dicentra eximia* it is found associated with cularimine (q.v.).

Manske., *Can. J. Res.*, **16B**, 81 (1938)
Manske., *J. Amer. Chem. Soc.*, **72**, 55 (1950)
Kametani, Fukumoto., *Chem. & Ind.*, 291 (1963)

Synthesis:
Ishiwata *et al., Chem. Pharm. Bull.,* **18,** 1850 (1970)
Jackson, Stewart., *J. Chem. Soc., D,* **3,** 149 (1971)

Biosynthesis:
Kametani, Fukumoto, Fujihara., *J. Chem. Soc., D,* **7,** 352 (1971)

CUPREINE

$C_{19}H_{22}O_2N_2$

M.p. 198°C

This alkaloid is found, together with quinine, in the bark of *Remija pedunculata* which is closely related to, but distinct from, the cinchonas. The base is prepared by converting the total alkaloids into the neutral sulphates when the sulphate of homoquinine (a molecular compound of cupreine and quinine) separates in needles or prisms, m.p. 177°C; $[\alpha]_D$ − 235.6° (dil. HCl). When a solution in H_2SO_4 is poured into NaOH with stirring, quinine is precipitated, the cupreine remaining in solution. The latter is obtained by passing CO_2 through the solution.

Cupreine crystallizes in concentrically grouped prisms of the dihydrate, becoming anhydrous at 120°C. It is readily soluble in EtOH but only sparingly so in $CHCl_3$ or Et_2O. Being a diacidic base it forms two series of salts. The acid sulphate crystallizes in prisms as the monohydrate. The normal sulphate formed colourless needles, m.p. 257°C (*dec.*). Various ethers have been prepared: the methyl ether is quinine (q.v.); the ethyl ether has m.p. 160°C and the propyl ether melts at 164°C. When heated with halogen acids, the alkaloid forms *apo*quinine, also produced by demethylation of quinine.

Paul, Cownley., *Pharm. J.,* **12,** 497 (1881)
Howard, Hodgkin., *J. Chem. Soc.,* **41,** 66 (1882)
Grimaux, Arnaud., *Bull. Soc. Chim.,* **7,** 308 (1892)
Giemsa, Halberkann., *Ber.,* **51,** 1325 (1918)

C-CURARINE I

$C_{40}H_{44}ON_4^{++}$

This quaternary alkaloid was originally named toxiferine when it was isolated by Wieland *et al.* from samples of curare from Urbana: It is one of the major constituents of calabash curare and is isolated from *Strychnos toxifera* bark. Crystalline salts have been prepared of which the chloride, originally formulated as $C_{20}H_{23}ON_2Cl$ forms colourless needles, m.p. $> 350°C$; $[\alpha]_D + 70-73°$ and the aurichloride which has m.p. $223-4°C$. The iodide has m.p. $> 320°C$ and the crystalline picrate, m.p. $308-9°C$ (*dec.*). The alkaloid decomposes slowly in acid media.

The chloride is converted by KOH into an ether base, m.p. $184°C$ which forms a dimethiodide, m.p. $301°C$ that is not amenable to Hofmann degradation. With bromine water, the chloride furnishes C-bromocurarine I chloride and with strong HNO_3 it forms C-nitrocurarine I nitrate which is 20 times more potent as a curarizing agent than the original base.

Wieland, Konz, Sonderhoff., *Annalen*, **527**, 160 (1937)
Wieland, Pistor, Bähr., *ibid*, **547**, 140 (1941)
Karrer *et al.*, *Helv. Chim. Acta*, **29**, 1853 (1946)
Karrer *et al.*, *ibid*, **30**, 2081 (1947)
Karrer *et al.*, *ibid*, **35**, 1864 (1952)
Wieland, Merz., *Chem. Ber.*, **85**, 731 (1952)
Philipsborn *et al.*, *Helv, Chim. Acta*, **38**, 1067 (1955)
Boekelheide *et al.*, *J. Amer. Chem. Soc.*, **81**, 2256 (1959)
Wieland, Reinshagen, Fritz., *Naturwiss.*, **48**, 50 (1961)
Nagvary *et al.*, *Tetrahedron*, **14**, 138 (1961)

C-CURARINE II (*Toxiferine IIA*)

$C_{38}H_{40}O_2N_4^{++}$

This quaternary alkaloid has been obtained from the bark of *Strychnos toxifera* indigenous to Venezuela and is best purified through the crystalline picrate which has m.p. $203-4°C$. The chloride, originally considered to be either $C_{20}H_{25}ON_2Cl$ or $C_{20}H_{23}N_2Cl.H_2O$ crystallizes as long, colourless needles which decompose at $220-230°C$ although a m.p. $274°C$ (*dec.*) has been reported. The chloride has $[\alpha]_D^{20} + 74.3°$. Both the iodide and the perchlorate (hemihydrate) are crystalline. The chloride is very readily nitrated or brominated and, as in the case of the preceding base, the monosubstituted derivatives are found to be more potent curarizing agents than the parent base.

Wieland, Pistor, Bähr., *Annalen*, **547**, 140 (1941)
Wieland, Bähr, Witkop., *ibid*, **547**, 156 (1941)
Wieland, Merz., *Chem. Ber.*, **85**, 731 (1952)
Wieland, Merz., *Annalen*, **580**, 204 (1953)
Asmis, Schmid, Karrer., *Helv. Chim. Acta*, **37**, 1983 (1954)

C-CURARINE III (*C-Fluorocurarine*)

$C_{20}H_{23}ON_2^+$

A curare alkaloid found in the bark of *Strychnos mitscherlischii,* the base was originally thought to be an isomeride of C-Curarine I but is now known to possess the simpler structure given above. It may be prepared by treatment of C-Curarine I with acid or by degradation of C-calebassine. With $Ce(SO_4)_2$ it produces a blue-violet colour that changes to yellow. The free quaternary base (as the hydroxide) forms colourless crystals from Et_2O-MeOH and has m.p. $212°C$ The chloride is also crystalline with m.p. $270-4°C$ and $[\alpha]_D^{20} - 936.9°$ (H_2O). A monoacetate is also formed with m.p. $294-6°C$ (*dec.*). The alkaloid is best purified through the picrate, m.p. $189°C$ or the β-anthraquinonesulphonate, m.p. $308-310°C$ (*dec.*).

Wieland, Pistor, Bähr., *Annalen,* **547**, 140 (1941)
Wieland *et al., Chem. Ber.,* **85**, 731 (1952)
Wieland *et al., ibid,* **604**, 1 (1957)
Wieland *et al., ibid,* **611**, 277 (1958)
Wieland *et al., ibid,* **617**, 166 (1958)
Wieland *et al., Angew. Chem.,* **71**, 126 (1959)
Karrer *et al., Helv. Chim. Acta.,* **41**, 1257 (1958)
Karrer *et al., Angew. Chem.,* **70**, 644 (1958)
Zurcher, Ceder, Boekelheide., *J. Amer. Chem. Soc.,* **80**, 1500 (1958)

(−)-CURINE

$C_{36}H_{38}O_6N_2$

M.p. $221°C$

The formula $C_{18}H_{19}O_3N$ was first assigned to this alkaloid, found in calabash-curare and also obtained from the bark of *Chondrodendron tomentosum* and *Radix Pareirae bravae,* by Boehm but later doubled by Späth and Kuffner, placing it among the bisbenzyl*iso*quinoline alkaloids. The base crystallizes from MeOH or C_6H_6 with one mole of solvent, the latter compound having m.p. $161°C$. The alkaloid has $[\alpha]_D^{20} - 328°$ (c 1.0, pyridine). Two monomethyl ether have been prepared of which one has m.p. $206-8°C$. The dimethyl ether methiodide has m.p. $257-8°C$. The nitrogen-free product from the Hofmann degradation of the alkaloid is O-methylbebeerilene, $C_{36}H_{32}O_6$, m.p. $198-9°C$ which, on oxidation with $KMnO_4$ gives an acid, $C_{34}H_{30}O_{16}$ and two isomeric acids, $C_{17}H_{14}O_9.2H_2O$. The former crystallizes from H_2O in minute needles, m.p. $283-4°C$ while the latter have been found to be 2:3-dimethoxy-5:6:4'-tricarboxydiphenyl ether and 2:2'-dimethoxy-dimethoxydiphenyl ether respectively.

Curine is generally said to have a comparatively low toxicity and not to exhibit the peripheral action which is characteristic of curare. Hauschild has found that it has some curarizing action in frogs but is primarily a central depressant with death occurring from heart failure. From this it is concluded that the alkaloid acts upon the exciting mechanism of the heart muscle but not through the vagus terminations of central nervous system.

Boehm., *Arch. Pharm.,* **235**, 660 (1897)
Späth, Leithe, Ladeck., *Ber.,* **61**, 1698 (1928)

Späth, Kuffner., *ibid*, **67**, 55 (1934)
King., *J. Chem. Soc.*, 1157 (1939)
Wieland, Pistor, Bähr., *Annalen*, **547**, 140 (1941)
King., *J. Chem. Soc.*, 936 (1947)

(+)-CURINE (*Bebeerine*)

$C_{36}H_{38}O_6N_2$

M.p. 221°C

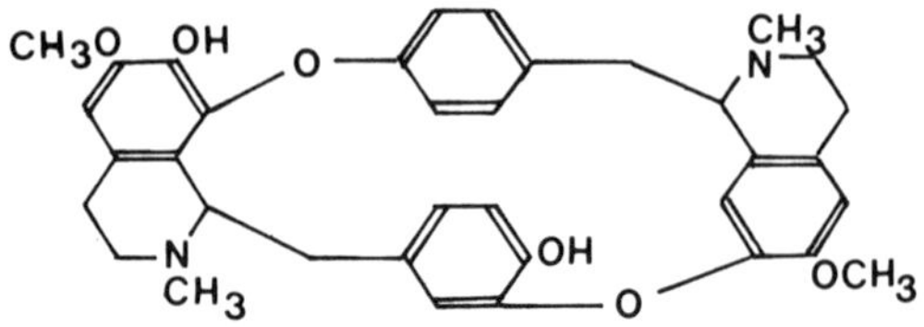

This form of the alkaloid also occurs in calabash-curare derived from *Strychnos toxifera*. It has $[\alpha]_D^{20} + 322°$ (c 1.0, pyridine). The chemical degradation products are those described above for the (−)-form. The (±)-form of the alkaloid has m.p. 299–300°C.

Späth, Leithe, Ladeck., *Ber.*, **61**, 1698 (1928)
Späth, Kuffner., *ibid*, **67**, 55 (1934)

(++)-CURINE 4″-METHYL ETHER

$C_{37}H_{40}O_6N_2$

M.p. 164°C

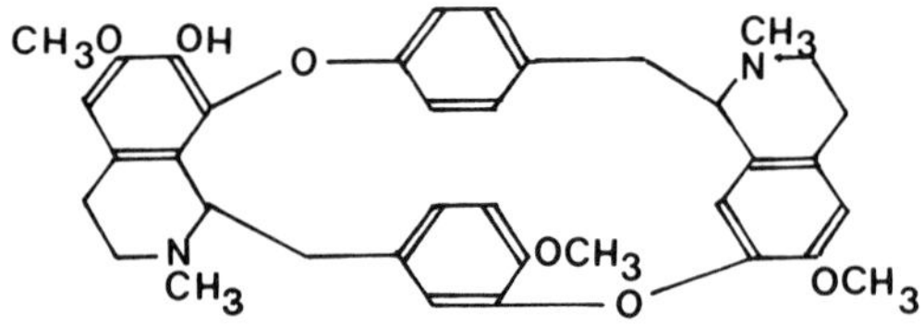

This derivative of curine occurs naturally in *Cissampelos pareira* L and forms colourless crystals from MeOH-pyridine. It has $[\alpha]_D + 273°$ (c 0.7, CHCl₃). Several crystalline derivatives have been prepared to characterize the base, e.g. dimethiodide, m.p. 200°C (*dec.*); dipicrate, m.p. 204–5°C; monoacetyl compound, m.p. 204–5°C and the ethyl ether, m.p. 125°C.

Hanes *et al.*, *J. Chem. Soc.*, C, 615 (1966)

CURRAYANGINE

$C_{23}H_{25}ON$

M.p. 260°C

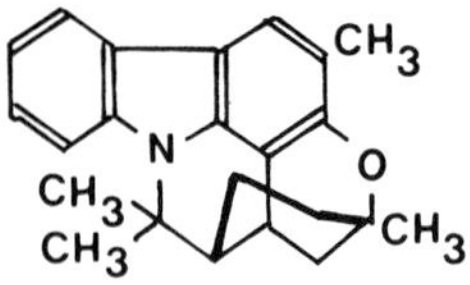

A pentacyclic base found in the stem bark of *Murraya koenigii*, the ultraviolet spectrum of the alkaloid shows absorption maxima at 228, 239, 266 and 308 mμ. The base is optically inactive in pyridine. It contains four C-methyl groups, two of which are *gem*-dimethyls.

Dutta *et al.*, *Ind. J. Chem.*, **7**, 1061 (1969)

366

CUSCAMIDINE

This uncharacterized alkaloid is stated to be a minor constituent of the bark of *Cinchona Pelletierana* Wedd.

Hesse., *Annalen,* **200**, 304 (1880)

CUSCAMINE

A second uncharacterized base found in the bark of *Cinchona Pelletierana* Wedd. this alkaloid forms colourless prisms, m.p. 218°C.

Hesse., *Annalen,* **200**, 304 (1880)

CUSKHYGRINE (*Bellarine, Cuscohygrine*)

$C_{13}H_{24}ON_2$

B.p. 169–170°/23 mm

A hygrine alkaloid first isolated from the leaves of *Erythroxylon truxillense* Rusby and subsequently discovered in *Convolvulus homadae*. The alkaloid is optically inactive and absorbs CO_2 from the air forming an unstable carbonate. It is completely miscible with H_2O and forms a crystalline hydrate with 3.5 H_2O, m.p. 40°C. The base forms crystalline salts and derivatives: hydrobromide, m.p. 234°C; nitrate, m.p. 209°C (*dec.*); oxime, m.p. 53–4°C; dipicrate, m.p. 200–215°C; distyphnate, m.p. 206–8°C; dipicrolonate, m.p. 218–220°C and dimethiodide, m.p. 244°C.

Chromic acid oxidizes the base to hygric acid and if allowed to stand over KOH in ethereal solution it is partially converted into *dl*-hygrine. Although it contains an active carbonyl group it does not form the usual condensation product with benzaldehyde. On reduction it furnishes two stereoisomeric alcohols which can be exhaustively methylated to yield n-undecane and n-undecan- -ol as the final products.

Liebermann, Cybulski., *Ber.*, **28**, 578 (1895)
Liebermann, Cybulski., *ibid*, **29**, 2050 (1896)
Hess, Bappert., *Annalen*, **441**, 137 (1925)
Sohl, Shriner., *J. Amer. Chem. Soc.*, **55**, 3828 (1933)
Späth, Tuppy., *Monatsh.*, **79**, 119 (1948)
Anet, Hughes, Ritchie., *Nature*, **163**, 289 (1949)
Galinovinsky *et al.*, *Monatsh.*, **82**, 551 (1951)
Tuppy, Faltaous., *ibid*, **91**, 167 (1960)

CUSPAREINE

$C_{20}H_{25}O_2N$

M.p. 32–5°C

Beckurts first reported the presence of this alkaloid in the rind of *Galipea officinalis* Hancock (Syn. *Cusparia trifoliata* Engler) although this was not confirmed by Tröger. It was later examined by Schläger and Leeb who found that the base has $[\alpha]_D^{20} - 2.76°$ (c 6.784, EtOH). The (±)-form has the same melting point.

Beckurts., *Apoth. Zeit.*, **18**, 697 (1903)
Tröger, Müller., *Arch. Pharm.*, **248**, 1 (1910)
Schläger, Leeb., *Monatsh.*, **81**, 714 (1950)

CUSPARIDINE

This alkaloid was also found by Beckurts in *Galipea officinalis* Hancock but its presence does not appear to have been confirmed.

Beckurts., *Arch. Pharm.*, **229**, 591 (1891)
Beckurts., *ibid*, **233**, 410 (1895)
Beckurts., *ibid*, **243**, 470 (1905)

CUSPARINE

$C_{19}H_{17}O_3N$

M.p. $91-2°C$

$(110-122°C)$

First isolated from the bark of *Galipea officinalis* Hancock, this alkaloid is also present in *Angostura cuspare,* Roem and Schult. It is stated to exist in three modifications, as yellow needles, m.p. $91-2°C$, colourless needles, m.p. $90-1°C$ and amber crystals, m.p. $110-122°C$. The salts are slightly soluble in H_2O and readily separated from those of the accompanying alkaloids. The hydrochloride forms a trihydrate, m.p. $185-7°C$ or $193-4°C$ *(dry)*; oxalate as yellow needles with 1.5 H_2O, m.p. $153-8°C$; platinichloride (3 H_2O), m.p. $210°C$ and the aurichloride, m.p. $190°C$. Salts are also formed with organic acids but all of these, on melting, give pyrocusparine, $C_{18}H_{15}O_3N$, m.p. $255°C$. The methiodide forms yellow prisms, m.p. $190°C$ which, on treatment with silver oxide, yields *iso*cusparine, m.p. $194°C$. On fusion with KOH, the alkaloid furnishes proto-catechuic acid. Cusparine gives a deep blue colour with Fröhde's reagent and a cherry-red colour with H_2SO_4.

Körner, Böhringer., *Ber.*, **16**, 2305 (1883)
Späth, Brunner., *ibid*, **57**, 1243 (1924)

CUSPIDALINE

$C_{37}H_{42}O_6N_2$

This bisbenzyl*iso*quinoline base is obtained as a colourless oil from *Limacia* *cuspidata* (Miers) Hook, f. et Thom. It has $[\alpha]_D - 48°$ ($CHCl_3$). The alkaloid contains one hydroxyl, three methoxyl and two methylimino groups in the molecule. The O,O-dimethyl ether is amorphous, yielding a crystalline methiodide, m.p. 181–4°C. The stereoisomeric mixture of this base has been synthesized and has m.p. 110°C after sintering at 85°C. Its O,O-dimethyl ether is identical with O-methyldauricine.

Tomita, Furukawa., *Tetrahedron Lett.*, 4293 (1966)

Kametani, Satoh., *Chem. Pharm. Bull. (Tokyo)*, **16**, 773 (1968)

CYCLANOLINE (*Cissamine*)

$C_{20}H_{24}O_4N^+$

This quaternary alkaloid occurs in *Cissampelos pareira* L. and also in *Stephania tetrandra* and is normally isolated as the chloride, m.p. 215–220°C with $[\alpha]_D^{26} - 129°$ (c 1.0, $CHCl_3$). The ultraviolet spectrum in NaOH-EtOH solution has absorption maxima at 218, 253 and 302 mμ whereas in absolute EtOH the maxima occur at 212, 235 and 285 mμ. The crystalline picrate has m.p. 154–6°C and the iodide, also crystalline, has m.p. 185°C (*dec.*). This protoberberine alkaloid contains two hydroxyl and two methoxyl groups.

Tomita *et al.*, *J. Pharm. Soc., Japan*, **87**, 316 (1967)

Anwer *et al.*, *Experientia*, **24**, 999 (1968)

CYCLEACURINE

$C_{35}H_{36}O_6N_2$

M.p. 205–8°C

A bisbenzyl*iso*quinoline alkaloid from *Cyclea peltata,* this base crystallizes as the dihydrate with the above melting point. It is laevorotatory with $[\alpha]_D^{25} -202°$ (c 1.0, MeOH) and yields a dibromide as colourless crystals from H_2O, m.p. 293–6°C. With CH_2N_2 it gives di-O-methyl(−)-curine, m.p. 117–9°C; $[\alpha]_D^{25} - 265°$ (c 1.0, $CHCl_3$).

Kupchan *et al.*, *J. Org. Chem.*, **38**, 1846 (1973)

CYCLEADRINE

$C_{37}H_{40}O_6N_2$

M.p. 160–2°C

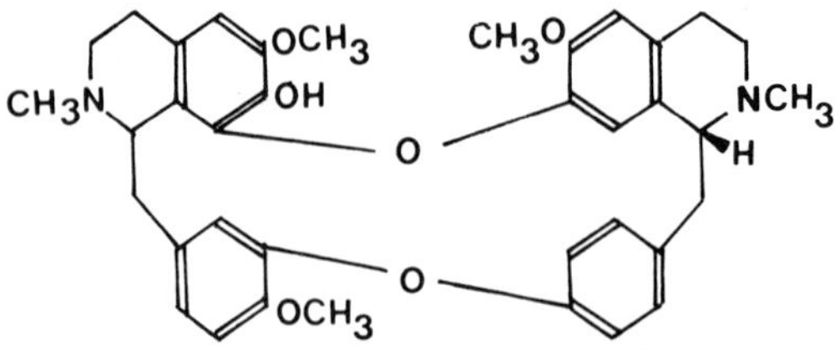

Also present in *Cyclea peltata,* this bisbenzyl*iso*quinoline alkaloid is optically inactive in $CHCl_3$ and has been characterized as the dihydriodide, m.p. 223–4°C, optically inactive in H_2O. Methylation with CH_2N_2 yields Isotetrandrine (q.v.).

Kupchan *et al., J. Org. Chem.,* **38,** 1846 (1973)

CYCLEAHOMINE

$C_{39}H_{45}O_6N_2^+$

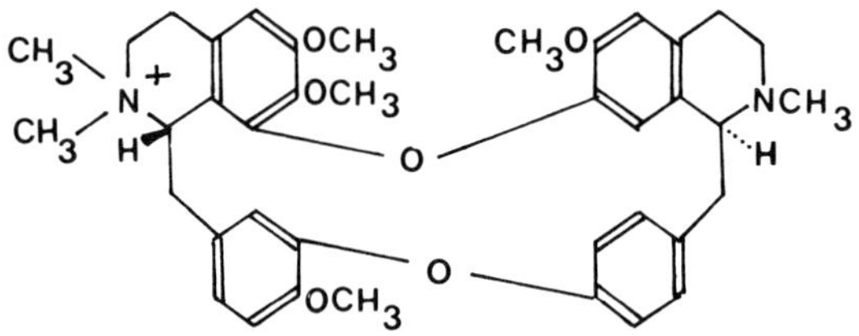

A quaternary alkaloid from *Cyclea peltata,* this base has been isolated as the chloride, m.p. 190–4°C which occurs as colourless crystals from CH_2Cl_2-EtOAc. This salt has $[\alpha]_D^{25} + 103°$ (c 0.15, $CHCl_3$). The ultraviolet spectrum of the chloride has a single absorption maximum at 284 mμ.

Kupchan *et al., J. Org. Chem.,* **38,** 1846 (1973)

CYCLEANINE

$C_{38}H_{42}O_6N_2$

M.p. 272–3°C

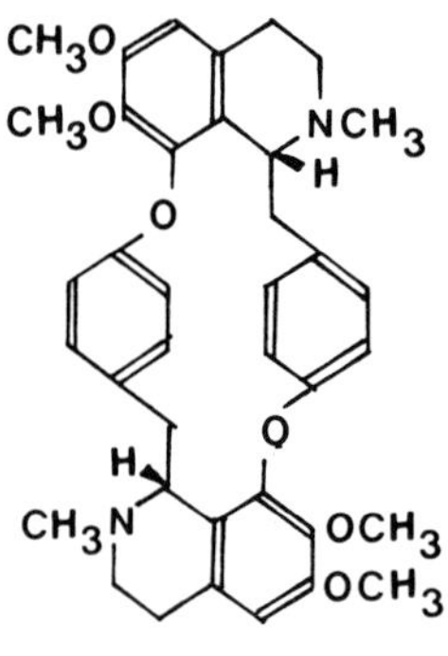

One of the bisbenzyl*iso*quinoline alkaloids isolated from the roots of *Cissampelos pareira* L., this base is also present in *Cyclea peltata* and *C. insularis* (Mak.) Diels and occurs as a minor constituent in *Stephania cepharantha* Hayata. It forms colourless needles or prisms and has $[\alpha]_D^{20} - 25.6°$ (EtOH) or $[\alpha]_D^{27} - 15.1°$ (CHCl$_3$). The methiodide has m.p. 280−2°C (300−1°C). The NMR and mass spectra show that the base belongs to the *iso*chondrodendrine group of alkaloids and earlier anomalies found in the NMR spectrum have been shown to be due to contamination, either with a closely related alkaloid or in the Me$_2$CO used as the solvent. The structure given has been confirmed by synthesis.

Kondo *et al.*, *J. Pharm. Soc., Japan,* **62**, 534 (1942)
Kondo, Tomita, Uyeo., *Ber.,* **70**, 1890 (1937)
Fujita, Murai., *J. Pharm. Soc., Japan,* **71**, 1043 (1951)
Tomita, Kunimoto., *ibid,* **58**, 4613 (1962)

Synthesis:
Tomita, Fujitani, Aoyagi., *Tetrahedron Lett.,* 4243 (1966)
Tomita, Fujitani, Aoyagi., *Chem. Pharm. Bull.,* **16**, 62 (1968)

NMR spectra:
Bhatnagar, Bhattacharji, Popli., *Ind. J. Chem.,* **6**, 125 (1968)

CYCLEANORINE

$C_{37}H_{40}O_6N_2$

M.p. 170−2°C

A further bisbenzyl*iso*quinoline alkaloid found in *Cyclea peltata,* the base is dextrorotatory with $[\alpha]_D^{25} + 308°$ (c 0.52, CHCl$_3$). It forms colourless needles from most organic solvents and on methylation gives the N-methyl derivative which is identical with tetrandrine.

Kupchan *et al.*, *J. Org. Chem.,* **38**, 1846 (1973)

CYCLEAPELTINE

$C_{37}H_{40}O_6N_2$

M.p. 232−4°C

This alkaloid from *Cyclea peltata* is obtained as colourless plates and is laevo-rotatory having $[\alpha]_D^{25} - 106°$ (c 1.0, CHCl$_3$). The O-methyl ether is identical with O-methylrepandine, m.p. 208−210°C; $[\alpha]_D^{25} - 71°$ (c 0.48, CHCl$_3$).

Kupchan *et al.*, *J. Org. Chem.,* **38**, 1846 (1973)

CYCLOBUXAMINE

$C_{24}H_{42}ON_2$

M.p. 209−211°C (*dec.*).

The *Buxaceae* yield a large number of steroidal type alkaloids based mainly upon the pregnane skeleton. This particular base is isolated from Buxus sempervirens L. and forms colourless crystals from C_6H_6. The alkaloid is dextrorotatory having $[\alpha]_D^{24} + 30°$ (c 1.08, $CHCl_3$). When crystallized from Me_2CO it is readily converted into the imine which has m.p. 248−250°C (*dec.*) and $[\alpha]_D^{25} + 67°$ (c 1.38, $CHCl_3$). The 3-N-acetyl derivative is an amorphous powder with no definite melting point. The O,N,N'-triacetyl compound, however, is crystalline, m.p. 261−3°C (*dec.*). The 3-N-isopropyl derivative has also been prepared with m.p. 267−9°C (*dec.*), forming a triacetyl compound with m.p. 280−1°C (*dec.*). A further crystalline derivative is the N,N,N'-trimethyl compound which has m.p. 217−8°C; $[\alpha]_D^{24} + 33°$ (c 0.5, $CHCl_3$).

Brown, Kupchan., *J. Amer. Chem. Soc.*, **86**, 4430 (1964)

CYCLOBUXINE

$C_{25}H_{42}ON_2$

M.p. 245−7°C (*dec.*).

Another of the numerous pregnane alkaloids obtained from *Buxus sempervirens* L. this base is also dextrorotatory having $[\alpha]_D^{23} + 98°$ ($CHCl_3$). It contains one hydroxyl and two methylimino groups and forms a crystalline dihydrobromide, m.p. 288−292°C (*dec.*). Of the acetyl derivative that have been prepared, the N,N-diacetyl compound is obtained as the dihydrate, m.p. 283−5°C (*dec.*) and the O,N,N'-triacetyl derivative has m.p. 256−8°C (*dec.*). The N,N'-dimethyl derivative is also known with m.p. 204−5°C (*dec.*); $[\alpha]_D^{25} + 99°$ ($CHCl_3$).

Heusler, Schlittler., *Helv. Chim. Acta*, **32**, 2226 (1949)
Brown, Kupchan., *J. Amer. Chem. Soc.*, **84**, 4590, 4593 (1962)

CYCLOBUXINE B

$C_{26}H_{44}ON_2$

M.p. 230–3°C

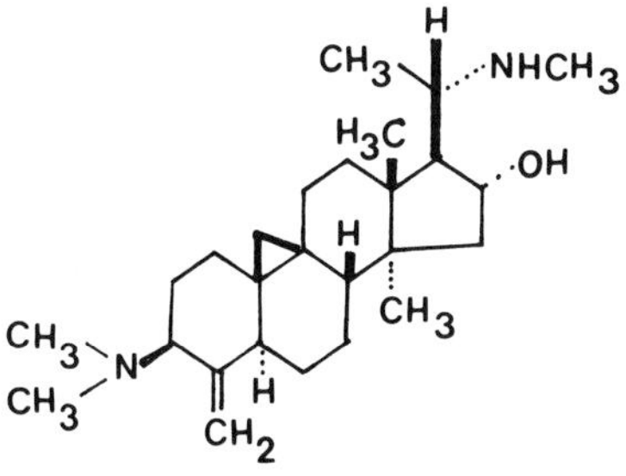

Obtained from *Buxus sempervirens* L. this base forms colourless prisms and has $[\alpha]_D^{24} + 119°$ (c 1.0, $CHCl_3$). The alkaloid contains one hydroxyl, one methyl-imino and one exocyclic methylene group in the molecule. The structure has been determined from chemical and spectroscopic investigations and comparison with other pregnane compounds.

Voticky, Paulik, Sedlak., *Chem. Zvesti.*, **23**, 702 (1969)

CYCLOBUXOMICREINE

$C_{25}H_{39}ON$

M.p. 195–7°C

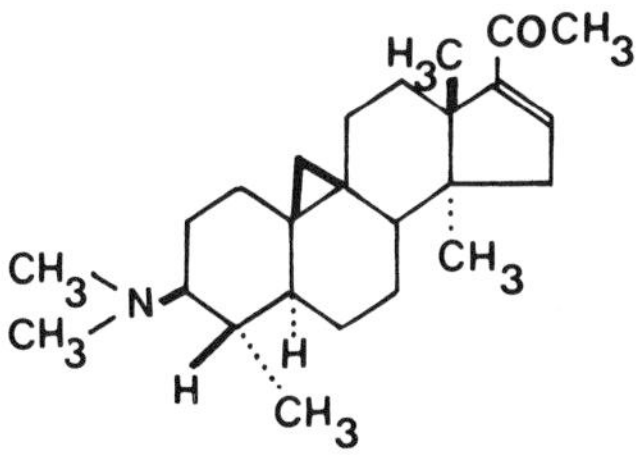

The species *Buxus microphylla* Sieb. et Zucc. var. *suffruticosa* Mak. yields this alkaloid which is obtained from EtOH in the form of colourless needles. It is dextrorotatory having $[\alpha]_D + 37°$ (c 1.62, $CHCl_3$). No derivatives have, as yet, been reported for this base.

Nakano, Terao, Saeki., *J. Chem. Soc.*, C, 1412 (1966)

CYCLOBUXOPHYLLINE

$C_{26}H_{41}ON$

M.p. 194–6°C

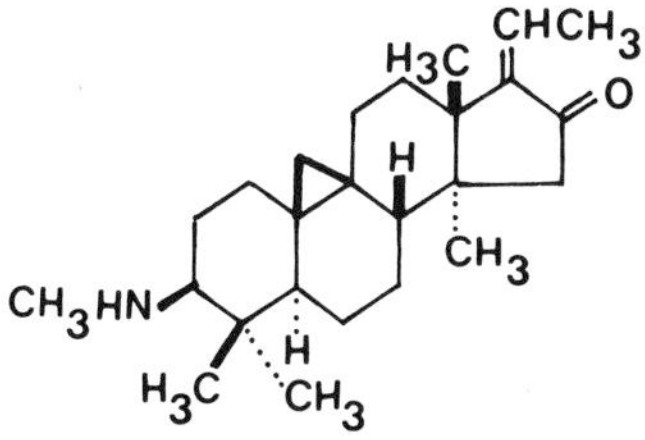

Also present in *Buxus microphylla* var. *suffruticosa,* this alkaloid is the 3-N-methyl derivative of cyclobuxophyllinine (q.v.). It is obtained as colourless needles when crystallized from EtOH and has $[\alpha]_D - 72°$ (c 0.52, $CHCl_3$). The ultraviolet spectrum has a single absorption maximum at 243 mμ.

Nakano, Terao, Saeki., *J. Chem. Soc., C*, 1412 (1966)

CYCLOBUXOPHYLLININE

$C_{25}H_{39}ON$

M.p. 181–2°C

This alkaloid from *Buxus microphylla* Sieb. et Zucc. var. *suffruticosa* Mak. is isomeric with cyclobuxomicreine. It may be crystallized as fine, colourless needles from light petroleum and is laevorotatory, $[\alpha]_D - 51°$ (c 0.49, $CHCl_3$). The N-acetyl derivative has m.p. 234–5°C with $[\alpha]_D - 114°$ (c 1.12, $CHCl_3$).

Nakano, Terao, Saeki., *J. Chem. Soc., C*, 1412 (1966)

CYCLOBUXOSUFFRINE

$C_{25}H_{39}ON$

M.p. 201–4°C

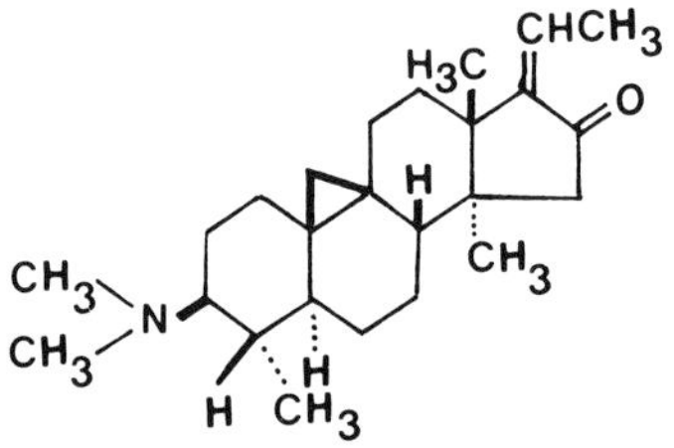

A pregnane-type alkaloid from *Buxus mircophylla* Sieb. et Zucc. *suffruticosa* Mak. this base is isomeric with cyclobuxomicreine and cyclobuxaphyllinine. It forms colourless needles when crystallized from EtOH and has $[\alpha]_D - 62°$ (c 0.52, $CHCl_3$). The ultraviolet spectrum is identical with that of the preceding alkaloid with one absorption maximum at 243 mμ.

Nakano, Terao, Saeki., *J. Chem. Soc., C*, 1412 (1966)

CYCLOBUXOVIRIDINE

$C_{26}H_{41}ON$

M.p. 182–3°C

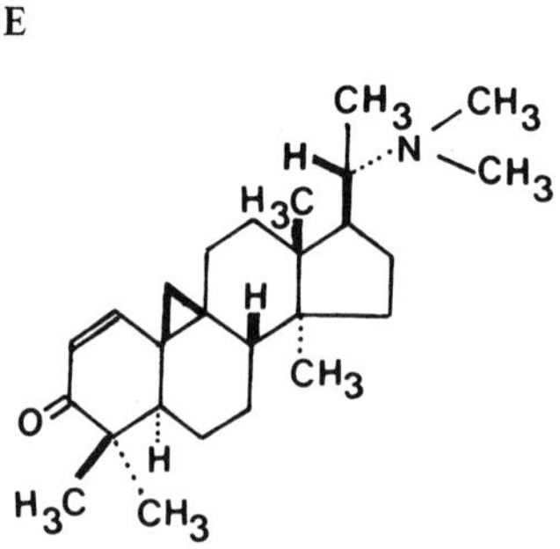

This base, also present in *Buxus microphylla* Sieb. et Zucc. var. suffruticosa Mak. is isomeric with cyclobuxophylline (q.v.) but is dextrorotatory with $[\alpha]_D$ +

16° (c 0.4, CHCl$_3$). The ultraviolet spectrum has one absorption maximum at 269 mμ.

Nakano, Terao, Saeki., *J. Chem. Soc., C,* 1412 (1966)

CYCLOBUXOXAZINE

C$_{27}$H$_{46}$O$_2$N$_2$

M.p. 245−6°C

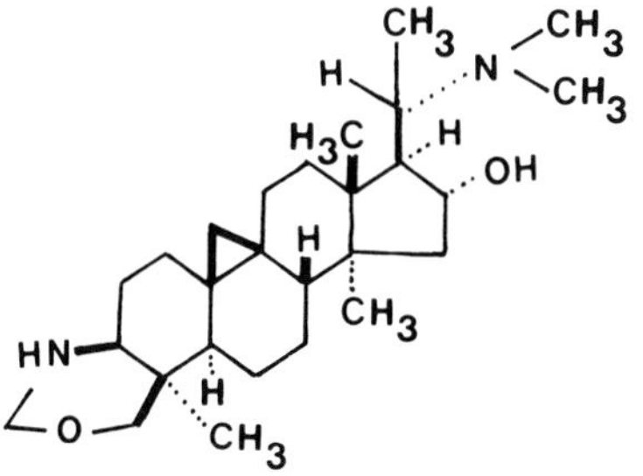

A further base isolated from *Buxus microphylla* Sieb. et Zucc. var *suffruticosa* Mak., this alkaloid has [α]$_D$ + 29° (CHCl$_3$). It forms an N-acetyl derivative, m.p. 283−5°C and an O,N-diacetyl compound, m.p. 240°C. The N-methyl derivative may be obtained as colourless needle-shaped crystals from Me$_2$CO-hexane, m.p. 201−2°C.

Nakano, Terao., *J. Chem. Soc.,* 4537 (1965)

CYCLOCLAVINE

C$_{16}$H$_{18}$N$_2$

M.p. 165−6°C

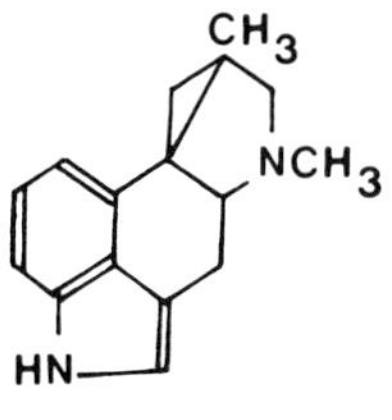

The seeds of *Ipomoea hildebrandtii* Vatke. contain this alkaloid which forms colourless crystals from MeOH. It is dextrorotatory with [α]$_D^{20}$ + 39° (c 1.0, pyridine) or + 63° (c 1.0, CHCl$_3$). The ultraviolet spectrum is typical of the lysergic acid type alkaloids with absorption maxima at 224, 275, 283 and 294.5 mμ in methanolic solution. The crystalline methiodide, m.p. 246°C (*dec.*) has been employed in the determination of the crystal structure by means of X-ray analysis.

Stauffacher, Niklaus, Tscherter, Weber, Hofmann., *Tetrahedron,* **25**, 5879 (1969)

CYCLOKOREANINE B

$C_{27}H_{46}ON_2$

M.p. 235–6°C

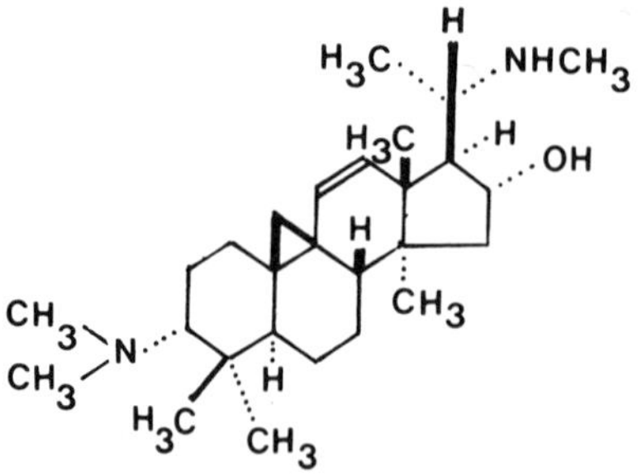

The bark and leaves of *Buxus koreana* Nakai yield this crystalline alkaloid which has $[\alpha]_D + 109°$ (c 1.65, $CHCl_3$). The ultraviolet spectrum exhibits an absorption maximum at 213 mμ. Of the crystalline derivatives that have been prepared, the N-methyl has m.p. 240–1°C; $[\alpha]_D + 92°$ (c 0.85, $CHCl_3$) and the O,N-diacetyl compound, m.p. 238–240°C.

Nakao *et al., J. Chem. Soc., C,* 1805 (1966)

CYCLOMAHANIMBIN

$C_{23}H_{25}ON$

M.p. 146°C

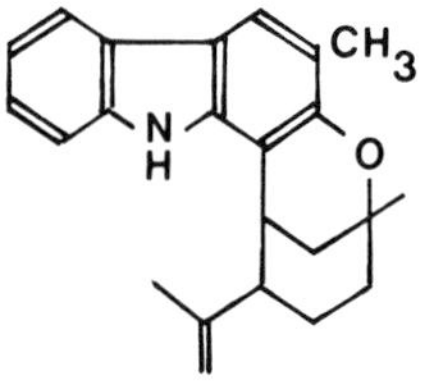

A carbazole base found in the leaves of *Murraya koenigii* Spreng. this alkaloid is optically inactive in $CHCl_3$. The ethanolic solution gives an ultraviolet spectrum with absorption maxima at 246, 251, 257, 307 and 341 mμ. The N-methyl derivative is also crystalline with m.p. 169–170°C. Hydrogenation with Pd-C yields the dihydro derivative, m.p. 136–7°C.

Kureel, Kapil, Popli., *Tetrahedron Lett.,* 3857 (1969)

CYCLOMICROBUXEINE

$C_{25}H_{37}ON$

M.p. 141–2°C

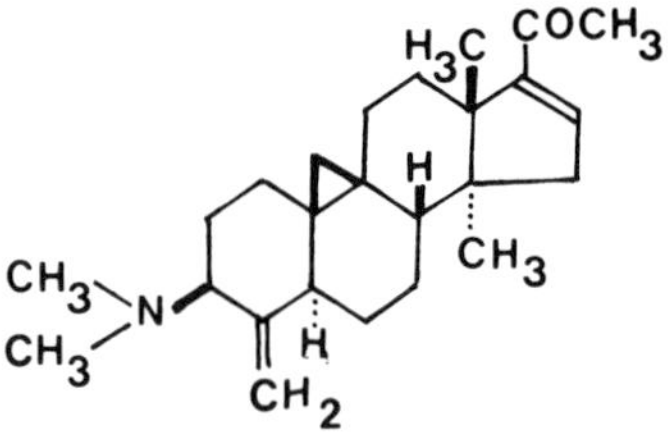

Nakano *et al.* have described this alkaloid which occurs in *Buxus microphylla* Sieb. et Zucc. var. *suffruticosa* Mak. It crystallizes from absolute MeOH as colourless needles and has $[\alpha]_D + 126°$ (c 1.2, $CHCl_3$). No derivatives have so far been reported.

Nakano, Terao, Saeki., *J. Chem. Soc., C,* 1412 (1966)

CYCLOMICROBUXINE (*Buxpiine*)

$C_{25}H_{39}O_2N$

M.p. 178–180°C

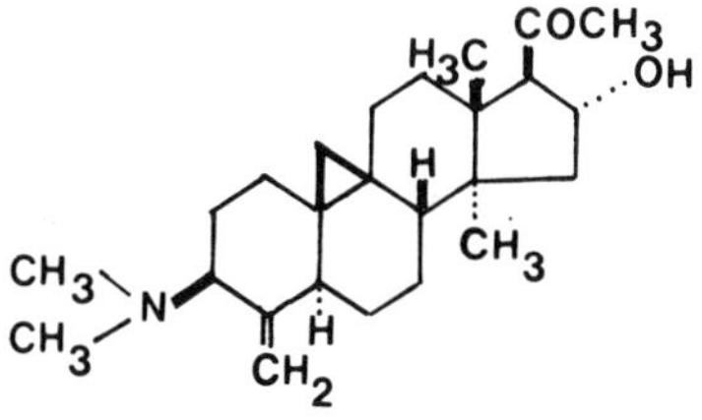

The leaves of two species, *Buxus microphylla* Sieb. et Zucc. and *B. sempervirens* L. yield this pregnane alkaloid which forms colourless crystals from Me_2CO. It is dextrorotatory with $[\alpha]_D + 172°C$ ($CHCl_3$). A figure of $+ 158°$ has also been reported. The 16-hydroxyl group is readily acetylated with Ac_2O in pyridine giving the acetate, m.p. 232–3°C. With $KMnO_4$ it yields acetaldehyde, indicative of an exocyclic methylene group in the molecule.

Nakano, Terao., *J. Chem. Soc.,* 4512 (1965)
Nakano, Hasegawa., *ibid,* 6688 (1965)
Voticky, Tomko., *Tetrahedron Lett.,* 3579 (1965)

CYCLOMICROBUXININE (*Buxtauine*)

$C_{24}H_{37}O_2N$

M.p. 178–181°C

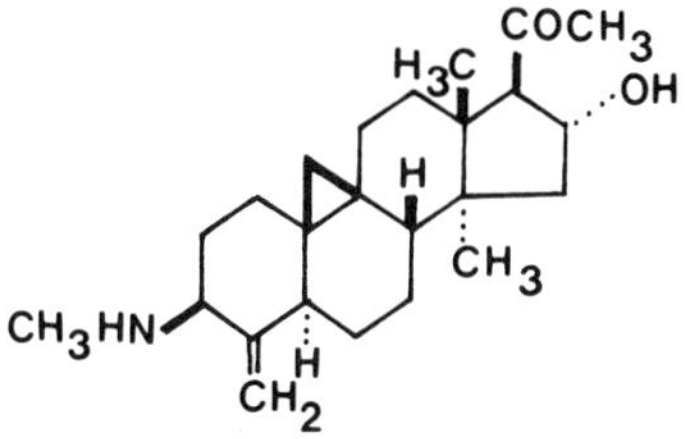

Also obtained from *Buxus microphylla* Sieb. et Zucc. and *B. sempervirens* L. this alkaloid is the N-demethyl analogue of the preceding base. It has $[\alpha]_D^{23} + 157°$ (c 0.237, EtOH) and $+ 154°$ (c 0.768, $CHCl_3$). The oxime may be obtained as colourless crystals from aqueous EtOH and has m.p. 235–8°C. The O,N-diacetyl derivative, also crystalline, has m.p. 213–5°C and $[\alpha]_D + 87°$ (c 0.67, $CHCl_3$). Voticky and Tomko have reported m.p. 193–7°C and $[\alpha]_D^{22} + 95°$ ($CHCl_3$) for this compound.

Nakano, Hasegawa., *J. Chem. Soc.,* 6688 (1965)
Voticky, Tomko., *Tetrahedron Lett.,* 3579 (1965)

CYCLOMICROPHYLLIDINE A

$C_{35}H_{52}O_3N_2$

M.p. Indefinite

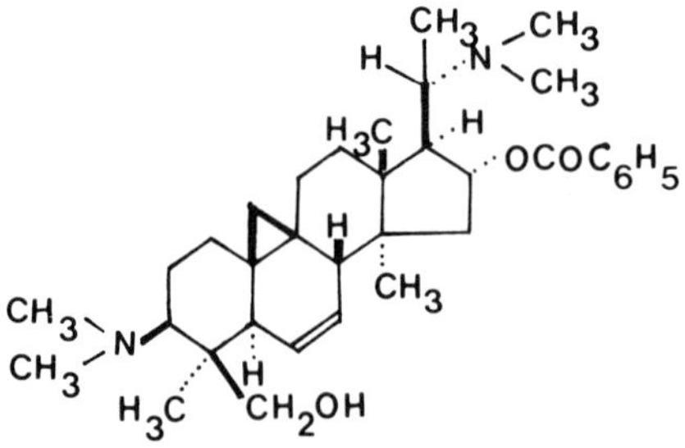

An amorphous alkaloid occurring in *Buxus microphylla* Sieb. et Zucc. var. *suffruticosa* Mak., this laevorotatory base has $[\alpha]_D - 160°$ (CHCl$_3$). The ultraviolet spectrum shows absorption maxima at 265, 273 and 280 mμ. The alkaloid may be hydrolyzed with dilute acid to yield benzoic acid and cyclomicrophylline A. The alkaloid contains two dimethylamine groups and one primary hydroxyl group.

Nakano, Terao., *J. Chem. Soc.*, 4512 (1965)

CYCLOMICROPHYLLINE A

$C_{28}H_{48}O_2N_2$

M.p. 232–3°C

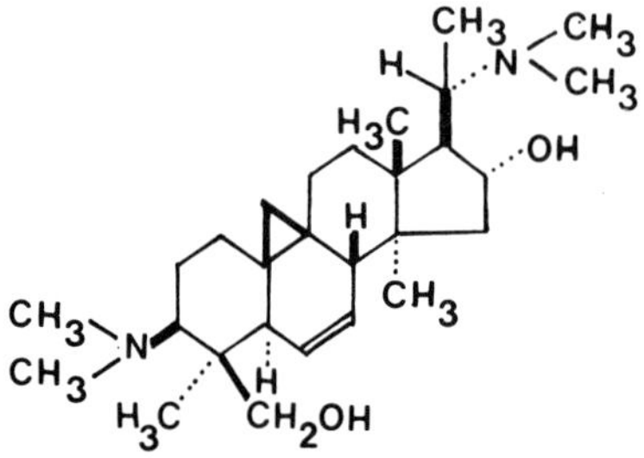

As mentioned above, this base is produced by hydrolysis of cyclomicrophyllidine A but it also occurs naturally in *Buxus microphylla* Sieb. et Zucc. var. *suffruticosa* Mak. From the available evidence it does not appear that the alkaloid is produced by hydrolysis during the extraction process. Both the diacetyl and dibenzoyl derivatives are amorphous, the latter having m.p. 105–113°C. Among the crystalline derivatives that have been prepared, the dimethiodide has m.p. > 320°C and the mono-*p*-toluenesulphonyl compound, m.p. 176–7°C. The dibenzoyl derivative forms a crystalline dipicrate with m.p. 253–4°C (*dec.*).

Nakano, Terao., *Tetrahedron Lett.*, 1035, 1045 (1964)
Nakano, Terao., *J. Chem. Soc.*, 4512 (1965)

CYCLOMICROPHYLLINE B (*Cyclobaleabuxine*)

$C_{27}H_{46}O_2N_2$

M.p. 251–2°C

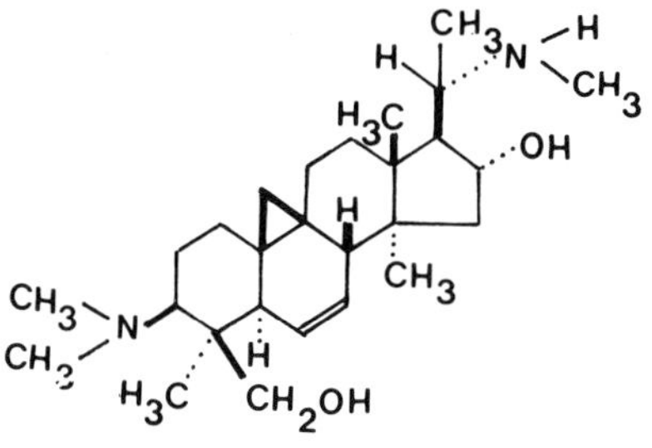

Another of the many steroidal alkaloids present in *Buxus microphylla* Sieb. et Zucc. var. *suffruticosa* Mak. this base forms colourless crystals from Me_2CO and has $[\alpha]_D - 65°$ (CHCl$_3$). The ultraviolet spectrum shows one absorption maximum at 204 mμ. The 16-O,N-diacetyl derivative is crystalline with m.p. 202–3°C; $[\alpha]_D - 151°$ (CHCl$_3$). Further investigation of *Buxus* species has shown that the alkaloid also occurs in *Buxus malayana* Ridl. and *B. balearica* Willd.

Nakano, Terao., *Tetrahedron Lett.*, 1035, 1045 (1964)
Nakano, Terao., *J. Chem. Soc.*, 4512 (1965)
Khuong-Huu-Laine *et al., Bull. Soc. Chim.*, 758 (1966)
Herlem-Gaulier *et al., ibid*, 657 (1965)

CYCLOMICROPHYLLINE C

$C_{27}H_{46}O_2N_2$

M.p. 283–4°C

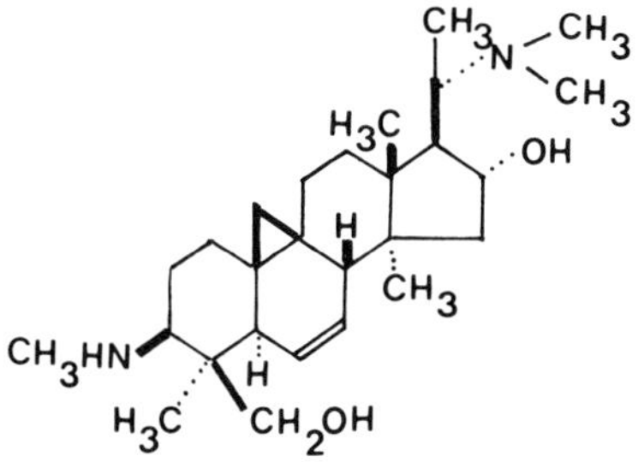

Isolated from *Buxus microphylla* Sieb. et Zucc. var. *suffruticosa* Mak., this alkaloid has $[\alpha]_D - 40°$ (CHCl$_3$) and exhibits a single absorption maximum in its ultraviolet spectrum at 204 mμ. It also forms an amorphous 16-O,N-diacetyl derivative with $[\alpha]_D - 132°$ (CHCl$_3$).

Nakano, Terao., *Tetrahedron Lett.*, 1035, 1045 (1964)
Nakano, Terao., *J. Chem. Soc.*, 4512 (1965)

379

CYCLOMICROSINE

$C_{34}H_{50}O_3N_2$

M.p. 282–4°C

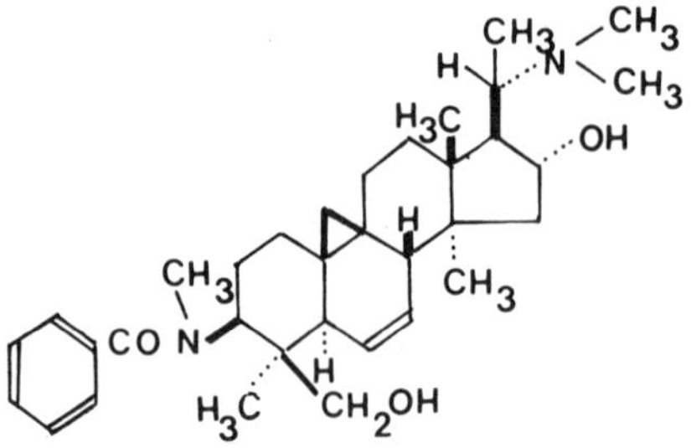

This alkaloid has been found to occur in *Buxus microphylla* Sieb. et Zucc. var. *suffruticosa* Mak. and also in *B. sempervirens* L. It may be crystallized in colourless needles from Me$_2$CO-hexane and has $[\alpha]_D$ − 33° (CHCl$_3$). Dilute acids and alkalies hydrolyze the base to benzoic acid and cyclomicrophyllline C (q.v.).

Döpke, Müller., *Naturwiss.*, **52**, 61 (1965)
Nakano, Terao, Saeki., *J. Chem. Soc.*, C, 1412 (1966)

CYCLOMIKURANINE

$C_{26}H_{43}O_2N$

M.p. 209–211°C

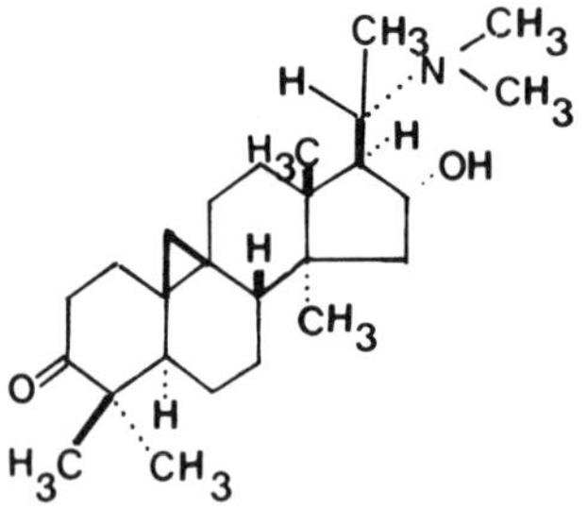

The shrub *Buxus microphylla* Sieb. et Zucc. var. *suffruticosa* Mak. *forma major* Mak. contains this alkaloid which may be obtained in the form of colourless plates from MeOH. The base has $[\alpha]_D$ − 3.0° (c 0.86, CHCl$_3$). It contains one hydroxyl and one dimethylimino group in the molecule.

Nakano, Terao, Saeki., *J. Chem. Soc.*, C, 1412 (1966)
Nakano *et al.*, *ibid*, 1805 (1966)

CYCLONEOSAMANDARIDINE

$C_{20}H_{32}O_3N$

M.p. 282°C

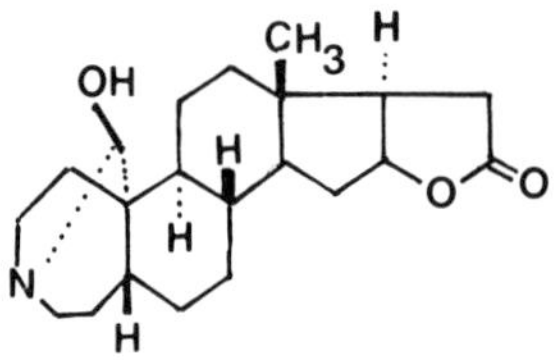

This alkaloid has been obtained from the skin gland secretion of *Salamandra*

maculosa. It is characterized as the crystalline hydrochloride, m.p. 250°C (*dec.*) and the N-acetyl derivative, m.p. 208°C.

Habermehl, Haaf., *Chem. Ber.,* **98**, 3001 (1965)

CYCLOPAMINE

An uncharacterized alkaloid isolated from the roots of *Veratrum californicum.* No salts or derivatives have yet been reported for this base.

Keeler., *Phytochem.,* **7**, 303 (1968)

CYCLOPOSINE

$C_{33}H_{50}O_7N$

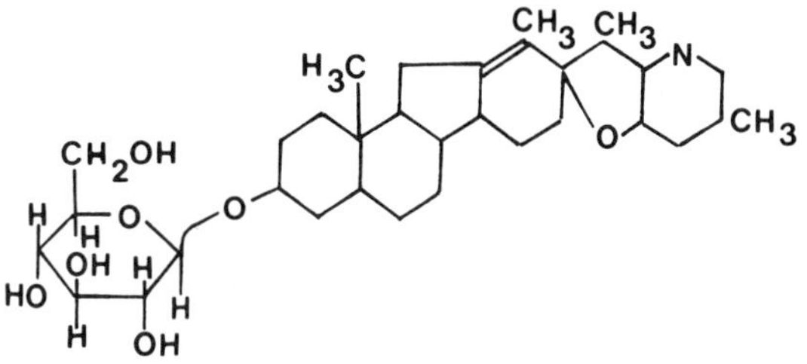

A glycosidic steroidal alkaloid, this base occurs in *Veratrum californicum.* It has been identified by infrared, NMR and mass spectrometry as 3-glucosyl-11-deoxojervine. Pharmacologically, the alkaloid produces fetal cyclopia and some related central nervous system malformations in sheep.

Keeler., *Steroids,* **13**, 579 (1969)

CYCLOPROTOBUXINE A

$C_{28}H_{50}N_2$

M.p. 207–8°C

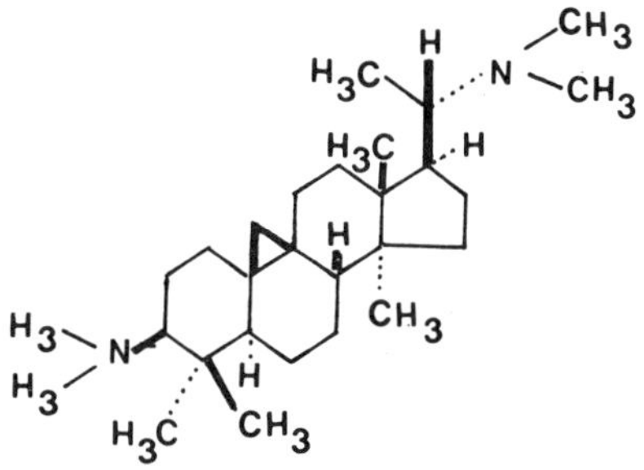

This oxygen-free alkaloid has been isolated from *Buxus balearica* Willd. and *B. malayana* Ridl. and forms colourless plates from Me_2CO. It is dextrorotatory with $[\alpha]_D$ + 75° (c 1.0, $CHCl_3$) or + 31° (c 0.54, $CHCl_3$). The methiodide has been prepared as colourless crystals, m.p. 262–3°C. The base contains two dimethylamino groups and recent work has shown that it is identical with the methyl derivative of Alkaloid L obtained originally by Schlittler and Friedrich.

381

Schlittler, Friedrich., *Helv. Chim. Acta*, **33**, 878 (1950)
Herlem-Gaulier *et al., Bull. Soc. Chim. Fr.*, 657 (1965)
Khuong Huu Laine *et al., ibid*, 758 (1966)

CYCLOPROTOBUXINE C (*Alkaloid L*)

$C_{27}H_{48}N_2$

M.p. 212°C

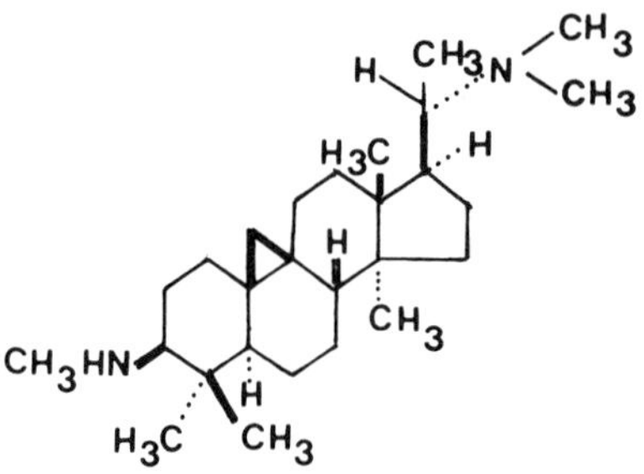

Originally isolated as Alkaloid L from *Buxus sempervirens* L., this alkaloid has also been obtained from *B. microphylla* Sieb. et Zucc. var. *suffruticosa* Mak. It is dextrorotatory with $[\alpha]_D + 76°$ (c 1.09, CHCl₃). Of the crystalline derivatives that have been prepared, the acetyl compound has m.p. 222–235°C and the benzoyl compound, m.p. 220–9°C.

Schlittler, Friedrich., *Helv. Chim. Acta*, **32**, 2209 (1949)
Schlittler, Friedrich., *ibid*, **33**, 878 (1950)
Nekano, Hasegawa., *Tetrahedron Lett.*, 3679 (1964)
Calame, Arigoni., *Chimia*, **18**, 185 (1964)
Nakano, Hasegawa., *J. Chem. Soc.*, 6688 (1965)
Herlem-Gaulier *et al., Bull. Soc. Chim. Fr.*, 657 (1965)
Nakano, Terao, Saeki., *J. Chem. Soc., C*, 1412 (1966)

CYCLOPROTOBUXINE D

$C_{26}H_{46}N_2$

M.p. 140–2°C

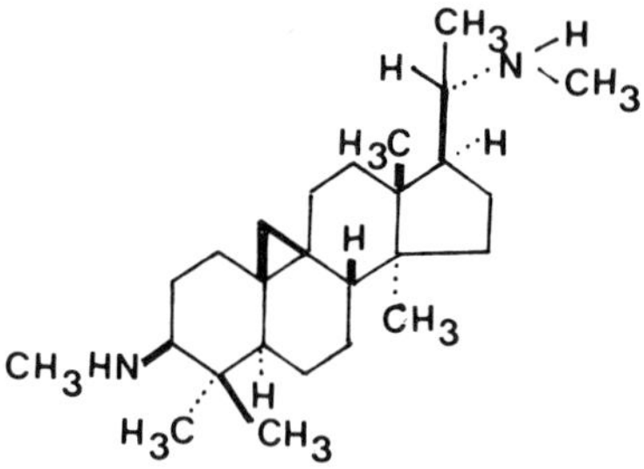

This alkaloid is obtained in the form of colourless needles when crystallized from Me₂CO. It is found in the leaves of *Buxus balearica* Willd. and also in *B. semper-virens* L. It is dextrorotatory having $[\alpha]_D^{28} + 112°$ (CHCl₃). It yields a crystalline diacetyl derivative with m.p. 276–8°C.

Kupchan, Kurosawa., *J. Org. Chem.*, **30**, 2046 (1965)
Khuong Huu Laine *et al., Tetrahedron*, **22**, 3321 (1966)

CYCLOPROTOBUXINE F

$C_{26}H_{46}N_2$

M.p. $163°C$

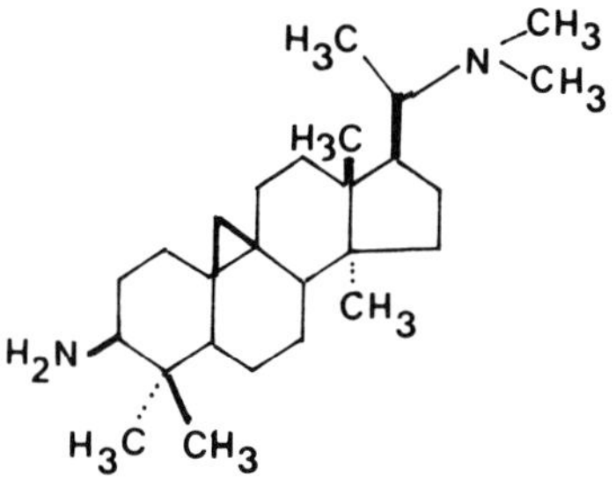

H_3C N CH_3 CH_3
H_3C
H_2N CH_3
H_3C CH_3

The roots of *Buxus madagascarica* yield this particular alkaloid which has $[\alpha]_D + 42°$ (CHCl$_3$). It contains an amino group and a dimethylamino group in the molecule and is isomeric with the preceding base.

Khuong Huu Laine *et al., Compt. Rend.,* **273**C, 558 (1971)

CYCLOSUFFROBUXINE

$C_{25}H_{37}ON$

M.p. $167-172°C$

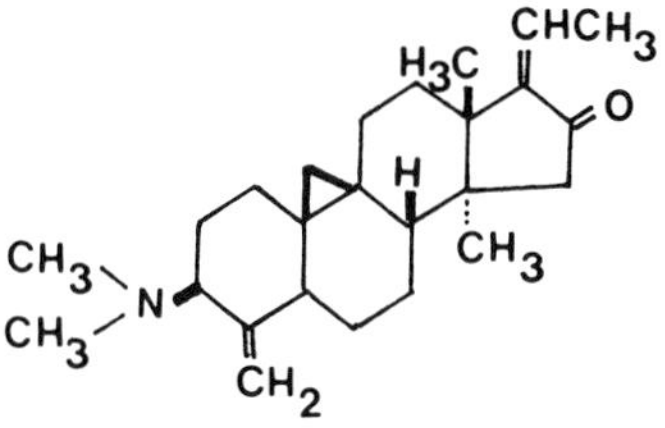

H_3C $CHCH_3$ O
H
CH_3 N CH_3
CH_3
CH_2

A further pregnane type alkaloid obtained from *Buxus microphylla* Sieb. et Zucc. var. *suffruticosa* Mak., this laevorotatory base has $[\alpha]_D - 92°$ (c 0.42, CHCl$_3$) and exhibits a single absorption maximum in the ultraviolet spectrum at 243 mμ.

Nakano, Terao, Saeki., *J. Chem. Soc., C,* 1412 (1966)

CYCLOSUFFROBUXININE

$C_{24}H_{35}ON$

M.p. $144-9°C$

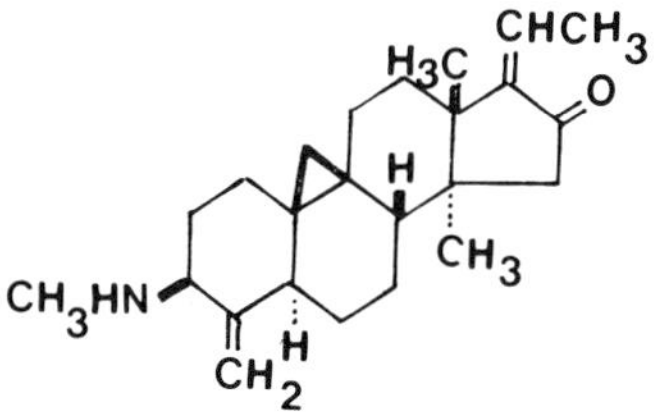

H_3C $CHCH_3$ O
H
CH_3
CH_3HN CH_3
H
CH_2

Buxus microphylla Sieb. et Zucc. var. *suffruticosa* Mak. also yields this alkaloid which is crystallizable from either light petroleum or Et$_2$O in the form of colourless needles. The base has $[\alpha]_D - 67°$ (c 0.64, CHCl$_3$) and shows a single absorption maximum at 243 mμ in the ultraviolet spectrum.

Nakano, Terao, Saeki., *J. Chem. Soc., C,* 1412 (1966)

CYCLOVIROBUXEINE A

$C_{28}H_{48}ON_2$

M.p. 220°C

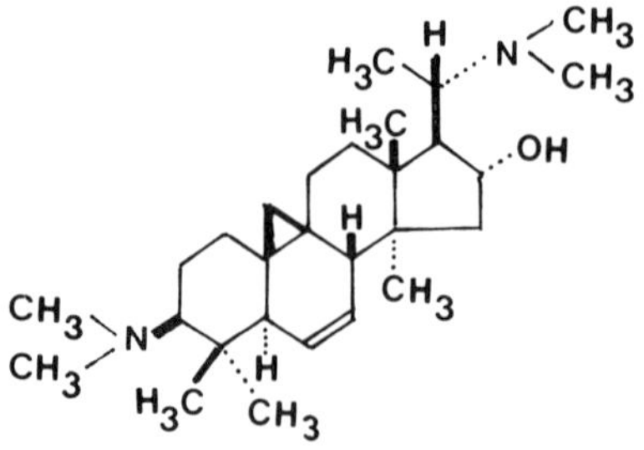

An unsaturated pregnene alkaloid found in both *Buxus sempervirens* L. and *B. malayana* Ridl. this base is obtained in the form of colourless prisms from Me₂CO. It is laevorotatory with $[\alpha]_D - 87°$ (c 1.0, CHCl₃). The alkaloid contains two dimethylamino groups and one hydroxyl group in the molecule.

Khuong-Huu-Laine *et al., Bull. Soc. Chim.*, 757 (1966)
Döpke, Muller, Jeffs., *Pharmazie*, **23**, 37 (1968)

CYCLOVIROBUXEINE B

$C_{27}H_{46}ON_2$

M.p. 203°C

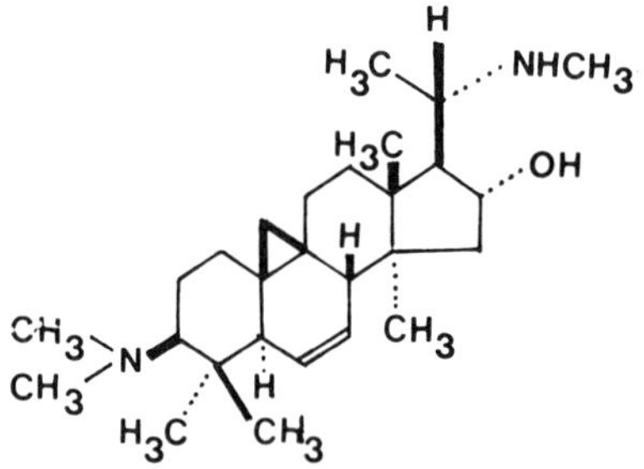

This alkaloid is isolated, together with the preceding base, from *Buxus semper-virens* L. and *B. malayana* Ridl. It is also crystallizable from Me₂CO as colourless crystals and has $[\alpha]_D - 75°$ (CHCl₃).

Friedrich, Schlittler., *Helv. Chim. Acta*, **33**, 873 (1950)
Kupchan, Ohta., *J. Org. Chem.*, **31**, 608 (1966)

CYCLOVIROBUXINE A

$C_{28}H_{50}ON_2$

M.p. 241–2°C

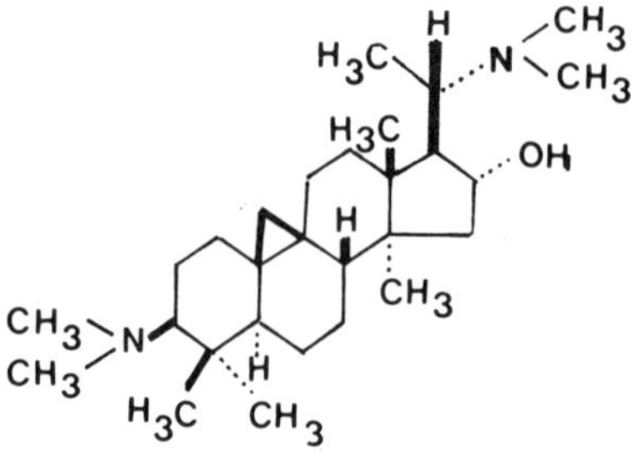

Nakano *et al.* obtained this alkaloid from *Buxus sempervirens* L. It is dextro-rotatory with $[\alpha]_D + 44°$ (c 0.73, CHCl$_3$). It may also be obtained by hydrogenation of cyclovirobuxeine A and is therefore the dihydro derivative of the latter.

Nakano, Terao, Saeki., *J. Chem. Soc., C,* 1412 (1966)
Nakano, Terao, Saeki, Jin., *ibid,* 1805 (1966)

CYCLOVIROBUXINE D

$C_{26}H_{46}ON_2$

M.p. 221–4°C

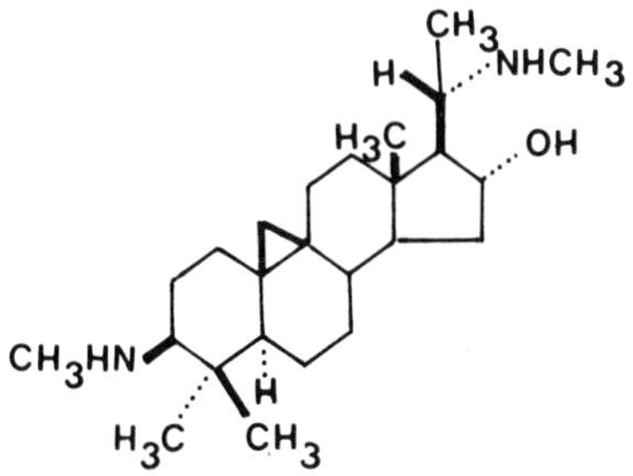

A minor constituent of both *Buxus malayana* Ridl. and *B. sempervirens* L. this dextrorotatory base has $[\alpha]_D + 63°$ (c 1.0, CHCl$_3$). Among the salts and derivatives that have been prepared are the diperchlorate, m.p. 249–252°C (*dec.*) and the dihydriodide, m.p. 313–5°C (*dec.*). A triacetyl derivative has also been obtained as the crystalline monohydrate with m.p. 237–9°C.

Brown, Kupchan., *Tetrahedron Lett.,* 2895 (1964)
Khuong-Huu-Laine *et al., Bull. Soc. Chim.,* 758 (1966)

CYGNINE

$C_{19}H_{22}O_3N_2$

This alkaloid has been reported as occurring in *Gastrolobium calycinum* Benth. It has not been examined further and its structure is unknown although it is stated to be a convulsant poison.

Mann, Ince., *Proc. Roy. Soc.,* **79B**, 488 (1907)

CYLINDROCARINE

$C_{21}H_{28}O_3N_2$

M.p. 204–5°C

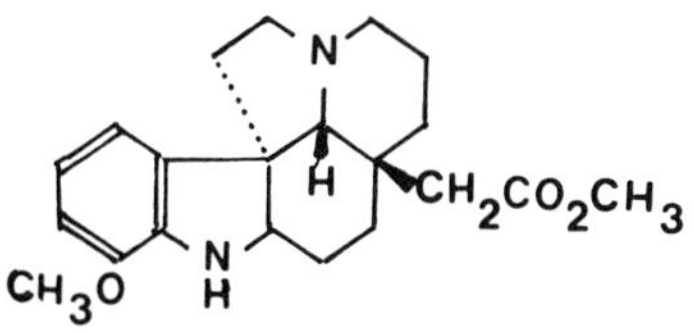

One of the alkaloids isolated from *Aspidosperma cylindrocarpon*, this laevo-rotatory base has $[\alpha]_D^{20} - 280°$ (c 0.0025, MeOH). In methanolic solution, the ultraviolet spectrum shows three absorption maxima at 215, 244 and 288 mμ.

The imino hydrogen is reactive and several derivatives have been prepared to characterize the alkaloid, e.g. the N-benzoyl compound, m.p. 126–9°C and the N-formyl derivative, m.p. 161–2°C.

Milborrow, Djerassi., *J. Chem. Soc., C*, 417 (1969)

CYLINDROCARPIDINE

$C_{23}H_{30}O_4N$

M.p. 118–118.5°C

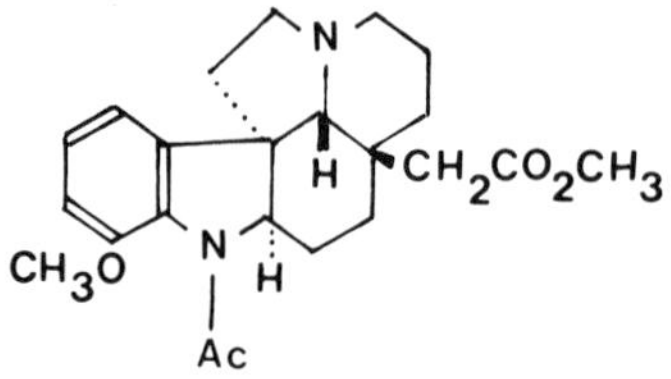

Djerassi *et al.* have investigated this alkaloid which is present in *Aspidosperma cylindrocarpon* and obtained it as colourless crystals from aqueous EtOH. It is laevorotatory in chloroform with $[\alpha]_D^{27} - 122°$ (c 0.72, CHCl$_3$). It contains a methoxyl and an N-acetyl group in the molecule.

Djerassi *et al.*, *Tetrahedron*, **16**, 212 (1961)
Milborrow, Djerassi., *J. Chem. Soc., C*, 417 (1969)

CYLINDROCARPINE

$C_{30}H_{34}O_4N_2$

M.p. 168–9°C

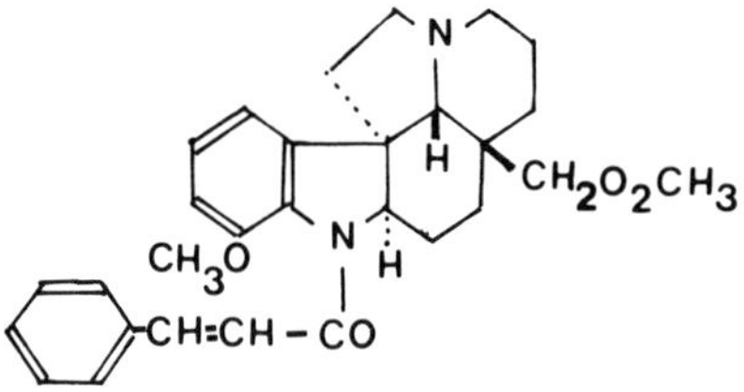

A yellow alkaloid which occurs in *Aspidosperma cylindrocarpon*, the base has $[\alpha]_D^{27} - 181°$ (c 0.41, CHCl$_3$). The crystalline perchlorate is obtained from MeOH and crystallizes with one mole of solvent, m.p. 243–5°C; $[\alpha]_D^{20} - 128°$ (c 0.41, CHCl$_3$). The picrate forms yellow needles, m.p. 137–9°C. Alkaline hydrolysis furnishes cinnamic acid.

Djerassi *et al.*, *Tetrahedron*, **16**, 212 (1961)

CYNAUSTRALINE

$C_{15}H_{27}O_4N$

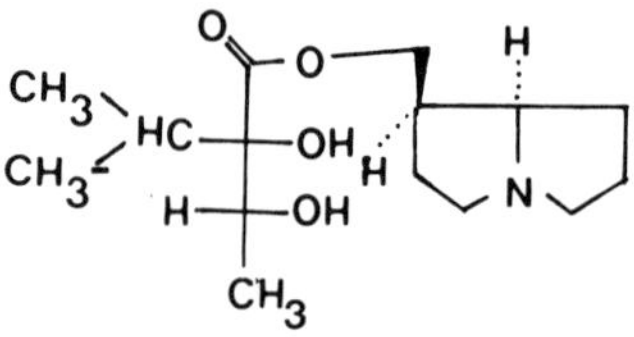

A pyrrolizidine base found in *Cynoglossum australe*, the structure of this alkaloid has been determined by chemical degradation and spectroscopic techniques.

Culvenor, Smith., *Austral. J. Chem.*, **20**, 2499 (1967)

CYNAUSTINE

$C_{16}H_{27}O_4N$

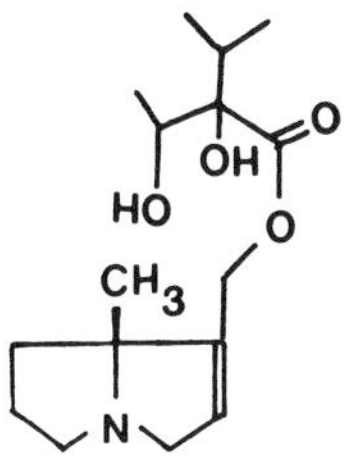

A further pyrrolizidine alkaloid isolated from *Cynoglossum australe*, this base yields the same necic acid as the preceding alkaloid but methylretronecine in place of platynecine.

Culvenor, Smith., *Austral. J. Chem.*, **20**, 2499 (1967)

CYNOCTONINE

$C_{36}H_{55}O_{13}N_2$

M.p. Indefinite

This aconite alkaloid was isolated from *Aconitum septentrionale* by Rosendahl. It is amorphous and dextrorotatory.

Rosendahl., *J. Pharm.*, **4**, 262 (1896)
Schultz, Ulfert., *Arch. Pharm.*, **260**, 230 (1922)
Wiedmann., *Arch. exp. Path. Pharm.*, **95**, 166 (1922)

CYNODINE

$C_{23}H_{23}O_3N_3$

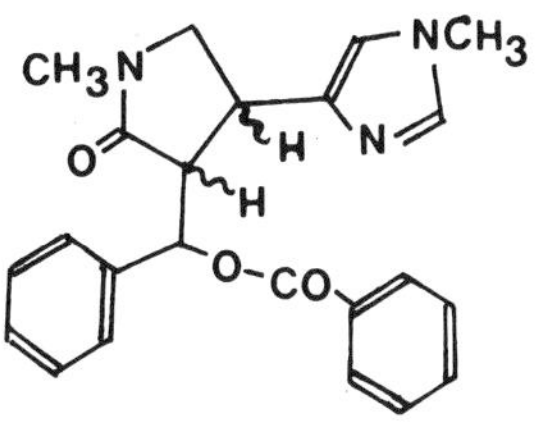

This novel alkaloid from the leaves of *Cynometra ananta* has recently been discovered. The structure has been shown to be that given above based upon spectroscopic evidence.

Khuong Huu Laine *et al.*, *Tetrahedron Lett.*, 1757 (1973)

CYNOGLOSSINE

An alkaloid described by Greiner as being present in *Anchusa officinalis* L., *Cynoglossum officinale* L. and *Echium vulgare* L., the base is stated to form a crystalline hydrochloride. Pharmacologically, it has a paralyzing effect upon the peripheral nerve terminations.

Greiner., *Arch. Pharm.*, **238**, 505 (1900)

CYNOMETRINE

$C_{16}H_{19}O_2N_3$

The leaves of *Cynometra ananta* also contain this novel alkaloid whose structure is very similar to that of Cynodine (q.v.).

Khuong Huu Laine *et al., Tetrahedron Lett.,* 1757 (1973)

CYTISINE

$C_{11}H_{14}ON_2$

M.p. 153°C;
B.p. 218°C/2 mm

This alkaloid, also described in the literature as baptitoxine, sophorine and ulexine, occurs widely among various species of Papilionaceae, e.g. *Anagyris foetida* L., *Baptisia australis, B. tinctoria* R. Br., *Cytisus Laburnum* L., *Euchresta Horsfieldii, Genista tinctoria, Sophora chrysophylla, S. microphylla, S. secundiflora, S. speciosa, S. tomentosum* and *Thermopsis rhombifolia* (Watt). It is a strongly alkaline base and forms well crystalline, although usually deliquescent, salts. The hydrochloride crystallizes as the monohydrate; the dihydrochloride occurs as yellow needles of the trihydrate; the perchlorate, m.p. 270°C; nitrate, m.p. 266°C; aurichloride, red-brown needles, m.p. 220°C (*dec.*); tartrate, m.p. 130–1°C; methiodide, m.p. 270°C and picrate, m.p. 277°C have been prepared. The formation of an N-nitroso derivative, m.p. 174°C, is indicative of a secondary nitrogen atom in the molecule. Cytisine also forms crystalline N-acyl derivative, e.g. the N-acetyl, m.p. 208°C; N-benzoyl, m.p. 116°C and the N-*p*-toluene-sulphonyl, m.p. 206–7°C.

On electrolytic reduction, the alkaloid furnishes tetrahydrodeoxycytisine, $C_{11}H_{20}N_2$, an oil with b.p. 270°C, characterized as the crystalline hydrochloride, m.p. 282°C and with phosphorus and hydriodic acid it gives NH_3 and cytosiline, m.p. 199°C. The latter has been shown to be 2-hydroxy-6:8-dimethylquinoline.

Cytisine falls in the same pharmacological group as nicotine and is a powerful poison causing nausea, then convulsions, and death due to respiratory failure. Numerous cases of poisoning due to the eating of laburnum seeds have been recorded.

Davy, Chu., *Chem. Abstr.,* **21**, 4025 (1927)
Ing., *J. Chem. Soc.,* 2195 (1931)
Ing., *ibid,* 2778 (1932)
Späth, Galinovsky., *Ber.,* **65**, 1526 (1932)
Orekhov *et al., ibid,* **66**, 625 (1933)
Orekhov *et al., ibid,* **67**, 1394 (1934)
Moisseva., *Trudy. Vostok Sibirsk Gosud. Univ.,* 148 (1940)
Tsarev., *C.R. Acad. Sci. URSS.,* **42**, 122 (1944)
Govindachari *et al., J. Chem. Soc.,* 3839 (1957)

D

DAMASCENINE

$C_{10}H_{13}O_3N$

M.p. 26°C;
B.p. 270°C

CO OCH$_3$
·NHCH$_3$
OCH$_3$

The history of this alkaloid is somewhat confused. Schneider isolated a crystal-line base from the seeds of *Nigella damascena* L. assigned the formula $C_{10}H_{15}O_3N$. This was subsequently examined by Pommerehne who gave it the formula $C_9H_{11}O_3N$ and stated that it could be converted into an isomeride, damasceninic acid, by the action of alkalies. Keller then obtained an alkaloid from the seeds of *Nigella aristata*, methyldamascenine, with the formula $C_{10}H_{13}O_3N$ which can also be obtained by the action of MeI on silver damasceninate. Ewins subsequently showed that the base examined by Pommerehne was a mixture of damascenine and damasceninic acid, while the alkaloids isolated by Schneider and Keller are identical.

Damascenine is soluble in most organic solvents, the solutions exhibiting a blue fluorescence. The hydrochloride forms prisms of the monohydrate, m.p. 122°C or 156°C (*dry*); the nitrate has m.p. 94—6°C; the platinichloride, m.p. 194°C and the picrate, lemon-yellow rhombic plates, m.p. 158—9°C. Hydrolysis with alkalies or acids yields MeOH and damasceninic acid, shown to be 2-methylamino-3-hydroxybenzoic acid. The alkaloid is therefore the correspond-ing methyl ester.

Schneider., *Pharm. Zent.*, **31**, 173 (1890)
Pommerehne., *Arch. Pharm.*, **238**, 531 (1900)
Keller., *ibid*, **242**, 299 (1904)
Keller., *ibid*, **246**, 1 (1908)
Ewins., *J. Chem. Soc.*, **101**, 544 (1912)
Kaufmann, Rothlin., *Ber.*, **49**, 578 (1916)
Keller, Schultz., *Chem. Zentr.*, **II**, 750 (1926)

DAMASCININE

$C_{10}H_{14}O_3N_2$

M.p. 75—9°C

CO$_2$CH$_3$
·NHCH$_3$
OH
NHCH$_3$

A second alkaloid isolated from the seeds of *Nigella damascena* L., this base forms colourless rhombic crystals from Me$_2$CO. It contains one hydroxyl group and two methylamino groups in the molecule.

Döpke, Fritsch., *Pharmazie*, **25**, 69 (1970)

DAPHMACRINE

$C_{32}H_{49}O_4N$

M.p. > 300°C

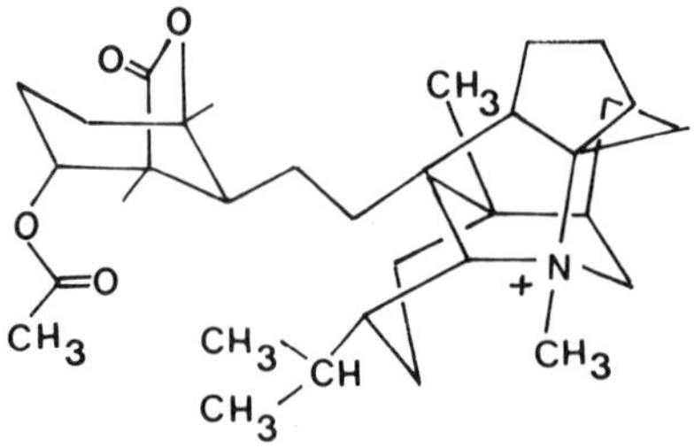

Isolated from *Daphniphyllum macropodum* Miquel, this complex alkaloid forms crystalline salts and derivatives. The hydrobromide is obtained as colourless crystals from Me_2CO-$CHCl_3$ and has m.p. > 300°C; $[\alpha]_D$ + 30.1° (c 1.79, MeOH). The methiodide has m.p. 174–5°C and forms orthorhombic crystals which have a = 14.23, b = 11.85 and c = 10.02 Å., Z 4 and space group $P2_12_12_1$. The structure of the alkaloid has been determined by ultraviolet, infrared, NMR and mass spectroscopy combined with X-ray analysis of the methiodide.

Nakano, Saeki., *Tetrahedron Lett.*, 4791 (1967)

Structure:
Nakano *et al.*, *Chem. Commun.*, 600 (1968)

DAPHMACROPODINE

$C_{32}H_{51}O_4N$

M.p. 214–5°C

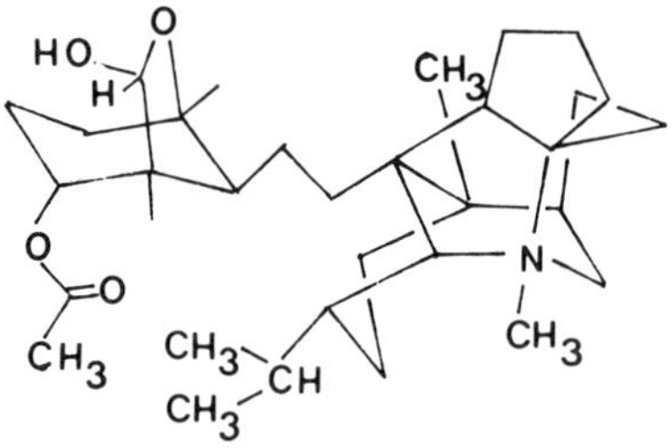

Also present in Daphniphyllum macropodum Miquel., this alkaloid is dextro-rotatory with $[\alpha]_D$ + 4.9° (c 1.11, $CHCl_3$). It forms a crystalline hydrobromide with m.p. 215–8°C.

Nakano, Saeki., *Tetrahedron Lett.*, 4791 (1967)

DAPHNANDRINE

$C_{36}H_{38}O_6N_2$

M.p. 280°C (*dec.*).

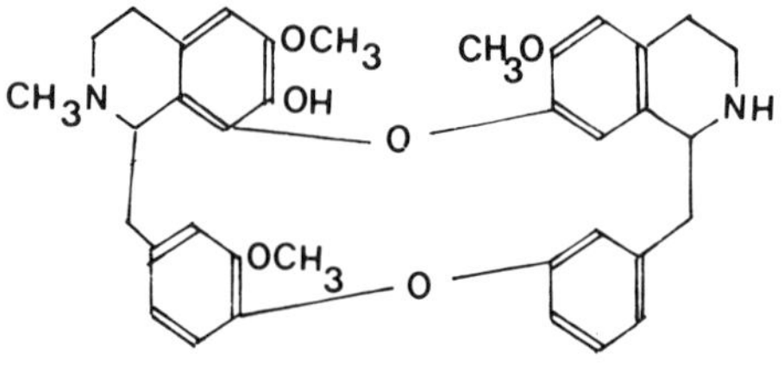

A bisbenzyl*iso*quinoline alkaloid obtained by Pyman from the bark of *Daphnandra*

micrantha, the base forms colourless needles from $CHCl_3$ with one mole of solvent that may be removed at 100°C with slight decomposition. The hydrochloride pentahydrate forms colourless prisms, m.p. 282°C (*dry, dec.*); $[\alpha]_D$ + 296–314° (c 3.9 to 1.1, H_2O); the hydrobromide hexahydrate, m.p. 291°C (*dry, dec.*) and the acid oxalate, m.p. 225°C have been prepared. The O,N-dimethyl dimethiodide has m.p. 255–265°C (*dec.*). The alkaloid is only slightly soluble in all organic solvents with the exception of boiling $CHCl_3$. It contains three methoxyl groups and one hydroxyl group.

Pyman., *J. Chem. Soc.,* **105**, 1679 (1914)
Bick, Ewen, Todd., *ibid,* 2767 (1949)

DAPHNARCINE

$C_{16}H_{17}O_4N$

M.p. 258–260°C

This base occurs in several *Narcissus* species and is obtained in the forms of colourless prisms from a 3:1 Me_2CO-MeOH mixture. It has $[\alpha]_D^{25}$ + 40° (c 0.1, dimethylformamide). The picrate is crystalline, m.p. 246°C (*dec.*).

Boit, Döpke, Beitner., *Chem. Ber.,* **90**, 2197 (1957)

DAPHNILACTONE A

$C_{23}H_{35}O_2N$

M.p. 194.5–195.5°C

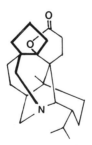

Daphniphyllum macropodum Miquel. yields this, and the following alkaloid, which have similar structures. Daphnilactone A contains one methyl and one isopropyl group and crystallizes from C_6H_6-hexane as colourless crystals. The crystal structure has been determined by X-ray analysis.

Toda *et al., Nippon Kagaku Zasshi.,* **91**, 103 (1970)
Sasaki, Hirata., *Tetrahedron Lett.,* 1275 (1972)

Structure:
Sasaki, Hirata., *J. Chem. Soc., Perkin II,* 1411 (1972)

DAPHNILACTONE B

$C_{22}H_{31}O_2N$

M.p. 92–4°C

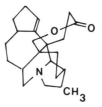

This base is found mainly in the fruit of *Daphniphyllum macropodium* Miquel and forms colourless rhombic crystals from C_6H_6-hexane. It contains one methyl group but no *iso*propyl groups in the molecule.

Sasaki, Hirata., *Tetrahedron Lett.*, 1891 (1972)
Niwa, Toda, Hirata., *ibid*, 2697 (1972)

DAPHNIMACRINE

$C_{27}H_{41}O_4N$

M.p. 75–84°C

This amorphous alkaloid was obtained from the bark of *Daphniphyllum macropodum* Miquel by Yagi. It is clearly not identical with Daphnimacropine (q.v.) with which it must not be confused.

Yagi., *Arch. Internat. Pharmacodyn.*, **20**, 117 (1910)

DAPHNIMACROPINE

$C_{31}H_{49}O_3N$

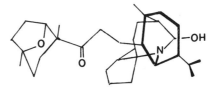

The bark of *Daphniphyllum macropodum* Miquel yields this alkaloid which has been examined by Nakano and Saeki. It forms a crystalline methiodide, m.p. 306–7°C.

Kamijo *et al.*, *Tetrahedron Lett.*, 2889 (1966)
Nakano, Saeki., *ibid*, 4791 (1967)

DAPHNIPHYLLAMINE

See Daphniphylline

DAPHNIPHYLLIDINE

$C_{30}H_{47}O_4N$

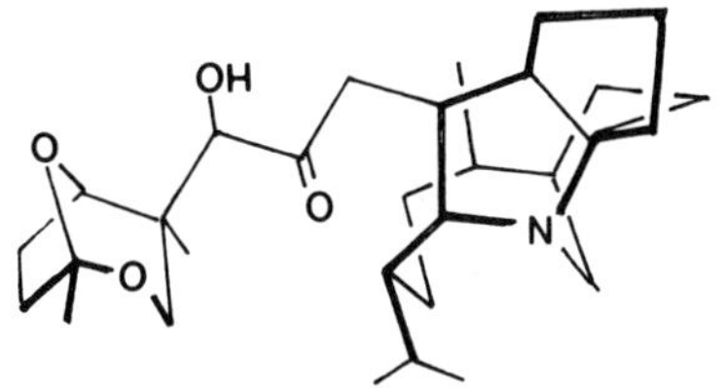

A further amorphous alkaloid found in *Daphniphyllum macropodum* Miquel, the above structure has been assigned to the base from chemical analysis and spectroscopic data.

Toda *et al., Tetrahedron Lett.,* **11**, 797 (1973)

DAPHNIPHYLLINE (*Daphniphyllamine*)

$C_{32}H_{49}O_5N$

M.p. 238–240°C

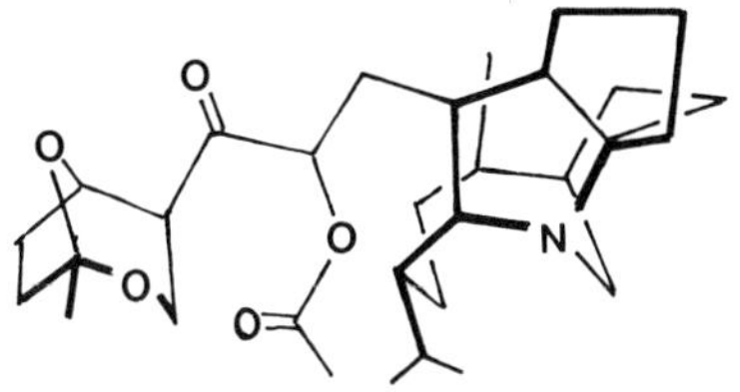

This alkaloid, under the name of daphniphyllamine, was isolated from the base fraction of the alkaloidal extract of the bark of *Daphniphyllum macropodum* and separated by chromatography on a neutralized silicic acid column. The alkaloid yields crystalline salts, e.g. the hydrochloride, m.p. 239–240°C; $[\alpha]_D$ + 43.7° (c 2.18, CHCl$_3$); hydrobromide, m.p. 228–230°C; $[\alpha]_D$ + 25.8° (c 1.34, MeOH) and the methiodide, m.p. 276–9°C. When treated with 6N HCl at 80°C, the alkaloid gives deacetyl*iso*daphniphylline which, with Ac$_2$O in pyridine, yields isodaphniphylline characterized as the hydrochloride, m.p. 197–198.5°C. An amorphous base of the same name was isolated from *Daphniphyllum bancanum* Kürz but it has not yet been established whether the two alkaloids are identical.

Plugge., *Arch. exp. Path. Pharm.,* **32**, 277 (1893)
Nakano, Saeki., *Tetrahedron Lett.,* 4791 (1967)
Yamamura, Irikawa, Hirata., *ibid,* 3361 (1967)
Irikawa *et al., Tetrahedron,* **24**, 5691 (1968)

NMR spectrum:
Sakebe *et al., Tetrahedron Lett.,* 963 (1966)

DAPHNOLINE (*Trilobamine*)

$C_{35}H_{36}O_6N_2$

M.p. 194–6°C

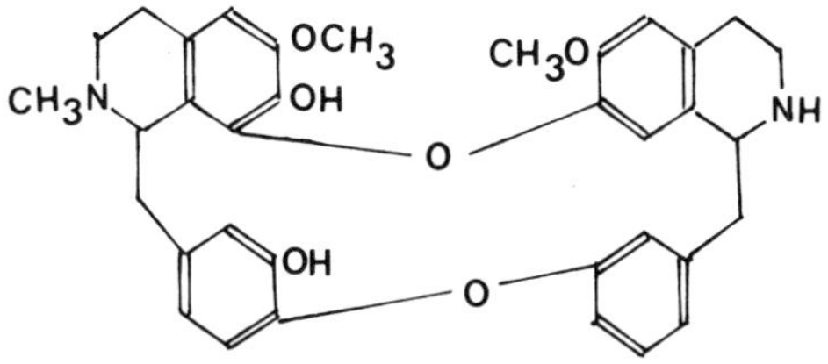

This base from *Daphnandra micrantha* Benth. also occurs in *Cocculus trilobus*

and crystallizes, with solvent, from $CHCl_3$ or EtOH in small hexahedral crystals. It is even less soluble than daphnandrine in ordinary solvents. It is dextrorotatory with $[\alpha]_D + 459°$ $(CHCl_3)$. The dihydrochloride crystallizes with 3.5 H_2O as large, colourless bipyramids, m.p. 290°C (*dry, dec.*) and the hydrobromide tetrahydrate forms microscopic needles, m.p. 286°C (*dec.*). The alkaloid is a phenolic base and contains one methylimino and two methoxyl groups. With Fröhde's reagent it gives a violet colour changing to red.

Pyman., *J. Chem. Soc.*, **105**, 1679 (1914)
Bick, Ewen, Todd., *ibid*, 2767 (1949)
Inubushi., *Pharm. Bull. Japan*, **3**, 384 (1955)

DARVASAMINE

$C_{15}H_{24}ON_2$

M.p. 102°C

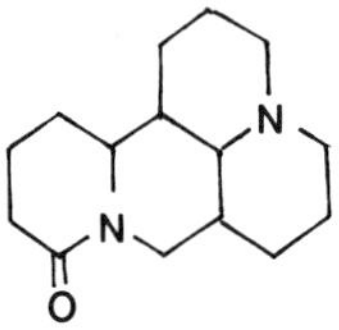

A tetracyclic alkaloid found in *Leontice darvasica*, this base has $[\alpha]_D + 72°$ (EtOH). The structure has been determined by chemical and spectroscopic examination.

Zunnunzhanov *et al., Khim. Prir. Soedin.*, **7**, 851 (1971)

DARVASOLINE

$C_{15}H_{24}O_2N_2$

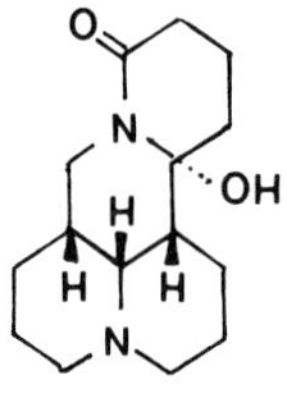

This alkaloid has recently been isolated from *Leontice darvasica*. Reduction with $LiAlH_4$ yields matridine and treatment with P_2O_5 at 200–210°C for 5 hours furnishes Sophoramine (q.v.). These reactions, coupled with infrared and mass spectrometry, confirm the above structure.

Zunnunzhanov, Iskandarov, Yunusov., *Khim. Prir. Soedin.*, **10**, 115 (1974)

DASYCARPIDOL

$C_{17}H_{22}ON_2$

M.p. 118–122°C

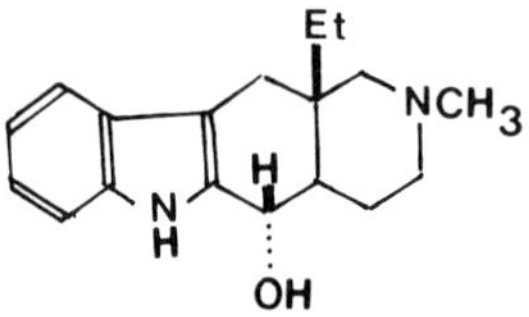

Isolated from *Aspidosperma dasycarpon* A. DC. this laevorotatory alkaloid has

$[\alpha]_D - 54°$ (EtOH). The ultraviolet spectrum in EtOH shows absorption maxima at 220, 282 and 290 mμ. Chromic acid oxidizes the secondary hydroxyl group to give Dasycarpidone (q.v.).

Ohashi *et al., Experientia*, **20**, 363 (1964)
Joule *et al., Tetrahedron*, **21**, 1717 (1965)

Stereochemistry:
Shamma *et al., Tetrahedron Lett.*, 2489 (1967)

DASYCARPIDONE

$C_{17}H_{20}ON_2$

M.p. Indefinite

An amorphous alkaloid found in *Aspidosperma dasycarpon* A. DC., having $[\alpha]_D^{26} + 64.7°$ (c 1.02, $CHCl_3$), this base has an ultraviolet spectrum with absorption maxima at 237 and 316 mμ. As already stated, it is also produced by oxidation of Dasycarpidol with chromic acid. The ($\pm$)-form is also amorphous and yields a crystalline picrate, m.p. 240°C (*dec.*).

Ohashi *et al., Experientia,* **20**, 363 (1964)
Joule *et al., Tetrahedron*, **21**, 1717 (1965)

Stereochemistry:
Shamma *et al., Tetrahedron Lett.*, 2489 (1967)
Gaskell, Joule., *Chem. & Ind.*, 1089 (1967)

DASYCARPINE

$C_{20}H_{35}N_3$

B.p. 160–5°C/0.5 mm

A liquid alkaloid isolated from *Ormosia dasycarpa* Jacks, this base has $[\alpha]_D^{20} +$ 12.5° (c 1.1, EtOH) and forms crystalline salts and derivatives, e.g. the hydrochloride, m.p. 270–4°C (*dec.*); perchlorate, m.p. 240°C (*dec.*); an amorphous picrate, m.p. 150–2°C and a methiodide hydriodide, m.p. 246–7°C (*dec.*). The N-methyl derivative is formed by the action of CH_2N_2 and has m.p. 120–1°C. Acetylation yields the N-acetyl compound, m.p. 155–7°C.

Clarke, Grundon., *J. Chem. Soc.*, 41 (1960)
Clarke, Grundon., *ibid*, 535 (1963)

2-epi-DASYCARPONE

$C_{17}H_{20}ON_2$

M.p. Indefinite

This amorphous base is a minor constituent of *Aspidosperma subincanum*. Its ultraviolet spectrum in EtOH has two absorption maxima at 238 and 314 mμ. The ($\pm$)-form has been synthesized by two groups of workers.

Gaskell, Joule., *Chem. & Ind.,* 1089 (1967)

Synthesis:
Dolby, Biere., *J. Amer. Chem. Soc.,* **90**, 2699 (1968)
Jackson *et al.,* *Chem. Commun.,* 364 (1968)

DATURINE

$C_{17}H_{23}O_3N$

This alkaloid from the leaves and seeds of *Datura arborea* was shown by von Planta to be identical with atropine (q.v.). The base of the same name isolated by Montesinos is also atropine.

von Planta., *Arch. Pharm.,* **74**, 245 (1850)
Montesinos., *Bol. Soc. Quim. Peru.,* **5**, 99 (1939)

DAUCINE

$C_{11}H_{18}N_2$

B.p. 240–250°C

An alkaloid found in *Daucus carota* L., this base has $[\alpha]_D$ + 7.8°. So far it has not been re-examined to determine the structure.

Pictet, Court., *Bull. Soc. Chim.,* **1**, 1001 (1907)

DAURICINE

$C_{38}H_{44}O_6N_2$

M.p. 115°C

One of the Menispermaceae alkaloids, this bisbenzy*iso*quinoline base is found in *Menispermum canadense* L. and *M. dauricum* DC. It is obtained as a bright yellow powder which is soluble in most organic solvents and has $[\alpha]_D^{11}$ − 139° (MeOH). It gives a blue-brown colour with $FeCl_3$. The hydrochloride has m.p. 213–4°C and the dimethiodide forms needles, m.p. 204°C; $[\alpha]_D^{22}$ − 110° (MeOH). Ethyl bromide in alkali yields ethyldauricine diethobromide, m.p. 136–9°C (*dec.*) which, on boiling with NaOK gives α-ethyldauricineethylmethine, of which the dimethiodide, m.p. 162–5°C (*dec.*) can be degraded to $C_{40}H_{44}O_6$, oxidized by $KMnO_4$ to 2-ethoxy-5:4'-dicarboxydiphenyl ether, m.p. 276–7°C.

The alkaloid contains one hydroxyl group which may be methylated to yield the O-methyl ether, m.p. 54–64°C. The (±)-form has m.p. 122–4°C and forms a stable hydrate, m.p. 110°C. It gives a dipicrate, m.p. 140–2°C and a distyphnate, m.p. 146–9°C.

Kondo, Narita., *J. Pharm. Soc. Japan,* **542**, 40 (1927)
Faltis, Frauendorfer., *Ber.,* **63**, 809 (1930)
Kondo, Narita, Uyeo., *ibid,* **68**, 519 (1935)
Kondo, Narita, Murakami., *J. Pharm. Soc. Japan,* **61**, 117 (1941)
Synthesis:
Kametani, Fukumoto., *Tetrahedron Lett.,* 2771 (1964)
Popp *et al., J. Org. Chem.,* **31**, 2296 (1966)

DAURICINOLINE

$C_{37}H_{42}O_6N_2$

M.p. Indefinite

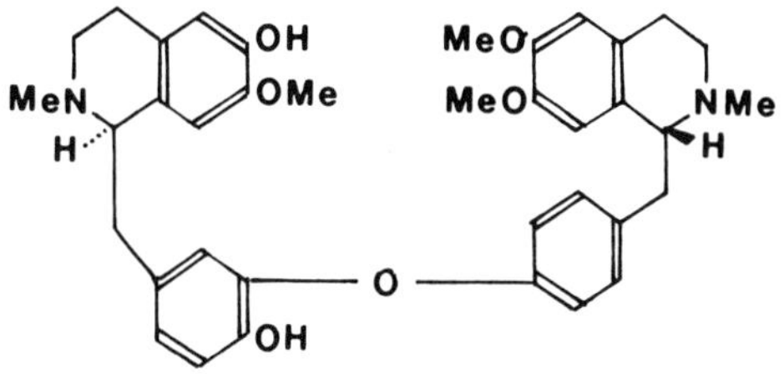

A bisbenzyl*iso*quinoline alkaloid which occurs in *Menispermum dauricum* DC., the base is obtained as a light yellow, amorphous powder. The O-methyl ether is dauricine (q.v.). The alkaloid contains three methoxyl groups, two hydroxyl groups and two methylimino groups in the molecule.

Tomita *et al., J. Pharm. Soc. Japan,* **90**, 1182 (1970)

DAURICOLINE

$C_{36}H_{40}O_6N_2$

M.p. Indefinite

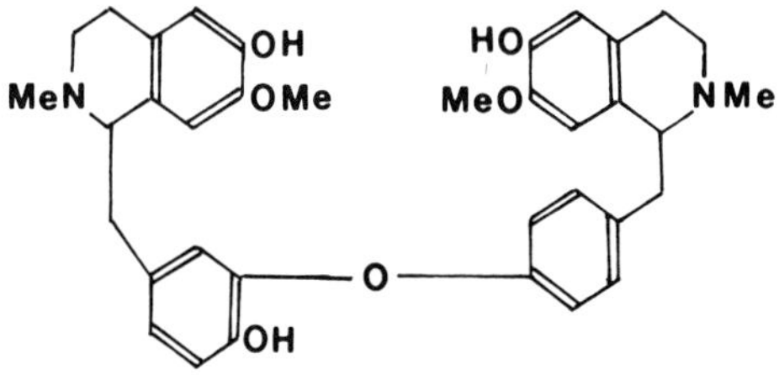

A second amorphous alkaloid found in *Menispermum dauricum* DC, this base is also a light yellow powder with no definite melting point. There are two methoxyl groups, three hydroxyl groups and two methylimino groups in the molecule. The O-methyl ether is identical with dauricinoline (q.v.) and the O,O-dimethyl ether with dauricine (q.v.).

Tomita *et al., J. Pharm. Soc. Japan,* **90**, 1178 (1970)

DAURINOLINE

$C_{37}H_{42}O_6N_2$

M.p. 103°C

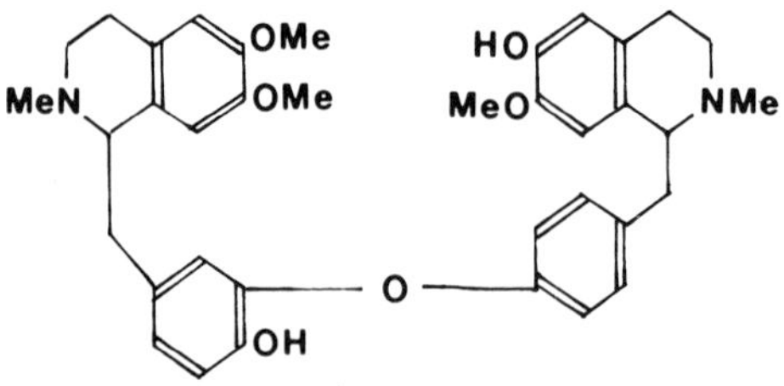

Menispermum dauricum DC also yields this alkaloid of the bisbenzyl*iso*quinoline type. The stereoisomeric mixture of the O,O-dibenzoyl derivatives, prepared synthetically by an Ullmann reaction between two tetrahydro*iso*quinoline derivatives, yields a dipicrate, m.p. 124–6°C. The dibenzoyl compound, when treated with excess CH_2N_2 furnishes O,O-dimethyldaurinoline (dipicrate, m.p. 143–5°C, *dec.*).

Tomita *et al., J..Pharm. Soc., Japan,* **90,** 1178 (1970)
Kametani *et al., Chem. Pharm. Bull. (Tokyo),* **16,** 1625 (1968)

DEACETYLAKUAMMILINE

$C_{20}H_{24}O_3N_2$

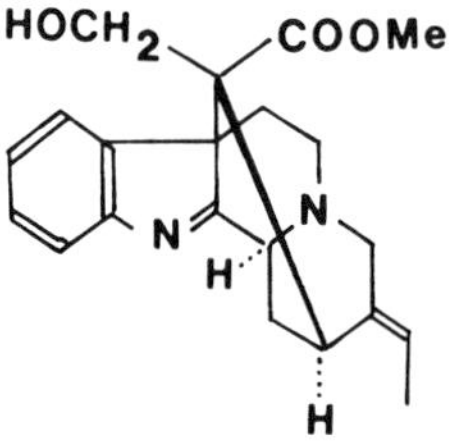

A carboline alkaloid, this base has recently been isolated from *Vinca minor.* It occurs together with the 10-methoxyl derivative (q.v.). The structure follows from spectroscopic determinations and chemical analysis.

Savaskan *et al., Helv. Chim. Acta,* **55,** 2861 (1972)

DEACETYLASPIDOSPERMINE

$C_{20}H_{28}ON_2$

M.p. 107–8°C

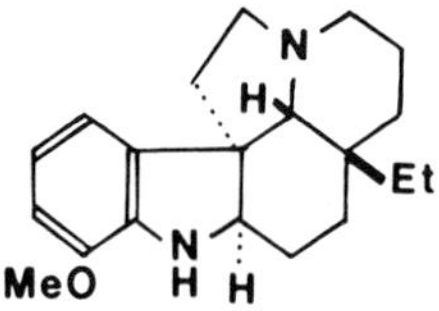

This alkaloid is a minor constituent of *Aspidosperma quebracho* Schlecht and also occurs in *A. polyneuron.* It yields a crystalline dihydriodide, m.p. > 280°C and the N-benzoyl derivative, m.p. 187–190°C. The N-formyl compound is Vallesine (q.v.) and the N-acetyl derivative is Aspidospermine (q.v.).

Ewins., *J. Chem. Soc.,* **105,** 2738 (1914)
Schlittler, Rottenburg., *Helv. Chim. Acta,* **31,** 446 (1948)
Paladini *et al., Anales Assoc. Quim. Argentina,* **50,** 352 (1962)

DEACETYLDEFORMYLAKUAMMILINE

$C_{19}H_{22}O_2N_2$

M.p. 140°C

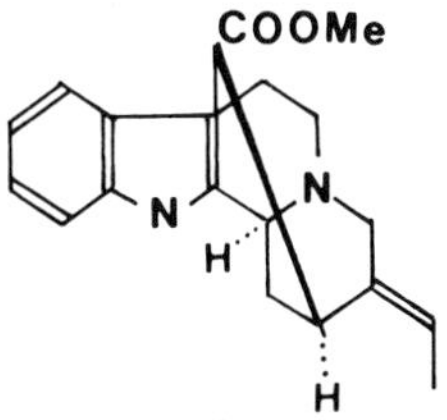

Isolated from the leaves of *Rauwolfia vomitora,* this alkaloid is dextrorotatory with $[\alpha]_D + 133°$ (CHCl$_3$).

Pousset., *Trav. Lab. Matiere Med. Pharm. Galenique Fac. Pharm. Paris,* **52**, II, 13 (1967)

DEACETYLDEFORMYLPICRALINE

$C_{20}H_{22}O_3N_2$

M.p. 216°C

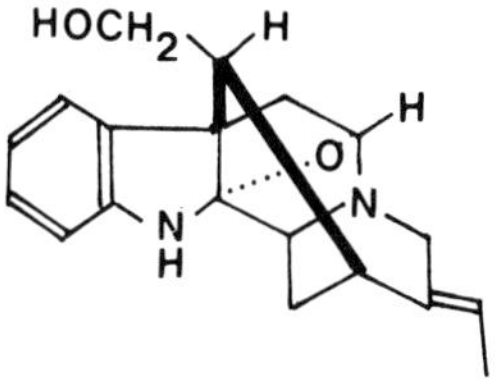

A further minor constituent of the leaves of *Rauwolfia vomitora,* this alkaloid is laevorotatory with $[\alpha]_D - 48°$ (CHCl$_3$).

Pousset., *Trav. Lab. Matiere Med. Pharm. Galenique Fac. Pharm. Paris,* **52**, II, 13 (1967)

2-DEACETYLEVONINE

$C_{34}H_{41}O_{16}N$

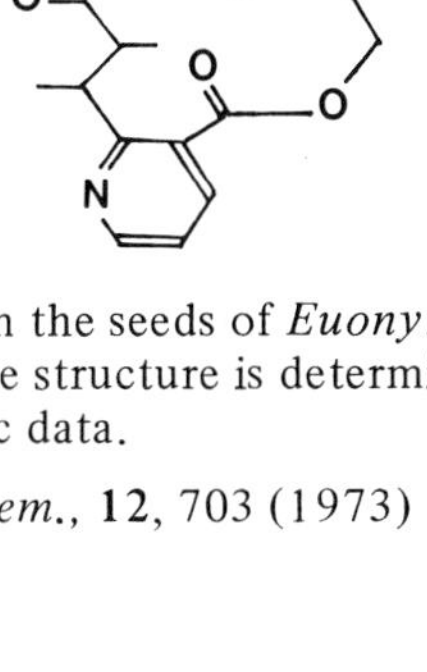

A minor alkaloid obtained from the seeds of *Euonymus europea,* the base has only recently been isolated. The structure is determined on the basis of chemical analysis and from spectroscopic data.

Crombie, Whiting., *Phytochem.,* **12**, 703 (1973)

DEACETYLFAWCETTIINE

$C_{16}H_{27}O_2N$

M.p. 205–7°C

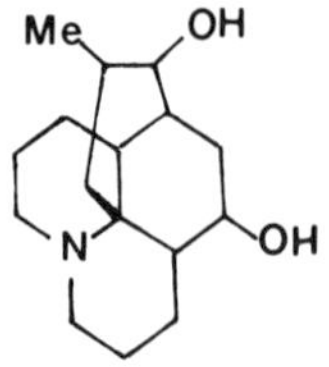

Lycopodium fawcettii yields this alkaloid which forms colourless needles from Me$_2$CO. It has also been discovered in *L. clavatum* grown in Jamaica. With ethyl chloroformate in pyridine it gives the dihydro derivative, m.p. 75–85°C; [α]$_D$ – 70° (c 1.18, EtOH), giving a methiodide, m.p. 263–5°C.

Burnell., *J. Chem. Soc.*, 3091 (1959)
Burnell, Mootoo, Taylor., *Can. J. Chem.*, **38**, 1927 (1960)
Burnell, Mootoo, Taylor., *ibid*, **39**, 1090 (1961)

N-DEACETYL-N-FORMYLCOLCHICINE

$C_{21}H_{23}O_6N$

M.p. 264–6°C

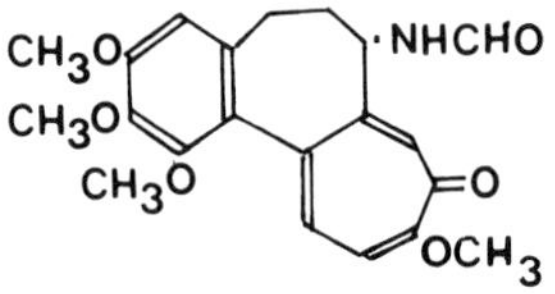

A colchicine alkaloid, this base occurs in *Androcymbium melanthioides* and has also been found in certain *Colchicum* species. It is laevorotatory with [α]$_D^{22}$ – 174° (c 1.03, CHCl$_3$). It contains four methoxyl groups in the molecule.

Santavy, Reichstein., *Helv. Chim. Acta.*, **33**, 1606 (1950)
Hrbek, Santavy., *Collect. Czech. Chem. Commun.*, **27**, 255 (1962)

DEACETYLGERMITETRINE

$C_{39}H_{61}O_{13}N$

M.p. 143–9°C (*dec.*).

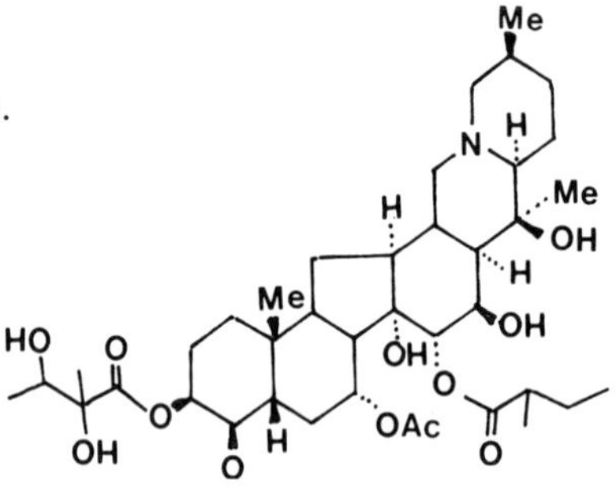

An alkaloid obtained from *Veratrum album,* this base forms white plates and is slightly laevorotatory with [α]$_D^{28}$ – 8° (c 1.0, pyridine). It is separated from the accompanying bases by countercurrent distribution methods. Alkaline hydrolysis furnishes Germine (q.v.), acetic acid and EtMeCH.COOH.

Myers *et al., J. Amer. Chem. Soc.*, **78**, 1621 (1956)

400

DEACETYLNEOPROTOVERATRINE

M.p. 181–3°C

A further constituent of *Veratrum album* which is obtained by countercurrent distribution methods. It has a specific rotation very similar to that of the preceding alkaloid, viz. $[\alpha]_D^{25} - 9°$ (c 1.0, pyridine).

Myers *et al.*, *J. Amer. Chem. Soc.*, **78**, 1621 (1956)

O-DEACETYLPACHYSANDRINE B

$C_{29}H_{50}O_2N_2$

M.p. 202°C

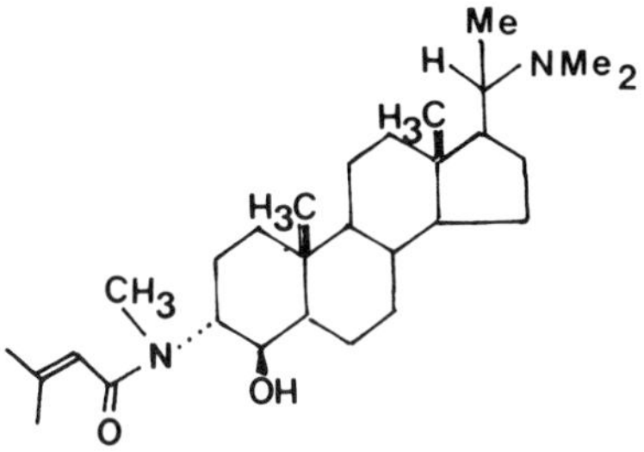

A minor alkaloid of *Pachysandra terminalis* Sieb. et Zucc., this alkaloid contains three methyl groups and one dimethylamino group in the molecule.

Tomita *et al.*, *Tetrahedron Lett.*, 1053 (1964)

DEACETYLPICRALINE

$C_{21}H_{24}O_4N_2$

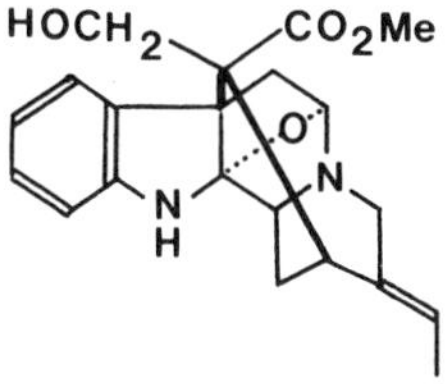

The bark of *Aspidosperma rigidum* contains this alkaloid as a minor constituent. No salts or derivatives have yet been reported.

Arndt *et al.*, *Phytochem.*, **6**, 1653 (1967)

DEACETYLPROTOVERATRINE

$C_{39}H_{61}O_{13}N$

M.p. 185–6°C (191–2°C)

A steroidal alkaloid found in *Veratrum album* and *V. viride*, the base crystallizes from C_6H_6 as colourless crystals. Various specific rotations have been recorded, e.g. $[\alpha]_D^{25} - 8°$ (c 1.0, pyridine); $[\alpha]_D^{25} - 15°$ (c 1.0, pyridine) and $+ 14°$ (c 1.0, $CHCl_3$). The methiodide is crystalline, m.p. 231–2°C. Alkaline hydrolysis with

NaOH in MeOH gives Protoverine. The alkaloid produces a lowering of blood pressure in anaesthetized dogs.

Myers *et al., J. Amer. Chem. Soc.,* **77**, 3348 (1955)
Myers *et al., ibid,* **78**, 1621 (1956)

DEACETYLSTRYCHNOSPERMINE

$C_{20}H_{26}O_2N_2$

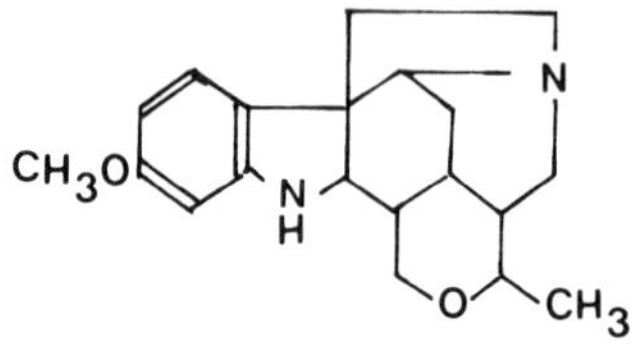

A minor alkaloid found in the leaves of *Strychnos psilosperma,* the structure of the base has been established from chemical analysis and comparison with the spectra of Strychnospermine (q.v.).

Anet, Hughes, Ritchie., *Austral. J. Chem.,* **6**, 58 (1953)

DEACETYLVINBLASTINE

$C_{44}H_{56}O_8N_4$

M.p. 205–210°C

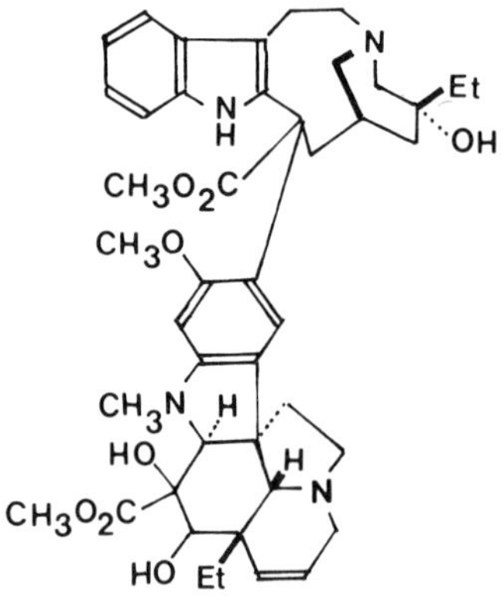

A dimeric alkaloid isolated from *Vinca Rosea* L., the base forms colourless leaflets from aqueous EtOH and gives an ultraviolet spectrum in EtOH with absorption maxima at 214, 266 and 295 mμ. It forms a crystalline sulphate, m.p. > 320°C (*dec.*). The alkaloid contains three hydroxyl groups, one methoxyl, two ethyl and one methylimino group.

Svoboda, Barnes., *J. Pharm. Sci.,* **53**, 1227 (1964)
Hargrove., *Lloydia,* **27**, 340 (1964)

DEACETYLVINDOLINE

$C_{23}H_{30}O_5N_2$

M.p. $163-5°C$

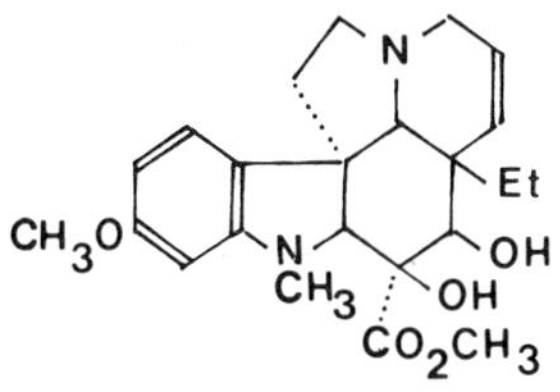

An imidazolidinocarbazole alkaloid present in the leaves of *Catharanthus roseus* G. Don. The base has two hydroxyl groups, one ethyl group and one methoxyl group.

Gorman et al., J. Amer. Pharm. Assoc., **48**, 256 (1959)
Moza et al., Collect. Czech. Chem. Commun., **29**, 1913 (1964)
Gröger, Stolle, Falshaw., Naturwiss., **52**, 132 (1965)

DECALINE

$C_{26}H_{31}O_5N$

M.p. $102-118°C$

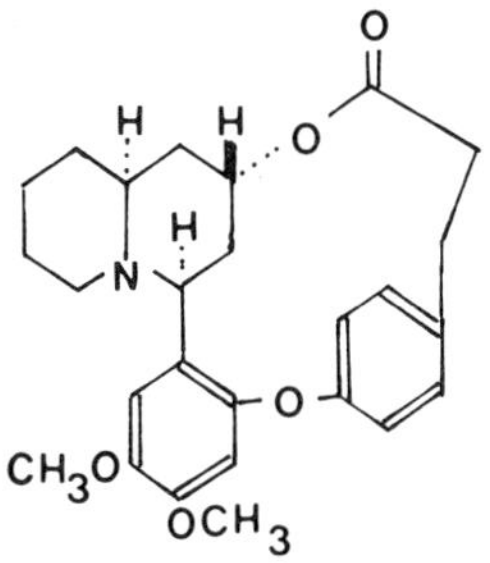

Isolated from *Decodon verticillatus* L., this base crystallizes with one mole of EtOH, m.p. $80-1°C$, the solvent being lost at $100°C$. The alkaloid has $[\alpha]_D -136°$ (CHCl$_3$). Preparation of the acetyl derivative has been attempted but without success, only unchanged material being obtained after prolonged treatment with Ac$_2$O.

Ferris., J. Org. Chem., **27**, 2985 (1962)
Ferris., ibid, **28**, 817 (1963)
Ferris et al., Tetrahedron Lett., 5125 (1966)

DECAMINE

$C_{26}H_{31}O_5N$

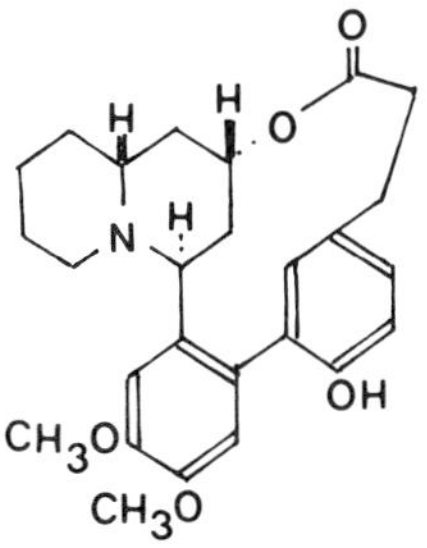

Also present in *Decodon verticillatus* L., this alkaloid has $[\alpha]_D -145°$ (CHCl$_3$).

The ultraviolet spectrum shows an absorption maximum at 294 mμ. The single hydroxyl group may be acetylated with Ac_2O in pyridine to yield the O-acetate, m.p. 197–8°C; $[\alpha]_D$ − 188° (c 1.16, pyridine).

Ferris., *J. Org. Chem.*, **27**, 2985 (1962)
Ferris., *ibid*, **28**, 817 (1963)
Ferris *et al.*, *Tetrahedron Lett.*, 3641 (1966)

DECARBOXYDIHYDROGAMBERTANNINE

$C_{19}H_{18}N_2$

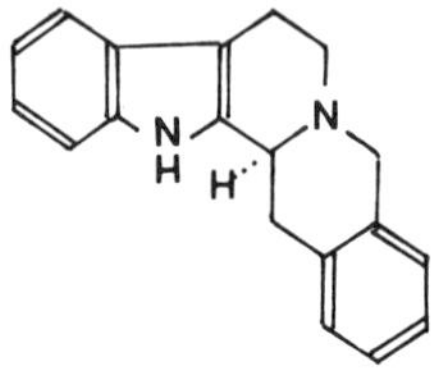

This indole alkaloid occurs in the leaves of *Ochrosia lifuana* and *O. miana*. The base has been identified by comparison of its spectra with those of Dihydro-gambertannine (q.v.).

Peube-Locou, Plat, Koch., *Phytochem.*, **12**, 199 (1973)

16-DECARBOMETHOXYDIHYDROVOBASINE
(*Alkaloid H100*)

$C_{19}H_{25}ON_2$

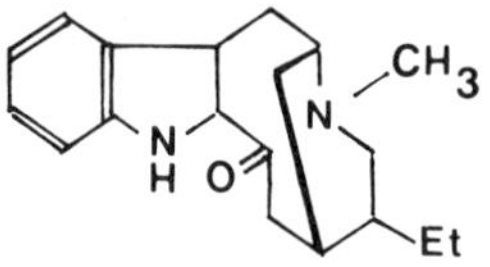

The structure of this alkaloid, obtained from species of *Rauwolfia* grown in Madagascar, has been established by chemical and clinical examination.

Combes *et al.*, *Phytochem.*, **7**, 477 (1968)

DECININE

$C_{26}H_{31}O_5N$

M.p. 222–4°C

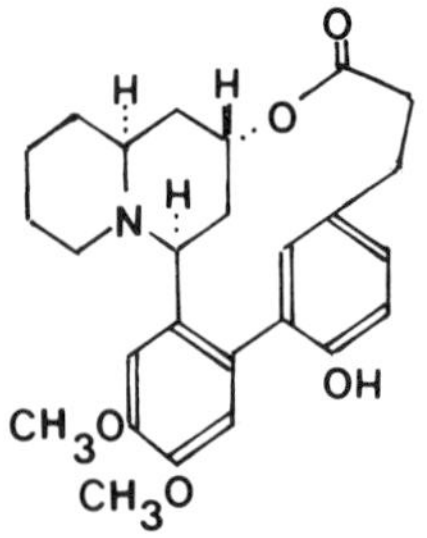

This particular alkaloid crystallizes as colourless rhombs from the MeOH extract

of *Decodon verticillatus* L. It is laevorotatory with $[\alpha]_D - 142°$ (c 1.37, CHCl$_3$).
Like Decamine (q.v.), the ultraviolet spectrum exhibits a single absorption
maximum at 294 mμ, with an inflexion at 251 mμ. A crystalline acetate has been
prepared with m.p. 197–8°C; $[\alpha]_D - 139°$ (c 1.59, CHCl$_3$). From the stereochemistry of the alkaloid it will be seen that the base and Decamine are
stereoisomers.

Ferris., *J. Org. Chem.*, **27**, 2985 (1962)
Ferris., *ibid*, **28**, 817 (1963)

Structure and stereochemistry:
Ferris *et al.*, *Tetrahedron Lett.*, 3641 (1966)
Zacharias *et al.*, *Experientia*, **21**, 247 (1965)

DECODINE

$C_{25}H_{29}O_5N$

M.p. 193–7°C

A further alkaloid obtained from *Decodon verticillatus* L. This base has $[\alpha]_D -$
97° (c 1.78, CHCl$_3$) and the ultraviolet spectrum shows absorption maxima at
287 and 312 mμ. There are two hydroxyl groups in the molecule and the alkaloid
forms crystalline derivative, e.g. the O-methyl ether, m.p. 227–8°C, characterized
as the acetate, m.p. 195.5–196.5°C and the O,O-dimethyl ether, m.p. 206–7°C.
The diacetate has m.p. 202–3°C.

Ferris., *J. Org. Chem.*, **27**, 2985 (1962)
Ferris., *ibid*, **28**, 817 (1963)
Ferris *et al.*, *Tetrahedron Lett.*, 3641 (1966)

DECORTICASINE

$C_{10}H_{16}O_2N_2$

This oily base is present in several *Adenocarpus* species and in particular in
A. decorticans. It forms a series of crystalline salts and derivatives: the dihydrobromide, m.p. 304°C (*dec.*); dihydriodide, m.p. 202°C; diplatinichloride, m.p.
250°C (*dec.*); diaurichloride, m.p. 250–3°C (*dec.*); dinitrate, m.p. 178–9°C;
dipicrate, m.p. 236–7°C (*dec.*) and the methiodide, m.p. 242°C. When hydrolyzed
with dilute HCl it furnishes propionic acid and depropionyldecorticasine. The
latter also yields crystalline salts, e.g. the dihydrochloride, m.p. 305–310°C and
the diperchlorate, m.p. 166–7°C.

Clark., *J. Amer. Chem. Soc.,* **54**, 3000 (1932)
Haller, Le Forge., *ibid,* **56**, 2415 (1934)
Boam *et al., J. Soc. Chem. Ind.,* **56**, 91 T (1937)
Fukami *et al., Agr. Biol. Chem.* (Japan), **25**, 252 (1961)

DEFORMYLTALBOTINIC ACID METHYL ESTER

$C_{20}H_{24}O_3N_2$

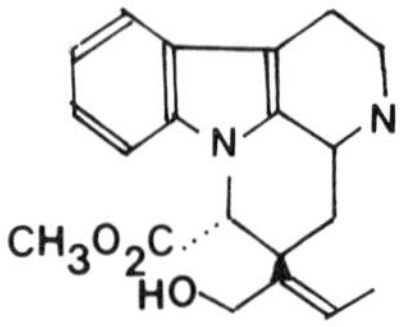

A recently isolated alkaloid from the leaves of *Pleiocarpa talbotii.* The structure has been established from the ultraviolet, infrared, NMR and mass spectra.

Pinar, Hesse, Schmid., *Helv. Chim. Acta,* **56**, 2719 (1973)

DEFORMYLVALLESINE

$C_{20}H_{28}ON_2$

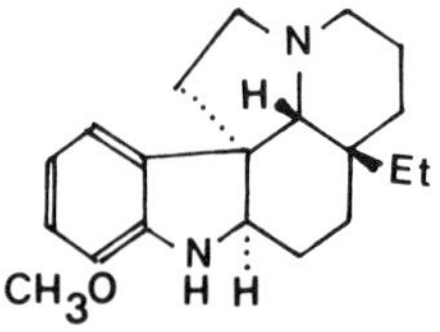

Walser and Djerassi have described this minor base, isolated from *Vallesia dichotoma.* It contains one methoxyl and one ethyl group in the molecule.

Walser, Djerassi., *Helv. Chim. Acta,* **47**, 2072 (1964)

DEHYDROALBINE

M.p. 50°C

This minor alkaloid occurs in the seeds of *Lupinus albus* and forms colourless needles from hexane. It is laevorotatory with $[\alpha]_D^{25} - 103°$ (c 1.6, MeOH). The base is characterized as the perchlorate, colourless crystals from H_2O, m.p. 252.5°C; $[\alpha]_D^{25} - 76°$ (c 1.0, H_2O).

Wiewiorowski, Wolinsku-Mocydlarz., *Bull. Acad. Polon. Sci.,* **12**, 217 (1964)

(+)-1:2-DEHYDROASPIDOSPERMIDINE

$C_{19}H_{24}N_2$

B.p. 155°C/0.01 mm

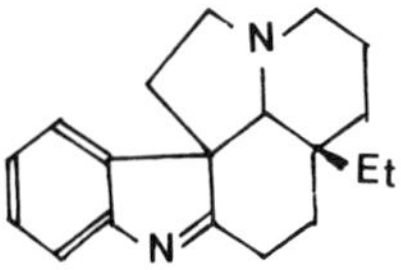

This alkaloid is present in *Aspidosperma quebracho blanco, Rhazya stricta* and

Amsonia tabernaemontana. As isolated it is a non-crystallizable syrup which has $[\alpha]_D^{20}$ + 243° (EtOH). The ultraviolet spectrum has absorption maxima at 222 and 263 mμ. With LiAlH$_4$ it yields (+)-Aspidospermidine and with NaBH$_4$ it also yields this base at 0°C, but the same reagent at 100°C furnishes (−)-Quebrachamine (q.v.).

Schnoes, Burlinghame, Biemann., *Tetrahedron Lett.,* 993 (1962)

Biemann *et al., ibid,* 484 (1963)

Smith, Wahid., *J. Chem. Soc.,* 4002 (1963)

Zsadon, Egry, Sarkosi., *Acta Chim.* (Budapest), **67**, 77 (1971)

(−)-1:2-DEHYDROASPIDOSPERMIDINE

$C_{19}H_{24}N_2$

B.p. 140°C/0.01 mm

This base occurs in the leaves of *Pleiocarpa tubicina* and has $[\alpha]_D^{23}$ − 212° ± 15° (c 0.15, EtOH). A scheme for the biosynthesis of the alkaloid has been advanced by Battersby and his colleagues.

Bycroft *et al., Helv. Chim. Acta,* **47**, 1147 (1964)

Biosynthesis:

Battersby *et al., Chem. Commun.,* 46 (1966)

DEHYDROBROWNIINE

$C_{25}H_{39}O_7N$

This minor alkaloid has been recorded in *Delphinium cardinale*. No salts or derivatives have been reported.

Benn., *Can. J. Chem.,* **44**, 1 (1966)

DEHYDROBUFOTENINE

$C_{12}H_{14}ON_2$

M.p. 199°C (*dec.*).

This alkaloidal base is found in the skin secretions of certain toads, including *Bufo bufo bufo* and *B. marinus*. The alkaloid forms colourless crystals from H$_2$O which contain water of crystallization. When obtained in the anhydrous form, the alkaloid has m.p. 218°C. The base forms a crystalline picrolonate, m.p. > 300°C and also the O,N-dimethyl derivative, characterized as the hydriodide, m.p. 208°C.

Wieland, Wieland., *Annalen*, **528**, 234 (1937)
Marki, Robertson, Witkop., *J. Amer. Chem. Soc.*, **83**, 3341 (1961)
Robinson *et al.*, *Proc. Chem. Soc.*, 310 (1961)

DEHYDROCAPAURIMINE

$C_{20}H_{21}O_5N$

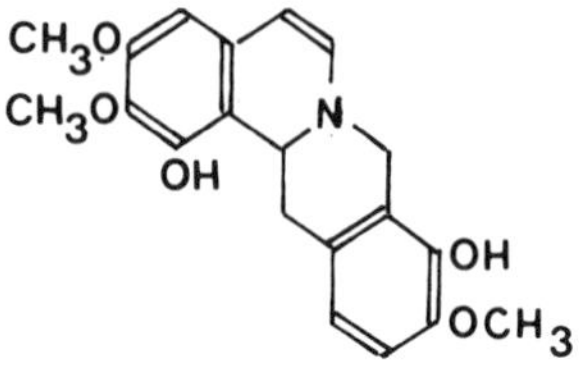

Although this alkaloid has not been isolated as such, it is considered to be present in *Corydalis platycarpa*. When the quaternary base fraction of the plant extract is reduced with $NaBH_4$ it yields (±)-Capaurimine and, since this is a reduction product, it is believed that it is present in the plant itself as the dehydro-base.

Tank *et al.*, *J. Pharm. Soc., Japan*, **90**, 903 (1970)

DEHYDROCHEILANTHIFOLINE (*Base A*)

$C_{19}H_{16}O_4N^+$

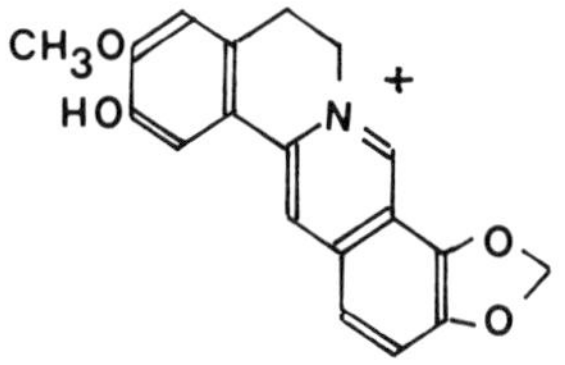

A quaternary alkaloid isolated as Base A from *Bocconia cordata*, the base has been shown to have the above structure.

Takao, Yasumoto, Kinuko., *J. Pharm. Soc., Japan*, **93**, 242 (1973)

DEHYDROCORYDALINE

$C_{22}H_{23}O_4N$

M.p. 112–3°C (*dec.*).

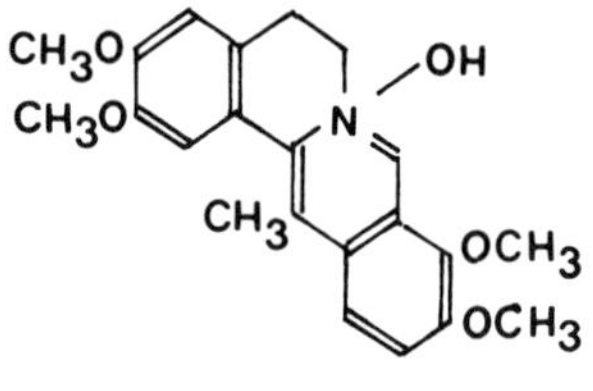

This alkaloid, which occurs naturally in *Corydalis ambigua* Cham. and Sch., *C. decumbens* Pers. and *C. tuberosa* DC. has also been obtained by oxidation of Corydaline (q.v.). It forms a yellow crystalline powder and yields a hydrochloride as the tetrahydrate, a hydriodide as small yellow needles of the dihydrate and an aurichloride as red-brown needles with m.p. 219°C. It resembles berberine in forming a stable compound with one mole of $CHCl_3$, m.p. 154°C. On reduction it forms two stereoisomerides of corydaline, m.p. 135°C and 158−9°C. The last of these may be partially separated into the (+)- and (−)-forms by crystallization of the (+)-camphorsulphonate whereas the former has not been resolved into optically active components.

Schmidt., *Arch. Pharm.*, **234**, 489 (1896)
Schmidt., *ibid*, **246**, 575 (1908)
Makoshi., *ibid*, **246**, 381, 401 (1908)
Asahina, Motigese., *J. Pharm. Soc., Japan*, **463**, 766 (1920)

DEHYDROCORYDALMINE

$C_{21}H_{22}O_4N^+$

A quaternary alkaloid, this base is isolated from the tubers of *Stephania glabra* as the crystalline chloride. When treated with methyl sulphate, this salt gives palmatine chloride.

Doskotch, Malik, Beal., *J. Org. Chem.*, **32**, 3253 (1967)

DEHYDRODECODINE

$C_{25}H_{27}O_5N$

M.p. 181−3°C

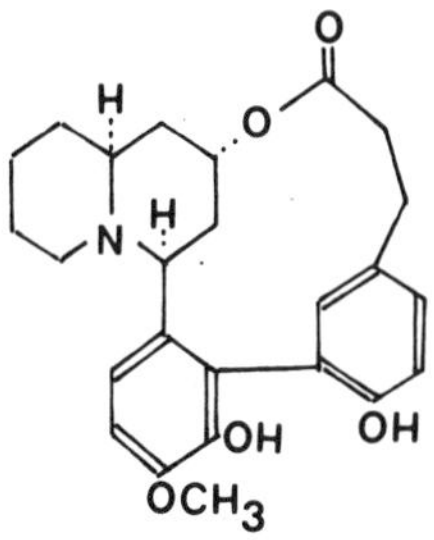

Found in *Heimia salicifolia* Link and Otto, this alkaloid contains one methoxyl and two hydroxyl groups and is closely related to the bases isolated from *Decodon verticillatus* L. The ultraviolet spectrum shows a single absorption maximum at 287 mμ.

Hörhammer, Schwarting, Edwards., *Z. Naturforsch.*, **26B**, 970 (1971)

DEHYDRODELCOSINE (*Shimoburo Base II*)

$C_{24}H_{37}O_7N$

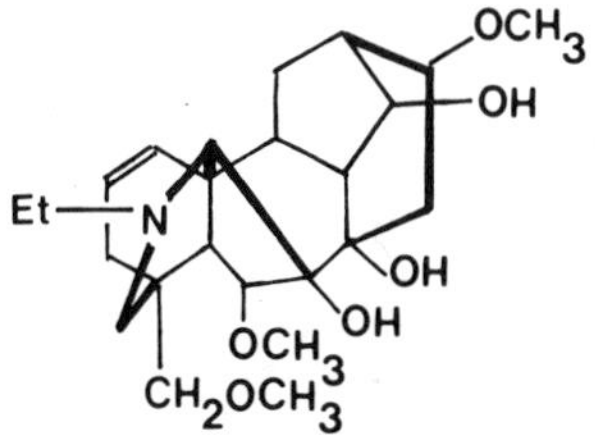

A minor alkaloid of Japanese *Delphinium* species, the identity of the two alkaloids has been proved by mixed melting point determinations, together with a comparison of their infrared spectra. The alkaloid forms a perchlorate, m.p. 225–6°C and an amorphous monoacetate. Reduction with $NaBH_4$ yields Delcosine (q.v.).

Ochiai, Okamoto, Kaneko., *Chem. Pharm. Bull.,* **6**, 730 (1958)

DEHYDRO-DE-N-METHYLULEINE

$C_{17}H_{18}N_2$

M.p. 220°C

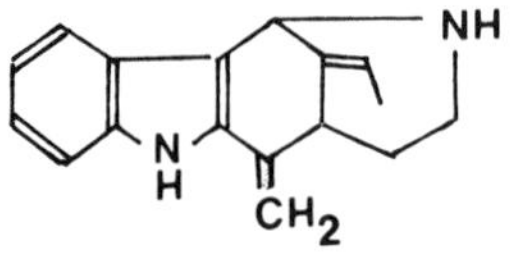

A minor constituent of *Aspidosperma dasycarpon* A. DC., this carbazole base contains two imino groups and one exocyclic methylene group. The ultraviolet spectrum has two absorption maxima at 303 and 310 mμ.

Joule *et al., Tetrahedron,* **21**, 1717 (1965)

DEHYDRODEOXYNUPHARIDINE

$C_{15}H_{21}ON$

M.p. Indefinite

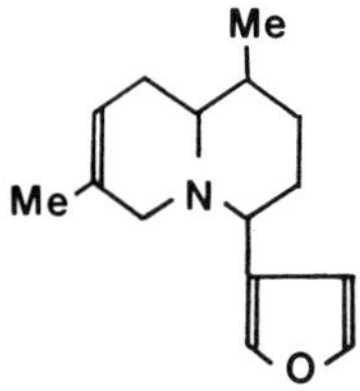

One of the alkaloids isolated from *Nuphar japonicum,* this base is unstable and is extremely difficult to obtain in a pure state.

Arata., *Chem. Pharm. Bull.,* **12**, 1394 (1964)

DEHYDRODICENTRINE

$C_{20}H_{19}O_4N$

M.p. 218°C

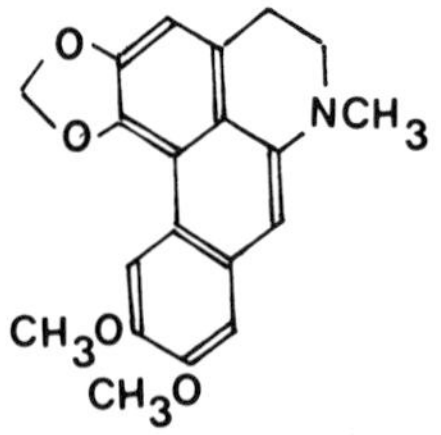

Obtained from *Ocotea macropoda* (H.B.K.) Mez., this alkaloid is best purified by recrystallization from $CHCl_3$ when it forms bright yellow needles. The ethanolic solution gives an ultraviolet spectrum with absorption maxima at 263, 302 and 340 mμ. It contains one methylenedioxy group, two methoxyl groups and a methylimino group in the molecule.

Cava *et al., Tetrahedron Lett.,* 2437 (1968)

(−)-3-DEHYDRO-*trans*-8:10-DIETHYLLOBELIDIOL
(*Alkaloid C-3*)

$C_{14}H_{27}O_2N$

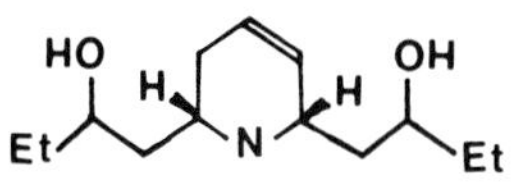

An alkaloid present in *Lobelia syphilitica* L., the base is a colourless oil which yields crystalline salts and derivative, e.g. the hydrochloride as long, colourless prisms from Me_2CO, m.p. 128°C; $[\alpha]_D^{25} - 14°$ (c 1.0, EtOH); perchlorate, m.p. 123°C; reineckate, m.p. 101−2°C and the tetraphenylborate derivative, m.p. 135−7°C. Hydrogenation over PtO_2 gives the dihydro derivative as an oil which crystallizes on standing, m.p. 84−5°C; $[\alpha]_D^{22} - 28°$ (c 1.0, EtOH).

Tschesche *et al.*, *Chem. Ber.*, 84, 3327 (1961)

19:20-DEHYDROERVATAMINE

$C_{21}H_{24}O_3N_2$

M.p. 198−200°C (*dec.*).

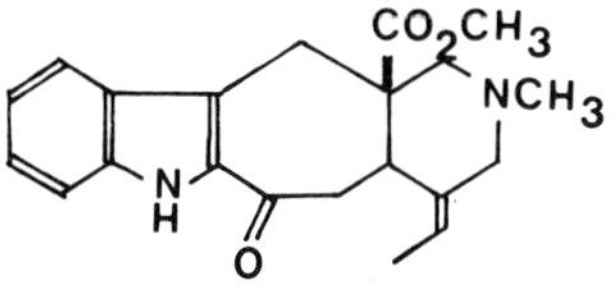

An indole alkaloid, the base occurs in *Ervatamia orientalis*. It is dextrorotatory with $[\alpha]_D + 53°$ ($CHCl_3$). It contains a vinyl group, an imino and a methylimino group.

Knox, Slobbe., *Tetrahedron Lett.*, 2149 (1971)

DEHYDROEVODIAMINE

$C_{19}H_{15}ON_3$

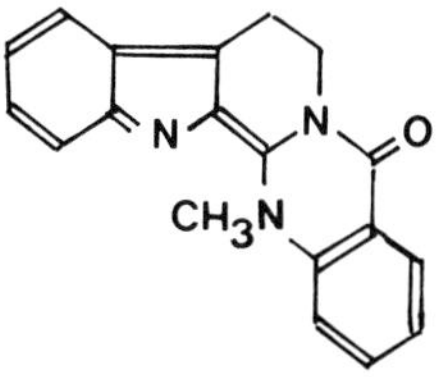

The leaves of *Evodia rutaecarpa* yield this base as the major alkaloid. It may be separated from the accompanying Hydroxyevodiamine (q.v.) by crystallization from C_6H_6. The base forms crystalline salts: the hydrochloride, m.p. 250−2°C; hydriodide, m.p. 252−3°C; picrate, m.p. 266°C (*dec.*) and the methiodide, m.p. 188°C. Reduction with $NaBH_4$ furnishes (±)-evodiamine, m.p. 267−270°C. Rutaecarpine (q.v.) is obtained on heating the hydrochloride *in vacuo* at 260−280°C.

Nakasato, Asada, Marui., *J. Pharm. Soc., Japan,* 82, 619 (1962)

DEHYDROGLAUCINE

$C_{21}H_{23}O_4N$

M.p. 133–4°C

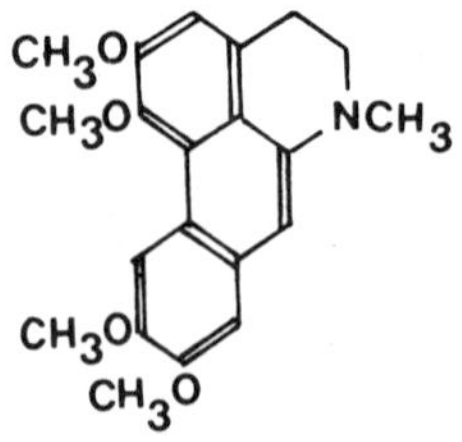

An optically inactive alkaloid found in *Glaucium flavum* Crantz, the base forms pale yellow prisms when recrystallized from EtOH. The ultraviolet spectrum in EtOH exhibits absorption maxima at 260.5 and 334 mμ. Catalytic hydrogenation yields Glaucine (q.v.).

Kiryakov., *Chem. & Ind.*, 1807 (1968)

5-DEHYDRO-13-HYDROXYMULTIFLORINE

$C_{15}H_{20}O_2N$

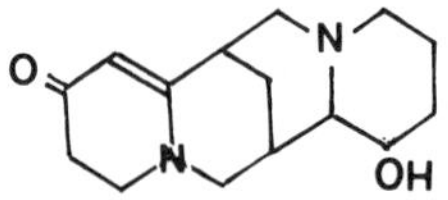

A minor alkaloid of *Lupinus albus,* this base is obtained from the high-boiling fraction by chromatography on an alumina column.

Wiewiorowski, Bartz, Wysocka., *Bull. Acad. Polon. Sci.,* 9, 715 (1961)

DEHYDROISOLONGISTROBINE

$C_{17}H_{17}O_3N_3$

M.p. 131°C

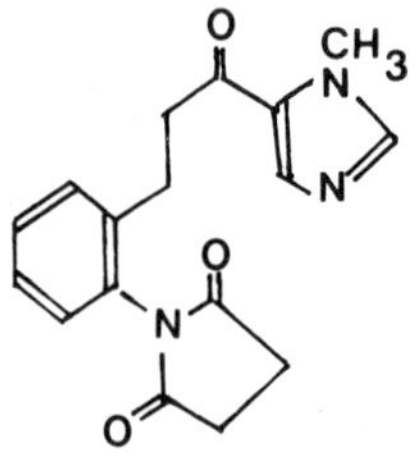

This alkaloid occurs in *Macrorungia longistrobus* and crystallizes from CH_2Cl_2-hexane as white needles. The structure has been deduced from the infrared spectrum and confirmed by synthesis from methyl-1-methylimidazole-5-carboxylate.

Arndt, Eggers, Jordaan., *Tetrahedron*, 25, 2767 (1969)

Synthesis:
Wuonola, Woodward., *J. Amer. Chem. Soc.*, 95, 284 (1973)

412

DEHYDROJOUBERTIAMINE

$C_{16}H_{19}O_2N$

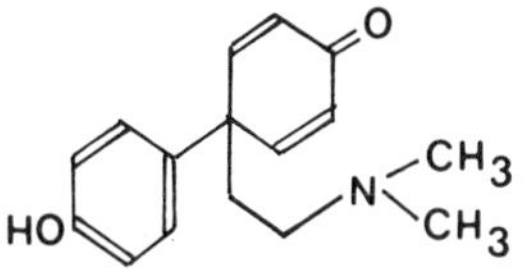

An amorphous base isolated from *Sceletium joubertii* L. Bol. The alkaloid contains one hydroxyl group and a dimethylaminoethyl group. The structure has been determined on the basis of spectroscopic data.

Arndt, Kruger., *Tetrahedron Lett.*, 3727 (1970)

5:6-DEHYDROLUPANINE

$C_{15}H_{22}ON_2$

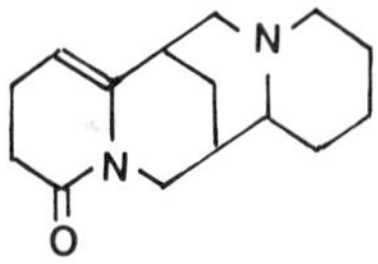

One of the bases present in *Thermopsis rhombifolia* Richards, this alkaloid is a colourless, slightly alkaline, liquid. The ultraviolet spectrum in EtOH has a single absorption maximum at 250 mμ. On catalytic hydrogenation with Pd-C, at room temperature and pressure, it is converted into Lupanine (q.v.).

Cho, Martin., *Can. J. Chem.*, **49**, 265 (1971)

DEHYDROLYCOPECURINE

$C_{16}H_{23}ON$

M.p. 57—9°C

A low-melting, minor alkaloid from *Lycopodium inundatum* L., the base has been shown to contain one methyl group. No salts or derivatives have been reported.

Braekman, Hootele, Ayer., *Bull. Soc. Chim. Belg.*, **80**, 83 (1971)

19:20-DEHYDRO-10-METHOXYDIHYDROCORYNANTHEOL

$C_{20}H_{26}O_2N_2$

M.p. 184—5°C

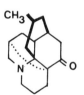

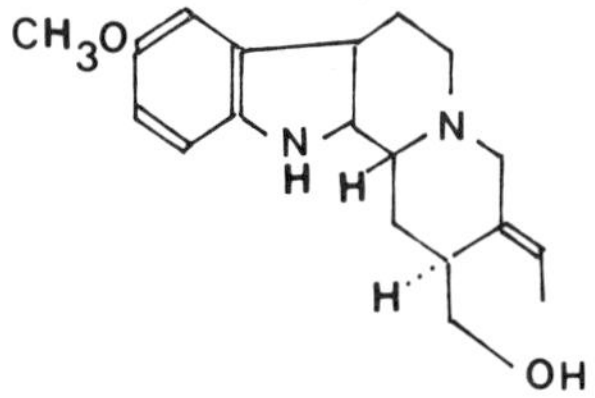

When first isolated, this alkaloid was provisionally named Alkaloid AD-VI. It occurs in *Aspidosperma discolor* A. DC. and also in *A. oblongum* A. DC. When recrystallized from EtOH it is obtained as colourless needles and has $[\alpha]_D^{26}$ − 42° (c 0.76, pyridine) or − 65° (c 1.0, pyridine). The ultraviolet spectrum exhibits absorption maxima at 225 and 280 mμ with inflexions at 297 and 308 mμ. The alkaloid forms crystalline derivatives, e.g. the picrate, m.p. 184−5°C (*dec.*) and the styphnate, m.p. 150−3°C (*dec.*). The O-acetate is amorphous.

Spiteller, Spiteller-Friedmann., *Monatsh.*, **93**, 795 (1962)
Spiteller, Spiteller-Friedmann., *ibid*, **94**, 779 (1963)
Dastoor, Schmid., *Experientia*, **19**, 297 (1963)
Gilbert *et al.*, *Tetrahedron*, **21**, 1141 (1965)

(−)-3-DEHYDRO-*trans*-8-METHYL-10-ETHYLLOBELIDIOL (*Alkaloid D-3*)

$C_{13}H_{25}O_2N$

Lobelia syphilitica L. yields this alkaloid which is characterized as the crystalline hydrochloride, m.p. 120°C; $[\alpha]_D^{28}$ − 110° (c 1.0, EtOH). Catalytic hydrogenation with PtO$_2$ gives the dihydro derivative as a colourless oil forming the aurichloride as colourless needles, m.p. 126−7°C.

Tschesche *et al.*, *Chem. Ber.*, **94**, 3327 (1961)

DEHYDRONORERYTHROSUAMINE

$C_{24}H_{35}O_6N$

M.p. Indefinite

An amorphous alkaloid present in *Erythrophleum guineense* and *E. chlorostachys*, the base is laevorotatory with $[\alpha]_D^{20}$ − 41° (c 0.3, EtOH). The original structure postulated for this alkaloid has recently been revised, on the basis of NMR data, to the amide form given above.

Friedrich, Fiechtl, Spiteller., *Chem. Ber.*, **104**, 3535 (1971)

Structure revision:
Loder *et al.*, *Tetrahedron Lett.*, 5069 (1972)

DEHYDRONUCIFERINE

$C_{19}H_{19}O_2N$

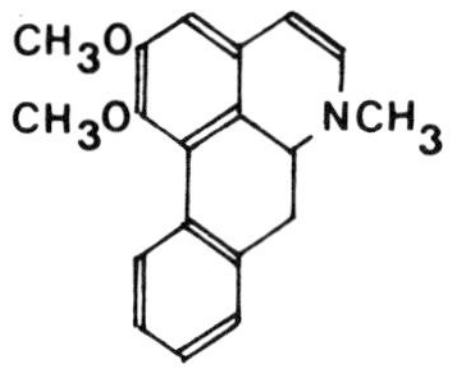

A minor base recently obtained from *Nelumbo nucifera,* the structure has been determined from chemical analysis and spectroscopic data.

Kunimoto *et al., Phytochem.,* **12,** 699 (1973)

DEHYDRO-3-OCHROLIFUANINE

$C_{29}H_{32}N_4$

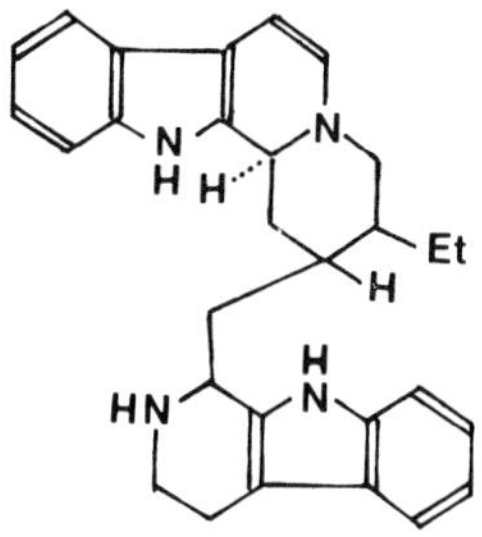

The leaves of *Ochrosia lifuana* yield this dimerica alkaloid as a minor constituent of the alkaloidal extract. The base is separated chromatographically and the structure has been established by chemical and spectroscopic methods.

Peube-Locou *et al., Ann. Pharm. Fr.,* **30,** 775 (1972)

DEHYDROOCOPODINE

$C_{21}H_{21}O_5N$

M.p. 113°C

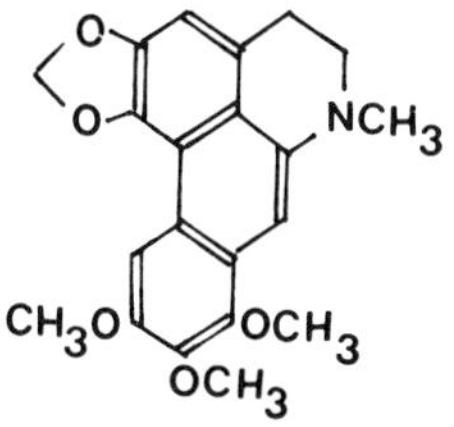

This alkaloid from *Ocotea macropoda* forms yellow platelets when recrystallized from EtOH. It is an aporphine base containing three methoxyl groups, one methylenedioxy group and a methylimino group. The ultraviolet spectrum in EtOH exhibits absorption maxima at 220, 267 and 340 mμ with a shoulder at 262 mμ.

Cava, Venkateswarlu., *Tetrahedron,* **27,** 2639 (1971)

DEHYDROOCOTEINE

$C_{21}H_{21}O_5N$

M.p. 203–4°C

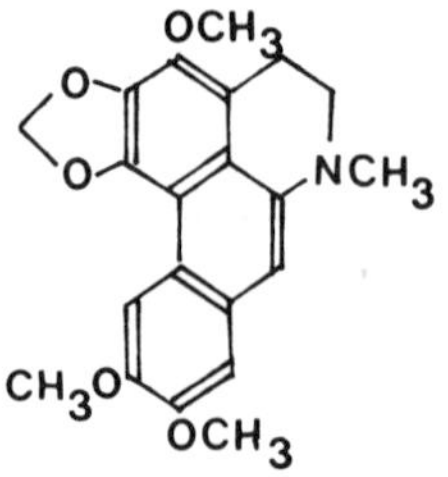

An isomer of the preceding alkaloid, this base occurs in *Ocotea puberula* and forms colourless crystals from AcOEt. It differs from dehydroocopodine only in the positions of the methoxyl groups.

Baralle *et al., Experientia,* **28**, 875 (1972)

2:3-DEHYDRO-O-(2-PYRROLYLCARBONYL)-VIRGILINE

$C_{20}H_{25}O_3N_3$

M.p. 186–193°C

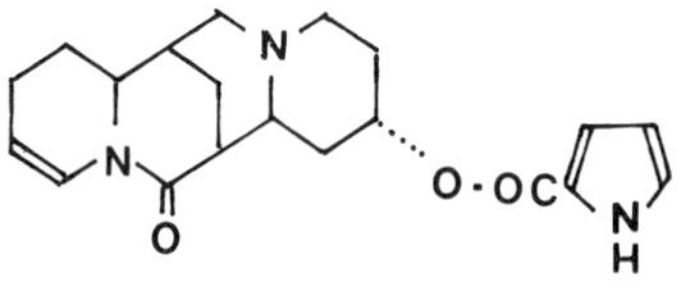

This alkaloid has been obtained from the leaves of the Fijian plant *Readea membranaceae* Gillespie. It is a lupanine type base and has $[\alpha]_D^{20} - 81.3°$ (c 0.46, $CHCl_3$). The ultraviolet spectrum in ethanol has an absorption maximum at 265 mμ. On hydrogenation it furnishes O-(2-pyrrolylcarbonyl)-virgiline.

Manchanda, Nabney, Young., *J. Chem. Soc., C,* 615 (1968)

DEHYDROROEMERINE

$C_{18}H_{15}O_2N$

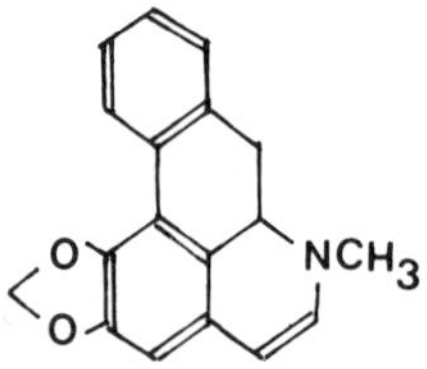

A recently isolated alkaloid, this base occurs in *Nelumbo nucifera*. The structure has been established from chemical analysis and comparison of the infrared, ultraviolet, NMR and mass spectra with those of Roemerine (q.v.).

Kunimoto *et al., Phytochem.,* **12**, 699 (1973)

416

DEHYDROSINOMENINE (*Disinomenine*)

$C_{38}H_{44}O_8N_2$

M.p. 222°C

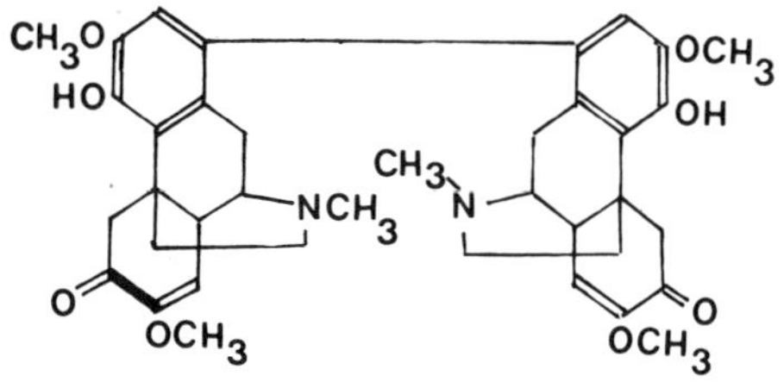

This alkaloid from *Sinomenium acutum* should, perhaps, be more correctly described as disinomenine which is more descriptive of its structure. It is also formed when sinomenine is gently oxidized, pseudosinomenine being produced at the same time, the latter not occurring naturally. The alkaloid forms colourless plates which decompose at 245°C. Crystalline salts and derivatives are known including the hydrochloride, m.p. > 290°C; oxime, m.p. 265°C (*dec.*); semi-carbazone, m.p. > 290°C and the methiodide which decomposes at 263°C. The alkaloid is dextrorotatory with $[\alpha]_D$ + 149.8°. When heated with Ac_2O in a sealed tube, the base yields methylamine and tetraacetyl-disinomenol, $C_{40}H_{34}O_{12}$, m.p. 253°C, from which disinomenol, m.p. > 310°C is readily obtained by hydrolysis.

Goto., *Proc. Imp. Acad. Tokyo*, **2**, 7, 167, 414 (1926)
Goto, Sudzuki., *Bull. Chem. Soc. Japan*, **4**, 107 (1929)

Δ⁵-DEHYDROSKYTANTHINE

$C_{11}H_{19}N$

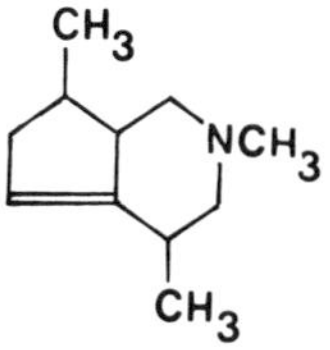

Closely related to the *Skytanthus* alkaloids, this base has recently been isolated from *Tecoma stans*. The structure has been assigned primarily on the basis of the NMR and mass spectra.

Gross *et al.*, *Phytochem.*, **12**, 201 (1973)

DEHYDROTHALICARPINE

$C_{41}H_{46}O_8N_2$

M.p. 186–7°C

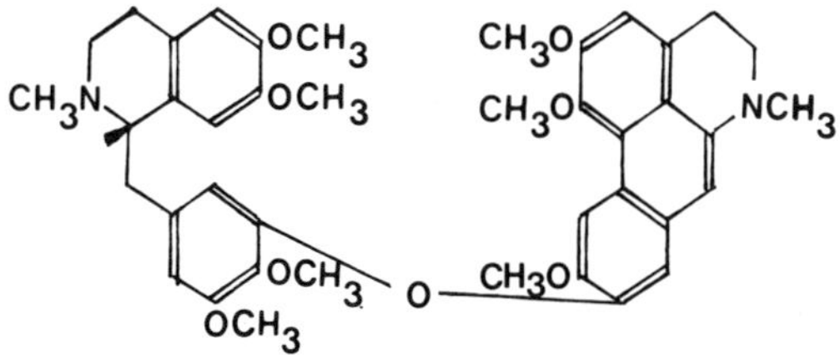

An aporphine-benzyl*iso*quinoline alkaloid present in both *Thalictrum dasycarpum*

Fisch. et Lall. and *T. minus* var. *elatum*. The base is obtained in the form of colourless crystals from MeOH or EtOH and has $[\alpha]_D^{22} + 54°$ (c 1.0, CHCl$_3$). The ultraviolet spectrum has absorption maxima at 268 and 331 mμ. The base gives a crystalline dimethiodide, m.p. 167–171°C and can be hydrogenated to Thalicarpine (q.v.). Sodium in liquid ammonia cleaves the base into 6'-hydroxylaudanosine and 2:10-dimethoxydehydroaporphine. The total synthesis was achieved by a route involving oxidation of thalicarpine with 2:3-dichloro-5:6-dicyano-1:4-benzoquinone.

Dutschewska, Mollov., *Chem. & Ind.*, 770 (1966)
Kupchan *et al.*, *J. Org. Chem.*, 33, 1052 (1968)

(+)-6:7-DEHYDROVINCADINE

$C_{21}H_{26}O_2N_2$

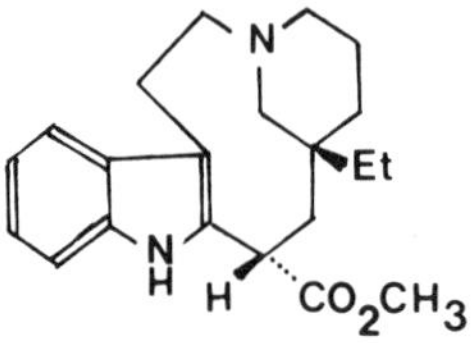

The leaves of *Amsonia tabernaemontana* have been shown to contain this minor alkaloid. The base gives typical indole reactions and the structure follows from the infrared, NMR and mass spectra.

Zsadon, Tamas, Szilasi., *Chem. Ind.*, 5, 229 (1973)

6:7-DEHYDRO-*epi*-VINCADINE

$C_{21}H_{26}O_2N_2$

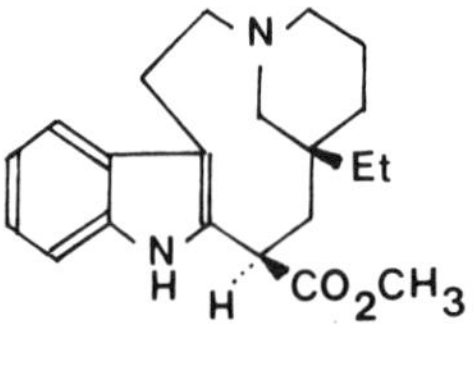

The epimer of the preceding base also occurs in the leaves of *Amsonia tabernaemontana* as a minor constituent.

Zsadon, Tamas, Szilasi., *Chem. Ind.*, 5, 229 (1973)

14:15-DEHYDROVINCAMINE

$C_{21}H_{24}O_3N_2$

M.p. 218°C

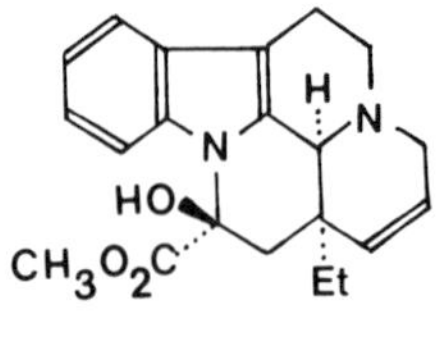

A carboline alkaloid present in *Crioceras longiflorus* Pierre, this base may be purified by recrystallization from either MeOH or Me$_2$CO when it forms colourless plates. It has $[\alpha]_D + 116°$ (c 0.75, $CHCl_3$). The ultraviolet spectrum shows absorption maxima at 222, 270, 279 and 289 mμ.

Cave *et al., Compt. Rend.,* **272C**, 1367 (1971)

16-*epi*-14:15-DEHYDROVINCAMINE

$C_{21}H_{24}O_3N_2$

M.p. 185°C

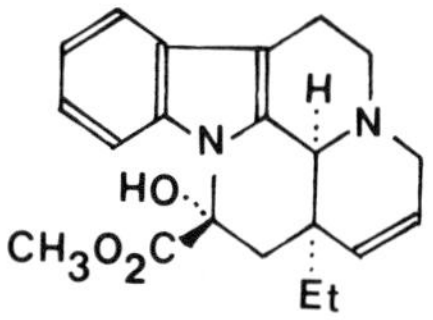

This epimer of the preceding alkaloid is also present in *Crioceras longiflorus* Pierre. It is also dextrorotatory with $[\alpha]_D + 30°$ (c 1.2, $CHCl_3$). The ultraviolet spectrum is almost identical with that of the epimer having absorption maxima at 222, 271, 278 and 290 mμ.

Cave *et al., Compt. Rend.,* **272C**, 1367 (1971)

DEHYDROVOACHOLINE

$C_{22}H_{24}O_3N_2$

M.p. 238–9°C

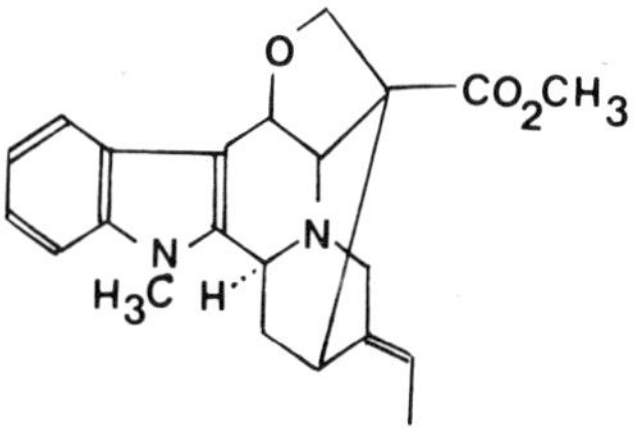

A minor alkaloid of *Voacanga chalotiana,* this base has been obtained from the countercurrent distribution fraction and is isolated therefrom by chromatography on silica gel. The alkaloid has $[\alpha]_D^{22} + 124°$ (c 0.9, MeOH) and may also be produced by oxidation of voachalotine with potassium dichromate.

Tirions *et al., Chimia,* **22**, 87 (1968)

19-DEHYDROYOHIMBINE

$C_{21}H_{24}O_3N_2$

M.p. 245°C

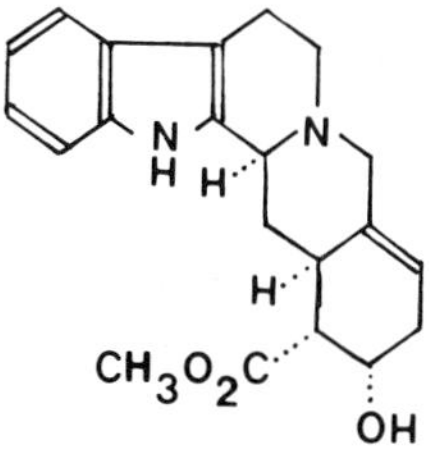

A minor base of *Corynanthe yohimbe,* this alkaloid is dextrorotatory with

$[\alpha]_D^{20} + 106°$ (c 0.53, pyridine). It gives an ultraviolet spectrum in EtOH with absorption maxima at 226, 283 and 293 mμ.

Arndt, Djerassi., *Experientia*, **21**, 566 (1965)

DELATINE

$C_{19}H_{25}O_3N$

M.p. 261–4°C

An atisine alkaloid present in the seeds of *Delphinium elatum* Linn, the base forms colourless prisms of the monohydrate from H_2O, m.p. 148°C; $[\alpha]_D^{23} + 13.5°$ (c N/HCl). The hydrochloride has m.p. 274–7°C and has $[\alpha]_D^{18} + 13.4°$ (H_2O). The base contains neither methoxyl nor methylimino groups in the molecule.

Goodson., *J. Chem. Soc.*, 139 (1943)

DELAVACONINE

$C_{23}H_{37}O_5N$

M.p. 150°C

A minor constituent of certain *Aconitum* species, this alkaloid forms crystalline salts, e.g. the perchlorate, m.p. 215°C; aurichloride, m.p. 184°C. The triacetate yields colourless crystals with m.p. 160°C; $[\alpha]_D - 53°$.

Chu *et al.*, *Hua Hseuh Hseuh Pao.*, **25**, 321 (1959)

DELAVACONITINE

$C_{30}H_{41}O_6N$

M.p. 147–9°C

This *Aconitum* base crystallizes from H_2O as the hemihydrate. The nitrate is also crystalline, m.p. 154°C, as is also the perchlorate, m.p. 241°C and the monoacetate, m.p. 106–110°C.

Chu *et al.*, *Hua Hseuh Hseuh Pao.*, **25**, 321 (1959)

DELAVAINE

$C_{20}H_{23}O_5N$

M.p. 149–150°C

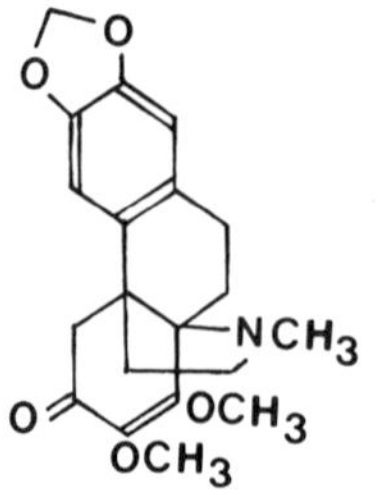

This morphine type alkaloid has recently been isolated from the grass *Stephania*

delavayi. It is laevorotatory with $[\alpha]_D - 240°$ and gives a hydrochloride, m.p. 203.5°C and a methiodide, m.p. 190–2°C. The structure has been deduced from chemical and spectroscopic evidence.

Fadeeva *et al.*, *Khim. Prir. Soedin.*, **6**, 140 (1970)
Fadeeva *et al.*, *ibid*, **7**, 784 (1971)

DELCORINE

$C_{26}H_{39}O_7N$

An atisine alkaloid obtained from the aerial parts of *Delphinium corumbosum*, the structure has been determined, together with the stereochemistry, from NMR and mass spectrometry.

Narzullaev, Yunusov, Yunusov., *Khim. Prir. Soedin.*, **9**, 497 (1973)

DELCOSINE (*Takao Base I*)

$C_{24}H_{39}O_7N$

M.p. 203–4°C

Present in both *Delphinium ajacis* and *D. consolida* Linn., this alkaloid forms colourless crystals from MeOH and has $[\alpha]_D^{25} + 56.8°$ (CHCl$_3$). It forms a series of crystalline salts, several of which crystallize with 2 moles of solvent. The hydrochloride dimethanolate has m.p. 89°C; hydrobromide dimethanolate, m.p. 103°C; hydriodide, m.p. 196–7°C; bitartrate, m.p. 217–8°C; perchlorate, m.p. 217–8°C; $[\alpha]_D + 32.0°$ (MeOH) and the dimethyl derivative, m.p. 203–6°C have been prepared. The alkaloid contains four hydroxyl groups, three methoxyl and an ethylimino group. The O-acetate occurs naturally, while the diacetate exists in two modifications; m.p. 127–8°C when crystallized from aqueous EtOH and with m.p. 167–171°C from MeOH. The triacetate has m.p. 203°C (*dec.*) and the dipropionate, m.p. 119–120°C.

Goodson., *J. Chem. Soc.*, 245 (1947)
Marion, Edwards., *J. Amer. Chem. Soc.*, **69**, 2010 (1947)
Taylor *et al.*, *Can. J. Chem.*, **32**, 780 (1954)
Anet *et al.*, *ibid*, **35**, 397 (1957)
Anet *et al.*, *ibid*, **36**, 766 (1958)
Ochiai, Okamoto, Kaneko., *Chem. Pharm. Bull.*, **6**, 730 (1958)
Skaric, Marion., *Can. J. Chem.*, **38**, 2433 (1960)
Biosynthesis:
Frost *et al.*, *Chem. & Ind.*, 320 (1967)

DELFLEXINE

$C_{24}H_{39}O_6N$

M.p. 191–2°C

A minor alkaloid of *Delphinium flexosum*, this base has been isolated by poly-buffer distribution of the alkaloidal extract. It forms colourless crystals from Me_2CO.

Brutko, Massagetov., *Khim. Prir. Soedin.*, **3**, 21 (1967)

DELFRENINE

$C_{27}H_{31}O_6N$

M.p. 246–7°C

This atisine alkaloid occurs in *Delphinium freynii* and has, like the preceding base, been obtained by polybuffer distribution of the total extract of the plant. It yields colourless crystals from a mixture of EtOH and Me_2CO and gives an ultraviolet spectrum with absorption maxima at 236, 274 and 281 mμ. Alkaline hydrolysis yields benzoic acid and an amino acid, $C_{20}H_{27}O_5N$, characterized as the hydrochloride, m.p. 250–1°C. Hydrogenation over Pt yields a decahydro derivative, m.p. 107–8°C, the ultraviolet spectrum of which consists of a single absorption maximum at 236 mμ.

Brutko, Massagetov., *Khim. Prir. Soedin.*, **3**, 21 (1967)

DELNUDINE

$C_{19}H_{23}O_3N$

M.p. 235–7°C

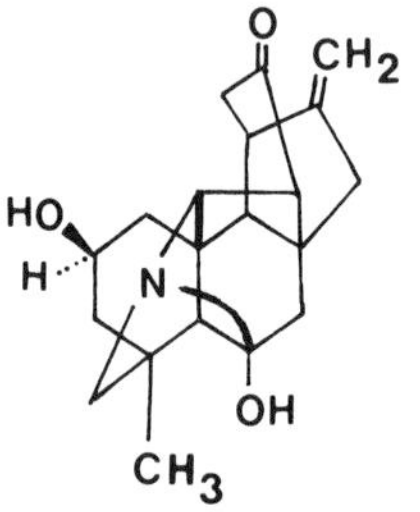

The seeds of *Delphinium denudatum* yield this alkaloid which, on acetylation with Ac_2O in pyridine gives a neutral diacetate, m.p. 282°C and a basic diacetate, m.p. 141–3°V. Oxidation with chromic acid in pyridine yields a hydroxy diketone, $C_{20}H_{23}O_3N$, m.p. 264–6°C. It has been postulated that the base may derive biogenetically from Hetisine (q.v.).

Goetz, Wiesner., *Tetrahedron Lett.*, 5335 (1969)

DELPHAMINE (*Shimoburo-Base II*)

$C_{25}H_{41}O_7N$

M.p. 195–8°C

This alkaloid was first isolated by Rabinovitch and Konovalova from an unidentified species of *Delphinium*. It has subsequently been discovered in other *Delphinium* species. From EtOH it crystallizes as colourless prisms and has $[\alpha]_D$ + 66.6°. It is only sparingly soluble in most organic solvents and yields crystalline salts, e.g. the acid tartrate, m.p. 160°C (*dec.*); the nitrate, m.p. 160°C (*dec.*); $[\alpha]_D$ + 33.5° and the methiodide, m.p. 180°C (*dec.*). A crystalline perchlorate, m.p. 181–6°C and the aurichloride, m.p. 171–2°C (*dec.*) have also been obtained. The base is stable to alkali and gives a diacetyl derivative, m.p. 118–121.5°C; $[\alpha]_D$ + 28.8°. On oxidation with $KMnO_4$ it yields acetaldehyde indicative of an ethylimino group.

Rabinovitch, Konovalova., *J. Gen. Chem., USSR*, **12**, 321 (1942)
Goodson., *J. Chem. Soc.*, 245 (1945)
Taylor *et al., Can. J. Chem.*, **32**, 780 (1954)
Skaric, Marion., *ibid*, **38**, 2433 (1960)

DELPHATINE

$C_{27}H_{45}O_7N$

M.p. 101–6°C

This alkaloid occurs in *Delphinium biternatum* and forms colourless crystals from Et O-light petroleum. It is dextrorotatory with $[\alpha]_D^{22}$ + 38.5° (CHCl₃). The hydriodide is crystalline with m.p. 199°C; $[\alpha]_D^{20}$ + 31.7° (EtOH); the perchlorate has m.p. 220–1°C; the picrate, m.p. 216°C; $[\alpha]_D^{19}$ + 20.6° (65% EtOH) and the methiodide, m.p. 197–8°C. The structure has been deduced from the NMR and mass spectra. Oxidation of the alkaloid with $KMnO_4$ in aqueous Me_2CO gives a compound, $C_{26}H_{41}O_8$, m.p. 94–5°C, containing a six-membered lactam ring.

Yunusov, Abubakirov., *J. Gen. Chem. USSR*, **19**, 869 (1949)
Abubakirov, Yunusov., *Sbornik Statei Obshchei Khim.*, **2**, 1453 (1953)
Structure:
Yunusov, Yunusov., *Dokl. Akad. Nauk SSSR*, **188**, 1077 (1969)
Yunusov, Yunusov., *Khim. Prir. Soedin.*, **6**, 334 (1970)

DELPHELATINE

$C_{30}H_{47}O_9N$

M.p. 188–9°C

A dextrorotatory alkaloid found in the roots of *Delphinium elatum*, this base has $[\alpha]_D^{17} - 26.32°$ (CHCl$_3$). A crystalline hydrochloride, m.p. 212–3°C and a nitrate, m.p. 169–171°C have been prepared. The alkaloid contains two hydroxyl groups, three methoxyl groups and one methylimino group.

Feofilaktov, Alekseeva., *J. Gen. Chem., USSR,* **24**, 738 (1954)
Kuzovkov, Platonova., *ibid,* **29**, 2782 (1959)
Carmack *et al., J. Amer. Chem. Soc.,* **81**, 4110 (1959)

DELPHELINE

$C_{25}H_{39}O_6N$

M.p. 227°C

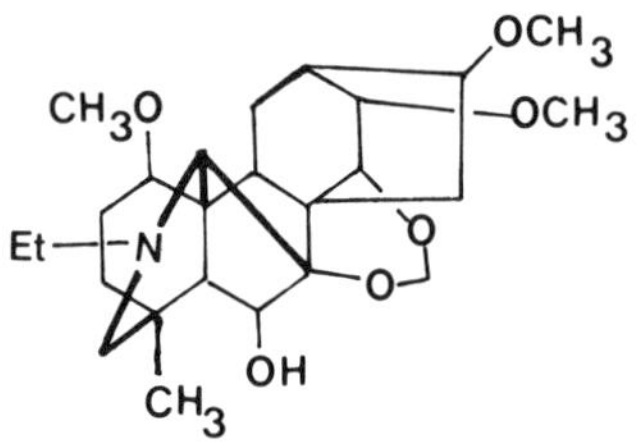

A minor alkaloid obtained from the seeds of *Delphinium elatum*, the base crystallizes from aqueous EtOH in colourless prisms. It has $[\alpha]_D^{15} - 25.8°$ (CHCl$_3$). The hydrochloride forms the monohydrate, m.p. 219°C (*dec.*); $[\alpha]_D^{20} - 42.8°$ (H$_2$O); nitrate, m.p. 191–3°C; $[\alpha]_D^{22} - 41.2°$ (H$_2$O). The alkaloid contains one hydroxyl group and forms an acetate, m.p. 125°C; $[\alpha]_D^{20} - 34.5°$ (EtOH). Delpheline is a weak base and the salts show a tendency to lose acid on drying.

Goodson., *J. Chem. Soc.,* 139 (1943)
Goodson., *ibid,* 665 (1944)

DELPHININE

$C_{33}H_{45}O_9N$

M.p. 198–200°C

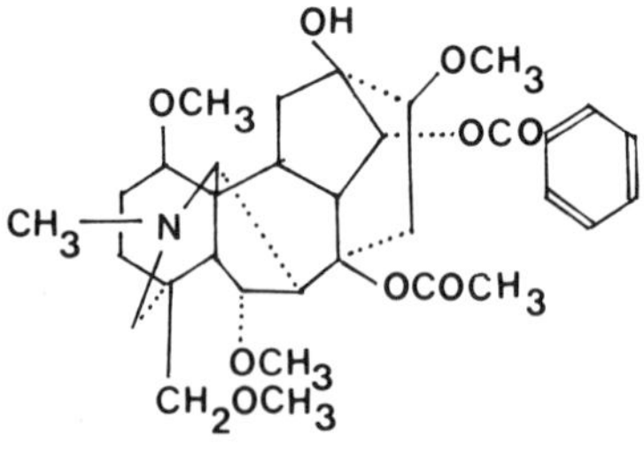

The earlier formula of $C_{34}H_{47}O_9N$ given to this alkaloid from *Delphinium Staphisagria* L. by Walz was altered to that given above by Jacobs and Craig. It crystallizes in hexagonal plates or rhombs and has $[\alpha]_D^{25} + 25°$ (EtOH) and exhibits mutarotation in ethanolic solution. It forms crystalline salts, e.g. the

424

acid oxalate, m.p. 168°C; hydrochloride, m.p. 208–210°C; monobenzoyl derivative, m.p. 171–3°C and the methochloride, m.p. 195°C (*dec.*). On alkaline hydrolysis it furnishes one mole each of acetic and benzoic acids and delphonine, $C_{24}H_{39}O_7N$, which is amorphous but can be distilled at 140°C/ 0.001–0.0001 mm. When distilled in this way a brittle, and possibly crystalline, resin remains which has m.p. 76–8°C; $[\alpha]_D^{24} + 37.5°$ (EtOH). Catalytic hydrogenation yields the hexahydro derivative, m.p. 192–3°C in which the benzoyl radical is reduced since hexahydrobenzoic acid is then produced on hydrolysis. When heated in MeOH, acetic acid is liberated with the formation of methylbenzoyldelphonine, m.p. 173–5°C; $[\alpha]_D^{25} + 27°$ (MeOH). The latter may, in turn, be oxidized with $KMnO_4$ to give methylbenzoyl-α-oxodelphonine, m.p. 221–3°C, melting again at 236–7°C after intermediate solidification.

When the alkaloid itself is oxidized with $KMnO_4$ it furnishes two isomerides, $C_{33}H_{43}O_{10}N$, designated α- and β-oxodelphinine with the former predominating. The former has m.p. 218–221°C; $[\alpha]_D^{20} - 62°$ (AcOH) and the latter, m.p. 228–9°C; $[\alpha]_D^{20} + 31°$ (AcOH). When the latter is heated at 100°C in MeOH with HCl it forms methylbenzoyl-α-oxodelphonine. This type of reaction also occurs with Aconitine and emphasizes the close similarity between the *Aconitum* and *Delphinium* alkaloids.

This parallelism between the two series of bases is found again in the action of heat on the alkaloid in an atmosphere of hydrogen when pyrodelphinine is produced, m.p. 208–212°C. In a similar way, -oxodelphinine loses acetic acid and gives pyro- -oxodelphinine, crystallizing from MeOH in colourless needles, m.p. 248–250°C. Treatment of delphinine with nitrous acid at 100°C furnishes a nitroso derivative, m.p. 240–1°C although the main product in this reaction is hydroxydelphinine, m.p. 180–2°C (*dec.*); $[\alpha]_D^{20} + 7°$ (EtOH).

Delphinine resembles aconitine in its pharmacological action, death being due to respiratory failure and cardiac and vasomotor damage. It also possesses an irritant action upon the skin.

Marquis., *Ann. Chim. Phys.,* **52**, 352 (1853)
Kara-Stojanov., *Pharm. Zeit. Russ.,* **29**, 641 (1890)
Ahrens., *Ber.,* 1581, 1669 (1899)
Keller., *Arch. Pharm.,* **248**, 648 (1910)
Walz., *ibid,* **260**, 9 (1922)
Keller., *Chem. Abstr.,* **19**, 2500 (1925)
Jacobs, Craig., *J. Biol. Chem.,* **127**, 361 (1939)
Jacobs, Craig., *ibid,* **128**, 431 (1939)
Jacobs, Craig., *ibid,* **136**, 303 (1940)
Jacobs, Huebner., *ibid,* **170**, 209 (1947)
Schneider., *Arch. Pharm.,* **283**, 281 (1950)
Backelor, Brown., *Tetrahedron Lett.,* **10**, 1 (1960)
Wiesner *et al., Tetrahedron,* **9**, 254 (1960)

Pharmacology:
Marsh, Clawson, Marsh., *Exp. Sta. Rec.* (USA), **35**, 770 (1916)
Jakobsen., *Norsk. Mag. Laegevidensk.,* **96**, 725 (1935)
Markwood., *J. Gen. Chem., USSR,* **12**, 321, 329 (1942)

Revised configuration:
Birnbaum *et al., Tetrahedron Lett.,* 867 (1971)

Synthesis:
Wiesner *et al., Experientia,* **27**, 363 (1971)

DELPHINOIDINE

$C_{25}H_{42}O_4N$

M.p. Indefinite

An amorphous alkaloid stated to occur in *Delphinium Staphisagria* L. The base has not been characterized, nor examined further since its isolation.

Kara-Stojanov., *Pharm. Zeit. Russ.*, **29**, 641 (1890)

DELPHISINE

$C_{33}H_{45}O_9N$

M.p. 189°C

This crystalline base has been isolated from *Delphinium Staphisagria* L. and is said to be isomeric with Delphinine (q.v.). It is not, however, well characterized and is possibly identical with this alkaloid.

Kara-Stojanov., *Pharm. Zeit. Russ.*, **29**, 641 (1890)

DELPHOCURARINE

This is a mixture of alkaloids obtained from *Delphinium bicolor* Nutt., *D. Mensiesii*, D.C., *D. Nelsonii*, Gr. and *D. scopulorum*, Gr. It is stated to possess pharmacological properties somewhat similar to the curare alkaloids. Heyl, however, has isolated a crystalline base, $C_{23}H_{33}O_7N$, m.p. 184–5°C, from this mixture.

Heyl., *Südd. Apoth. Zeit.*, **43**, 28 (1903)

DELPHONINE

$C_{24}H_{39}O_7N$

M.p. 78.5°C

This alkaloid occurs in *Delphinium* species and is also produced by hydrolysis of Delphinine (q.v.). It has $[\alpha]_D^{26} + 37.7°$ (EtOH). The acetyl derivative is Delphinine (q.v.). The benzoyl compound is amorphous with $[\alpha]_D^{27} + 33°$ (c 1.0, MeOH).

Jacobs, Craig., *J. Biol. Chem.*, **136**, 303 (1940)
Schneider., *Arch. Pharm.*, **283**, 281 (1950)
Schneider., *ibid*, **288**, 365 (1955)
Schneider., *Chem. Ber.*, **89**, 768 (1956)
Jacobs, Pelletier., *J. Org. Chem.*, **22**, 1428 (1957)
Abubakirov, Yunusov., *J. Gen. Chem.*, *USSR*, **26**, 1798 (1956)

DELPYRINE

$C_{49}H_{82}O_{17}N_2$

M.p. 76°C

This complex alkaloid is obtained from *Delphinium pyramidatum* and may be obtained crystalline by trituration with absolute EtOH. It is dextrorotatory with $[\alpha]_D$ + 58° (EtOH) and yields a hydrochloride, $[\alpha]_D$ + 22° (EtOH) and a reineckate, m.p. 179–180°C. The base contains two hydroxyl groups and on hydrolysis yields an unidentified acid and an amorphous compound, $C_{46}H_{74}O_{15}N_2$, with $[\alpha]_D$ + 46.6° (EtOH).

Brutko, Massagetov., *Khim. Prir. Soedin.*, **3**, 21 (1967)

DELSEMIDINE

$C_{37}H_{50}O_{10}N_2$

M.p. 122–130°C (*dec.*).

An alkaloid of *Delphinium semibarbatum*, the base is non-crystallizable. It yields a hydriodide trihydrate, m.p. 199–202°C (*dry*) and a perchlorate, m.p. 194–5°C.

Yunusov, Abubakirov., *J. Gen. Chem., USSR,* **22**, 1461 (1952)

DELSINE

This uncharacterized alkaloid has been obtained *Delphinium oreophilum* and *D. semibarbatum.*

Yunusov, Abubakirov., *J. Gen. Chem., USSR,* **21**, 967 (1951)

DELSOLINE

$C_{25}H_{41}O_7N$

M.p. 213–216.5°C

Obtained from *Delphinium colsolida* L., this alkaloid has $[\alpha]_D^{28}$ + 51.7° (CHCl$_3$) and yields a perchlorate, m.p. 192.5–193.5°C; $[\alpha]_D^{27}$ + 28.1° (MeOH) and a hydrobromide which crystallizes from Me$_2$CO with 0.5 Me$_2$CO, m.p. 83°C. The alkaloid is not affected by KOH in EtOH.

Markwood., *J. Amer. Pharm. Assoc.,* **13**, 696 (1924)
Cionga, Iliescu., *Ber.,* **74**, 1031 (1941)
Marion, Edwards., *J. Amer. Chem. Soc.,* **69**, 2010 (1947)
Marion *et al., Tetrahedron,* **4**, 157 (1958)
Suginome, Furusawa., *Chem. Abstr.,* **54**, 19736 (1960)
Skaric, Marion., *Can. J. Chem.,* **38**, 2433 (1960)

DELSONINE

$C_{24}H_{41}O_6N$

M.p. Indefinite

A further base isolated from *Delphinium consolida* L., this alkaloid is amorphous. When boiled with KOH in EtOH it is readily isomerized to *iso*delsonine, m.p. 108–111°C. The following crystalline salts of the alkaloid have been prepared to characterize the base, perchlorate, m.p. 216°C (*dec.*); $[\alpha]_D^{32} + 23°$ (MeOH) and the hydriodide, m.p. 202°C.

Marion, Edwards., *J. Amer. Chem. Soc.*, **69**, 2010 (1947)
Abubakirov, Yunusov., *Sbornik Statei Obshchei Khim.*, **2**, 1453 (1953)

DELTALINE (*Eldeline*)

$C_{27}H_{41}O_8N$

M.p. 193.5–194°C
(*in vac.*)

The main component of *Delphinium barbeyi* and *D. occidentale*, the alkaloid is also found in *D. elatum*. The alkaloid has $[\alpha]_D^{23} - 28.5°$ (MeOH) and $[\alpha]_D^{24} - 27.8°$ (EtOH). It forms a crystalline aurichloride as the trihydrate, m.p. 120–5°C, a monoacetyl derivative, m.p. 155–6°C; $[\alpha]_D^{25} - 31°$ (CHCl$_3$) and an amorphous triacetyl compound, m.p. 270–2°C.

Couch., *J. Amer. Chem. Soc.*, **58**, 684 (1936)
Rabinovitch., *J. Gen. Chem.*, USSR, **22**, 1702 (1952)
Kuzovkov, Platonova., *ibid*, **29**, 2782, 3840 (1959)
Carmack *et al.*, *J. Amer. Chem. Soc.*, **81**, 4110 (1959)

DEMECOLCINE

$C_{21}H_{25}O_5N$

M.p. 186°C

A colchicine alkaloid, this base is found in *Colchicum autumnale* and *C. speciosum*. It is best purified from AcOEt when it crystallizes as light yellow prisms. It has $[\alpha]_D^{23} - 129°$ (c 1.0217, CHCl$_3$). The alkaloid contains four methoxyl groups and one methylimino group in the molecule.

Masinova, Santavy., *Collect. Czech. Chem. Commun.*, **19**, 1283 (1954)
Uffer *et al.*, *Helv. Chim. Acta*, **37**, 18 (1954)

DEMERARINE

$C_{36}H_{38}O_6N_2$

M.p. 222–3°C

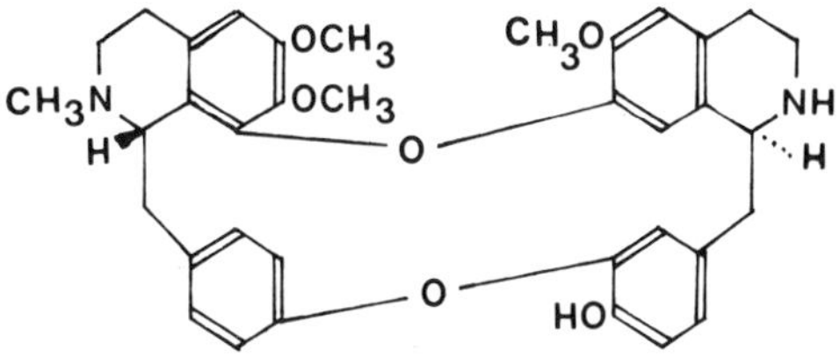

This alkaloid present in *Ocotea rodiaei* forms colourless needles from MeOH and has $[\alpha]_D^{25} - 162°$ (c 0.35, CHCl$_3$). It is characterized as the hydrochloride which is laevorotatory with $[\alpha]_D^{25} - 181°$ (c 1.0, H$_2$O). The complete structure is not yet known with certainty.

Hearst., *J. Org. Chem., 29*, 466 (1964)
Hearst *et al., ibid, 33*, 1229 (1966)

DEMETHOXYASPIDOSPERMINE

$C_{21}H_{28}ON_2$

M.p. Indefinite

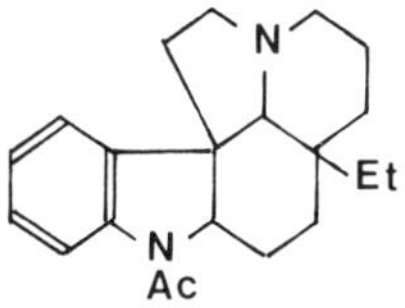

Ferreira and his colleagues have isolated this base from *Aspidosperma discolor* A. DC. and *A. eburneum* Fr. All, while Arndt has found it in *A. marcgravianum*. It is an amorphous powder with no definite melting point and has $[\alpha]_D^{25} - 15°$ (c 1.8, CHCl$_3$). The ultraviolet spectrum shows absorption maxima at 253, 280 and 289 mμ. The alkaloid may be characterized as the perchlorate which crystallizes as the hemihydrate from H$_2$O, $[\alpha]_D^{35} + 21°$ (c 1.3, MeOH).

Ferreira *et al., Experientia, 19*, 585 (1963)
Arndt *et al., Phytochem., 6*, 1653 (1967)

DEMETHOXYCYLINDROCARPIDINE

$C_{22}H_{28}O_3N_2$

B.p. 120°C/0.001 mm

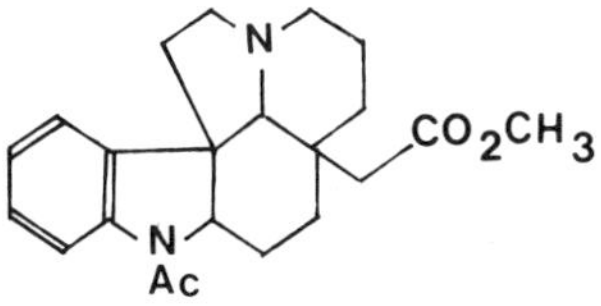

A liquid alkaloid present in *Aspidosperma cylindrocarpon* and *Tabernaemontana amygdalifolia*, the base is laevorotatory with $[\alpha]_D^{30} - 49°$. The structure has been assigned on the basis of high-resolution mass spectral analysis.

Achenbach., *Z. Naturforsch., B, 22*, 955 (1967)
Milborrow, Djerassi., *J. Chem. Soc., C*, 417 (1969)

3-DEMETHOXYERYTHRATIDINONE

$C_{18}H_{21}O_3N$

M.p. 111–2°C

An erythrina alkaloid present in *Erythrina lithosperma*, the base forms yellow prisms from EtOH. It is strongly dextrorotatory with $[\alpha]_D$ + 325° (c 0.249, CHCl$_3$) and yields a crystalline picrate, m.p. 200–2°C. It contains two methoxyl and one hydroxyl group in the molecule.

Barton *et al., J. Chem. Soc., Perkin I,* 874 (1973)

DEMETHOXYPALOSINE

$C_{22}H_{30}ON_2$

M.p. 117–120°C

Several *Aspidosperma* species contain this alkaloid which has $[\alpha]_D$ – 20° (CHCl$_3$). The ultraviolet spectrum shows absorption maxima at 253 and 289 mμ which are characteristic of this group of bases.

Gilbert *et al., Chem. & Ind.,* 1949 (1962)
Ferreira *et al., Experientia,* **19**, 585 (1963)

DEMETHOXYVINDOLINE

This minor constituent of the aerial parts of *Vinca pusilla* has been characterized on the basis of infrared, ultraviolet, NMR and mass spectroscopic data.

Chatterjee, Biswas, Kundu., *Ind. J. Chem.,* **11**, 7 (1973)

DEMETHYLASPIDOSPERMINE

$C_{21}H_{28}O_2N_2$

This particular alkaloid, obtained from *Aspidosperma discolor* A. DC. and *A. eburneum* Fr. All., is an oily liquid whose ultraviolet spectrum exhibits absorption maxima at 220, 258 and 293 mμ. It forms a crystalline perchlorate from MeOH containing one mole of solvent, m.p. 170°C (*dec.*); $[\alpha]_D^{25}$ + 94° (c 0.98, MeOH). It resembles the preceding in structure but has one less hydroxyl group.

Witkop, Patrick., *J. Amer. Chem. Soc.,* **76**, 5603 (1954)
Ferreira *et al., Experientia,* **19**, 585 (1963)

430

DEMETHYLCEPHAELINE

$C_{27}H_{36}O_4N_2$

M.p. 147–9°C

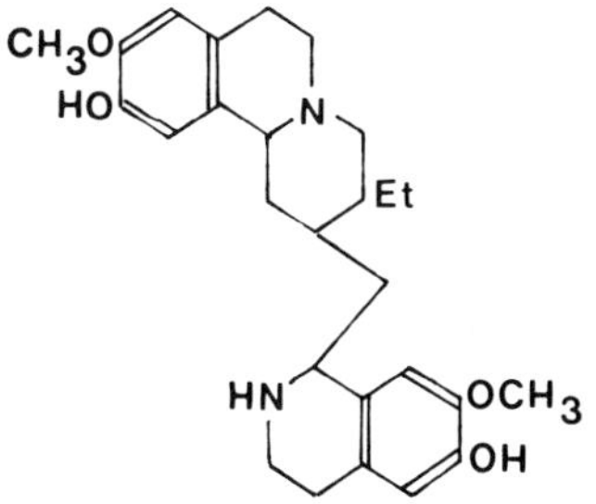

Isolated from *Alangium lamarckii* Thw., this alkaloid is laevorotatory with $[\alpha]_D - 53.5°$ (CHCl$_3$). The ultraviolet spectrum has absorption maxima at 211 and 286 mμ with a shoulder at 225 mμ. The base forms a crystalline hydrochloride, m.p. 262–5°C (*dec.*). It contains two hydroxyl, two methoxyl, an ethyl and an imino group.

Pakrashi, Achari., *Experientia,* **26,** 933 (1970)

DEMETHYLCEPHALOTAXINE

$C_{17}H_{19}O_4N$

M.p. 109–111°C

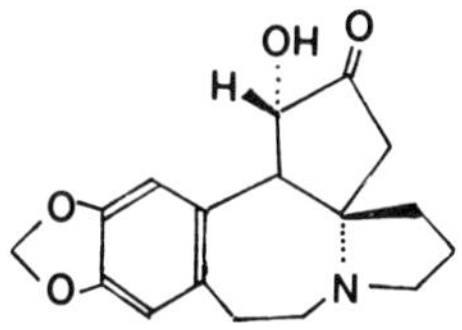

A minor alkaloid of *Cephalotaxus fortunei,* the base is laevorotatory, having $[\alpha]_D^{25} - 110°$ (c 0.28, CHCl$_3$). The structure given above has been established from spectroscopic data.

Paundler, McKay., *J. Org. Chem.,* **38,** 2110 (1973)

2-DEMETHYLCOLCHICINE

$C_{21}H_{23}O_6N$

M.p. 176–182°C

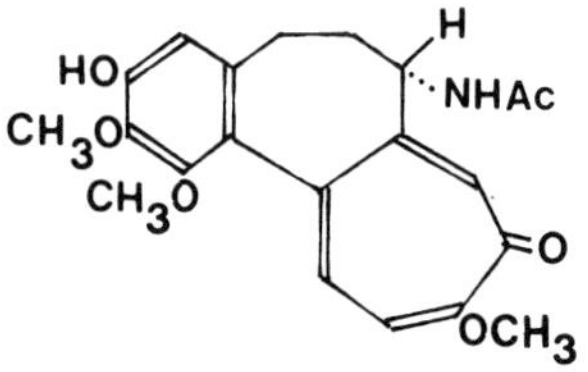

A minor colchicine alkaloid found in *Colchicum autumnale* L., this laevorotatory base has $[\alpha]_D^{22} - 130.7°$ (CHCl$_3$). The methyl ether is identical with Colchicine (q.v.). The ethyl ether is crystalline with m.p. 232–4°C; $[\alpha]_D^{23} - 135.8°$ (CHCl$_3$).

Santavy, Reichstein., *Helv. Chim. Acta,* **33,** 1606 (1950)
Santavy *et al., Collect. Czech. Chem. Commun.,* **18,** 710 (1953)

3-DEMETHYLCOLCHICINE

$C_{21}H_{23}O_6N$

M.p. 140–180°C

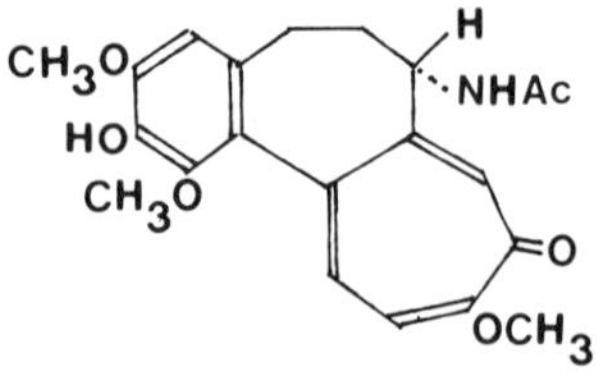

Isomeric with the preceding alkaloid, this base is also found in *Colchicum autumnale* L. It melts over a very wide range and has $[\alpha]_D^{22} - 130°$ (CHCl$_3$). Treatment with CH_2N_2 also yields Colchicine (q.v.).

Santavy, Reichstein., *Helv. Chim. Acta,* **33**, 1606 (1950)
Santavy *et al., Collect. Czech. Chem. Commun.,* **15**, 552 (1950)
Santavy *et al., ibid,* **18**, 710 (1953)

DE-N-METHYLDASYCARPIDONE

$C_{16}H_{18}ON_2$

M.p. 208–210°C

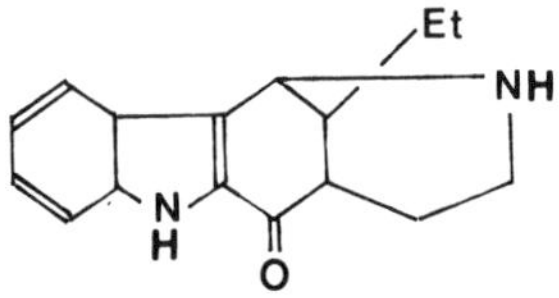

One of the minor alkaloids isolated from *Aspidospermum dasycarpon* A. DC., the base contains two imino groups and one ethyl group. Treatment with CH_2N_2 yields Dasycarpidone (q.v.).

Ohashi *et al., Experientia,* **20**, 363 (1964)
Joule *et al., Tetrahedron,* **21**, 1717 (1965)

2-DEMETHYLDEMECOLCINE

$C_{20}H_{23}O_5N$

M.p. 220–2°C

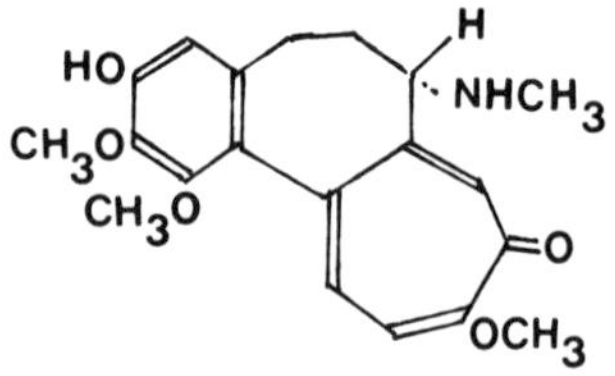

Colchicum cornigerum contains this base as a minor constituent. It is laevo-rotatory with $[\alpha]_D^{20} - 128° \pm 3°$ (c 0.888, CHCl$_3$).

Saleh *et al., Collect. Czech. Chem. Commun.,* **28**, 3413 (1963)

432

O²-DEMETHYL-N-FORMYLDEACETYLCOLCHICINE

$C_{20}H_{21}O_6N$

M.p. 229–230°C

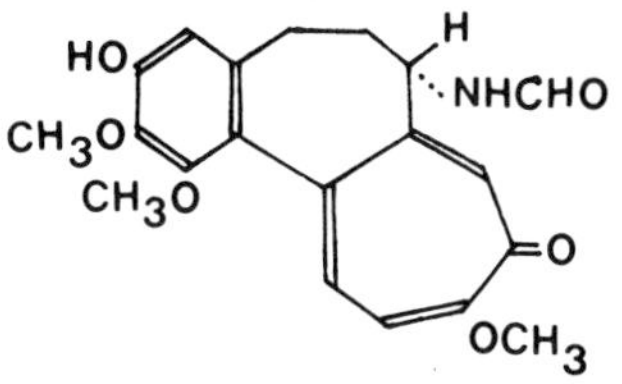

This alkaloid has been isolated from *Gloriosa superba* by chromatography of the $CHCl_3$ extract of the acid fraction. The structure has been ascertained from chemical reactions and the NMR spectrum.

Canonica *et al.*, *Chem. Ind.* (Milan), **49**, 1304 (1967)

O²-DEMETHYL-N-FORMYLDECAETYL-β-LUMICOLCHICINE

$C_{21}H_{23}O_6N$

M.p. 230–1°C

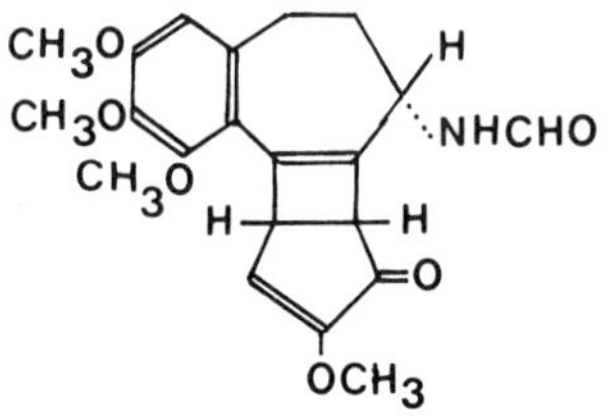

A further alkaloid present in *Gloriosa superba,* this base has also been isolated by chromatographic analysis of the $CHCl_3$ extract of the acid fraction. The structure has been determined from a series of chemical reactions.

Canonica *et al.*, *Chem. Ind.* (Milan), **49**, 1304 (1967)

DEMETHYLGARDNERAMINE

$C_{22}H_{26}O_5N_2$

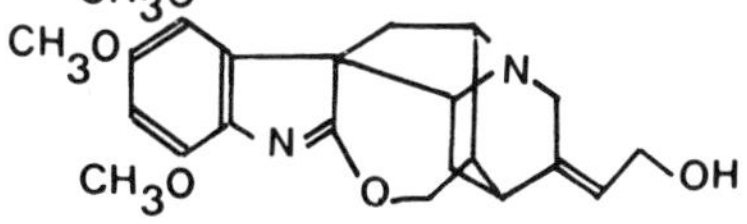

This alkaloid has only recently been isolated from *Gardneria multiflora* Mak. The structure has been determined from chemical and spectroscopic evidence.

Haginiwa *et al.*, *J. Pharm. Soc., Japan,* **90**, 219 (1970)
Sakai *et al.*, *Tetrahedron Lett.*, 2057 (1971)

4-DEMETHYLHASUBONINE

$C_{20}H_{25}O_5N$

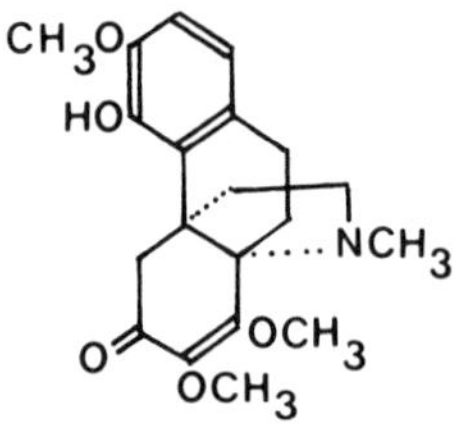

The structure of this alkaloid from *Stephania hernandifolia* has been deduced by chemical, and confirmed by spectroscopic, methods. Methylation with CH_2N_2 yields Hasubonine (q.v.).

Kupchan *et al., J. Org. Chem.*, **33**, 4529 (1968)

3-O-DEMETHYLHERNANDIFOLINE

$C_{28}H_{31}O_9N$

M.p. 149°C

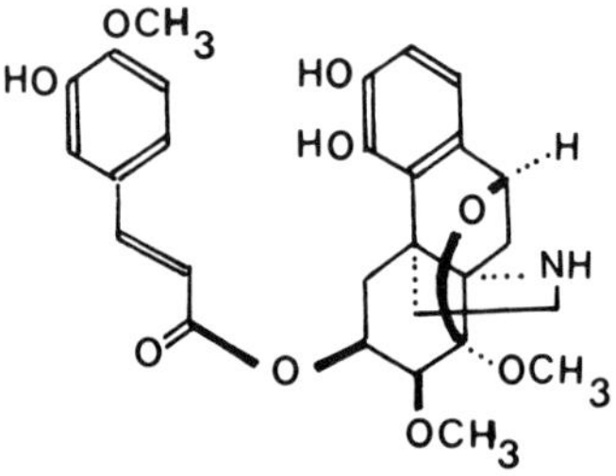

A complex morphine alkaloid, this base has recently been obtained from *Stephania hernandifolia*. It contains three methoxyl group and three hydroxyl groups and the structure has been elucidated primarily from the infrared, NMR and mass spectra.

Fadeeva *et al., Khim. Prir. Soedin.*, **8**, 130 (1972)

9-DEMETHYLHOMOLYCORINE

$C_{17}H_{19}O_4N$

M.p. 213–4°C

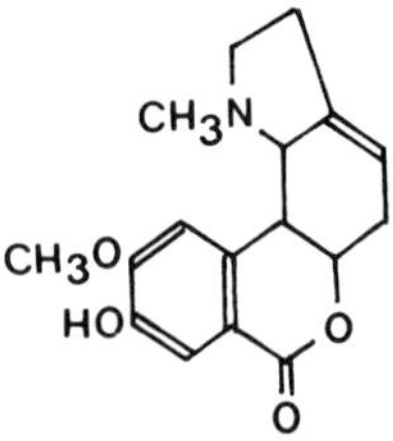

This alkaloid is stated by Uyeo to occur in *Lycoris radiata* and to have the structure given above. No salts have yet been prepared.

Uyeo., See Wildman., *The Alkaloids*, Ed. Manske, **3**, 333 (1960)

434

2-DEMETHYL-β-LUMICOLCHICINE

$C_{22}H_{25}O_6N$

M.p. 183–4°C

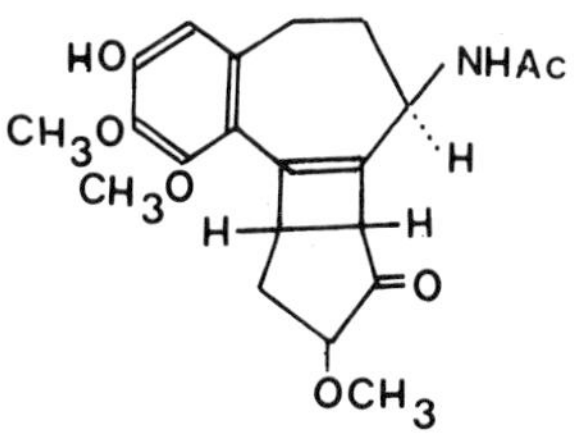

A minor constituent of *Colchicum kesselringii* and *Gloriosa superba,* this alkaloid forms colourless needles from methyl ethyl ketone.

Canonica *et al., Chem. Ind.* (Milan), **49**, 1304 (1967)
Turdikulov, Yusupov, Sadykov., *Khim. Prir. Soedin.,* 7, 541 (1971)

3-DEMETHYL-β-LUMICOLCHICINE

$C_{22}H_{25}O_6N$

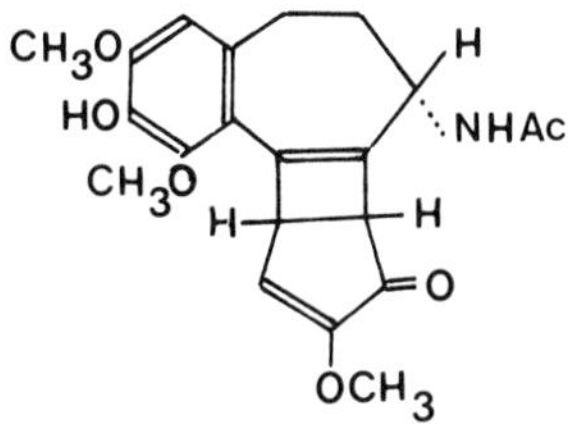

A recently discovered alkaloid, the base is a minor constituent of the bulbs of *Colchicum kesselringii.* The structure has been established spectroscopically.

Turdikulov, Yusupov, Sadykov., *Khim. Prir. Soedin.,* 7, 541 (1971)

3-DEMETHYL-γ-LUMICOLCHICINE (*Alkaloid L-6*)

$C_{20}H_{23}O_6N$

M.p. 291–3°C

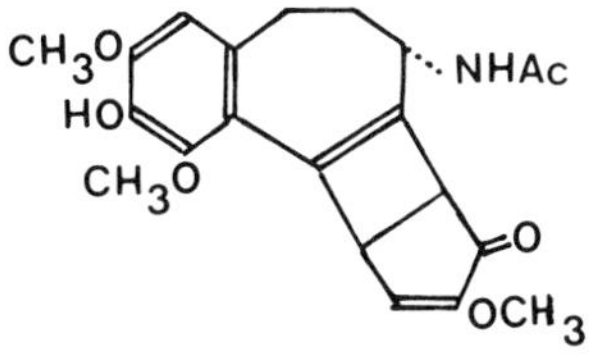

First isolated as Alkaloid L-6 from *Colchicum luteum,* the base has been assigned the above structure on the basis of the NMR and mass spectra. It is strongly laevorotatory with $[\alpha]_D^{20} - 410°$. The O-methyl ether, m.p. 275–6°, is identical with -lumicolchicine.

Chommadov, Yusupov, Sadykov., *Khim. Prir. Soedin.,* 6, 275 (1970)
Trozyan, Yusupov, Sadykov., *ibid,* 7, 541 (1971)

N-DEMETHYLNORACRONYCINE

$C_{18}H_{15}O_3N$

M.p. 245–6°C

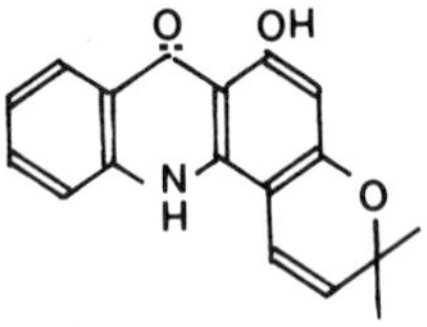

An acridone alkaloid present in *Glycosmis pentaphylla* (Retz.) Correa, the base forms yellow needles when recrystallized from C_6H_6-AcOEt. The ultraviolet spectrum shows absorption maxima at 275, 295 and 410 mμ, with a shoulder at 252 mμ. With $FeCl_3$ in EtOH it gives a deep green colour (cf. des-N-methylacronycine). It contains one hydroxyl group and a *gem*-dimethyl group.

Govindachari *et al.*, *Tetrahedron*, **22**, 3245 (1966)

O-DEMETHYLNUCIFERINE

$C_{18}H_{19}O_2N$

M.p. 214–5°C

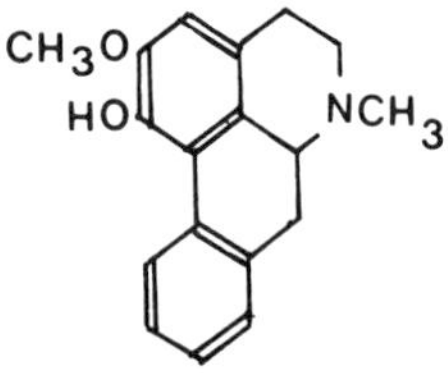

This aporphine alkaloid has been isolated from *Papaver persicum*. It has been characterized as the crystalline hydrochloride, m.p. 256–7°C and the oxalate, m.p. 225–7°C (*dec.*). The alkaloid also occurs in trace amounts in *P. caucasicum*.

Preininger *et al.*, *Collect. Czech. Chem. Commun.*, **32**, 2682 (1967)

DE-N-METHYL-α-OBSCURINE

$C_{16}H_{24}ON_2$

M.p. 266–8°C

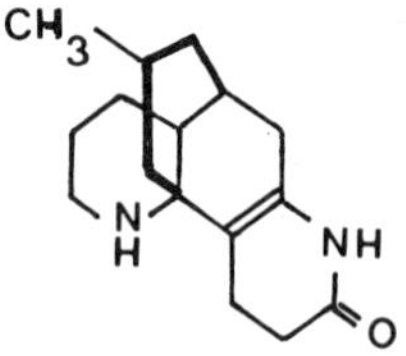

A minor constituent of *Lycopodium clavatum* L. and *L. flabbeliforme*, this alkaloid is obtained as colourless needles when crystallized from Me_2CO. The ultraviolet spectrum shows one absorption maximum at 255 mμ.

Ayer, Berezowsky, Iverach., *Tetrahedron*, **18**, 567 (1962)
Alam, Adams, MacLean., *Can. J. Chem.*, **42**, 2456 (1964)

O-DEMETHYLPALOSINE

$C_{22}H_{30}O_2N_2$

M.p. 169°C

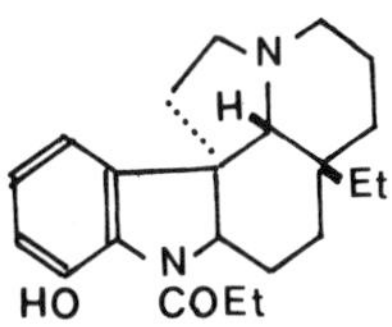

The roots of *Tabernaemontana amygdafolia* yield this alkaloid which has $[\alpha]_{578}^{20} + 118°$ (c 0.36, $CHCl_3$). It contains one hydroxyl group and the O-methyl ether is Palosine (q.v.).

Achenbach., *Tetrahedron Lett.*, 5027 (1966)

DEMETHYLPSYCHOTRINE

$C_{27}H_{34}O_4N_2$

M.p. 166–8°C

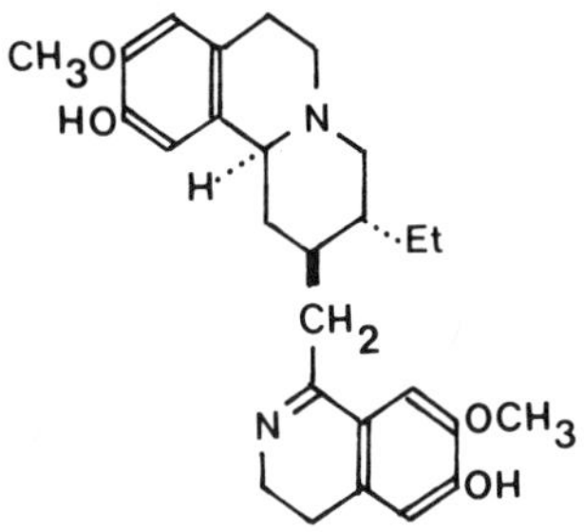

This alkaloid from *Alangium lamarckii* Thw. is obtained from EtOH in the form of deep yellow cubic granules. It has $[\alpha]_D + 67.9°$ (c 0.5, MeOH). In methanol, the ultraviolet spectrum exhibits absorption maxima at 223, 277, 310 and 410 mμ, while in 0.1 N/NaOH, the maxima occur at 243, 307 and 325 mμ. The alkaloid contains two methoxyl groups and two hydroxyl groups. The 7-O-methyl ether is Psychotrine (q.v.).

Pakrashi, Ali., *Tetrahedron Lett.*, 2143 (1967)

N_1-DEMETHYLSEREDAMINE

$C_{20}H_{24}O_2N_2$

M.p. 242–5°C

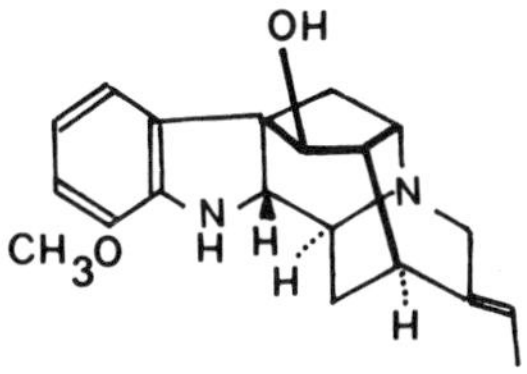

Isolated from *Rauwolfia sumatrana* Jack, this alkaloid forms colourless needles from $CHCl_3$ and has $[\alpha]_D^{22} + 32.6°$ (MeOH). The ultraviolet spectrum shows absorption maxima at 246 and 287 mμ. The O-acetate is a glassy solid; the O,N_1-diacetyl derivative has m.p. 172–5°C; the N_1-acetyl compound has m.p. 295–8°C; the O,N_1-diformyl compound, m.p. 201–3°C and the N_1-formyl derivative, m.p. 320–4°C (*dec.*).

Hanaoka *et al.*, *Helv. Chim. Acta.*, 53, 1723 (1970)

437

DEMETHYLTETRANDRINE

See Fangchinoline

12-DEMETHYLTRILOBINE

$C_{34}H_{32}O_5N_2$

M.p. 256–8°C

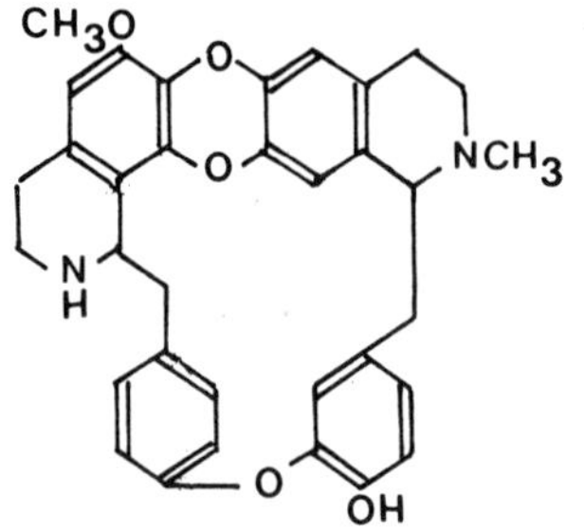

A bisbenzyl*iso*quinoline type base, this alkaloid is found in *Anisocyclea grandidieri*. It forms colourless crystals from Me$_2$CO-MeOH and has $[\alpha]_D^{20} + 332°$ (c 1.5, pyridine). It contains one hydroxyl, one methoxyl and two ether bridges across the *iso*quinoline radicals.

Schlittler, Weber., *Helv. Chim. Acta*, 55, 2061 (1972)

DEMETHYLTUBULOSINE

$C_{28}H_{35}O_3N_3$

M.p. 198–200°C

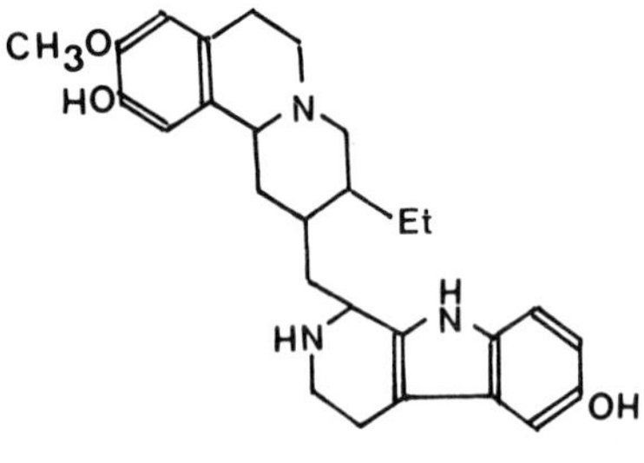

A further alkaloid isolated from *Alangium lamarckii* Thw., this base forms colourless crystals from MeOH-CHCl$_3$. It has $[\alpha]_D^{23} - 51.9°$ (c 1.0, pyridine). The ultraviolet spectra have been extensively studied. In MeOH, there is one broad absorption maximum at 278–280 mμ; in 0.1 N/NaOH the absorption maximum occurs at 280–285 mμ with shoulders at 305 and 320–323 mμ. In acid solution (0.1 N/HCl), the absorption maximum is found at 275 mμ.

Popelak, Haack, Spingler., *Tetrahedron Lett.*, 1081 (1966)

DE-N-METHYLULEINE

$C_{17}H_{20}N_2$

M.p. 143–5°C

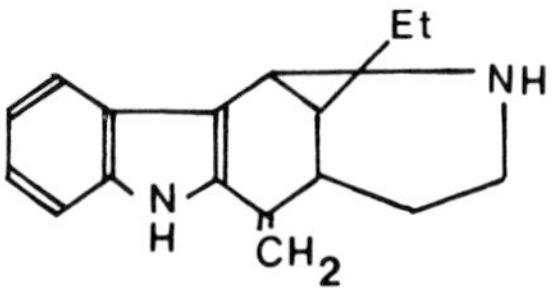

Obtained from *Aspidosperma dasycarpon* A. DC., this alkaloid may be purified

438

by crystallization from $CHCl_3$ when it forms colourless prisms. It is laevorotatory with $[\alpha]_D^{26} - 20°$ (c 1.18, EtOH). The ultraviolet spectrum exhibits two absorption maxima at 305 and 312 mμ. It forms a crystalline N-acetyl derivative, m.p. 214–5°C. The N-ethyl derivative is obtained as a clear, glassy solid which forms a crystalline methiodide, m.p. 190–1°C.

Ohashi et al., Experientia, 20, 363 (1964)
Joule et al., Tetrahedron, 21, 1717 (1965)

DEMETHYLVOBTUSINE

$C_{42}H_{48}O_6N_4$

Dec. 297°C

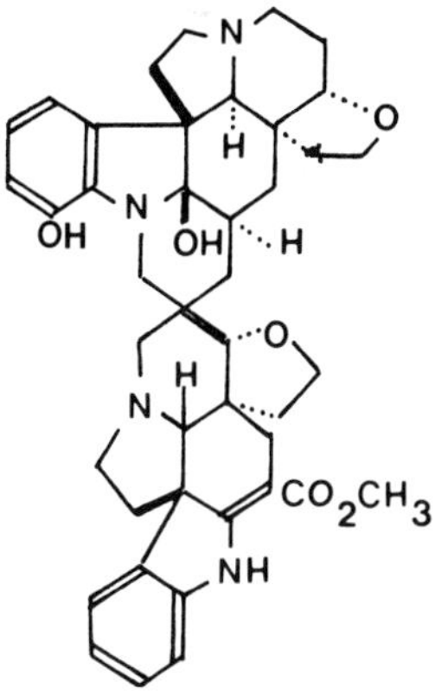

The leaves of *Hedranthera barteri* contain this alkaloid which decomposes over a range from 293–299°C. It is laevorotatory with $[\alpha]_D^{25} - 273°$ (c 0.035, MeOH). In ethanolic solution, the ultraviolet spectrum exhibits absorption maxima at 263, 300 and 326 mμ. The base contains a phenolic and a tertiary hydroxyl group.

Naranjo, Hesse, Schmid., Helv. Chim. Acta, 55, 1849 (1972)

DEMISSIDINE (*Solanine-D*)

$C_{27}H_{45}ON$

M.p. 219–220°C

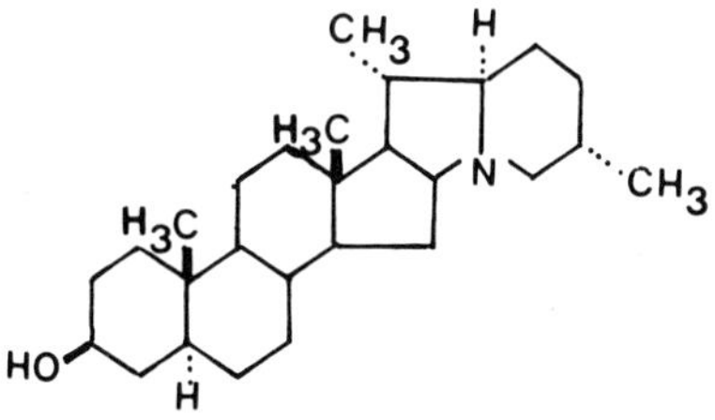

This base is obtained by the hydrolysis of demissine (q.v.) and is also present in minute amounts in the leaves of *Solanum demissum* although it is probable that it is produced during the extraction process and does not exist as such in the plant. It has $[\alpha]_D^{18} + 28°$ (MeOH) and contains four methyl groups and one hydroxyl group. The O-acetate has m.p. 194°C. On dehydrogenation with Se it yields 2-ethyl-5-methylpyridine.

Kuhn, Löw., *Ber.*, **80**, 406 (1947)
Kuhn *et al.*, *Angew. Chem.*, **64**, 397 (1954)
Schreiber., *ibid*, **67**, 127 (1955)

DEMISSINE

$C_{50}H_{83}O_{20}N$

M.p. 276–9°C

A complex glucoalkaloid present in the leaves of *Solanum demissum*, the base is obtained as fine, colourless needles when crystallized from either EtOH or MeOH. It decomposes above its m.p. at 305–8°C and has $[\alpha]_D^{10} - 20°$ (c 1.0, pyridine). On hydrolysis it yields demissidine, galactose, glucose and xylose.

Kuhn, Löw., *Ber.*, **80**, 406 (1947)
Prokoshev *et al.*, *Dokl. Akad. Nauk. SSSR*, **74**, 339 (1950)

DENDRAMINE

$C_{16}H_{25}O_3N$

M.p. 186–8°C

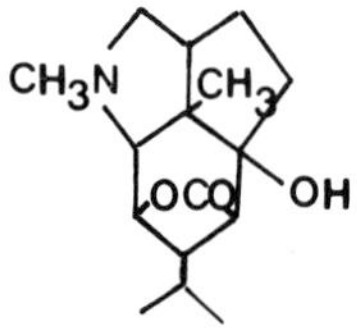

This alkaloid from *Dendrobium nobile* Lindl. is 6-hydroxydendrobine. It has $[\alpha]_D - 27°$ (CHCl$_3$) and contains one hydroxyl group, one *iso*propyl group and a methylimino group in the molecule. It forms a crystalline O-acetate, m.p. 156–8°C.

Inubishi *et al.*, *Chem. Pharm. Bull.* (Tokyo), **12**, 1175 (1964)
Inubushi *et al.*, *ibid*, **14**, 668 (1966)
Okamoto *et al.*, *ibid*, **14**, 676 (1966)

DENDRINE

$C_{19}H_{29}O_4N$

M.p. 191–2°C

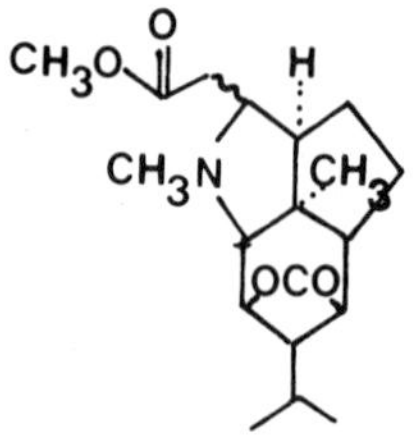

The Chinese drug 'Chin-Shih-Hu', known to be derived from *Dendrobium nobile* Lindl. contains this alkaloid which is laevorotatory with $[\alpha]_D^{11} - 114°$

(c 0.85, CHCl$_3$). The above structure has been determined from chemical and spectroscopic examination.

Inubushi, Nakano., *Tetrahedron Lett.*, 2723 (1965)

DENDROBINE

C$_{16}$H$_{25}$O$_2$N

M.p. 135–6°C

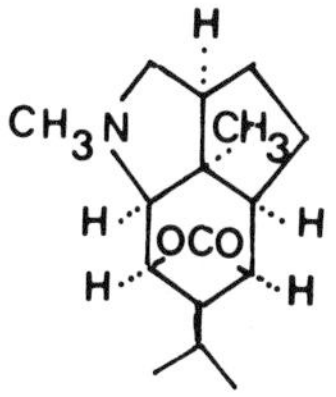

An alkaloid present in *Dendrobium nobile* Lindl., the base crystallizes in colourless prisms or needles and has $[\alpha]_D^{16}$ – 51.5° (EtOH). It gives well-crystallized salts; the hydrochloride, m.p. 246°C (*dec.*); $[\alpha]_D^{14}$ – 41° (H$_2$O); hydriodide, m.p. 223°C (*dec.*); $[\alpha]_D^{14}$ – 34.5° (H$_2$O); aurichloride, m.p. 181°C and the methiodide, m.p. 231°C (*dec.*); $[\alpha]_D^{15}$ – 30.9° (MeOH). The alkaloid acts as a β-lactone giving dendrobinic acid, C$_{16}$H$_{27}$O$_3$N, m.p. 227°C (*dec.*); $[\alpha]_D^{31}$ – 27.5° (EtOH). This acid yields an unstable hydrochloride, an amorphous aurichloride, m.p. 85°C (*dec.*) and a crystalline methiodide, m.p. 211°C (*dec.*). The methyl ester has m.p. 94°C; $[\alpha]_D^{14.5}$ – 17.5° (EtOH). Dendrobine methiodide is readily converted to the methohydroxide, m.p. 251°C (*dec.*). With cyanogen bromide, the alkaloid furnishes cyano*nor*dendrobine, m.p. 188°C from which *nor*dendrobine may be prepared via the carbamide. The latter has m.p. 117–8°C; $[\alpha]_D^{10}$ – 21.6° (EtOH).

Dendrobine diminishes cardiac activity in large doses and produces a moderate hyperglycemia. It also lowers the blood pressure, depresses the respiration and exhibits a weak analgesic, antipyretic action. The convulsions induced by injection of the alkaloid appear to be central in origin due to the action on the cord and medulla and may be controlled by sodium *iso*amylethylbarbiturate.

Suzuki *et al.*, *J. Pharm. Soc., Japan*, **52**, 162 (1932)
Yamamura, Hirata., *Tetrahedron Lett.*, 79 (1964)
Inubushi *et al.*, *Tetrahedron*, **20**, 2007 (1964)

Absolute configuration:
Inubushi *et al.*, *Chem. & Ind.*, 1689 (1964)
Inubushi *et al.*, *Tetrahedron Lett.*, 1519 (1965)

Total synthesis:
Inubushi *et al.*, *J. Chem. Soc., Commun.*, 1252 (1972)

Biosynthesis:
Edwards, Douglas, Mootoo., *Can. J. Chem.*, **48**, 2517 (1970)

Pharmacology:
Chen *et al.*, *J. Biol. Chem.*, **111**, 653 (1935)
Chen *et al.*, *J. Pharm. exp. Ther.*, **55**, 319 (1935)
Chen, Rose., *Proc. Soc. Exp. Biol. Med.*, **34**, 553 (1936)

DENDROBINE N-OXIDE

$C_{16}H_{25}O_3N$

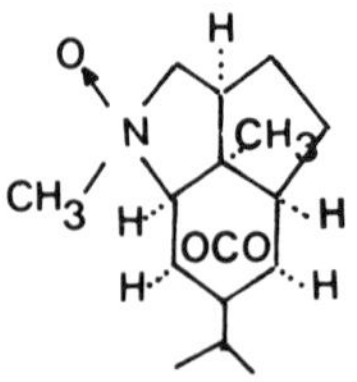

This alkaloid occurs in *Dendrobium nobile* Lindl. It has been identified by chemical analysis, spectroscopic methods and comparison with a specimen produced by oxidation of Dendrobine (q.v.).

Hedman, Leander., *Acta Chem. Scand.*, **26**, 3177 (1972)

cis-DENDROCHRYSINE

$C_{21}H_{28}O_2N_2$

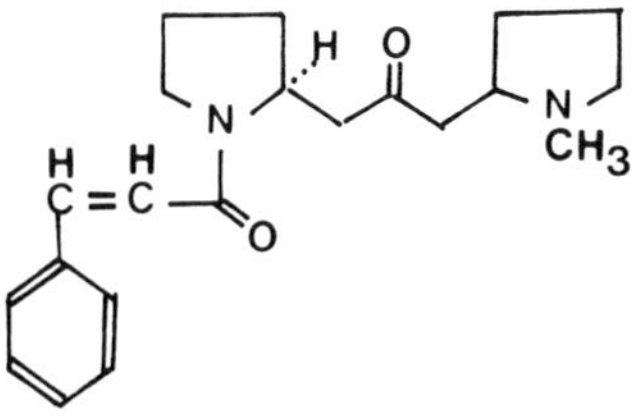

A minor alkaloid of *Dendrobium crysanthum*, the structure has been assigned on the basis of spectroscopic measurements and classical degradation reactions.

Ekevag *et al.*, *Acta Chem. Scand.*, **27**, 1982 (1973)

trans-DENDROCHRYSINE

$C_{21}H_{28}O_2N_2$

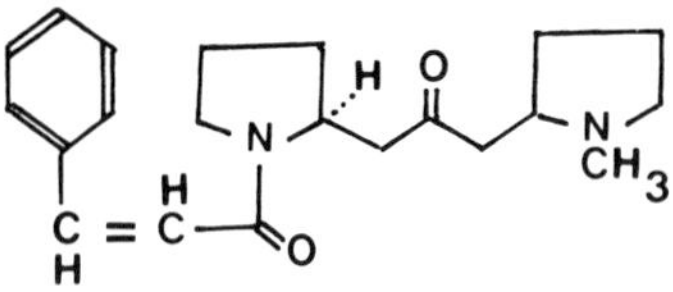

This form of the alkaloid also occurs in *Dendrobium crysanthum*. In addition to the chemical reactions and spectroscopic investigations on which the structure has been based, this has also been confirmed by total synthesis.

Ekevag *et al.*, *Acta Chem. Scand.*, **27**, 1982 (1973)

Synthesis:
Elander., *Chem. Commun. Univ. Stockholm*, No. 6 (1973)

DENDROCREPINE

$C_{33}H_{45}O_3N_2$

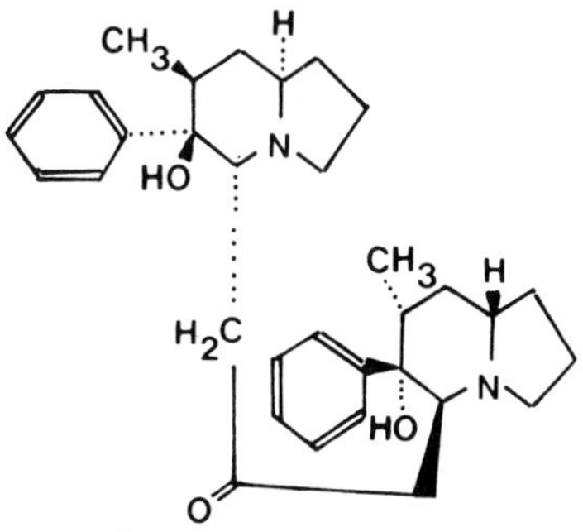

A dimeric alkaloid found in *Dendrobium crepidatum*, the crystal structure of the dihydrobromide has recently been determined by X-ray crystallographic analysis. The salt forms monoclinic crystals with space group P_n and $a = 15.720$, $b = 8.933$, $c = 11.837$ Å and $Z = 2$.

Elander *et al.*, *Acta Chem. Scand.*, **27**, 1907 (1973)

Crystal structure:
Pilotte, Wiehager., *Acta Cryst.*, **29B**, 1563 (1973)

DENDROPRIMINE

$C_{10}H_{19}N$

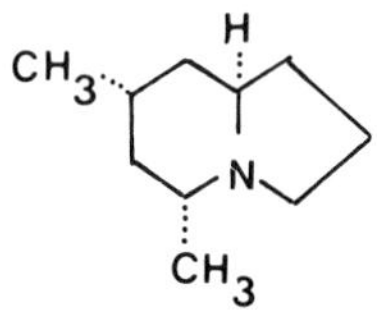

This alkaloid occurs in *Dendrobium primulinum*. The structure has been determined by its conversion through three successive Hofmann degradations into (+)-4-methylnonane.

Blomqvist *et al.*, *Acta Chem. Scand.*, **26**, 3203 (1972)

DENDROWARDINE

$C_{19}H_{32}O_4N^+$

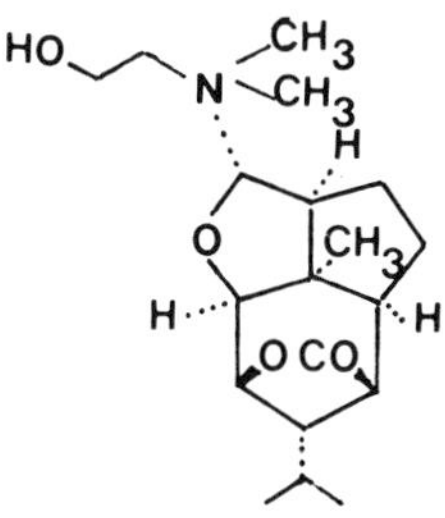

A quaternary alkaloid isolated from *Dendrobium wardianum*, the structure of this base has been shown to be that given above based upon spectroscopic and chemical studies.

Blomqvist *et al.*, *Acta Chem. Scand.*, **27**, 1439 (1973)

DENDROXINE

$C_{17}H_{25}O_3N$

M.p. 114–5°C

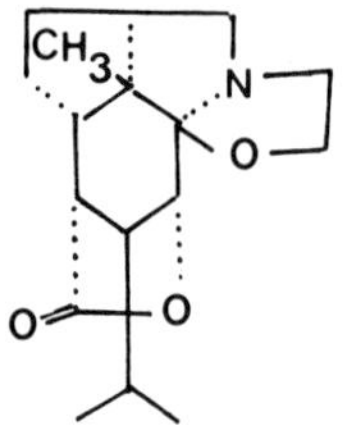

Isolated from *Dendrobium nobile* Lindl., this alkaloid is laevorotatory with $[\alpha]_D - 30.1°$ (EtOH). It has a β-lactone ring but no hydroxyl groups. Catalytic reduction in AcOH in the presence of PtO_2 yields an amorphous base characterized as the methiodide, m.p. 190–3°C. The amorphous base is also obtained by the action of ethylene oxide in MeOH on *nor*dendrobine and is therefore 2-hydroxymethyl*nor*dendrobine.

Okamoto *et al.*, *Chem. Pharm. Bull.*, **14**, 672 (1966)

DENUDATINE

$C_{21}H_{33}O_2N$

M.p. 248–9°C

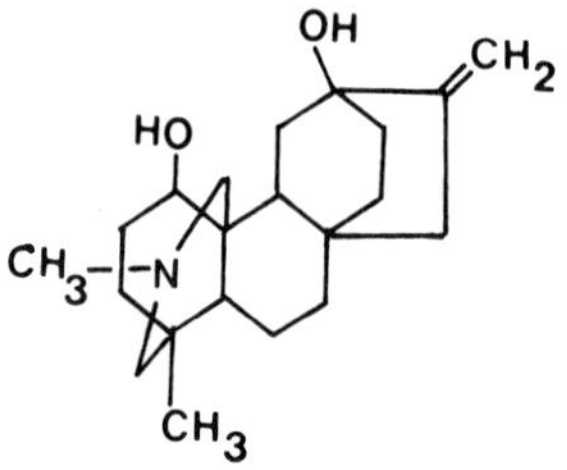

One of the aconite alkaloids present in certain *Delphinium* species, the base has $[\alpha]_D^{21} + 0.154°$ (EtOH). Although this value of the specific rotation is very small it nevertheless appears to be real and not due to experimental error. The ultra-violet spectrum consists of a single absorption maximum at 210 mμ. The alkaloid contains two hydroxyl groups and forms a crystalline O,O-diacetate, m.p. 130°C. Oxidation with $KMnO_4$ yields formaldehyde indicative of an exocyclic methylene group. With chromic acid in pyridine, the alkaloid yields oxodenudatine, m.p. 327°C and the N-deethyl derivative, m.p. 282°C. Reduction with Pd in EtOH yields isodenudatine, m.p. 192°C.

Singh, Singh, Malik., *Chem. & Ind.*, 1909 (1961)

Structure:
Goetz, Wiesner., *Tetrahedron Lett.*, 4369 (1969)

11-DEOXOJERVINE

$C_{27}H_{41}O_2N$

M.p. 237–8°C

The roots of *Veratrum album* var. *grandiflorum* Maxim. contain this alkaloid which forms colourless crystals from MeOH or EtOH. It is laevorotatory with $[\alpha]_D - 44.2°$ (95% EtOH). The base contains two active hydrogens on the hydroxyl and imino groups and forms an O,N-diacetyl derivative which has two melting points, 163–4°C and 195–7°C with intermediate solidification. This compound is slightly dextrorotatory with $[\alpha]_D^{23} + 1.1°$.

Masamune *et al.*, *Tetrahedron Lett.*, 913 (1964)
Masamune *et al.*, *Bull. Chem. Soc., Japan*, **38**, 1374 (1965)

Absolute configuration:
Kupchan, Suffness., *J. Amer. Chem. Soc.*, **90**, 2730 (1968)

10-DEOXYADIFOLINE

$C_{22}H_{20}O_6N_2$

The heartwood of *Adina cordifolia*, on extraction with AcOEt, yields this alkaloid belonging to the indole group, together with 10-deoxycordifoline (q.v.). The structure of the base has been elucidated by chromatographic separation, first by paper chromatography of the AcOEt extract followed by elution on a cellulose column. The alkaloid forms a methylated acetyl derivative as colourless crystals, m.p. 253–5°C and the structure has been confirmed from the NMR spectrum of this derivative. Like the accompanying alkaloid, this base contains a carboxylic acid group in the molecule, together with a methyl group and a methoxycarbonyl group.

Merlini, Nasini., *Gazz. Chim. Ital.*, **98**, 974 (1968)

DEOXYANIFLORINE

$C_{20}H_{21}O_2N_3$

M.p. 168–172°C

Present in *Anisotes sessiliflorus* C.B.Cl., this alkaloid may be crystallized from

MeOH. The ultraviolet spectrum in ethanolic solution has absorption maxima at 211, 232, 285, 315 and 324 mμ. In EtOH-HCl solution, the absorption maxima are at 211, 237, 285, 315 and 320 mμ. The alkaloid contains one methoxyl group and one dimethylimino group.

Arndt, Eggers, Jordaan., *Tetrahedron*, 23, 3521 (1967)

DEOXYASPIDODISPERMINE

$C_{19}H_{24}O_2N_2$

M.p. Indefinite

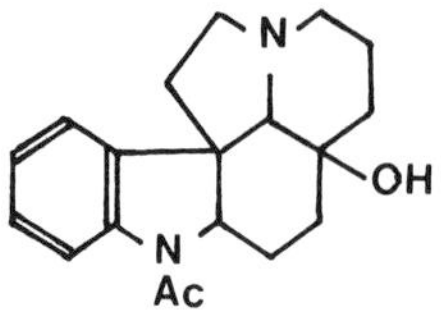

This alkaloid has been isolated from *Aspidosperma dispermum* and is obtained as an amorphous powder with no definite melting point. It has $[\alpha]_D - 20°$ (MeOH) and the ultraviolet spectrum in MeOH has absorption maxima at 207, 252, 279 and 289 mμ. The O-acetate is also amorphous.

Ikeda, Djerassi., *Tetrahedron Lett.*, 5837 (1968)

16-DEOXYBUXIDIENINE C

$C_{27}H_{46}ON_2$

M.p. 200–1 °C

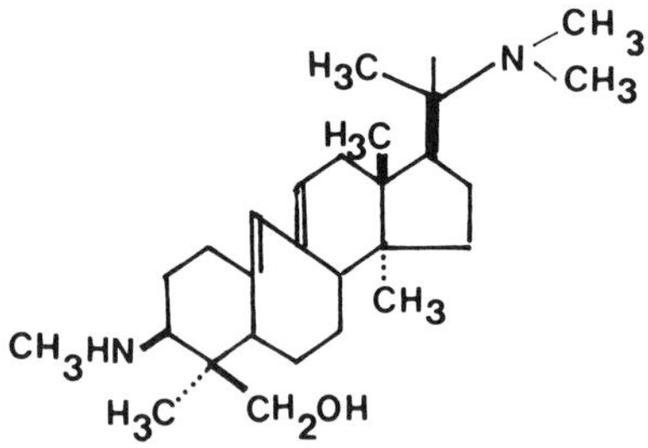

One of the numerous *Buxus* alkaloids, this base is found in *Buxus madagascarica*. It is dextrorotatory with $[\alpha]_D + 55°$. The ultraviolet spectrum exhibits absorption maxima at 238, 246 and 254 mμ. The alkaloid contains a methyl and a dimethylimino group in the molecule.

Khuong Huu Laine *et al.*, *Compt. Rend.*, 273C, 558 (1971)

DEOXYCORDIFOLINE

$C_{28}H_{30}O_{11}N_2$

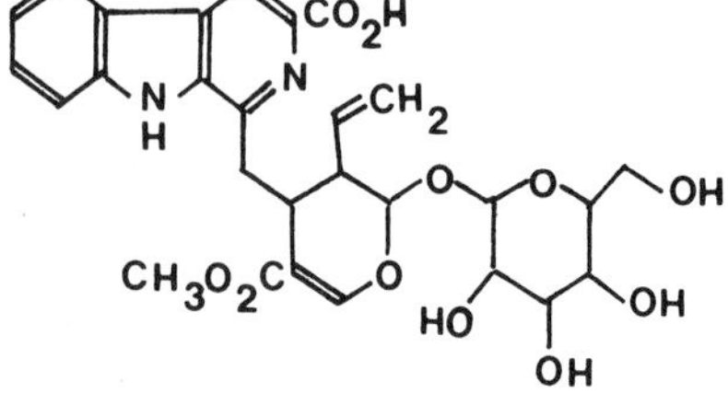

A glucosidic alkaloid present in the heartwood of *Adina cordifolia*, the base has been obtained by extraction with AcOEt followed by paper chromatography and further purification by column chromatography on a cellulose column. The structure has been established from the NMR spectrum of the tetraacetate methyl ether, m.p. 91–3°C.

Merlini, Nasini., *Gazz. Chim. Ital.*, **98**, 974 (1968)

DEOXYCORDIFOLINE LACTAM

$C_{27}H_{26}O_{10}N_2$

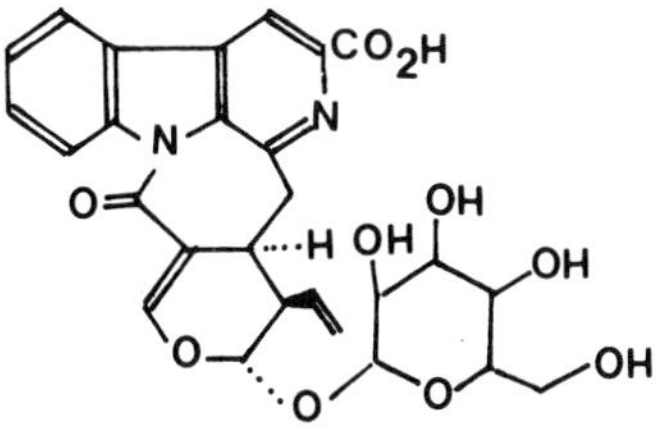

This base is one of the *Adina* alkaloid and occurs in *Adina rubescens*. The structure has been determined by means of chemical and spectroscopic techniques.

Brown, Fraser., *Tetrahedron Lett.,* 841 (1973)

DEOXYCORDIFOLINE LACTAM METHYL ESTER

$C_{28}H_{28}O_{10}N_2$

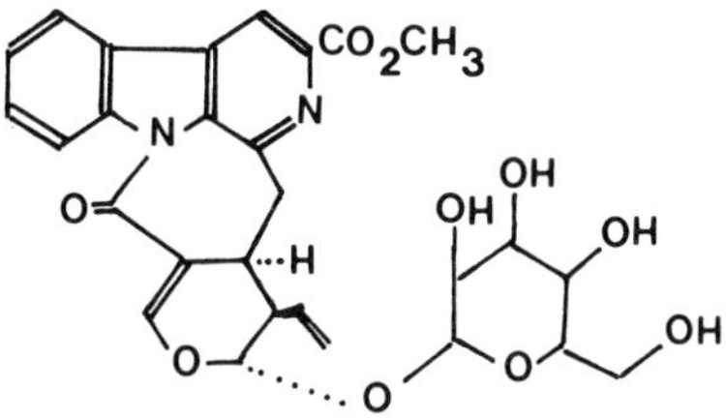

The methyl ester of the preceding base has also been found as a constituent of *Adina rubescens.* Its structure follows directly from that of the former base from which it may also be prepared by the action of CH_2N_2.

Brown, Fraser., *Tetrahedron Lett.,* 841 (1973)

DEOXYCYCLOBUXOXAZINE A

$C_{28}H_{48}ON_2$

M.p. 161–2°C

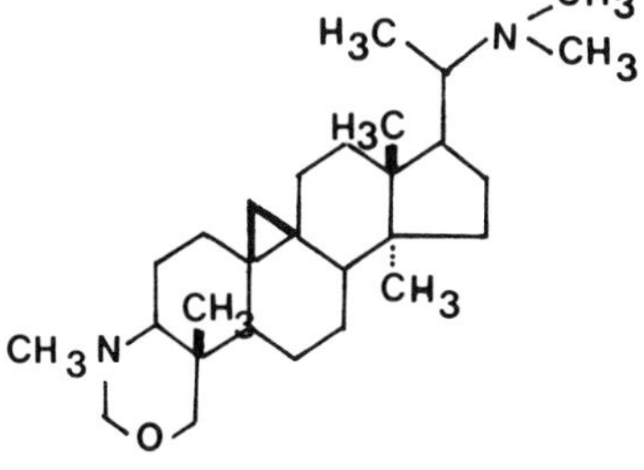

A further *Buxus* alkaloid, this base occurs in *Buxus sempervirens* L. It is dextrorotatory with $[\alpha]_D + 56°$ (c 0.2, $CHCl_3$). The structure has been elucidated by spectroscopic methods and comparison with Cyclobuxoxazine A.

Härtel et al., Tetrahedron Lett., 2741 (1971)

4-DEOXYEVONINE

$C_{36}H_{43}O_{16}N$

M.p. 150–8°C

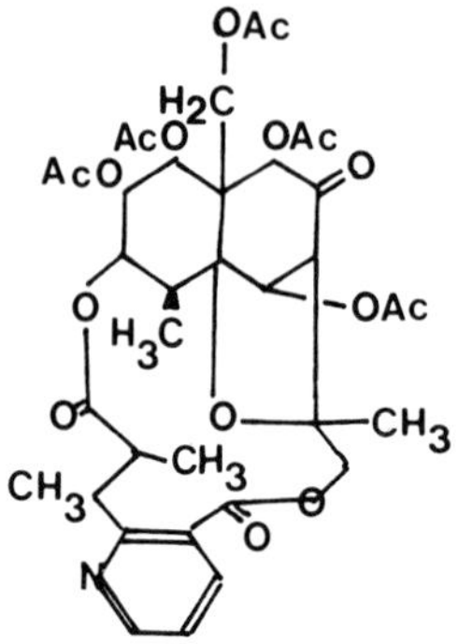

A complex and highly substituted alkaloid, this base is found in Euonymus europea L. It forms small, colourless crystals from a mixture of Me_2CO and light petroleum. The ultraviolet spectrum in EtOH has absorption maxima at 226 and 256 mμ. The base contains five acetoxy groups and a pyridine ring in the molecule.

Budzikiewicz, Romer, Taraz., Naturforsch., 27B, 800 (1972)

DEOXYHARRINGTONINE

$C_{28}H_{37}O_8N$

M.p. Indefinite

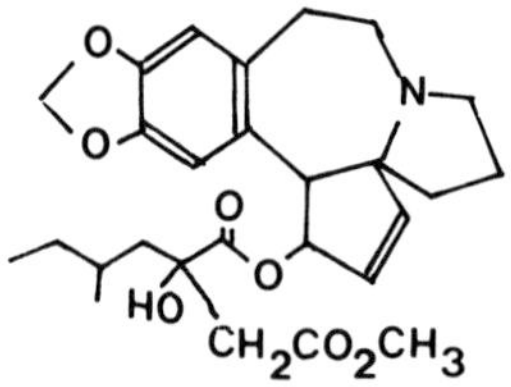

This amorphous alkaloid occurs in Cephalotaxus harringtonia K. Koch. It is laevorotatory with $[\alpha]_D^{26} - 151°$ (c 0.03, EtOH) or $- 119°$ (c 0.6, $CHCl_3$). The ultraviolet spectrum in ethanol exhibits absorption maxima at 261 and 291 mμ. Pharmacologically, it has a marked antitumour effect.

Mikolajczak, Powell, Smith., Tetrahedron, 28, 1995 (1972)

448

DE(OXYMETHYLENE)LYCOCTONINE

$C_{24}H_{39}O_6N$

B.p. 160°C/0.00005 mm

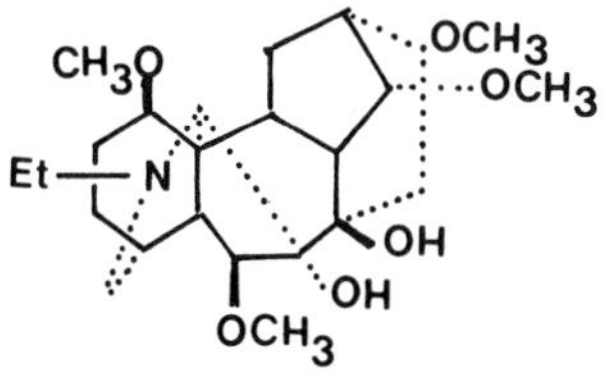

Possibly present in small quantities in *Aconitum lycoctonum* roots, this alkaloid has $[\alpha]_D^{25} + 27.8°$ (c 2.19, EtOH). It forms a crystalline hydriodide monohydrate, m.p. 173–4°C (*dry, dec.*) and a perchlorate, m.p. 146°C (*dec.*).

Edwards, Marion., *Can. J. Chem.*, **30**, 627 (1952)

DEOXYPEGANIDINE

$C_{14}H_{16}ON_2$

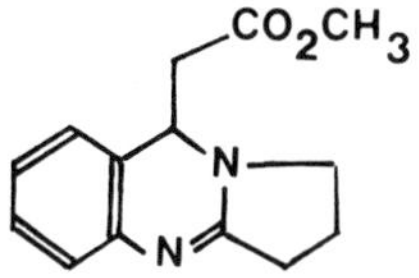

An alkaloid recently isolated from *Peganum harmala*, the structure of the base has been determined spectroscopically. Oxidation with $KMnO_4$ yields Vasicinone (q.v.).

Zharekeev, Telezhenetskaya, Yunusov., *Khim. Prir. Soedin.*, 279 (1973)

(−)-DEOXYTUBULOSINE

$C_{29}H_{37}O_2N_3$

M.p. 230–2°C

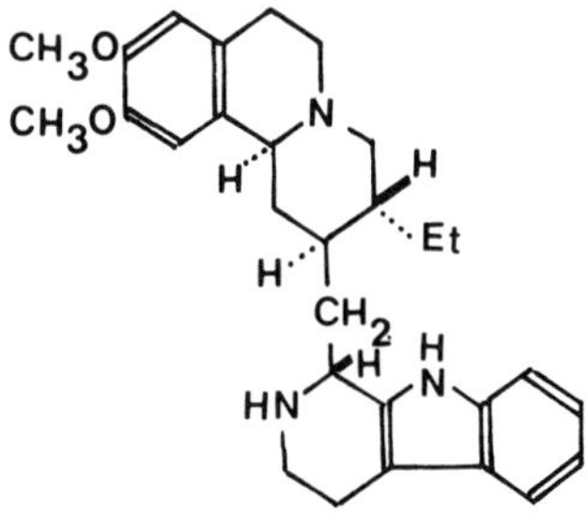

The fruit of *Alangium lamarckii* and *Cassinopsis ilicifolia* Kuntze yield this alkaloid which forms colourless crystals from EtOH. It has $[\alpha]_D - 24°$ (CHCl$_3$). The alkaloid is characterized as the *p*-toluenesulphonate, m.p. 145–150°C.

Battersby *et al.*, *J. Chem. Soc.*, 3899 (1961)
Battersby *et al.*, *Chem. Commun.*, 315 (1965)
Monteiro *et al.*, *ibid*, 317 (1965)

DEOXYVASICINONE

$C_{11}H_{10}ON_2$

M.p. 109–110°C

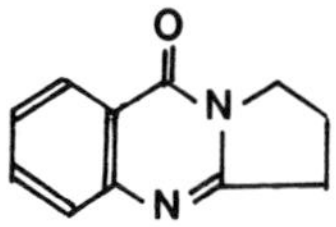

A minor constituent of *Peganum harmala* L. and *Mackinlaya macrosciadia*, the alkaloid occurs in the EtOH or petroleum ether extract of the seeds together with Harmine (q.v.) and Harmaline (q.v.). The alkaloid has been synthesized by refluxing γ-aminobutyric acid and anthranilic acid with P_2O_5 in xylene for 3 hours at 170–180°C.

Chatterjee, Ganguly., *Phytochem.*, 7, 307 (1968)

Hart, Johns, Lamberton., *Austral. J. Chem.*, 24, 223 (1971)

DEOXYVINBLASTINE A (*Isoleurosine*)

$C_{46}H_{58}O_8N_4$

M.p. 202–6°C (*dec.*).

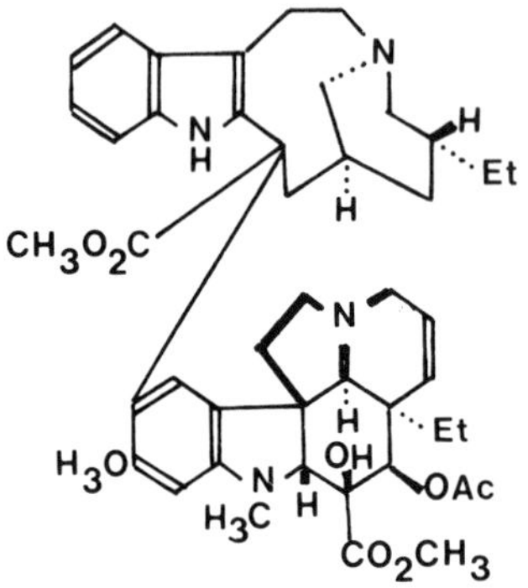

A dimeric base which occurs in *Vinca rosea* L., this alkaloid contains two acetoxy groups, one methoxyl and two ethyl groups in the molecule. It has $[\alpha]_D^{25} + 61.2°$. The ultraviolet spectrum has absorption maxima at 214, 261 and 287 mμ. The original structure proposed for the base has recently been revised to that given above.

Svoboda *et al.*, *J. Pharm. Sci.*, 50, 409 (1961)

Structure revision:
Neuss *et al.*, *Tetrahedron Lett.*, 783 (1968)

DEOXYVOBTUSINE

$C_{43}H_{50}O_5N_4$

M.p. 305°C (*dec.*).

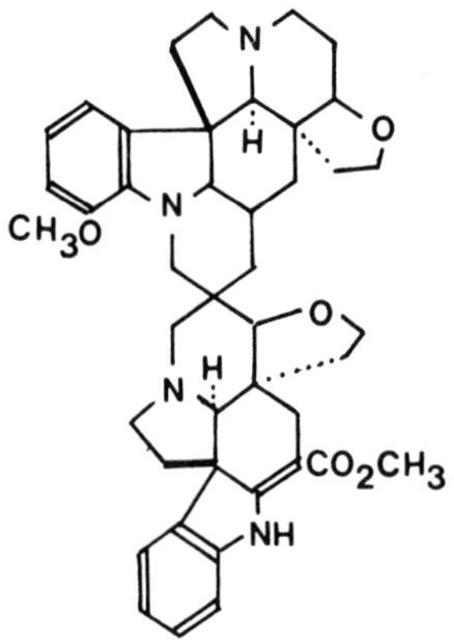

This dimeric alkaloid is obtained from *Voacanga africana* Stapf. where it occurs mainly in the leaves. It is laevorotatory with $[\alpha]_{578} - 355°$ and the ultraviolet spectrum has absorption maxima at 224, 267, 303 and 327 mμ. The base contains one methoxyl group.

Kunesch, Das, Poisson., *Bull. Soc. Chim. Fr.,* 4370 (1970)

DEOXYVOBTUSINE LACTONE

$C_{43}H_{48}O_6N_4$

M.p. 305°C (*dec.*).

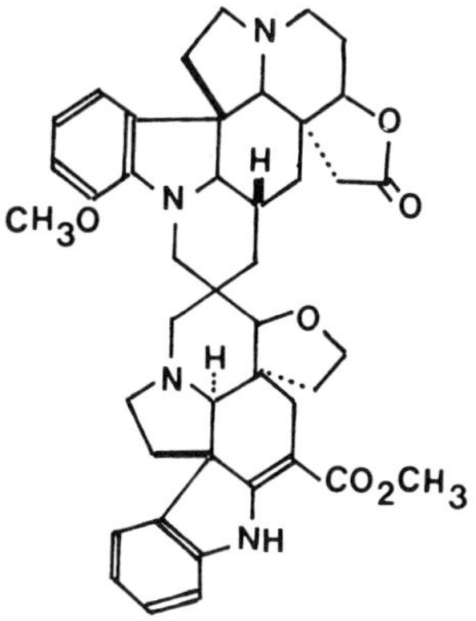

Like the preceding base, this alkaloid is present in *Voacanga africana* Stapf. but here it is found chiefly in the flowers rather than in the leaves. It is also laevorotatory with $[\alpha]_{578}^{22} - 348°$ (CHCl$_3$). The ultraviolet spectrum in EtOH is very similar to that of deoxyvobtusine with absorption maxima at 222, 262, 302 and 326 mμ. It differs from the latter only in the lactam structure of one of the rings.

Kunesch, Poisson., *Tetrahedron Lett.,* 1745 (1968)

N-DEPROPIONYLDECORTICASINE

$C_7H_{12}ON_2$

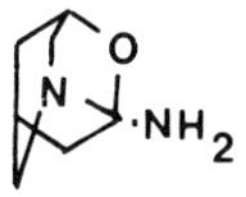

This alkaloid has been shown to be present in *Adenocarpus decorticans* together with the three following bases. All of the evidence shows that the alkaloid is not a hydrolysis product of the accompanying amides.

Landa Velon., *Acta Cient. Compostela.,* 8, 171 (1971)

N-DEPROPIONYLCORTICASINE BUTYRAMIDE

$C_{11}H_{18}O_2N_2$

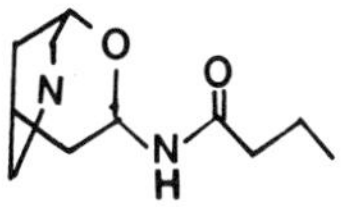

Also present in *Adenocarpus decorticans,* the structure of this alkaloid has been confirmed by synthesis.

Landa Velon., *Acta Cient. Compostela.,* 8, 171 (1971)

N-DEPROPIONYLCORTICASINE ISOBUTYRAMIDE

$C_{11}H_{18}O_2N_2$

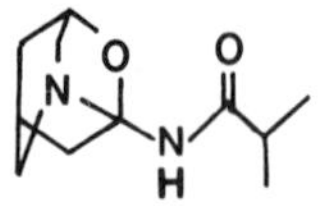

Adenocarpus decorticans contains this isomer of the preceding alkaloid, the structure again having been proved by synthesis.

Landa Velon., *Acta Cient. Compostela.*, **8**, 171 (1971)

N-DEPROPIONYLCORTICASINE ISOVALERAMIDE

$C_{12}H_{20}O_2N_2$

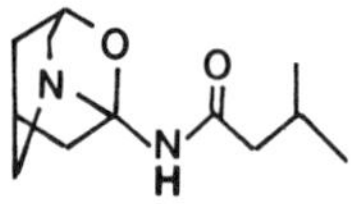

A fourth base occurring in *Adenocarpus decorticans*, the structure has been confirmed by synthesis.

Landa Velon., *Acta Cient. Compostela.*, **8**, 171 (1971)

DESEMINE

A minor alkaloid of *Delphinium oreophilum* and *D. semibarbatum*. When hydrolyzed with 10 per cent HCl at 100°C, the base furnishes methylsuccinic acid and anthranyldelsine, m.p. 166°C; $[\alpha]_D^{32} + 49.2°$ (EtOH).

Yunusov, Abubakirov., *J. Gen. Chem., USSR*, **21**, 967 (1951)

DESERPIDEINE

$C_{32}H_{36}O_8N_2$

M.p. 149–152°C
(*dec.*)

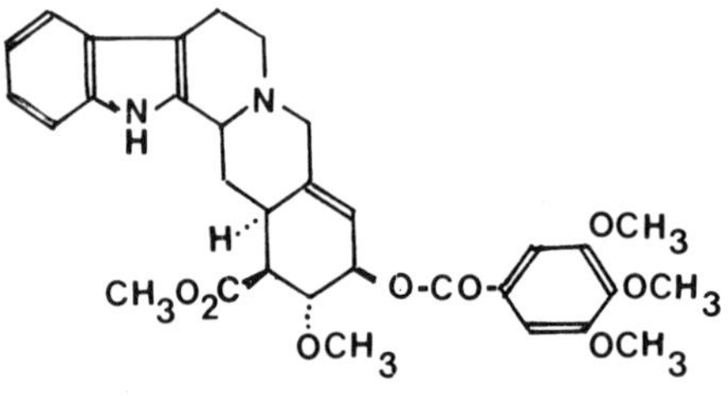

The roots of *Rauwolfia nitida* Jacq. yield this alkaloid which forms colourless crystals from Et_2O. It is laevorotatory with $[\alpha]_D - 133°$ (c 1.0, pyridine). Some crystalline salts have been prepared including the hydrochloride, m.p. 277°C (*dec.*); $[\alpha]_D^{25} - 98.5°$ (c 9.50, $CHCl_3$); and the methiodide, m.p. 246–8°C (*dec.*).

Smith *et al.*, *Lloydia*, **27**, 440 (1964)
Smith *et al.*, *J. Amer. Chem. Soc.*, **86**, 2083 (1964)
Smith *et al.*, *ibid*, **89**, 2469 (1967)

DESERPIDINE (*Canescine*)

$C_{32}H_{38}O_8N_2$

M.p. 228–232°C

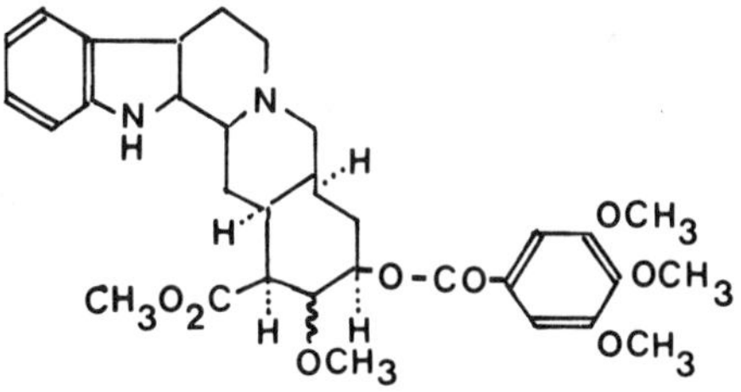

A *Rauwolfia* alkaloid, this base is found in *Rauwolfia canescens*. When recrystallized from Et_2O it is obtained as colourless needles or prisms. It has $[\alpha]_D^{24.5}$ – 137° ($CHCl_3$) and has been described in the literature under various names including recanescine, harmonyl or 11-demethoxyreserpine.

MacPhillamy *et al., J. Amer. Chem. Soc.*, **75**, 4335 (1953)
Neuss *et al., ibid*, **77**, 4087 (1955)
Huebner *et al., Experientia*, **11**, 303 (1955)
Schlittler *et al., ibid*, **11**, 64 (1955)
Saxton., *Quart. Rev.*, **10**, 133 (1956)
Weichet *et al., Collect. Czech. Chem. Commun.*, **26**, 1529, 1537 (1961)

DES-N-METHYLACRONYCINE

$C_{19}H_{17}O_3N$

M.p. 268–270°C (*dec.*).

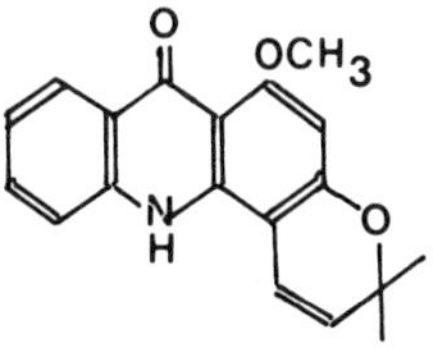

This alkaloid from *Glycosmis pentaphylla* (Retz.) Correa is obtained as yellow needles when recrystallized from Me_2CO. The ultraviolet spectrum shows absorption maxima at 265, 295 and 395 mμ with an inflexion at 333 mμ. The hydrochloride forms orange needles, m.p. 137–141°C; the perchlorate, orange needles, m.p. 251–2°C (*dec.*) and the picrate, orange needles, m.p. 222–4°C (*dec.*). The alkaloid gives no colour with $FeCl_3$ (cf. N-demethyl*nor*acronycine).

Govindachari, Pai, Subramanian., *Tetrahedron*, **22**, 3245 (1966)

DESMETHYLDECALINE

$C_{24}H_{27}O_5N$

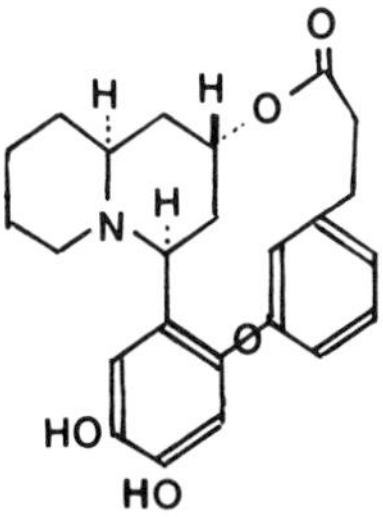

453

Obtained from *Decodon verticillatus* L. this alkaloid gives Decaline (q.v.) with CH_2N_2. The structure has been confirmed by comparison with the latter base.

Ferris *et al.*, *Tetrahedron Lett.*, 5125 (1966)

12-O'-DESMETHYLTRILOBINE

$C_{34}H_{32}O_5N_2$

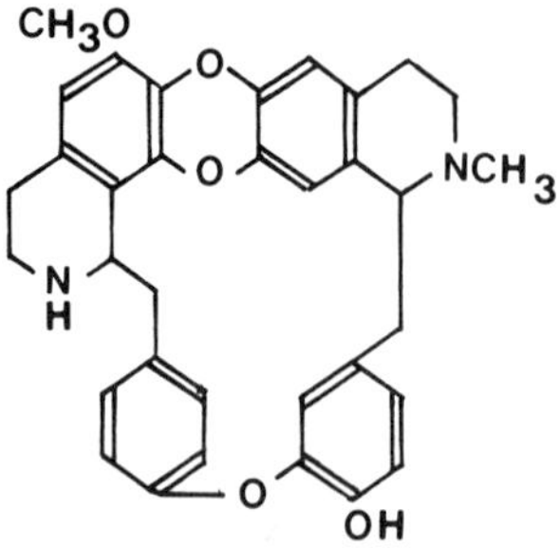

A bisbenzyl*iso*quinoline alkaloid found in *Anisocyclea grandidieri*, the structure has been deduced from the ultraviolet, infrared, NMR and mass spectra. One methoxyl group, one phenolic hydroxyl group and a methylimino group are present.

Schlittler, Weber., *Helv. Chim. Acta*, 55, 2061 (1972)

DES-N-METHYLULEINE

$C_{17}H_{20}N_2$

M.p. 143–5°C

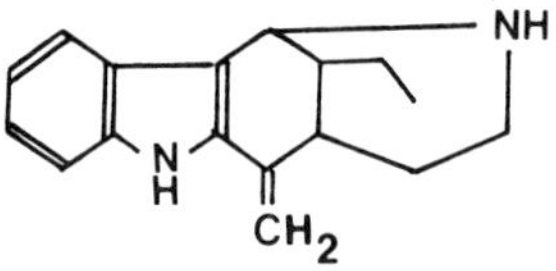

This alkaloid from *Aspidosperma dasycarpon* crystallizes from $CHCl_3$ as colourless needles. It is laevorotatory with $[\alpha]_D^{26} - 20°$ (c 1.18, EtOH).

Joule *et al.*, *Tetrahedron*, 21, 1717 (1965)

DESMETHYLVERTALINE

Present in *Decodon verticillatus* L., this alkaloid reacts with CH_2N_2 to yield Vertaline (q.v.), thereby confirming the structure.

Ferris *et al.*, *Tetrahedron Lett.*, 5125 (1966)

DIABOLINE

$C_{21}H_{24}O_3N_2$

M.p. 187–9°C

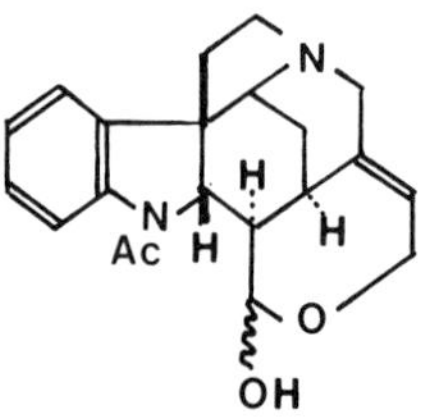

A curare alkaloid occurring in *Strychnos diaboli* Sandwith, this base is the

N-acetyl derivative of Caracurine VII (q.v.). It forms crystalline salts, e.g. the hydrochloride, m.p. > 360°C; nitrate, m.p. 244°C (*dec.*) and the picrate, m.p. 234–240°C.

King., *J. Chem. Soc.*, 955 (1949)
Bader *et al.*, *Helv. Chim. Acta*, **36**, 1256 (1953)
Battersby, Hodson., *Proc. Chem. Soc.*, 126 (1959)

DIACETYLLYCOFOLINE

$C_{20}H_{29}O_4N$

M.p. 113–8°C

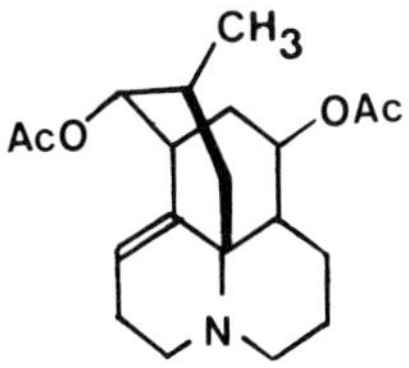

A *Lycopodium* alkaloid, this base is found in *L. fawcettii*. It yields colourless crystals from Et_2O. The structure has been elucidated from the infrared, NMR and mass spectra.

Anet, Kuhn., *Can. J. Chem.*, **37**, 1589 (1959)
Anet, Ahmed, Khan., *ibid*, **40**, 236 (1962)

DIACETYLMACRANTHINE

$C_{20}H_{23}O_7N$

M.p. 219–221°C

An alkaloid of *Crinium macrantherium* Engl., the base forms colourless crystals from a mixture of Me_2CO and Et_2O. It is dextrorotatory with $[\alpha]_D^{22} + 38°$ (c 0.203, EtOH) and + 44° (c 0.284, CHCl$_3$). Acetylation with Ac_2O in pyridine yields the O,O,N-tracetyl derivative, m.p. 190–2°C; $[\alpha]_D^{22} - 2°$ (c 0.220, CHCl$_3$). Alkaline hydrolysis furnishes acetic acid and Macranthine (q.v.).

Hauth, Stauffacher., *Helv. Chim. Acta*, **47**, 185 (1964)

DIBROMOPHAKELLIN

$C_{11}H_{13}ON_5Br_2$

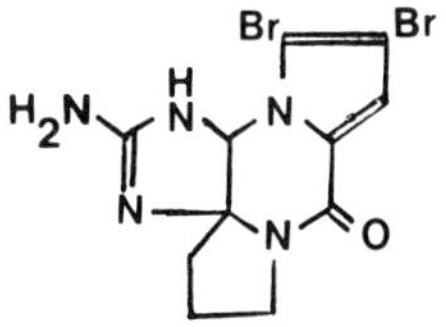

A bromine-containing alkaloid isolated from the marine sponge *Phakellia flabellata*, the base has been shown to possess the structure given above on the basis of chemical degradation and spectroscopic investigation. Catalytic hydrogenation furnishes phakellin.

Sharma, Burkholder., *J. Chem. Soc., D*, **3**, 151 (1971)

DICENTRINE

$C_{20}H_{21}O_4N$

M.p. 168–9°C

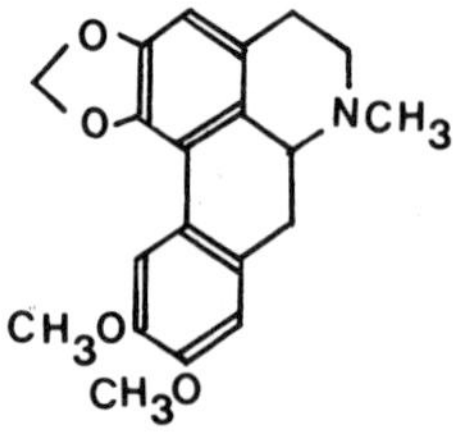

This aporphine alkaloid is present in *Dicentra eximia* (Ker) Torr., *D. formosa* Walp., *D. oregana* Eastwood and *D. pusilla* Sieb. et Zucc. It crystallizes in colourless prisms from EtOH, Et_2O or AcOEt and has $[\alpha]_D$ + 62.1° ($CHCl_3$). The methiodide monohydrate has m.p. 224°C and yields a methine base, m.p. 158–9°C. The monoacetyl derivative is also crystalline, m.p. 202°C. The synthetic (±)-form has m.p. 178–9°C and forms crystalline salts, e.g. the hydrochloride, m.p. 263–5°C (*dec.*); methiodide, m.p. 228–9°C and the picrate, m.p. 188–9°C. On demethylation, the alkaloid yields a phenolic base which may be methylated to give Glaucine (q.v.).

Asahina, Osada., *J. Pharm. Soc., Japan*, **48**, 85 (1928)
Manske., *Can. J. Res.*, **10**, 521, 765 (1934)
Manske., *ibid*, **14B**, 348 (1936)

DICENTRINONE

$C_{19}H_{13}O_5N$

M.p. 300°C (*dec.*).

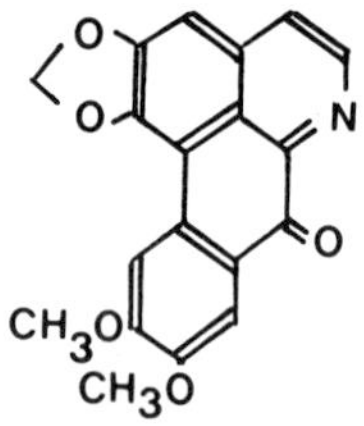

This keto base corresponding to decentrine occurs in *Ocotea macropoda* and forms yellow crystals from EtOH-$CHCl_3$. The ethanolic solution gives an ultraviolet spectrum with absorption maxima at 213, 250, 272, 352, 396 and 433 mμ with a shoulder at 310 mμ. It contains two methoxyl groups and one methylenedioxy group.

Cava, Venkateswarlu., *Tetrahedron*, **27**, 2639 (1971)

DICHOTAMINE

$C_{21}H_{24}O_4N_2$

M.p. 262–3°C (*dec.*).

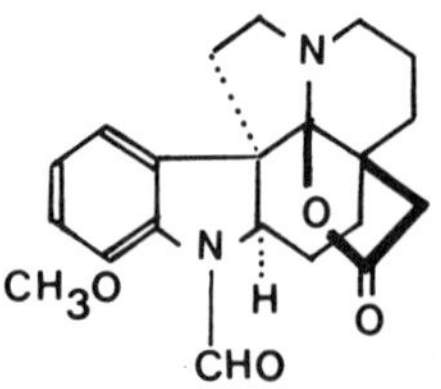

A base found in *Vallesia dichotoma* Ruiz et Pav., this alkaloid is laevorotatory

with $[\alpha]_D - 116°$ (CHCl₃). The ultraviolet spectrum has absorption maxima at
217 and 257 mμ.

Holker *et al., J. Org. Chem.*, **24**, 314 (1959)
Brown *et al., Tetrahedron Lett.*, 1731 (1963)

DICHOTINE (*Alkaloid 26*)

$C_{22}H_{26}O_6N_2$

M.p. 209–211°C (*dec.*).

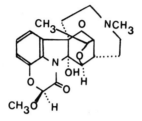

A reduced carbazole alkaloid, this base has been isolated from *Vallesia dichotoma*
Ruiz. et Pav. It has $[\alpha]_D + 88°$ (CHCl₃) and gives an ultraviolet spectrum
which shows absorption maxima at 222 and 292 mμ with an inflexion at 253
mμ. The O-acetate may be crystallized from Me₂CO and has m.p. 247–8°C.

Walser, Djerassi., *Helv. Chim. Acta,* **48**, 391 (1965)
Ling, Djerassi., *J. Amer. Chem. Soc.,* **92**, 6019 (1970)
Crystal structure:
Ling *et al., J. Amer. Chem. Soc.,* **92**, 222 (1970)

DICHROIDINE

$C_{18}H_{25}O_3N_3$

M.p. 213°C

This alkaloid has been isolated from *Dichroa febrifuga* Lour. which is a member
of the family Saxifragaceae and from which the antimalarial drug Ch'ang Shan is
obtained. No further details of this base are available.

Jang *et al., Nature,* **161**, 400 (1948)

DICHROINE A

M.p. 230°C (*dec.*).

This, and the following alkaloid, were stated to occur in the Chinese drug
Ch'ang-Shan from *Dichroa febrifuga* Lour. although subsequent examination by
Tonkin and Work failed to substantiate this observation.

Jang *et al., Science,* **103**, 59 (1946)
Tonkin, Work., *Nature,* **161**, 400 (1948)

DICHROINE B

M.p. 237–8°C (*dec.*).

The second alkaloid said to occur in *Dichroa febrifuga* Lour., this base exhibited some activity against chick malaria, particularly against a trophozoite-induced infection of *Plasmodium gallinaceum.* Tonkin and Work showed that although aqueous and acid extracts of the plant produced this anti-malarial activity, they did not exhibit alkaloidal reactions.

Jang *et al., Science,* **103**, 59 (1946)
Tonkin, Work., *Nature,* **161**, 400 (1948)

DICHROINE-α

$C_{16}H_{21}O_3N_3$

M.p. 136°C

A quinazoline alkaloid present in *Dichroa febrifuga* Lour., the base yields crystalline salts, e.g. the hydrochloride, m.p. 210°C and the sulphate, m.p. 230°C (*dec.*). It is interconvertible and isomeric with the two succeeding alkaloids.

Jang *et al., Nature,* **161**, 400 (1948)

DICHROINE-β

$C_{16}H_{21}O_3N_3$

M.p. 145°C

A second quinazoline alkaloid isolated from *Dichroa febrifuga* Lour. the following crystalline salts have been prepared; sulphate, m.p. 224°C (*dec.*); hydrochloride, m.p. 219°C (*dec.*) and dihydrochloride, m.p. 238°C (*dec.*).

Jang *et al., Nature,* **161**, 400 (1948)

DICHROINE-γ

$C_{16}H_{21}O_3N_3$

M.p. 161°C

The third alkaloid isolated from *Dichroa febrifuga* Lour. and isomeric with the preceding bases, this alkaloid yields crystalline salts, e.g. the sulphate, m.p. 224°C (*dec.*); hydrochloride, m.p. 219°C (*dec.*) and dihydrochloride, m.p. 238°C (*dec.*).

Jang *et al., Nature,* **161**, 400 (1948)

DICINCHONINE (*Dicinchonicine*)

$C_{38}H_{44}O_2N_4$

M.p. 40°C

A minor alkaloid obtained from *Cinchona rosulenta* and *C. succirubra,* this base is an amorphous solid with $[\alpha]_D^{15} + 65.6°$ (EtOH). It forms a crystalline dihydrochloride.

Hesse., *Annalen,* **227,** 154 (1885)

DICONQUININE

$C_{40}H_{46}O_3N_4$

M.p. Indefinite

This alkaloid is said to occur to a small extent in *Cinchona succirubra.* It is an amorphous powder which is dextrorotatory.

Hesse., *Ber.,* **10,** 2155 (1877)

DICROTALINE

$C_{14}H_{19}O_5N$

M.p. 170°C (*dec.*).

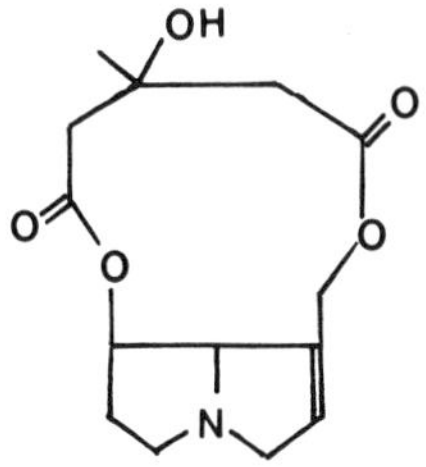

A hepatotoxic alkaloid found in *Crotalaria dura,* Wood and Evans, *C. globifera,* Mey, this base is unstable and decomposes on keeping. It forms a crystalline hydrochloride, m.p. 258–260°C (*dec.*); $[\alpha]_D^{27} + 25.7°$ (H$_2$O) and a picrate, m.p. 238–240°C (*dec.*). Alkaline hydrolysis furnishes retronecine and dibasic dicrotalic acid, $C_6H_{10}O_5$, m.p. 109°C.

Marais., *Onderstepoort J.,* **20,** 61 (1944)

DICTAMNINE

$C_{12}H_9O_2N$

M.p. 132–3°C

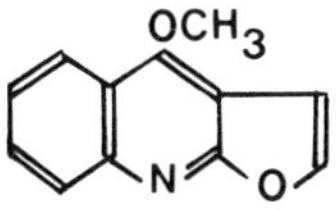

This furoquinoline base was first obtained from *Dictamnus albus* L. by Thoms and subsequently discovered in *Skimmia repens.* It forms colourless prisms and gives crystalline salts; the hydrochloride, m.p. 195°C; aurichloride, m.p. 152°C; platinichloride, m.p. > 250°C; picrate, m.p. 163°C and the picrolonate, m.p.

178°C. Methyl iodide at 80°C converts the alkaloid into isodictamnine, m.p. 188°C which contains no methoxyl group. With benzoyl chloride and benzoic anhydride it gives N-benzoyl*nor*dictamnine, m.p. 165°C from which *nor*dictamnine, m.p. 248°C, is obtained by hydrolysis.

The alkaloid is oxidized with $KMnO_4$ in Me_2CO to dictamnal, m.p. 259–260°C and dictamnic acid, m.p. 260°C (*dec.*). The former may be converted by HBr in AcOH into *nor*dictamnal which has been shown to be 2:4-dihydroxy-quinoline-3-aldehyde.

Thoms., *Ber. deut. Pharm. Ges.*, **33**, 68 (1923)
Thoms, Dambergis., *Arch. Pharm.*, **268**, 39 (1930)
Asahina, Ohta, Inubuse., *Ber.*, **63**, 2045 (1930)
Asahina, Inubuse., *ibid*, **65**, 61 (1932)
Kovalenko., *Farmatsiya*, **9**, 20 (1946)

DICTYOCARPINE

$C_{26}H_{39}O_8N$

M.p. 210–2°C

A minor constituent of *Delphinium dictyocarpum*, this alkaloid has only recently been isolated. The structure has not yet been fully determined.

Narzullaev, Yunusov, Yunusov., *Khim. Prir. Soedin.*, 8, 498 (1972)

DICTYOLUCIDAMINE

$C_{23}H_{41}O_2N$

M.p. 205°C

A steroidal alkaloid present in *Dictyophleba lucida*, this base is slightly dextrorotatory with $[\alpha]_D + 6°$ ($CHCl_3$). The O-acetate is crystalline with m.p. 228–9°C; $[\alpha]_D + 30°$ ($CHCl_3$). The structure as an androstane derivative has been determined from infrared, NMR, mass spectral and circular dichroism determinations.

Janot *et al.*, *Bull. Soc. Chim. Fr.*, **11**, 3472 (1966)

DICTYOLUTIDINE

$C_{22}H_{39}O_2N$

M.p. 198°C

A further androstane type alkaloid found in *Dictyophleba lucida*, this base has

$[\alpha]_D + 30°$ (CHCl$_3$). The O,N-diacetyl derivative has m.p. 220°C; $[\alpha]_D + 18°$ (CHCl$_3$). The structure has been determined from circular dichroism data and the infrared, NMR and mass spectra.

Janot *et al., Bull. Soc. Chim. Fr.,* **11**, 3472 (1966)

6α:7-DIDEHYDROAPORHEINE

C$_{12}$H$_{15}$O$_3$N

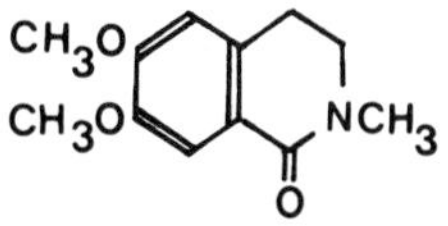

This alkaloid has been isolated from *Papaver urbanianum* but it is possible that it may be an artifact produced during the isolation procedure.

Preininger, Tosnarova., *Planta Med.,* **23**, 233 (1973)

6:6α-DIDEHYDROGLAUCINE (*Alkaloid GF-A*)

C$_{20}$H$_{23}$O$_4$N

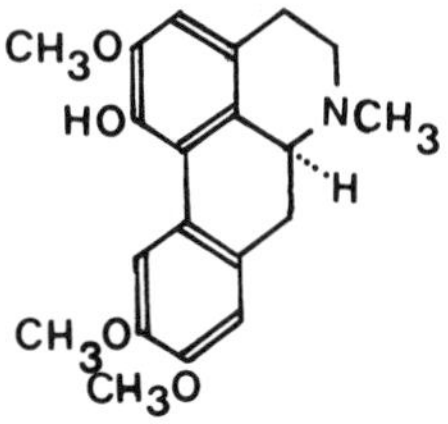

This aporphine alkaloid has recently been discovered in *Glaucium flavum*. Three methoxyl groups, one phenolic hydroxyl group and a methylimino group are present in the molecule.

Duchevska, Orahovats, Mollov., *Dokl. Bolg. Akad. Nauk.,* **26**, 899 (1973)

DIDEHYDROTALBOTINE

C$_{21}$H$_{22}$O$_4$N$_2$

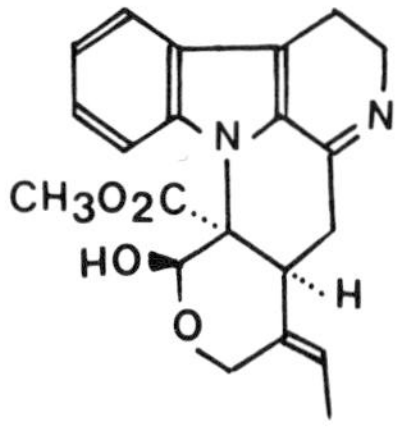

A dihydrocarboline alkaloid found in the leaves of *Pleiocarpa talbotii,* the structure of this newly-discovered base has been determined spectroscopically.

Pinar, Hesse, Schmid., *Helv. Chim. Acta,* **56**, 2719 (1973)

(−)-cis-8:10-DIETHYLLOBELIONOL (*Alkaloid D-2b*)

$C_{14}H_{27}O_2N$

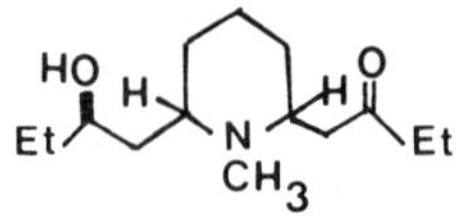

This base from *Lobelia syphilitica* L. has been characterized as the crystalline hydrochloride, m.p. 120–1°C and the aurichloride, m.p. 133–4°C.

Tschesche *et al.*, *Chem. Ber.*, **94**, 3327 (1961)

8:10-DIETHYLNORLOBELIDONE

$C_{13}H_{23}O_2N$

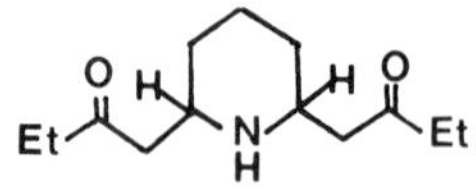

A further base from *Lobelia syphilitica* L. The crystalline hydrochloride has two melting points, 154–7°C and 183–4°C. Treatment with formic acid and formaldehyde gives *cis*-8:10-Diethyllobelidone.

Tschesche *et al.*, *Chem. Ber.*, **94**, 3327 (1961)

cis-8:10-DIETHYLNORLOBELIONOL (*Alkaloid C-1*)

$C_{13}H_{25}O_2N$

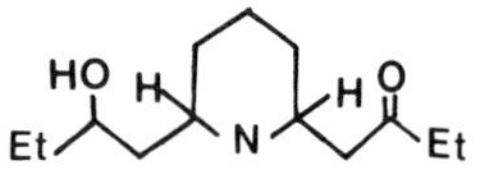

Also present in *Lobelia syphilitica* L., this alkaloid is characterized as the hydrochloride, m.p. 183–4°C.

Tschesche *et al.*, *Chem. Ber.*, **94**, 3327 (1961)

DIHYDROAGROCLAVINE (*Festuclavine*)

$C_{16}H_{20}N_2$

M.p. 242°C (*dec.*).

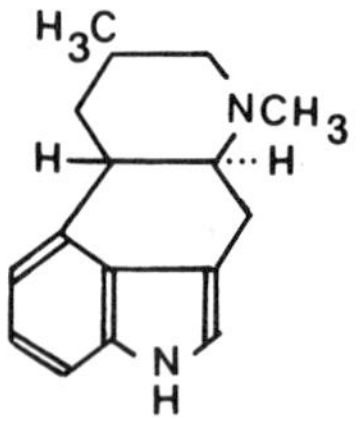

One of the ergot alkaloids isolated from *Claviceps purpurea* grown on *Elymus*, *Phragmites*, *Phalaris* and *Apropyrum* in Japan. The base crystallizes from most organic solvents as long, colourless needles with $[\alpha]_D^{20} - 69°$ (c 0.5, $CHCl_3$), − 115° (c 0.5, pyridine). It is insoluble in petroleum ether, moderately so in toluene, C_6H_6 or Et_2O and dissolves readily in $CHCl_3$, Me_2CO, AcOEt, MeOH, EtOH and pyridine. The succinate crystallizes as colourless prisms from H_2O, m.p. 213°C (*dec.*); $[\alpha]_D^{17} - 87°$ (c 0.13, pyridine).

Abe *et al., J. Agr. Chem. Soc., Japan,* **24**, 416 (1951)
Abe *et al., ibid,* **25**, 458 (1952)
Abe *et al., ibid,* **27**, 18, 614, 617 (1953)
Abe *et al., ibid,* **28**, 44, 501 (1954)
Abe *et al., ibid,* **29**, 364 (1955)
Abe *et al., Bull. Agr. Chem. Soc., Japan,* **19**, 92, 94 (1955)

19:20-DIHYDROAKUAMMICINE

$C_{20}H_{24}O_2N_2$

M.p. 173–5°C

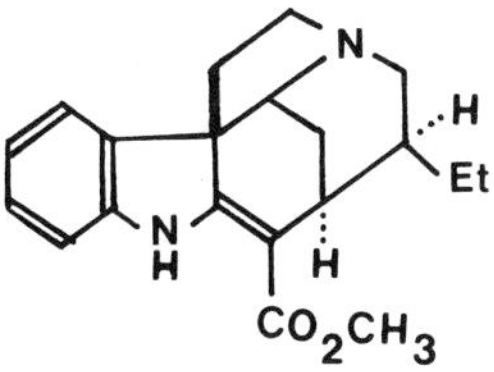

This base is present in the leaves of *Pleiocarpa pycnantha* (K. Schum) Stapf. var. *tubicina* (Stapf) Pichon. It contains an ethyl and an imino group in the molecule.

Weissmann *et al., Helv. Chim. Acta,* **44**, 1877 (1961)
Kump *et al., ibid,* **47**, 1497 (1964)

1:2-DIHYDROASPIDOSPERMIDINE

$C_{19}H_{28}N_2$

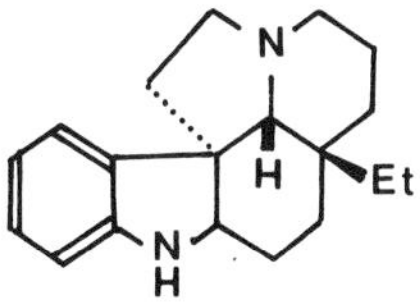

This alkaloid from *Amsonia tabernaemontana* is a colourless oil which is dextro-rotatory with $[\alpha]_D$ + 265° (c 0.25, EtOH).

Zsadon, Kaposi., *Acta Chim.* (Budapest), **71**, 115 (1972)

F-DIHYDROATISINE

This alkaloid is stated to be present in the strong base fraction of *Aconitum heterophyllum.* It had previously been prepared as a reduction product of both Atisine (q.v.) and *iso*atisine.

Pelletier, Aneja, Gopinath., *Phytochem.,* **7**, 625 (1968)

DIHYDROAUSTAMIDE

$C_{21}H_{23}O_3N_3$

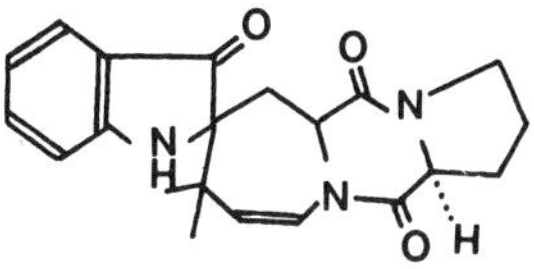

A dioxopiperazine base isolated from *Aspergillus ustus,* both the structure and absolute configuration of this alkaloid have been established.

Steyn., *Tetrahedron,* **29**, 107 (1973)

DIHYDROCORYNANTHEINE

$C_{22}H_{30}O_3N_2$

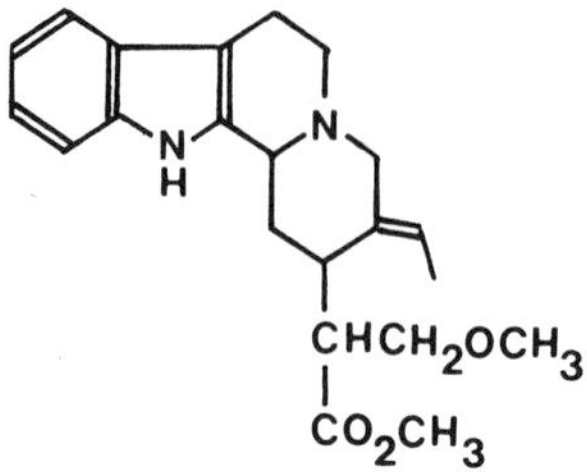

An alkaloid recently isolated from *Uncaria rhyncophylla,* the base most probably possesses the structure given above.

Haginawa *et al., J. Pharm. Soc., Japan,* **93**, 448 (1973)

DIHYDROCORYNANTHEOL

$C_{19}H_{26}ON_2$

M.p. 185–6°C

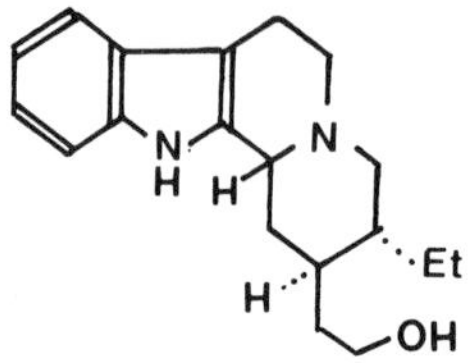

The bark of certain *Aspidosperma* species including *A. auriculatum* Mgf., *A. discolor* A. DC. and *A. marcgravianum* Woodson, yield this alkaloid which forms colourless crystals from aqueous MeOH. It has $[\alpha]_D - 369°$ (c 0.453, pyridine) or $[\alpha]_D^{27} - 18°$ (c 0.92, $CHCl_3$). The ultraviolet spectrum exhibits absorption maxima at 226, 281 and 290 mμ. The base contains one primary hydroxyl group and forms an acetate, m.p. 125–8°C, the latter yielding a crystalline hydrochloride in the form of pale yellow needles, m.p. 253–260°C (*dec.*).

Vamvacas *et al., Helv. Chim. Acta,* **40**, 1793 (1957)
Gilbert *et al., J. Org. Chem.,* **27**, 4702 (1962)
Gilbert *et al., Tetrahedron,* **21**, 1141 (1965)

Synthesis:
Sawa, Matsumura., *Chem. Commun.,* 679 (1968)

464

DIHYDROCUPREINE (*Hydrocupreine*)

$C_{19}H_{24}O_2N_2$

M.p. 230°C (*dec.*).

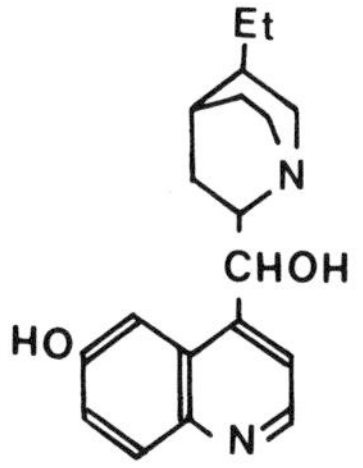

This base has been known synthetically for almost a century but has only recently been found to occur naturally in *Timonius kaniensis*. As obtained from the plant, it is described as a glassy solid with $[\alpha]_D - 143°$ (EtOH). It may be prepared by demethylating dihydroquinine or by the reduction of Cupreine (q.v.). In this case it crystallizes from aqueous EtOH in minute, colourless needles and is readily soluble in EtOH, $CHCl_3$ or hot C_6H_6, less so in AcOEt and insoluble in light petroleum. The hydrochloride has m.p. 280°C (*dec.*); $[\alpha]_D^{22.5} - 132.2°$ (H_2O); the dihydrobromide dihydrate, m.p. 180–190°C and the nitrate, m.p. 220–2°C. With CH_2N_2 it yields dihydroquinine.

Hesse., *Annalen.*, **241**, 281 (1887)
Heidelberger, Jacobs., *J. Amer. Chem. Soc.*, **41**, 817 (1919)
Giemsa, Halberkann., *Ber.*, **51**, 1325 (1918)
Heidelberger, Jacobs., *J. Amer. Chem. Soc.*, **44**, 1091 (1922)
Johns, Lamberton., *Austral. J. Chem.*, **23**, 211 (1970)

DIHYDROCYCLOMICROPHYLLIDINE A

$C_{35}H_{54}O_3N_2$

M.p. Indefinite

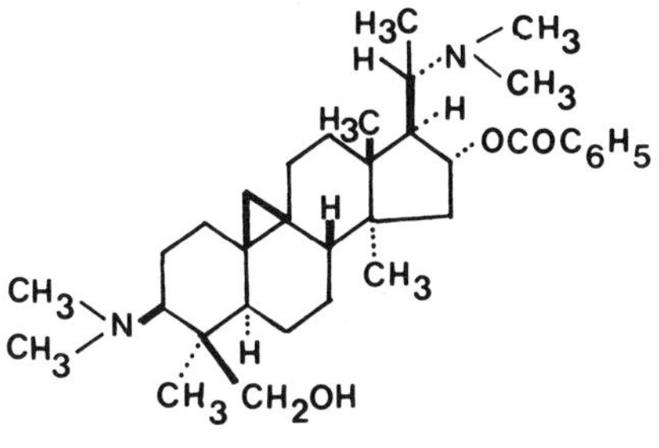

An amorphous steroidal alkaloid, this base is a constituent of *Buxus microphylla* Sieb. et Zucc. var. *suffruticosa* Mak. It is laevorotatory with $[\alpha]_D - 33°$ ($CHCl_3$). The ultraviolet spectrum shows absorption maxima at 265, 273 and 280 mμ. The base contains two dimethylamino groups, a primary hydroxyl group and a benzoyl radical in the molecule.

Nakano, Terao., *J. Chem. Soc.*, 4512 (1965)

DIHYDROCYCLOMICROPHYLLINE A

$C_{28}H_{50}O_2N_2$

M.p. 271–2°C

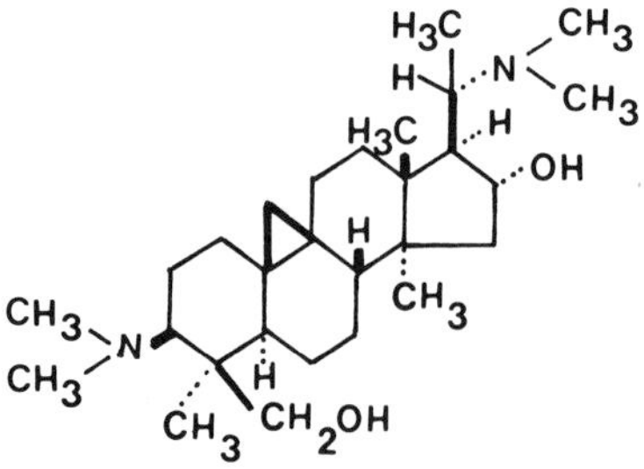

A further alkaloid found in *Buxus microphylla* Sieb. et Zucc. var *suffruticosa* Mak., this base forms colourless crystals when crystallized from Me$_2$CO. It has $[\alpha]_D + 37°$ (CHCl$_3$). The alkaloid contains two hydroxyl groups and forms a crystalline O,O-diacetyl derivative, m.p. 156–7°C.

Nakano, Terao., *J. Chem. Soc.*, 4512 (1965)

DIHYDROCYCLOMICROPHYLLINE F

$C_{26}H_{46}O_2N_2$

M.p. 260°C

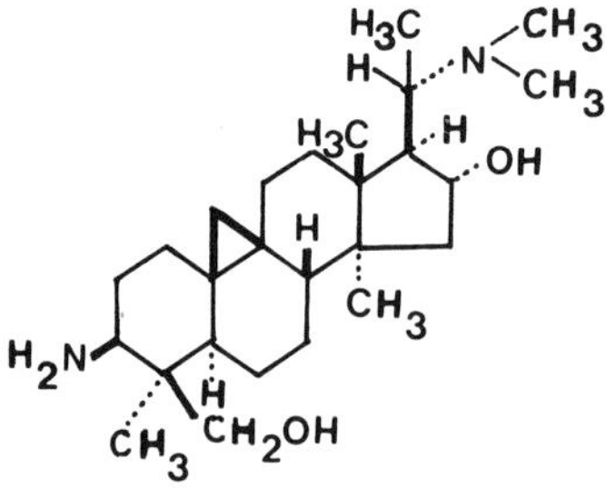

Also present in *Buxus microphylla* Sieb. et Zucc. var. *suffruticosa* Mak., this alkaloid crystallizes from MeOH as small, colourless crystals. It has $[\alpha]_D + 4.6°$ (CHCl$_3$). The base is soluble in Me$_2$CO but only sparingly so in most other organic solvents.

Nakano, Terao., *J. Chem. Soc.*, 4512 (1965)

DIHYDRODECAMINE

$C_{26}H_{32}O_5N$

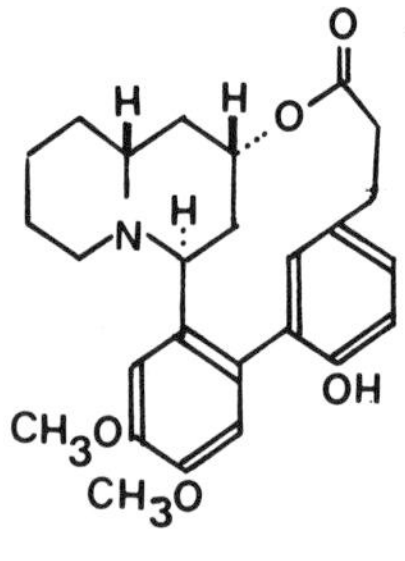

This alkaloid is said to be present in *Decodon verticullatus* L (Ell.). The structure given, however, is identical with that of decamine (q.v.).

Ferris., *J. Org. Chem.*, **27**, 2985 (1962)

Ferris., *ibid*, **28**, 817 (1963)

DIHYDROELLIPTICINE

$C_{17}H_{16}N_2$

M.p. 293–6°C (*dec.*).

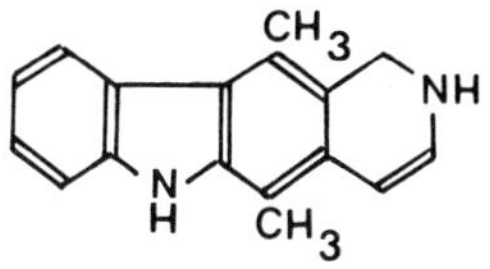

A minor constituent of *Aspidosperma subincanum*, this alkaloid contains two methyl groups and two imino groups. The structure has been determined mainly from spectroscopic evidence.

Buechi, Mayo, Hochstein., *Tetrahedron*, **15**, 167 (1961)

DIHYDROERGOSINE

$C_{30}H_{39}O_5N_5$

M.p. 212°C (*dec.*).

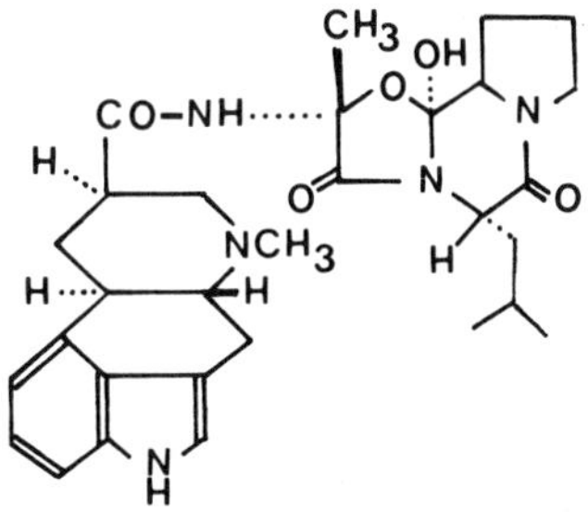

This alkaloid was first prepared by the hydrogenation of ergosine and subsequently isolated from the sclerotia of *Sphacelia sorghi* (McRae) grown in Nigeria, probably related to *Claviceps*. The alkaloid has $[\alpha]_D^{20} - 52°$ (c 0.5, pyridine) or $+ 10.1°$ (c 1.5, $CHCl_3$). Acid hydrolysis furnishes leucine and proline which are known to be components of the polypeptide side-chain of ergosine. The identity of the naturally occurring alkaloid and that prepared synthetically has been proved by chromatography and comparison of their infrared and NMR spectra and mass fragmentation pattern.

Stoll, Hoffmann., *Helv. Chim. Acta*, **26**, 2070 (1943)

Mantle, Waight., *Nature*, **218**, 581 (1968)

6:7-DIHYDROFLAVEPEREIRINE

$C_{17}H_{16}N_2$

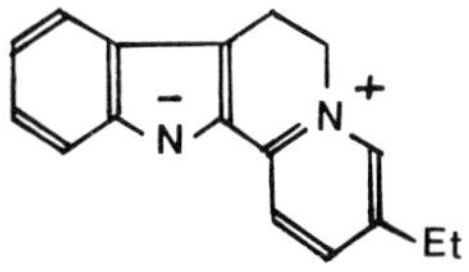

This anhydronium base has recently been discovered in Strychnos usambarensis and its structure assigned on the basis of spectroscopic data and comparison with a synthetic specimen.

Angenot, Denoel., *Planta Med.*, **23**, 226 (1973)

(−)-DIHYDROGAMBIRTANNINE

$C_{21}H_{20}O_2N_2$

M.p. 163°C

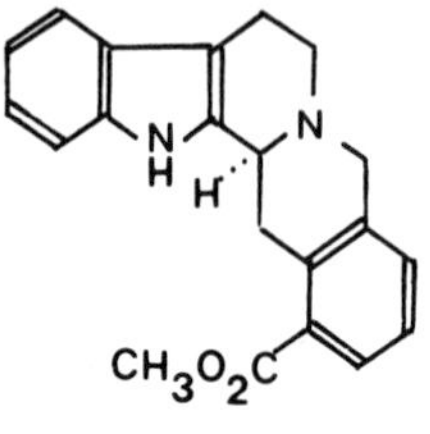

This protoberberine type alkaloid occurs in *Ourouparia Gambir* Baill. (Syn. *Uncaria Gambir* Roxb.) and is obtained in the form of yellow crystals from Et_2O-hexane. It has $[\alpha]_D^{20} - 270°$ (c 0.088, $CHCl_3$) and the ultraviolet spectrum in EtOH shows absorption maxima at 225, 283 and 290 mμ.

The (+)-form has m.p. 174−6°C; $[\alpha]_D^{25} + 288°$ (pyridine) and a similar ultraviolet spectrum with absorption maxima at 223 and 282 mμ. The corresponding (±)-form melts at 176−8°C and forms a crystalline hydrochloride with m.p. 248−250°C.

Merlini *et al.*, *Tetrahedron*, **23**, 3129 (1967)
Smith *et al.*, *J. Amer. Chem. Soc.*, **86**, 2083 (1964)
Wenkert *et al.*, *ibid*, **90**, 5251 (1968)

DIHYDROHARMINE

$C_{13}H_{14}ON_2$

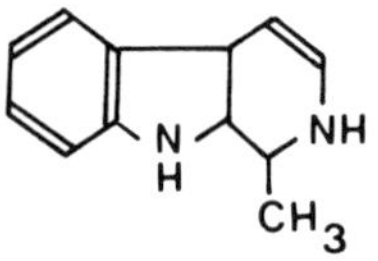

Isolated from the woody stem of a liana of the *Melphighiaceae* family, both the genus and species of which are still undetermined, this alkaloid is isomeric with, but not identical with, harmaline (q.v.). The probable constitution is that given above.

Biocca, Galeffi, Montalvo., *Ann. Chim.* (*Rome*), **54**, 1175 (1964)

5:6-DIHYDRO-6-HYDROXY-4-METHOXYCARBONYL-7-METHYL-7H-CYCLOPENTAPYRIDINE

$C_{11}H_{13}O_3N$

M.p. 132−3°C

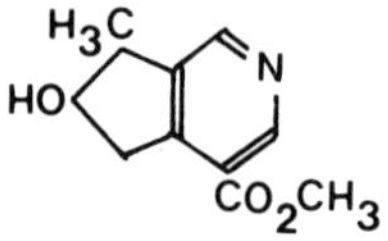

This comparatively simple monoterpenoid alkaloid occurs in some *Jasminium*

species and forms colourless needles when crystallized from C_6H_6. It is laevo-rotatory with $[\alpha]_D - 34°$ (c 1.2, $CHCl_3$) and gives an ultraviolet spectrum in which the absorption maxima occur at 271 and 278 mμ.

Hart, Johns, Lamberton., *Austral. J. Chem.*, **22**, 1283 (1969)

6:7-DIHYDRO-6-HYDROXY-7-METHYL-5H-2-PYRINDINE (*RW 47*)

$C_9H_{11}ON$

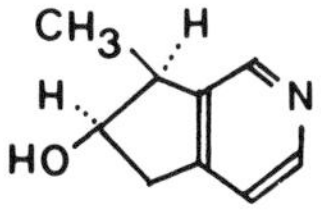

A novel monoterpenoid base found in *Rauwolfia verticillata* grown in Hong Kong, the alkaloid has been shown to be related to the known alkaloids of the actinidine group and appears to have the structure given above.

Arthur *et al.*, *Austral. J. Chem.*, **20**, 2505 (1967)

6:7-DIHYDRO-2-[2-(4-HYDROXYPHENYL)-ETHYL]-4:7-DIMETHYL-5H-CYCLOPENTAPYRIDINIUM

$C_{17}H_{20}ON^+$

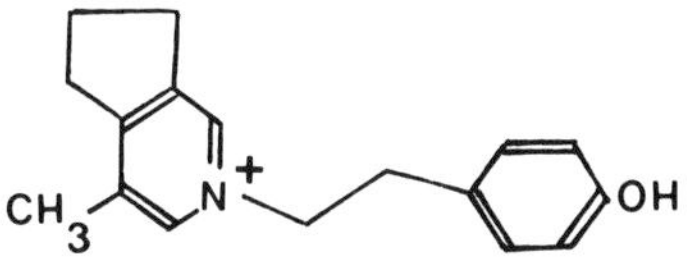

This pyridinium base has recently been isolated from *Valleriana officinalis* and shown to possess the above structure. No derivatives have yet been prepared.

Gross *et al.*, *Arch. Pharm.*, **304**, 19 (1971)

1:13-DIHYDRO-13-HYDROXYULEINE

$C_{18}H_{24}ON_2$

M.p. Indefinite

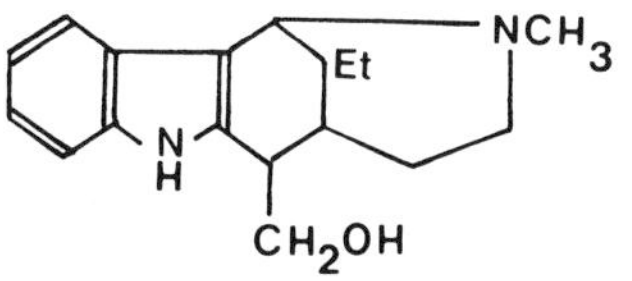

An amorphous alkaloid found in *Aspidosperma dasycarpon* A. DC, this alkaloid has $[\alpha]_D - 96°$ (c 0.25, EtOH). The ultraviolet spectrum exhibits absorption maxima at 221, 282 and 289 mμ. It contains one primary hydroxyl group in the molecule.

Ohashi *et al.*, *Experientia*, **20**, 363 (1964)
Joule *et al.*, *Tetrahedron*, **21**, 1717 (1965)

DIHYDROIPALBIDINE

C$_{15}$H$_{21}$ON

B.p. 156–8°C/3 mm

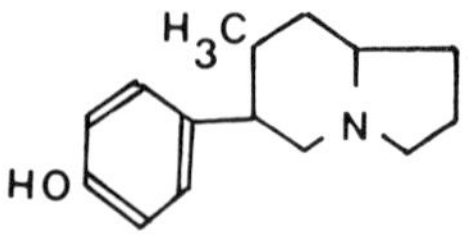

A minor constituent of *Ipomoea alba* L., this alkaloid is a light yellow oil which forms an O-acetyl derivative, m.p. 76–7°C. The ultraviolet spectrum shows absorption maxima at 223, 277 and 283 mμ.

Gourley *et al.*, *Chem. Commun.*, 709 (1969)

DIHYDROISOHISTRIONICOTOXIN

C$_{19}$H$_{26}$ON

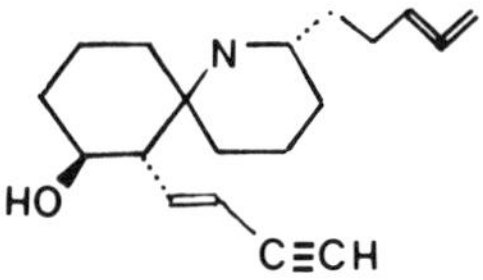

This unique highly-unsaturated alkaloid has recently been obtained from the Colombian frog *Dendrobates histrionicus* and characterized as the hydrochloride which crystallizes in space group $P2_12_12_1$ with $a = 11.438 \pm 0.004$; $b = 14.598 \pm 0.004$; $c = 11.379 \pm 0.004$ Å. Structural and conformational parameters have been determined both for the allene and vinylacetylene substituents in the solid state and the configuration compared with those already established for other cholinergic agonists and antagonists. The alkaloid is a potent and selective inhibitor of cholinergic mechanisms.

Karle., *J. Amer. Chem. Soc.*, **95**, 4036 (1973)

DIHYDROJOUBERTIAMINE

C$_{16}$H$_{23}$O$_2$N

M.p. Indefinite

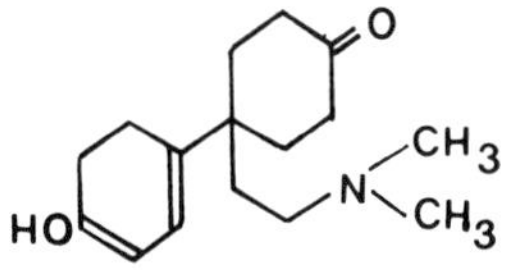

An alkaloid isolated from *Scleletium joubertii* L. Bol. The ultraviolet spectrum shows two absorption maxima at 226 and 278 mμ.

Arndt, Kruger., *Tetrahedron Lett.*, 3237 (1970)

DIHYDROKREYSIGINONE

C$_{20}$H$_{25}$O$_4$N

M.p. 217–222°C

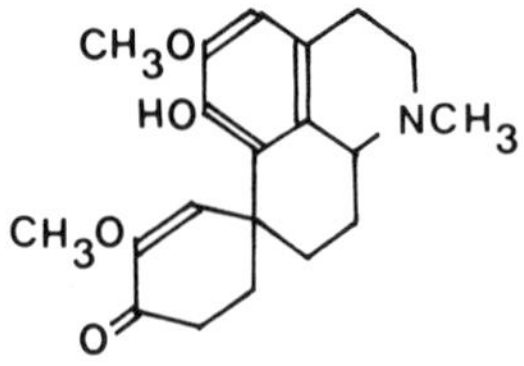

One of the alkaloids obtained from *Kreysigia multiflora,* this base contains one methoxyl and one phenolic hydroxyl group in the *iso*quinoline portion of the molecule and a further methoxyl group in the spiroquinone ring. The ultraviolet spectrum exhibits absorption maxima at 220 and 269 mμ.

Battersby *et al.*, *Chem. Commun.*, 934 (1967)

(+)-DIHYDROLYSERGOL

A minor base obtained from *Claviceps gigantea* found in Mexico. No salts or derivatives have been reported for this alkaloid.

Agunell, Ramstad., *Acta Pharm. Suecica.*, **2**, 231 (1965)

DIHYDROLYTHRINE

$C_{26}H_{31}O_5N$

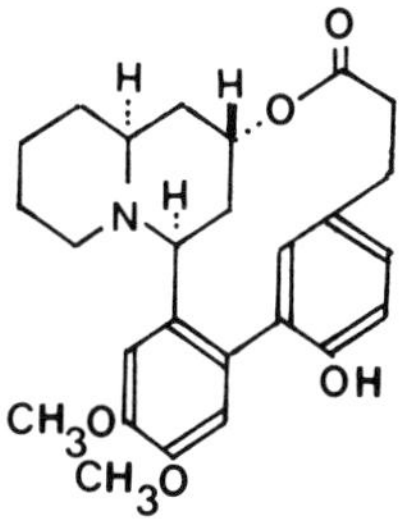

A minor constituent of *Decodon verticillatus* L., the alkaloid contains two methoxyl groups and one hydroxyl group.

Ferris., *J. Org. Chem.*, **27**, 2985 (1962)
Ferris., *ibid*, **28**, 817 (1963)

14:19-DIHYDRO-11-METHOXYCONDYLOCARPINE

$C_{21}H_{26}O_3N_2$

M.p. Indefinite

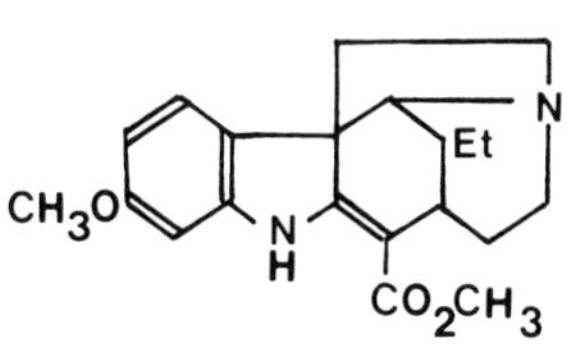

An amorphous alkaloid which is present in the bark of *Aspidosperma populifolium* A. DC, the base has $[\alpha]_D^{29} + 213°$ (c 0.49, CHCl$_3$). In ultraviolet light the alkaloid exhibits a marked blue fluorescence. The ultraviolet spectrum in EtOH shows absorption maxima at 255, 286 and 327 mμ.

Gilbert *et al.*, *Tetrahedron*, **21**, 1141 (1965)

1:2-DIHYDRO-9-METHOXYELLIPTICINE

$C_{18}H_{18}ON_2$

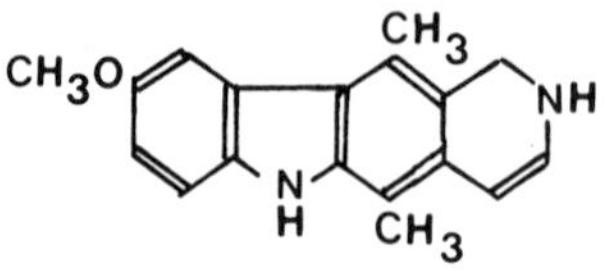

A minor alkaloid isolated from the dried leaves of *Ochrosia balansae*. The structure assigned to this alkaloid has been determined from the infrared, NMR and mass spectra.

Bruneton *et al.*, *Ann. Pharm. Fr.*, **30**, 629 (1972)

8:14-DIHYDRONORSALUTARIDINE

$C_{18}H_{21}O_4N$

M.p. 208–212°C

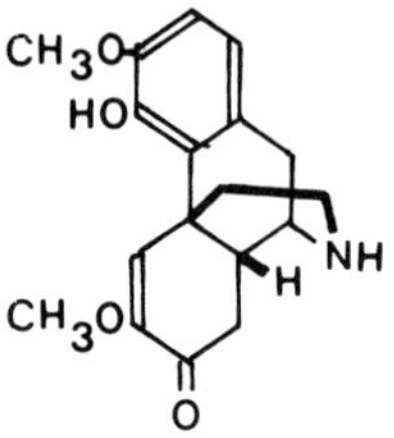

A morphine type alkaloid found in *Croton linearis* Jacq., the base forms colourless crystals from AcOEt which crystallize with solvent. The alkaloid has $[\alpha]_D^{15}$ − 69.1° (MeOH) and contains two active hydrogens as a phenolic hydroxyl and an imino group. The N-acetyl derivative is crystalline with m.p. 250–5°C, whereas the O,N-diacetyl compound is amorphous.

Haynes *et al.*, *Chem. Commun.*, 15 (1967)
Haynes *et al.*, *J. Chem. Soc., C*, 951 (1968)

DIHYDRONOR-c-TOXIFERINE I

$C_{19}H_{20-22}N_2$

A minor constituent of *Strychnos toxifera*, this alkaloid yields dihydro-C-toxiferine I when methylated with methyl iodide.

Asmis *et al.*, *Helv. Chim. Acta*, **38**, 1661 (1955)

DIHYDROOBSCURINERVIDINE

$C_{24}H_{30}O_5N_2$

M.p. 189–190°C

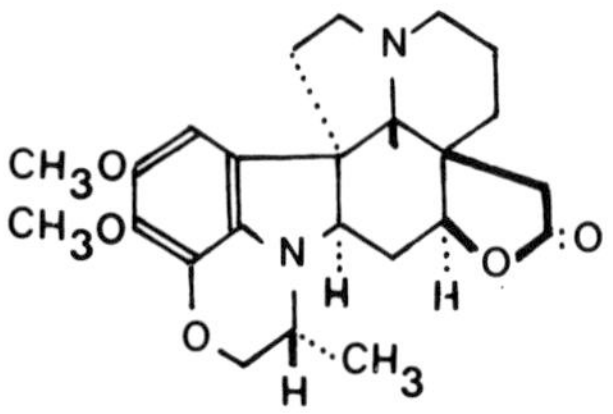

One of the numerous *Aspidosperma* alkaloids, this base occurs in *A. obscurinerv-*

ium Azembuja. It is obtained in the form of colourless needles from Me$_2$CO-hexane and is laevorotatory with $[\alpha]_D^{27} - 44°$ (c 0.85, CHCl$_3$). It contains two methoxyl groups and a lactam ring in the molecule.

Brown, Djerassi., *J. Amer. Chem. Soc.*, 86, 2451 (1964)

DIHYDROOBSCURINERVINE

C$_{25}$H$_{32}$O$_5$N$_2$

M.p. 184–5°C (*dec.*).

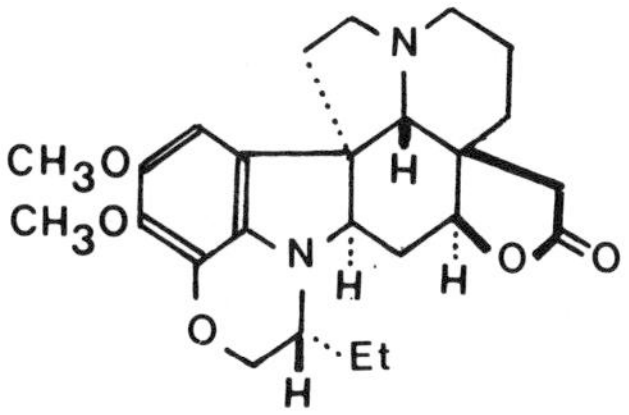

A second alkaloid occurring in *Aspidosperma obscurinervium* Azembuja, this base also crystallizes from Me$_2$CO-hexane. It has $[\alpha]_D^{26} - 61°$ (c 0.92, CHCl$_3$). The structure is similar to that of the preceding base but with the methyl group replaced by an ethyl.

Brown, Djerassi., *J. Amer. Chem. Soc.*, 86, 2451 (1964)

DIHYDROORIENTALINONE

C$_{19}$H$_{23}$O$_4$N

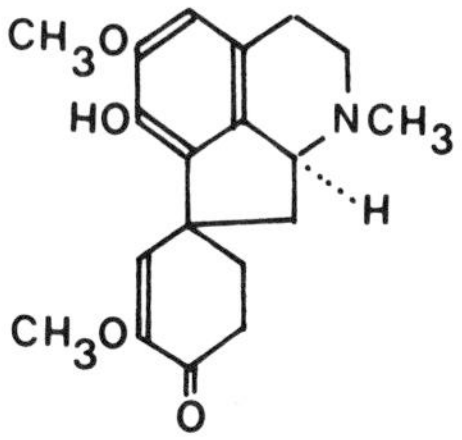

This minor alkaloid from *Papaver orientale* has been described by Battersby and Brown. It is dextrorotatory with $[\alpha]_D + 50°$ (CHCl$_3$).

Battersby, Brown., *Chem. Commun.*, 170 (1966)

αβ-DIHYDROPIPERINE

C$_{17}$H$_{21}$O$_3$N

M.p. 78°C

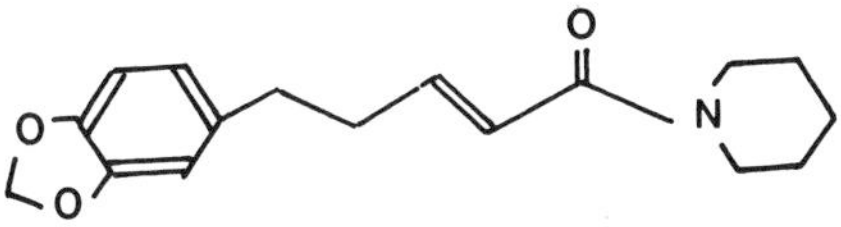

A piperylpiperidine base, this alkaloid is found in the wood of *Piper novae-hollandiae*. It crystallizes from light petroleum in the form of slender, colourless needles. In EtOH, the ultraviolet spectrum exhibits absorption maxima at 232 and 285 mμ. The structure has been determined by chemical degradation and spectroscopic examination.

Loder, Moorhouse, Russell., *Austral. J. Chem.*, 22, 1531 (1969)

DIHYDROPROTOEMETINE

$C_{19}H_{29}O_3N$

A minor constituent of *Alangium lamarckii* Thw., this alkaloid has been characterized as the crystalline perchlorate which forms colourless prisms from aqueous EtOH, m.p. 199–200°C. The structure has been elucidated from the infrared, NMR and mass spectra and direct comparison with other emetine alkaloids.

Battersby, Harper., *J. Chem. Soc.,* 1748 (1959)
Battersby *et al., Tetrahedron Lett.,* 4965 (1966)

DIHYDROQUINIDINE (*Hydroquinidine*)

$C_{20}H_{26}O_2N_2$

M.p. 169.5°C

This alkaloid accompanies Quinidine (q.v.) in most *Cinchona* barks but is found particularly in those of *C. amygdalifolia, C. Calisaya* and *C. pitayensis*. It may be prepared from commercial quinidine, after removal of cinchonine by the mercuric acetate process but is more readily obtained by the catalytic reduction of quinidine. The alkaloid forms thick, colourless tablets from Et_2O or needles from EtOH. It gives the thalleioquin reaction and fluoresces in dilute H_2SO_4 solution. The base is dextrorotatory with $[\alpha]_D^{15} + 299°$ (c 0.25, 0.1 N/H_2SO_4). The hydrochloride has m.p. 273–4°C (*dry, dec.*); the dihydrobromide forms a crystalline trihydrate with m.p. 244–7°C; $[\alpha]_D^{15} + 200.4°$ (c 0.25, H_2O); the platinichloride, orange needles, and the sulphate with 12 H_2O have also been prepared. On demethylation, the alkaloid furnishes dihydrocupreidine.

Forst, Böhringer., *Ber.,* **14**, 1954 (1881)
Forst, Böhringer., *ibid,* **15**, 520, 1656 (1882)

DIHYDROQUININE

$C_{20}H_{26}O_2N_2$

M.p. 173.5°C

First isolated by Hesse from the mother liquors of quinine sulphate manufacture, the alkaloid is present to the extent of between 5 and 6 per cent in commercial sulphate of quinine. It is best obtained therefrom by the mercuric acetate process. In addition, it may also be obtained by catalytic reduction of Quinine (q.v.). The alkaloid gives the thalleioquin reaction and the solution in dilute H_2SO_4 in fluorescent but it may be distinguished from the similar solution given by quinine by its resistance to $KMnO_4$. The alkaloid crystallizes from Et_2O or C_6H_6 in colourless needles and has $[\alpha]_D^{15} - 235.7°$ (c 0.25, 0.1 N/H_2SO_4) or $- 142.2°$ (EtOH). The hydrochloride forms a dihydrate, m.p. 206–8°C (*dry*); $[\alpha]_D^{21} - 123.9°$ (H_2O); the dihydrobromide has $[\alpha]_D^{15} - 152.5°$ (c 0.25, H_2O); the acid sulphate trihydrate forms long needles, readily soluble in H_2O or EtOH. The base also gives a crystalline benzoyl derivative, m.p. 102–7°C. It readily forms crystalline addition compounds with cinchonidine, cupreine and quinidine. On demethylation it furnishes dihydrocupreine.

Hesse., *Ber.*, **15**, 854 (1882)
Hesse., *Annalen*, **241**, 257 (1887)
Skita *et al.*, *Ber.*, **44**, 2866 (1911)
Skita *et al.*, *ibid*, **49**, 1597 (1916)

8:14-DIHYDROSALUTARIDINE

$C_{19}H_{23}O_4N$

M.p. 198–203°C

This alkaloid occurs in *Croton discolor* Willd. and *C. linearis* Jacq. and forms colourless crystals from MeOH. It has $[\alpha]_D^{15} - 76.1°$ (MeOH) and the ultraviolet spectrum in EtOH has absorption maxima at 206, 238 and 265 mμ.

Haynes *et al.*, *Chem. Commun.*, 15 (1967)
Haynes *et al.*, *J. Chem. Soc.*, C, 951 (1968)

DIHYDROSANGUINARINE

$C_{20}H_{15}O_4N$

M.p. 191°C

This alkaloid was first prepared by hydrogenation of sanguinarine (q.v.) and subsequently discovered in *Bocconia arborea*. It contains two methylenedioxy groups and one methylimino group.

Späth, Kuffner., *Ber.*, **64**, 2034 (1931)

MacLean *et al.*, *Can. J. Chem.*, **47**, 1951 (1969)

16:17-DIHYDROSECODINE

$C_{21}H_{28}O_2N_2$

M.p. Indefinite

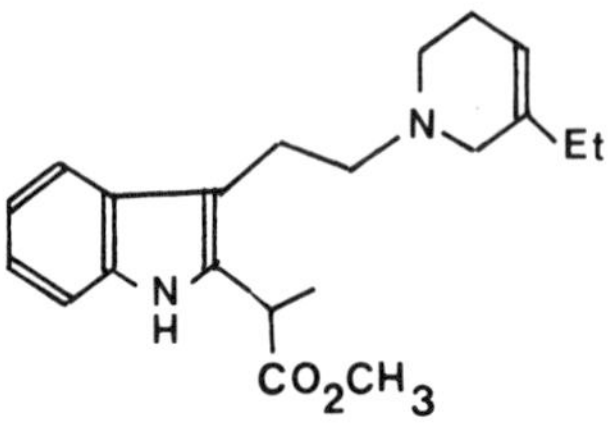

An indole base, this alkaloid has been found in the leaves of *Rhazya stricta*. When purified, it forms a colourless gum with no definite melting point. The site of reduction has been shown to be in the side chain and not in the tatrahydropyridine ring.

Cordell, Smith, Smith., *Chem. Commun.*, 189 (1970)

Synthesis:
Cordell, Smith, Smith., *Chem. Commun.*, 191 (1970)

DIHYDROSITSIRIKINE

$C_{21}H_{28}O_3N_2$

M.p. 215°C

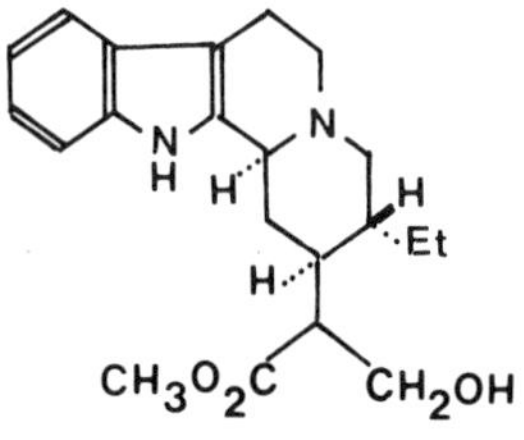

A carboline type alkaloid, isolated from *Pausinystalia yohimbe* Pierre and *Vinca rosea* L., the base forms colourless crystals from MeOH and is laevorotatory with $[\alpha]_D^{26} - 55°$ (MeOH). When crystallized from Me_2CO, the alkaloid contains solvent of crystallization and the crystals have m.p. 180°C. The ultraviolet spectrum shows absorption maxima at 226, 282 and 290 mμ. The alkaloid contains one primary hydroxyl group and forms a crystalline acetate as slender needles from Me_2CO-light petroleum, m.p. 174°C. The picrate, amber-yellow prisms, has m.p. 228–230°C and the *p*-bromobenzoyl derivative, m.p. 187°C; $[\alpha]_D^{26} - 31°$ (MeOH).

Kutney, Brown., *Tetrahedron Lett.*, 1815 (1963)
van der Meulen, van der Kirk., *Rec. Trav. Chim.*, **83**, 148, 154 (1964)
Kutney, Brown., *Tetrahedron Lett.*, **22**, 321 (1966)

476

C-DIHYDROTOXIFERINE I

$C_{40}H_{46}N_4^{++}$

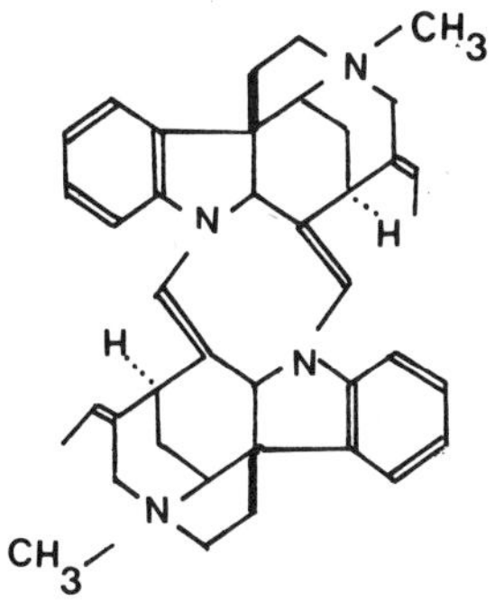

A dimeric alkaloid isolated from calabash curare from Caracas in which it is invariably accompanied by C-curarine I. The chloride crystallizes in rectangular leaflets or as needles, $[\alpha]_D - 610.6°$ (H_2O). The picrate has m.p. $183-5°C$ and a crystalline bromide and sulphate have also been prepared.

Karrer, Schmid., *Helv. Chim. Acta*, **29**, 1853 (1946)
Grdinic, Nelson, Boekelheide., *J. Amer. Chem. Soc.*, **86**, 3357 (1964)

C-*iso*DIHYDROTOXIFERINE I

$C_{40}H_{46}N_4^{++}$

This alkaloid occurs in several curares accompanied by C-curarine I. It forms a crystalline chloride as needles of the trihydrate; $[\alpha]_D^{20} - 566°$ (H_2O); a perchlorate and a picrate, the latter having m.p. $242°C$ (*dec.*).

Karrer, Schmid., *Helv. Chim. Acta,* **29**, 1853 (1946)

3:4-DIHYDROUSAMBARENSINE

$C_{29}H_{30}N_4$

M.p. Indefinite

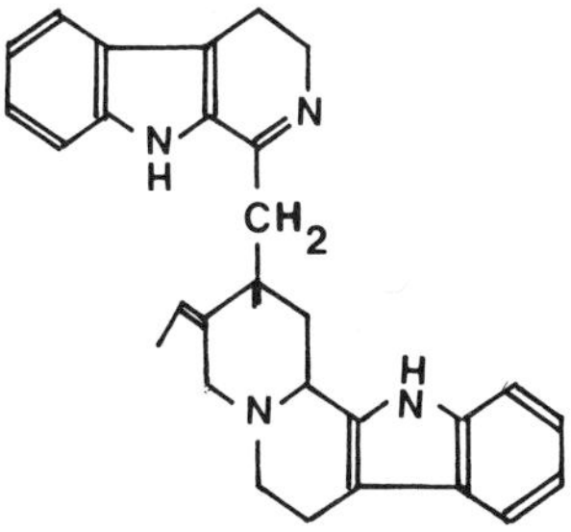

The roots of *Strychnos usambarensis* yield this alkaloid which forms a light yellow powder with no definite melting point. The ultraviolet spectrum shows absorption maxima at 229, 284, 291 and 318 mμ.

Angenot, Bisset., *J. Pharm. Belg.*, **26**, 585 (1971)

DIHYDROVERTICILLATINE

$C_{25}H_{29}O_5N$

M.p. 258–9°C

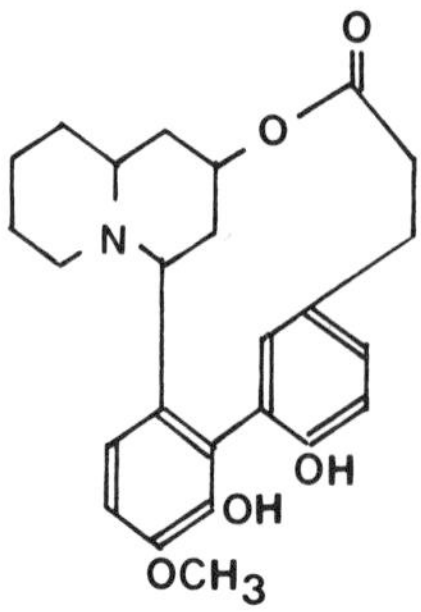

This base, related to the alkaloids obtained from *Decodon verticillatus,* is found in *Lagerstroemia indica* L. It forms colourless crystals from MeOH. The above structure has been confirmed by synthesis.

Ferris *et al., J. Amer. Chem. Soc.,* **93**, 2958 (1971)

Synthesis:
Ferris., *J. Org. Chem.,* **27**, 2985 (1962)

2:11-DIHYDROXY-1:10-DIMETHOXYAPORPHINE

$C_{19}H_{21}O_4N$

M.p. 198–200°C

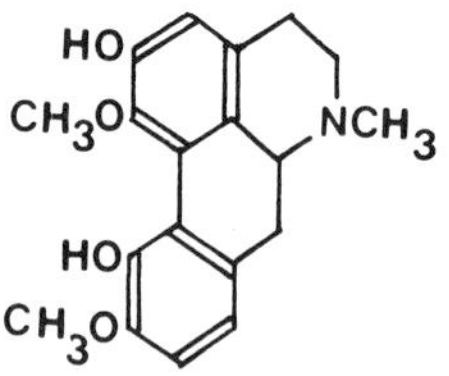

An aporphine alkaloid present in the leaves of *Phoebe clemensii* Allen., this base crystallizes from C_6H_6 or MeOH in the form of colourless prisms. The alkaloid has $[\alpha]_D + 160°$ (c 0.21, $CHCl_3$) and its ultraviolet spectrum exhibits absorption maxima at 270 and 303 mμ. The O,O-dimethyl ether is *iso*corydine and the O,O-diacetate is an amorphous solid which cannot be crystallized.

Johns, Lamberton., *Austral. J. Chem.,* **20**, 1277 (1967)

DIHYDROXYHELIOTRIDANE

$C_8H_{15}O_2N$

M.p. 76–7°C

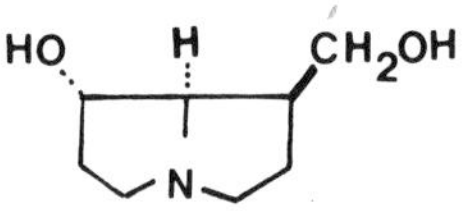

One of the Senecio alkaloids, this base is found in several *Senecio* species. It is laevorotatory with $[\alpha]_D - 34°$ (c 1.0, EtOH). It contains two hydroxyl groups, one primary and one secondary. The crystalline picrate has m.p. 157–8°C.

Men'shikov, Kuzovkov., *J. Gen. Chem., USSR,* **19**, 1702 (1949)

(R)(−)-3:5-DIHYDROXY-6-METHOXYAPORPHINE

$C_{18}H_{19}O_3N$

M.p. 149−152°C (*dec.*).

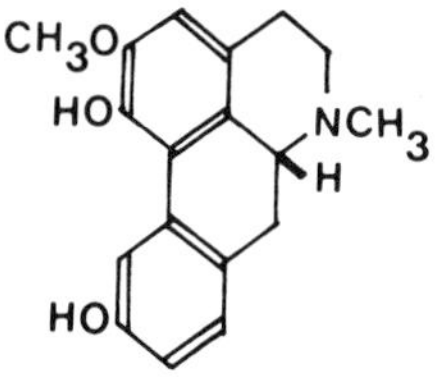

The leaves of *Ocotea glaziovii* contain this alkaloid of the aporphine type which forms colourless crystals of the monohydrate from aqueous EtOH. It has $[\alpha]_D^{26} - 35°$ (c 0.2, $CHCl_3$) and forms crystalline salts and derivatives, e.g. the hydrochloride, m.p. > 300°C (*dec.*); the methiodide which occurs as the monohydrate, m.p. 226−9°C or 251−3°C (*dry*). The O-methyl derivative is characterized as the methosulphate, m.p. 189−202°C (*dec.*). The structure has been determined from spectroscopic evidence and direct comparison with other aporphine bases.

Gilbert *et al., J. Amer. Chem. Soc.*, **86**, 694 (1964)

6:6′-DIHYDROXYTHIONUPHLUTINE A

$C_{30}H_{42}O_4N_2S$

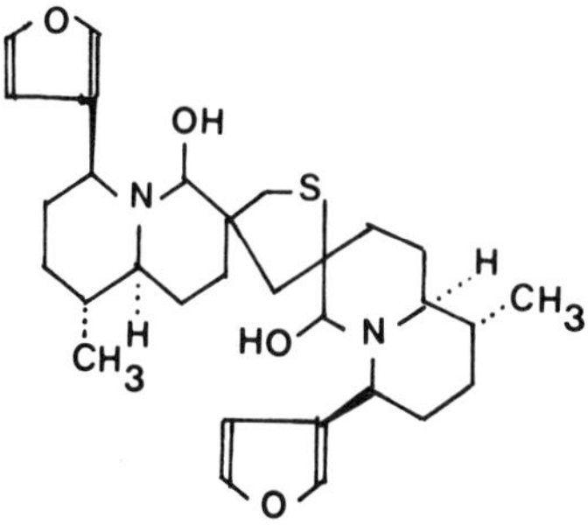

This, and the following alkaloid have been isolated from *Nuphar luteum* and shown to be stereoisomers of the above structure.

LaLonde, Wong, Cullen., *Tetrahedron Lett.*, 4477 (1970)

6:6′-DIHYDROXYTHIONUPHLUTINE B

$C_{30}H_{42}O_4N_2S$

A second alkaloid found in *Nuphar luteum*, stereoisomeric with the preceding base.

LaLonde, Wong, Cullen., *Tetrahedron Lett.*, 4477 (1970)

DIHYDROXYTROPANE

$C_8H_{15}O_2N$

M.p. 209–209.5°C

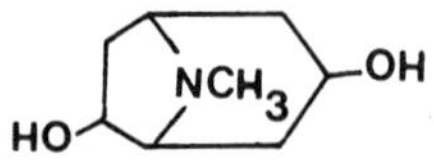

This base has been obtained from the mixture of hydrolyzed bases found in *Erythroxylon coca* Lam. grown in Java. It is laevorotatory with $[\alpha]_D^{27} - 22°$ (EtOH) and furnishes a crystalline hydrochloride with $[\alpha]_D^{27} + 1.75°$ (H_2O); a picrate, m.p. 253–4°C (*dec.*) and a dibenzoyl derivative which forms a hydrochloride (dihydrate), m.p. 115°C or 205°C (*dry*); $[\alpha]_D^{22} + 41.8°$ (aqueous EtOH) and a nitrate, m.p. 197°C. Reduction with HI and red phosphorus furnishes tropane. The dibenzoyl derivative has been found to possess local anaesthetic properties.

Wolfes, Hromatka., *Merck's Jahresb.*, **47**, 45 (1934)
Kreitmair., *ibid*, **47**, 54 (1934)

DILUPINE

$C_{16}H_{26}O_2N_2$

An alkaloid which occurs in *Lupinus barbiger* S. Wats., the base is an oil which has $[\alpha]_D^{26} + 65.6°$ (H_2O). The derivatives contain one less oxygen atom than the parent alkaloid. The hydrobromide has m.p. 233–4°C and the methiodide, m.p. 253°C.

Couch., *J. Amer. Chem. Soc.*, **54**, 1691 (1932)
Couch., *ibid*, **58**, 686, 1296 (1936)
Soine, Jenkins., *Pharm. Arch.*, **12**, 65 (1941)

6:8-DIMETHOXYDICTAMNINE

$C_{14}H_{13}O_4N$

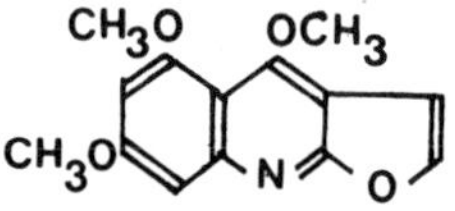

Recently isolated from *Dictamnus caucasicus*, this alkaloid has the structure given above based upon chemical degradative and spectroscopic data.

Kikvidze *et al.*, *Khim. Prir. Soedin.*, **5**, 675 (1971)

DIMETHOXYEBURNAMONINE

$C_{22}H_{30}O_2N_2$

M.p. 219–220°C

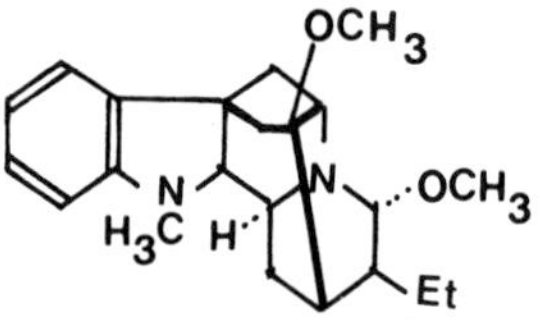

This alkaloid is present in the weakly basic fraction from the isolation of

11-Methoxyeburnamonine (q.v.) from *Vinca minor.* The structure has been established from the infrared and ultraviolet spectra.

Dopke, Meisel, Spiteller., *Pharmazie,* **23**, 99 (1968)

2:9-DIMETHOXY-3-HYDROXYPAVINANE

$C_{19}H_{21}O_3N$

M.p. 197–8°C

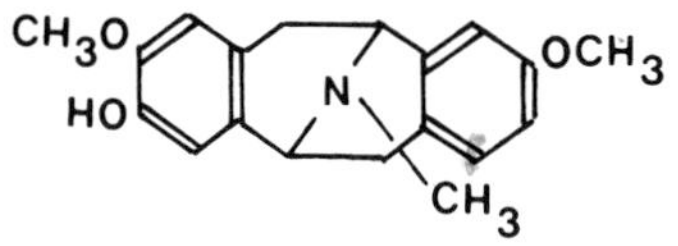

An alkaloid present in *Argemone munita* subsp. *rotundata,* the base is laevo-rotatory with $[\alpha]_D^{27} - 254°$ (c 1.59, MeOH). The structure has been confirmed by synthesis of the optically inactive form, m.p. 162°C.

Coomes *et al., J. Org. Chem.,* **38**, 3701 (1973)

6:8-DIMETHOXYISODICTAMNINE

$C_{14}H_{13}O_4N$

A minor alkaloid of *Dictamnus caucasicus,* the base is found in the non-phenolic fraction of the alkaloidal extract.

Asatiani *et al., Soobshch. Akad. Nauk. Gruz SSR,* **64**, 85 (1971)

10:11-DIMETHOXYISOMITRAPHYLLINE

$C_{23}H_{28}O_6N_2$

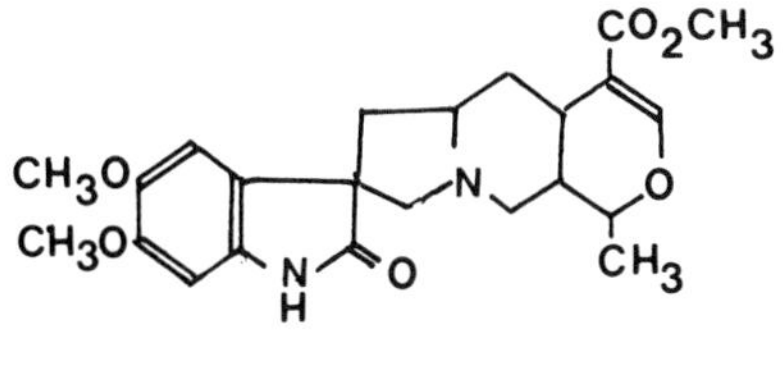

An alkaloid isolated from the aerial parts of *Cabucala madagascariensis,* the structure is determined from spectroscopic evidence and the ready isomerization of the base to 10:11-dimethoxymitraphylline.

Kan-Fan *et al., Phytochem.,* **11**, 435 (1972)

1:3-DIMETHOXY-10-METHYL-9-ACRIDONE

$C_{16}H_{15}O_3N$

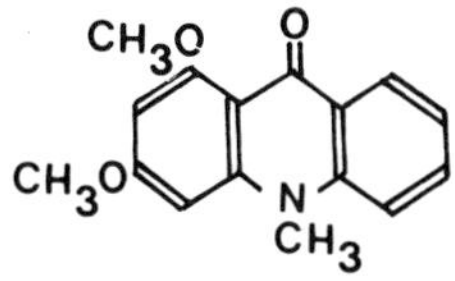

The leaves of *Acronychia baueri* yield this alkaloid as a minor constituent. The base forms colourless crystals of the dihydrate. The structure follows from chemical and spectroscopic data.

Lamberton, Price., *Austral. J. Chem.*, **6**, 66 (1953)

7:8-DIMETHOXY-2:3-METHYLENEDIOXYBENZO-PHENANTHRIDINE

$C_{20}H_{15}O_4N$

M.p. 220–1°C

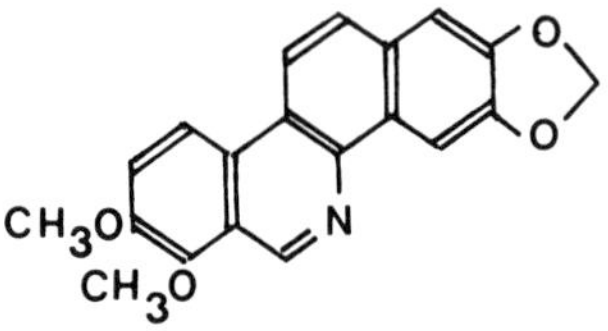

Isolated from the mother liquors obtained from the root bark extract of *Toddalia aculeata* after removal of chelerythrine and dihydrochelerythrine, this alkaloid is purified by chromatography on a silica gel column when it forms colourless crystals from C_6H_6-$CHCl_3$. The structure has been established from ultraviolet, NMR and mass spectral data.

Govindachari, Visvanathan., *Ind. J. Chem.*, **5**, 280 (1967)

1:2-DIMETHOXY-9:10-METHYLENEDIOXY-NORAPORPHINE

$C_{19}H_{19}O_4N$

M.p. 163–4°C

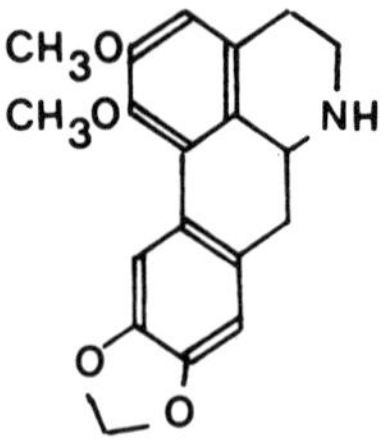

This alkaloid, also given the name *nornantenine*, occurs in *Cassytha racemosa* Nees. It crystallizes from Me_2CO-light petroleum in the form of colourless needles and has $[\alpha]_D + 85°$ (c 0.75, $CHCl_3$). The ultraviolet spectrum has absorption maxima at 218, 282 and 308 mμ with inflexions at 272 and 318 mμ. The N-methyl derivative is nantenine (q.v.) and the N-acetyl compound forms colourless needles from EtOH, m.p. 294°C; $[\alpha]_D + 349°$(c 0.44, $CHCl_3$).

Johns, Lamberton, Sioumis., *Austral. J. Chem.*, **20**, 1457 (1967)

1:2-DIMETHOXY-9:10-METHYLENEDIOXY-7-OXOAPORPHINE

$C_{19}H_{13}O_5N$

M.p. 215–8°C (dec.).

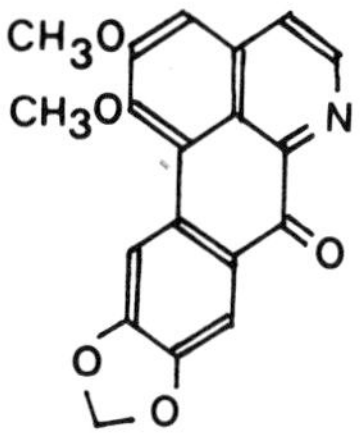

Also isolated from *Cassytha racemosa* Nees, this alkaloid forms yellow needles when crystallized from EtOH. The ultraviolet spectrum has absorption maxima at 243, 272, 317 and 358 mμ with inflexions at 288 and 380 mμ.

Johns, Lamberton, Sioumis., *Austral. J. Chem.*, 20, 1457 (1967)

3:4-DIMETHOXYPHENETHYLAMINE

$C_{10}H_{15}O_2N$

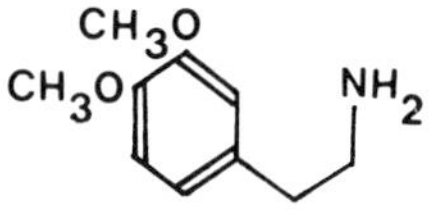

An alkaloidal amine present in *Echinocereus merkeri*, this cactus base possesses the hallucinatory properties of most of these simple amines.

Agurell, Lundstrom, Masoud., *J. Pharm. Sci.*, 58, 1413 (1969)

DIMETHOXYPICRAPHYLLINE

$C_{24}H_{30}O_6N_2$

M.p. 183–5°C

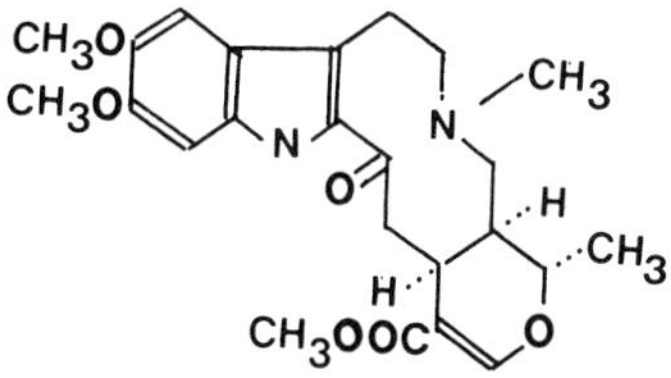

The leaves of *Ochrosia balansae* Guill. contain this protopine type alkaloid which forms colourless crystals from Et_2O. It has $[\alpha]_D - 50°$ (c 1.0, $CHCl_3$) and an ultraviolet spectrum with absorption maxima at 214 and 342 mμ with a shoulder at 240 mμ.

Bruneton, Pousset, Cave., *Compt. Rend.*, 273C, 442 (1971)

3:4-DIMETHOXY-2-(2-PIPERIDYL)ACETOPHENONE

$C_{15}H_{21}O_3N$

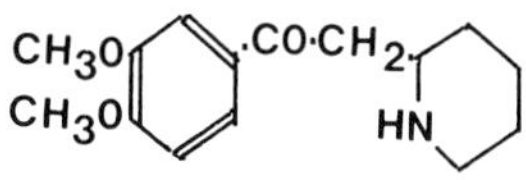

From the alkaloidal fraction of *Boehmeria platyphylla*, this alkaloid has been isolated as the major component. It is identical with the compound obtained by O-methylation of pleurospermine (q.v.).

Hart, Johns, Lamberton., *Austral. J. Chem.*, 21, 1397 (1968)

10:11-DIMETHOXYSTRYCHNOBRASILINE

$C_{24}H_{30}O_5N_2$

M.p. 168–175°C

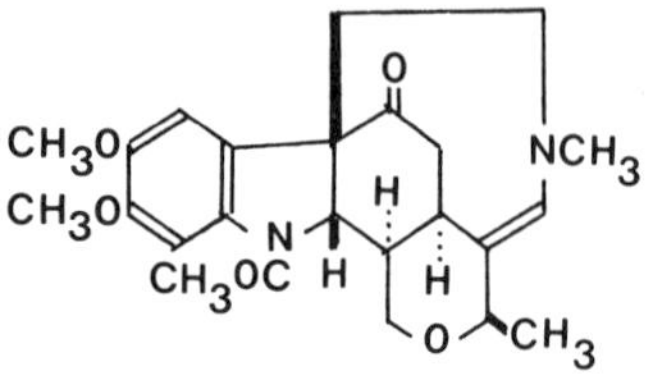

This alkaloid occurs in the bark of *Strychnos brasiliensis* Mart. and yields colourless crystals from either EtOH or AcOEt. It has $[\alpha]_D^{20} + 148°$ (c 0.61, $CHCl_3$) and the ultraviolet spectrum of the ethanolic solution exhibits absorption maxima at 217, 258 and 297 mμ.

Iwataki, Comin., *Tetrahedron*, 27, 2541 (1971)

4:7-DIMETHOXY-1-VINYL-β-CARBOLINE

$C_{15}H_{14}O_2N_2$

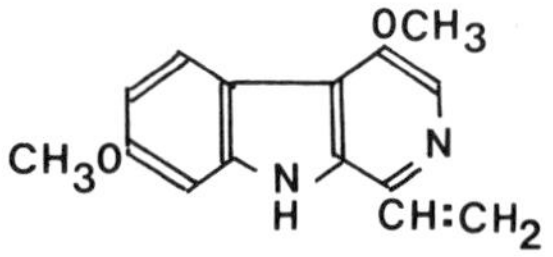

This comparatively simple carboline alkaloid has been isolated from the bark and wood of Pereira madagascariensis. No derivatives have yet been prepared.

Bourgaigynon-Zylber, Polonsky., *Chim. Ther.*, 5, 396 (1970)

3α-(β,β-DIMETHYLACRYLYL)AMINO-20α-DIMETHYLAMINO-5α-PREGNANE (*Alkaloid A*)

$C_{28}H_{48}ON_2$

M.p. 148–150°C

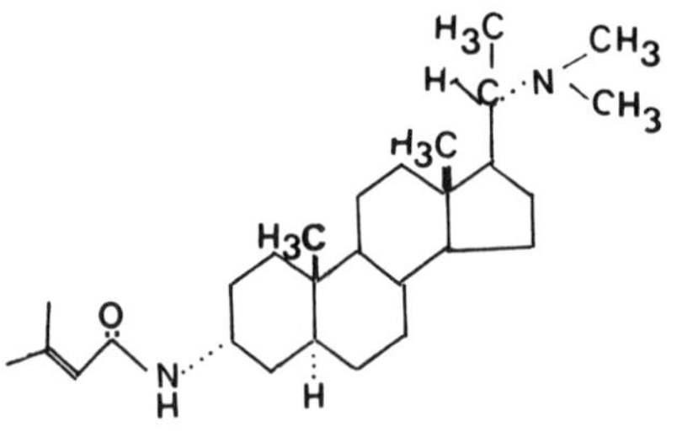

A steroidal alkaloid present in *Sarcococca pruniformis* Lindl. The base has $[\alpha]_D^{25} + 46°$ ($CHCl_3$).

Chatterjee, Mukherjee., *Chem. & Ind.*, 769 (1966)

3β-(β,β-DIMETHYLACRYLOXY)-20α-DIMETHYLAMINO-5α-PREGNANE (*Alkaloid B*)

$C_{28}H_{47}O_2N$

M.p. 274–6°C

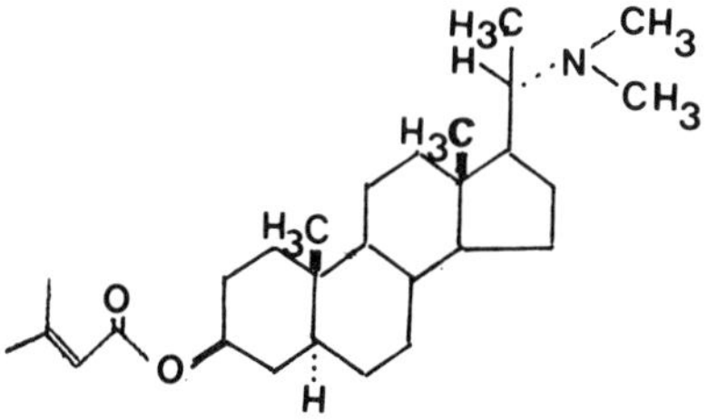

A second alkaloid found in *Sarcococca pruniformis* Lindl., the base has a similar structure to that of the preceding alkaloid. It also has $[\alpha]_D^{25} + 10°$ (CHCl$_3$).

Chatterjee, Mukherjee., *Chem. Ind.*, 769 (1966)

3-DIMETHYLALLYL-4-DIMETHYLALLYLOXY-2-QUINOLONE

$C_{19}H_{23}O_3N$

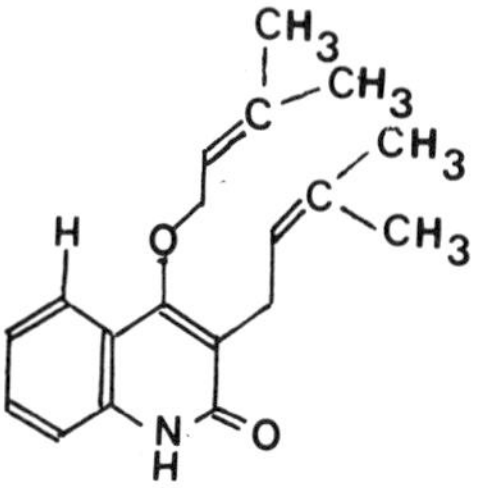

A novel quinolone type alkaloid isolated from *Haplophyllum tuberculatum*. The base has been characterized by NMR and mass spectrometry and the structure confirmed by conversion into the known dihydroflindersine.

Lavie *et al.*, *Tetrahedron*, 24, 3011 (1968)

N:N-DIMETHYLAMINOETHYL-3:4-DIMETHOXYPHENANTHRENE

$C_{20}H_{23}O_2N$

M.p. 199–200°C

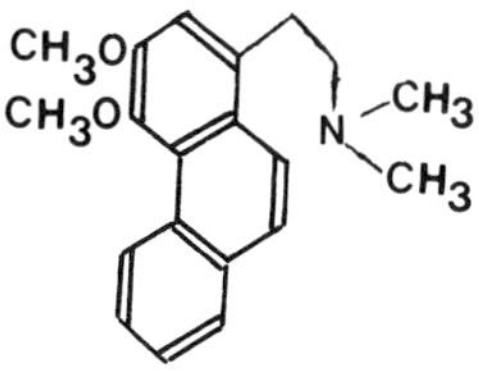

This alkaloid has been found in *Atherosperma moschatum* Labill. and *Cryptocarya angulata* C.T. White. It may be obtained as colourless needles from a mixture of Me$_2$CO and light petroleum although, as yet, it has not been found possible to recrystallize the base. It forms a series of crystalline salts and derivatives: the hydrochloride has m.p. 234–5°C (*dec.*); the hydriodide, m.p. 234–5°C (*dec.*); the perchlorate, m.p. 195–6°C and the picrate, yellow needles, m.p. 186–8°C. The methiodide, which may be used to characterize the alkaloid, has m.p. 274.5–276.5°C and its ultraviolet spectrum shows absorption maxima at 257, 279, 302 and 312 mμ with a shoulder at 250 mμ.

Yunusov, Konovalova, Orekhov., *Bull. Soc. Chim.*, **7**, 70 (1946)
Cooke, Haynes., *Austral. J. Chem.*, **7**, 99 (1954)
Bick, Clezy, Crow., *ibid*, **9**, 111 (1956)
Bick, Douglas., *ibid*, **18**, 1997 (1965)

1-DIMETHYLAMINOETHYL-3-HYDROXY-4-METHOXYPHENANTHRENE

$C_{19}H_{21}O_2N$

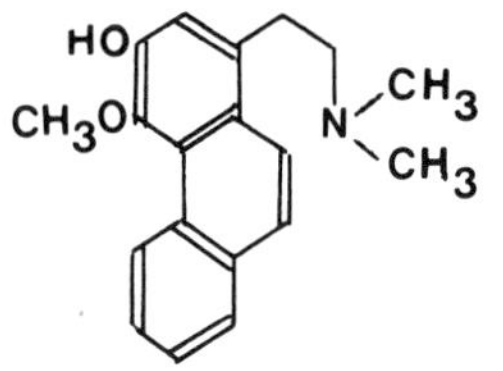

A non-crystallizable oil, this base is present in *Aristolchia argentina* Gris. It forms a crystalline oxalate, m.p. 176–7°C and an ethyl ether, characterized as the oxalate, m.p. 202–3°C and the methiodide, m.p. 289°C.

Priestap *et al.*, *Chem. Commun.*, 754 (1967)

3-DIMETHYLAMINOETHYL-1:5-(DIMETHOXY)INDOLE

$C_{13}H_{18}O_2N_2$

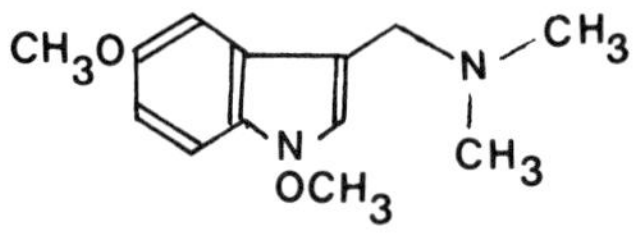

An indole alkaloid which occurs in the leaves of *Gymnacranthera paniculata* (A. DC.) Warb. var. *zippeliana* (Miq.) J. Sinclair. The alkaloid is a colourless oil whose ultraviolet spectrum exhibits two absorption maxima at 276 and 304 mμ. The picrate exists in two modifications, as yellow crystals or bronze needles, both having m.p. 154–5°C.

Johns, Lamberton, Occolowitz., *Austral. J. Chem.*, **20**, 1737 (1967)

DIMETHYLCROTONOSINE

$C_{19}H_{21}O_3N$

M.p. 127–8°C

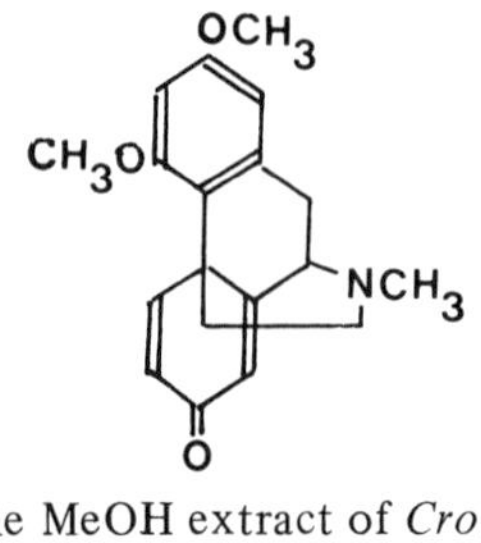

This alkaloid occurs in the MeOH extract of *Croton linearis* and is isolated by countercurrent distribution methods. It is dextrorotatory having $[\alpha]_D^{24} + 111.2°$ (c 1.24, EtOH) and yields a crystalline methiodide, m.p. 244–5°C.

Haynes, Stuart., *J. Chem. Soc.*, 1784 (1963)

O,N-DIMETHYLCROTSPARINE

$C_{19}H_{21}O_3N$

M.p. 125–7°C

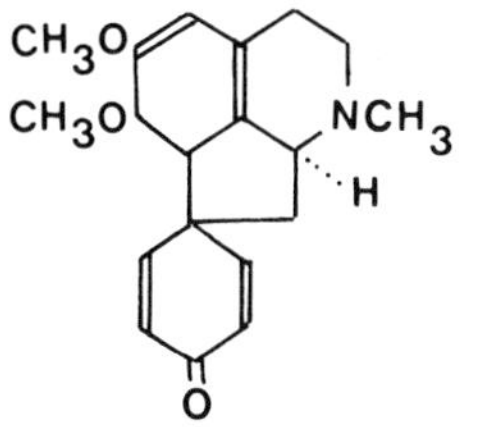

A proaporphine alkaloid found in *Croton sparsiflorus,* the structure has been confirmed from the infrared, ultraviolet, NMR and mass spectra.

Bhakuni, Satish, Dhar., *Phytochem.,* **9**, 2573 (1970)

N,N-DIMETHYL-3:4-DIMETHOXYPHENETHYLAMINE

$C_{12}H_{19}O_2N$

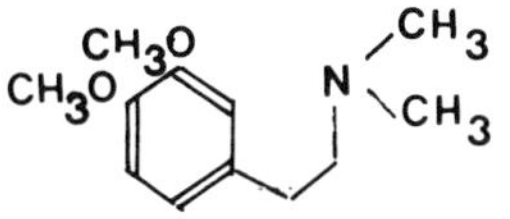

An alkaloidal amine present in the cactus *Echinocereus Merkeri,* the structure of this base has been determined by chemical degradation and spectroscopic evidence. Like most of these amines, it possesses pronounced hallucinatory properties.

Agurell, Lundstrom, Masoud., *J. Pharm. Sci.,* **58**, 1413 (1969)

DIMETHYLFUNTUMINE

$C_{23}H_{39}ON$

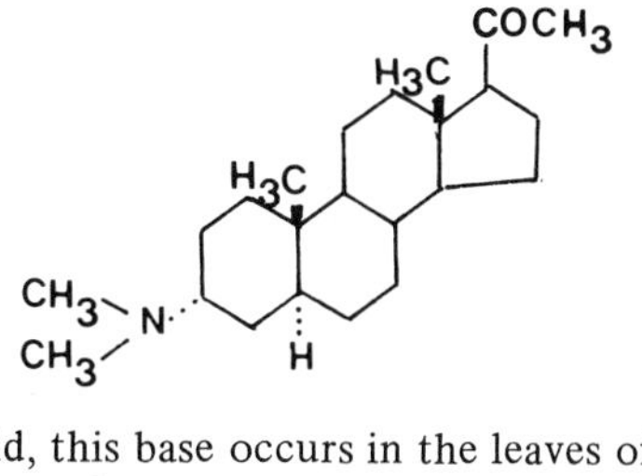

A pregnane type alkaloid, this base occurs in the leaves of *Holarrhena febrifuga.* The structure follows from the spectroscopic evidence and comparison with Funtumine (q.v.).

Conreur, Cave., *Phytochem.,* **12**, 923 (1973)

N-DIMETHYLMESCALINE

See Trichocereine

O,N-DIMETHYLMICRANTHINE

$C_{36}H_{36}O_5N_2$

M.p. 210–4°C

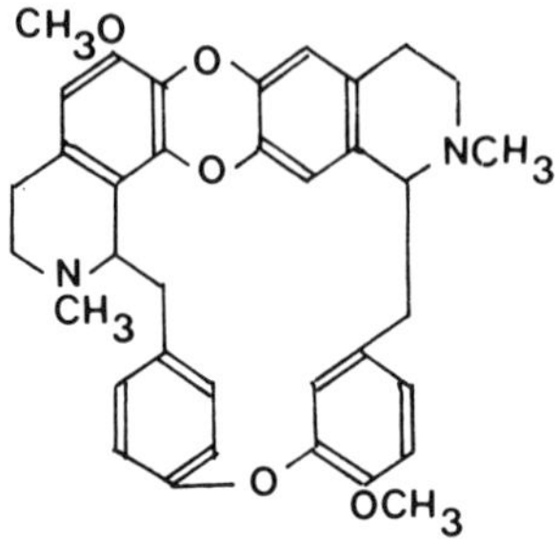

A minor constituent of several species of *Daphnandra*, particularly *D. micrantha* Benth. The base is strongly laevorotatory with $[\alpha]_D^{19} - 230°$ (CHCl$_3$).

Bick, Todd., *J. Chem. Soc.*, 1606 (1950)

2:9-DIMETHYL-6-METHOXY-1:2:3:4-TETRAHYDRO-CARBOLINE

$C_{14}H_{18}ON_2$

M.p. 214°C (*dec.*).

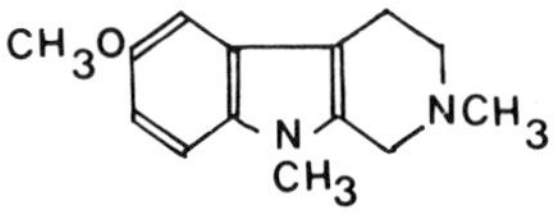

This alkaloid from *Philaris arundinacea* L. var. *Ottawa* yields colourless needles from MeOH. The structure has been established from the infrared, ultraviolet, NMR and mass spectra.

Audette, Vijayanagar, Bolan., *Can. J. Chem.*, 48, 149 (1970)

5:7-DIMETHYLOCTAHYDROINDOLIZINE

$C_{10}H_{19}N$

A minor base of *Dendrobium primulinum,* this alkaloid is a colourless oil and is laevorotatory with $[\alpha]_D - 38°$ (c 1.0, CHCl$_3$).

Luning, Leander., *Acta Chem. Scand.*, 19, 1607 (1965)

1:2-DIMETHYLQUINOL-4-ONE

$C_{11}H_{12}ON^+$

M.p. 178–9°C

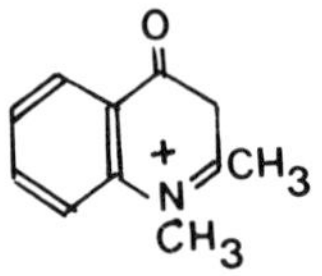

The leaves of *Acronychia baueri* contain this minor alkaloid which has been characterized as the picrate, pale yellow needles, m.p. 234–8°C. The structure has been established spectroscopically.

Lamberton., *Austral. J. Chem.*, **19**, 1995 (1966)

DIMETHYLTRYPTAMINE

$C_{12}H_{16}N_2$

M.p. 45°C

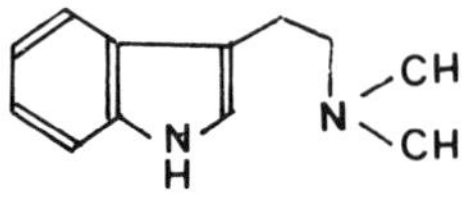

This tryptamine derivative has been isolated from *Phalaris arundinacea* and *P. tuberosa*. It forms colourless crystals from petroleum ether. The picrate is also crystalline with m.p. 168.5°C.

Culvenor, Dal Bon, Smith., *Austral. J. Chem.*, **17**, 1301 (1964)

DIMETHYLTRYPTAMINE-N$_6$-OXIDE

$C_{12}H_{16}ON_2$

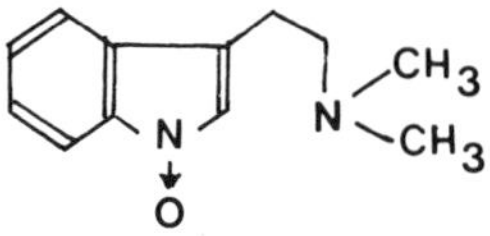

The leaves of *Banisteriopsis argentea* have recently been found to contain this alkaloid. The structure follows from comparison with Dimethyltryptamine (q.v.).

Ghosal, Mazumder., *Phytochem.*, **10**, 2840 (1971)

S-(+)-N(b)-DIMETHYLTRYPTOPHAN METHYL ESTER

$C_{14}H_{18}O_2N_2$

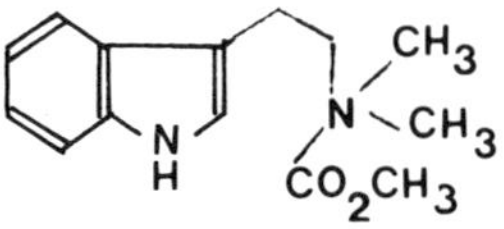

This ester alkaloid occurs in *Aotus subglauca* and *Pultenacea altissima*. The structure has been determined by comparison with known tryptophan derivatives.

Johns, Lamberton, Sioumis., *Austral. J. Chem.*, **24**, 439 (1971)

DIOSCINE

$C_{13}H_{21}O_2N$

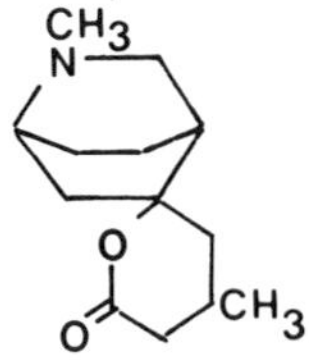

A minor component of the alkaloidal extract from the tubers of *Dioscorea dumetorum* Pax. and *D. sanziborensis*. The alkaloid is an oil and has $[\alpha]_D^{18}$ –

42.2° (c 3.4, CHCl₃). It forms crystalline salts, e.g. the hydrochloride, m.p. 209°C; picrate, m.p. 189°C and methiodide, m.p. 258°C. The (±)-form yields a picrate with m.p. 164−5°C and a methiodide, m.p. 229−230°C.

Pinder., *J. Chem. Soc.*, 2236 (1952)
Bevan, Broadbent, Hirst., *Chem. & Ind.*, 103 (1958)

DIOSCORINE

$C_{13}H_{19}O_2N$

M.p. 43.5°C

This alkaloid was first isolated from the tubers of *Dioscorea hirsuta* Blume by Boorsma and subsequently investigated by Schutte and Gorter. It is obtained as greenish-yellow plates and is soluble in EtOH, CHCl₃ or H₂O but only sparingly so in C_6H_6 or Et₂O. The hydrochloride has m.p. 204°C; $[\alpha]_D$ + 4.6°; the aurichloride forms yellow needles, m.p. 171°C (*dry*) and the platinichloride, orange-yellow tablets, m.p. 199−200°C (*dry*). Its presence in the tubers of *D. hispida* has been reported by Zevya and Gutierrez.

The alkaloid is bitter and toxic, producing paralysis of the central nervous system and in general it behaves like picrotoxin (q.v.).

Boorsma., *Meded. uit's Lands Plant.*, 13 (1894)
Schutte., *Chem. Zentr.*, 130 (1897)
Gorter., *Ann. Jard. Bot. Buit.*, Suppl. 3, 385 (1909)
Zevya, Gutierrez., *J. Phil. Isl. Med. Assoc.*, 17, 349 (1937)

10:22-DIOXOKOPSANE

$C_{20}H_{20}O_2N_2$

M.p. 298°C

The stem bark of *Pleiocarpa mutica* Benth. yields this alkaloid which is obtained as slender, colourless needles from MeOH. It has $[\alpha]_D^{28}$ + 156° (c 0.32, CHCl₃) and the ultraviolet spectrum shows absorption maxima at 242 and 294 mμ.

Achenbach, Biemann., *J. Amer. Chem. Soc.*, 87, 4944 (1965)

(−)-cis-8:10-DIPHENYLLOBELIDIOL

$C_{22}H_{29}O_2N$

M.p. 117°C

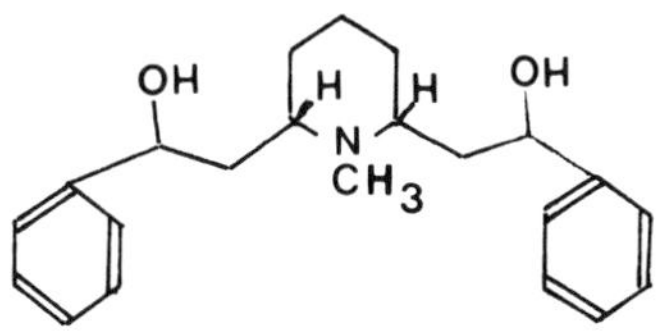

The herb *Isotoma longiflora* yields this alkaloid which crystallizes from Et_2O. It has $[\alpha]_D^{20} - 71.8°$ (c 1.16 $CHCl_3$) and, by repeated treatment with moist Et_2O, yields a hydrate, m.p. 216–8°C (*dec.*). The crystalline nitrate has m.p. 216–7°C and the dibenzoyl derivative, m.p. 141–2°C. Oxidation with chromic acid yields (−)-lobeline (q.v.). Oxidation with $KMnO_4$ furnishes benzoic acid.

Arthur, Chan., *J. Chem. Soc.*, 750 (1963)

DIPTERINE (*N-methyltryptamine*)

$C_{11}H_{14}N_2$

M.p. 87–8°C

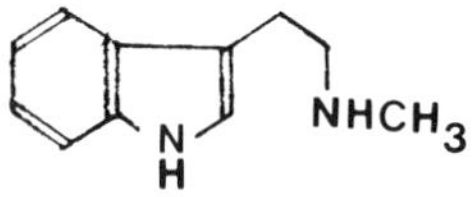

This alkaloid has been isolated from *Girgensohnia diptera* Bge. together with N-methylpiperidine. It is optically inactive and yields a crystalline hydrochloride, m.p. 177–8°C; a picrate, m.p. 189–190°C and a picrolonate, m.p. 242–3°C.

Juraschevski, Stepanova., *J. Gen. Chem. USSR*, 9, 2203 (1939)

DIQUINICINE

See Diconquinine

DISCARINE A

$C_{33}H_{43}O_4N_5$

M.p. 229–231°C

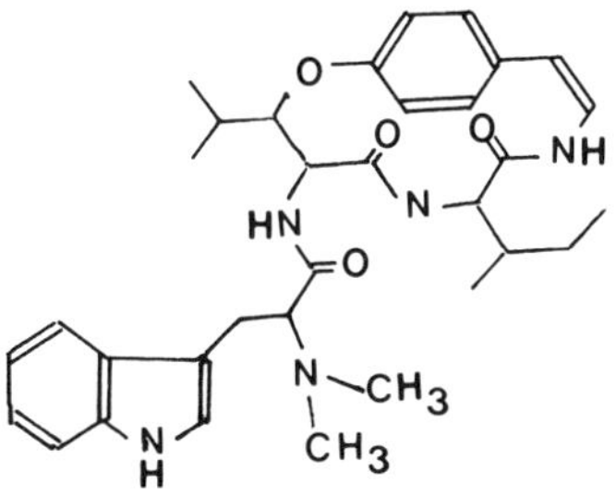

A peptide alkaloid present in *Discaria longispina*, the base forms colourless crystals from Et_2O-CH_2Cl_2 and is laevorotatory with $[\alpha]_D - 282°$ (c 0.05, $CHCl_3$). The structure given is still somewhat in doubt since it has also been assigned to Amphibin A.

Mascaretti *et al.*, *Phytochem.*, 11, 1133 (1972)

DISCARINE B

$C_{33}H_{43}O_4N_5$

M.p. 235–6°C

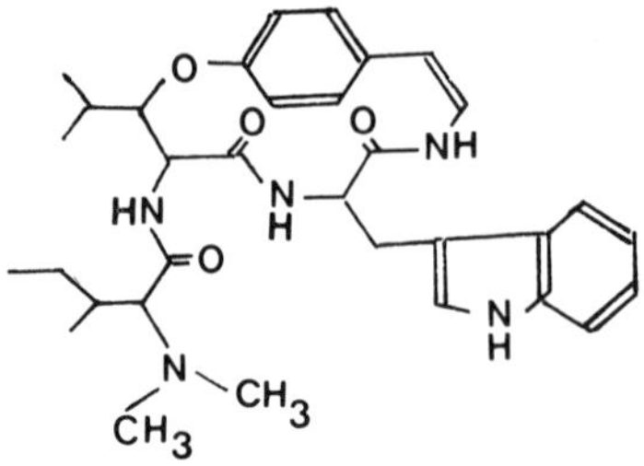

A second peptide alkaloid obtained from *Discaria longispina*, this base is also laevorotatory with $[\alpha]_D - 172°$ (c 1.0, CHCl$_3$).

Mascaretti *et al., Phytochem.,* **11**, 1133 (1972)

DISCRETINE

$C_{20}H_{23}O_4N$

M.p. 180–1°C

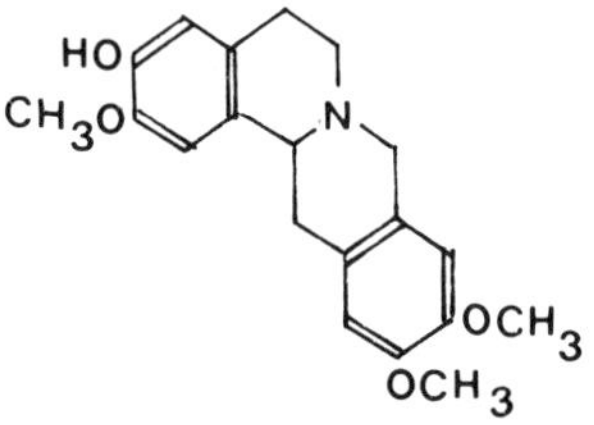

A protoberberine alkaloid occurring in *Xylopia discreta*. The base is laevo-rotatory with $[\alpha]_D - 300°$ (CHCl$_3$). It is characterized as the crystalline hydrochloride, m.p. 212–3°C. The alkaloid contains three methoxyl groups and one hydroxyl group in the molecule. The structure has been confirmed by synthesis.

Schmutz., *Helv. Chim. Acta,* **42**, 335 (1959)
Bernoulli, Linde, Meyer., *ibid,* **46**, 323 (1963)

Synthesis:
Kametani, Takeshita, Takano., *J. Chem. Soc., Perkin I,* 2834 (1972)

DISCOLORINE

$C_{18}H_{23}O_3N$

M.p. 206–8°C

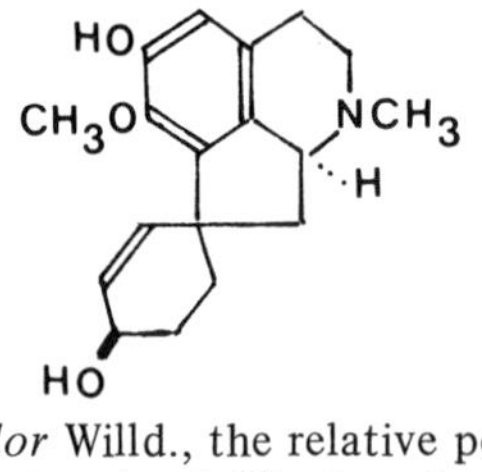

Isolated from *Croton discolor* Willd., the relative positions of the methoxyl and hydroxyl groups is still undetermined. The base has $[\alpha]_D + 99°$ (c 0.5, EtOH) and the ultraviolet spectrum has absorption maxima at 229 and 287 mμ with a shoulder at 210 mμ.

Stuart *et al., J. Chem. Soc., C,* 1228 (1970)

DITAMINE

$C_{16}H_{19}O_2N$

According to Hesse, this alkaloid accompanies Echitamine in the bark of *Alstonia scholaris* and *A. spectabilis*. It is, however, still ill-defined and is probably a mixture of bases.

Hesse., *Annalen,* **176**, 326 (1875)

DI(TETRAHYDROPYRIDOIMIDAZOLIUM)

$C_{11}H_{17}N_2^+$

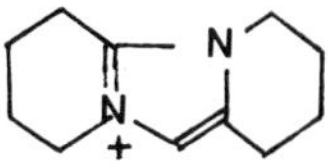

A quaternary alkaloid of *Dendrobium anosmum* and *D. parishii,* the base is characterized as the chloride, hygroscopic crystals, m.p. 86–88.5° and 153–6°C with intermediate solidification and the bromide which forms colourless crystals, m.p. 164–6°C. Catalytic reduction with Raney Ni gives the saturated base, $C_{11}H_{20}N_2$. The structure has been deduced from spectroscopic data and confirmed by synthesis.

Leander, Luning., *Tetrahedron Lett.,* 905 (1968)

DITHERMAMINE

$C_{30}H_{40}O_2N_4$

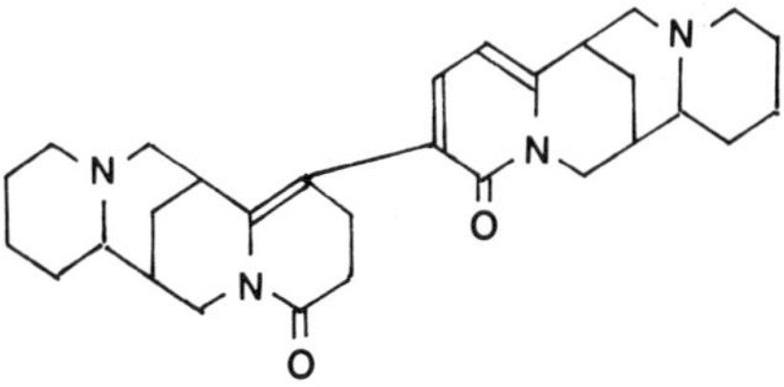

This alkaloid is present in *Thermopsis lanceolata* and is isolated as the crystalline perchlorate, m.p. 211–2°C or the picrate, m.p. 203–4°C.

Vinogradova, Iskandarov, Yunusov., *Khim. Prir. Soedin.,* 8, 87 (1972)

DITIGLOYLTROPANE

$C_{18}H_{27}O_4N$

M.p. Indefinite

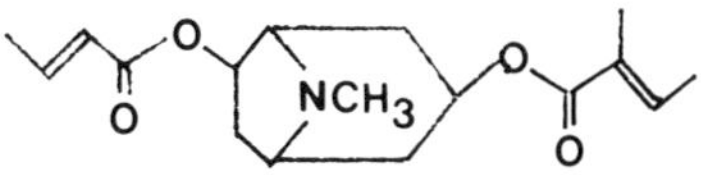

The roots of several *Datura* species contain this alkaloid which forms a colourless gum that cannot be crystallized. It has $[\alpha]_D^{20} - 21.5°$ (c 3.1, EtOH). The platinichloride forms orange rosettes, m.p. 230°C (*dec.*) and the picrate has m.p. 150–1°C.

Schrecker, Hartnell., *J. Amer. Chem. Soc.,* **77**, 432 (1955)

(−)-3β,6α-DITIGLOYLOXYTROPANE

$C_{18}H_{27}O_4N$

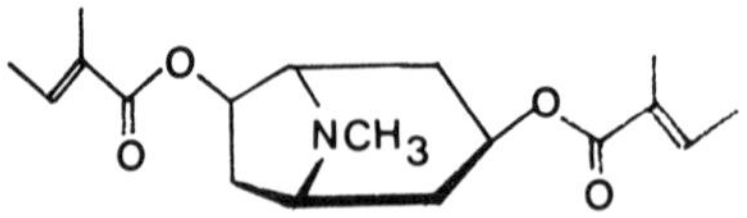

An alkaloid present in the roots of *Datura meteloides*. The structure has been determined spectroscopically, particularly from NMR and mass spectral data.

Evans, Woolley., *J. Chem. Soc.*, 4936 (1965)

3β,6α-DITIGLOYLOXYTROPAN-7β-OL

$C_{18}H_{27}O_5N$

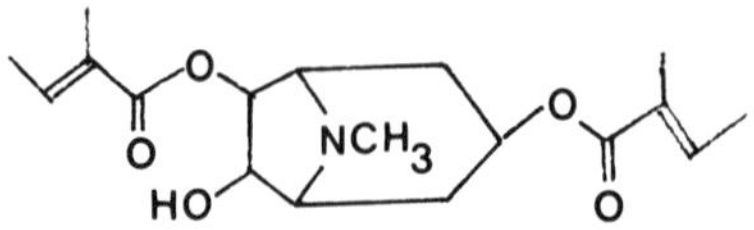

First discovered in the roots of *Datura meteloides*, this base has more recently been found in the aerial parts of *D. discolor*. The structure follows from the infrared, NMR and mass spectra.

Evans, Woolley., *J. Chem. Soc.*, 4936 (1965)
Evans, Somanabandhu., *Phytochem.*, **13**, 304 (1974)

DOLICHOTHELINE

$C_{10}H_{17}ON_3$

M.p. 130−1°C

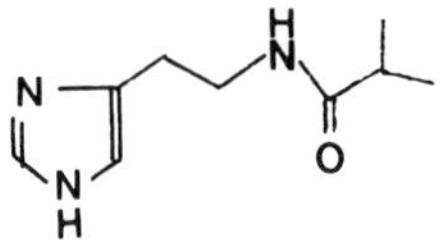

This alkaloid occurs in *Dolichothela sphaerica*, a small cactus which is indigenous to Texas and North Mexico. It forms a crystalline picrate, m.p. 150−2°C and an N-acetyl derivative, m.p. 76−8°C. Acid hydrolysis yields histamine, isolated as the dihydrochloride, m.p. 227−231°C and *iso*valeric acid, thereby establishing the structure as N-isovalerylhistamine. The alkaloid may be synthesized by refluxing histamine with *iso*valeryl anhydride.

Rosenberg, Paul., *Tetrahedron Lett.*, 1039 (1969)

DOMESTICINE

$C_{19}H_{19}O_4N$

M.p. 115−7°C

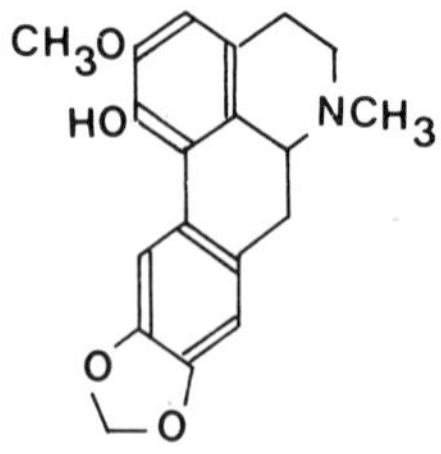

First isolated from *Nandina domestica* Thunb. by Kitasato, this alkaloid is also present in *Cassytha pubescens* R. Br. From aqueous MeOH it crystallizes as the monohydrate with the above melting point. From MeOH-C_6H_6 it has m.p. 84–5°C while the anhydrous base melts at 152–3°C (*dec.*). It is dextrorotatory with $[\alpha]_D$ + 60.51°. The phenolic hydroxyl group may be methylated with CH_2N_2 to give Nantenine (q.v.). The alkaloid gives a blue colour with HNO_3 vapour, a reddish-violet colour with H_2SO_4 and a green colour with $FeCl_3$.

Kitasato., *J. Pharm. Soc., Japan,* **535**, 71 (1926)
Takese, Ahashi., *ibid,* **535**, 70 (1926)
Tomita, Kitamura., *ibid,* **79**, 1092 (1959)
Kitamura., *ibid,* **90**, 1140 (1960)

DONAXARINE

$C_{13}H_{16}O_2N_2$

M.p. 217°C

This alkaloid has been isolated from the grass *Arundo donax* L. It crystallizes from Me_2CO and is optically inactive. It contains one active hydrogen and one methylimino group but no methoxyl group. It gives no colour reaction with the glyocylic acid or dimethylaminobenzaldehyde reagents but the vapour does give the pyrrole reaction with pine-wood.

Madinaveitia., *J. Chem. Soc.,* 1927 (1937)

DONAXINE

See Gramine

DORYAFRINE

M.p. 92–4°C

The leaves of *Doryphora sassefras* yield two closely related alkaloids. This particular base forms colourless plates from Me_2CO and has $[\alpha]_D^{27}$ + 41.5° (c 2.12, $CHCl_3$). The ultraviolet spectrum exhibits two absorption maxima at 225 and 286 mμ.

Gharbo *et al., Lloydia,* **28**, 237 (1965)

DORYANINE

M.p. 160–2°C

The second minor alkaloid obtained from the leaves of *Doryphora sassefras,* this base forms colourless prisms and gives an ultraviolet spectrum consisting of a single absorption maximum at 231 mμ.

Gharbo *et al., Lloydia,* **28**, 237 (1965)

495

DORYPHORINE

$C_{18}H_{21}O_4N$

M.p. 115–7°C

An alkaloid also said to be present in *Doryphora sassefras*, this base is so far uncharacterized and its structure is unknown.

Petrie., *Proc. Linn. Soc., N.S.W.*, 37, 139 (1912)

DOURADINE

M.p. 235°C

This crystalline alkaloid is stated to occur in *Palicourea rigida* H.B.K. So far it has not been characterized beyond the determination of the melting point.

Santesson., *Arch. Pharm.*, 235, 143 (1897)

DREGAMINE

$C_{21}H_{26}O_3N_2$

M.p. 180–2°C

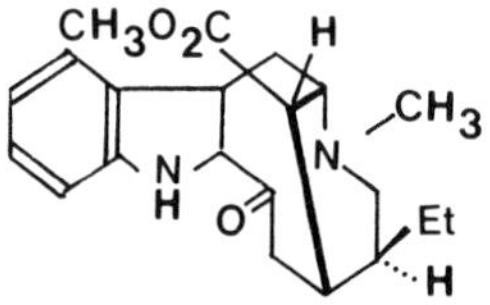

An alkaloid present in *Ervatamia coronaria* and *Voacanga dregei* E.M. From the latter plant it is obtained from the C_6H_6 extract of the powdered bark and purified by elution chromatography with C_6H_6-$CHCl_3$. It is laevorotatory with $[\alpha]_D^{26} - 93.1°$ (c 1.0, $CHCl_3$) and forms a hydrochloride, m.p. 249–250°C (*dec.*). The ultraviolet spectrum of the free base in EtOH shows two absorption maxima at 239 and 316 mμ.

Neuss, Cone., *Experientia*, 15, 414 (1959)
Gorman *et al.*, *J. Amer. Chem. Soc.*, 82, 1141 (1960)
Renner, Prins., *Experientia*, 17, 209 (1961)
Renner *et al.*, *Helv. Chim. Acta*, 46, 2186 (1963)
Cava *et al.*, *Tetrahedron Lett.*, 53 (1963)

DRYADINE

$C_{37}H_{40}O_6N_2$

M.p. 249–250°C

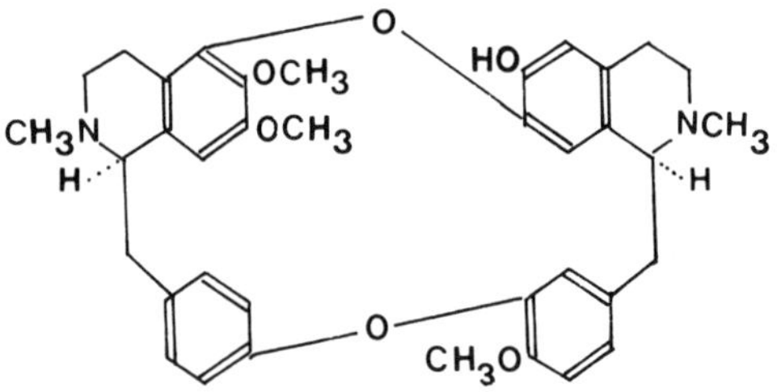

The bark of *Dryadodaphne novo-guineensis* yields two closely related bisbenzyl-

*iso*quinoline alkaloids. This particular base is obtained in the form of colourless needles from C_6H_6, Me_2CO or $CHCl_3$-MeOH. It is dextrorotatory with $[\alpha]_D^{16}$ + 490° (c 1.5, $CHCl_3$). The ultraviolet spectrum shows one absorption maximum at 285 mμ. The alkaloid contains three methoxyl groups, one hydroxyl and two methylimino groups in the molecule.

Bick, Douglas, Taylor., *J. Chem. Soc., C,* 1627 (1969)

DRYADODAPHNINE

$C_{36}H_{38}O_6N_2$

M.p. Indefinite

The second bisbenzyl*iso*quinoline alkaloid found in the bark of *Dryadodaphne novo-guineensis* is amorphous and has not been obtained in the crystalline form. It is also dextrorotatory with $[\alpha]_D$ + 390° (MeOH). The ultraviolet spectrum in EtOH is identical with that of the preceding base with an absorption maximum at 285 mμ. In the presence of base (EtOH-KOH), the absorption maxima are located at 288 and 305 mμ. The alkaloid contains one more hydroxyl and one less methoxyl group than Dryadine.

Bick, Douglas, Taylor., *J. Chem. Soc., C,* 1627 (1969)

DUBAMINE

$C_{14}H_{19}O_2N$

M.p. 96–7°C

Obtained from *Haplophyllum dubium,* this alkaloid may be crystallized from MeOH or light petroleum when it forms colourless needles. The hydrochloride is crystalline with m.p. 201–2°C, as is also the nitrate, m.p. 157–8°C. Oxidation with $KMnO_4$ in Me_2CO gives oxalylanthranilic acid whereas oxidation with $KMnO_4$ in H_2SO_4 yields quinaldinic acid, m.p. 152–3°C, characterized as the methyl ester, m.p. 78–80°C. The structure, as α-piperonylquinoline, has been confirmed by synthesis.

Yunusov., *J. Gen. Chem., USSR,* **25,** 2009 (1955)
Sidyakin *et al., ibid,* **32,** 4091 (1962)
Sidyakin, Pastukhova, Yunusov., *Uzbeksk. Khim. Zh.,* **6,** 56 (1962)

DUBINIDINE

$C_{15}H_{17}O_4N$

M.p. 132–3°C

This alkaloid occurs in several *Haplophyllum* species, particularly *H. foliosum*. It may be obtained from the aerial parts of the latter plant by extraction with $CHCl_3$ followed by thin-layer chromatography on alumina and determined quantitatively by polarpgraphy after extraction from the absorbent. It is laevo-rotatory with $[\alpha]_D^{26.5} - 62.95°$ and forms several crystalline salts and derivatives, e.g. the hydrochloride, m.p. 195–6°C; $[\alpha]_D^{18} - 53.92°$; hydro-bromide, m.p. 197–8°C; hydriodide, m.p. 161–2°C; nitrate, m.p. 176–7°C; methiodide, m.p. 153–4°C and picrate, m.p. 155–6°C. The base contains both a primary and secondary hydroxyl group and forms a monoacetate, m.p. 186–186.5°C and a diacetate, m.p. 108–9°C.

Yunusov., *J. Gen. Chem., USSR*, 25, 2009 (1955)
Sidyakin, Eskairov, Yunusov., *Dokl. Akad. Nauk. Uzbek SSR*, 8, 27 (1958)
Polieutsev., *Izv. Akad. Nauk. Uzbek. SSR., Ser. Med.*, 6, 66 (1959)
Sidyakin *et al., J. Gen. Chem., USSR*, 32, 4091 (1962)
Bessonova, Sidyakin, Yunusov., *Dokl. Akad. Nauk. Uzbek. SSR.*, 19, 50 (1962)
Rakhimov, Dobronravova, Shakirov., *Khim. Prir. Soedin.*, 6, 778 (1970)

DUBININE

$C_{16}H_{17}O_5N$

M.p. 185–6°C

An alkaloid occurring in *Haplophyllum* species, the base crystallizes from EtOH or MeOH as colourless prisms. It is laevorotatory with $[\alpha]_D - 73.1°$ (Me_2CO). It forms a crystalline hydrochloride, m.p. 170–1°C; nitrate, m.p. 148–150°C (*dec.*) and a methiodide, m.p. 212°C.

Yunusov., *J. Gen. Chem., USSR*, 25, 2009 (1955)

DUBIRHEINE

$C_{22}H_{23}O_6N$

M.p. 236–7°C

A minor alkaloid of *Papaver dubium*, the base has $[\alpha]_D^{24} + 236°$ and has been shown to be ethylrhoeagenine, previously prepared by treatment of Rhoeadine (q.v.) with absolute EtOH at room temperature. It has been suggested that this alkaloid may be formed by ethanolysis of rhoeadine during the working up of the natural material.

Slavik *et al., Collect. Czech. Chem. Commun.*, 30, 2464 (1965)

E

α-EARLEINE

This alkaloid was obtained from *Astralagus earlei* by Pease and Elderfield and later found in *A. wootoni*. It was subsequently shown to be betaine.

Pease, Elderfield., *J. Org. Chem.*, **5**, 192 (1940)
Stempel, Elderfield., *ibid*, **7**, 432 (1942)

β-EARLEINE

A second base isolated from *Astralagus earlei* and *A. wootoni*, this compound was later identified as choline.

Pease, Elderfield., *J. Org. Chem.*, **5**, 192 (1940)
Stempel, Elderfield., *ibid*, **7**, 432 (1942)

EBURCINE

$C_{23}H_{30}O_4N_2$

M.p. Indefinite

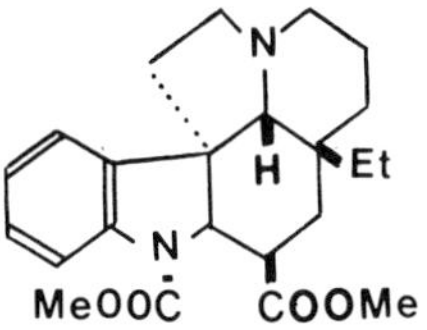

An amorphous alkaloid found in *Hunteria eburnea* Pichon, this base has not been obtained crystalline. It has $[\alpha]_D - 61°$ (c 1.0, CHCl$_3$). The ultraviolet spectrum exhibits two absorption maxima at 242 and 285 mμ. It contains two methoxycarbonyl groups and one ethyl group.

Olivier *et al.*, *Compt. Rend.*, **270C**, 1667 (1970)

EBURINE

$C_{21}H_{28}O_2N_2$

M.p. Indefinite

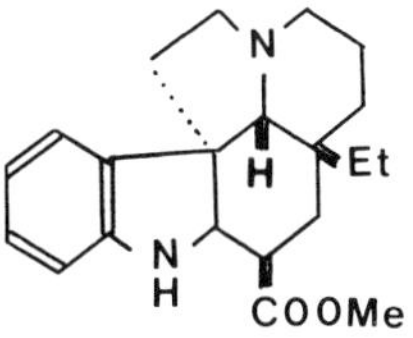

A further amorphous, non-crystallizable alkaloid obtained from *Hunteria eburnea* Pichon, this base has $[\alpha]_D - 18°$ (CHCl$_3$) and the ultraviolet spectrum shows two absorption maxima at 245 and 310 mμ. The N-methoxycarbonyl derivative is Eburcine (q.v.).

Olivier *et al.*, *Compt. Rend.*, **270C**, 1667 (1970)

EBURNAMENINE

$C_{19}H_{24}N_2$

M.p. Indefinite

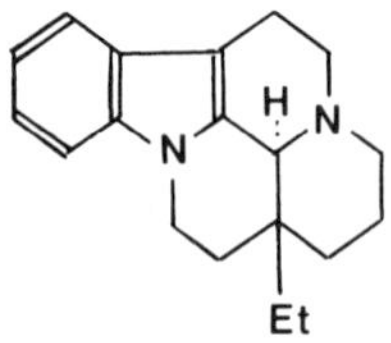

Also present in *Hunteria eburnea* Pichon, this alkaloid is amorphous but forms a crystalline methiodide, m.p. 274°C (*dec.*) and picrate, m.p. 186–196°C with $[\alpha]_D^{25} + 183°$ (CHCl₃). The absolute configuration has been determined by Trojanek *et al.*

Bartlett, Taylor, Raymond-Hamet., *Compt. rend.,* **249**, 1259 (1959)
Bartlett, Taylor., *J. Amer. Chem. Soc.,* **82**, 5941 (1960)
Trojanek, Koblicova, Blaha., *Chem. & Ind.,* 1261 (1965)

EBURNAMINE

$C_{19}H_{24}ON_2$

M.p. 181°C

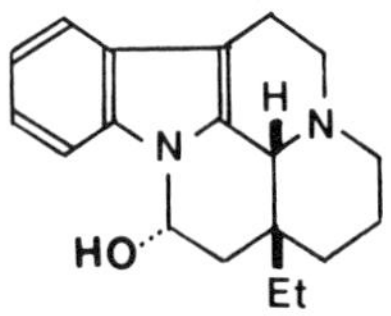

This alkaloid occurs in *Haplophyton cimicidum* and also in *Hunteria eburnea* Pichon. It is normally obtained as the monohydrate, m.p. 105–110°C; $[\alpha]_D^{26} - 93°$ (CHCl₃). The picrate is crystalline, melts at 152–166°C and again at 186°C after resolidifying. The O-methyl derivative is found in *H. cimicidum* (q.v.); the O-ethyl compound is also crystalline with m.p. 147–8°C; $[\alpha]_D + 64°$. The structure has been confirmed by the synthesis of the (±)-form.

Bartlett, Taylor, Raymond-Hamet., *Compt. rend.,* **249**, 1259 (1959)
Bartlett, Taylor., *J. Amer. Chem. Soc.,* **82**, 5941 (1960)
Cava *et al.*, *Chem. & Ind.,* 1242 (1963)

Synthesis:
Barton, Harley-Mason., *Chem. Commun.,* 298 (1965)

Absolute configuration:
Trojanek, Koblicova, Blaha., *Chem. & Ind.,* 1261 (1965)

EBURNAMONINE

$C_{19}H_{22}ON_2$

M.p. 183°C

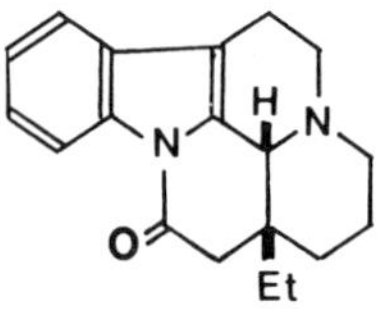

A constituent of *Hunteria eburnea* Pichon, this alkaloid has $[\alpha]_D^{26} + 89°$ (CHCl₃). It contains one carbonyl group and an ethyl group in the molecule. The (−)-form, although not occurring naturally is encountered as a degradation product of Vincamine (q.v.).

Bartlett, Taylor, Raymond-Hamet., *Compt. rend.*, **249**, 1259 (1959)
Bartlett, Taylor., *J. Amer. Chem. Soc.*, **82**, 5941 (1960)
Trojanek *et al.*, *Tetrhaedron Lett.*, 702 (1961)
Mokry *et al.*, *Collect. Czech. Chem. Commun.*, **28**, 1309 (1963)
Trojanek, Koblicova, Blaha., *Chem. & Ind.*, 1261 (1965)

(±)-EBURNAMONINE

See Vincanorine

EBURNAPHYLLINE

$C_{21}H_{24}O_4N_2$

M.p. 237°C

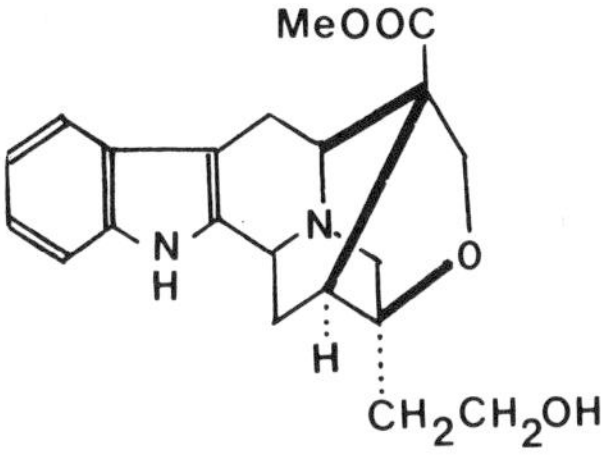

The leaves of *Hunteria eburnea* Pichon contain this alkaloid which is obtained as colourless crystals from EtOH or MeOH. It contains one methoxycarbonyl group and a hydroxyethyl group. The monoacetate is also crystalline with m.p. 215°C. The structure and absolute configuration have been determined by correlation with akuammidine and polyneuridine.

Morfaux, Olivier, Le Men., *Bull. Soc. Chim. Fr.*, 3967 (1971)
Morfaux *et al.*, *Tetrahedron Lett.*, 1939 (1973)

ECBOLINE

This basic product was obtained from the mycelia of *Claviceps purpurea* by Wenzell together with ergotine. Recent work indicates that it is identical with ergometrine (q.v.).

Wenzell., *Amer. J. Pharm.*, **36**, 193 (1864)

ECHINATINE

$C_{15}H_{25}O_5N$

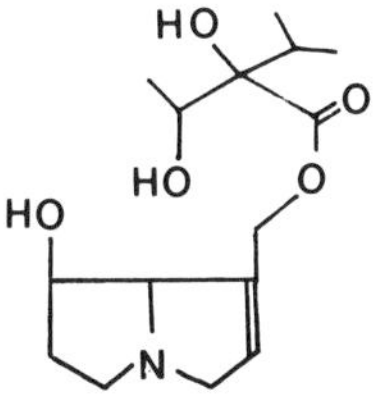

A pyrrolizidine alkaloid present in *Eupatorium maculatum* L. and *Rindera*

501

echinata, this base is an oil which forms a crystalline methopicrate as yellow needles, m.p. 153–5°C and a picrolonate, m.p. 214–6°C. When hydrolyzed with aqueous NaOH it yields heliotridine and viridifloric acid. Catalytic reduction over Pt furnishes hydroxyheliotridane and viridifloric acid.

Men'shikov, Kuzuvkov., *J. Gen. Chem. USSR,* **19**, 1702 (1949)
Men'shikov, Denisova., *Sbornik Statei Obshchei Khim.,* **2**, 1458 (1953)
Warren, Klemperer., *J. Chem. Soc.,* 4574 (1958)
Tsuda, Marion., *Can. J. Chem.,* **41**, 1919 (1963)

ECHINOPSEINE

This uncharacterized alkaloid has been obtained from the seeds of *Echinops Ritro.* It does not appear to have been examined further since its original isolation.

Greshoff., *Rec. trav. Chim.,* **19**, 360 (1900)

ECHINOPSINE

$C_{10}H_9ON$

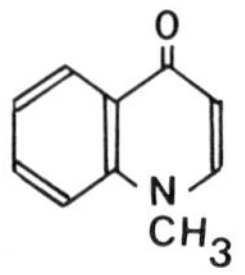

Also present in the seeds of *Echinops Ritro,* this alkaloid forms colourless crystals from EtOH. It forms a crystalline hydrochloride, m.p. 185–6°C; platinichloride, m.p. 210–2°C and a picrate, m.p. 223–4°C. The base, shown to be N-methyl-γ-quinolone, is freely soluble in EtOH, $CHCl_3$ and H_2O but only sparingly so in Et_2O.

Greshoff., *Rec. trav. Chim.,* **19**, 360 (1900)
Späth, Kolbe., *Monatsh.,* **43**, 469 (1923)

ψ-ECHINOPSINE

M.p. 135°C

This uncharacterized alkaloid has also been isolated from the seeds of *Echinops Ritro.* It forms colourless crystals from EtOH.

Greshoff., *Rec. trav. Chim.,* **19**, 360 (1900)

ECHINORINE

$C_{11}H_{12}ON^+$

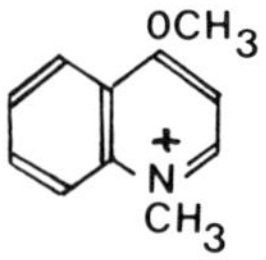

Isolated from the fruit of *Echinops Ritro* and *E. sphaerocephalus* as the crystalline perchlorate, m.p. $251-3°C$, the latter has been shown by synthesis and its ultraviolet spectrum to be 1-methyl-4-methoxyquinolinium perchlorate. The synthesis employs quinoline as the starting material.

Schreoder, Luckner., *Arch. Pharm.*, **301**, 39 (1968)

ECHITAMIDINE

$C_{20}H_{22}O_3N_2$

M.p. $244°C$ (*dec.*).

A minor alkaloid of *Alstonia congensis* and *A. scholaris,* the base was assigned the formula $C_{20}H_{26}O_3N_2$ by Goodson who also showed that the ultraviolet spectrum is almost identical with that of akuammicine (q.v.). The empirical formula was later modified to that given above by Chatterjee and Ghosal. The alkaloid crystallizes from moist Et_2O in rosettes of hexagonal plates, m.p. $135°C$ with softening at $122°C$. The anhydrous form has the m.p. given above. It is a monoacidic base with $[\alpha]_D^{16} - 515°$ (EtOH). The hydrochloride forms colourless prisms of the tetrahydrate, m.p. $179°C$ (*dec. dry*); the hydrobromide, m.p. $181°C$ (*dec.*); the sulphate, rosettes of needles with 11 H_2O, m.p. $169°C$ (*dec. dry*) and the picrate, m.p. $226-7°C$.

The alkaloid is not catalytically hydrogenated over prereduced PtO_2 but the acetate, m.p. $220°C$, may be reduced with Zn and HCl and dihydroechitamidine obtained therefrom. Rationalization of the fragmentation formed by mass spectrometry of both the alkaloid and the dihydro derivative, combined with NMR evidence, indicate that the hydroxyl group is situated in the side chain and not in the nucleus.

Goodson., *J. Chem. Soc.*, 2628 (1932)

Chatterjee, Ghosal., *Naturwiss.*, **48**, 219 (1961)

Djerassi *et al., Tetrahedron Lett.*, 653 (1962)

ECHITAMINE

$C_{22}H_{28}O_4N_2^+$

M.p. $206°C$

This alkaloid is the major constituent of the bark of *Alstonia congensis.* The free base is said to have been obtained by Hesse as a crystalline tetrahydrate which loses 3 H_2O at $100°C$, forming a stable monohydrate with $[\alpha]_D^{20} - 28.8°$ (EtOH). The hydrochloride forms short, colourless prisms of the monohydrate when crystallized slowly from H_2O with m.p. 292°C or as long anhydrous needles when crystallized rapidly, m.p. 195°C (dec.); $[\alpha]_D^{15} - 58°$ (H_2O); the hydrobromide occurs in colourless prisms of the monohydrate, m.p. 183°C or 268°C (dec. dry); the sulphate, monohydrate decomposes from 275°C; $[\alpha]_D^{15} - 51.6°$ (H_2O) and the picrate, dihydrate, has m.p. 98°C. The alkaloid also yields several crystalline derivatives, e.g. the diacetate, which yields a hydrochloride, m.p. 271°C (dec.); the nitroso-derivative, yellow needles, m.p. 157°C (dec.) and a dinitro-compound in the form of minute red needles, m.p. 184°C (dec. dry).

The alkaloid contains one methylimino group and one methoxyl group. The latter is present as a methoxycarbonyl group since any attempt to produce free echitamine results in the formation of demethylechitamine, $C_{21}H_{26}O_4N_2$, m.p. 268°C (dec. dry) which yields a hydrochloride as colourless prisms, m.p. 306°C (dec.). The salts of demethylechitamine are acid to litmus whereas those of the alkaloid itself are neutral.

Harnack., Ber., 13, 1648 (1880)
Hesse., Annalen, 203, 144 (1880)
Bacon., Phil. J. Sci., 1, 1007 (1906)
Goodson., J. Chem. Soc., 127, 1640 (1925)
Birch et al., Proc. Chem. Soc., 62 (1961)
Govindachari, Rajappa., Tetrahedron, 16, 132 (1961)
Hamilton et al., Proc. Chem. Soc., 63 (1961)
Hamilton et al., J. Chem. Soc., 5061 (1962)
Manohar, Ramseshan., Tetrahedron Lett., 814 (1961)

ECHITENINE

$C_{20}H_{27}O_4N$

According to Hesse, this alkaloid accompanies echitamine in the bark of *Alstonia scholaris* and *A. spectabilis*. It is, however, a very ill-defined product and may be a mixture of alkaloids.

Hesse., Annalen, 203, 144 (1880)

ECHITOVENALDINE

$C_{24}H_{30}O_5N_2$

M.p. Indefinite

COOMe

This amorphous alkaloid occurs in *Alstonia venenata*. The base contains one methoxyl group. The structure has been determined from chemical degradation and infrared, NMR and mass spectrometry.

Majumder, Chanda, Dinda., Chem. & Ind., 21, 1032 (1973)

ECHITOVENIDINE

$C_{26}H_{32}O_4N_2$

M.p. 162–3°C

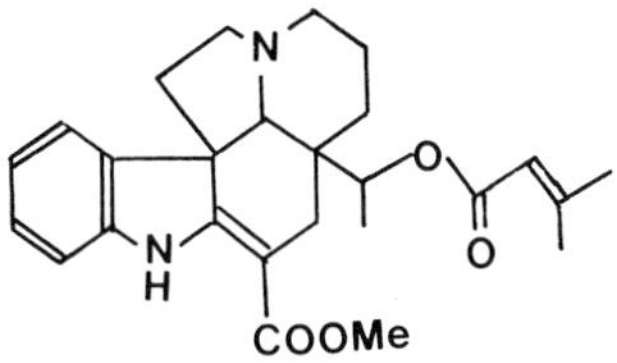

A further alkaloid isolated from *Alstonia venenata,* this alkaloid is laevorotatory with $[\alpha]_D - 580°$ (CHCl$_3$). The ultraviolet spectrum has absorption maxima at 219, 302 and 327 mμ.

Das, Biemann, Chatterjee, Ray, Majumder., *Tetrahedron Lett.,* 2483 (1966)

ECHITOVENINE

$C_{23}H_{28}O_4N_2$

M.p. 168–170°C

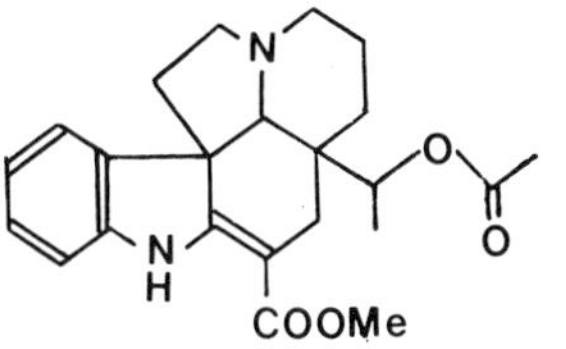

Also present in *Alstonia venenata,* this alkaloid is dextrorotatory with $[\alpha]_D^{30} + 640°$ (CHCl$_3$). The ultraviolet spectrum has absorption maxima at 228, 298 and 328 mμ. The structure has been determined mainly from spectroscopic data.

Das, Biemann, Chatterjee, Ray, Majumder., *Tetrahedron Lett.,* 2239 (1965)

ECHIUMINE

$C_{20}H_{31}O_6N$

M.p. 99–100°C

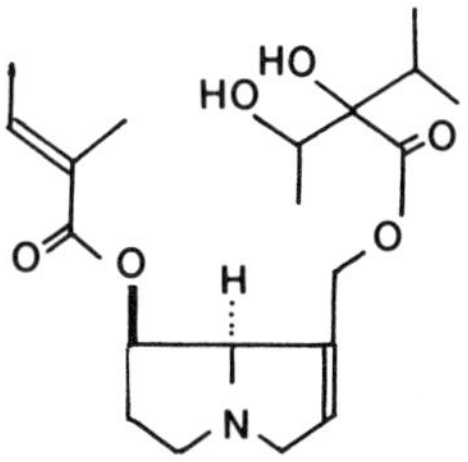

A pyrrolizidine alkaloid present in the leaves of *Amsinckia intermedia* Fisch. & Mey and *Echium plantagineum* L. The base is obtained in the form of colourless needles from light petroleum and has $[\alpha]_D + 14.4°$ (c 2.02, EtOH). The crystalline picrate forms yellow prisms from aqueous EtOH, m.p. 131–2°C. Alkaline hydrolysis furnishes retronecine, angelic acid and trachelanthic acid.

Culvenor., *Austral. J. Chem.,* **9**, 512 (1956)
Culvenor, Smith., *ibid,* **19**, 1955 (1966)

EDPETILIDINE

$C_{27}H_{45}O_2N$

M.p. 269–271°C

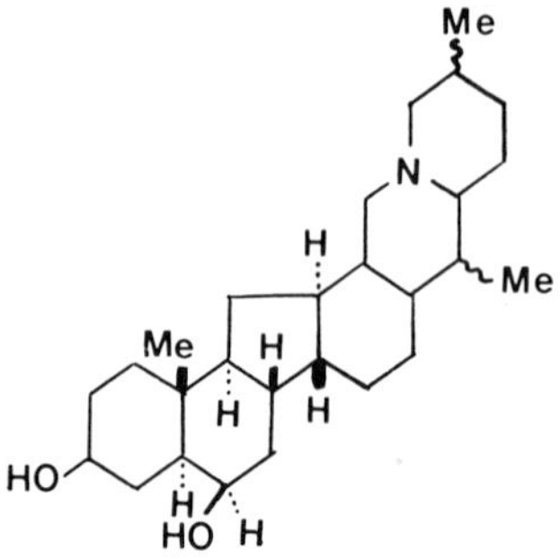

A steroidal alkaloid of *Petilium eduardi,* this base crystallizes from MeOH as colourless needles. It is dextrorotatory with $[\alpha]_D + 42.48°$ (c 0.306, EtOH) and gives a hydrochloride, m.p. 283°C (*dec.*) and a hydrobromide, m.p. 281–2°C. The structure, as cevan-3:5-diol, has been determined from the infrared and NMR spectra of the O-acetate.

Shakirov, Nuriddinov, Yunusov., *Khim. Prir. Soedin., Akad. Nauk. Uzbek. SSR,* **6,** 384 (1965)

Nuriddinov, Yunusov., *Khim. Prir. Soedin.,* **5,** 333 (1969)

EDPETILINE

$C_{33}H_{53}O_8N$

M.p. 272–6°C

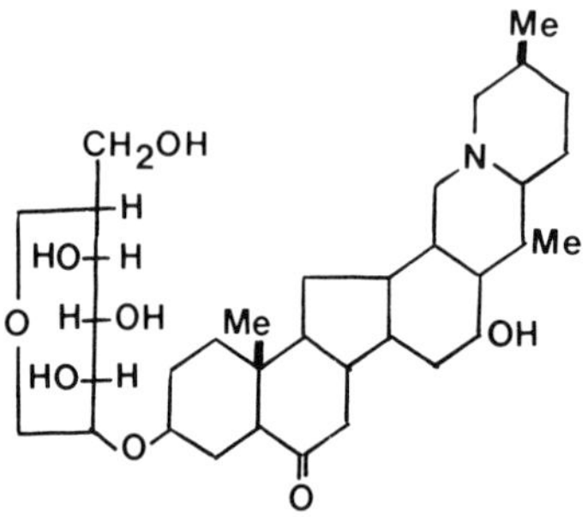

An alkaloid occurring in *Petilium eduardi,* this base forms colourless needles from MeOH. It has $[\alpha]_D - 57.89°$ (c 0.449, MeOH). The hydrochloride forms colourless prisms from Me_2CO, m.p. 220°C; the hydrobromide has m.p. 226°C; the hydriodide, m.p. 228°C; the oxime, m.p. 259–262°C (*dec.*) and the tetraacetate, m.p. 224–6°C. The position of the hydroxyl group in the nucleus has not yet been firmly established.

Shakirov, Nuriddinov, Yunusov., *Uzbeksk. Khim. Zh.,* **9,** 38 (1965)

EDPETINE

$C_{27}H_{41}O_4N$

M.p. 314–5°C

Petilium eduardi also yields this steroidal alkaloid which forms colourless crystals from EtOH. It contains two hydroxyl groups, three methyl groups and one exocyclic methylene group in the molecule.

Nuriddinov, Yunusov., *Khim. Prir. Soedin.*, **5**, 603 (1969)

EDULININE

$C_{16}H_{21}O_4N$

M.p. 140–2°C

Isolated from the bark of *Casimiroa edulis* Llave et Lex., this alkaloid forms colourless plates when crystallized from AcOEt. The ultraviolet spectrum has absorption maxima at 228, 274, 282 and 324 mμ. The structure has been determined from the NMR and mass spectra.

Iriarte *et al.*, *J. Chem. Soc.*, 4170 (1956)
Toube, Murphy, Cross., *Tetrahedron*, **23**, 2061 (1967)

EDULITINE

$C_{11}H_{11}O_3N$

M.p. 235–6°C

The trunk bark of *Casimiroa edulis* Llave et Lex. yields this alkaloid which has been shown to be 4:8-dimethoxycarbostyril. The alkaloid is best crystallized from AcOEt when it forms fine, colourless needles. The ultraviolet spectrum exhibits absorption maxima at 222, 248, 280 and 320 mμ.

The picrate forms minute yellow needles when crystallized from MeOH, m.p. 189–191°C and the N-acetyl derivative has m.p. 200–201°C. The base has been synthesized from *o*-anisidine and malonic acid in the presence of POCl₃ to give 4-hydroxy-8-methoxycarbostyril which is then esterified with CH₂N₂ in MeOH.

Iriarte *et al.*, *J. Chem. Soc.*, 4170 (1956)

Synthesis:
Kappe, Ziegler., *Tetrahedron Lett.*, 1947 (1968)
Venturella, Bellino, Piozzi., *Chim. Ind.* (Milan), **50**, 451 (1968)
Narasimhan, Alurkar., *Chem. & Ind.*, 515 (1968)

Spectra:
Toube, Murphy, Cross., *Tetrahedron*, **23**, 2061 (1967)

EFIRINE

$C_{34}H_{32}O_4N_2$

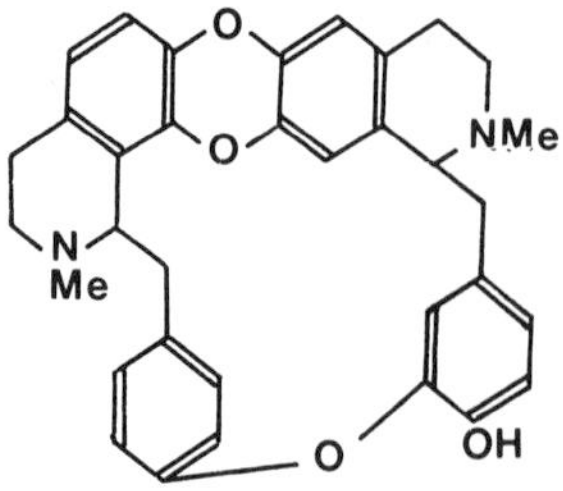

This alkaloid has recently been isolated from *Triclisia gilletii*. The structure has been determined from spectroscopic evidence and the fact that O-methylation yields isotrilobine.

Huls, Detry., *Bull. Soc. Roy. Sci. Liege*, **42**, 73 (1973)

ELAEOCARPIDINE

$C_{17}H_{21}N_3$

M.p. 229–230°C

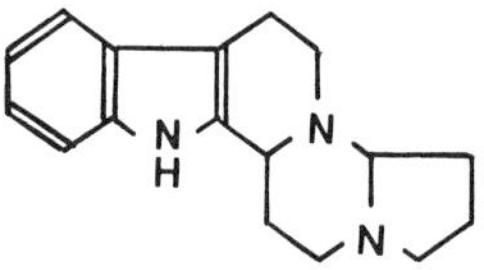

The major constituent of the leaves of *Elaeocarpus archboldianus* A.C. Sm. This base is optically inactive and the ultraviolet spectrum shows absorption maxima at 226, 283 and 290 mμ the latter being present as an inflexion on the spectrum.

Johns, Lamberton, Sioumis., *Chem. Commun.*, 410 (1968)

Stereochemistry:
Gribble., *J. Org. Chem.*, **35**, 1944 (1970)

ELAEOCARPILINE

$C_{16}H_{21}O_2N$

M.p. 165–6°C

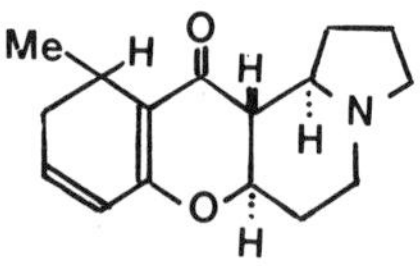

This alkaloid occurs in the leaves of *Elaeocarpus dolichostylis* Schl. It is dextrorotatory with $[\alpha]_D + 395°$ (CHCl$_3$). The ultraviolet spectrum exhibits absorption maxima at 221 and 323 mμ with aninflexion at 241 mμ. The base has been shown to be 15:16-dihydroelaeocarpine.

Johns, Lamberton, Sioumis., *Chem. Commun.*, 1324 (1968)

Absolute configuration:
Johns *et al.*, *Chem. Commun.*, 804 (1970)

508

epiallo-ELAEOCARPILINE

$C_{16}H_{21}O_2N$

M.p. 136–7°C

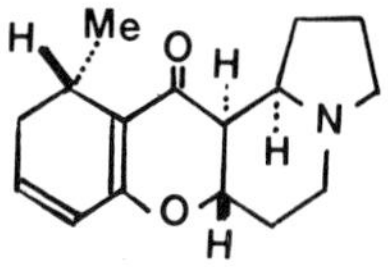

Found in *Elaeocarpus sphaericus*, this alkaloid has $[\alpha]_D$ + 139° ($CHCl_3$) and the ultraviolet spectrum shows absorption maxima at 228, 239 and 325 mμ.

Johns *et al., Chem. Commun.*, 804 (1970)

epi-ELAEOCARPILINE

$C_{16}H_{21}O_2N$

M.p. 70–4°C

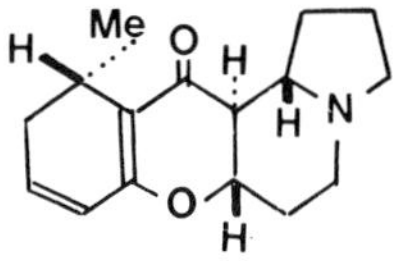

A further stereoisomeric alkaloid from *Elaeocarpus sphaericus*, this base has $[\alpha]_D$ − 396° ($CHCl_3$).

Johns *et al., Chem. Commun.*, 804 (1970)

ELAEOCARPINE

$C_{16}H_{19}O_2N$

M.p. 81–2°C

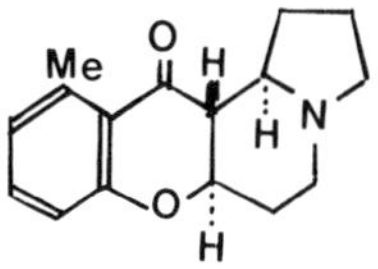

Isolated from the leaves of *Elaeocarpus polydactylus* Schl., this base has only a small optical rotation of $[\alpha]_D$ + 0.1° ($CHCl_3$). From the values obtained, however, this rotation appears to be real and not due to experimental error.

Johns *et al., Chem. Commun.*, 290 (1968)

Total synthesis:
Tanaka, Iijima., *Tetrahedron Lett.*, 3963 (1970)

ELAEOKANIDINE A

$C_{12}H_{20}ON_2$

M.p. 38–38.5°C

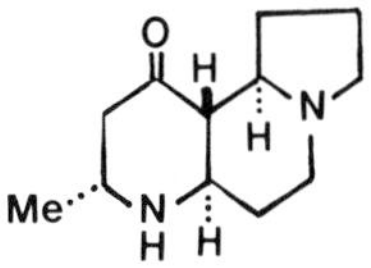

This low-melting alkaloid occurs in *Elaeocarpus kaniensis* Schltr. and forms colourless crystals. It is dextrorotatory with $[\alpha]_D$ + 90° ($CHCl_3$). It forms a crystalline dipicrate, m.p. 153–5°C.

Hart, Johns, Lamberton., *Chem. Commun.*, 460 (1971)

ELAEOKANIDINE B

$C_{12}H_{20}ON_2$

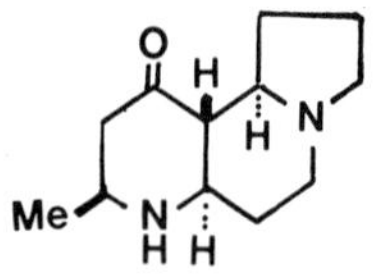

A further alkaloid isolated from *Elaeocarpus kaniensis* Schltr. This base is optically inactive in $CHCl_3$.

Hart, Johns, Lamberton., *Chem. Commun.*, 460 (1971)

ELAEOKANIDINE C

$C_{12}H_{20}ON_2$

M.p. 56–8°C

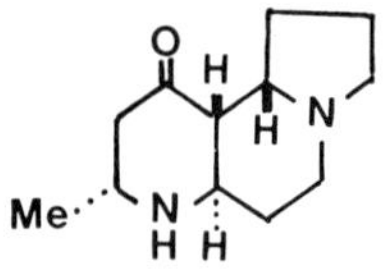

Elaeocarpus kaniensis Schltr. also yields this alkaloid which is stereoisomeric with the two preceding bases. It has $[\alpha]_D + 1°$ ($CHCl_3$).

Hart, Johns, Lamberton., *Chem. Commun.*, 460 (1971)

ELAEOKANINE A

$C_{12}H_{19}ON$

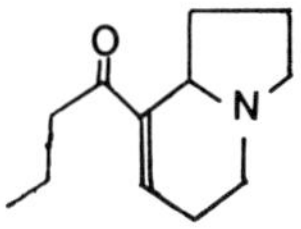

A hexahydroindolizine alkaloid present in *Elaeocarpus kaniensis* Schltr., this base is a colourless oil which has $[\alpha]_D + 13°$ ($CHCl_3$). The ultraviolet spectrum exhibits one absorption maximum at 229 mμ. The crystalline picrate has m.p. 163–5°C.

Hart, Johns, Lamberton., *Chem. Commun.*, 460 (1971)

ELAEOKANINE B

$C_{12}H_{21}ON$

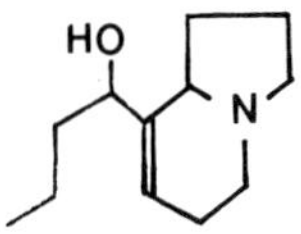

Also present in *Elaeocarpus kaniensis* Schltr. This alkaloid is closely related to the preceding base. The structure is identical with the exception that here the carbonyl group in the side chain has been reduced to a secondary alcoholic group. The alkaloid forms a colourless gum which cannot be crystallized. It has $[\alpha]_D - 72°$ ($CHCl_3$).

Hart, Johns, Lamberton., *Chem. Commun.*, 460 (1971)

ELAEOKANINE C

$C_{12}H_{21}O_2N$

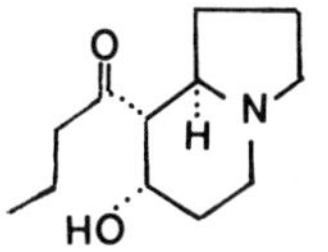

A third closely-related alkaloid from *Elaeocarpus kaniensis* Schltr. this alkaloid is also a colourless, non-crystallizable gum. It is laevorotatory with $[\alpha]_D - 14°$ (CHCl$_3$). The structure has been shown to be 8-butyryl-7-hydroxyindolizidine.

Hart, Johns, Lamberton., *Chem. Commun.*, 460 (1971)

ELAEOKANINE D

$C_{12}H_{19}O_2N$

M.p. 76–8°C

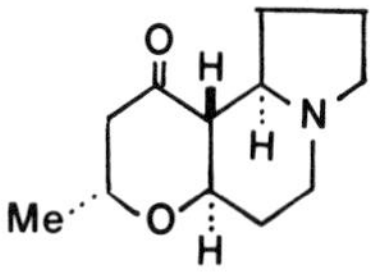

A crystalline alkaloid obtained from *Elaeocarpus kaniensis* Schltr. this alkaloid has $[\alpha]_D + 51°$ (CHCl$_3$).

Hart, Johns, Lamberton., *Chem. Commun.*, 460 (1971)

ELAEOKANINE E

$C_{12}H_{19}O_2N$

M.p. 57–8°C

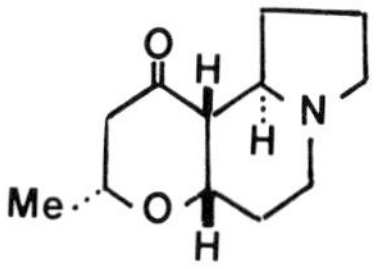

A stereoisomer of the preceding base, this alkaloid also occurs in *Elaeocarpus kaniensis* Schltr. It is dextrorotatory with $[\alpha]_D + 35°$ (CHCl$_3$).

Hart, Johns, Lamberton., *Chem. Commun.*, 460 (1971)

ELATINE

$C_{38}H_{50}O_{10}N_2$

M.p. 233–5°C

An aconite alkaloid obtained from *Delphinium elatum*, the base forms colourless crystals from either MeOH or EtOH. It has $[\alpha]_D + 3.4°$ (CHCl$_3$). The alkaloid forms crystalline salts, e.g. the hydrochloride m.p. 180–210°C (*dec.*) and the perchlorate, m.p. 175–200°C (*dec.*). Alkaline hydrolysis yields elatidine and elatinic acid. The former crystallizes from Me$_2$CO with m.p. 172–

4°C and forms crystalline salts and derivatives: hydrobromide as the hemihydrate, m.p. 206–207.5°C; hydriodide, m.p. 197–198.5°C. With phloroglucinol and HCl it yields lycoctonine. Elatinic acid, m.p. 154–5°C may be further hydrolyzed with dilute HCl to give anthranilic acid and methylsuccinic acid, thereby establishing its constitution as methylsuccinylanthranilic acid.

Rabinovitch., *J. Gen. Chem., USSR*, **24**, 2242 (1954)
Kuzovkov., *ibid*, **25**, 422 (1955)
Kuzovkov, Platonova., *ibid*, **29**, 2782 (1959)

ELATRINE

$C_{40}H_{56}O_6N_3$

M.p. 180–3°C (*dec.*).

This alkaloid is found in *Thabitrum minus* var. *elatum*. It is obtained as colourless needles from EtOH and is dextrorotatory with $[\alpha]_D^{26} + 229°$ (EtOH). It forms a crystalline picrate with m.p. 174–5°C (*dec.*) and an amorphous picrolonate, m.p. 178–182°C (*dec.*).

Nakajima., *J. Pharm. Soc., Japan*, **65B**, 422 (1945)

ELDELIDINE

$C_{27}H_{41}O_8N$

M.p. 184°C

An atisine type alkaloid isolated from *Delphinium elatum* and subsequently discovered in *D. dictylocarpum*. The structure is not yet known with certainty.

Narzullaev, Yunusov, Yunusov., *Khim. Prir. Soedin.*, **8**, 498 (1972)

ELEAGNINE

$C_{12}H_{14}N_2$

M.p. 180–181.5°C

A constituent of the bark of several species of *Eleagnus*, this alkaloid forms colourless crystals which are sparingly soluble in H_2O but readily so in most organic solvents. The crystalline hydrochloride has m.p. 253–254.5°C. When heated slowly, the base sublimes below its melting point.

Massagetov., *J. Gen. Chem., USSR*, **16**, 139 (1946)
Men'shikov *et al.*, *ibid*, **20**, 1927 (1950)

ELEGANTINE

$C_{23}H_{28}O_6N_2$

M.p. 202–4°C

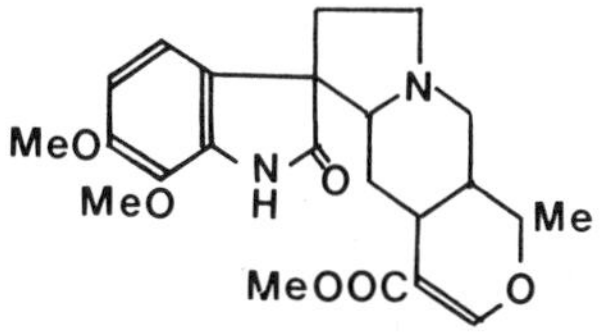

One of the numerous *Vinca* alkaloids, this base has been isolated from *V. elegantissima* Hort. The ultraviolet spectrum of the solution in EtOH shows one absorption maximum at 228 mμ. The alkaloid contains two methoxyl groups, one methyl and one methoxycarbonyl group in the molecule. The structure given has been established from chemical and spectroscopic data.

Bhattacharya, Pakrashi., *Tetrahedron Lett.*, 159 (1972)

ELLIPTAMINE

$C_{24}H_{30}O_5N_2$

M.p. Indefinite

This alkaloid, obtained from the leaves and root bark of *Ochrosia* species, particularly from *O. poweri* Bailey, is unstable to light and air. The picrate is obtained as the monohydrate from aqueous MeOH, m.p. 170°C (*dec.*) and in the anhydrous form from absolute MeOH has m.p. 215–7°C (*dec.*).

Doy, Moore., *Austral. J. Chem.*, 15, 548 (1962)
Douglas *et al., ibid,* 17, 246 (1964)

ELLIPTICINE

$C_{17}H_{14}N_2$

M.p. 311–5°C (*dec.*).

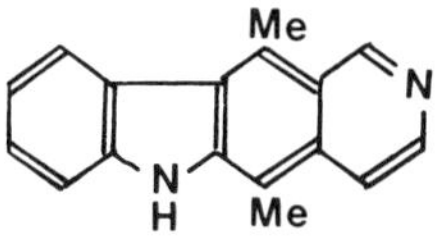

A highly unsaturated alkaloid found in *Ochrosia elliptica* Labill., the base forms orange rods when crystallized from CHCl$_3$ or AcOEt and light yellow needles from MeOH. The crystalline methiodide decomposes at 355–360°C.

Goodwin, Smith, Horning., *J. Amer. Chem. Soc.*, 81, 1903 (1959)
Woodward, Jacobucci, Hochstein., *ibid,* 81, 4434 (1959)
Buccli, Mayo, Hochstein., *Tetrahedron,* 15, 167 (1961)
Cranwell, Saxton., *J. Chem. Soc.*, 3482 (1962)
Govindachari, Rajappa, Sudaranam., *Ind. J. Chem.*, 1, 247 (1963)
Synthesis:
Dalton *et al., Austral. J. Chem.*, 20, 2715 (1967)

ELLIPTICINE METHONITRATE

$C_{18}H_{17}O_3N_3$

M.p. 293–304°C (dec.).

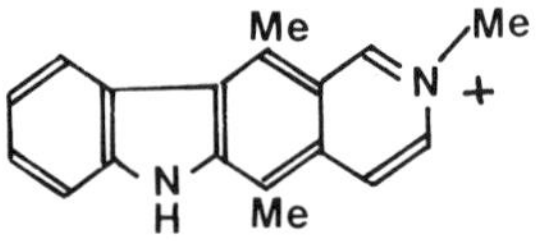

A minor component of *Aspidosperma subincanum*, this alkaloid forms colourless crystals which melt over a wide range of temperature.

Goodwin, Smith, Horning., *J. Amer. Chem. Soc.*, **81**, 1903 (1959)
Woodward, Jacobucci, Hochstein., *ibid*, **81**, 4434 (1959)

ELLIPTININE

$C_{20}H_{24}O_2N_2$

M.p. 231–2°C

This alkaloid occurs in *Ochrosia elliptica* Labill. It is strongly laevorotatory with $[\alpha]_{589}^{24} - 255°$ and $[\alpha]_{436}^{24} - 593°$ (c 0.2, MeOH). The ultraviolet spectrum in EtOH has a broad maximum at 311 mμ with a shoulder at 272 mμ. On acidification with HCl there is a slight hypsochromic shift to 308 mμ. The alkaloid is very soluble in C_6H_6, $CHCl_3$ and AcOEt, slightly soluble in EtOH or MeOH and insoluble in H_2O.

Goodwin, Smith, Horning., *J. Amer. Chem. Soc.*, **81**, 1903 (1959)

ELWESINE (*Dihydrocrinine*)

$C_{16}H_{19}O_3N$

M.p. 218–9°C

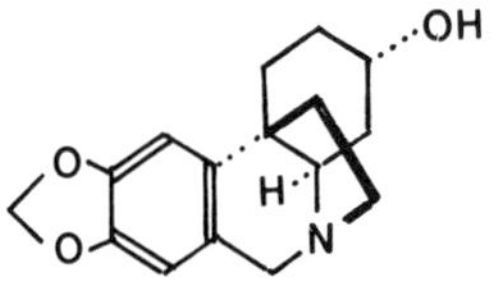

Present in *Galanthus elwesi* Hook, this alkaloid is laevorotatory with $[\alpha]_D^{25} - 32°$ (c 0.4, $CHCl_3$). It contains one methylenedioxy group and one hydroxyl group. The O-acetate is crystalline with m.p. 149–150°C. The above structure has been confirmed by synthesis.

Boit, Döpke., *Naturwiss.*, **48**, 406 (1961)
Synthesis:
Stevens, DuPree, Loewenstein., *J. Org. Chem.*, **37**, 977 (1972)

ELYMOCLAVINE

$C_{16}H_{18}ON_2$

M.p. 250–2°C (*dec.*).

One of the ergot alkaloids, this base is present in the mycelia of *Claviceps purpurea* which has *Elymus mollis* as its host. It forms colourless prisms when recrystallized from a wide variety of solvents. The alkaloid is laevorotatory with $[\alpha]_D^{20} - 152°$ (c 1.0, pyridine) or $- 59°$ (c 0.1, EtOH). The mode of biosynthesis of this alkaloid has been studied by Preininger and his colleagues.

Abe *et al., J. Agr. Chem. Soc., Japan,* **25**, 458 (1952)
Yamatodani, Abe., *Bull. Agr. Chem. Soc., Japan,* **19**, 94 (1955)
Stoll *et al., Helv. Chim. Acta,* **37**, 1815 (1954)
Hofmann *et al., ibid,* **40**, 1358 (1957)

Biosynthesis:
Preininger, Fischer, Liede., *Annalen,* **672**, 223 (1964)

EMETAMINE

$C_{29}H_{36}O_4N_2$

M.p. 153–4°C

One of the Ipecacuanha alkaloids present in the roots of *Psychotria ipecacuanha,* this base forms colourless needles when crystallized from AcOEt. If it is formed in Et_2O from its salts, however, it crystallizes with 0.5 mole of solvent and then has m.p. 138–9°C or 142–3°C (*dry*). It has $[\alpha]_D^{20} + 13.6°$ (EtOH) and is insoluble in H_2O or alkalies, sparingly soluble in Et_2O but readily so in most other organic solvents.

The hydrochloride forms glistening needles from dilute HCl with 8.5 H_2O, m.p. 77–80°C or 218–223°C (*dry*); $[\alpha]_D - 17.5°$ (H_2O); the hydrobromide heptahydrate forms colourless prismatic needles, m.p. 210–215°C (*dry*); the hydriodide, microscopic needles, m.p. 274°C with frothing; the nitrate (dihydrate) has m.p. 165–6°C; the hydrogen oxalate forms a trihydrate, m.p. 172°C (*dec.*); $[\alpha]_D - 6.1°$ (H_2O) and the picrate softens at 147°C gradually melting up to 173°C.

The (±)-form crystallizes from Et_2O, m.p. 132–3°C and forms a crystalline oxalate, m.p. 168–9°C (*dec.*). The alkaloid contains four methoxyl groups and both nitrogen atoms are tertiary. With Fröhde's reagent it gives a deep emerald-green colour.

Pyman., *J. Chem. Soc.,* **111**, 428 (1917)
Brindley, Pyman., *ibid,* 1067, 1071 (1927)
Karrer, Eugster, Rüttner., *Helv. Chim. Acta,* **31**, 1219 (1948)
Battersby, Davidson, Turner., *J. Chem. Soc.,* 3899 (1961)

EMETINE

$C_{29}H_{40}O_4N_2$

M.p. 74°C

The principal constituent of the roots of *Cephaelis ipecacuanha,* this alkaloid is also present in *C. acuminata* Karsten. Fries has also stated that the alkaloid may be found in certain Rubiaceous species which are not normally regarded as sources of this and related alkaloids, while the roots of *Bourreria verticillata* contain 0.1 per cent of alkaloids including emetine but not cephaeline. Dultz has shown that ipecacuanha seed from plants grown in Nicaragua contain this alkaloid and Wagenaar has demonstrated that in the roots of these plants, the alkaloids are to be found in the peripheral cells just beneath the cork.

The alkaloid forms an amorphous powder and has $[\alpha]_D - 25.8°$ (c 1.8, 50% EtOH) or $- 50°$ (CHCl$_3$). It is readily soluble in CHCl$_3$, EtOH or Et$_2$O, less so in C$_6$H$_6$ or light petroleum and only sparingly soluble in H$_2$O. It is somewhat sensitive to light. The hydrochloride forms colourless needles of the heptahydrate from hot H$_2$O or thick prisms from concentrated, cold solutions, m.p. 235–55°C (*dry*); $[\alpha]_D + 11°$ (c 1.0, H$_2$O) or $+ 53°$ (CHCl$_3$); the hydrobromide tetrahydrate forms slender, colourless needles, m.p. 250–260°C; $[\alpha]_D + 12°$ (c 1.4, H$_2$O); the hydriodide, trihydrate, crystallizes from EtOH in colourless needles, m.p. 235–8°C; the nitrate forms a trihydrate which sinters at 188°C and gradually melts up to 245°C and the sulphate heptahydrate has m.p. 205–245°C and in extremely soluble in H$_2$O. The platinichloride is amorphous with m.p. 253–265°C although a lower figure of 213–7°C (*dec.*) has been given for this salt. The aurichloride has m.p. 127–9°C and the N-acetyl derivative, m.p. 97–9°C.

When emetine is fully methylated with MeI it furnishes a mixture of α- and β-N-methylemetine methiodides with m.p. 225–6°C and 262°C respectively which both give the same N-methylemetinemethine (oxalate m.p. 82–3°C) indicating that the methiodides are stereoisomeric. Gentle oxidation with iodine in EtOH yields O-methylpsychotrine while more vigorous oxidation by boiling with FeCl$_3$ furnishes rubremetine (dehydroemetine) which may be isolated as the hydrochloride (rubremetinium chloride) in brilliant scarlet needles of the hexahydrate, m.p. 127–8°C or 166–173°C (*dry*).

Oxidation with KMnO$_4$ in Me$_2$CO yields 6:7-dimethoxy*iso*quinoline-1-carboxylic acid and *meta*hemipinic acid thereby confirming the presence of an *iso*quinloine nucleus in this, and the closely related, alkaloids. The observation that oxidation with a faintly alkaline solution of KMnO$_4$ yields 1-keto-6:7-

dimethoxy-1:2:3:4-tetrahydroisoquinoline (corydaldine) implies the presence of a second isoquinoline nucleus in the molecule, this containing the secondary nitrogen atom.

Emetine is sometimes employed as an emetic, and in small doses as an expectorant although for the latter purposes it is more common to use ipecacunha itself or one of its galenical preparations. The chief use for the alkaloid is as a remedy for amoebic dysentry owing to its direct toxic action on *Entamoeba histolytica*.

Pelletier, Magendie., *Ann. Chim. Phys.*, **4**, 172 (1817)
Pelletier, Magendie., *ibid*, **24**, 180 (1823)
Paul, Cownley., *Pharm. J.*, **25**, 111, 373, 641, 690 (1894–5)
Carr, Pyman., *J. Chem. Soc.*, **105**, 1599 (1914)
Dultz., *Pharm. Zentr.*, **75**, 598 (1934)
Fries., *Pharm. Zent.*, **36**, 223 (1935)
Wagenaar., *Pharm. Weekbl.*, **72**, 513 (1935)
Orazi., *Rev. facultad. cienc. quim.*, **19**, 17 (1946)

Synthesis:
Szantay, Töke, Kolonits., *J. Org. Chem.*, **31**, 1447 (1966)

Absolute configuration:
Battersby, Binks, Davidson., *J. Chem. Soc.*, 2704 (1959)
Battersby, Garratt., *ibid*, 3512 (1959)

Pharmacology:
Dobell *et al.*, *Parasitology*, **20**, 207 (1928)
Fischl, Schlossberger., *Handb. Chemother.*, 224 (1932)
Sapeika., *S. Afr. J. Med.*, **2**, 10 (1937)
Manson-Bahr., *Brit. Med. J.*, 255 (1941)
Boyd, Scharf., *J. Pharm. exp. Ther.*, **71**, 362 (1941)
Kile, Welch., *Arch. Dermat. Syphilol.*, **45**, 550 (1942)
Jones., *Brit. J. Pharmacol.*, **2**, 217 (1947)
Goodwin, Hoare, Sharp., *ibid*, **3**, 44 (1948)

EMILINE

$C_{19}H_{27}O_6N$

M.p. 105–7°C

A pyrrolizidone alkaloid isolated from *Emilia flammea* Cass., the base forms colourless needles when crystallized from Et_2O. It has $[\alpha]_D^{20} - 13.1°$ ($CHCl_3$). The alkaloid forms crystalline salts and derivatives, e.g. the hydrochloride as colourless needles from EtOH, m.p. 248–251°C and the methiodide, colourless needles from MeOH-AcOEt, m.p. 194–7°C.

Kohlmuenzer, Tomczyk, Saint-Firmin., *Diss. Pharm. Pharmacol.*, **23**, 419 (1971)

Tomczyk, Kohlmuenzer., *Herba. Pol.*, **17**, 226 (1971)

EPHEDRINE

$C_{10}H_{15}ON$

M.p. 38.1°C

The major alkaloid isolated from *Ephedra* species, this base occurs in *Ephedra sinica* Stapf., *E. helvetica* C.A. Meyer, *E. equisetina* and in five species indigenous to India, namely *E. foliata* Boiss., *E. gerardiana* Wall, *E. intermedia* Schrenk and Mayer, *E. nebrodensis* Tineo and *E. pachyclada* Boiss.

The alkaloid usually occurs in the anhydrous form with the melting point given above although it may be obtained as the hemihydrate, m.p. 40°C; b.p. 225°C. It has $[\alpha]_D^{20} - 6.3°$ (EtOH) or $+ 11.2°$ (H_2O). The hydrochloride forms colourless needles, m.p. 217–8°C or 220–1°C (*corr.*); $[\alpha]_D - 34°$ (H_2O); the hydrobromide, m.p. 205°C; the sulphate as hexagonal plates, m.p. 243°C; $[\alpha]_D^{22} - 30°$ (H_2O); the oxalate, prismatic needles, m.p. 249°C (*dec.*); the aurichloride, m.p. 128–131°C; the platinichloride, yellow needles, m.p. 186°C (*dec.*); the dibenzoyl derivative, m.p. 134°C and the nitrosamine, m.p. 92°C.

When boiled with 25 per cent HCl, the alkaloid is partially changed into pseudoephedrine which crystallizes from Et_2O in colourless rhombs, m.p. 118–9°C; $[\alpha]_D^{20} + 51.2°$ (EtOH) and is, unlike ephedrine itself, only sparingly soluble in H_2O. The hydrochloride has m.p. 181–2°C; $[\alpha]_D^{20} + 62.05°$ (H_2O); the oxalate, m.p. 218°C (*dec.*) and the aurichloride, m.p. 126.5–127.5°C. The nitroso-derivative has m.p. 86°C and the dibenzoyl compound, m.p. 119–120°C. The conversion of ephedrine into pseudoephedrine is reversible with an equilibrium mixture of the two bases being formed.

The accepted formula for the alkaloid was first suggested by Ladenburg and Oelschägel who found that on oxidation, under certain conditions, benzoic acid and methylamine is produced. Support for this structure was provided by Schmidt and Bümming who found that the hydrochlorides of ephedrine and pseudoephedrine, when distilled in CO_2 yield methylamino hydrochloride and propiophenone. *dl*-Ephedrine has been resolved into its optically active components by treatment with D-arabonic acid or D-arabonolactone.

Ephedrine was originally employed as a mydriatic until 1924 when Chen and Schmidt reported its similarity to adrenaline in pharmacological action. Its properties in this respect resemble those of other sympathomimetic amines, namely dilatation of the pupil, a rise in arterial blood pressure, contraction of the plain muscle of the orbit, inhibition of the rhythm and tone of the muscular walls of mammalian intestine and the production of saliva and tears which are not readily abolished by atropine.

The mydriatic action of *l*-ephedrine is greater than that of *d*-ephedrine and the same is true of its pressor action in pithed cats. According to Schultz, the alkaloid exerts some local anaesthetic effect.

Merck., *Merck's Jahresb.*, 1 (1888)
Ladenburg, Oelschägel., *Ber.*, **22**, 1823 (1889)
Miller., *Arch. Pharm.*, **240**, 481 (1902)
Schmidt., *ibid*, 244, **239**, 251 (1906)
Emde., *ibid*, **245**, 662 (1907)
Schmidt, Bümming., *ibid*, **247**, 141 (1909)
Chen, Schmidt., *Proc. Soc. Exp. Biol. Med.*, **21**, 351 (1924)
Chavezt., *Bol. Soc. Quim. Peru.*, **3**, 198 (1937)
Mitchell., *J. Chem. Soc.*, 1153 (1940)

Pharmacology:
Chen, Schmidt., *J. Pharm. Exp. Ther.*, **24**, 339 (1924)
Gaddum., *Brit. Med. J.*, 713 (1938)
Schultz., *J. Pharm. exp. Ther.*, **70**, 283 (1940)
Kole, Ergang., *Arch. exp. Path. Pharm.*, **199**, 577 (1942)

(−)-EPIBAPTIFOLINE

$C_{15}H_{20}O_2N_2$

M.p. 215°C

An alkaloid of *Retama sphaerocarpa*, this base is separated from the accompanying alkaloids by chromatography of the picrates. It has $[\alpha]_D^{21} - 138.88°$ and the ultraviolet spectrum has two absorption maxima at 234 and 308 mμ. Several crystalline salts are known including the hydrochloride monohydrate, m.p. 270°C; $[\alpha]_D - 165.28°$ (H$_2$O); hydrobromide, m.p. 208°C; $[\alpha]_D^{20} - 137.40°$ (H$_2$O); hydriodide, m.p. 250−280°C (*dec.*); perchlorate, m.p. 276−7°C; $[\alpha]_D^{16} - 123.84°$ (H$_2$O) and the picrate dihydrate, m.p. 250°C. Partialy hydrogenation with PtO$_2$ as catalyst in AcOH gives (−)-epihydroxylupanine, m.p. 192−3°C; $[\alpha]_D^{23} - 57.5°$ (EtOH).

Bohlmann *et al.*, *Chem. Ber.*, **95**, 944 (1962)

EPICEPHALOTAXINE

$C_{18}H_{21}O_4N$

M.p. 136−7°C

This alkaloid has been isolated from *Cephalotaxus fortunei* and has $[\alpha]_D^{35} - 150°$ (c 0.8, CHCl$_3$). The structure of this minor base has been determined from spectroscopic data.

Paudler, McKay., *J. Org. Chem.*, **38**, 2110 (1973)

(+)-14-EPICORYNOLINE

$C_{21}H_{21}O_5N$

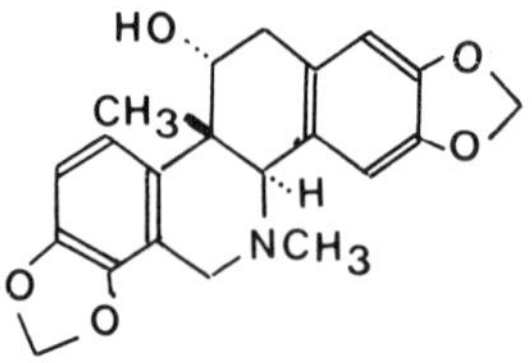

A minor constituent of *Corydalis incisa*, this base has only recently been isolated. The structure has been established from chemical and spectroscopic determinations. No salts or derivatives have yet been reported.

Takao, Bersch, Takao., *Chem. Pharm. Bull.*, 21, 1096 (1973)

EPIELWESINE

$C_{16}H_{19}O_3N$

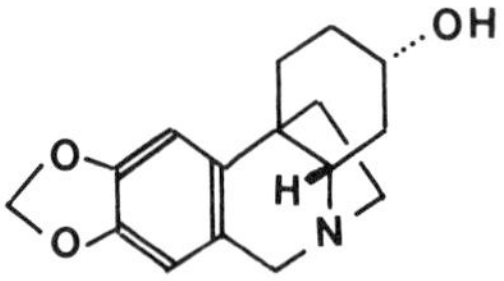

This spimer of Elwesine (q.v.) occurs in small quantities in *Galanthus elwesi* Hook. It has been synthesized from piperonyl cyanide and 1:2-dibromoethane with lithium amide in a six-stage synthesis which gives an overall yield of the base of 65 per cent.

Stevens, Velman, DuPree., *J. Chem. Soc.*, 1585 (1970)

EPIGUAIPYRIDINE

$C_{15}H_{21}N$

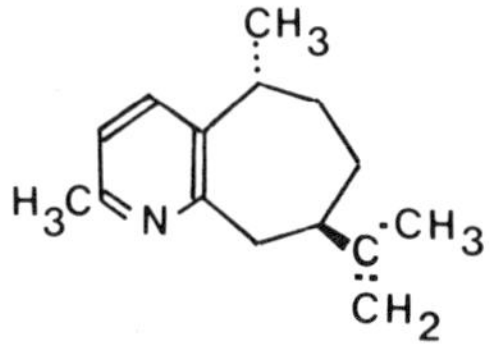

An oily alkaloid obtained from Patchouli oil (*Pogostemon patchouli* Pellet). The base is laevorotatory with $[\alpha]_D^{25.5} - 34.5°$ (c 2.69, EtOH). The ultraviolet spectrum exhibits absorption maxima at 270 mμ with shoulders at 215, 273 and 278 mμ. The alkaloid forms a crystalline perchlorate as wax-like plates from Et_2O-MeOH, m.p. 105–105.5°C; $[\alpha]_D^{29} - 17°$ (c 8.0, MeOH).

Büchi, Goldman, Mayo., *J. Amer. Chem. Soc.*, 88, 3109 (1966)

EPIIBOGAMINE

$C_{19}H_{24}N_2$

M.p. 194–6°C

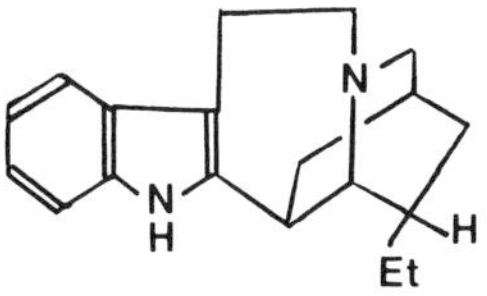

A minor constituent of *Tabernanthe iboga,* this base forms colourless needles from EtOH. The structure has been determined from chemical and spectroscopic evidence, comparison with ibogamine, and confirmed by total synthesis of the (±)-form. The base contains an ethyl group and one imino group, the second nitrogen atom being tertiary.

Ban *et al., Tetrahedron Lett.,* 3383 (1968)

3-EPINUPHAMINE

$C_{15}H_{23}O_2N$

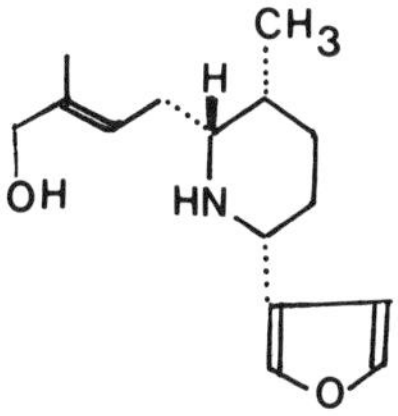

This alkaloid has recently been isolated from *Nuphar luteum* subsp. variegatum. The structure has been determined from the infrared, NMR and mass spectra.

Wong, LaLonde., *Phytochem.,* **9,** 1851 (1970)

3-EPINUPHARAMINE

$C_{15}H_{25}O_2N$

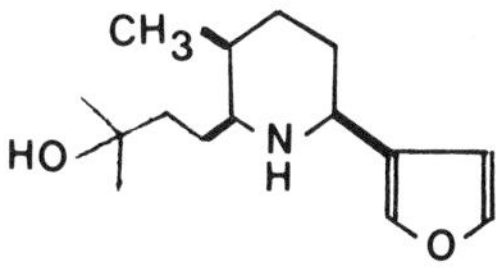

A pale yellow oil isolated from *Nuphar luteum* subsp. *variegatum,* this base is laevorotatory with $[\alpha]_D^{23} - 24.8°$ (c 1.45, MeOH). Its ultraviolet spectrum shows one absorption maximum at 263 mμ. The picrolonate is crystalline with m.p. 83–5°C and the alkaloid also forms a crystalline N-acetyl derivative, m.p. 107–9°C.

Forrest, Ray., *Can. J. Chem.,* **49,** 1774 (1971)

521

EPIPACHYSAMINE B

$C_{29}H_{45}ON_3$

M.p. 260–2°C

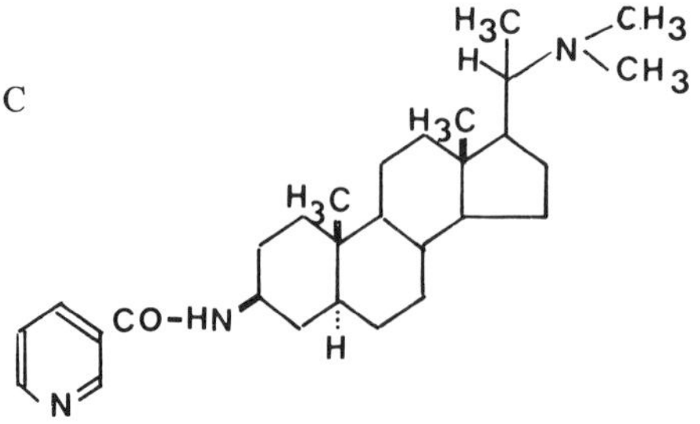

One of a series of steroidal alkaloids occurring in *Pachysandra terminalis* Sieb. et Zucc. This base is dextrorotatory with $[\alpha]_D + 16°$ (CHCl$_3$). It should be noted that this alkaloid is not epimeric with Pachysamine B (q.v.), nor are it and the four alkaloids following, epimers. The name is therefore somewhat misleading in this respect.

Kikuchi, Uyeo, Nishinaga., *Tetrahedron Lett.*, 1993 (1965)

EPIPACHYSAMINE C

$C_{23}H_{46}N_2$

M.p. 242–3°C

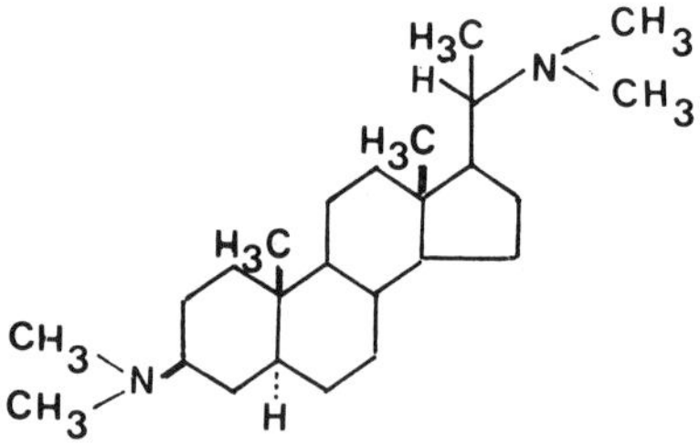

Also present in *Pachysandra terminalis* Sieb. et Zucc., this pregnane alkaloid has $[\alpha]_D − 16°$ (CHCl$_3$). The structure 3β:20α-bisdimethylamino-5α-pregnane has been established by chemical and spectroscopic data.

Kikuchi, Uyeo, Nishinga., *Tetrahedron Lett.*, 1993 (1965)

EPIPACHYSAMINE D

$C_{30}H_{46}ON_2$

M.p. 245–8°C

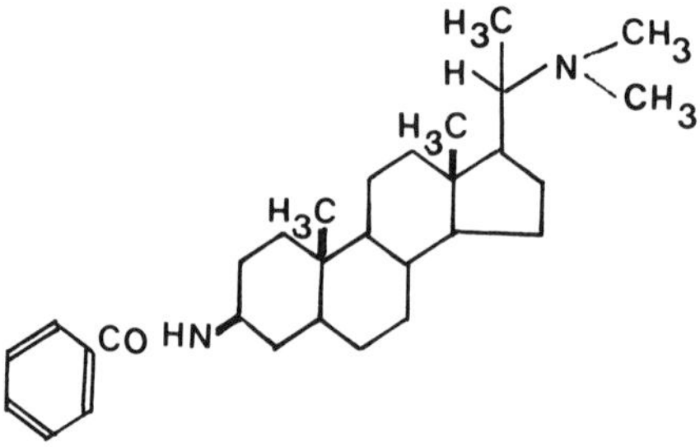

Pachysandra terminalis Sieb. et Zucc. also yields this pregnane base which has

522

$[\alpha]_D + 13°$ (CHCl$_3$). It contains a dimethylamino and also a benzoylamino group and on alkaline hydrolysis yields chonemorphine.

Kikuchi, Uyeo, Nishinga., *Tetrahedron Lett.*, 3169 (1965)

EPIPACHYSAMINE E

C$_{28}$H$_{48}$ON$_2$

M.p. 210–2°C

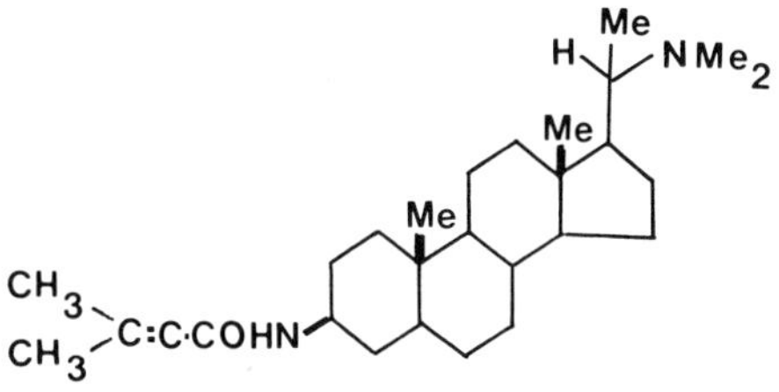

A fourth in the series of closely-related pregnane alkaloids obtained from *Pachysandra terminalis* Sieb. et Zucc., this base also yields chonemorphine on alkaline hydrolysis. It is dextrorotatory with $[\alpha]_D + 20°$ (CHCl$_3$).

Kikuchi, Uyeo, Nishinga., *Tetrahedron Lett.*, 3169 (1965)

EPIPACHYSAMINE F

C$_{23}$H$_{42}$N$_2$

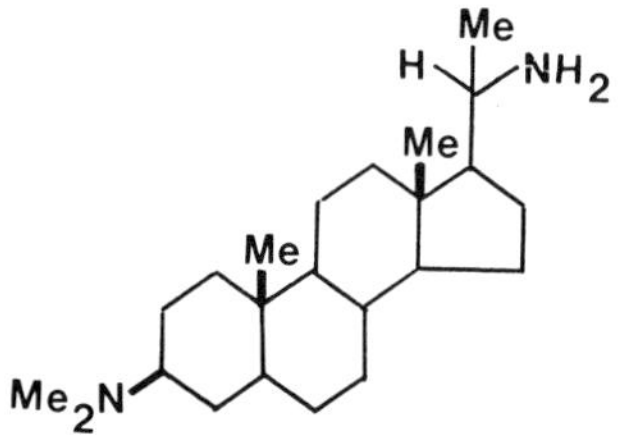

This base is isomeric with Epipachysamine C and is also present in *Pachysandra terminalis* Sieb. et Zucc. It forms an N-acetyl derivative with m.p. 250–3°C; $[\alpha]_D + 6°$ (CHCl$_3$).

Kikuchi, Uyeo, Nishinga., *Tetrahedron Lett.*, 3169 (1965)

EPIPACHYSANDRINE A

C$_{30}$H$_{46}$O$_2$N$_2$

M.p. > 295°C

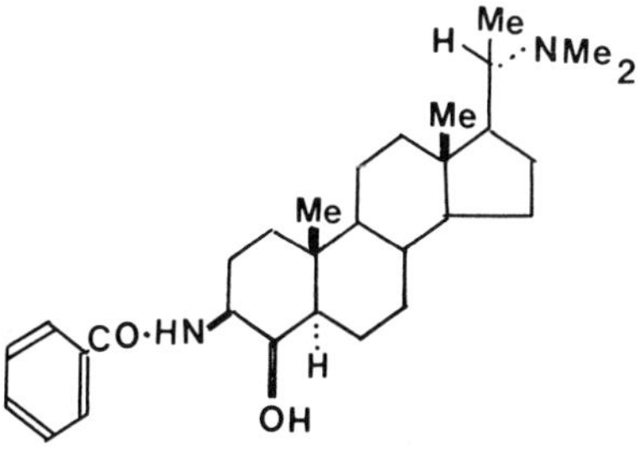

This alkaloid occurs in small amounts in *Pachysandra terminalis* Sieb. et Zucc.

and is a high-melting solid. It has $[\alpha]_D + 12°$ (1:1-MeOH-CHCl$_3$). It contains a dimethylamino group, a benzoylamino group and a hydroxyl group in the molecule, the latter capable of acetylation to yield the O-acetate, m.p. 280–5°C; $[\alpha]_D + 21°$ (CHCl$_3$).

Kikuchi, Uyeo, Nishinga., *Tetrahedron Lett.,* 1749 (1966)

EPIVINCADINE

$C_{21}H_{28}O_2N_2$

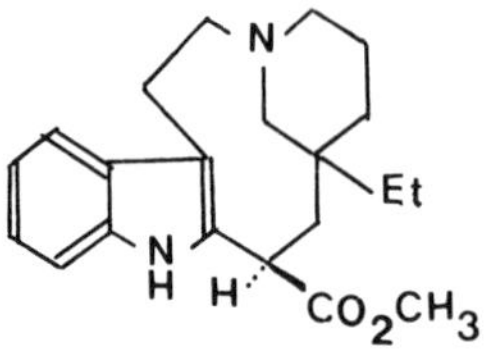

This epimer of Vincadine (q.v.) has recently been discovered in *Amsonia tabernaemontana.* The structure follows from the NMR and mass spectra.

Zsadon, Tamas, Szilasi., *Chem. Ind.,* 5, 229 (1973)

1β,2β-EPOXY-1α-HYDROXYMETHYL-8α-PYRROLIZIDINE

$C_8H_{13}O_2N$

M.p. 66–7°C;
B.p. 80°C/0.04 mm

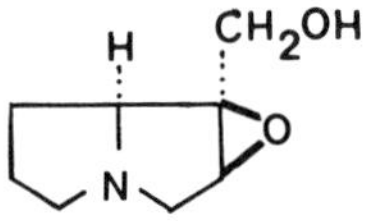

One of two simple bases occurring in *Crotalaria trifoliastrum* Willd. and *C. aridicola* Domin., this alkaloid crystallizes from Me$_2$CO in colourless prisms. It is laevorotatory with $[\alpha]_D^{20} - 60.1°$ (c 2.2, EtOH). It forms a crystalline picrate with m.p. 173–4°C; $[\alpha]_D^{20} - 8.0°$ (c 4.97, Me$_2$CO). The methyl ether (q.v.) also occurs naturally.

Culvenor, O'Donovan, Smith., *Austral. J. Chem.,* **20**, 757 (1967)

EPOXYKOPSINONE

$C_{21}H_{22}O_3N_2$

M.p. 123–4°C

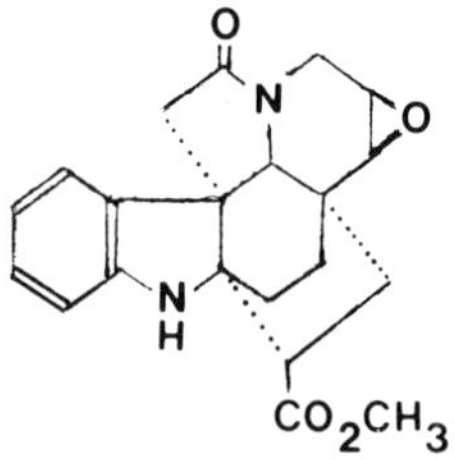

An alkaloid of *Vinca erecta,* the base is purified by thin-layer chromatography and identified by infrared, ultraviolet, NMR and mass spectrometry.

Rakhimov *et al., Khim. Prir. Soedin.,* 5, 677 (1971)

1β,2β-EPOXY-1α-METHOXYMETHYL-8α-PYRROLIZIDINE

$C_9H_{15}O_2N$

B.p. 53°C/0.1 mm

This alkaloid is a colourless oil obtained from *Crotalaria aridicola* Domin. and *C. trifoliastrum* Willd. It is laevorotatory having $[\alpha]_D^{18} - 63°$ (c 1.08, EtOH) and forms crystalline salts and derivatives, e.g. the hydrochloride, m.p. 232–4°C; picrate, m.p. 166–8°C and the picrolonate, m.p. 164–5°C.

Culvenor *et al.*, *Austral. J. Chem.*, **16**, 131 (1963)
Culvenor, O'Donovan, Smith., *ibid*, **20**, 757 (1967)

21:22-α-EPOXY-N-METHYL-*sec*-PSEUDOBRUCINE

$C_{24}H_{28}O_6N_2$

M.p. 239–241°C

This alkaloid was first isolated from the leaves of *Strychnos icaja* Baill. as Alkaloid C. The base is obtained as colourless hexagonal plates from MeOH. It has $[\alpha]_D + 12°$ (c 1.09, $CHCl_3$) and the ultraviolet spectrum shows absorption maxima at 215.5, 265 and 301 mμ. The structure has been established on the basis of chemical and spectroscopic data. The alkaloid undergoes an unusual *cis*-opening of the epoxy ring, on treatment with refluxing AcOH to yield the dihydroxy compound which is also obtained from novacine by hydroxylation with osmium tetroxide in pyridine. It appears that the stereochemistry of the epoxide ring is responsible for the *cis*-opening, probably there also being anchimeric aid from the oxygen in the seven-membered ring.

Jaminet., *J. Pharm. Belg.*, **8**, 449 (1953)
Bisset., *Tetrahedron Lett.*, 3107 (1968)

ERGOBASINE

See Ergometrine

ERGOCLAVINE

This compound, isolated from *Claviceps purpurea* by Kussner, has been shown to be an equimolecular mixture of ergosine and ergosinine.

Kussner., *Arch. Pharm.*, **272**, 503 (1934)

ERGOCORNINE

$C_{31}H_{39}O_5N_5$

M.p. 182–4°C (*dec.*).

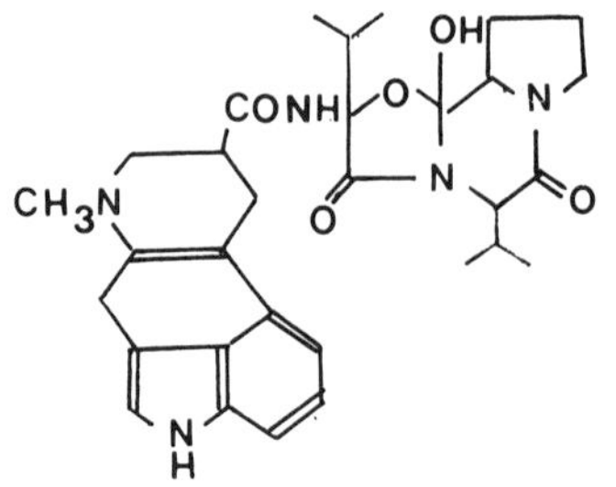

This ergot alkaloid was first prepared by Stoll and Hofmann by the fractional crystallization of the di-(*p*-toluoyl-)-(−)-tartrates of commercial ergotoxine. It forms colourless polyhedra when crystallized from MeOH and has $[\alpha]_D^{20} - 188°$ (CHCl$_3$) or − 105° (pyridine). The base forms a series of crystalline salts and derivatives including the hydrochloride, m.p. 223°C (*dec.*); hydrobromide, m.p. 225°C (*dec.*); phosphate, m.p. 190–5°C; ethanesulphonate, m.p. 209°C (*dec.*) and the di-*p*-toluoyl hydrogen (−)-tartrate, m.p. 180–1°C (*dec.*); $[\alpha]_D^{20} + 103°$ (c 0.2, EtOH).

Stoll, Hofmann., *Helv. Chim. Acta,* **26**, 1570 (1943)
Stoll, Hofmann, Petrzilka., *ibid,* **34**, 1544 (1951)

ERGOCORNININE

$C_{31}H_{39}O_5N_5$

M.p. 228°C (*dec.*).

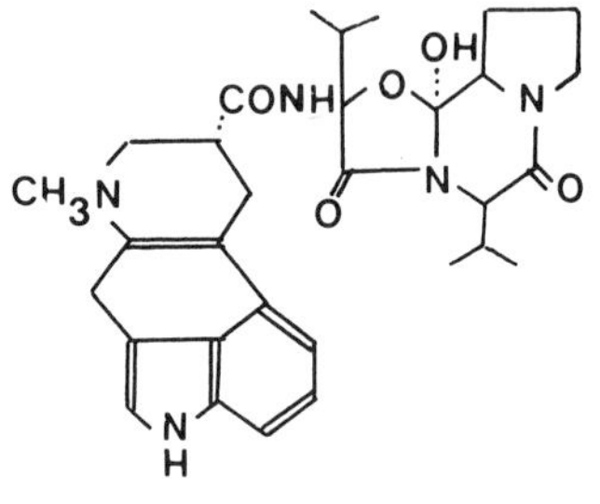

This alkaloid occurs as a minor constituent of *Claviceps purpurea* but is best obtained from ergocornine on standing in aqueous alcoholic KOH. It crystallizes from boiling aqueous EtOH in massive prisms and has $[\alpha]_D^{20} + 409°$ (c 1.0, EtOH).

Stoll, Hofmann., *Helv. Chim. Acta,* **26**, 1570 (1943)
Stoll, Hofmann, Petrzilka., *ibid,* **34**, 1544 (1951)

ERGOCRISTINE

$C_{35}H_{39}O_5N_5$

M.p. 165–170°C (*dec.*).

One of the alkaloids of *Claviceps purpurea*, this base was isolated by Stoll and Burckhardt from the double compound with Ergocristinine (q.v.) which has m.p. 172–5°C (*dec.*); $[\alpha]_D^{20} + 105°$ (c 0.92, CHCl$_3$), as the hydrochloride. The free base crystallizes from Me$_2$CO as colourless prisms with 1 mole of solvent and has $[\alpha]_D^{20} - 183°$ (c 1.0, CHCl$_3$). It has also been obtained from commercial ergotoxine as the di-(*p*-toluoyl-)-(−)-tartrate, m.p. 191°C (*dec.*); $[\alpha]_D^{20} + 58°$ (c 0.2, EtOH). The hydrochloride has m.p. 205°C; $[\alpha]_D^{20} + 105.7°$ (c 0.2, EtOH); the phosphate, m.p. 195°C (*dec.*); the tartrate, m.p. 185–190°C and the ethanesulphonate, m.p. 207°C (*dec.*). On boiling with MeOH, the alkaloid is converted into its isomeride Ergocristinine (q.v.).

Stoll, Burckhardt., *Zeit. Physiol. Chem.,* **250,** 1 (1937)
Stoll, Burckhardt., *ibid,* **251,** 287 (1938)
Stoll, Hofmann., *Helv. Chim. Acta,* **26,** 1570 (1943)
Stoll, Hofmann, Petrzilka., *ibid,* **34,** 1544 (1951)

ERGOCRISTININE

$C_{35}H_{39}O_5N_5$

M.p. 214°C (*dec.*).

A further ergot alkaloid obtained from *Claviceps purpurea*, this base is also produced by the action of boiling MeOH on ergocristine. It has $[\alpha]_D^{20} + 366°$ (c 1.0, CHCl$_3$) and is reconverted into ergocristine by boiling with 1 per cent phosphoric acid in EtOH. Unlike most of the ergot alkaloid it possesses little physiological action.

Stoll, Burckhardt., *Z. Physiol. Chem.,* **250,** 1 (1937)
Stoll, Burckhardt., *ibid,* **251,** 287 (1938)
Stoll, Hofmann, Petrzilka., *Helv. Chim. Acta,* **34,** 1544 (1951)

α-ERGOCRYPTINE (*Ergokryptine*)

$C_{32}H_{41}O_5N_5$

M.p. 212–4°C

This alkaloid of *Claviceps purpurea* occurs together with ergotoxine and was originally named ergocryptine until the recent discovery of its isomeride β-ergocryptine (q.v.). The alkaloid crystallizes in colourless prisms from MeOH or boiling C_6H_6 and has $[\alpha]_D^{20} - 187°$ (c 1.0, $CHCl_3$). It forms crystalline salts and derivatives, e.g. the hydrochloride, m.p. 208°C (*dec.*); phosphate, m.p. 198–200°C (*dec.*); tartrate, m.p. 209°C (*dec.*); ethanesulphonate, m.p. 204°C (*dec.*) and the di-(p-toluoyl-)-l-tartrate, m.p. 186°C (*dec.*); $[\alpha]_D^{20} + 103°$ (c 0.2, EtOH). On boiling in MeOH it is converted into its ergotinine analogue, ergocryptinine (q.v.). The structure of the alkaloid has been confirmed by synthesis.

Stoll, Hofmann., *Helv. Chim. Acta*, **26**, 1570 (1943)
Stoll, Hofmann, Petrzilka., *ibid*, **34**, 1544 (1951)

Synthesis:
Stadler *et al.*, *Helv. Chim. Acta*, **52**, 1549 (1969)

β-ERGOCRYPTINE

$C_{32}H_{41}O_5N_5$

M.p. 174–7°C (*dec.*).

An isomer of α-ergocryptine from *Claviceps purpurea*, this alkaloid is separated from the former base by chromatography on dimethyl phthalate impregnated paper as the stationary phase using 20 per cent formamide and 80 per cent citrate buffer as the mobile phase. The natural base is laevorotatory with $[\alpha]_D^{20} - 174°$ (c 1.5, $CHCl_3$) and its ultraviolet spectrum in MeOH exhibits one absorption maximum at 312 mμ. Alkaline hydrolysis yields lysergic acid, proline, leucine, ammonia and dimethylpyruvic acid. Catalytic hydrogenation gives the 9:10-dihydro derivative, m.p. 194–5°C (*dec.*); $[\alpha]_D^{20} - 31°$ (pyridine). Epimerization furnishes the (+)-form, m.p. 220°C (*dec.*); $[\alpha]_D^{20} + 492°$ (pyridine) or + 424° ($CHCl_3$). The structure has been determined from infrared and NMR data and confirmed by synthesis.

528

Schlientz *et al.*, *Experientia,* **23**, 991 (1967)

Synthesis:

Stadler *et al.*, *Helv. Chim. Acta,* **52**, 1549 (1969)

ERGOCRYPTININE

$C_{32}H_{41}O_5N_5$

M.p. 240–2°C (*dec.*).

It has not yet been firmly established that this alkaloid occurs naturally in *Claviceps purpurea*. It is formed by the action of alcoholic alkalies or boiling MeOH on α-ergocryptine. It forms colourless prisms from EtOH and has $[\alpha]_D^{20} + 408°$ (CHCl$_3$) or $+ 396°$ (Me$_2$CO).

Stoll, Hofmann., *Helv. Chim. Acta,* **26**, 1570 (1943)

ERGOMETRINE

$C_{19}H_{23}O_2N_3$

M.p. 162–3°C (*dec.*).

One of the major alkaloids of *Claviceps purpurea*, this base has been described under various names before its common identity was recognised, e.g. ergobasine, ergoclinine, ergonovine, ergostetrine, ergotocine and ergotrate. It is one of the simpler of the ergot alkaloids having the structure of (+)-lysergic-(+)-β-hydroxy-*iso*propylamide. The base crystallizes as prisms from MeEtCO or needles from C_6H_6 with 1 mole of solvent in each case. From AcOEt it may be obtained in the anhydrous form, m.p. 160–1°C (*dec.*) by crystallization at − 4°C. From Me$_2$CO, Grant and Smith have obtained a second, more stable form, m.p. 212°C (*dec.*) into which the other forms pass on long standing. The alkaloid has $[\alpha]_D^{20} + 91°$ (H$_2$O), − 44° (CHCl$_3$) or + 42.2° (c 1.7, EtOH). It is somewhat unstable, darkening in air.

The hydrochloride forms colourless needles, m.p. 245–6°C (*dec.*); $[\alpha]_D^{25} + 63°$ (H$_2$O); the hydrobromide, needles, m.p. 236–7°C (*dec.*); the oxalate, m.p. 193°C (*dec.*); $[\alpha]_D + 55.4°$ (H$_2$O), while the picrate exists in two interconvertible forms, a hydrate as yellow needles, m.p. 148°C (*dec.*) and the anhydrous form as ruby-red prismatic columns which decompose abruptly at 188–9°C. Catalytic hydrogenation furnishes the dihydro derivative, m.p. 225–230°C (*dec.*). On hydrolysis the alkaloid yields lysergic acid and 1-(+)-β-aminopropyl alcohol.

Ergometrine exhibits action on smooth muscle, e.g. blood vessels, intestine and uterus but does not inhibit the sympathetic functions of the vegetative system.

Dudley., *Proc. Roy. Soc.*, **118B**, 478 (1935)
Thompson., *J. Amer. Pharm. Assoc.*, **24**, 748 (1935)
Dudley, Moir., *Brit. Med. J.*, **520**, 798 (1935)
Dudley, Moir., *Science*, **81**, 559 (1935)
Kharasch, Legault., *Brit. Med. J.*, **81**, 388 (1935)
Stoll, Burckhardt., *Compt. rend.*, **200**, 1680 (1935)
Stoll, Hofmann., *Zeit. Physiol. Chem.*, **251**, 155 (1938)
Craig *et al.*, *J. Biol. Chem.*, **125**, 289 (1938)
Jacobs, Craig., *J. Amer. Chem. Soc.*, **60**, 1701 (1938)
Woodward *et al.*, *ibid*, **76**, 5256 (1954)

Pharmacology:
Stoll., *Experientia*, **1**, 250 (1945)

ERGOMETRININE

$C_{19}H_{23}O_2N_3$

M.p. 195–7°C (*dec.*).

A further alkaloid of *Claviceps purpurea*, this base is isomeric with ergometrine and crystallizes as colourless prisms from Me_2CO. It has $[\alpha]_D^{20} + 414°$ ($CHCl_3$) or $+ 413°$ (MeOH). The salts are crystalline, the hydrochloride forming a dihydrate, m.p. 175–180°C (*dec.*); hydrobromide, needles of the monohydrate, m.p. indefinite (between 130 and 190°C); nitrate, colourless prisms from Et_2O-MeOH, m.p. 235°C (*dec.*), sulphate, decomposes at 250°C and the perchlorate which darkens at 210°C and decomposes at 225°C.

Hydrolysis yields lysergic acid and *l*-(+)-aminopropyl alcohol as does ergometrine.

Pharmacologically, the alkaloid possesses only a slight action on uterus.

Smith, Timmis., *J. Chem. Soc.*, 1166, 1440 (1936)
Craig *et al.*, *J. Biol. Chem.*, **125**, 289 (1938)
Stoll, Hofmann., *Zeit. Physiol. Chem.*, **251**, 155 (1938)
Jacobs, Craig., *J. Amer. Chem. Soc.*, **60**, 1701 (1938)

ERGOMOLLININE

$C_{32}H_{41}O_5N_5$

M.p. 241°C (*dec.*).

This alkaloid has been isolated from *Claviceps purpurea* growing on *Elymus mollis* and forms colourless crystals from EtOH. It is dextrorotatory with $[\alpha]_D^{17} + 420°$ (CHCl$_3$). On heating it yields ergomolline, C$_{32}$H$_{41}$O$_5$N$_5$, m.p. 215°C (*dec.*); $[\alpha]_D^{25} - 176.9°$ (CHCl$_3$). When heated with phosphoric acid it furnishes ergomolline phosphate, characterized as the ethanolate, m.p. 198–9°C.

Hashimoto., *J. Pharm. Soc. Japan*, **66**, 22 (1946)

ERGOMONAMINE

C$_{19}$H$_{19}$O$_4$N

M.p. 132–132.5°C

This alkaloid was obtained from *Claviceps purpurea* by Holden and Diver. It furnishes a crystalline picrate, m.p. 163–4°C and differs from the other ergot bases in not giving indole colour reactions. The structure is not yet known.

Holden, Diver., *Quart. J. Pharm.*, **9**, 230 (1936)

ERGONOVINE

See Ergometrine

ERGOSECALININE

C$_{24}$H$_{28}$O$_4$N$_4$

M.p. 217°C (*dec.*).

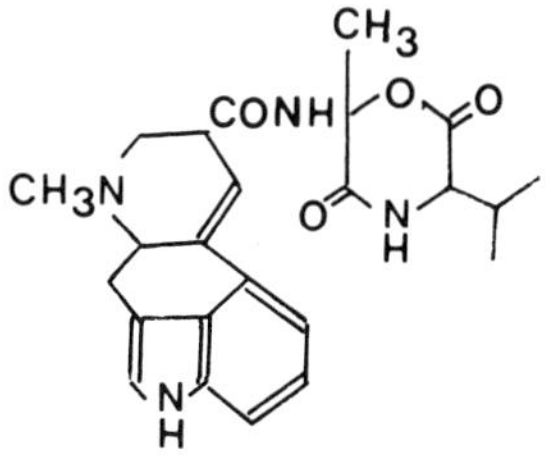

A further alkaloid of *Claviceps purpurea*, this base forms colourless crystals. It is dextrorotatory with $[\alpha]_D^{18} + 298°$ (c 0.2, CHCl$_3$).

Abe *et al.*, *Bull. Agr. Chem. Soc. Japan*, **23**, 246 (1959)

ERGOSINE

C$_{30}$H$_{37}$O$_5$N$_5$

M.p. 228°C (*dec.*).

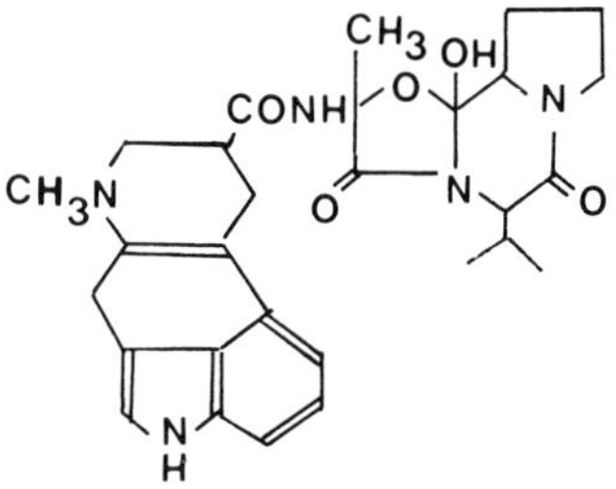

This, and the following alkaloid, were isolated from *Claviceps purpurea* by Smith and Timmis. Mixtures of the two bases are normally obtained and require special methods of separation. The alkaloid crystallizes from AcOEt in colourless prisms. It has $[\alpha]_D^{20} - 161°$ (CHCl$_3$). The hydrochloride forms from Me$_2$CO in diamond-shaped plates with 1 mole of solvent, m.p. 235°C (*dec.*); the hydrobromide also contains 1 mole of Me$_2$CO, m.p. 230°C (*dec.*); the nitrate crystallizes from Me$_2$CO, again with 1 mole of solvent and darkens at 185°C, decomposing at 215°C while the methiodide decomposes at 215°C.

Smith, Timmis., *J. Chem. Soc.*, 396 (1937)
Stoll, Hofmann, Petrzilka., *Helv. Chim. Acta*, **34**, 1544 (1951)

ERGOSININE

$C_{30}H_{37}O_5N_5$

M.p. 228°C (*dec.*).

Obtained from *Claviceps purpurea*, normally as the molecular compound with ergosine, m.p. 200°C (*dec.*), this alkaloid crystallizes readily from various solvents in colourless prisms, or from MeOH in needles with 0.5 MeOH, m.p. 220°C. The base has $[\alpha]_D^{20} + 420°$ (CHCl$_3$) or $+ 380°$ (Me$_2$CO). Acid hydrolysis yields leucine while heating with phosphoric acid in a mixture of EtOH and Me$_2$CO gives ergosine. The hydrochloride is amorphous, darkens at 200°C and decomposes at 206°C. Unlike the preceding base, it exerts only a weak action on uterus.

Smith, Timmis., *J. Chem. Soc.*, 396 (1937)

ERGOSTINE

M.p. 204–8°C

This alkaloid is found in *Claviceps purpurea* and crystallizes readily from AcOEt or Me$_2$CO. It has $[\alpha]_D^{20} - 1.69°$ (CHCl$_3$) or $- 38°$ (pyridine). The acid maleate has m.p. 191–2°C. Catalytic hydrogenation furnishes the dihydro derivative which has m.p. 224–6°C and $[\alpha]_D^{20} - 30°$ (CHCl$_3$) or $- 59°$ (pyridine).

Schlientz *et al.*, *Helv. Chim. Acta*, **47**, 1921 (1964)

ERGOTAMINE

$C_{33}H_{35}O_5N_5$

M.p. 213–4°C (*dec.*).

According to Stoll, there are two strains of ergot, one providing ergotamine and the other ergotoxine. The latter is the source of commercial ergot and comes from Russia and Spain whereas the former occurs in the material from Bulgaria and Hungary and also from that collected from fescue grass in New Zealand.

Ergotamine may be crystallized from a variety of solvents but always contains solvent of crystallization. The recommended medium is aqueous Me_2CO from which it forms rectangular plates with 2 moles of Me_2CO, decomposing at 180°C.

The solvent free base has $[\alpha]_D^{20} - 160°$ (c 1.0, $CHCl_3$) or $- 12.7°$ (c 1.0, pyridine). It behaves as a weak, monoacidic base forming crystalline salts, e.g. the hydrochloride, m.p. 212°C (*dec.*); hydrobromide, m.p. 213°C (*dec.*); sulphate, m.p. 205°C (*dec.*); phosphate crystallizing with 1 mole of EtOH, m.p. 200°C (*dec.*) and tartrate with 2 moles of MeOH, m.p. 203°C (*dec.*). The methanesulphonate has m.p. 210°C (*dec.*) and the ethanesulphonate, m.p. 207°C (*dec.*). The alkaloid is unstable, particularly its aqueous salt solutions when exposed to light. When boiled with MeOH it furnishes ergotaminine (q.v.) while alcoholic KOH yields ergine.

The alkaloid exhibits oxytocic activity on the isolated rabbit uterus *in situ* and is comparatively toxic, particularly in comparison to its dihydro derivative, the respective figures for L.D.50, in mgms/kilo by intravenous injection in rabbits being 3.55 for ergotamine and 25.00 for dihydroergotamine. The tartrate is official in the U.S. Pharmacopoeia XIII. Both it, and the dihydro salt are employed in the relief of migraine.

Smith, Timmis., *J. Chem. Soc.*, 1390 (1930)
Smith, Timmis., *ibid*, 1543 (1932)
Soltys., *Ber.*, **65**, 553 (1932)
Stoll., *Helv. Chim. Acta*, **28**, 1283 (1945)
Stoll, Hofmann, Pretzilka., *ibid*, **34**, 1544 (1951)
Hofmann, Frey, Ott., *Experientia*, **17**, 206 (1961)
Synthesis:
Hoffmann *et al.*, *Helv. Chim. Acta*, **46**, 2306 (1963)
Pharmacology:
Stoll., *Experientia*, **1**, 250 (1945)
Rothlin, Brügger., *Helv. Physiol. Pharm. Acta*, **3**, 117 (1945)

ERGOTAMININE

$C_{33}H_{35}O_5N_5$

M.p. 252°C (*dec.*).

This isomer of ergotamine is a further constituent of the ergot alkaloids. It may be crystallized from boiling MeOH and forms rhombic plates. It has $[\alpha]_D^{20} + 369°$ (c 0.5, $CHCl_3$) or $+ 397°$ (c 0.5, pyridine). It is freely soluble in pyridine, moderately so in $CHCl_3$, sparingly soluble in EtOH, MeOH, AcOEt, C_6H_6 or Me_2CO and insoluble in petroleum ether, dilute alkalies or alkali carbonates. It does not form crystalline salts. With alcoholic KOH it yields ergine.

Smith, Timmis., *J. Chem. Soc.*, 1390 (1930)
Smith, Timmis., *ibid*, 1543 (1932)
Soltys., *Ber.*, **65**, 553 (1932)
Stoll., *Helv. Chim. Acta*, **28**, 1283 (1945)

ERGOTOXINE (*Hydroergotinine*)

M.p. $190-200°C$

This alkaloid from Claviceps purpurea was first described in detail by Barger and Carr who assigned to it the formula $C_{35}H_{41}O_6N_5$. This was later modified to $C_{31}H_{39}O_5N_5$, making it isomeric with ψ-ergotinine. The alkaloid separates from C_6H_6 in rhombic crystals having $[\alpha]_{5461}^{19} - 226°$ (c 1.0, $CHCl_3$). The phosphate crystallizes in colourless needles of the monohydrate, m.p. $186-7°C$; the methanesulphonate, m.p. $214°C$ and the ethanesulphonate, m.p. $209°C$ (*dec.*); the hydrochloride occurs as diamond-shaped plates, m.p. $205°C$; the hydrobromide, as acicular prisms, m.p. $208°C$ and the acid oxalate as minute prisms, m.p. $179°C$.

Barger, Carr., *Chem. News.*, **94**, 89 (1906)
Smith, Timmis., *J. Chem. Soc.*, 1390 (1930)
Foster., *Analyst*, **70**, 132 (1945)
Foster, Smith, Timmis., *Pharm. J.*, **157**, 43 (1946)

ERGOVALIDE

$C_{21}H_{28}O_2N_4$

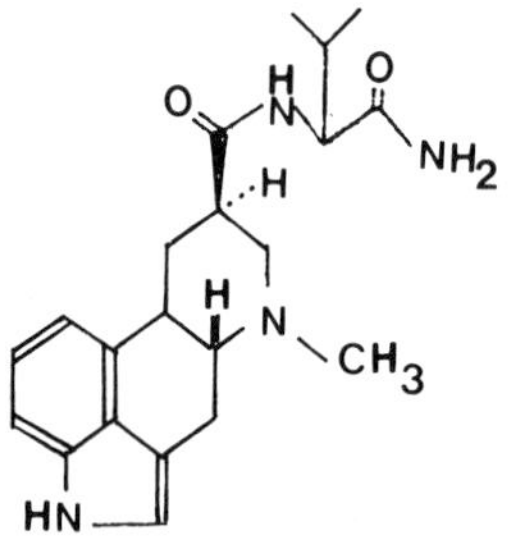

This alkaloid has recently been isolated from *Claviceps purpurea* and its structure determined by infrared, NMR and mass spectrometry. Hydrolysis of the base furnishes lysergic acid and valine.

Ban'kovskaya *et al.*, *Khim. Prir. Soedin.*, **9**, 134 (1973)

ERINICINE

$C_{22}H_{23}O_4N_2$

M.p. $210-2°C$

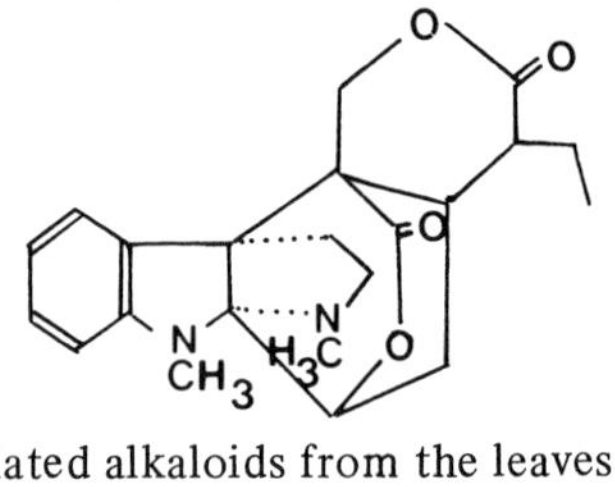

One of two closely related alkaloids from the leaves of *Hunteria umbellata*, this base forms colourless crystals. The structure has been established from chemical and spectroscopic data.

Bycroft, Hesse, Schmid., *Helv. Chim. Acta*, **48**, 1598 (1965)

534

ERININE

$C_{22}H_{21}O_4N_2$

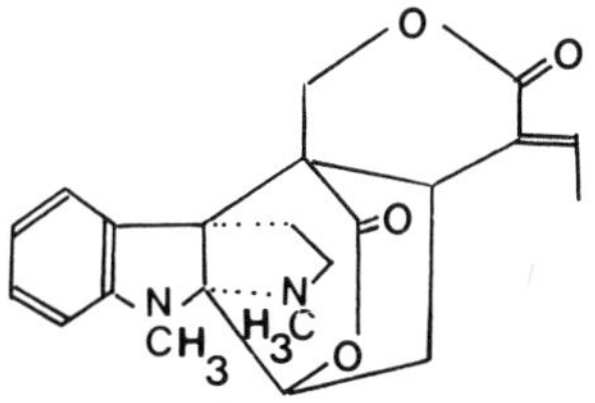

The second base obtained from the leaves of *Hunteria umbellata,* this indole alkaloid is difficult to crystallize. Hydrogenation with PtO_2 as catalyst yields Erinicine (q.v.), whereas $LiAlH_4$ gives 19:20-dihydroerininediol.

Bycroft, Hesse, Schmid., *Helv. Chim. Acta,* 48, 1598 (1965)

ERIPINE

$C_{23}H_{28}O_5N_2$

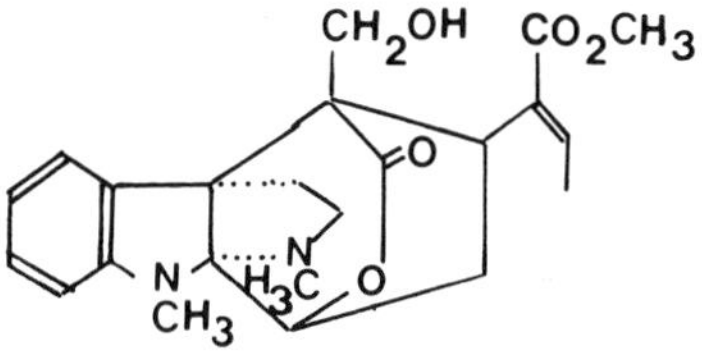

An indole alkaloid present in the leaves of *Hunteria umbellata,* the structure has been established from spectroscopic data. When heated the base yields a mixture of erinine and its stereoisomer, erininine.

Morita, Hesse, Schmid., *Helv. Chim. Acta,* 51, 138 (1968)

ERITADENINE

$C_9H_{13}O_4N_4$

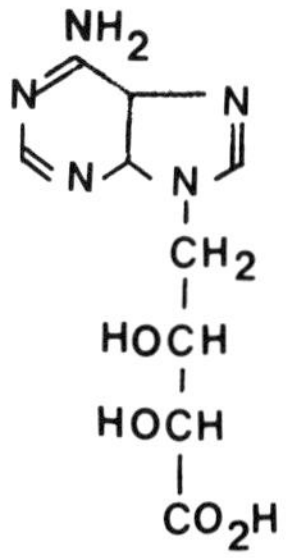

A hypocholesterolenic alkaloid, this base occurs in *Lentinus edodes.* The structure has been deduced from chemical studies and confirmed by the total synthesis of the alkaloid.

Kamiya *et al., Tetrahedron,* 28, 899 (1972)

535

ERUCIFOLINE

$C_{17}H_{21}O_6N$

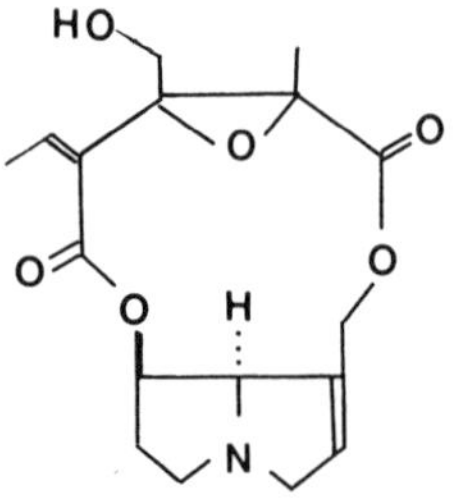

A pyrrolizidine alkaloid present in *Senecio erraticus*, the structure has been determined from chemical reactions, NMR and mass spectra. Hydrolysis furnishes erucifolinecic acid, $C_{10}H_{16}O_7$.

Sedmera *et al., Collect. Czech. Chem. Commun.*, **37**, 4112 (1972)

ERVAMYCINE

$C_{22}H_{26}O_3N_2$

M.p. Indefinite

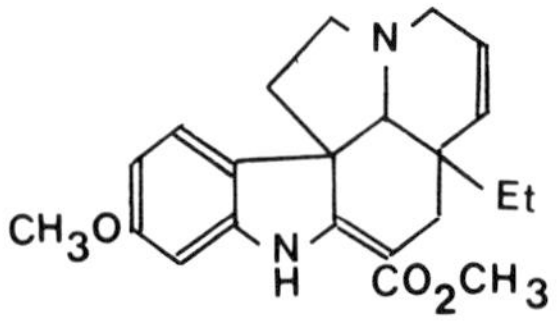

This alkaloid has been obtained as the hydrochloride, m.p. 213–4°C from the C_6H_6 extract of *Vinca erecta* after removal of Ervinceine (q.v.). The free base is an amorphous solid with no definite melting point. It yields a hydriodide, m.p. 207–8°C (*dec.*).

Rakhimov, Malikov, Yunusov., *Khim. Prir. Soedin.*, **5**, 332 (1969)

Structure:
Rakhimov *et al., Khim. Prir. Soedin.*, **6**, 226 (1970)

ERVATAMINE

$C_{21}H_{26}O_3N_2$

M.p. 92–8°C

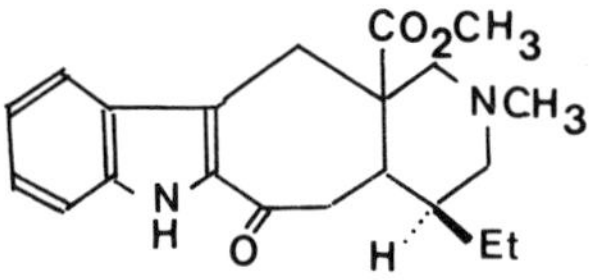

This indole alkaloid occurs in *Ervatamia orientalis* and forms colourless crystals from MeOH containing 1 mole of solvent. It is laevorotatory with $[\alpha]_D - 3.7°$. The alkaloid contains one imino and one methylimino group, together with an ethyl and a methoxycarbonyl group.

Knox, Slobbe., *Tetrahedron Lett.*, 2149 (1971)

20-*epi*-ERVATAMINE

$C_{21}H_{26}O_3N_2$

M.p. 185–7°C (*dec.*).

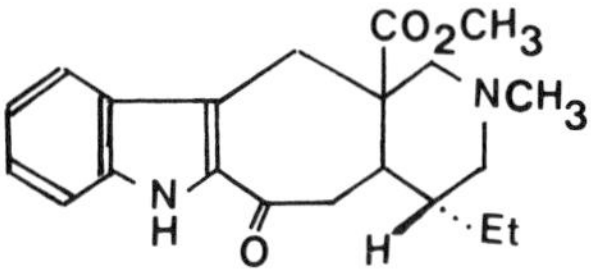

Ervatamia orientalis also contains this alkaloid. It is, like the preceding base, laevorotatory with $[\alpha]_D - 22°$. The structure has been determined from the infrared and NMR spectra.

Knox, Slobbe., *Tetrahedron Lett.*, 2149 (1971)

ERVINCEINE

$C_{22}H_{28}O_3N_2$

M.p. 99–100°C

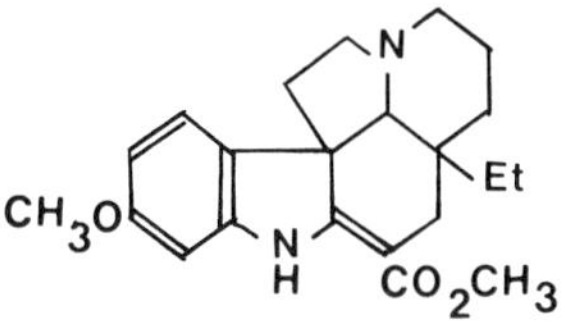

An alkaloid occurring in *Vinca erecta,* this base forms colourless crystals from MeOH. It is strongly laevorotatory with $[\alpha]_D^{12} - 448°$ (MeOH). No crystalline salts have yet been reported although it contains one imino group in the molecule.

Rakhimov, Malikov, Yunusov., *Khim. Prir. Soedin.*, 5, 330 (1969)

ERVINCINE

$C_{21}H_{24}O_3N_2$

M.p. 157°C

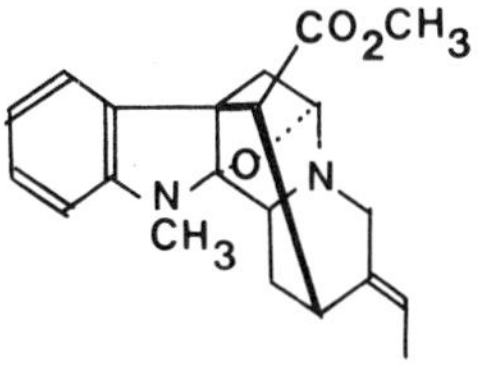

A further alkaloid present in *Vinca erecta,* this base contains a methylimino group, a methoxycarbonyl group and an ether bridge. The second nitrogen atom is tertiary.

Rakhimov, Malikov, Yunusov., *Khim. Prir. Soedin.*, 5, 330 (1969)

ERVINCININE

$C_{22}H_{26}O_4N_2$

M.p. 247–8°C

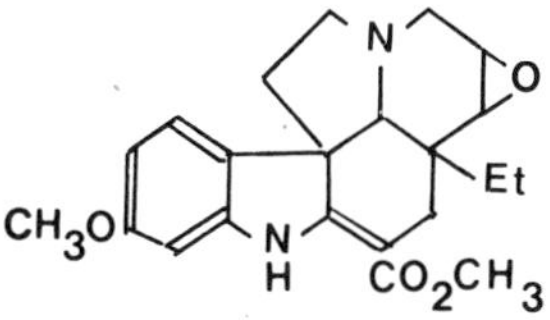

Also present in Vinca erecta, this alkaloid has $[\alpha]_D^{22} - 80.5°$ (c 0.39, CHCl$_3$).

Reduction with Zn and H_2SO_4 gives the dihydro derivative, m.p. 206.5–207.5°C. The structure given above has been established on the basis of the ultraviolet, infrared, NMR and mass spectra.

Rakhimov, Malikov, Yunusov., *Khim. Prir. Soedin.,* **4**, 331 (1968)
Rakhimov *et al., ibid,* **6**, 226 (1970)

ERVINE

$C_{21}H_{26}O_3N_2$

Present in *Vinca erecta,* the structure of this heteroyohimbine alkaloid has been established from spectroscopic data. The C and D rings are *trans*-linked, the D and E rings *cis*-linked and the C-19 methyl group has a α-axial configuration.

Malikov, Yunusov., *Khim. Prir. Soedin,* **6**, 346 (1970)

ERVINIDINE

$C_{22}H_{26}O_4N_2$

M.p. 283–4°C (*dec.*).

One of the number of bases isolated from *Vinca erecta,* this alkaloid crystallizes as colourless needles from MeOH. It has $[\alpha]_D - 17.3°$ ($CHCl_3$). With $NaBH_4$, the alkaloid is reduced to ervindiol which is amorphous and exhibits typical indole ultraviolet and infrared spectra. The alkaloid is a 2-acylindole base of the picraphylline type.

Malikov, Yunusov., *Khim. Prir. Soedin.,* **3**, 142 (1967)

ERVINIDININE

$C_{21}H_{24}O_3N_2$

M.p. 255–8°C (*dec.*).

A further alkaloid isolated from *Vinca erecta,* this base forms colourless crystals from MeOH. It is laevorotatory with $[\alpha]_D^6 - 160.6°$ (MeOH) and is reduced with Zn and H_2SO_4 to the dihydro derivative, m.p. 215–6°C. The alkaloid has been shown to possess an epoxy ring in the molecule. In a later paper, Malikov and Yunusov give a melting point of 265–6°C for the alkaloid.

Malikov, Yunusov., *Khim. Prir. Soedin.,* **3**, 142 (1967)
Malikov, Yunusov., *ibid,* **5**, 65 (1969)

538

ERYBIDINE

$C_{20}H_{25}O_4N$

M.p. 178–180°C

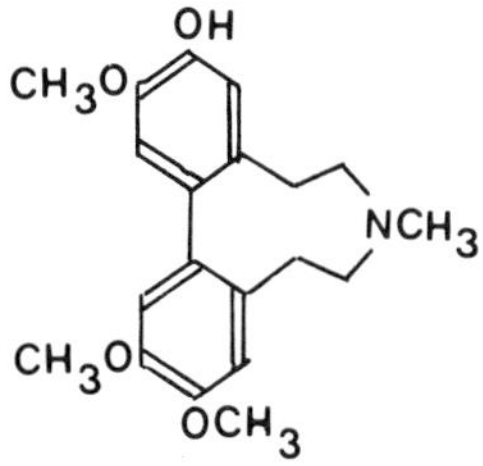

From the leaves of *Erythrina x bidwilli* Lindl., Ito and his colleagues have isolated this alkaloid which forms colourless needles from MeOH. The base has been characterized as the crystalline 3-methyl ether which has m.p. 139–140°C.

Ito, Furukawa, Tanaka., *Chem. Pharm. Bull.*, **19**, 1509 (1971)

ERYCININE

$C_{21}H_{24}O_4N_2$

M.p. 206–7°C

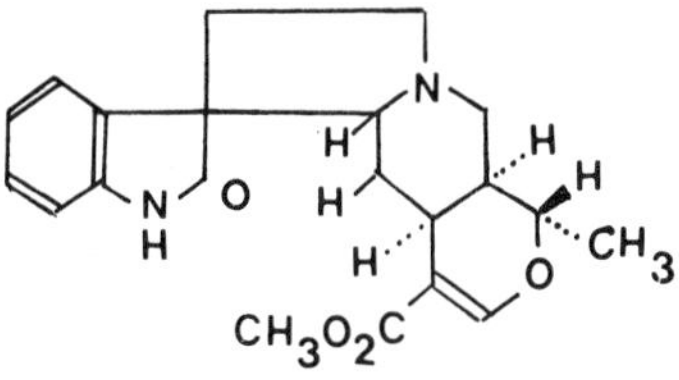

The aerial parts of *Vinca erecta* yield this alkaloid which is isomeric with Vinerine and Vineridine (q.v.). The base had $[\alpha]_D^{18} + 43.8°$ (Me$_2$CO). It forms a methobromide, m.p. 237–8°C and an N-acetyl derivative, m.p. 158–9°C; $[\alpha]_D^{18} - 98°$ (Me$_2$CO) which is identical with N-acetylvinerine. Epimerization with pyridine gives a compound, m.p. 200–1°C; $[\alpha]_D^{20} - 98°$ (Me$_2$CO) which is identical with hydroxyindolereserpinine. The structure has been established from the ultraviolet, infrared and NMR spectra.

Abdurakhimova, Kasymov, Yunusov., *Khim. Prir. Soedin.*, **4**, 135 (1968)

ERYSOCINE

$C_{18}H_{21}O_3N$

M.p. 162°C

This compound has been isolated from several Erythrina species and occurs as needles from Et$_2$O. It is soluble in CHCl$_3$, moderately so in Et$_2$O and EtOH. It has $[\alpha]_D + 238.1°$ and is only weakly basic. Later work indicates that it is, in reality, a mixture of erysodine and erysovine.

Folkers, Koniuszy., *J. Amer. Chem. Soc.*, **62**, 1677 (1940)

ERYSODINE

$C_{18}H_{21}O_3N$

M.p. 204–5°C

An alkaloid obtained from *Erythrina* species, particularly *E. americana* Mill. and *E. crista* galli. The base is extracted from the plant material only after acid hydrolysis and it appears probable that it is liberated from some more complex base during this process (cf. erysopine and erysovine). The alkaloid forms colourless needles from EtOH and has $[\alpha]_D^{27} + 248°$ (EtOH). It is freely soluble in $CHCl_3$ and moderately so in Et_2O and EtOH. It possesses a curare-like action similar to the majority of the *Erythrina* bases. The structure has been determined by spectroscopic techniques and confirmed by synthesis of the (±)-form.

Folkers *et al.*, *J. Amer. Chem. Soc.*, **62**, 1677 (1940)
Folkers *et al.*, *ibid*, **64**, 1892 (1942)
Koniuszy, Wiley, Folkers., *ibid*, **71**, 875 (1949)
Prelog *et al.*, *Helv. Chem. Acta*, **32**, 453 (1949)
Folkers, Koniuszy, Shavel., *J. Amer. Chem. Soc.*, **73**, 589 (1951)
Kenner, Khorana, Prelog., *Helv. Chim. Acta*, **34**, 1969 (1951)
Carmack, Koniuszy, Prelog., *ibid*, **34**, 1601 (1951)
Belleau., *Chem. & Ind.*, 410 (1956)
Prelog *et al.*, *Helv. Chim. Acta.*, **39**, 498 (1956)
Prelog *et al.*, *ibid*, **42**, 1301 (1959)

Structure:
Barton *et al.*, *Chem. Commun.*, 294 (1966)

Synthesis:
Mondon, Ehrhardt., *Tetrahedron Lett.*, 2557 (1966)

ERYSONINE

$C_{17}H_{19}O_3N$

M.p. 236–7°C

A further Erythrina alkaloid obtained from *E. costaricensis* Micheli, this base crystallizes from EtOH in colourless needles. It is dextrorotatory with $[\alpha]_D^{25} + 286°$ (aqueous HCl) and + 272° (morpholine).

Folkers *et al.*, *J. Amer. Chem. Soc.*, **63**, 1544 (1941)
Prelog *et al.*, *Helv. Chim. Acta*, **42**, 1301 (1959)
Mondon, Ehrhardt., *Tetrahedron Lett.*, 2557 (1966)

540

ERYSOPINE

$C_{17}H_{19}O_3N$

M.p. 241–2°C

This alkaloid is obtained from the acid hydrolysis product of several *Erythrina* species and forms colourless crystals from EtOH. It is only sparingly soluble in $CHCl_3$, H_2O and hydroxylic solvents and has $[\alpha]_D^{25} + 265.2°$ (EtOH-glycerol). It is only a weak base and is unstable in alkaline solution. In the plant, it occurs as the sulphoacetic ester, erysothiopine (q.v.) from which it is liberated during the extraction process.

Folkers, Koniuszy., *J. Amer. Chem. Soc.*, **62**, 1677 (1940)
Folkers, Koniuszy, Shavel., *ibid*, **66**, 1083 (1944)
Koniuszy, Wiley, Folkers., *ibid*, **71**, 875 (1949)
Folkers, Koniuszy, Shavel., *ibid*, **73**, 589 (1951)
Carmack, McKusick, Prelog., *Helv. Chim. Acta*, **34**, 1601 (1951)
Kenner, Khorana, Prelog., *ibid*, **34**, 1969 (1951)
Labriola, Deulofeu, Berinzaghi., *J. Org. Chem.*, **16**, 90 (1951)
Belleau., *Chem. & Ind.*, 410 (1956)
Prelog *et al.*, *Helv. Chim. Acta*, **39**, 498 (1956)

ERYSOSALINE

$C_{18}H_{23}O_4N$

An alkaloid recently isolated from *Erythrina folkersii* and *E. salviiflora*. The base has the typical skeleton common to this group of alkaloids. Two methoxyl groups, a phenolic and a non-phenolic hydroxyl group are present in the molecule.

Millington, Steinman, Ruchat., *J. Amer. Chem. Soc.*, **96**, 1909 (1972)

ERYSOTHIOPINE

$C_{18}H_{19}O_7NS$

M.p. 168–9°C

A sulphur-containing alkaloid found in the seeds of *Erythrina* species, particularly *E. glauca* Willd. The base is dextrorotatory with $[\alpha]_D^{25} + 194°$ (EtOH). Hydrolysis yields erysopine and sulphoacetic acid and the most probable linkage appears to

541

be between the sulphonyl radical and the base, leaving a free carboxylic acid group in the molecule.

Folkers, Koniuszy, Shavel., *J. Amer. Chem. Soc.*, **66**, 1083 (1944)

ERYSOTHIOVINE

$C_{20}H_{23}O_7NS$

M.p. 187°C

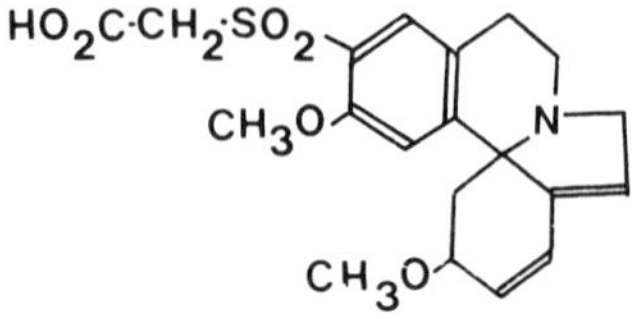

The second sulphur-containing alkaloid to be isolated from *Erythrina glauca* Willd., this base has $[\alpha]_D^{25} + 208°$ (EtOH). Hydrolysis yields erysovine and sulphoacetic acid. The linkage is believed to be the same as in the preceding alkaloid.

Folkers, Koniuszy, Shavel., *J. Amer. Chem. Soc.*, **66**, 1083 (1944)

ERYSOTINONE

$C_{18}H_{21}O_4N$

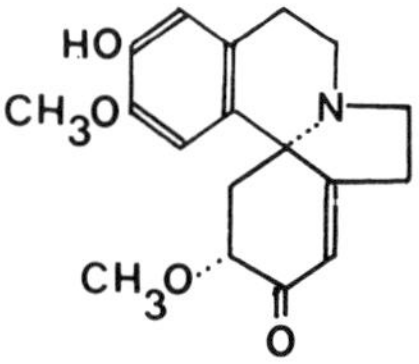

Recently isolated from *Erythrina folkersii* and *E. salviiflora*, this base contains two methoxyl groups and a phenolic hydroxyl group. The structure has been determined from the infrared, NMR and mass spectra.

Millington, Steinman, Rinehart., *J. Amer. Chem. Soc.*, **96**, 1909 (1974)

ERYSOTRAMIDINE

$C_{19}H_{21}O_4N$

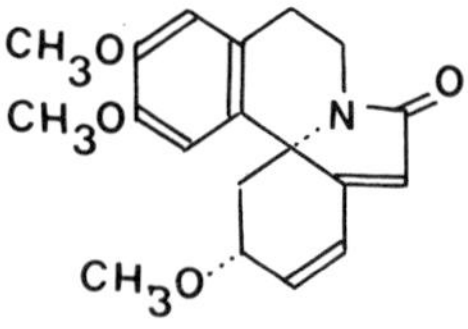

An *Erythrina* alkaloid recently obtained from *E. arborescens* Roxb., this base contains three methoxyl groups in the molecule. The structure has been elucidated from chemical and spectroscopic evidence.

Ito, Furukawa, Haruna., *J. Pharm. Soc., Japan,* **93**, 1617 (1973)

542

ERYSOTRINE

$C_{19}H_{23}O_3N$

M.p. 95-7°C

This alkaloid from the leaves of *Erythrina lysistemon* is closely related to the preceding base. It forms colourless crystals from light petroleum and its ultra-violet spectrum exhibits absorption maxima at 228 and 280 mμ.

Ito, Furukawa, Haruna., *J. Pharm. Soc., Japan,* **93**, 1617 (1973)

ERYSOVINE

$C_{18}H_{21}O_3N$

M.p. 178-9°C

Obtained from the leaves of several *Erythrina* species, this alkaloid forms colourless prisms when crystallized from Et$_2$O. It is dextrorotatory with $[\alpha]_D$ + 252° (EtOH) and is a weak base. It is readily soluble in CHCl$_3$ and moderately so in Et$_2$O and EtOH. It contains one hydroxyl group and two methoxyl groups in the molecule. Since it is obtained from the acid hydrolysis product of the plant, it is believed to be derived from Erysothiovine (q.v.) during the extraction process.

Folkers, Koniuszy., *J. Amer. Chem. Soc.,* **62**, 1677 (1940)
Koniuszy, Wiley, Folkers., *ibid,* **71**, 875 (1949)
Folkers, Koniuszy, Shavel., *ibid,* **73**, 589 (1951)
Carmack, McKusick, Prelog., *Helv. Chim. Acta,* **34**, 1601 (1951)
Kenner, Khorana, Prelog., *ibid,* **34**, 1969 (1951)

ERYSTEMINE

$C_{20}H_{25}O_4N$

M.p. 127-9°C

This alkaloid is isolated from *Erythrina lysistemon* together with Erysodine (q.v.) and is present in 0.0024 per cent yield. It crystallizes from light petroleum as pale yellow prisms and has $[\alpha]_D^{22}$ + 189°. The picrate has m.p. 145-150°C and the 2-bromo-4:6-dinitrophenolate, m.p. 144-6°C has been used for the X-ray determination of the structure. The ultraviolet and infrared spectra are almost identical with those of Erythraline (q.v.).

Ito, Furukawa, Haruna., *J. Pharm. Soc., Japan,* **93**, 1617 (1973)

ERYTHARBINE

$C_{19}H_{21}O_4N$

This alkaloid has recently been isolated from *Erythrina arborescens* Roxb. The structure has been determined primarily from chemical and spectroscopic data.

Ito, Furukawa, Haruna., *J. Pharm. Soc., Japan*, **93**, 1617 (1973)

ERYTHRALINE

$C_{18}H_{19}O_3N$

M.p. 106–7°C

This alkaloid was first obtained, together with erythratine, from *Erythrina glauca* Willd. but have since been isolated from other species of this genus. It has $[\alpha]_D^{27} + 211-8°$ (EtOH) and furnishes the following crystalline salts: hydrobromide, m.p. 243°C; $[\alpha]_D^{27} + 216.6°$ (H_2O); hydriodide, m.p. 252–3°C (*dec.*); $[\alpha]_D^{23} + 177°$ (H_2O) and the methiodide as light yellow crystals from MeOH-C_6H_6, m.p. 185–7°C. On hydrogenation in dilute HCl in the presence of prereduced PtO_2 it yields the dihydro derivative. Pharmacologically, the threshold dose for curare-like action in frogs in 7–8 mgm per kilo.

Folkers, Koniuszy., *J. Amer. Chem. Soc.*, **62**, 436, 1673 (1940)
Folkers, Koniuszy., *ibid*, **64**, 2146 (1942)
Prelog *et al.*, *Helv. Chim. Acta*, **32**, 453 (1949)
Carmack, McKusick, Prelog., *ibid*, **34**, 1601 (1951)
Kenner, Khorana, Prelog., *ibid*, **34**, 1969 (1951)
Folkers, Koniuszy, Shavel., *J. Amer. Chem. Soc.*, **73**, 589 (1951)
Prelog *et al.*, *Helv. Chim. Acta*, **39**, 498 (1956)
Novacki, Bonsma., *Z. Krist.*, **110**, 89 (1958)
Biosynthesis:
Barton, Boar, Widdowson., *J. Chem. Soc.*, C, 1213 (1970)

ERYTHRAMINE

$C_{18}H_{21}O_3N$

M.p. 103–4°C;
B.p. 125°C/0.0039 mm

Both *Erythrina sandwicensis* Deg. and *E. subumbrans* (Hassk.) Merrill yield this alkaloid which occurs with hypaphorine (q.v.). It is normally isolated as the hydriodide, orange-yellow needles from EtOH, m.p. 249°C (*dec.*); $[\alpha]_D^{25} + 220°$ (H_2O). The free base is dextrorotatory with $[\alpha]_D^{29.5} + 227.6°$ (EtOH). It also forms a crystalline hydrochloride, m.p. 250°C (*dec.*); hydrobromide, m.p. 228°C; $[\alpha]_D^{26} + 203.2°$ (H_2O); methiodide, m.p. 96–8°C; $[\alpha]_D^{28} + 176°$ (H_2O). Catalytic hydrogenation over PtO_2 in dilute HCl under 2 atmospheres pressure yields the dihydro derivative, m.p. 89–90°C also furnishing crystalline salts, e.g. the hydrobromide monohydrate, m.p. 240°C; hydriodide, m.p. 214–5°C which is optically inactive and the methiodide hemihydrate, m.p. 160–1°C. The hydrobromide exhibits curare-like activity in the frog at 7 mgm per kilo.

Folkers *et al.*, *J. Amer. Chem. Soc.*, **61**, 1232 (1939)
Folkers *et al.*, *ibid*, **62**, 436, 1673 (1940)
Folkers *et al.*, *ibid*, **64**, 2146 (1942)
Folkers, Koniuszy, Shavel., *ibid*, **73**, 589 (1951)
Carmack, McKusick, Prelog., *Helv. Chim. Acta*, **34**, 1601 (1951)

ERYTHRASCINE

$C_{21}H_{25}O_5N$

M.p. 138–140°C

This alkaloid occurs in the seeds of *Erythrina arborescens* Roxb. It crystallizes from Me_2CO-EtOH as cream-coloured needles and has $[\alpha]_D^{25} + 152°$ (c 0.51, $CHCl_3$). The ultraviolet spectrum exhibits absorption maxima at 210–2, 233–5 and 284–8 mμ. It contains three methoxyl groups and one methoxycarbonyl group in the molecule.

Ghosal, Chakraborti, Srivastava., *Phytochem.*, **11**, 2101 (1972)

ERYTHRATIDINE

$C_{19}H_{25}O_4N$

M.p. 120–1°C

An *Erythrina* alkaloid isolated from *E. falcata,* the base crystallizes from aqueous EtOH as colourless needles of the hemihydrate. It is dextrorotatory with $[\alpha]_D^{20} + 222.5°$ (c 0.508, H_2O). It forms a crystalline methiodide as colourless needles, m.p. 183°C; $[\alpha]_D^{20} + 193.8°$ (c 0.358, H_2O) and a picrate as rhombic yellow plates, m.p. 222–4°C. It contains three methoxyl groups and one hydroxyl group.

Deulofeu., *Ber.*, **85**, 620 (1952)

ERYTHRATINE

$C_{18}H_{21}O_4N$

M.p. 170–5°C

This alkaloid was first isolated from the seeds of *Erythrina glauca* Willd. together with erythraline and has since been discovered in other *Erythrina* species. The base crystallizes from Et_2O-petroleum ether as the hemihydrate and has $[\alpha]_D^{28}$ + 145.5° (EtOH). It forms several well-crystalline salts, e.g. the hydrobromide, m.p. 241°C; $[\alpha]_D^{25}$ + 158.7° (H_2O); hydriodide, m.p. 242–242.5°C; $[\alpha]_D^{25}$ + 109° (H_2O). The methiodide hemihydrate has m.p. 121–5°C; $[\alpha]_D^{25}$ + 109.7° (H_2O) or m.p. 135–6°C (*dry*). The latter readily yields an amorphous methine base, $C_{19}H_{23}O_4N$.

In very dilute HBr, in the presence of PtO_2, the alkaloid yields the dihydro derivative hydrobromide, m.p. 249°C. The alkaloid contains a methoxyl, a hydroxyl and one methylenedioxy group. The structure has been determined by spectroscopic techniques.

Folkers *et al.*, *J. Amer. Chem. Soc.*, **62**, 436 (1940)
Folkers *et al.*, *ibid*, **64**, 2146 (1942)
Folkers, Koniuszy, Shavel., *ibid*, **73**, 589 (1951)

Structure:
Barton *et al.*, *Chem. Commun.*, 294 (1966)

Biosynthesis:
Barton *et al.*, *Chem. Commun.*, 266 (1967)
Barton, Boar, Widdowson., *J. Chem. Soc., C*, 1213 (1970)

ERYTHRATINIDONE

$C_{19}H_{23}O_4N$

M.p. 119–120°C

An alkaloid from *Erythrina lithosperma*, this base contains three hydroxyl groups and one keto group. The structure has been established from the infrared, ultraviolet, NMR and mass spectra.

Barton *et al.*, *J. Chem. Soc., Perkin Trans.*, I, 874 (1973)

ERYTHRAVINE

$C_{18}H_{21}O_3N$

A further alkaloid just recently obtained from *Erythrina* species, e.g. *E. folkersii* and *E. salviiflora.* The structure has been determined mainly from spectroscopic data and contains two methoxyl groups and a non-henolic hydroxyl group.

Millington, Steinman, Rinehart., *J. Amer. Chem. Soc.*, **96**, 1909 (1974)

ERYTHRININE

Two alkaloids of this name have recently been isolated from *Erythrina* species and, since these do not appear to be identical, these are described below.

$C_{30}H_{36}O_5N_4$

This alkaloid has been isolated from *Erythrina lithosperma* seeds. All four nitrogen atoms are present in ring systems, the base containing four methoxyl groups and one amide group.

Tandon, Tiwari, Gupta., *Proc. Nat. Acad. Sci., India, Sect. A*, **39**, 263 (1969)

$C_{18}H_{19}O_4N$

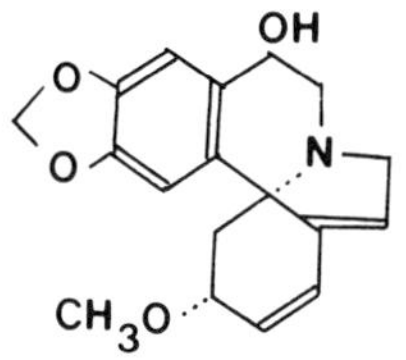

The second alkaloid of this name occurs in the leaves of *Erythrina indica* Lam. It has m.p. 197–200°C (*dec.*) and occurs together with erysodine and de-N-methylorientaline. It is dextrorotatory with $[\alpha]_D + 204°$ (CHCl₃) and the ultraviolet spectrum has absorption maxima at 209, 230 and 289 mμ. From chemical and spectral data (infrared, mass and NMR), the above structure has been determined.

Ito, Furukawa, Tanaka., *J. Chem. Soc., D,* 1076 (1970)

ERYTHRISTEMINE

$C_{20}H_{25}O_4N$

M.p. 127–9°C

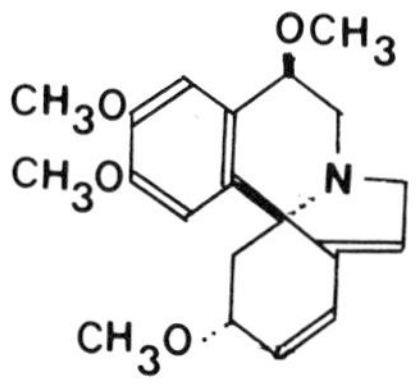

Obtained from the leaves and seeds of *Erythrina lysistemon,* this alkaloid is dextrorotatory with $[\alpha]_D^{22} + 189°$ (c 0.4, CHCl₃). The ultraviolet spectrum shows absorption maxima at 235 and 283 mμ in ethanol solution. It forms a crystalline picrate, m.p. 145–150°C. The base contains four methoxyl groups.

Barton *et al., Chem. Commun.,* 391 (1970)
Barton *et al., J. Chem. Soc., Perkin Trans.,* I, 874 (1973)

ERYTHROCULINE

$C_{20}H_{25}O_4N$

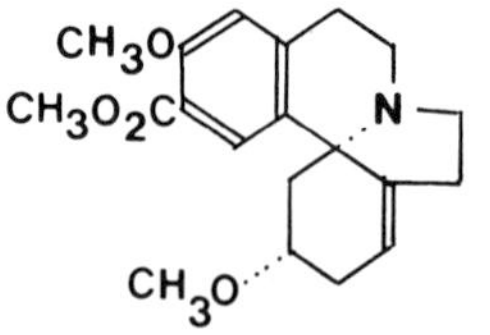

An amorphous base found in *Cocculus laurifolius* where it occurs mainly in the leaves, this dextrorotatory base has $[\alpha]_D + 194°$ (c 2.02, $CHCl_3$). The ultraviolet spectrum shows one absorption maximum at 304 mμ. A crystalline styphnate, m.p. 193–6°C has been prepared. The alkaloid contains two methoxy groups and one methoxycarbonyl group. The presence of the latter on the benzene ring in the molecule is biosynthetically unusual. The structure has been elucidated from degradative and spectroscopic data and by a chemical correlation with tetrahydroerysotrine whose stereochemistry has already been established.

Inubushi, Furukawa, Ju-ichi., *Tetrahedron Lett.*, 153 (1969)

Structure:
Inubushi, Furukawa, Ju-ichi., *Chem. Pharm. Bull.*, **18**, 1951 (1970)

ERYTHROCULINOL

$C_{19}H_{25}O_3N$

M.p. 150–2°C

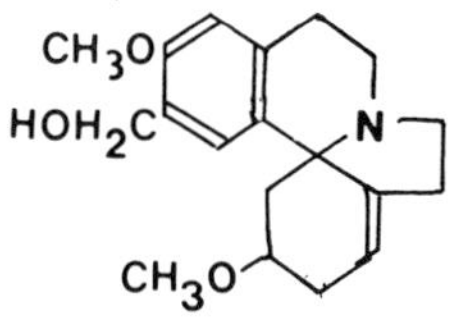

A minor constituent of the leaves of *Cocculus laurifolius*, this base has $[\alpha]_D + 210°$ (c 1.02, $CHCl_3$) and its ultraviolet spectrum shows two absorption maxima at 280 and 284 mμ. It contains two methoxyl groups and one hydroxymethyl group.

Inubushi, Furukawa, Ju-ichi., *Tetrahedron Lett.*, 153 (1969)

ERYTHROIDINE

$C_{16}H_{19}O_3N$

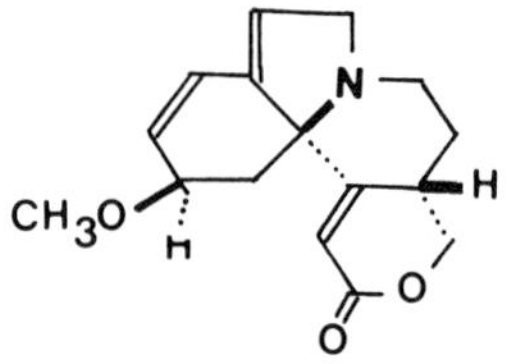

First obtained from the seeds of *Erythrina americana* Mill. this alkaloid was described as having m.p. 94–6°C, giving a hydrochloride, m.p. 228–9°C (*dec.*); $[\alpha]_D^{31} + 109.7°$ (H_2O), the base was subsequently discovered in several other *Erythrina* species and shown to be a mixture of two thereoisomers, described below.

α-ERYTHROIDINE

M.p. 94–5°C

This alkaloid yields a series of crystalline salts and derivatives, e.g. the hydrochloride, m.p. 227–8°C; $[\alpha]_D$ + 118°; hydrobromide as the hemihydrate, m.p. 224°C or 220–2°C (dry); hydriodide, m.p. 210–2°C; perchlorate, m.p. 208–208.5°C and the flavianate, m.p. 216°C.

β-ERYTHROIDINE

M.p. 98.5–99.5°C

This stereoisomeric alkaloid is also dextrorotatory with $[\alpha]_D$ + 88.8° (H_2O) and yields the following crystalline salts: hydrochloride hemihydrate, m.p. 229.5–230°C (dec.) or 232°C (dry, dec.); $[\alpha]_D^{25}$ + 109° (H_2O); hydrobromide, crystallizing with 0.5 EtOH, m.p. 227°C or 222–4°C (dry); $[\alpha]_D^{25}$ + 111.2° (H_2O); hydriodide monohydrate, m.p. 206°C; $[\alpha]_D^{25}$ + 108.1° (H_2O); perchlorate, m.p. 203–203.5°C; $[\alpha]_D^{25}$ + 96.3° (H_2O) and the flavianate, m.p. 216–216.5°C.

The mixture of the two isomers, on hydrogenation as the hydrochloride, yields tetrahydroerythroidine hydrochloride hemihydrate, m.p. 215–7°C from which the tetrahydro base may be obtained as an oil, b.p. 70–100°C/0.0001 mm. The hydrobromide has m.p. 215–8°C (dry).

β-erythroidine behaves as a lactone and catalytic hydrogenation of one of its salts with an alkali under pressure yields a mixture from which the pure dihydro compound may be obtained as the hydrobromide. Dihydro-β-erythroidine has m.p. 85–6°C (dec.); $[\alpha]_D^{25}$ + 102.5° and yields crystalline salts, e.g. the hydrochloride, m.p. 238°C (dec.); $[\alpha]_D^{25}$ + 124.7°; hydrobromide, m.p. 231°C (dec.); $[\alpha]_D^{25}$ + 106°; hydriodide, m.p. 230°C (dec.); $[\alpha]_D^{25}$ + 95.5° and the perchlorate, m.p. 235–6°C (dec.); $[\alpha]_D^{25}$ + 102.5°.

Dihydro-β-erythroidine is a potent curarizing agent with a potency of 0.5 mgm per kilo in frogs.

Folkers, Major., J. Amer. Chem. Soc., 59, 1580 (1937)
Koniuszy, Folkers., ibid, 72, 5579 (1950)
Koniuszy, Folkers., ibid, 73, 333 (1951)
Lapiere, Robinson., Chem. & Ind., 650 (1951)
Boekelheide, Grundon, Weinstock., J. Amer. Chem. Soc., 74, 1866 (1952)
Godfrey, Tarbell, Boekelheide., ibid, 77, 3342 (1955)
Hanson., Proc. Chem. Soc., 52 (1963)
Wenzinger, Boekelheide., ibid, 53 (1963)
Weiss, Ziffer., Experientia, 19, 108 (1963)

ERYTHROPHAMINE

$C_{25}H_{39}O_6N$

M.p. 149–151°C

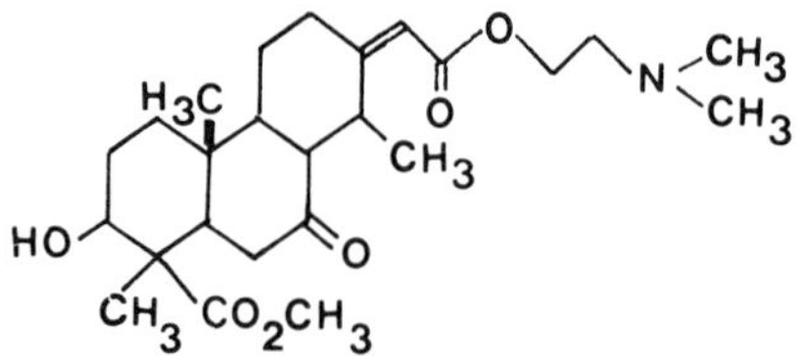

This alkaloid has been isolated from *Erythrophleum guineense* E. Don. It is laevorotatory with $[\alpha]_D^{20} - 62.5°$ (c 0.91, EtOH). The ultraviolet spectrum exhibits one absorption maximum at 222 mμ. The base is characterized as the crystalline picrate which forms slender needles, m.p. 184–7°C (*dec.*). The nitrogen atom is present as a terminal dimethylamino group in the side chain.

Ruzicka, Plattner, Engel., *Experientia*, **1**, 160 (1945)
Engel, Tondeur., *Helv. Chim. Acta*, **32**, 2364 (1949)
Mathieson *et al.*, *Experientia*, **16**, 404 (1960)

ERYTHROPHLEGUINE

$C_{25}H_{41}O_6N$

M.p. 77–8°C

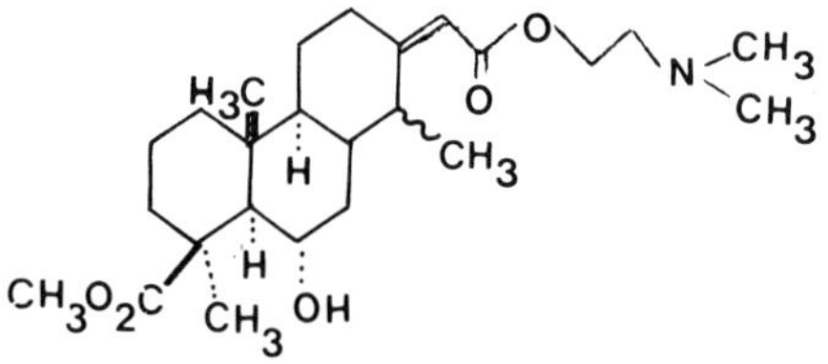

A further alkaloid obtained from *Erythrophleum guineense* G. Don. The base has $[\alpha]_D - 38°$ (c 1.6, EtOH) and the ultraviolet spectrum is almost identical with that of the preceding base having a single absorption maximum at 221 mμ. Acid hydrolysis yields dimethylaminoethanol and an acid, m.p. 194–6°C; $[\alpha]_D + 54°$ (c 2.2, EtOH) which may be catalytically reduced to yield dihydrocessamic acid. The latter observation, coupled with spectroscopic examination of the alkaloid, its *p*-nitrobenzoate and the acid formed on hydrolysis, give the structure shown above.

Lindwall *et al.*, *Tetrahedron Lett.*, 4203 (1965)
Sandberg *et al.*, *Herba Hung.*, **5**, 61 (1966)

ERYTHROPHLEINE

$C_{24}H_{39}O_5N$

M.p. Indefinite

This amorphous alkaloid was first isolated from the bark of *Erythrophleum guineense* G. Don. by Gallois and Hardy. It also appears to be present in the Australian species, *E. chlorostachys, E. lasianthum* from South Africa and an unidentified species from Mozambique.
   The free base has not been crystallized and is characterized as the sulphate

which is commercially available as a cream-coloured amorphous powder although a crystalline specimen has been described by Chen *et al.* The sulphate is freely soluble in H_2O and also in several organic solvents including C_6H_6. The alkaloid itself contains one hydroxyl, one methoxyl and one methylimino group, while the presence of a carbonyl group is indicated by the positive test with 2:4-dinitrophenylhydrazine. Acid hydrolysis with H_2SO_4 under carefully controlled conditions, gives β-methylaminoethanol and erythrophleic acid, $C_{21}H_{32}O_5$, m.p. 218°C; $[\alpha]_D^{20} - 40°$ ($CHCl_3$). On selenium dehydrogenation, the acid furnishes 1:7:8-trimethylphenanthrene, m.p. 143–4°C and a selenium derivative, $C_{19}H_{16}Se$, m.p. 161–2°C.

It has been known for several decades that the alkaloid possesses local anaesthetic properties and was the only alkaloid known exhibiting digitalis-like action. It produces emesis in cats and, like other cardiac drugs increases the blood pressure in cats and stimulates rabbit intestine and guinea-pig uterus. Erythrophleic acid is, however, devoid of any characteristic action on the heart in a dosage at least 100 times as large as the minimal dosage of erythrophleine sulphate.

Gallois, Hardy., *Bull. Soc. Chim.*, **26**, 39 (1876)
Harnack, Zabrocki., *Arch. exp. Path. Pharm.*, **15**, 403 (1881)
Harnack., *Arch. Pharm.*, **234**, 561 (1896)
Laborde., *Ann. Mus. Col. Marseille*, **5**, 305 (1907)
Power, Salway., *Amer. J. Pharm.*, **84**, 337 (1912)
Petrie., *Proc. Linn. Soc., N.S.W.*, **46**, 333 (1921)
Kamerman., *S. Afr. J. Sci.*, **23**, 179 (1926)
Chen, Chen, Anderson., *J. Amer. Pharm. Assoc.*, **25**, 579 (1936)
Ruzicka, Dalma, Scott., *Helv. Chim. Acta*, **22**, 1516 (1939)
Blount, Openshaw, Todd., *J. Chem. Soc.*, 286 (1940)

Pharmacology:
Chen, Chen, Anderson., *J. Amer. Pharm. Assoc.*, **25**, 579 (1936)
Trabucchi., *Arch. Farm. sperim.*, **64**, 97 (1937)
Santi, Zweifel., *Arch. exp. Path. Pharm.*, **193**, 152 (1939)
Rothlin, Raymond-Hamet., *Arch. int. Pharmacodyn.*, **63**, 10 (1939)
Maling, Krayer., *J. Pharm. exp. Ther.*, **86**, 66 (1946)

ESCHOLAMINE

$C_{18}H_{18}O_4N^+$

A quaternary alkaloid found in *Eschscholtzia oregana*, this base is isolated as the crystalline iodide, m.p. 265–6°C which yields colourless crystals from H_2O and has $[\alpha]_D^{22} 0° \pm 3°$ (c 0.20, H_2O). On reduction with Zn and HCl at 80–90°C, this salts gives tetrahydroescholamine, m.p. 96–7°C, which on heating at 90°C with HNO_3 yields hydrastinine and with $KMnO_4$ furnishes 3:4-methylenedioxy-benzoic acid, m.p. 227–8°C. The structure has been determined from spectroscopic evidence.

Slavikova, Slavik., *Collect. Czech. Chem. Commun.*, **31**, 3362 (1966)

ESCHOLERINE

$C_{41}H_{61}O_{13}N$

M.p. $235-235.5°C$ (dec.).

A steroidal hypotensive alkaloid present in *Veratrum escholtzii*, the base forms colourless plates from aqueous Me_2CO and has $[\alpha]_D^{25} - 30°$ (c 1.0, pyridine). The aurichloride crystallizes from aqueous Me_2CO with m.p. $191.4°C$ (dec.) and the picrate as pale yellow needles from Et_2O-Me_2CO, m.p. $259.5°C$ (dec.). Acid hydrolysis furnishes protoverine, acetic acid, angelic acid and L-β-methylbutyric acid.

Klohs *et al., J. Amer. Chem. Soc.*, **74**, 1871 (1952)
Klohs *et al., ibid*, **76**, 1152 (1954)

ESCHOLIDINE

$C_{20}H_{22}O_4N$

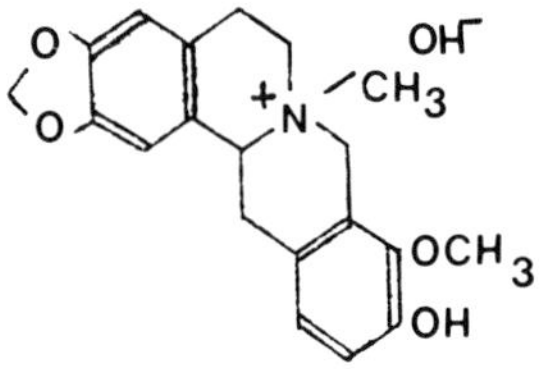

This alkaloid is the principal quaternary alkaloid of the roots of *Eschscholtzia californica, E. douglasi* and *E. glauca.* The structure, as (−)-tetrahydrothalifendine methohydroxide, has been established from infrared, ultraviolet and NMR spectra and on the identification of the Hofmann degradation products.

Slavik, Dolejs, Sedmera., *Collect. Czech. Chem. Commun.*, **35**, 2597 (1970)

ESCHOLINE

This alkaloid, isolated from *Eschscholtzia californica*, has been shown to be identical with Magnoflorine (q.v.).

Slavik, Dolejs., *Collect. Czech. Chem. Commun.*, **38**, 3514 (1973)

ESCHOLININE

$C_{21}H_{26}O_4N^+$

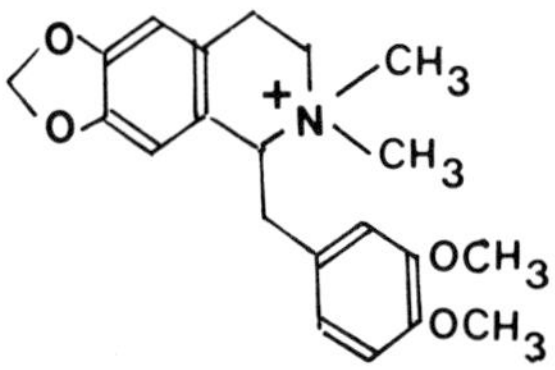

A quaternary alkaloid found in *Eschscholtzia californica*, this base has been isolated as the crystalline perchlorate. The structure has been determined from chemical degradations and spectroscopic data.

Slavik, Dolejs., *Collect. Czech. Chem. Commun.*, **38**, 3514 (1973)

(−)-ESCHSCHOLTZIDINE

$C_{20}H_{21}O_4N$

M.p. Indefinite

An amorphous alkaloid obtained from *Eschscholtzia californica* Chan., this base is non-crystallizable. It is dextrorotatory with $[\alpha]_D^{24} + 194.2°$ (c 1.56, MeOH). The ultraviolet spectrum shows one absorption maximum at 291 mμ. It contains two methoxyl, one methylenedioxy and one methylimino group in the molecule.

Manske, Shin., *Can. J. Chem.*, **44**, 1259 (1966)

Absolute configuration:
Barker, Battersby., *J. Chem. Soc.*, C, 1317 (1967)

(−)-ESCHSCHOLTZINE

$C_{19}H_{17}O_4N$

M.p. 128°C

Also isolated from *Eschscholtzia californica* Chan., this alkaloid crystallizes from MeOH or Et$_2$O as stout, colourless prisms. It is laevorotatory with $[\alpha]_D^{20} -$ 202° (c 1.0, MeOH) and the ultraviolet spectrum closely resembles that of the preceding alkaloid is exhibiting one absorption maximum at 295 mμ. The alkaloid forms a crystalline methiodide, m.p. 286−7°C (*dec.*) and an oxalate, m.p. 140°C following sintering and effervescence. The (±)-form yields a crystalline picrolonate, m.p. 223−5°C. The structure has been confirmed by synthesis of the latter form of the alkaloid.

Manske, Shin., *Can. J. Chem.*, **43**, 2180 (1965)
Manske *et al.*, *ibid*, **43**, 2183 (1965)

Synthesis:
Barker, Battersby., *J. Chem. Soc.*, C, 1317 (1967)

Absolute configuration:
Barker, Battersby., *J. Chem. Soc.*, C, 1317 (1967)

ESERAMINE

$C_{16}H_{22}O_3N_4$

M.p. 245°C (*dec.*).

An alkaloid from the calabar bean (*Physostigma venenosum*), this base was first isolated by Ehrenberg and subsequently by Salway. It forms colourless needles from EtOH and has $[\alpha]_D^{23} - 289°$ (EtOH). The ultraviolet spectrum shows absorption maxima at 256 and 311 mμ. The base is only sparingly soluble in $CHCl_3$, Et_2O or C_6H_6 but readily so in hot EtOH. The ($\pm$)-form crystallizes from EtOH as fine white needles, m.p. 197–201°C with slight decomposition.

Ehrenberg., *Verh. Ges. Deut. Nat. Aerzte*, **2**, 102 (1893)
Salway., *J. Chem. Soc.*, **99**, 2148 (1911)
Robinson, Spiteller., *Chem. Ind.*, 459 (1964)

Synthesis:
Robinson., *Chem. Ind.*, 87 (1965)
Robinson., *J. Chem. Soc.*, 3339 (1965)

ESERIDINE

$C_{15}H_{23}O_3N_3$

M.p. 132°C

This alkaloid was obtained by Böhringer and Söhne and subsequently examined by Eber. It was stated to revert to eserine when heated with dilute mineral acids. Its presence in *Physostigma venenosum* was questioned by Salway who was unable to detect it. Recent evidence suggests that it is identical with geneserine (q.v.).

Böhringer, Söhne., *Pharm. Post.*, **21**, 663 (1888)
Eber., *Pharm. Zeit.*, **37**, 483 (1892)
Merck., *Merck's Berichte*, **40**, 37 (1926)

ESERINE (*Physostigmine*)

$C_{15}H_{21}O_2N_3$

M.p. 86–7°C
and 105–6°C

The major alkaloid of *Physostigma venenosum*, this base exists in two crystalline forms with the above melting points, the higher melting form being the more stable. It is freely soluble in EtOH, Et_2O or $CHCl_3$. The solutions are all markedly alkaline and laevorotatory with $[\alpha]_D$ − 75.8° ($CHCl_3$) or − 120° (C_6H_6). The salts are well crystalline: the hydrochloride forms colourless needles, m.p. 221–3°C; the hydrobromide, m.p. 224–6°C; sulphate, microcrystalline deliquescent powder, m.p. 145°C; aurichloride, yellow leaflets, m.p. 163–5°C; platinichloride, orange-yellow needles, m.p. 180°C; picrate, m.p. 114°C; methiodide, m.p. 188°C; salicylate, colourless acicular crystals, m.p. 186–7°C; benzoate, prisms, m.p. 115–6°C and the derivative with mercuric iodide, m.p. 170°C.

On treatment with alkali, the alkaloid is converted into eseroline, $C_{13}H_{18}ON_2$, CO_2 and methylamine. With EtONa, the products are eseroline and methyluretane while, on heating at its melting point, methylcarbimide is evolved. Eseroline forms colourless needles, m.p. 129°C; $[\alpha]_D$ − 107° (EtOH) and, like eserine, behaves as a monoacidic tertiary base. On exposure to the atmosphere it is oxidized to rubreserine which crystallizes from H_2O in deep red needles, m.p. 152°C (*dry*), while under certain conditions, eserine blue, $C_{17}H_{23}O_2N_3$ results from the oxidation, this compound being apparently a combination of eseroline with one of the degradation products.

The action of eserine on the parasympathetic nervous system was recognised a long time ago and as early as 1873, its potentiating effect on the stimulation of such nerves was observed, e.g. on the cardiac vagus. More recently, its antagonistic effect on the action of curare was discovered and it has recently been suggested that the action of the alkaloid on the heart is due to the inhibition of the destruction of acetylcholine by an esterase normally present there. It has been demonstrated that the normal destruction of acetylcholine is largely enzymic in nature and is specifically inhibited by eserine.

Jobst, Hesse., *Annalen,* **129**, 115 (1864)
Jobst, Hesse., *ibid,* **141**, 913 (1867)
Vee., *Jahresb.,* 456 (1865)
Polonovski, Polonovski., *Bull. soc. chim.,* **37**, 744 (1925)
King, Liguori, Robinson., *J. Chem. Soc.,* 1475 (1933)
Julian, Pikl., *J. Amer. Chem. Soc.,* **57**, 755 (1935)
Harley-Mason, Jackson., *J. Chem. Soc.,* 3651 (1954)

Pharmacology:
Pal., *Zbl. Physiol.,* **14**, 255 (1900)
Hunt, Taveau., *J. Pharm. exp. Ther.,* **1**, 303 (1910)
Dale., *ibid,* **6**, 147 (1914–5)
Loewi, Nevratil., *Pfluger's Archiv.,* **214**, 689 (1926)
Cowan., *J. Physiol.,* **93**, 215 (1938)

ESPINIDINE

$C_{37}H_{42}O_6N_2$

M.p. Indefinite

An amorphous bisbenzylisoquinoline alkaloid found in *Berberis laurina* Billb. The alkaloid has $[\alpha]_D + 31°$ (CHCl$_3$) and contains three methoxyl, two hydroxyl and two methylimino groups. Chemical and spectroscopic data have established its constitution as the 4″-methyl ether of espinine (q.v.).

Falco *et al.*, *Experientia*, **25**, 1236 (1969)

ESPININE

$C_{36}H_{40}O_6N_2$

M.p. 123–5°C

A further bisbenzylisoquinoline alkaloid isolated from *Berberis laurina* Billb., this base forms colourless crystals from MeOH and has $[\alpha]_D + 25°$ (CHCl$_3$). It forms a trimethyl ether with $[\alpha]_D + 14°$ (CHCl$_3$). The alkaloid contains two methylimino groups, two methoxyl and three hydroxyl groups in the molecule.

Falco *et al., Experientia,* **25**, 1236 (1969)

ETHYLBENZOYLECGONINE

See Methylcocaine

2-ETHYL-3-[2-(3-ETHYLPIPERIDINO)ETHYL]-INDOLE

$C_{19}H_{28}N_2$

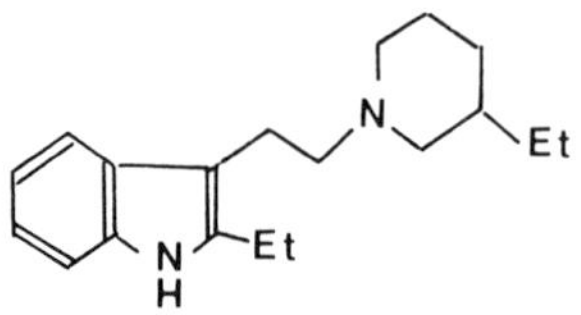

This alkaloid may be separated from the Et$_2$O-soluble bases of *Tabernaemontana cumminsii* by chromatography on alumina followed by thin layer chromatography with an Et$_2$O-ligroine mixture. It forms a crystalline picrate, m.p. $137-8°$C. The structure of the alkaloid has been confirmed by synthesis from 2-ethylindole which is reacted with oxaloyl chloride followed by reaction with 3-ethylpiperidine. The resulting compound, on reduction with LiAlH$_4$ yields the alkaloid.

Crooks, Robinson, Smith., *Chem. Commun.,* **20**, 1210 (1968)

ETIOLINE

$C_{27}H_{43}O_2N$

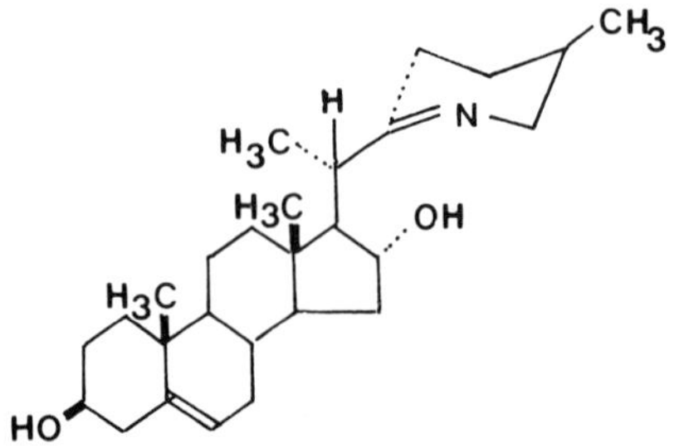

This steroidal alkaloid from *Veratrum grandiflorum* has a cholestadiene skeleton and forms colourless crystals from Me$_2$CO. It contains two hydroxyl groups and four methyl groups. The crystalline triacetyl derivative has m.p. $194-6°$C.

Kaneko *et al., Tetrahedron Lett.,* 4251 (1971)

EUCURARINE

$C_{20}H_{23}ON_2$

M.p. $135-144°$C

Freise has obtained this alkaloid from the old bark of an undetermined *Strychnos* species. The base is said to be toxic to frogs at a dosage of 0.13 mgm per kilo.

556

Freise., *Pharm. Zeit.*, **78**, 852 (1933)

Freise., *ibid*, **81**, 241 (1936)

Freise., *ibid*, **82**, 577 (1937)

EUONYMINE

$C_{38}H_{47}O_{18}N$

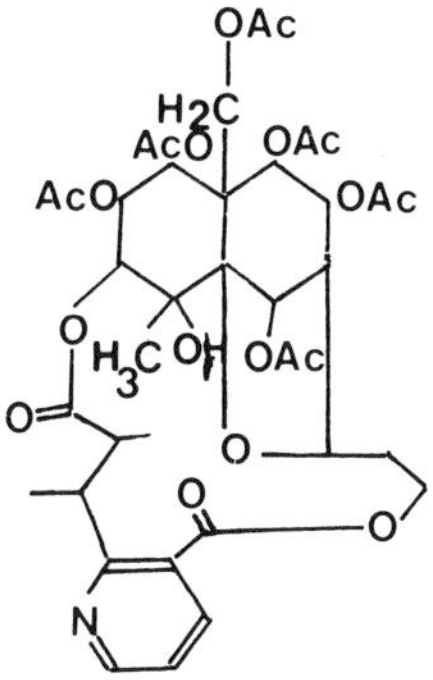

An amorphous macrocyclic alkaloid found in *Euonymus sieboldiana* Blume. The base forms a crystalline picrate from C_6H_6, m.p. 140–6°C. It contains six acetoxy groups, four methyl groups, one hydroxyl group and a pyridine ring.

Sugiura *et al.*, *Tetrahedron Lett.*, 2733 (1971)

Stereochemistry:

Wada *et al.*, *Tetrahedron Lett.*, 3131 (1971)

EUXYLOPHORICINE A

$C_{20}H_{17}O_3N_3$

M.p. 295–8°C

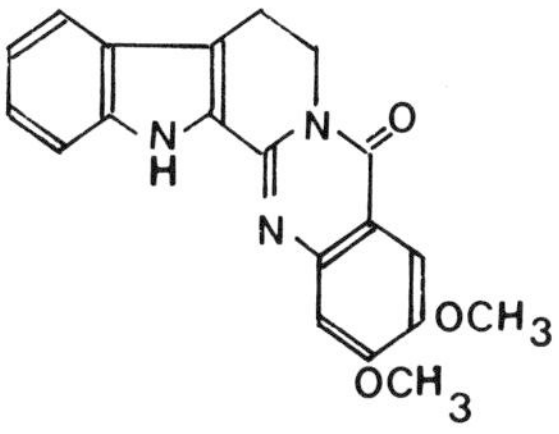

The bark of the Brazilian plant *Euxylophora paraensis* yields five closely-related quinazolinocarboline alkaloids. This particular base crystallizes from $CHCl_3$-MeOH in colourless needles. The ultraviolet spectrum in MeOH solution has absorption maxima at 255, 337, 353 and 360 mμ. The alkaloid contains two methoxyl groups, a keto group and one imino group.

The alkaloid may by hydrolyzed by KOH in amyl alcohol to give tetrahydro-carbolinone and 2-amino-4:5-domethoxybenzoic acid and may be synthesized by condensation of these two products.

Canonica *et al.*, *Tetrahedron Lett.*, 4865 (1968)

EUXYLOPHORICINE B

C$_{20}$H$_{15}$O$_3$N$_3$

M.p. 310–2°C

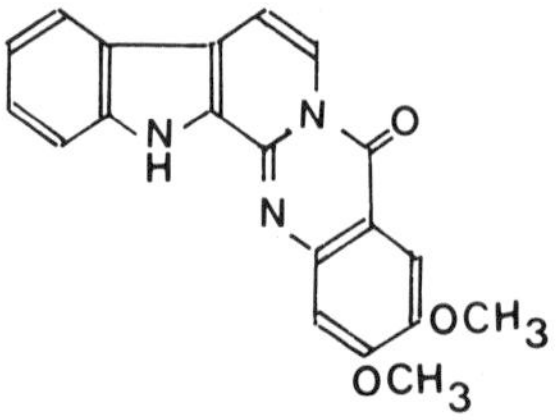

This alkaloid extracted from the bark of *Euxylophora paraensis* forms pale yellow prisms when crystallized from CHCl$_3$-MeOH. The ultraviolet spectrum in ethanolic solution exhibits absorption maxima at 256, 294, 303, 330, 353, 372 and 392 mμ.

Canonica *et al.*, *Tetrahedron Lett.*, 4865 (1968)

EUXYLOPHORICINE C

C$_{19}$H$_{13}$O$_3$N$_3$

M.p. 310–2°C

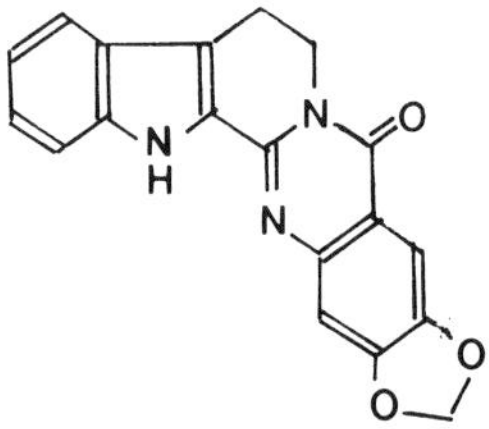

Also present in the bark of *Euxylophora paraensis,* this alkaloid forms yellow crystals from EtOH and its ultraviolet spectrum has absorption maxima at 232, 337, 350 and 368 mμ in acrylonitrile. The structure is that of euxylophoricine A with a methylenedioxy group replacing the two methyl groups.

Danieli *et al.*, *Phytochem.*, **11**, 1833 (1972)

EUXYLOPHORINE

C$_{21}$H$_{19}$O$_3$N$_3$

M.p. 227–230°C

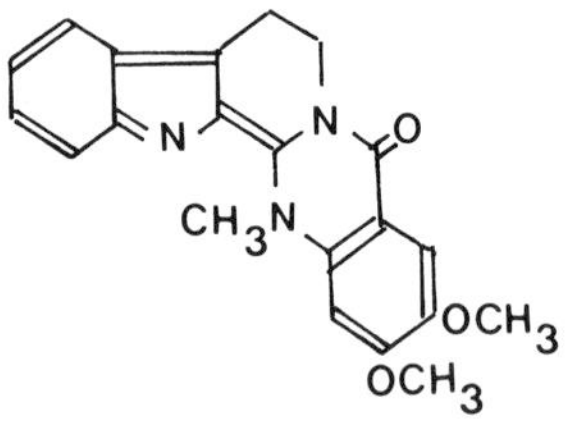

Obtained from the bark of *Euxylophora paraensis*, this alkaloid crystallizes from C$_6$H$_6$ as orange-red needles. The ultraviolet spectrum in acrylonitrile solution shows two absorption maxima at 253 and 402 mμ. When hydrolyzed with KOH in amyl alcohol it yields 1-tetrahydronorharmanone (tetrahydro-carbolinone) and 6-methylaminoveratric acid.

Canonica *et al.*, *Tetrahedron Lett.*, 4865 (1968)

EUXYLOPHORINE B

$C_{21}H_{17}O_3N_3$

M.p. 268–271°C

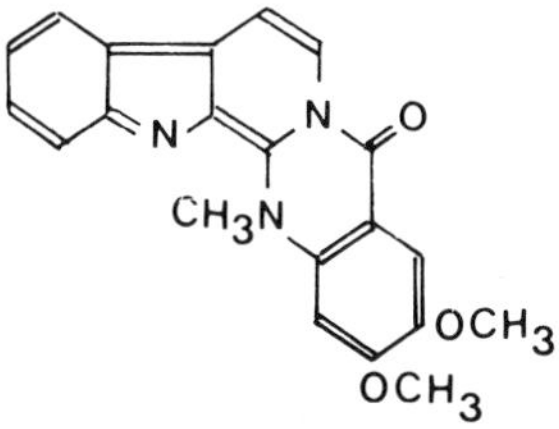

This alkaloid also occurs in the bark of *Euxylophora paraensis*. The ultraviolet spectrum in acrylonitrile shows absorption maxima at 278 and 352 mμ.

Danieli *et al., Phytochem.*, **11**, 1833 (1972)

EVELLERINE

$C_{17}H_{19}O_5N$

M.p. 149–150°C

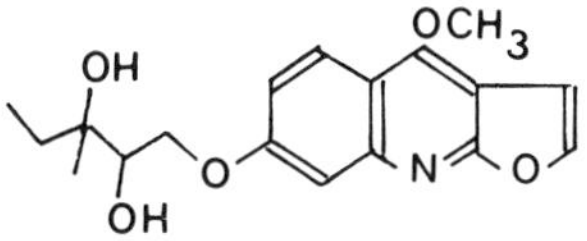

A furanoquinoline alkaloid isolated from the leaves of *Evodia elleryana* F. Muell. The base crystallizes from Me$_2$CO as colourless prisms and has $[\alpha]_D + 21°$ (c 0.3, CHCl$_3$). The ultraviolet spectrum has absorption maxima at 245, 307 and 329 mμ with an inflexion at 295 mμ. The base contains one secondary and one tertiary hydroxyl group and forms a crystalline acetate as colourless needles from MeOH, m.p. 163–4°C.

Johns, Lamberton, Sioumis., *Austral. J. Chem.*, **24**, 1897 (1968)

EVOCARPINE

$C_{23}H_{33}ON$

M.p. 34–8°C

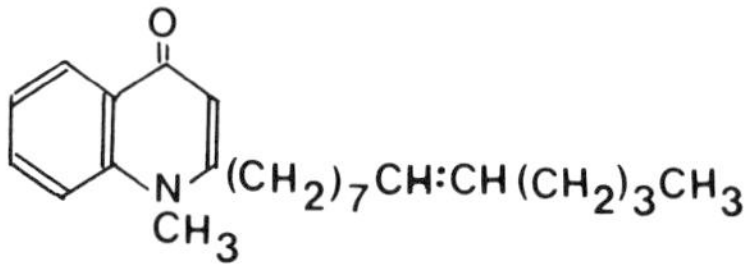

From the fruit of *Evodia rutaecarpa*, Tschesche and Werner have isolated this methylquinolone alkaloid as colourless crystals from MeOH. The ultraviolet spectrum in neutral MeOH has absorption maxima at 215, 240, 322 and 335 mμ, while in an acid medium (0.1 N/HCl-MeOH), the absorption maxima are at 232 and 305 mμ. A crystalline picrate, m.p. 96–96.5°C and a picrolonate, m.p. 128–9°C have been prepared.

Tschesche, Werner., *Tetrahedron*, **23**, 1873 (1967)

EVODIAMINE (*Rhetsine*)

$C_{19}H_{17}ON_3$

M.p. 278°C

A major component of the Chinese drug 'Wou-chou-yu' which is the dried fruit of *Evodia rutaecarpa* Benth., this alkaloid was first isolated by Asahina *et al.* The alkaloid forms yellowish leaflets from EtOH and has $[\alpha]_D^{15} + 352°$ (Me$_2$CO). It is only a weak base and insoluble in mineral acids. It is readily soluble in Me$_2$CO, sparingly so in Et$_2$O, AcOH, CHCl$_3$ and EtOH and insoluble in C$_6$H$_6$, petroleum ether and H$_2$O.

When heated with EtOH in dilute HCl it takes on 1 mole of H$_2$O to form the hydrate, *iso*evodiamine, $C_{19}H_{19}O_2N_3$, which forms rhombic leaflets, m.p. 146–7°C and is optically inactive. The latter forms a hydrochloride, m.p. 265–7°C (*dry*) and a nitrosamine, m.p. 120°C. The alkaloid is decomposed by boiling alcoholic KOH into dihydro*nor*harman and N-methylanthranilic acid. Under the same conditions, *iso*evodiamine yields CO$_2$, N-methylanthranilic acid and a base shown to be 3-β-aminoethylindole.

Asahina, Ohta., *Ber.*, **61**, 319 (1928)
Asahina *et al.*, *Chem. Zentr.*, **III**, 249 (1923)
Chatterjee, Bose, Ghosh., *Tetrahedron*, **7**, 257 (1959)
Gopinath, Govindachari, Rao., *ibid*, **8**, 293 (1960)

Biosynthesis:
Yamazaki, Ikuta., *Tetrahedron Lett.*, 3221 (1966)
Yamazaki *et al.*, *ibid*, 3317 (1967)

EVODINE

$C_{18}H_{19}O_5N$

M.p. 153–4°C

A furoquinoline alkaloid found in *Evodia xanthoxyloides* F. Muell., this base is laevorotatory with $[\alpha]_{4358}^{20} - 56°$ (c 1.66, CHCl$_3$). The ultraviolet spectrum has absorption maxima at 245, 323 and 335 mμ. It contains a secondary hydroxyl group in the side chain and forms a crystalline O-acetate as colourless plates from aqueous EtOH, m.p. 126–7°C.

Hughes, Neill, Ritchie., *Austral. J. Sci. Res.*, **5A**, 401 (1952)
Prager *et al.*, *Austral. J. Chem.*, **15**, 301 (1962)

EVOEUROPINE (*Alkaloid D*)

An uncharacterized alkaloid found in *Euonymus europeus* grown in Poland. The base was originally designated Alkaloid D.

Bishey, Kowalewski., *Herba Pol.*, **17**, 233 (1971)

EVOEVOLINE (*Alkaloid A*)

A second alkaloid isolated from a Polish specimen of *Euonymus europeus.* No salts or derivatives have been reported for this base.

Bishey, Kowalewski., *Herba Pol.*, **17**, 233 (1971)

EVOLATINE

$C_{18}H_{21}O_6N$

M.p. 201−2°C

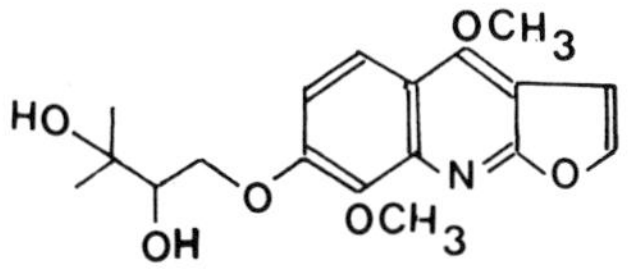

A furoquinoline base present in *Evodia alata,* occurring chiefly in the bark and leaves. The base crystallizes as colourless needles from Me_2CO and has $[\alpha]_D^{24} +$ 17.5° (c 0.3, EtOH). With methyl iodide at 100°C for 4 hours, it forms *iso*evolatine, m.p. 233−4°C; $[\alpha]_D^{24} + 29°$ (c 0.3, EtOH). The structure has been determined as 7-(2:3-dihydrox-3-methylbutoxy)-4:8-dimethoxyfuro 2,3-b quinoline.

Gell, Hughes, Ritchie., *Austral. J. Chem.*, 8, 114 (1955)

EVOLITRINE

$C_{13}H_{11}O_3N$

M.p. 114−5°C

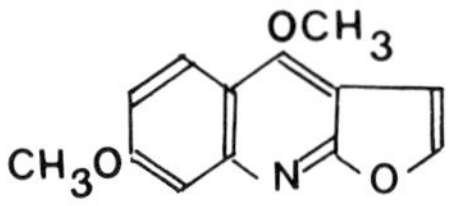

Found in the leaves and bark of *Eyodia littoralis,* this alkaloid forms colourless crystals from petroleum ether. It yields a crystalline hydrochloride, m.p. 150−1°C (*dec.*) and a picrate, m.p. 201−2°C.

Cooke, Haynes., *Austral. J. Chem.*, 7, 273 (1954)
Cooke, Haynes., *ibid*, 22, 225 (1958)
Ohta, Mori., *J. Pharm. Soc., Japan*, 78, 446 (1958)
Sato, Ohta., *Bull. Chem. Soc., Japan*, 31, 161 (1958)

EVOMINE

M.p. 232−5°C

This alkaloid from *Evonymus europaea* L. has been described by Bishay and Kowalewski. It forms colourless needles when crystallized from Et_2O.

Bishay, Kowalewski., *Herba Pol.*, **17**, 233 (1971)

EVONINE

$C_{36}H_{43}O_{17}N$

M.p. 184–190°C

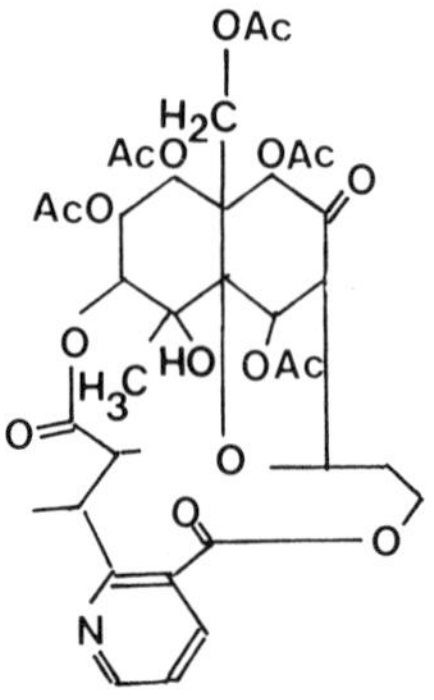

Also present in *Evonymus europaea* L., this macrocyclic alkaloid has subsequently been discovered in *E. sieboldiana* Blume. It is obtained as colourless crystals from EtOH and has $[\alpha]_D + 8.4°$ (c 1.5, CHCl$_3$). The ultraviolet spectrum has two absorption maxima at 227 and 267 mμ. It contains four acetoxy groups, one acetoxymethyl group, four methyl groups, one hydroxyl group and a pyridine nucleus.

Pailer, Libiseller., *Monatsh.*, **93**, 403, 511 (1962)
Wada *et al., Tetrahedron Lett.*, 2655 (1971)
Shizuri *et al., ibid,* 2659 (1971)

Stereochemistry:
Klasek *et al., Helv. Chim. Acta*, **54**, 2144 (1971)
Wada *et al., Tetrahedron Lett.*, 3131 (1971)

EVONOLINE

$C_{36}H_{43}O_{16}N$

M.p. Indefinite

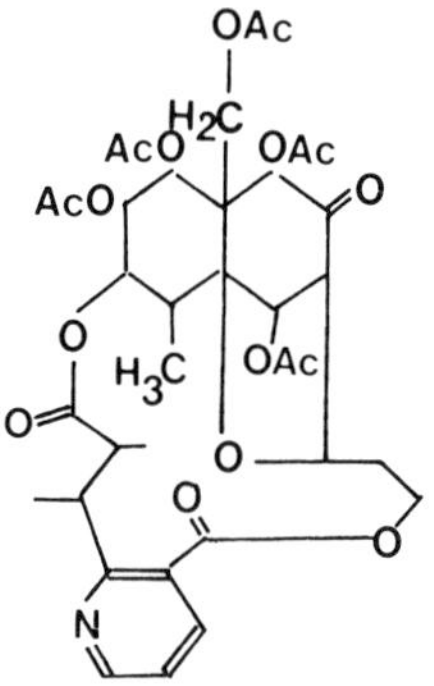

An amorphous alkaloid from *Evonymus europaea* L., the alkaloid has $[\alpha]_D^{20} + 6.0°$ (c 3.2, CHCl$_3$). The ultraviolet spectrum closely resembles that of the preceding base with absorption maxima at 225 and 265 mμ.

Wada *et al., Tetrahedron Lett.*, 2655 (1971)

EVOPRENINE

$C_{20}H_{21}O_4N$

M.p. 143°C

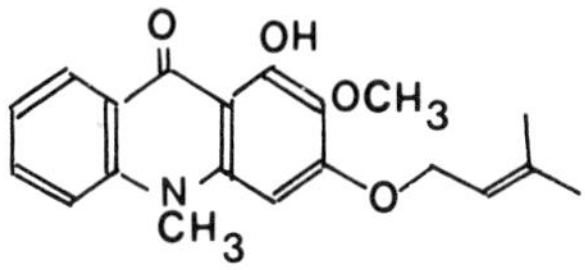

Isolated from the bark of *Evodia alata* F. Muell., this alkaloid crystallizes as light yellow needles from EtOH. The ultraviolet spectrum has absorption maxima at 274 and 400 mμ with an inflexion at 325 mμ. The structure has been demonstrated to be 1-hydroxy-2-methoxy-3-[(3-methylbut-2-enyl)oxy]-10-methylacridan-9-one.

Diment, Ritchie, Taylor., *Austral. J. Chem.*, **20**, 1719 (1967)

EVORINE

$C_{34}H_{41}O_{16}N$

M.p. 257–9°C

The seeds of *Evonymus europaea* L. yield this macrocyclic alkaloid which forms colourless crystals from MeOH. It has $[\alpha]_D^{22} + 20°$ (c 1.11, CHCl$_3$).

Klasek *et al.*, *Helv. Chim. Acta*, **54**, 2144 (1971)

EVOXANTHIDINE

$C_{15}H_{11}O_4N$

M.p. 312–3°C

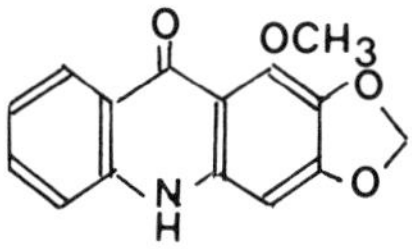

An acridone alkaloid which occurs in *Evodia xanthoxyloides*, this base contains one methoxyl, one methylenedioxy and a methylimino group. The structure has been determined by chemical and spectroscopic techniques.

Hughes, Neill, Ritchie., *Austral. J. Sci. Res., Ser. A*, **5**, 401 (1952)
Cannon *et al.*, *ibid*, **5**, 406 (1952)

EVOXANTHINE

$C_{16}H_{13}O_4N$

M.p. 217–8°C

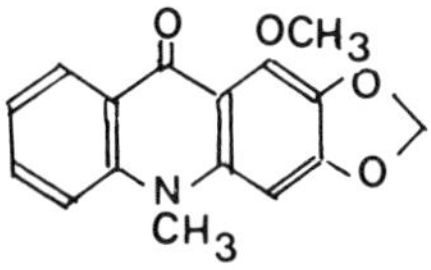

Isolated from the bark of *Balfourodendron riedolanium* and *Evodia xanthoxyloides*, this acridone alkaloid crystallizes as pale yellow needles from EtOH. The ultraviolet spectrum has absorption maxima at 275 and 400 mμ with shoulders at 240 and 320 mμ. The structure has been established as 1-methoxy-2:3-methylenedioxy-10-methylacridone.

Hughes *et al.*, *Nature*, **162**, 223 (1948)
Hughes, Neill, Ritchie., *Austral. J. Sci. Res.*, **3A**, 497 (1950)
Cannon *et al.*, *ibid*, **3A**, 497 (1950)
Rapoport, Holden., *J. Amer. Chem. Soc.*, **82**, 4395 (1960)
Synthesis:
Govindachari *et al.*, *Tetrahedron*, **23**, 1827 (1967)

EVOXINE

$C_{18}H_{21}O_6N$

M.p. 154–5°C

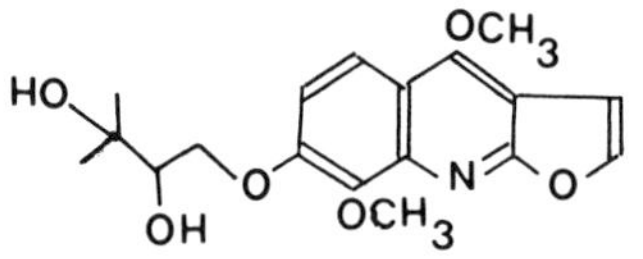

The bark of *Evodia xanthoxyloides* yields this alkaloid of the furoquinoline type. It crystallizes from aqueous MeOH as colourless crystals and has $[\alpha]_D^{22}$ + 14.6° (EtOH). It contains a secondary and tertiary hydroxyl group and forms a di-acetate, m.p. 101.5°C; $[\alpha]_D^{21}$ 0° (c 1.0, EtOH) and a crystalline picrate, m.p. 159–160°C.

Hughes, Neill, Ritchie., *Austral. J. Sci. Res.*, **5A**, 401 (1952)
Eastwood, Hughes, Ritchie., *Austral. J. Chem.*, **7**, 87 (1954)

EVOXOIDINE

$C_{18}H_{19}O_5N$

M.p. 136–7°C

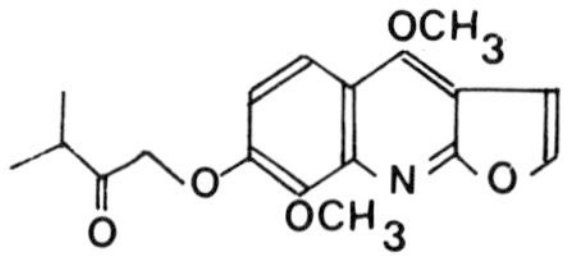

Evodia xanthoxyloides also yields this furoquinoline alkaloid which crystallizes in colourless prisms from EtOH. It is optically inactive in EtOH and forms a crystalline picrate, m.p. 162°C. The oxime has m.p. 185°C and the semicarbazone, m.p. 210°C (*dec.*).

Hughes, Neill, Ritchie., *Austral. J. Sci. Res.*, **5A**, 401 (1952)
Eastwood, Hughes, Ritchie., *Austral. J. Chem.*, **7**, 87 (1954)

564

EVOZINE

$C_{32}H_{39}O_{15}N$

M.p. 288–290°C

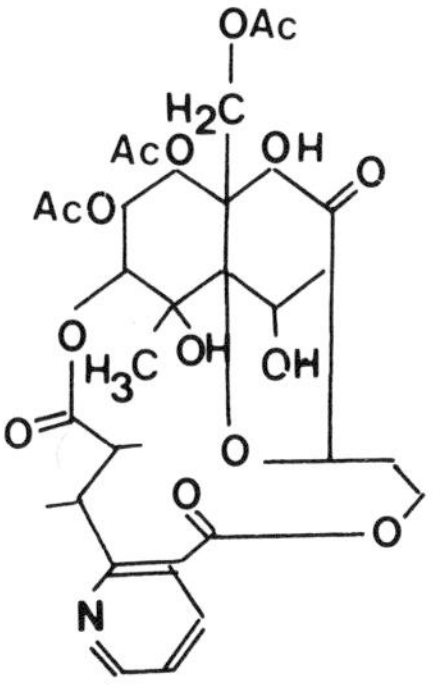

A macrocyclic alkaloid isolated from the seeds of *Evonymus europaea* L., this base has $[\alpha]_D^{22} + 13°$ (c 0.92, $CHCl_3$). It contains two acetoxy groups, one acetoxymethyl group, three hydroxyl groups, four methyl groups and a pyridine ring in the molecule.

Klasek *et al., Helv. Chim. Acta,* **54**, 2144 (1971)

Structure:
Klasek *et al., Tetrahedron Lett.,* 941 (1972)

EXCELSINE

$C_{22}H_{33}O_6N$

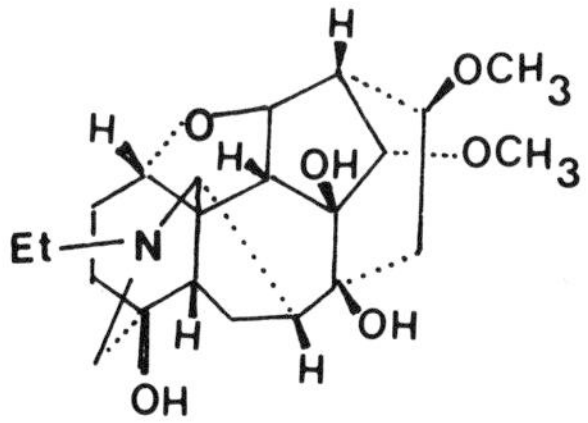

This aconite alkaloid has recently been isolated from the roots of *Aconitum excelsum.* The structure has been determined by NMR and mass spectrometry and by reduction with Raney Ni to give lappaconidine. When treated with HCl and then H_2SO_4, followed by acetylation, it gives dehydroaconitane tetraacetate.

Tel'nov, Yunusov, Yunusov., *Khim. Prir. Soedin,* **9**, 129 (1973)

EXCELSININE

$C_{21}H_{26}O_3N_2$

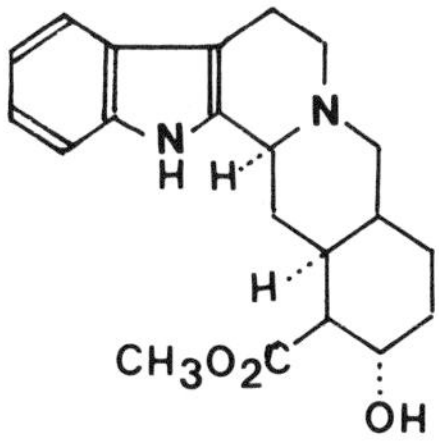

A yohimbine type alkaloid found in *Aspidosperma excelsum,* the structure given above is based upon infrared, NMR and mass spectrometry.

Burnell, Medina., *Can. J. Chem.,* **45**, 725 (1967)

EXIMIDINE

$C_{20}H_{23}O_4N$

M.p. $133°C$

This phenolic alkaloid is present in *Dicentra eximia* (Ker) Torr. It is isomeric with Corydine (q.v.) and yields a crystalline methiodide, m.p. $218°C$ (*dec.*).

Manske., *Can. J. Res.*, 8, 592 (1933)

EXIMINE

This alkaloid is identical with (+)-Corydine (q.v.).

F

FABIANINE

$C_{14}H_{21}ON$

B.p. $74°C/0.05$ mm

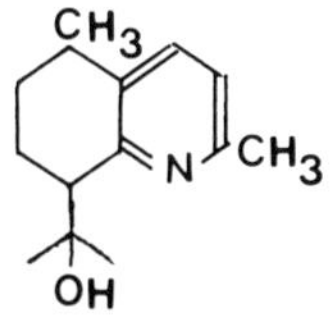

This oily alkaloid occurs in *Fabiana imbricata*. Its optical activity is still some-what in doubt with $[\alpha]_D$ certainly less than $1°$. It contains a tertiary hydroxyl group and forms an acetyl derivative, also an oil, b.p. $70-5°C/0.01$ mm. The picrate is crystalline, however, forming needles from AcOEt, m.p. $114-6°C$. It contains two methyl groups and the nitrogen atom is tertiary.

Edwards, Elmore., *Can. J. Chem.*, **40**, 256 (1962)

FAGARAMIDE

$C_{14}H_{17}O_3N$

M.p. $119.5°C$

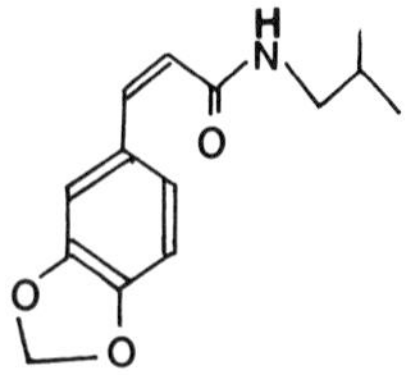

This base occurring in the bark of *Xanthoxylum macrophyllum* Oliver, is a member of the group of pungent acid amides and is not an alkaloid in the strict sense of the term since it is a neutral substance and exerts little, if any, pharma-cological action. It forms a hydrochloride, however, m.p. $137°C$ and a dibromide, m.p. $134-5°C$. Alkaline hydrolysis furnishes *iso*butylamine and methylene-dioxycinnamic acid. Oxidation with $KMnO_4$ gives first piperonal and then piperonylic acid. The structure has been established as the *iso*butylamide of piperonylacrylic acid.

Thoms, Thümen., *Ber.*, **44**, 3717 (1911)
Goodson., *Biochem. J.*, **15**, 123 (1921)

α-FAGARINE

$C_{21}H_{23}O_5N$

M.p. $169-170°C$;
B.p. $170-5°C/0.001$ mm

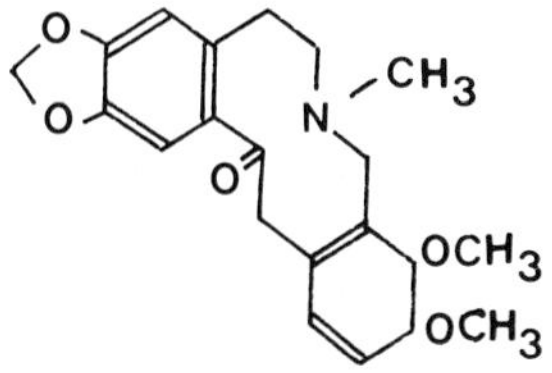

Isolated by Stuckert from the leaves of *Fagara coco* (Gill), England, this alkaloid distils unchanged at low pressures and is optically inactive. It forms crystalline salts and derivatives, e.g. the hydrochloride, m.p. 192–3°C; hydrobromide, m.p. 186–8°C (*dec.*); hydriodide, m.p. 190–2°C; methiodide, m.p. 205°C (*dec.*) and picrate, m.p. 208–9°C. Two methoxyls, one methylimino group and one methylenedioxy group are present. The base cannot be hydrogenated in the presence of PtO_2 even at a pressure of 4 atmospheres and is stable to boiling dilute acids and alkalies. On distilling with soda lime, it yields methylamine while oxidation with $KMnO_4$ under acid conditions gives formaldehyde and *m*-methoxybenzaldehyde.

Pharmacologically, it has been employed as a substitute for quinidine in the treatment of auricular fibrillation. It is identical to fagarine-I.

Stuckert., *Invest. Labor. Quim. biol. Univ. nac. Cordoba,* **1**, 69 (1933)
Deulofeu *et al., Science,* **102**, 69 (1945)
Berinzaghi *et al., J. Org. Chem.,* **10**, 181 (1945)
Deulofeu, Labriola, Berinzaghi., *ibid,* **12**, 217 (1947)
Yunusov., *J. Gen. Chem.,* **25**, 2009 (1955)

β-FAGARINE

See Skimmianine

γ-FAGARINE (*Aegelenine*)

$C_{13}H_{11}O_3N$

M.p. 139–142°C

The original formula of this alkaloid of $C_{15}H_{15}O_3N$ was altered to that given above by *Deulofeu et al,* thereby representing it as a furoquinoline base. It is present in *Fagara coco, Aegle marmelos* grown in Bihar and several Haplophyllum species. The alkaloid forms a platinichloride, orange needles, m.p. > 200°C (*dec.*); a picrate, m.p. 177°C and a picrolonate, m.p. 174–5°C.

$KMnO_4$ in Me_2CO oxidizes the base first to 2-hydroxy-4:8-dimethoxy-quinoline-3-aldehyde (γ-fagaraldehyde), m.p. 185°C and then to fagaric acid, m.p. 215°C. In boiling, dilute HCl, the latter is decarboxylated to give 2:4-dihydroxy-8-methoxyquinoline, m.p. 250°C. With MeI at 100°C the base is converted into γ-*iso*fagarine.

Stuckert., *Invest. Labor. Quim. biol. Univ. nac. Cordoba,* **1**, 69 (1933)
Chakravarty., *J. Ind. Chem. Soc.,* **21**, 401 (1944)
Berinzaghi *et al., J. Org. Chem.,* **10**, 181 (1945)
Yunusov., *Dokl. Akad. Nauk. Uzbek SSR,* **12**, 22 (1953)
Yunusov., *J. Gen. Chem. USSR,* **25**, 2009 (1955)

FAGARINE

M.p. 136°C

This uncharacterized alkaloid was obtained by Stuckert from *Fagara coco*, occurring mainly in the leaves. So far, its physical and chemical constants, except for the melting point, have not been determined.

Stuckert., *Invest. Labor. Quim. biol. Univ. nac. Cordoba,* 1, 69 (1933)

FAGARINE II

$C_{21}H_{23}O_5N$

M.p. 200–1°C

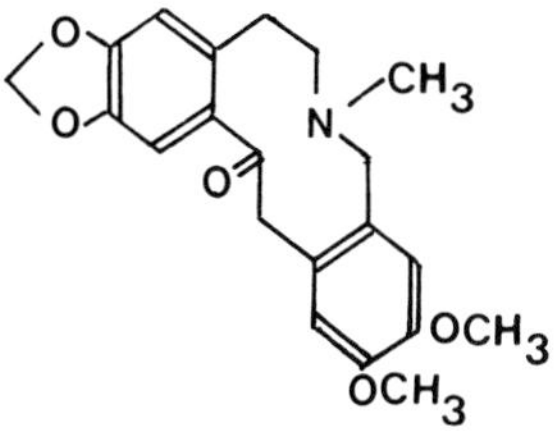

An alkaloid found in *Fagara coco,* this base forms colourless crystals from EtOH. The ultraviolet spectrum exhibits two absorption maxima at 232 and 286 mμ. The alkaloid contains two methoxyl, one methylenedioxy and one methylimino group in the molecule. The structure has been confirmed by synthesis.

Comin, Deulofeu., *Tetrahedron,* 16, 63 (1959)
Giacopello, Deulofeu, Comin., *ibid,* 20, 2971 (1964)

FAGARINE III

$C_{22}H_{26}O_4N$

M.p. 181–3°C

A further alkaloid of *Fagara coco,* this base is strongly laevorotatory with $[\alpha]_D^{27} - 300°$ (CHCl$_3$). The hydrochloride is also crystalline with m.p. 232–4°C (*dec.*).

Redemann, Wisegarver, Alles., *J. Amer. Chem. Soc.,* 71, 1030 (1949)

FAGARONINE

$C_{21}H_{20}O_4N^+$

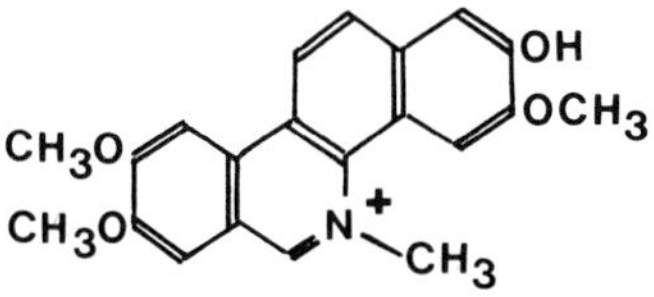

A quaternary alkaloid isolated from *Fagara zanthoxyloides* as the crystalline chloride, m.p. 202°C and 255°C with intermediate solidification. The salt is a tumour inhibitor with a high order of activity against P-388 leukaemia in mice.

The structure has been determined from ultraviolet, infrared, NMR and mass spectral data.

Messmer *et al.*, *J. Pharm. Sci.*, **61**, 1858 (1972)

FALCATINE

$C_{17}H_{19}O_4N$

M.p. 127–8°C

Present in *Nerine falcata* and *N. laticonia*, this alkaloid may be purified by recrystallization from Et_2O when it forms colourless prisms. It is laevorotatory with $[\alpha]_D^{22} - 197.8°$ (c 1.05, $CHCl_3$). It is somewhat unstable, developing a pale yellow colour on exposure to air and light. The hydrochloride is a microcrystalline powder, m.p. 220–235°C (*dec.*); the picrate forms crystals from aqueous EtOH, m.p. 182–5°C (*dec.*); the methiodide, m.p. 250–2°C and the O-acetate has m.p. 201–2°C. Hydrogenation with Pd yields the dihydro derivative as colourless crystals from Et_2O, m.p. 128.5–129.5°C. One hydroxyl group, one methoxyl group and a methylenedioxy group are present.

Wildman, Kaufman., *J. Amer. Chem. Soc.*, **77**, 4807 (1955)
Fales, Wildman., *ibid*, **80**, 4395 (1958)
Torssell., *Acta Chem. Scand.*, **15**, 947 (1961)

FANGCHININE

M.p. 218°C

This alkaloid has been described by King and Shih who obtained it from the Chinese drug 'Feng-fan-chi', whose botanical origin is still somewhat obscure. The alkaloid is stated to be dextrorotatory with $[\alpha]_D^{18} + 267°$. The structure is not yet known.

King, Shih., *Bull. Nat. Acad. Peiping.*, **6**, 13 (1935)

FANGCHINOLINE

$C_{37}H_{40}O_6N_2$

M.p. 237–8°C

This bisbenzyl*iso*quinoline alkaloid was first isolated from the Chinese drug 'Han-fang-chi' and later shown to be present in *Cyclea peltata* Diels and *Stephania hernandifolia* Willd. It forms colourless crystals from Me_2CO or

570

EtOH with the above melting point. It is dextrorotatory with $[\alpha]_D^{19} + 255.2°$ (CHCl$_3$). The ultraviolet spectrum shows a single absorption maximum at 283 mμ. With alcoholic FeCl$_3$ it gives a blue-green colour. The crystalline picrate has m.p. 242°C (*dec.*) when crystallized from Me$_2$CO. When obtained crystalline from EtOH, however, it has m.p. 186°C (*dec.*). The base forms an ethyl ether as colourless needles from aqueous EtOH, m.p. 116–7°C and a methyl ether, m.p. 252°C, which is identical with Tetrandrine (q.v.).

Chuang *et al.*, *Ber.*, **72**, 519 (1939)
Hsing, Chang., *Sci. Sinica* (Peking), **7**, 59 (1958)
Kupchan, Yokoyama, Thyagarajan., *J. Pharm. Sci.*, **50**, 164 (1961)
Kupchan, Asbun, Thyagarajan., *ibid*, **50**, 819 (1961)

FASTUDINE

$C_{16}H_{21}O_3N$

The basic fraction of the EtOH extract of *Datura fastuosa* seeds (Syn. *D. Metel*) contains, besides Atropine (q.v.), three minor bases, fastudine, fastunine and fastunidine. This particular alkaloid is isomeric with *Nor*hyoscyamine (q.v.) and is separated from the accompanying bases on a basic alumina column followed by further purification by countercurrent distribution methods.

Khaleque *et al.*, *Sci. Res.* (Dacca), **3**, 212 (1966)

FASTUNIDINE

A further minor constituent of the seeds of *Datura fastuosa,* this alkaloid has been characterized as the picrate, m.p. 161–2°C. The infrared spectrum shows an ester carbonyl absorption at 1723 cm^{-1}.

Khaleque *et al.*, *Sci. Res.* (Dacca), **3**, 212 (1966)

FASTUNINE

$C_{17}H_{23}O_3N$

M.p. 88–90°C

Also present in the EtOH extract of the seeds of *Datura fastuosa*, this alkaloid forms colourless crystals from EtOH. It is isomeric with Atropine (q.v.) but the melting point, ultraviolet and infrared spectra are distinctly different.

Khaleque *et al.*, *Sci. Res.* (Dacca), **3**, 212 (1966)

FASTUSINE

$C_{15}H_{19}O_2N$

M.p. 75–6°C

Isolated from *Datura fastuosa* by the combined technique of alumina chroma-tography and countercurrent distribution, this alkaloid is crystalline but hygroscopic. It has $[\alpha]_D^{30} + 55°$ (EtOH) and gives a picrate, m.p. 210–1°C and a picrolonate, m.p. 195–7°C. The base occurs primarily in the seeds but has also been obtained from the roots of this plant.

Khaleque *et al.*, *Sci. Res.* (Dacca), 2, 147 (1965)

FASTUSININE

$C_{18}H_{12}O_5N$

M.p. Indefinite

This base from *Datura fastuosa* forms a semi-solid mass which cannot be crystallized. It has been purified via the crystalline picrate, m.p. 235–5°C.

Khaleque *et al.*, *Sci. Res.* (Dacca), 2, 147 (1965)

FAWCETTIDINE

$C_{16}H_{23}ON$

B.p. 125°C/0.1 mm

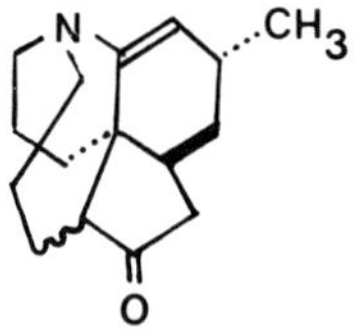

One of the *Lycopodium* alkaloids found in *L. fawcettii* Lloyd and Underwood, this base is a colourless oil which has $[\alpha]_D + 161°$ (c 0.6, EtOH). It may be characterized as the methiodide, colourless crystals from Me$_2$CO-MeOH, m.p. 224–6°C and the picrate, m.p. 223–5°C. One methyl group is present in the molecule.

Burnell., *J. Chem. Soc.*, 3091 (1959)
Burnell *et al.*, *Can. J. Chem.*, 41, 3091 (1963)
Ishii *et al.*, *Tetrahedron Lett.*, 6215 (1966)

FAWCETTIINE

$C_{18}H_{29}O_3N$

M.p. Indefinite

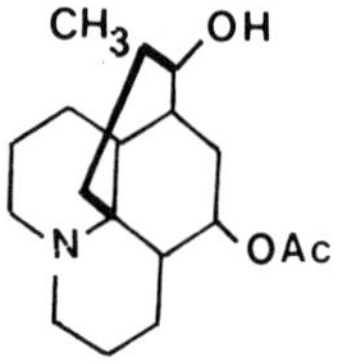

Present in several *Lycopodium* species, this alkaloid forms a crystalline

572

perchlorate which crystallizes as the monohydrate from H_2O or Me_2CO, m.p. 272–5°C (*dec.*). The methiodide also forms a crystalline monohydrate, m.p. 279–280°C. The alkaloid contains an acetyl group, a methyl group and a hydroxyl group. The O-acetate, m.p. 116–7°C is a minor constituent of *L. fawcettii*. Acid hydrolysis of the base yields deacetylfawcettiine, also present in *L. fawcettii*.

Burnell., *J. Chem. Soc.*, 3091 (1959)
Anet, Khan., *Can. J. Chem.*, **37**, 1589 (1959)
Burnell, Mootoo, Taylor., *ibid,* **38**, 1927 (1960)
Burnell, Mootoo, Taylor., *ibid,* **39**, 1090 (1961)
Burnell, Taylor., *Tetrahedron,* **15**, 173 (1961)

FAWCETTIMINE

$C_{16}H_{25}O_2N$

M.p. Indefinite

This alkaloid is a constituent of *Lycopodium clavatum* L. and is obtained as a glassy varnish with no definite melting point. The hydrochloride is crystalline, m.p. 235°C (*dec.*); the perchlorate forms colourless crystals from Me_2CO-isopropanol, m.p. 225–6°C and the methiodide, colourless prisms from Me_2CO-EtOH has m.p. 240–2°C. The alkaloid almost certainly exists in tautomeric forms and the imino modification yields an N-acetyl derivative, m.p. 144–5°C.

Burnell, Mootoo., *Can. J. Chem.*, **39**, 1090 (1961)
Burnell *et al.*, *ibid,* **41**, 3091 (1963)

FEBRIFUGINE

$C_{16}H_{19}O_3N_3$

M.p. 139–140°C

Dichroa febrifuga Lour. is a member of the botanical family Saxifragaceae and the source of the Chinese anti-malarial drug 'Ch'ang Shan'. The roots and leaves of this plant contain this alkaloid which has $[\alpha]_D^{25} + 6°$ ($CHCl_3$). It yields a crystalline dihydrochloride, m.p. 220–2°C (*dec.*). The alkaloid is approximately 100 times as effective as quinine against *Plasmodia lophurae* in ducks.

Koepfli, Mead, Brockman., *J. Amer. Chem. Soc.*, **69**, 1837 (1947)

isoFEBRIFUGINE

$C_{16}H_{19}O_3N_3$

M.p. 129–130°C

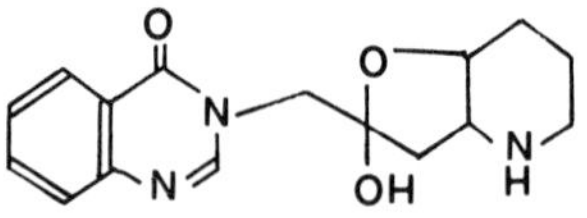

This alkaloid is isomeric with febrifugine and is also present in the roots and leaves of *Dichroa febrifuga* Lour. It is dextrorotatory with $[\alpha]_D^{23} + 131°$ (CHCl$_3$) and forms a hygroscopic hydrochloride. When heated it passes into febrifugine. The ultraviolet spectrum is identical with that of the preceding alkaloid with absorption maxima at 225, 266, 275 and 302 mμ

Koepfli, Mead, Brockman., *J. Amer. Chem. Soc.,* **69**, 1837 (1947)

FEDAMAZINE

$C_{20}H_{21}ON_2^+$

M.p. 185–6°C

A quaternary alkaloid from the bark of *Strychnos toxifera,* the base has been characterized as the picrate which forms light yellow crystals from aqueous Me$_2$CO.

Asmis, Schmid, Karrer., *Helv. Chim. Acta,* **37**, 1983 (1954)

FENDLERIDINE

$C_{19}H_{24}ON_2$

M.p. 185–6°C

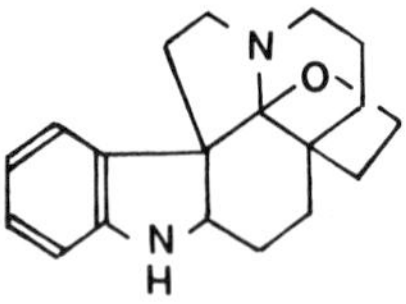

One of the minor alkaloids isolated from the seeds of *Aspidosperma fendleri* Woodson, this imidazolidinocarbazole base has an ultraviolet spectrum showing two absorption maxima at 242.5 and 292.5 mμ. The alkaloid contains one imino group.

Burnell, Medina, Ayer., *Chem. & Ind.,* **33** (1964)

FENDLERINE

$C_{23}H_{30}O_4N_2$

M.p. 179–181°C

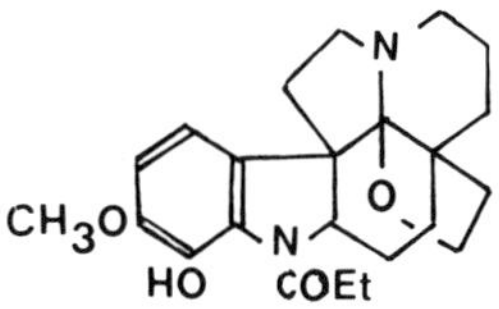

A further alkaloid of *Aspidosperma fendleri* Woodson, this base occurs mainly in the bark and fruit of the plant. Its ultraviolet spectrum also shows two absorption maxima at 225 and 258 mμ.

Burnell, Medina, Ayer., *Chem. & Ind.*, 235 (1964)

FENDLISPERMINE

$C_{19}H_{26}ON_2$

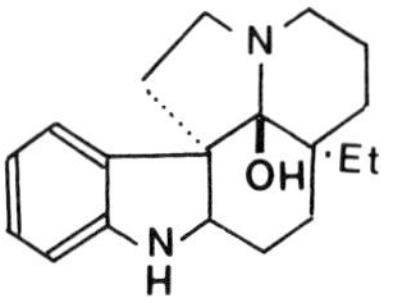

A recently discovered alkaloid, this base is found in the root bark of *Aspidosperma fendleri* Woodson. The structure has been established from the infrared, NMR and mass spectra.

Medina, Hurtardo, Burnell., *Rev. latinoamer. Quim.*, **4**, 73 (1973)

FESTUCINE

$C_8H_{14}ON_2$

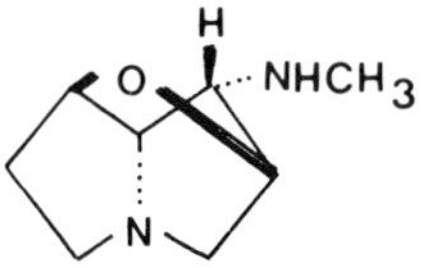

This pyrrolizidine alkaloid has been isolated from the Tall Fescue grass of Australia, *Festuca arundinacea* Schreb. It forms a non-crystallizable oil which does, however, yield crystalline salts and derivatives, e.g. the hydrochloride, colourless needles from EtOH, m.p. 237−242°C (*dec.*); the picrate which may be crystallized from EtOH or H_2O with m.p. 252−7°C (*dec.*); the N-acetyl derivative forming a hydrochloride, m.p. 202−3°C; $[\alpha]_D^{25}$ + 5.4° (c 1.106, H_2O) and the N-nitroso compound, m.p. 64−65.5°C. The base contains one methylamino group and an ether bridge across the two rings.

Yates, Tookey., *Austral. J. Chem.*, **18**, 53 (1965)

FETIDINE

$C_{40}H_{46}O_8N_2$

M.p. 132−5°C

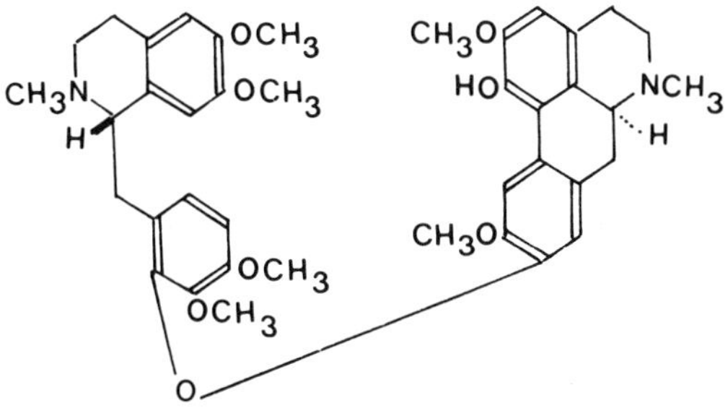

An aporphine-benzyl*iso*quinoline alkaloid, this base occurs in *Thalictrum foetidum*. As usually obtained it is amorphous but may be crystallized from

AcOEt. It is dextrorotatory with $[\alpha]_D + 121.4°$ (MeOH). When treated with sodium in liquid ammonia at $-45°C$ it yields (+)-Laudanosine (q.v.). The alkaloid forms a dihydrochloride, m.p. $229-230°C$; $[\alpha]_D - 30.93°$ (H_2O). There are six methoxyl, two methylimino and one hydroxyl group in the molecule, the structure of which has been determined by chemical degradation and spectroscopic evidence.

Sargazakov, Ismailov, Yunusov., *Dokl. Akad. Nauk. Uzbek SSR*, **20**, 28 (1963)
Ismailov, Yunusov., *Khim. Prir. Soedin.*, **2**, 43 (1966)
Cava, Wakisaka., *Tetrahedron Lett.*, 2309 (1972)

FIBRAMININE

$C_{18}H_{19}O_8N$

M.p. $192-3°C$

One of two alkaloids found in *Fibrauria tinctoria,* this base yields yellow prisms and is dextrorotatory with $[\alpha]_D^{15} + 28.33°$ ($CHCl_3$). The hydrobromide also forms yellow needles, m.p. $202-3°C$. Four methoxyl groups are present in the molecule.

Chu, Ch'en, Skeng., *Hua Hseuh Hseuh Pao.*, **28**, 89 (1962)

FIBRANINE

$C_{25}H_{29}O_7N$

A further alkaloid from *Fibrauria tinctoria,* this amorphous base forms crystalline salts and derivatives, e.g. the hydrochloride monohydrate as red prismatic needles, m.p. $196-8°C$; $[\alpha]_D^{15} + 273.3°$ (EtOH); hydriodide, yellow needles, m.p. $217-8°C$; perchlorate, yellow needles, m.p. $273-4°C$; aurichloride, green-yellow needles, m.p. $185-192°C$ and the picrate, red needles, m.p. $212-3°C$. With Zn and H_2SO_4 the alkaloid yields the dihydro derivative as colourless needles, m.p. $184-6°C$; $[\alpha]_D^{15} + 141.6°$ ($CHCl_3$).

Chu, Ch'en, Skeng., *Hua Hseuh Hseuh Pao.*, **28**, 89 (1962)

FICINE

$C_{20}H_{19}O_4N$

M.p. $235°C$

A coumarin type alkaloid present in *Ficus pantoniana* King, this base has an ultraviolet spectrum with two absorption maxima at 275 and 329 mμ. It contains two hydroxyl and one methylimino group in the molecule.

Johns, Russell, Hefferman., *Tetrahedron Lett.*, 1987 (1965)

FLABELLIDINE

$C_{18}H_{28}ON_2$

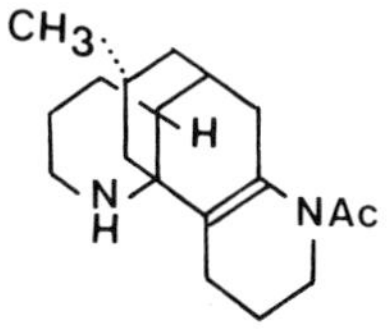

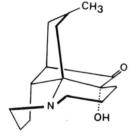

This alkaloid was first isolated from *Lycopodium flabelliforme* as Alkaloid L-5 by Manske and Marion and given the formula $C_{18}H_{28}O_2N_2$. The perchlorate has m.p. 281–2°C and the ultraviolet spectrum has an absorption maximum at 237 mμ. The N-acetyl derivative has m.p. 150–2°C.

Manske, Marion., *Can. J. Res.*, **20B**, 87 (1942)
Alam, Adams, MacLean., *Can. J. Chem.*, **42**, 2456 (1964)

FLABELLIFORMINE

$C_{16}H_{25}O_2N$

M.p. 210–1°C

Lycopodium flabelliforme also contains this alkaloid which has one hydroxyl and one methyl group present. On heating, the crystal form changes at about 150°C. The base is characterized as the hydrobromide, m.p. > 337°C (*dec.*) or the methiodide which also has m.p. > 337°C (*dec.*).

Curcumelli-Rodostamo, Muchean., *Can. J. Chem.*, **40**, 1068 (1962)

FLABELLINE

$C_{18}H_{28}ON_2$

M.p. 185–187.5°C

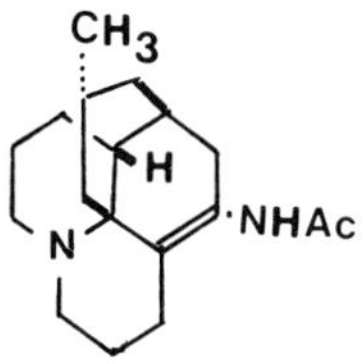

A further *Lycopodium* alkaloid found in *L. flabelliforme*, this base crystallizes from a mixture of Et_2O and Me_2CO as pale yellow rhombic crystals. The structure has been established from spectroscopic evidence, particularly the mass spectrum. It yields a perchlorate, m.p. 280–2°C and a methiodide, m.p.

281–2°C. One nitrogen atom is tertiary while the other is present as an acetyl-amino group. Acid hydrolysis yields acetic acid and lycopodine (q.v.).

Young, MacLean., *Can. J. Chem.,* **41**, 2731 (1963)

Mass spectrum:
Alam, Adams, MacLean., *Can. J. Chem.,* **42**, 2456 (1964)

FLAVINANTINE

$C_{19}H_{21}O_4N$

M.p. 130–2°C

This morphine-type alkaloid occurs in *Croton flavens* L. and is laevorotatory with $[\alpha]_D$ − 14.5° (EtOH). In ethanolic solution, the ultraviolet spectrum has absorption maxima at 239 and 286 mμ. It contains two methoxyl groups and one hydroxyl group, forms a methiodide, m.p. 201–3°C; an O-acetyl derivative, m.p. 196–7°C and an O-methyl ether which is obtained as a light yellow glassy solid with no definite melting point. The latter may be characterized as the crystalline methiodide, m.p. 222–3°C (*dec.*). The structure has been confirmed by synthesis.

Chambers, Stuart., *Chem. Commun.,* 328 (1968)

Synthesis:
Kametani *et al., Chem. Commun.,* 1398 (1968)

FLAVININE

$C_{18}H_{19}O_4N$

M.p. 130–2°C

Also present in *Croton flavens* L., this alkaloid crystallizes with 1 mole of Me_2CO from this solvent. It is laevorotatory with $[\alpha]_D^{16}$ − 6.1° (EtOH). The ultraviolet spectrum is almost identical with that of the preceding base, having absorption maxima at 238 and 285 mμ. The N-methyl ether is flavinantine (q.v.). The O,N-dimethyl ether has been obtained as the crystalline methiodide, m.p. 250–2°C (*dec.*) and is identical with flavinantine O-methyl ether.

Stuart, Chambers., *Tetrahedron Lett.,* 2879 (1967)
Chambers, Stuart., *Chem. Commun.,* 328 (1968)

578

FLAVOPEREIRINE (*Melinonine G*)

$C_{17}H_{14}N_2$

M.p. 233–5°C

Isolated from *Geissospermum laeve* (Vellozo) Baill., this alkaloid also occurs in the bark of *G. vellosii* and *Strychnos melinoniana* Baill. It forms yellow-white crystals from Me_2CO and furnishes crystalline salts and derivatives of which the following have been prepared and characterized: perchlorate, m.p. 330°C (*dec.*); methiodide, m.p. 321–3°C (*dec.*) and the picrate, m.p. 229.5–230.5°C. The compound with tetraphenylboron has m.p. 222–4°C. The alkaloid contains one ethyl group and from the structure it will be seen that there is a distribution of charge on the two nitrogen atoms in the molecule.

Bejar *et al., Compt. rend.*, **244**, 2066 (1957)
Hughes, Rapoport., *J. Amer. Chem. Soc.*, **80**, 1604 (1958)
Prasad, Swan., *J. Chem. Soc.*, 2024 (1958)
Bächli *et al., Helv. Chim. Acta*, **40**, 1167 (1959)
Thesing, Festag., *Experientia*, **15**, 127 (1959)
Kaneko., *J. Pharm. Soc. Japan*, 1374 (1960)
Ban, Seo., *Tetrahedron*, **16**, 5 (1961)
Wenkert *et al., J. Amer. Chem. Soc.*, **84**, 3732 (1962)
Wenkert, Kilzer., *J. Org. Chem.*, **27**, 2283 (1962)

FLEXININE

$C_{16}H_{17}O_4N$

M.p. 232–4°C

This alkaloid has been isolated from *Crinium erubescens* and *Nerine flexuosa* and is obtained as colourless prisms from EtOH. A melting point of 221–2°C has also been recorded for this base. It is laevorotatory with $[\alpha]_{589}^{25} - 12.7°$. The salts and derivatives are crystalline, including the perchlorate, m.p. 250°C (*dec.*); the methiodide, m.p. 223–4°C and the O-acetyl compound, m.p. 206–7°C. The base contains one hydroxyl, one methylenedioxy group and an epoxy ring.

Boit, Ehmko., *Ber.*, **90**, 369 (1957)
Fales, Wildman., *J. Org. Chem.*, **26**, 181 (1961)

FLINDERSIAMINE

$C_{14}H_{11}O_5N$

M.p. 212°C

This furoquinoline alkaloid is quite widely distributed. It is present in several

Flindersia species, particularly *F. maculosa,* in *Balfourodendron redelsamia* and *Vepris bicocularis.* The alkaloid may be characterized as the crystalline picrate, m.p. 200–1°C. It contains two methoxyl groups and one methylenedioxy group in the molecule.

Anet *et al., Austral. J. Sci. Res.,* **5A**, 412 (1952)
Brown *et al., Austral. J. Chem.,* 7, 181 (1954)

Mass spectrum:
Clugston, MacLean., *Can. J. Chem.,* **43**, 2516 (1965)

Synthesis:
Govindachari, Prabhakar., *Ind. J. Chem.,* 1, 348 (1963)

FLINDERSINE

$C_{14}H_{13}O_2N$

M.p. 185–6°C (*dec.*).

This alkaloid was first obtained from the wood of *Flindersia australis* R. Br. by Matthes and Schreiber who assigned to it the formula $C_{23}H_{26}O_7N_2$. The base is obtained in the form of colourless needles from several organic solvents. It yields a picrate, m.p. 174–8°C and a platinichloride, m.p. 262°C. It is optically inactive.

Matthes, Schreiber., *Ber. deut. Pharm. Ges.,* **24**, 385 (1914)
Brown *et al., Austral. J. Chem.,* 7, 348 (1954)
Brown, Hughes, Ritchie., *ibid,* 9, 277 (1956)
Brown, Hughes, Ritchie., *Chem. & Ind.,* 1385 (1955)

FLORAMULTINE

$C_{21}H_{25}O_5N$

M.p. 230°C (*dec.*).

A homoaporphine alkaloid present in *Kreysigia multiflora* Reichb., this base is laevorotatory with $[\alpha]_D^{18} - 77°$ (c 1.19, CHCl$_3$). It forms colourless crystals from Et$_2$OH or C$_6$H$_6$. The ultraviolet spectrum has absorption maxima at 220, 259 and 287 mμ. Three methoxyl groups and two hydroxyls are present and the alkaloid forms an O,O-dimethyl ether which cannot be crystallized but does form a crystalline hydrobromide, m.p. 243°C (*dec.*).

Badger, Bradbury., *J. Chem. Soc.,* 445 (1960)

Structure:
Battersby *et al., Chem. Commun.,* 450 (1967)

Absolute configuration:
Beecham *et al., Austral. J. Chem.,* 21, 2829 (1968)

580

FLORAMULTININE

$C_{21}H_{27}O_6N$

M.p. 165°C

Also occurring in *Kreysigia multiflora* Reichb., this base forms colourless crystals from C_6H_6-light petroleum. Unlike the preceding alkaloid from the same plant, it is dextrorotatory with $[\alpha]_D^{20} + 118°$ (c 0.17, EtOH). The ultraviolet spectrum contains two absorption maxima at 217 and 275 mμ.

Badger, Bradbury., *J. Chem. Soc.*, 445 (1960)

FLORIBUNDINE

$C_{18}H_{19}O_2N$

M.p. 193–5°C

An alkaloid from *Papaver floribundum*, this base occurs in the non-phenolic fraction together with floripavidine (q.v.). It crystallizes from Me_2CO in colourless prisms and has $[\alpha]_D - 204.28°$ (CHCl$_3$). One methoxyl and one methylimino group are present. The alkaloid forms a methiodide, m.p. 178–180°C and a tartrate, m.p. 181–3°C.

Konovalova, Yunusov, Orekhov., *Ber.*, **68**, 2277 (1935)

FLORICALINE (*Acetylfloridanine*)

$C_{23}H_{33}O_{10}N$

M.p. 177–8°C

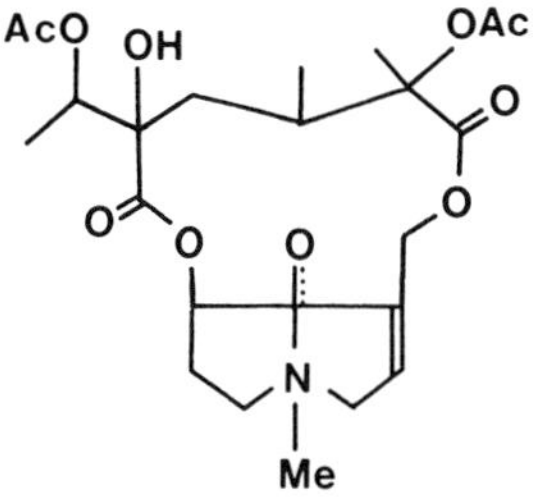

A pyrrolizidone alkaloid present in *Cacalia floridana*, the base crystallizes from C_6H_6 with 1 mole of solvent, m.p. 120–2°C. The solvent can only be removed by prolonged drying at 90–100°C when the anhydrous base is obtained as a white, microcrystalline powder. It is dextrorotatory with $[\alpha]_D + 74.3°$ (c 1.10, CHCl$_3$). The structure has been determined on the basis of chemical interconversions and spectroscopic evidence.

Cava *et al.*, *J. Org. Chem.*, **33**, 3570 (1968)

FLORIDANINE

$C_{21}H_{31}O_9N$

M.p. 195–6°C

A further pyrrolizidone alkaloid found in *Cacalia floridana,* this base forms colourless prisms from $CHCl_3$ containing 1 mole of solvent. It has $[\alpha]_D + 66.5°$ (c 0.8, $CHCl_3$). It contains one acetyl group and a secondary and a tertiary hydroxyl group. The 18-O-acetyl derivative is floricaline (q.v.).

Cava *et al., J. Org. Chem.,* **33**, 3570 (1968)

FLORIPAVIDINE

$C_{21}H_{29}O_5N$

M.p. 241–2°C

This alkaloid occurs in the crude mixture of non-phenolic bases obtained from *Papaver floribundum* and may be separated from floribundine by repeated crystallization of the hydrochlorides in H_2O. It is laevorotatory with $[\alpha]_D -$ 156.25° (MeOH). It yields a crystalline hydrochloride, m.p. 209–210°C; a hydriodide and a methiodide, the last having m.p. 228–230°C. A Zerewitinoff determination shows that no hydroxyl group is present, but the alkaloid does contain a methoxyl, a methylenedioxy and a methylimino group.

Konovalova, Yunusov, Orekhov., *Ber.,* **68**, 2277 (1935)

FLORIPAVINE

$C_{19}H_{21}O_4N$

M.p. 200–1°C

This alkaloid from *Papaver floribundum* is present in the phenolic mixture of bases and crystallizes from EtOH as long, thin needles. It has $[\alpha]_D^{18} + 88°$ (c 1.9, $CHCl_3$) or + 110° (c 1.66, EtOH). The following salts and derivatives have been prepared: hydrochloride, m.p. 235–6°C; methiodide, 215–6°C, oxime, m.p. 222°C and a picrate, m.p. 223–4°C. The O-acetate, m.p. 171–2°C; $[\alpha]_D^{18} + 129°$ (c 0.66, EtOH) is identical with salutaridine (q.v.).

When hydrogenated over Pt black it yields the hexahydro derivative, m.p. 218°C; $[\alpha]_D^{18} + 49°$ (c 0.91, EtOH). Treatment with CH_2N_2 in MeOH furnishes O-methylfloripavine, m.p. 147–8°C; $[\alpha]_D^{21} + 79°$ (c 1.21, $CHCl_3$), yielding a picrate, m.p. 206–8°C. Reduction with $NaBH_4$ in MeOH yields floripavinol, m.p. 228–9°C (*dec.*); $[\alpha]_D^{18} \pm 5°$ (c 0.89, EtOH) which, on treatment with 2N

HCl for 1 hour gives thebaine (q.v.), m.p. $191-2°$C. Oxidation with $KMnO_4$ in Me_2CO gives hemipinic acid, m.p. $176-8°$C, characterized as the ethylimide, m.p. $86-7°$C

Konovalova, Yunusov, Orekhov., *Ber.*, **68**, 2277 (1935)

Mndzhoyan, Mnatsakanyan, Mkrtchyan., *Arm. Khim. Zh.*, **20**, 376 (1967)

FLOROSENINE (*Acetylotosenine*)

$C_{21}H_{29}O_8N$

M.p. $100-3°$C

A third pyrrolizidone alkaloid present in *Cacalia floridana*. The base forms colourless flakes with 1 mole of solvent when crystallized from C_6H_6. It is dextrorotatory with $[\alpha]_D + 31.9°$ (c 1.12, $CHCl_3$). The structure given above has been proposed on the basis of spectroscopic data and chemical interconversions.

Cava *et al.*, *J. Org. Chem.*, **33**, 3570 (1968)

C-FLUOROCURINE

$C_{20}H_{25}O_2N_2^+$

This quaternary curare alkaloid has been obtained by Karrer and Schmid from calabash curare whose origin appears to be the middle Orinoco region of South America. The base was isolated as the picrate, m.p. $178°$C and originally formulated as $C_{20}H_{21}ON_2.H_2O$. The picrate may be converted into the chloride, a yellow powder containing $0.5\ H_2O$ which exhibits a yellow-green fluorescence in aqueous solution and gives an intense, although unstable, red-violet colour with ceric sulphate in 50 per cent H_2SO_4. The iodide, also made from the picrate, forms yellow platelets and has $[\alpha]_D + 326°$ (MeOH). On hydrogenation, the alkaloid absorbs 2 molecules of hydrogen rapidly without losing its yellow colour, followed by the absorption of a further 1.4 molecules, becoming colourless and losing the quaternary nature. So far, no crystalline hydro derivatives has been prepared. The ultraviolet spectrum of the chloride shows absorption maxima at 235, 263, 305 and 423 mμ.

Karrer, Schmid., *Helv. Chim. Acta,* **29**, 1853 (1946)

Karrer, Schmid., *ibid,* **30**, 1162, 2081 (1947)

Structure:

Hesse *et al., Helv. Chim. Acta,* **47**, 878 (1964)

FOLICANGINE

$C_{42}H_{46}O_5N_4$

M.p. 200°C (*dec.*).

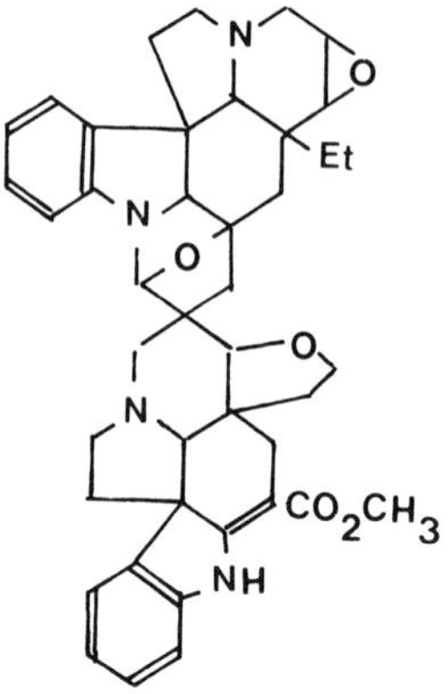

This complex alkaloid occurs in the leaves of *Voacanga africana* Stapf. It may be crystallized from MeOH when it forms colourless plates. It is laevorotatory with $[\alpha]_{578} - 271°$ (CHCl$_3$). The ultraviolet spectrum of the base in EtOH shows absorption maxima at 210, 255, 298 and 328 mμ with a shoulder at 225 mμ. The structure has been elucidated from infrared, ultraviolet, NMR and mass spectrometry.

Kunesch, Das, Poisson., *Bull. Soc. Chim. Fr.,* 4370 (1970)

FOLICANTHINE

$C_{24}H_{30}N_4$

M.p. 169°C

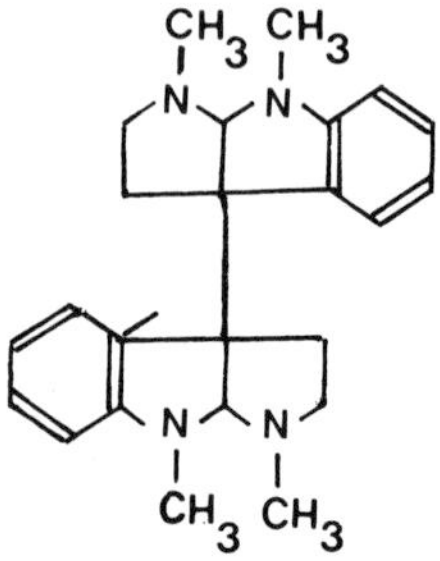

Present in *Calycanthus floridus* and *C. occidentalis,* this alkaloid is dimeric and contains four methylimino groups. It forms a crystalline methiodide, m.p. 219–220°C and a picrate, m.p. 178–9°C. The mode of biosynthesis of the base has been examined by O'Donovan and Keogh.

O'Donovan, Keogh., *J. Chem. Soc., C,* 1570 (1966)

584

FOLIFIDINE

$C_{11}H_{11}O_3N$

M.p. 226–7°C

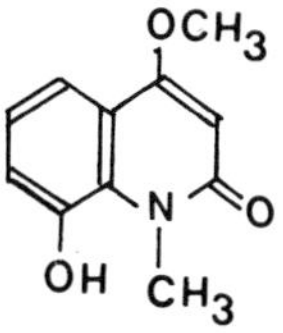

An alkaloid of *Haplophyllum bucharicum* and *H. foliosum,* this alkaloid is separated from the accompanying bases by chromatography on an alumina column. The base forms a hydrochloride, m.p. 232°C and a picrate, m.p. 218°C. The alkaloid has been shown to be 1-methyl-4-methoxy-8-hydroxy-2-quinolone by comparison with an authentic sample.

Faizutdinova, Bessonova, Yunusov., *Khim. Prir. Soedin.,* **3**, 257 (1967)

FOLIFINE

$C_{15}H_{17}O_3N$

M.p. 225–6°C

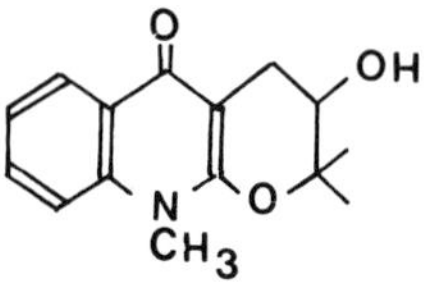

Also present in *Haplophyllum foliosum,* this base is present in the non-phenolic portion of the extract. It has $[\alpha]_D$ + 14.4° (c 2.772, MeOH) and gives a hydrochloride, m.p. 230–1°C; nitrate, m.p. 148–9°C; picrate, m.p. 189–190°C and the O-acetate, m.p. 154–5°C. The base gives Me_2CO on oxidation with $KMnO_4$.

Faizutdinova, Bessonova, Yunusov., *Khim. Prir. Soedin.,* **3**, 257 (1967)

FOLIMIDINE

$C_{17}H_{15}O_3N$

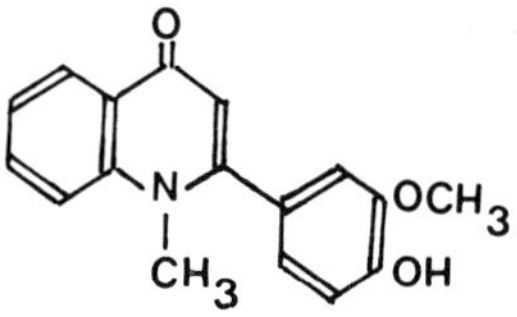

This quinolone alkaloid has been isolated from the aerial parts of *Haplophyllum foliosum* and is present in the phenolic fraction of the alkaloidal extract. The structure has been determined from the infrared, NMR and mass spectra of the base and its deuterated product.

Razzakova, Bessonova, Yunusov., *Khim. Prir. Soedin.,* **6**, 755 (1972)

FOLIMININE

$C_{17}H_{17}O_3N$

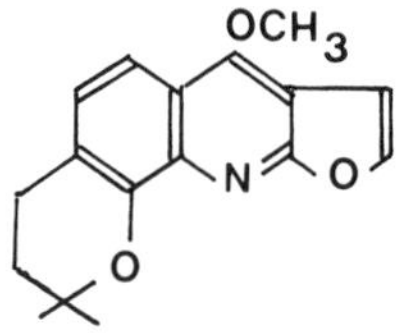

A furoquinoline alkaloid, also present in the aerial portions of *Haplophyllum foliosum,* the structure has been established by NMR, infrared, ultraviolet and mass spectrometry. In the presence of Pt, the base yields the tetrahydro derivative and with methyl iodide, it is converted into *iso*foliminine.

Bessonova, Yunusov., *Khim. Prir. Soedin.,* **10**, 52 (1974)

FOLIOSIDINE

$C_{16}H_{21}O_4N$

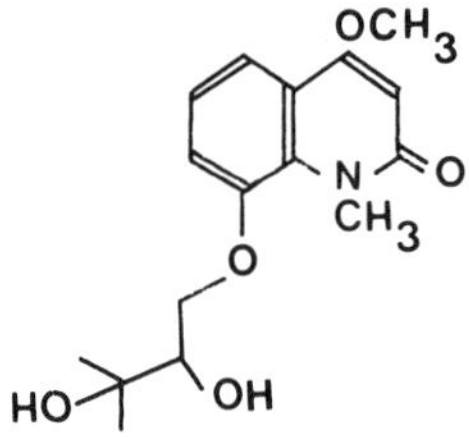

This alkaloid has recently been isolated from *Haplophyllum foliosum* and has the structure given above based upon chemical and spectroscopic evidence.

Kurbanov *et al., Khim. Prir. Soedin.,* **4**, 58 (1968)

FOLIOSIDINE ACETONIDE

$C_{19}H_{25}O_5N$

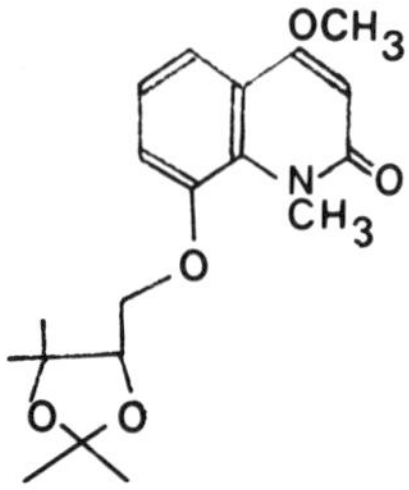

A further alkaloid of *Haplophyllum foliosum.* On hydrolysis the base furnishes Foliosidine (q.v.) and it may be synthesized by treatment of an acetone solution of foliosidine with H_2SO_4.

Tel'nov, Bessonova, Yunusov., *Khim. Prir. Soedin.,* **6**, 724 (1970)

FOLIOSINE

A recently discovered alkaloid present in *Haplophyllum foliosum,* this base has been studied by Kurbanov and his co-workers.

Kurbanov *et al., Khim. Prir. Soedin.,* **4**, 58 (1968)

586

FOLIOZIDINE

$C_{16}H_{21}O_5N$

M.p. 141–2°C

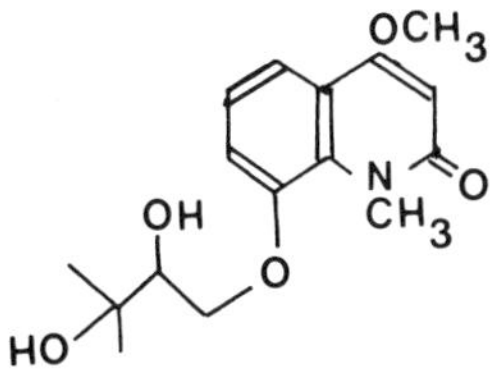

A quinolone alkaloid found in *Haplophyllum foliosum,* this base has $[\alpha]_D$ + 41.6° (EtOH) and forms a crystalline diacetyl derivative, m.p. 142–3°C; $[\alpha]_D$ + 5.4° (EtOH). With periodic acid it furnishes Me_2CO and foliozidinal which is optically inactive.

Pastukhova, Sidyakin, Yunusov., *Dokl. Akad. Nauk. Uzbek SSR,* **21**, 31 (1964)

FONTAPHILLINE

$C_{18}H_{17}O_5N$

M.p. 80–1°C
and 121–2°C

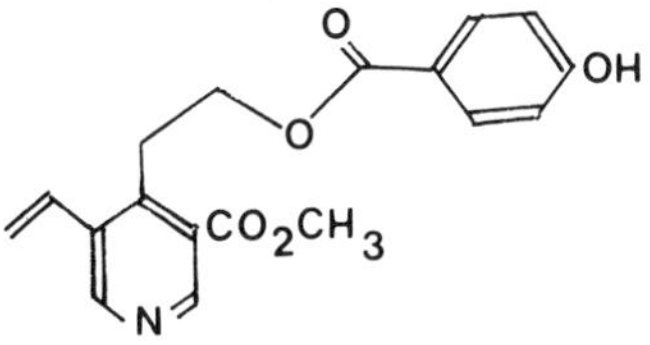

The leaves of *Fontanesia phillyreoidea* Labill. when extracted with methanolic ammonia, yield this pyridine alkaloid. The base may be crystallized from aqueous MeOH when it forms fine, colourless needles which have the double melting point given above. The ultraviolet spectrum shows two absorption maxima at 212 and 257 mμ. The base slowly decolorizes $KMnO_4$ due to the presence of the vinyl group in the molecule.

Budzikiweicz *et al., Chem. Ber.,* **100**, 2798 (1967)

FORMYLCINEGALLINE

$C_{25}H_{32}O_7N_2$

M.p. 188–9°C

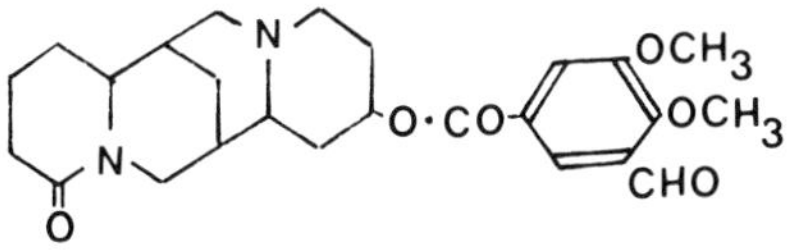

A sparteine type alkaloid present in *Genista cinerea* DC. Acid hydrolysis yields formylveratric acid. The structure has been established from chemical and spectroscopic evidence.

Faugeras, Paris., *Compt. Rend.,* **271D**, 1219 (1970)
Faugeras, Paris., *Plant. Med. Phytother.,* **5**, 134 (1971)

N-FORMYLCONKURCHINE (*N-Formylirehline*)

$C_{22}H_{32}ON_2$

M.p. 247°C

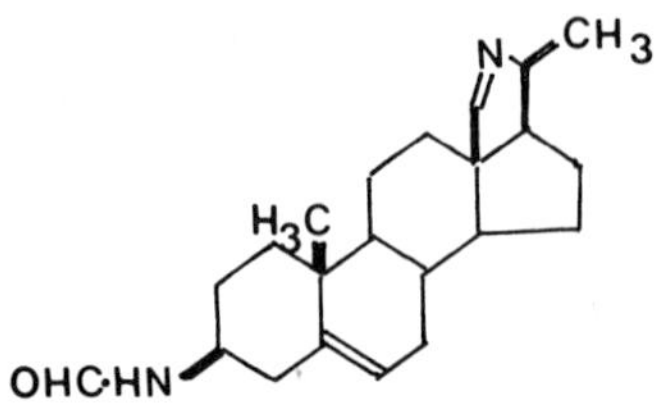

This steroidal alkaloid occurs in the leaves of *Holarrhena crassifolia* and forms colourless crystals from Me_2CO. It is laevorotatory with $[\alpha]_D - 50°$ (CHCl₃). It contains one secondary and one tertiary nitrogen atom.

Einhorn, Monneret, Khuong Huu., *Phytochem.*, **11**, 769 (1972)

N-FORMYLCORYDAMINE

$C_{21}H_{18}O_5N_2$

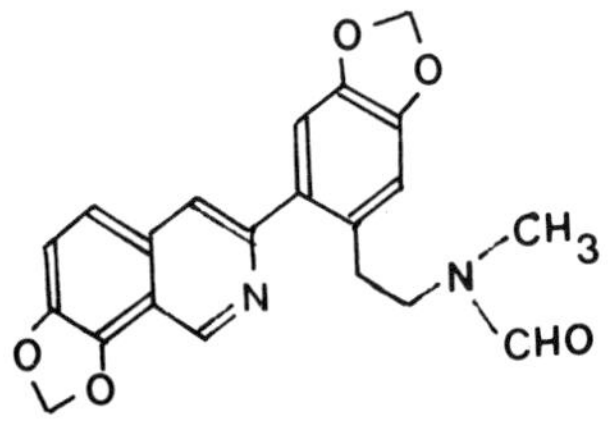

An *iso*quinoline alkaloid recently obtained from *Corydalis incisa,* the structure of this base has been elucidated from spectroscopic data.

Nonaka, Nishioka., *Chem. Pharm. Bull.,* **21**, 1410 (1973)

N-FORMYLCYCLOVIROBUXEINE C

$C_{28}H_{45}O_2N_2$

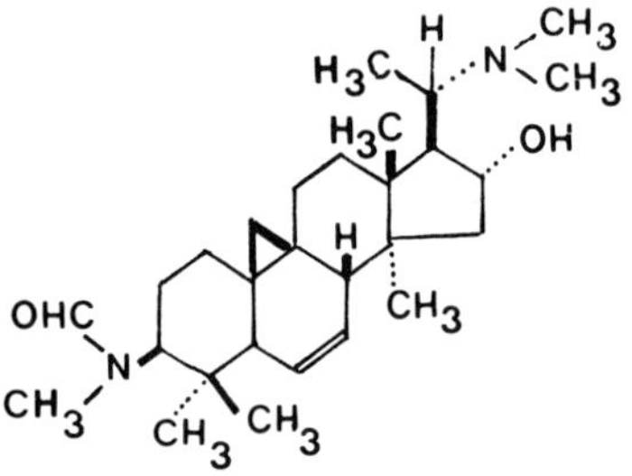

This alkaloid occurs in the leaves, bark and stem of *Buxus malayana*. The structure has been established from spectroscopic data and comparison with other *Buxus* alkaloids.

Khuong Huu Laine, Magdaleine., *Ann. Pharm. Fr.*, **28**, 211 (1970)

588

N-FORMYLCYLINDROCARPINOL

$C_{21}H_{28}O_3N_2$

M.p. 101–5°C

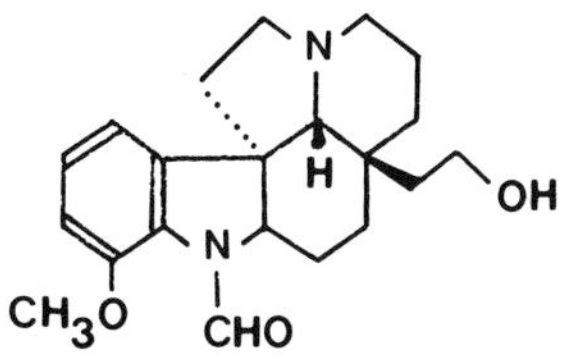

Present in *Aspidosperma cylindrocarpon*, this base forms colourless crystals from EtOH and is laevorotatory with $[\alpha]_D^{20} - 150°$ (c 0.0016, MeOH). The ultraviolet spectrum exhibits absorption maxima at 220, 260 and a shoulder at 292 mμ.

Milborrow, Djerassi., *J. Chem. Soc., C,* 417 (1969)

N-FORMYLDEACETYLCOLCHICINE

$C_{21}H_{23}O_6N$

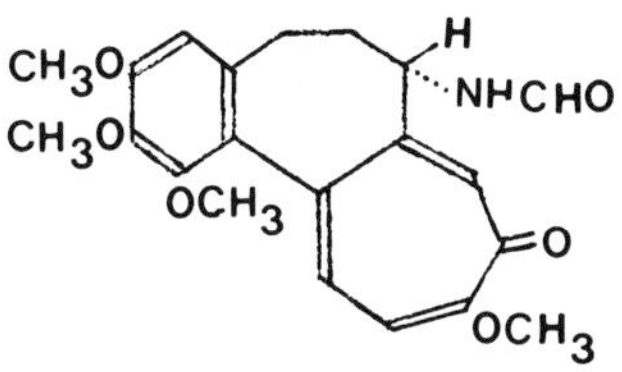

A colchicine alkaloid found in the neutral fraction of the alkaloidal extract from *Merendera raddeana*. The structure given above has been determined on the basis of chemical analysis, comparison with Colchicine (q.v.) and spectroscopic data.

Trozyan, Yusupov, Sadykov., *Khim. Prir. Soedin.,* 7, 541 (1971)

N-FORMYLDEACETYL-β-LUMICOLCHICINE

$C_{21}H_{23}O_6N$

M.p. 214–5°C

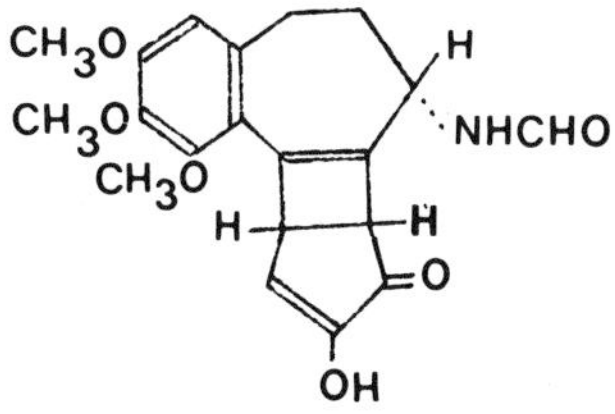

One of a series of alkaloids isolated from *Gloriosa superba,* this base crystallizes as colourless needles from MeOH-AcOEt. It is dextrorotatory with $[\alpha]_D^{20} + 340°$ (c 1.0, CHCl$_3$).

Canonica., *Chem. Ind.* (Milan), **49**, 1304 (1967)

N-FORMYLDEACETYL-γ-LUMICOLCHICINE

$C_{21}H_{23}O_6N$

M.p. 255–6°C

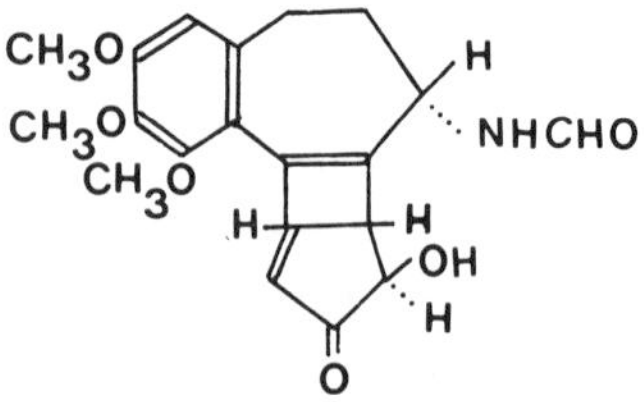

Also present in *Gloriosa superba,* this alkaloid crystallizes as colourless needles from MeOH-CHCl₃. The structure has been determined from spectroscopic evidence and intercomparison with other colchicine alkaloids.

Canonica., *Chem. Ind.* (Milan), **49**, 1304 (1967)

N-FORMYL-16:17-DIMETHOXYASPIDOFRACTININE

$C_{22}H_{28}O_3N_2$

M.p. Indefinite

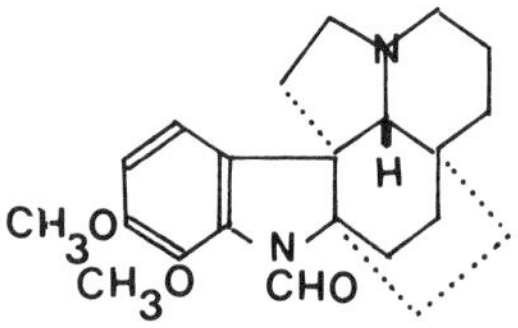

An amorphous base occurring in the bark of *Aspidosperma populifolium* A. DC. The alkaloid contains two methoxyl groups and one N-formyl group. The ultraviolet spectrum in MeOH shows absorption maxima at 253 and 287 mμ. Alkaline hydrolysis of the base furnishes 16:17-dimethoxy-aspidofractinine.

Gilber *et al., Tetrahedron,* **21**, 1141 (1965)

N-FORMYLKOPSANOL

$C_{21}H_{24}O_2N_2$

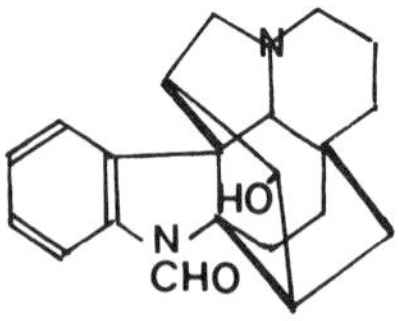

This dihydroindole alkaloid has been discovered during a study of *Aspidosperma verbascifolium.* The structure given above has been elucidated from a comparison with other alkaloids of this type.

Braekman *et al., Bull. Soc. Chim. Belg.,* **78**, 63 (1969)

590

N-FORMYL-17-METHOXYASPIDOFRACTININE

$C_{21}H_{26}O_2N_2$

M.p. Indefinite

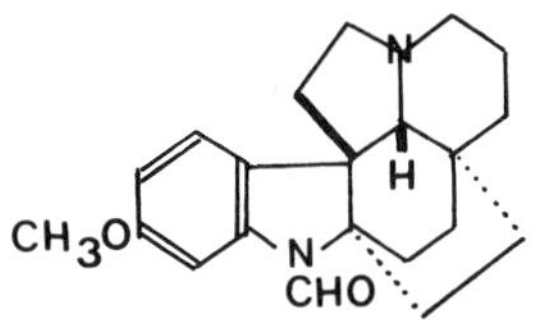

A second amorphous base found in the bark of *Aspidosperma populifolium* A. DC. The alkaloid undergoes a similar hydrolysis to the dimethoxy analogue (q.v.), yielding 17-methoxyaspidofractinine. The ultraviolet spectrum is also similar with an absorption maximum at 255 mμ and an inflexion at 288 mμ.

Gilbert *et al., Tetrahedron,* **21**, 1141 (1965)

N-FORMYLNORMACROMERINE

$C_{11}H_{15}O_4N$

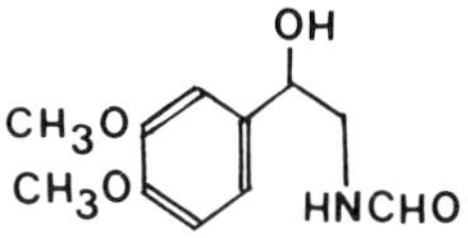

This base has recently been discovered in *Coryphantha macromeris* var. *runyonii.* No salts or derivatives have yet been reported for the alkaloid.

Keller, McLaughlin, Brady., *J. Pharm. Sci.,* **62**, 408 (1973)

FORMOSANINE

$C_{21}H_{24-26}O_4N_2$

M.p. 202–218°C

This alkaloid from *Ourouparia formosana* Mats. has been described by Raymond-Hamet. It is dextrorotatory with $[\alpha]_D$ + 91.3°. No salts or derivatives have yet been prepared and the structure is not yet fully determined.

Raymond-Hamet., *Compt. rend.,* **203**, 1383 (1936)
Raymond-Hamet., *Arch. Int. Pharmocodyn.,* **63**, 336 (1939)

FRANGANINE

$C_{28}H_{44}O_4N_4$

M.p. 248°C

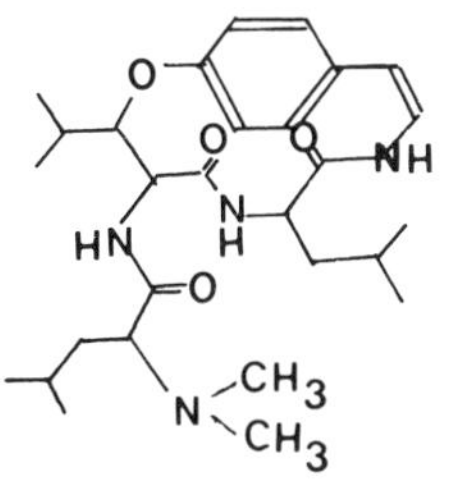

The bark of *Rhamnus frangula* L. yields this peptide alkaloid which may be crystallized from light petroleum when it forms colourless slender needles. It is laevorotatory having $[\alpha]_D^{22} - 302°$ (c 0.1, $CHCl_3$). Three of the nitrogen atoms are present as peptide groups and the fourth as a dimethylamino group. The structure has been established mainly from the mass spectrum.

Tschesche, Last., *Tetrahedron Lett.*, 2993 (1968)
See also:
Tschesche, Reutel., *Tetrahedron Lett.*, 3817 (1968)

FRANGUFOLINE

$C_{31}H_{42}O_4N_4$

M.p. 244°C

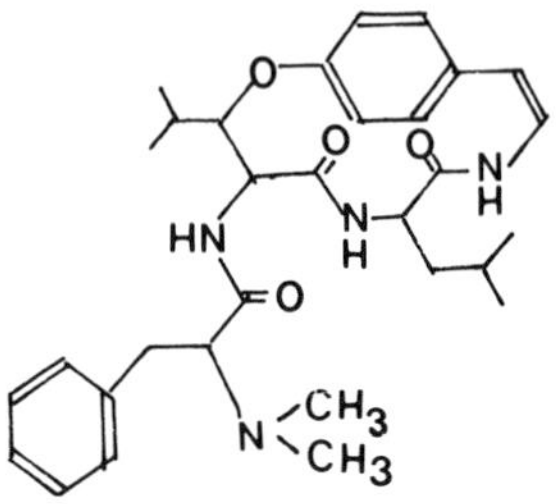

A second peptide alkaloid found in the leaves of *Rhamnus frangula* L., this base also occurs in *Melochia corchorifolia*. It forms colourless needles from aqueous EtOH and is also laevorotatory with $[\alpha]_D^{22} - 299°$ (c 0.1, $CHCl_3$). The structure, determined from the mass spectrum differs from that of the preceding alkaloid only in having a benzene ring in place of an *iso*propyl group.

Tschesche, Last., *Tetrahedron Lett.*, 2993 (1968)
Tschesche, Reutel., *ibid*, 3817 (1968)

FRANGULANINE

$C_{28}H_{44}O_4N_4$

M.p. 275–6°C

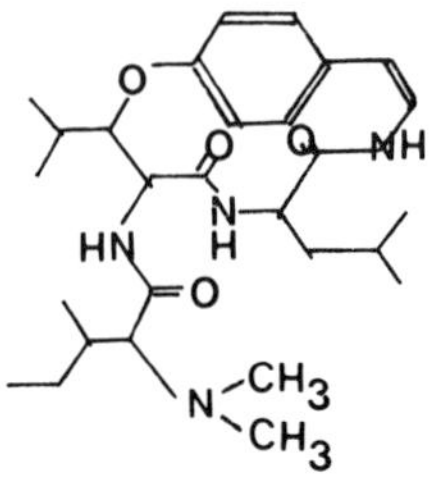

This peptide alkaloid isolated from the bark of *Rhamnus frangula* L. is identical with Ceanothamine A. It crystallizes as colourless needles from $CHCl_3$-light petroleum and is laevorotatory with $[\alpha]_D - 288°$ (c 0.1, $CHCl_3$). The ultraviolet spectrum exhibits absorption maxima at 252 (shoulder) and 279 mμ. The structure has been determined mainly from the fragmentation pattern of the mass spectrum.

Tschesche, Last, Fehlhaber., *Chem. Ber.*, **100**, 3937 (1967)
Servis, Kosak., *J. Amer. Chem. Soc.*, **90**, 4179, 6895 (1968)

FRITILLARINE

$C_{19}N_{33}O_2N$

M.p. 130–1°C

An amorphous alkaloid present in the residual bases extracted from *Fritillaria verticillata* var. *Thunb.* The base is normally isolated as the perchlorate.

Chou, Chen., *Chin. J. Physiol.*, 7, 41 (1933)

FRITIMINE

$C_{38}H_{62}O_3N_2$

M.p. 167°C

This alkaloid has been obtained from the Chinese drug 'Pei-mu' originating in Szechuan, the source of which is, according to Read, *Fritillaria Roylei* Hook. The alkaloid is laevorotatory with $[\alpha]_D^{22} - 50°$ (EtOH) and forms a crystalline hydrochloride, m.p. 230°C.

Chou, Chen., *Chin. J. Physiol.*, 7, 41 (1933)
Read., *Chinese Medicinal Plants from the Pen Ts'ao Kang Mu, A.D. 1596* (Pekin, 1936)

FRUTICOSAMINE

$C_{22}H_{24}O_4N_2$

M.p. 181°C

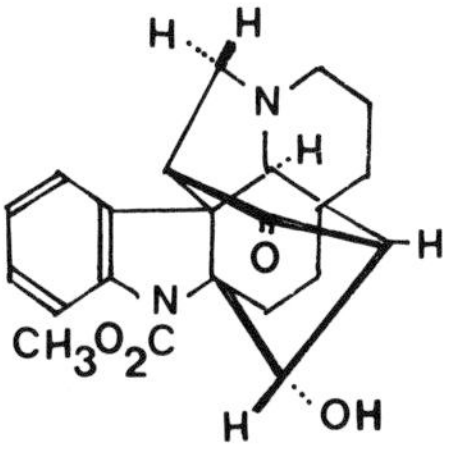

This crystalline alkaloid is widespread in occurrence among *Kopsia* species. It forms a picrate, m.p. 212–3°C (*dec.*) by means of which it may be characterized. The structure has been established by infrared, ultraviolet, NMR and mass spectrometry.

Battersby *et al.*, *Chem. Commun.*, 786 (1966)
Battersby *et al.*, *J. Chem. Soc.*, C, 813 (1967)

FRUTICOSINE

$C_{22}H_{24}O_4N_2$

M.p. 225–6°C

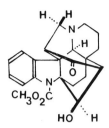

A further minor *Kopsia* alkaloid, this base occurs chiefly in *K. fruticosa* from whence it may be isolated as the crystalline picrate, m.p. 163–4°C. The structure has, as before, been determined by various spectroscopic techniques.

Battersby *et al., Chem. Commun.,* 786 (1966)
Battersby *et al., J. Chem. Soc., C,* 813 (1967)

FUCHSISENECIONINE

$C_{12}H_{21}O_3N$

A hepatotoxic alkaloid of the pyrrolizidine group isolated from *Senecio Fuchsii,* this base has been characterized as the crystalline hydrochloride, m.p. 225–7°C.

Muller., *Chem. Zentr.,* ii, 1049 (1925)

FUGAPAVINE

$C_{18}H_{17}O_3N$

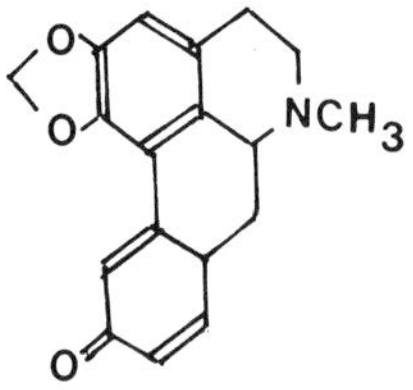

An alkaloid of *Papaver fugax* Poir, this oxoaporphine base yields a crystalline semicarbazone, m.p. 237°C. Hydrogenation with Pt as catalyst affords the hexahydro derivative, m.p. 267–9°C; $[\alpha]_D$ − 38.2°. Heating the alkaloid with mineral acid converts it into *iso*fugapavine, a phenolic base, m.p. 238–240°C; $[\alpha]_D$ + 88.8° (MeOH), shown to be 3-hydroxy-5:6-methylenedioxyaporphine.

Mnatsakanyan, Yunusov., *Dokl. Akad. Nauk. Uzbek SSR,* 12, 36 (1961)

FULVINE

$C_{16}H_{23}O_5N$

M.p. 212–3°C

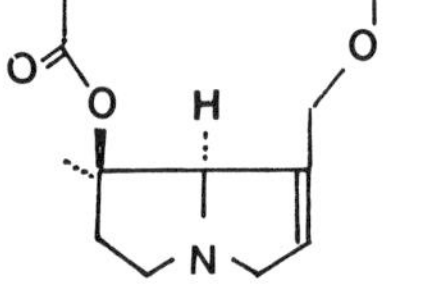

An alkaloid of the pyrrolizidine group present in *Crotalaria crispata* F. Muell. ex

Benth and also in *C. fulva* Roxb. The base is laevorotatory having $[\alpha]_D^{20} - 50.8°$ (CHCl$_3$). It yields a hydrochloride as colourless prisms, m.p. 285°C (*dec.*) and a yellow crystalline picrate, m.p. 250°C (*dec.*). Hydrolysis with dilute acids furnishes retronecine and fulvinic acid, the latter being 3-hydroxy-2:3:4-trimethylglutaric acid.

Culvenor, Smith., *Austral. J. Chem.,* **16**, 239 (1963)
Schoental., *ibid,* **16**, 233 (1963)

FULVINE N-OXIDE

$C_{16}H_{23}O_6N$

M.p. 198°C (*dec.*).

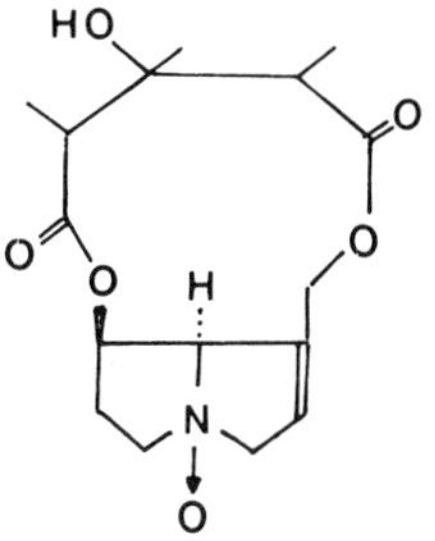

This derivative of fulvine occurs in *Crotalaria fulva* Roxb. It crystallizes as white needles from Me$_2$CO and forms a picrate, yellow needles, m.p. 185°C (*dec.*).

Schoental., *Austral. J. Chem.,* **16**, 233 (1963)
Culvenor, Smith., *ibid,* **16**, 239 (1963)

FUMARAMINE

$C_{21}H_{20}O_5N_2$

M.p. 223–4°C

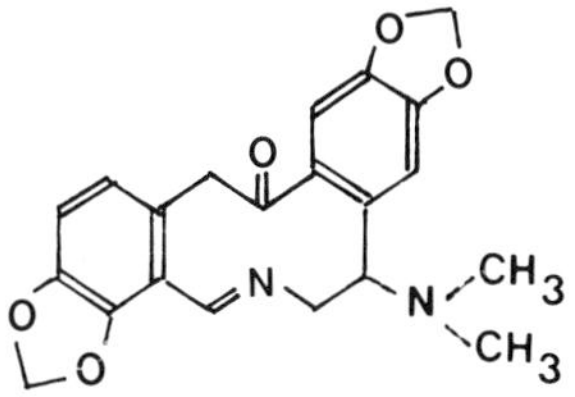

The roots of *Fumaria micrantha* and *F. schleicheri* contain this alkaloid. It may be characterized as the crystalline hydrobromide, m.p. 258–260°C or the tartrate, m.p. 200°C. The alkaloid contains two methylenedioxy groups and one dimethylamino group in the molecule. The structure has been deduced from infrared, NMR and mass spectrometry.

Platonova *et al., J. Gen. Chem., USSR,* **26**, 181 (1956)
Israilov, Yunusov, Yunusov., *Khim. Pir. Soedin.,* **6**, 588 (1970)

FUMARICINE (*Alkaloid F-37*)

$C_{21}H_{23}O_5N$

M.p. 177°C

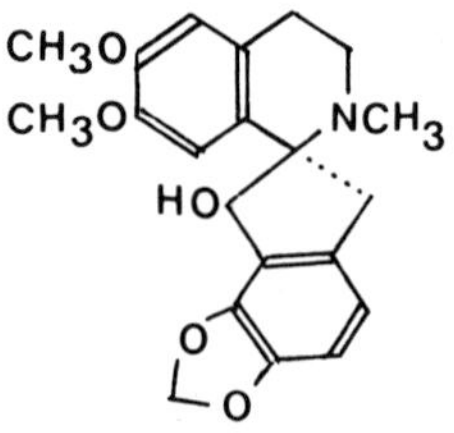

Another *Fumaria* alkaloid, this base is isolated from *F. officinalis* L., and is laevorotatory with $[\alpha]_D - 31°$ (c 0.97 CHCl$_3$). The ultraviolet spectrum has absorption maxima at 208, 235 and 288 mμ. The structure has been established by spectroscopic methods and confirmed by synthesis of the (±)-form.

Saunders *et al., Can. J. Chem.,* **46**, 2873 (1968)
Saunders *et al., ibid,* **46**, 2876 (1968)

Synthesis:
Kishimoto, Uyeo., *J. Chem. Soc., C,* 2600 (1969)

FUMARIDINE

$C_{22}H_{24}O_5N_2$

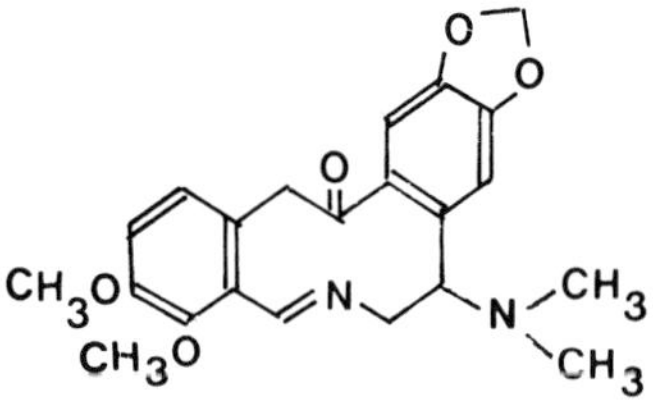

This base occurs in *Fumaria parviflora* and *F. vaillantii.* The structure is similar to that of Fumaramine (q.v.) with one of the methylenedioxy groups replaced by two methoxyl groups. The structure has been determined by spectroscopic methods and comparison with other *Fumaria* alkaloids.

Israilov, Yunusov, Yunusov., *Khim. Prir. Soedin.,* **6**, 588 (1970)

FUMARILINE

$C_{20}H_{17}O_5N$

M.p. 138°C

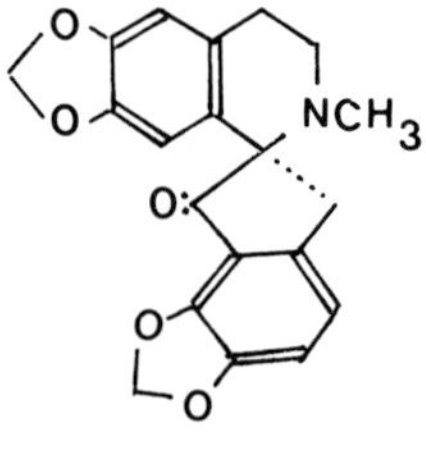

An alkaloid present in *Fumaria officinalis* L., this base has $[\alpha]_D + 138°$ (c 1.05, CHCl$_3$) and give an ultraviolet spectrum in ethanolic solution with absorption maxima at 203, 237, 263, 294 and 355 mμ. The structure and absolute configuration have been determined and the optically inactive form synthesized.

Saunders *et al.*, *Can. J. Chem.*, **46**, 2873 (1968)
Saunders *et al.*, *ibid*, **46**, 2876 (1968)

Absolute configuration:
Shamma *et al.*, *Chem. Commun.*, 310 (1970)

Synthesis:
Kishimoto, Uyeo., *J. Chem. Soc.*, *C*, 1644 (1971)

FUMARINE

See Protopine

FUMARININE

$C_{16}H_{15}O_4N$

M.p. 189–190°C

This alkaloid occurs in *Fumaria schleicheri* and forms colourless crystals from MeOH. It yields a hydrochloride, m.p. 157–9°C and an oxalate, m.p. 213°C. One methylimino group is present in the molecule.

Platonova *et al.*, *J. Gen. Chem.*, *USSR*, **26**, 181 (1956)

FUMARITINE

$C_{20}H_{21}O_5N$

M.p. 157–9°C

A further minor constituent of *Fumaria schleicheri*, this alkaloid is characterized as the hydrochloride, m.p. 224°C and the hydrobromide, m.p. 219°C. It contains one methylimino group in the molecule.

Platonova *et al.*, *J. Gen. Chem.*, *USSR*, **26**, 181 (1956)

FUMARITRIDINE

$C_{21}H_{23}O_5N$

M.p. 198–200°C

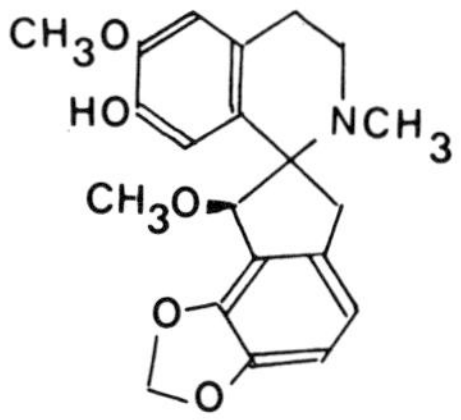

Several species of *Fumaria* contain this alkaloid which crystallizes from MeOH or EtOH as slender, colourless needles. It is dextrorotatory with $[\alpha]_D^{22} + 18°$ (c 1.0,

CHCl$_3$). The ultraviolet spectrum in EtOH has absorption maxima at 215, 230 and 285 mμ. Two methoxyl, one hydroxyl, one methylenedioxy and one methylimino group are present.

Mollov, Kirjakov, Yakimov., *Phytochem.*, **11**, 2331 (1972)

FUMARITRINE

C$_{20}$H$_{21}$O$_5$N

M.p. 153–5°C

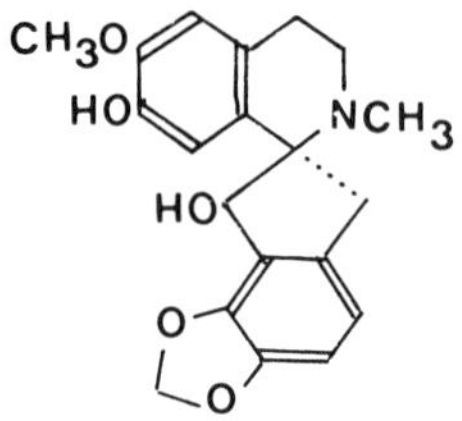

The O-methyl ether of Fumaritridine (q.v.), this alkaloid also occurs in several *Fumaria* species. It crystallizes from EtOH as colourless needles and contains two methoxyl, one hydroxyl, one methylenedioxy and one methylimino group in the molecule.

Mollov, Kirjakov, Yakimov., *Phytochem.*, **11**, 2331 (1972)

FUMAROFINE

C$_{20}$H$_{19}$O$_6$N

M.p. 256°C (*dec.*).

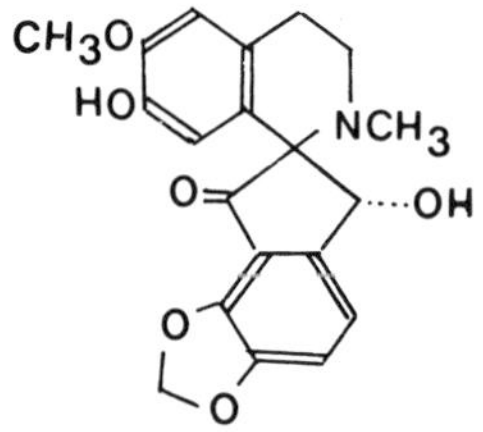

A further alkaloid present in *Fumaria officinalis* L., this base may be crystallized from a mixture of MeOH and dioxan when it forms clusters of colourless prisms. It was originally obtained by Manske and provisionally designated Alkaloid F-38.

Manske., *Can. J. Res.*, **16B**, 438 (1938)
Yu *et al.*, *Can. J. Chem.*, **49**, 3020 (1971)

FUMAROPHYCINE

C$_{22}$H$_{23}$O$_6$N

M.p. 108–9°C

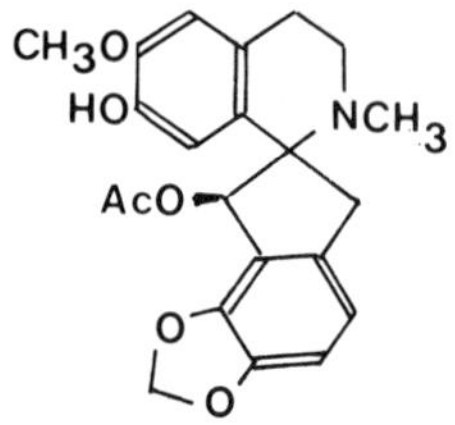

Present in *Fumaria officinalis* L. of Bulgarian origin, this alkaloid is, like the preceding base, a member of the spiro*iso*quinoline group. It yields colourless prisms from MeOH and is laevorotatory having $[\alpha]_D^{20} - 67.5°$ (c 1.0, CHCl$_3$). The structure has been established as 14-O-acetylfumaritine. A hydroxyl group is still present in the molecule and the base form an O-acetate as a colourless oil and a methyl ether, colourless crystals, m.p. 124−6°C.

Mollov, Yakimov, Panov., *Compt. Rend. Acad. Bulg. Sci.*, **20**, 557 (1967)
Castillo *et al., Can. J. Chem.*, **49**, 139 (1971)

FUMJUDAINE

$C_{19}H_{17}O_4N$

An amorphous base isolated from the leaves, stems and roots of *Fumaria judaica*. The alkaloid is optically inactive and yields a hydrochloride, m.p. 248°C and a picrate, m.p. 128°C. A methylenedioxy group is present but no methoxyl, methylimino or phenolic hydroxyl groups.

Saleh, Gabr., *J. Pharm. Sci. U. Arab. Repub.*, **6**, 61 (1965)

FUMVAILINE

$C_{20}H_{19}O_6N$

M.p. 180.5−181.5°C

A *Fumaria* alkaloid, this base occurs in *F. vaillantii*. It crystallizes from Me$_2$CO and is laevorotatory with $[\alpha]_D - 44.4°$. The hydrochloride is crystalline with m.p. 212°C. The alkaloid is non-phenolic and contains two methoxyl groups.

Platonova *et al., J. Gen. Chem., USSR*, **26**, 181 (1956)

FUNGIPAVINE (*Mecambrine*)

$C_{18}H_{17}O_3N$

M.p. 178.5−179.5°C

This spiro*iso*quinoline alkaloid occurs in *Meconopsis cambrica, Papaver caucasicum* Marsch. Bieb and in *P. fugax*. It crystallizes from Et$_2$O as colourless prismatic crystals and has $[\alpha]_D - 116°$ (CHCl$_3$). The base forms crystalline salts and derivative including the hydrochloride, m.p. 269−270°C; oxime, m.p. > 285°C; picrate, m.p. 165°C; semicarbazone, m.p. 237°C and the 2:4-dinitrophenylhydrazone, m.p. > 285°C.

Mnatsakanyan, Yunusov., *Dokl. Akad. Nauk. Uzbek SSR*, 36 (1961)
Yunusov, Mnatsakanyan, Akramov., *ibid*, 43 (1961)
Slavik, Slavikova., *Collect. Czech. Chem. Commun.*, **28**, 1720 (1963)
Kühn *et al., Naturwiss.*, **51**, 556 (1964)
Bick., *Experientia*, **20**, 362 (1964)

FUNIFERINE (*Alkaloid TC-100*)

$C_{36}H_{40}O_6N_2$

M.p. 232°C

An alkaloid isolated from the root bark of *Tiliacora funifera*, the base has $[\alpha]_D^{32} + 184.3°$ (CHCl$_3$) or $[\alpha]_D^{27} + 171.4°$ (MeOH) and has been shown to be homogeneous by thin-layer chromatography on alumina. It is soluble in Me$_2$CO and CHCl$_3$. Three methoxyl groups, two methylimino groups and one hydroxyl group are present. The ultraviolet spectrum, with a single absorption maximum at 290 mμ is similar to that of Tiliacorine and Tiliarine (q.v.) found in similar plant species but the colour reactions and physical characteristics of this base differ from those of these two alkaloids.

Tackie, Thomas., *Ghana J. Sci.*, **5**, 11 (1965)

FUNTADIENINE

$C_{22}H_{31}ON$

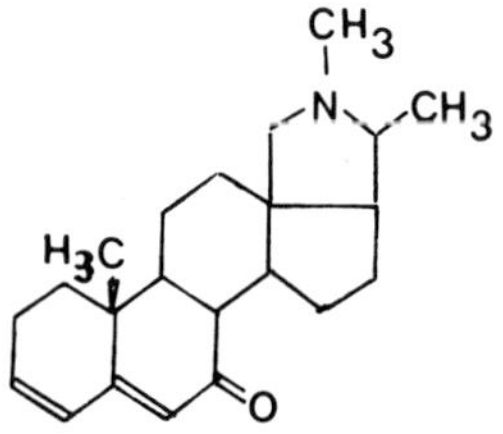

This amorphous alkaloid occurs in the bark of *Funtumia latifolia* and has $[\alpha]_D -247°$ (CHCl$_3$). It yields a crystalline oxime, m.p. 190°C; $[\alpha]_D - 228°$ (c 1.0, CHCl$_3$). Hydrogenation with Pd-C gives the tetrahydro derivative while reduction with NaBH$_4$ gives conadienol. The latter may be acetylated with Ac$_2$O in pyridine to 7β-acetoxy-3:5-conadiene, m.p. 104°C; $[\alpha]_D + 60°$ (c 0.9, CHCl$_3$).

Khuong Huu *et al.*, *Bull. Soc. Chim. Fr.*, 2169 (1964)

FUNTAMAFRINE C

$C_{23}H_{39}ON$

M.p. 168–170°C

An alkaloid isolated from *Chonemorpha macrophylla*, this base is dextrorotatory with $[\alpha]_D^{25} + 33.4°$ (CHCl$_3$). No salts or derivatives have been reported.

Chatterjee, Banerji., *Ind. J. Chem.*, **10**, 1197 (1972)

FUNTESSINE

C$_{22}$H$_{38}$ON$_2$

M.p. 194–5°C

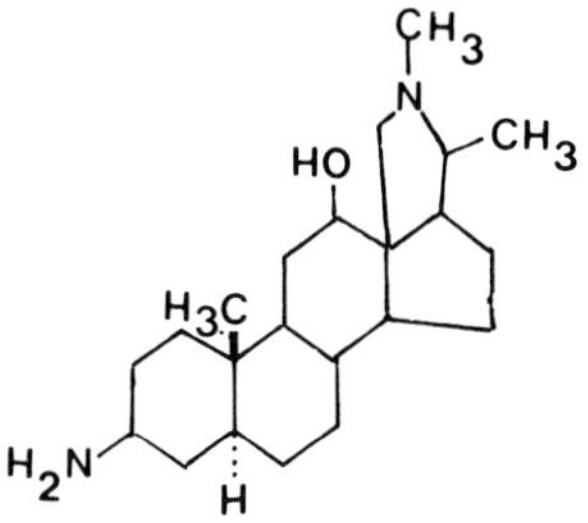

The bark of *Funtumia latifolia* yields this crystalline alkaloid which forms colourless needles from MeOH. It has $[\alpha]_D + 50°$ (c 1.0, CHCl$_3$) and yields the N-*iso*propylidene derivative, m.p. 215–6°C; $[\alpha]_D + 45°$ (c 1.0, CHCl$_3$) and the N,N-dimethyl compound, m.p. 186°C; $[\alpha]_D + 42°$ (c 1.25, CHCl$_3$). The base has been identified as 3β-amino-5α-conan-12β-ol.

Khuong-Huu-Qui *et al., Bull. Soc. Chim. Fr.*, 1831 (1965)

FUNTULINE

C$_{22}$H$_{35}$O$_2$N

M.p. 235°C

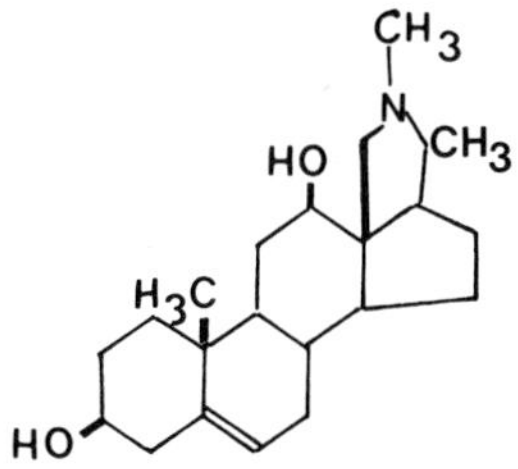

This conanene alkaloid is a constituent of *Funtumia latifolia* and yields colourless crystals from Et$_2$O-MeOH. It has $[\alpha]_D - 6°$ (CHCl$_3$-MeOH). It contains two hydroxyl groups and forms a diacetate as colourless crystals, m.p. 237°C; $[\alpha]_D - 15°$ (c 1.0, CHCl$_3$).

Janot *et al., Bull. Soc. Chim. Fr.*, 787 (1964)

FUNTUMIDINE

C$_{21}$H$_{37}$ON

M.p. 182°C

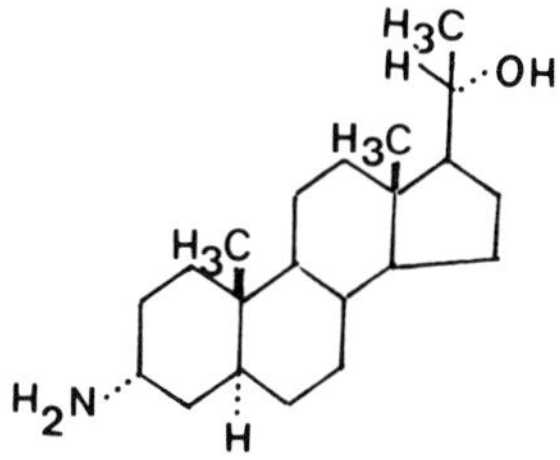

A steroidal alkaloid of the pregnane type, this base also occurs in *Funtumia latifolia*. It has $[\alpha]_D + 10°$ (CHCl$_3$). The structure has been established by spectroscopic methods as 3α-amino-20-α-hydroxy-5α-pregnane.

Janot, Khuong Huu, Goutarel., *Compt. rend.*, **246**, 3076 (1958)
Janot, Khuong Huu, Goutarel., *ibid*, **248**, 982 (1959)

FUNTUMINE

$C_{21}H_{35}ON$

M.p. 126°C

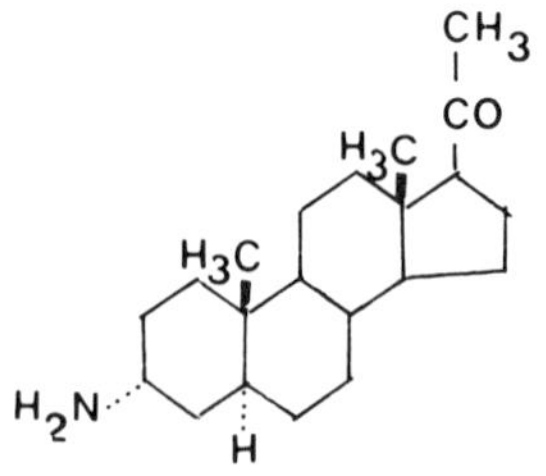

A further pregnane type alkaloid from *Funtumia latifolia,* this dextrorotatory base has $[\alpha]_D + 95°$ (CHCl₃). The structure is similar to that of the preceding alkaloid, being 3α-amino-2-oxo-5α-pregnane.

Janot, Khuong Huu, Goutarel., *Compt. rend.,* **246**, 3076 (1958)
Janot, Khuong Huu, Goutarel., *ibid,* **248**, 982 (1959)

FUNTUMUFRINE B

$C_{22}H_{37}ON$

M.p. 160°C

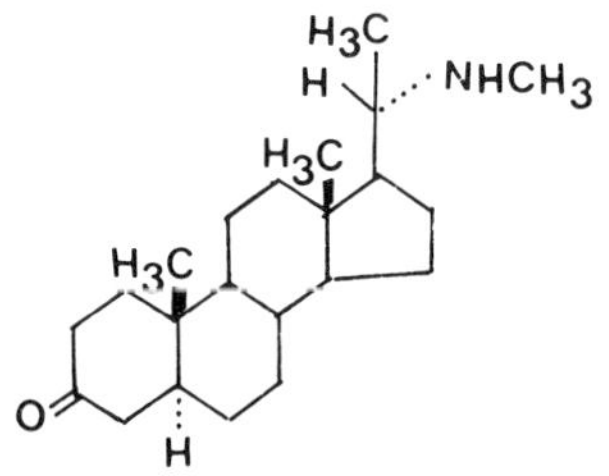

Isolated from *Funtumia africana,* this steroidal alkaloid is also of the pregnane type and is dextrorotatory with $[\alpha]_D + 43°$. The structure has been established as 20α-methylamino-3-oxo-5α-pregnane.

Janot, Khuong-Huu, Goutarel., *Compt. rend.,* **250**, 2445 (1960)

FUNTUMUFRINE C

$C_{23}H_{39}ON$

M.p. 174°C

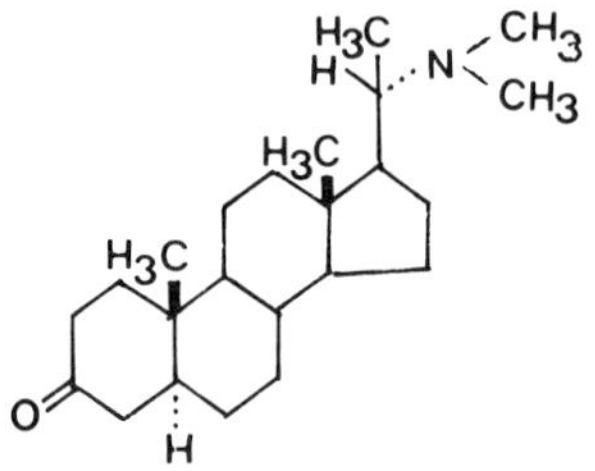

A further pregnane type alkaloid isolated from *Funtumia latifolia* Stapf and *Malouetia bequaertiana,* this base has $[\alpha]_D + 45°$. The constitution of this alkaloid is very similar to that of the preceding base, being 20α-dimethylamino-3-oxo-5α-pregnane.

Janot, Khuong-Huu, Goutarel., *Compt. rend.,* **250**, 2445 (1960)
Janot *et al., Bull. Soc. Chim. Fr.,* 111 (1962)

FUNTUPHYLLAMINE A

$C_{21}H_{37}ON$

M.p. 173°C

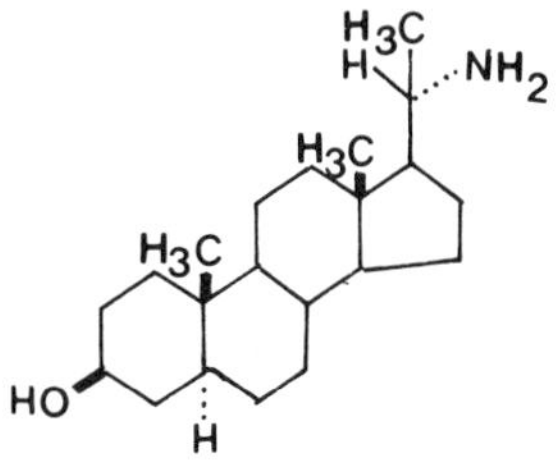

Another alkaloid in the series which have been isolated from various *Funtumia* species, this base occurs in *F. africana*. It has $[\alpha]_D + 13°$ and has the structure of 20α-amino-3β-hydroxy-5α-pregnane.

Janot, Khuong-Huu, Goutarel., *Compt. rend.,* **250**, 2445 (1960)

FUNTUPHYLLAMINE B

$C_{22}H_{39}ON$

M.p. 214°C

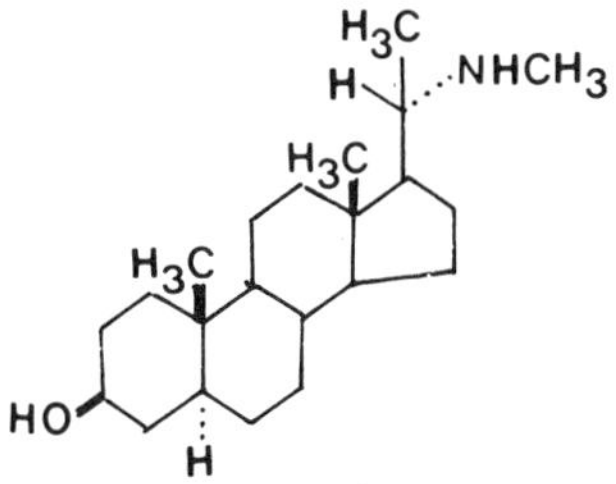

This closely-allied pregnane base is found in *Funtumia africana* and also in *Malouetia bequaertiana*. It is also dextrorotatory with $[\alpha]_D + 24°$. Its structure is 20α-methylamino-3β-hydroxy-5α-pregnane.

Janot, Khuong-Huu, Goutarel., *Compt. rend.,* **250**, 2445 (1960)

FUNTUPHYLLAMINE C

$C_{23}H_{41}ON$

M.p. 172°C

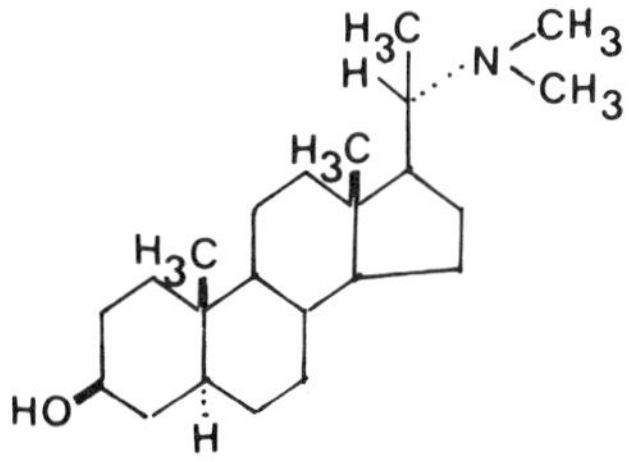

The dimethylamino derivative of the three closely-related bases from *Funtumia africana* has $[\alpha]_D + 24°$. By comparison with funtuphyllamines A and B, the structure is established as 20α-dimethylamino-3β-hydroxy-5α-pregnane.

Janot, Khuong-Huu, Goutarel., *Compt. rend.,* **250**, 2445 (1960)

G

GABONINE

$C_{42}H_{54}O_8N_4$

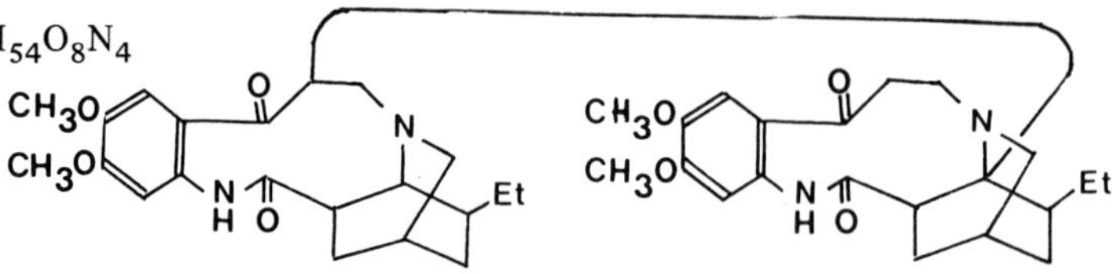

This alkaloid from *Tabernanthe iboga* Baillon has been shown to be dimeric from high resolution mass spectrometry determinations. The mode of linkage between the two moieties is most probably that given above.

Dickel *et al., J. Amer. Chem. Soc.*, **80**, 123 (1958)
Taylor., *J. Org. Chem.*, **30**, 309 (1965)

GABUNINE

$C_{42}H_{50}O_5N_4$

M.p. 244–6°C

(*dec.*).

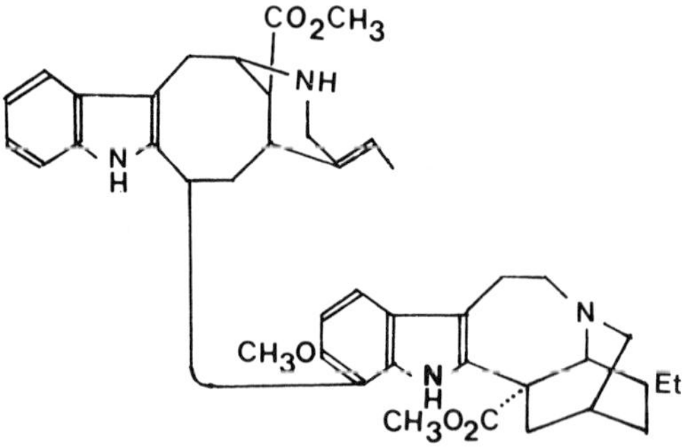

This very complex alkaloid is found in *Gabunia odoratissima* Stapf. It is most readily crystallized from EtOH or MeOH when it yields colourless needles. The base is strongly laevorotatory with $[\alpha]_D^{20} - 105°$ (c 0.62, CHCl$_3$). The crystalline hydrobromide, obtained as needles from Me$_2$CO, has m.p. 280°C (*dec.*). The ultraviolet spectrum of the free base in EtOH has absorption maxima at 266, 287 and 295 mμ. The alkaloid forms an N-methyl derivative which is identical with Conodurine (q.v.).

Cava *et al., Tetrahedron Lett.*, 931 (1965)

GAGAMININE

$C_{36}H_{43}O_7N$

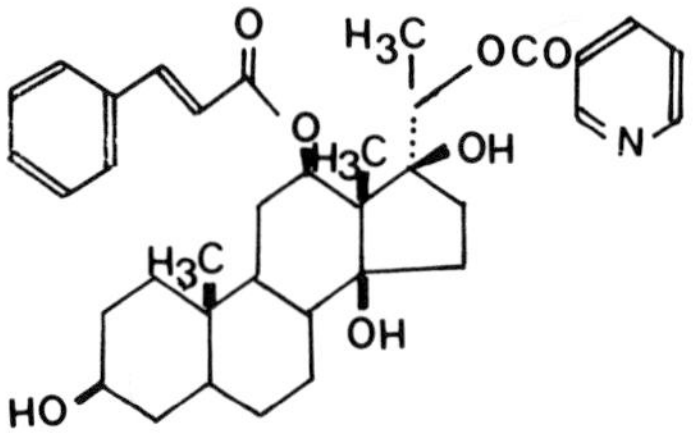

A recently discovered alkaloid of *Cynanchium caudatum*, the structure of this

604

pregnene base has been established by chemical reactions and a study of the NMR and mass spectra.

Yamagishi, Hayashi, Mitsuhashi., *Chem. Pharm. Bull.*, **20**, 2289 (1972)

GALANTHAMIDINE

$C_{18}H_{23}O_5N$

M.p. 211–3°C

The roots of *Galanthus woronovi* yield this crystalline alkaloid which forms colourless crystals from MeOH. It is laevorotatory with $[\alpha]_D$ – 94.2°. The methiodide is also crystalline, m.p. 219°C with almost complete decomposition at the melting point. One methylenedioxy group and a tertiary nitrogen are present but no methoxyl groups.

Proskurnina, Yakovleva., *J. Gen. Chem., USSR,* **26,** 172 (1956)

GALANTHAMINE (*Lycorenine, Lycorimine*)

$C_{16}H_{19}O_3N$

M.p. 130–1°C

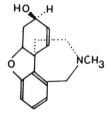

An alkaloid present in *Galanthus elwesii, G. woronovi, Leudojum vernum* and *Lycoris radiata,* the base forms colourless needles from EtOH or MeOH and is laevorotatory with $[\alpha]_D^{22}$ – 122° (c 0.60, EtOH) or $[\alpha]_D^{26}$ – 120° (c 0.99, EtOH). The ultraviolet spectrum contains absorption maxima at 234 and 290 mμ. The alkaloid yields crystalline salts and derivatives including the hydrochloride, m.p. 254–5°C (*dec.*); hydriodide, m.p. 260–1°C (*dec.*); perchlorate, m.p. 225–7°C (*dec.*); O-acetate, m.p. 129–130°C and the methiodide, m.p. 289–291°C; $[\alpha]_D^{22}$ – 94.4° (c 0.67, 75% EtOH), the last being useful in the characterization of the base. When hydrogenated over Pd-C, the alkaloid yields the dihydro derivative, m.p. 122–4°C which is identical with Lycoramine (q.v.). The alternative name, Lycorenine, sometimes given to this alkaloid in the literature is misleading as it may be confused with another alkaloid of the same name but with the empirical formula $C_{18}H_{23}O_4N$ (q.v.).

Kondo, Tomiura, Ishiwata., *J. Pharm. Soc., Japan,* **52,** 433 (1930)
Uyeo, Kobayashi., *Chem. Pharm. Bull.,* **1,** 139 (1953)
Uyeo, Koizumi., *ibid,* **1,** 202 (1953)
Proskurnina, Yakovleva., *J. Gen. Chem., USSR,* **25,** 1035 (1955)
Proskurnina, Yakovleva., *ibid,* **26,** 172 (1956)
Fales, Guiffrida, Wildman., *J. Amer. Chem. Soc.,* **78,** 4145 (1956)
Kobayashi, Shingu, Uyeo., *Chem. & Ind.,* 177 (1956)
Kobayashi, Uyeo., *J. Chem. Soc.,* 638 (1957)

Crystal structure:
Williams, Rogers., *Proc. Chem. Soc.*, 357 (1964)

Synthesis:
Kametani *et al.*, *J. Chem. Soc., C,* 2602 (1969)
Kametani *et al.*, *ibid*, 1043 (1971)
Kametani *et al.*, *J. Org. Chem.*, **36**, 1295 (1971)

GALANTHINE

$C_{18}H_{23}O_4N$

M.p. 134–6°C

This alkaloid is of widespread occurrence being found in *Crinum* species,
Galanthus woronovi, Hippeastrum aulicum, Hymenocallis species, *Narcissus
pseudonarcissus, N. incomparabilis.* The alkaloid crystallizes as pale green prisms
of the hydrate from EtOH or Me_2CO with the above melting point. The
anhydrous form has m.p. 162–4°C; $[\alpha]_D^{22} - 84.5°$ (c 0.23, $CHCl_3$), or $- 81°$
(c 0.21, EtOH). The hydrochloride has m.p. 198–9°C; hydrobromide, m.p.
208°C (*dec.*); hydriodide, m.p. 165–7°C; perchlorate, m.p. 199–201°C and
decomposing at 218°C, and the picrate, m.p. 199–200°C. (*dec.*).

Proskurnina, Yakovleva., *J. Gen. Chem., USSR,* **22**, 1899 (1952)
Proskurnina., *Dokl. Akad. Nauk., SSSR,* **90**, 565 (1953)
Boit, Ehmke., *Chem. Ber.,* **89**, 163 (1956)
Proskurnina, Yakovleva., *J. Gen. Chem., USSR,* **26**, 172 (1956)
Fales, Guiffrida, Wildman., *J. Amer. Chem. Soc.,* **78**, 4145 (1956)
Boit, Döpke., *Naturwiss.,* **48**, 406 (1961)

GALANTHUSINE

$C_{18}H_{23}O_5N$

A methylindole alkaloid found in *Galanthus caucasicus*, the base contains one
methoxyl, one methylenedioxy and one hydroxyl group. A methylimino group
and a hydroxymethyl group are also present. The structure has been deduced
from infrared, NMR and mass spectrometry.

Tsakadze *et al., Khim. Prir. Soedin.,* **6**, 773 (1970)

606

GALANTIDINE

$C_{14}H_{17}O_3N$

M.p. 235–8°C

This alkaloid occurs in the bulbs and leaves of *Galanthus Woronovi*. It forms crystalline salts, e.g. the hydrochloride, m.p. 197–9°C; hydrobromide, m.p. 213–213.5°C; $[\alpha]_D + 32.3°$ and the methiodide, m.p. 232–3°C.

Proskurnina, Areshkina., *J. Gen. Chem., USSR,* **17**, 1216 (1947)

GALANTINE

$C_{16}H_{23}O_4N$

M.p. 132–3°C

A second base found in *Galanthus Woronovi,* this alkaloid crystallizes with 1 H_2O having the melting point given above. When dried for a prolonged period at 100°C it forms the anhydrous base, m.p. 160–4°C. It is laevorotatory with $[\alpha]_D - 87°$ and forms crystalline salts with mineral acids: the hydrochloride, m.p. 198–9°C; hydrobromide, m.p. 201–3°C and the perchlorate, m.p. 199–201°C. It contains three methoxyl groups and one hydroxyl group.

Proskurnina, Areshkina., *J. Gen. Chem., USSR,* **17**, 1216 (1947)

GALBULIMINA ALKALOIDS

The species *Galbulimina,* found mainly in Australia, yields a series of eighteen closely-related alkaloids. As yet, these have not been named, but are designated by numbers.

GALBULIMINA ALKALOID G.B.1

$C_{33}H_{39}O_9N$

M.p. 242°C

This base crystallizes from $CHCl_3$-MeOH as colourless prisms and is dextrorotatory with $[\alpha]_D + 8°$ ($CHCl_3$). The ultraviolet spectrum in neutral solution (EtOH) has absorption maxima at 228, 272 and 280 mμ. In acid solution (HCl-EtOH), the absorption maxima remain in the same positions. When heated with MeOH, the alkaloid furnishes the tetrahydroxy compound which has m.p. 176–7°C; $[\alpha]_D^{23} + 40°$ (c 0.9, $CHCl_3$).

GALBULIMINA ALKALOID G.B.2

$C_{30}H_{39}O_{10}N$

M.p. $238°C$

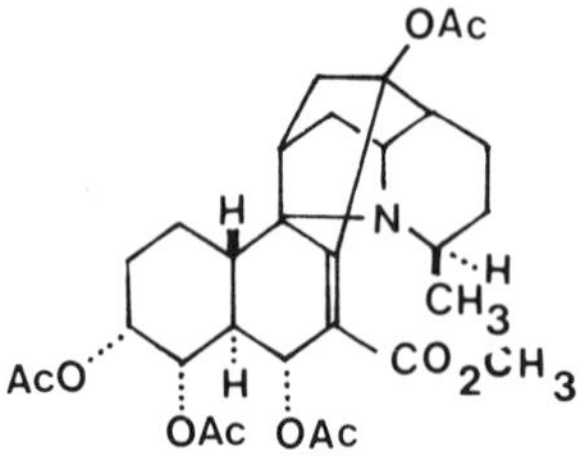

This alkaloid, when crystallized from AcOEt-cyclohexane, forms colourless prisms and has $[\alpha]_D + 38°$ (CHCl$_3$). The ultraviolet spectrum in ethanolic solution has two absorption maxima at 215 and 245 mμ. Heating with MeOH yields the same tetrahydroxy compound as the previous base.

GALBULIMINA ALKALOID G.B.3

$C_{26}H_{35}O_8N$

M.p. $237°C$

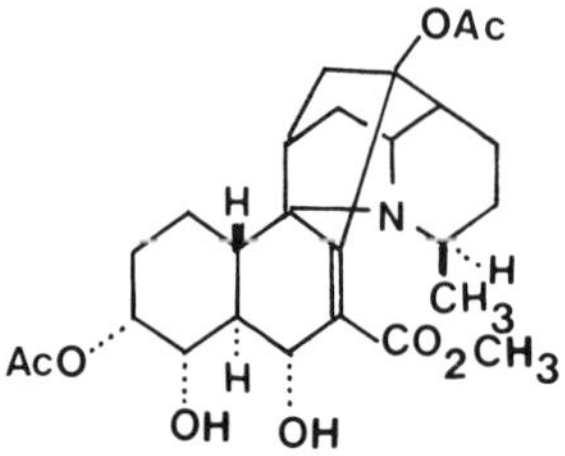

This alkaloid crystallizes from AcOEt as colourless prisms and is dextrorotatory with $[\alpha]_D + 97°$ (CHCl$_3$). The ultraviolet spectrum in EtOH is identical with that of the preceding base with absorption maxima at 215 and 245 mμ. Methanolysis again yields the tetrahydroxy derivative, m.p. 176–7°C.

GALBULIMINA ALKALOID G.B.4

$C_{31}H_{37}O_8N$

M.p. $238°C$

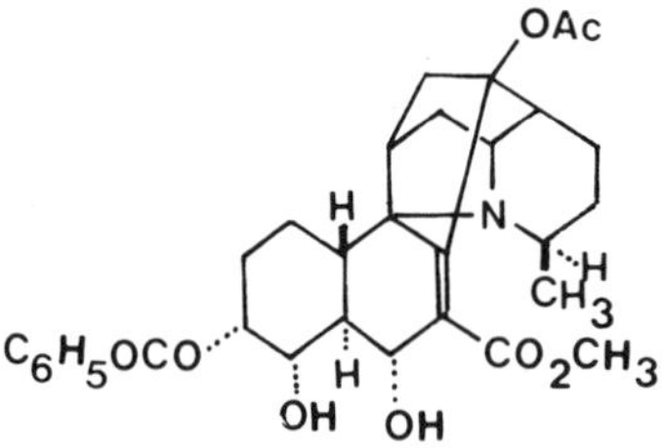

When crystallized from CHCl$_3$-MeOH, the alkaloid is obtained as colourless prisms and has $[\alpha]_D + 63°$ (CHCl$_3$). The ultraviolet spectrum in neutral solution (EtOH) has absorption maxima at 226, 273 and 280 mμ. In acid solution (HCl-EtOH), the maxima are at the same wavelengths. When heated with MeOH it yields alkaloid G.B.5 (q.v.).

608

GALBULIMINA ALKALOID G.B.5

$C_{24}H_{33}O_7N$

M.p. 234°C

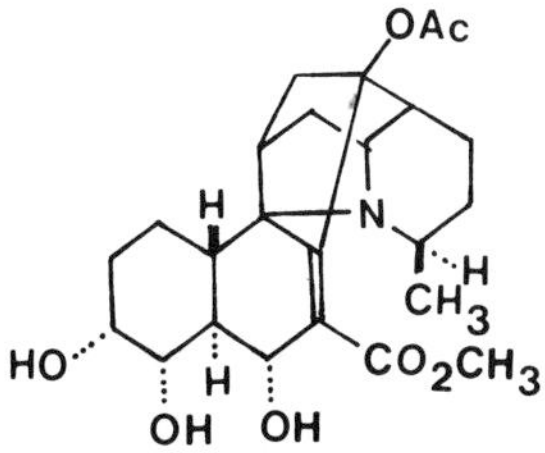

This alkaloid contains two acetoxy groups and three hydroxyl groups and forms colourless prisms from AcOEt. It has $[\alpha]_D + 60°$ (CHCl$_3$) and the ultraviolet spectrum in EtOH exhibits two absorption maxima at 215 and 254 mμ.

GALBULIMINA ALKALOID G.B.6

$C_{32}H_{39}O_8N$

M.p. 170°C

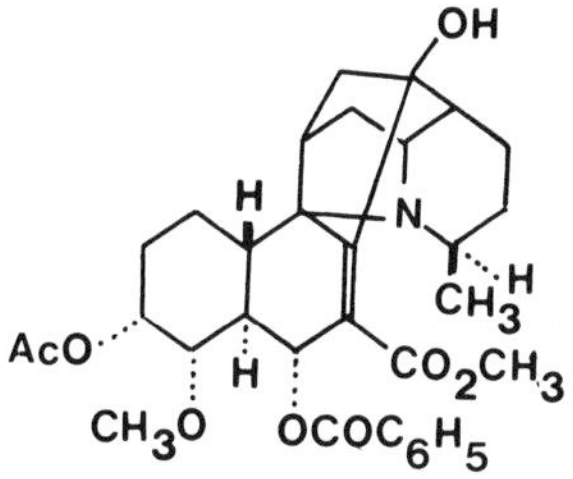

Obtained as colourless prisms from Me$_2$CO, the base has $[\alpha]_D - 12°$ (CHCl$_3$) and is identical with 13-acetylhimandridine. It contains two acetoxy groups, one methoxyl and one benzoyl group in the molecule. The ultraviolet spectrum in EtOH has absorption maxima at 230, 272 and 280 mμ and in HCl-EtOH solution, at 228, 272 and 280 mμ.

GALBULIMINA ALKALOID G.B.7

$C_{32}H_{39}O_8N$

M.p. 183°C

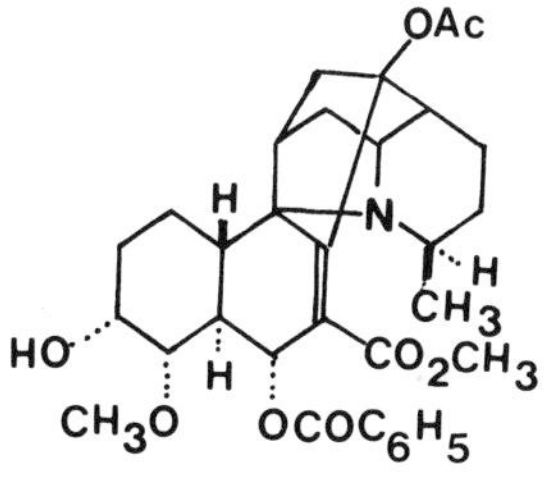

An isomer of the preceding alkaloid, this base is 20-acetylhimandridine and is obtained as prisms from n-heptane. It is dextrorotatory with $[\alpha]_D + 35°$ (CHCl$_3$) and the ultraviolet spectra in EtOH and HCl-EtOH are identical with those of the foregoing alkaloid. Heating with MeOH furnishes himandridine (q.v.).

609

GALBULIMINA ALKALOID G.B.8

$C_{23}H_{33}O_5N$

M.p. 188°C

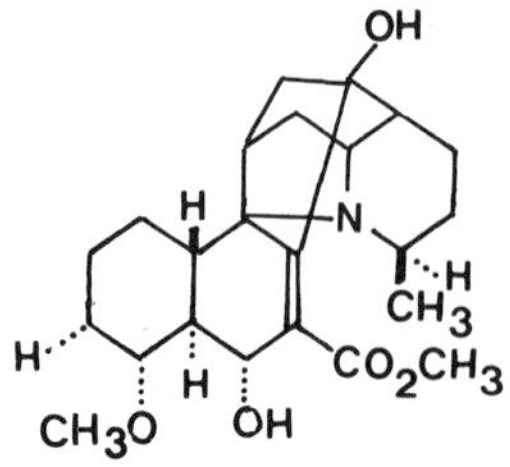

The alkaloid crystallizes from cyclohexane as colourless prisms and is also dextrorotatory with $[\alpha]_D + 63°$ (CHCl$_3$). Two hydroxyl groups, one methoxyl and one methoxycarbonyl group are present. The ultraviolet spectrum has absorption maxima at 215 and 245 mμ.

GALBULIMINA ALKALOID G.B.9

$C_{25}H_{35}O_6N$

M.p. 168°C

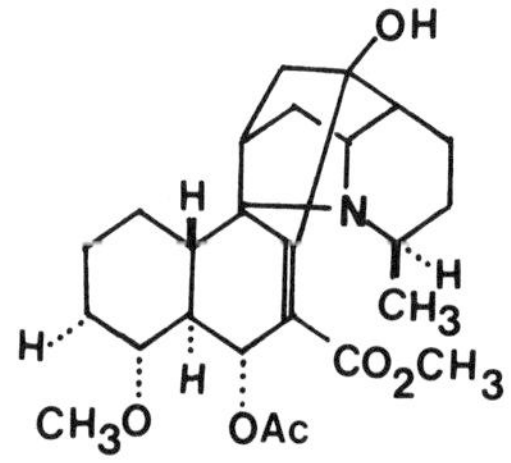

This alkaloid is best crystallized from *n*-heptane when it forms colourless prisms. It is dextrorotatory with $[\alpha]_D + 23°$ (CHCl$_3$) and exhibits three absorption maxima in the ultraviolet spectrum in ethanolic solution at 215, 230 and 245 mμ. One methoxyl, one hydroxyl, an acetoxy and a methoxycarbonyl group are present in the molecule.

GALBULIMINA ALKALOID G.B.10

$C_{27}H_{37}O_7N$

M.p. 162°C

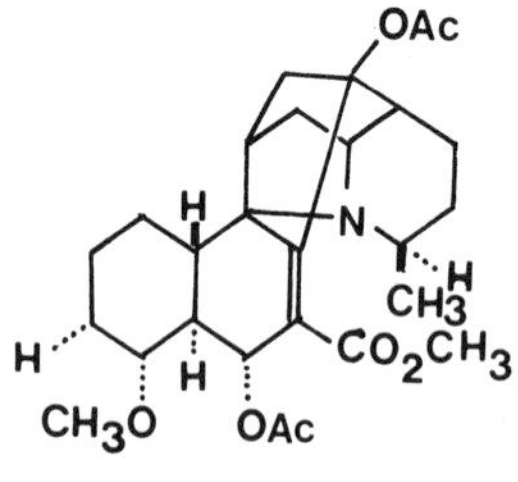

A dextrorotatory alkaloid with $[\alpha]_D + 19°$ (CHCl$_3$), the base is obtained in the form of prisms from a mixture of AcOEt and cyclohexane. The ultraviolet spectrum is similar to that of most of this series of alkaloids with absorption maxima at 215 and 245 mμ.

610

GALBULIMINA ALKALOID G.B.11

$C_{24}H_{33}O_6N$

M.p. 239°C

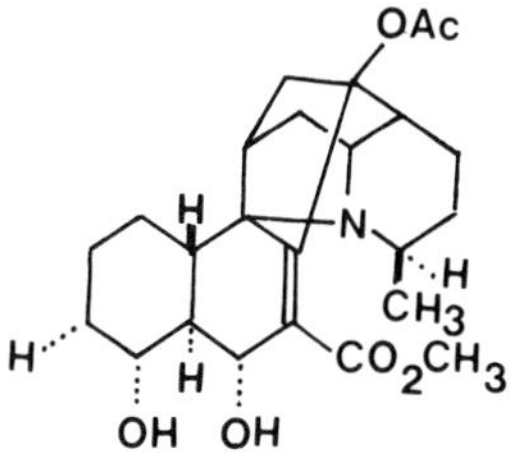

Like the majority of these alkaloids, this particular base forms colourless prisms when crystallized from AcOEt. It has $[\alpha]_D + 64°$ (CHCl$_3$) and the ultraviolet spectrum exhibits absorption maxima at 215 and 245 mμ. With Ac$_2$O in pyridine it gives the di-O-acetyl derivative identical with Galbulimina alkaloid G.B.12.

GALBULIMINA ALKALOID G.B.12

$C_{28}H_{37}O_8N$

M.p. 222°C

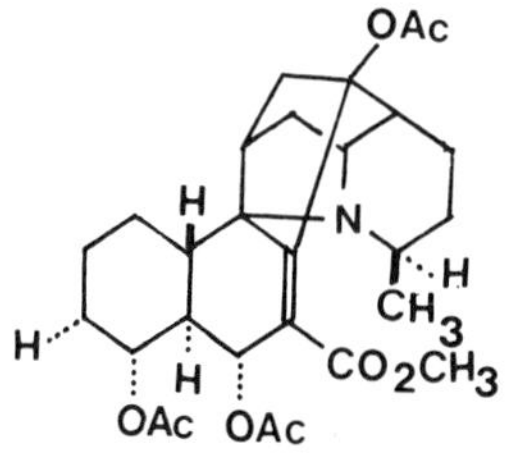

Colourless prisms from AcOEt-cyclohexane, this alkaloid has $[\alpha]_D + 23°$ (CHCl$_3$). The ultraviolet spectrum is identical with those of the majority of these bases with maxima at 215 and 245 mμ.

GALBULIMINA ALKALOID G.B.13

$C_{20}H_{29}O_2N$

M.p. 185°C

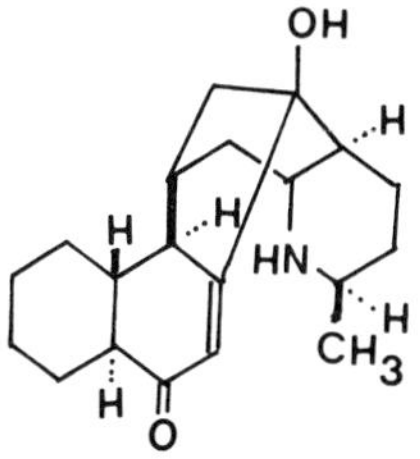

This alkaloid crystallizes as prisms from n-heptane and is laevorotatory with $[\alpha]_D - 84°$ (CHCl$_3$). The ultraviolet spectrum has an absorption maximum at 246 mμ in ethanolic solution which shifts to 237 mμ in HCl-EtOH. The structure of this alkaloid differs somewhat from those of the preceding bases containing only two oxygen atoms, one present as a hydroxyl group and the other as a keto group. The alkaloid forms a crystalline hydrochloride as rectangular prisms, m.p. 275–7°C and an N-acetyl derivative, m.p. 220°C; $[\alpha]_D^{25} - 119°$ (c 2.4, CHCl$_3$). The N-methyl compound is identical with himbadine (q.v.).

GALBULIMINA ALKALOID G.B.14

$C_{24}H_{33}O_5N$

M.p. $106°C$

A further alkaloid from this species, this base is obtained as colourless prisms from an aqueous mixture of Me_2CO-heptane. The structure has not yet been fully established.

GALBULIMINA ALKALOID G.B.15

$C_{22}H_{35}O_3N$

M.p. $230°C$

Formed as white needles from C_6H_6, this base is dextrorotatory with $[\alpha]_D +58°$ ($CHCl_3$). Once again, its structure has to be definitely established.

GALBULIMINA ALKALOID G.B.16

$C_{20}H_{27}O_2N$

M.p. $203°C$

Colourless prisms when crystallized from AcOEt, this alkaloid is strongly dextrorotatory with $[\alpha]_D + 550°$ ($CHCl_3$). The structure has not been determined although it may possibly be a dehydro-form of Alkaloid G.B.13.

GALBULIMINA ALKALOID G.B.17

$C_{21}H_{31}O_3N$

M.p. $115°C$

This alkaloid forms colourless needles of the monohydrate from aqueous MeOH. It is laevorotatory and has $[\alpha]_D - 21°$ ($CHCl_3$). The structure is still not known with certainty.

GALBULIMINA ALKALOID G.B.18

$C_{22}H_{33}O_3N$

M.p. $120°C$

The last alkaloid in this series forms colourless prisms from n-heptane and has $[\alpha]_D + 37°$ ($CHCl_3$). Its structure has still to be determined.

Binns *et al.*, *Austral. J. Chem.*, **18**, 569 (1965)

Structures:
Guise *et al.*, *Austral. J. Chem.*, **20**, 1029 (1967)
Mander, Prager, Rasmussen, Ritchie, Taylor., *ibid*, **20**, 1473 (1967)

GALEGINE

$C_6H_{13}N_3$ $(NH_2)_2C:N\cdot CH_2\cdot CH:C(CH_3)_2$

M.p. 60–5°C

This alkaloid was first isolated from the seeds of *Galega officinalis* Linn and considered to be a 3-methylpyrrolidine derivative. It was subsequently shown to be a guanidine derivative of the above structure by Barger and White. The base forms several crystalline salts and derivatives, e.g. the sulphate, m.p. 227°C; nitrate, m.p. 108°C; oxalate, m.p. 192–5°C; bicarbonate, m.p. 138°C; platinichloride, m.p. 123°C; N-benzoyl derivative, m.p. 95–6°C and the N:N′-di-*m*-nitrobenzoyl compound, m.p. 163–4°C. A crystalline picrate, m.p. 180–1°C has also been prepared.

Tanret., *Compt. rend.*, **158**, 1182, 1426 (1914)
Tanret., *Bull. Soc. Chim.*, **35**, 404 (1924)
Barger, White., *Biochem. J.*, **17**, 827 (1923)
Späth, Spitzy., *Ber.*, **58**, 2273 (1925)
Babor, Jezo., *Chem. Zvesti.*, **8**, 18 (1954)

GALIPIDINE

The presence of this alkaloid in the bark of *Galipea officinalis* Hancock was reported by Beckurts but this discover was not confirmed by later work carried out by Tröger. It is possible that the compound is a mixture of alkaloids and no physical constants of the supposed alkaloid have been reported.

Beckurts., *Arch. Pharm.*, **229**, 591 (1891)
Beckurts., *ibid*, **233**, 410 (1895)
Tröger., *ibid*, **248**, 1 (1910)

GALIPINE

$C_{20}H_{21}O_3N$

M.p. 115–6°C

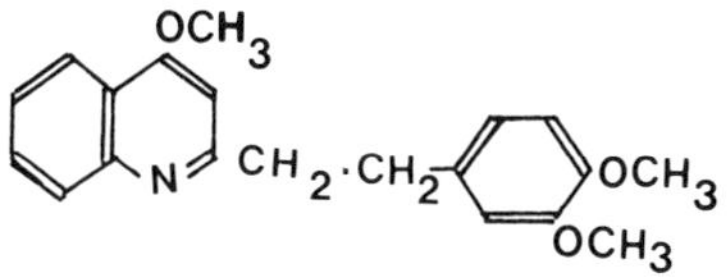

Occurring in the bark of *Galipea officinalis* Hancock, this alkaloid forms prisms from either EtOH or Et$_2$O. It yields crystalline salts which are, in general, more soluble in H$_2$O than those of cusparine with which it is usually found. The hydrochloride tetrahydrate forms colourless leaflets, m.p. 165°C; the hydriodide, m.p. 178°C; aurichloride, m.p. 174–5°C; platinichloride, m.p. 174–5°C; picrate, m.p. 194°C and the methiodide, yellow needles, m.p. 146°C.

The alkaloid contains three methoxyl groups and on oxidation with chromic acid yields veratric acid and a second acid, $C_{11}H_9O_3N$ as the crystalline dihydrate, m.p. 194°C, shown by Späth and Brunner to be 4-methoxyquinoline-2-carboxylic acid. Destructive distillation with Zn dust furnishes quinoline.

Körner, Böhringer., *Ber.*, **16**, 2305 (1883)
Späth, Brunner., *ibid*, **57**, 1243 (1924)
Späth, Papaioanou., *Monatsh.*, **52**, 134 (1929)
Schläger, Leeb., *ibid*, **81**, 714 (1950)

GALIPOIDINE

$C_{19}H_{15}O_4N$

M.p. 231–3°C

This quinoline alkaloid is present in the bark of *Galipea officinalis* Hancock and is only sparingly soluble in most organic solvents. It forms a normal platini-chloride, thick yellow prisms with 2.5 H_2O, m.p. 158°C (*dec.*) and an unusual aurichloride, $(B.HCl)_2.AuCl_3.1.5$ H_2O crystallizing as bright yellow needles, m.p. 170°C (*dec.*).

Tröger, Müller., *Arch. Pharm.*, **248**, 1 (1910)
Tröger, Rimne., *ibid*, **249**, 174 (1911)
Späth, Pikl., *Monatsh.*, **55**, 352 (1930)

GALIPOLINE

$C_{19}H_{19}O_3N$

M.p. 193°C

Späth and Papaioanou isolated this quinoline alkaloid from the mixture of phenolic bases extracted from *Galipea officinalis* Hancock. It crystallizes from H_2O and contains two methoxyl groups and one hydroxyl group. With CH_2N_2 it furnishes galipine (q.v.). The alkaloid may be synthesized by the condensation of 4-chloro-2-methylquinoline with 3:4-dimethoxy-benzaldehyde followed by treatment with sodium benzyl oxide which replaced the chlorine by a benzyloxy group. The resulting 4-benzyloxy-2:3':4'-dimethoxystyrylquinoline is then reduced and hydrolyzed to remove the benzyl group, forming galipoline.

Späth, Eberstaller., *Ber.*, **57**, 1687 (1924)
Späth, Papaioanou., *Monatsh.*, **52**, 129 (1929)

GAMBIRDINE

$C_{21}H_{26}O_4N_2$

M.p. 199–201°C

This alkaloid is present in the stem of *Uncaria gambir* (*Uncaria gambier* Roxb.). It forms colourless crystals and has $[\alpha]_D^{21}$ + 84.8° (c 0.02, $CHCl_3$). In the plant it occurs together with mitraphylline (q.v.) and spectroscopic data shows that the two alkaloids are stereoisomers.

Chan., *Tetrahedron Lett.*, 3403 (1968)

*iso*GAMBIRDINE

$C_{21}H_{26}O_4N_2$

M.p. 202–3°C

Also present in the stem of *Uncaria gambier* Roxb. this alkaloid forms colourless crystals and has $[\alpha]_D^{21} + 115.5°$ (c 0.2, $CHCl_3$). It has also been shown spectroscopically to be stereoisomeric with mitraphylline.

Chan., *Tetrahedron Lett.*, 3403 (1968)

GAMBIRINE

$C_{22}H_{28}O_4N_2$

M.p. 163–5°C

A hypotensive alkaloid found in *Uncaria gambier* Roxb., this base was originally assigned the empirical formula $C_{22}H_{26}O_4N_2$, later altered to that given above. The alkaloid forms pale orange-yellow crystals from $CHCl_3$-hexane or petroleum ether and has $[\alpha]_D^{20} + 28.6°$ (c 0.077, $CHCl_3$). The ultraviolet spectrum exhibits absorption maxima at 226.5, 285 and 294 mμ with a shoulder at 250 mμ. It is insoluble in H_2O or cold alkalies, sparingly so in petroleum ether and readily dissolves in $CHCl_3$, C_6H_6, EtOH or Et_2O. The solution in H_2SO_4 or hot alkalies shows a marked green fluorescence. The crystalline hydrochloride has m.p. 256–7°C and the aurichloride forms yellow crystals, m.p. 112–4°C. The alkaloid contains one hydroxyl group which is phenolic in character, yielding an O-methyl derivative identical with speciogynine (q.v.).

Raymond-Hamet., *Bull. acad. med.*, **112**, 645 (1935)
Pavolini, Gambarin, Monteechis., *Ann. chim.* (Rome), **40**, 654 (1950)
Spectra:
Merlini *et al.*, *Tetrahedron Lett.*, 1571 (1967)

GAMBIRTANNINE

$C_{21}H_{18}O_2N_2$

M.p. 150–3°C (*dec.*).

Isolated from the bark of *Uncaria gambier* Roxb., this alkaloid forms orange needle-shaped crystals from Et_2O-hexane. The base is optically inactive and contains one methoxycarbonyl group. The ultraviolet spectrum in neutral solution (EtOH) has absorption maxima at 314, 340 and 410 $m\mu$ with a shoulder at 266 $m\mu$. In HCl-EtOH solution, the spectrum has an absorption maximum at 358 $m\mu$ with a shoulder present at 250 $m\mu$.

Merlini et al., Tetrahedron, **23**, 3129 (1967)

GANIARINE

So far, this amorphous alkaloid from the stem bark of *Premna integrifolia* Linn. (Verbenaceae) has been characterized only as the crystalline platinichloride, m.p. 239–241°C. The structure is unknown.

Basu, Dandiya., J. Amer. Pharm. Assoc., **36**, 389 (1947)

GARDNERAMINE

$C_{23}H_{28}O_5N_2$

M.p. 134–5°C

A hydroindole alkaloid present in *Gardneria nutans* Sieb. et Zucc., this base has $[\alpha]_D - 287.7°$ ($CHCl_3$). The ultraviolet spectrum shows absorption maxima at 264, 270 and 324 $m\mu$. The alkaloid contains three methoxyl groups in the benzene ring.

Haginiwa et al., J. Pharm. Soc., Japan, **87**, 1484 (1967)
Sakai et al., Tetrahedron Lett., 2057 (1971)

Crystal structure:
Aimi et al., Tetrahedron Lett., 2061 (1971)

GARDNERINE

$C_{20}H_{24}O_2N_2$

M.p. 243–4°C

Gardneria nutans Sieb. et Zucc. also yields this alkaloid which is found mainly in the stems and roots of the plant. It is laevorotatory with $[\alpha]_D^{25} - 29.4°$. The ultraviolet spectrum of the methanolic solution exhibits absorption maxima at 228.5, 268.5 and 298 $m\mu$. One methoxyl group and a hydroxymethyl group are present. The acetyl derivative is crystalline with m.p. 218–9°C.

Sakai, Kubo, Haginiwa., Tetrahedron Lett., 1485 (1969)

Absolute configuration:
Sakai et al., Tetrahedron Lett., 1489 (1969)

GARDNUTINE

$C_{20}H_{22}O_2N_2$

M.p. 319–320°C

A further constituent of the stem and roots of *Gardneria nutans* Sieb. et Zucc. The ultraviolet spectrum in MeOH shows absorption maxima at 223.5, 260 and 295 mμ with an inflexion at 302 mμ. The base is dextrorotatory having $[\alpha]_D^{25} +$ 30.3°.

Sakai, Kubo, Haginiwa., *Tetrahedron Lett.*, 1485 (1969)

GARRYFOLINE (*Laurifoline*)

$C_{22}H_{33}O_2N$

M.p. 130–3°C

One of the *Garrya* alkaloids which are closely related to the *Aconitum* and *Delphinium* bases, this alkaloid is present in *Garrya laurifolia* Hartw. It forms colourless crystals from *n*-hexane or Et₂O and has $[\alpha]_D - 60°$. On heating in MeOH, the alkaloid furnishes isolaurifoline, m.p. 140–4°C; $[\alpha]_D - 57°C$ while aqueous HCl gives cuauchicicine (q.v.). The base contains one methyl, one hydroxyl and an exocyxlic methylene group.

Djerassi *et al., J. Amer. Chem. Soc.*, 77, 4801 (1955)
Djerassi, Vorbrüggen., *ibid*, 84, 2990 (1962)

GARRYINE

$C_{22}H_{34}O_2N$

M.p. 96°C

This *Garrya* alkaloid occurs in *G. veatchii* bark and forms colourless crystals from EtOH which shrink at 88°C and then have the melting point given above. The natural alkaloid is laevorotatory with $[\alpha]_D^{27.5} - 84.23°$ (c 1.0, EtOH). The following crystalline salts have been described: hydrochloride, m.p. 251–2°C (*dec.*); hydrobromide, m.p. 229–230°C (*dec.*); hydriodide, m.p. 203–4°C (*dec.*) and the sulphate which decomposes over a wide range of temperature. The structure has been confirmed by the total synthesis of the (±)-form of the alkaloid.

Oneto., *J. Amer. Pharm. Assoc.*, **35**, 204 (1946)

Total synthesis:
Masamune., *J. Amer. Chem. Soc.*, **86**, 290 (1964)
Nagata *et al., ibid*, **86**, 929 (1964)
Valenta, Wiesner, Wong., *Tetrahedron Lett.*, 2437 (1964)
Nagata *et al., J. Amer. Chem. Soc.*, **89**, 1499 (1967)

GEISSOLOSIMINE

$C_{38}H_{44}ON_4$

M.p. $140^\circ C$

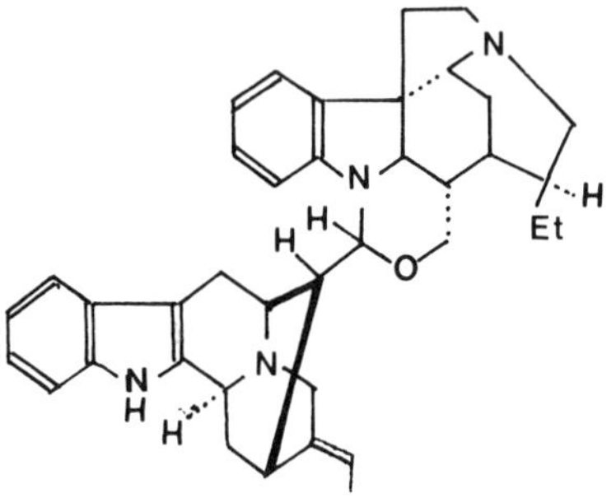

When first isolated from *Geissospermum vellosii* this alkaloid was provisionally designated Alkaloid D_2. It yields colourless crystals from aqueous MeOH and has $[\alpha]_D^{22} + 70.4^\circ$. The ultraviolet spectrum has absorption maxima at 250, 284 and 292 mμ. Three tertiary nitrogen atoms are present, the fourth being an imino group.

Rapoport *et al., J. Amer. Chem. Soc.*, **80**, 1601 (1958)
Rapoport, Moore., *J. Org. Chem.*, **27**, 2981 (1962)

GEISSOSCHIZINE

$C_{21}H_{24}O_3N_2$

M.p. $194-6^\circ C$

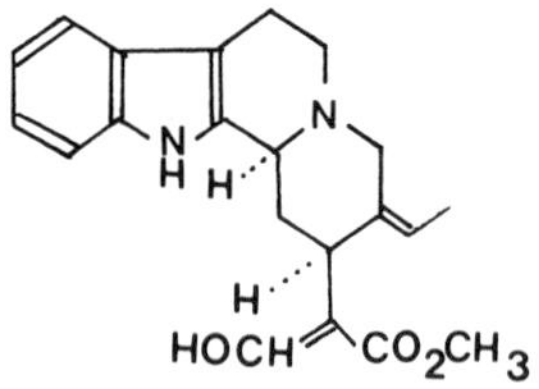

There is still some doubt as to whether this base occurs naturally in *Geissospermum vellosii* (*Tabernaemontana laevis* Vell.) or is an artifact produced by hydrolysis of geissospermine (q.v.) during extraction. It is dextrorotatory with $[\alpha]_D^{21} + 115^\circ$ (EtOH) and forms a 2:4-dinitrophenylhydrazone hydrochloride, m.p. $198^\circ C$.

Janot., *Tetrahedron*, **14**, 113 (1961)

618

GEISSOSCHIZOLINE

$C_{19}H_{26}ON_2$

M.p. 84–7°C

This alkaloid, which is also produced during the hydrolysis of geissospermine, does occur naturally in *Geissospermum vellosii*. It has $[\alpha]_D + 32°$ (c 1.0, EtOH) and a melting point of 126°C has been recorded for it in addition to that given above. The ultraviolet spectrum shows two absorption maxima at 247 and 301 mμ. It forms a crystalline compound with $CHCl_3$ with m.p. 105–8°C; $[\alpha]_D^{25} + 24°$ (c 1.0, EtOH) and the O,N-diacetyl derivative which forms colourless crystals from Me_2CO, m.p. 196–7°C.

Rapoport *et al., J. Amer. Chem. Soc.,* **80**, 1602 (1958)
Janot., *Tetrahedron,* **14**, 113 (1961)

GEISSOSPERMINE

$C_{40}H_{48}O_3N_4$

M.p. 217–9°C (*dry*)

The bark of *Geissospermum vellosii,* used in Brazil as a febrifuge, contains this alkaloid which forms two crystalline hydrates. When obtained from aqueous MeOH it yields the sesquihydrate, m.p. 145–7°C (*dec.*); $[\alpha]_D^{20} - 101.9°$ (EtOH) which is soluble in most organic solvents but only slightly so in H_2O, CCl_4 or Et_2O. Crystallization from AcOEt gives the dihydrate, m.p. 213–4°C (*dec.*) after sintering at 160°C. This form has $[\alpha]_D^{20} - 101°$ (EtOH). The alkaloid forms a series of crystalline salts and derivatives including the hydrochloride, m.p. 148°C; the oxalate pentahydrate, m.p. 193°C (*dec.*); sulphate (hexahydrate), m.p. 226°C (*dec.*); $[\alpha]_D - 84.2°$ (H_2O); the tartrate, m.p. 158°C and the dimethiodide which crystallizes as the tetrahydrate, m.p. 261–2°C (*dec.*); $[\alpha]_D^{20} - 61.5°$ (EtOH). The base contains a labile, basic methylimino group, two active hydrogens as shown by the Zerewitinoff test and one methoxyl group. It yields a colourless solution with H_2SO_4, a blue colour on the addition of ferric sulphate and a purple colouration with HNO_3.

Cold, strong HCl hydrolyzes the base into geissoschizine and geissoschizoline (q.v.). With phosphorus and HI in boiling AcOH it furnishes a deoxy-base, $C_{20}H_{26}ON_2$, m.p. 212–3°C (*dec.*). Distillation with Zn dust gives 2-methyl-4-ethylpyridine.

Bertho, Moog., *Annalen,* **509,** 241 (1934)
Raymond-Hamet., *Bull. Sci. Pharmacol.,* **44,** 449 (1937)
Bertho, Sarx., *Annalen,* **556,** 22 (1944)
Wiesner, Rideout, Marson., *Experientia,* **9,** 369 (1953)
Rapoport *et al., J. Amer. Chem. Soc.,* **80,** 1001 (1958)
Janot., *Tetrahedron,* **14,** 113 (1961)

GEISSOVELLINE

$C_{23}H_{32}O_3N_2$

M.p. 188–190°C

The bark of *Geissospermum vellosii* yields this dihydroindole alkaloid which is obtained as a white powder having $[\alpha]_D^{25} - 125°$ (c 1.15, $CHCl_3$). Acid hydrolysis yields acetic acid and deacetylgeissovelline as pale yellow crystals, m.p. 158–159.5°C; $[\alpha]_D^{25} - 6°$ (c 1.07, $CHCl_3$). The structure given is based upon proton and C-13 NMR spectra of this derivative. The deacetyl compound is readily pyrolyzed to 1-ethyl-6:7-dimethoxycarbazole, m.p. 136–8°C and 159–160°C with intermediate solidification. On catalytic hydrogenation, the base forms the dihydro derivative, m.p. 50–70°C.

Moore, Rapoport., *J. Org. Chem.,* **38,** 215 (1973)

GELSEDINE

$C_{19}H_{24}O_3N_2$

M.p. 172.5–174°C

One of the *Gelsemium* alkaloids, this base occurs in *G. sempervirens* and forms colourless rhombic crystals from AcOEt. It is laevorotatory with $[\alpha]_D^{25} - 159°$ (c 1.35, $CHCl_3$). It yields a crystalline perchlorate, m.p. 183°C; $[\alpha]_D^{25} - 96°$ (c 0.73, $CHCl_3$); a picrate, m.p. 224–6°C (*dec.*); an acetyl derivative, m.p. 165–6°C; $[\alpha]_D^{25} - 139°$ (c 0.72, $CHCl_3$) and a benzoyl compound, m.p. 251–2°C; $[\alpha]_D^{25} - 116°$ (c 0.99, $CHCl_3$).

Janot, Goutarel, Sneedon., *Helv. Chim. Acta,* **34,** 1205 (1951)
Wenkert, Reid., *Chem. & Ind.,* 1390 (1953)
Schwartz, Marion., *J. Amer. Chem. Soc.,* **75,** 4372 (1953)
Schwartz, Marion., *Can. J. Chem.,* **31,** 958 (1953)

GELSEMICINE

$C_{20}H_{26}O_4N_2$

M.p. 171°C

This alkaloid from *Gelsemium sempervirens*, Ait., crystallizes from Me_2CO in broad, orthorhombic prisms and has $[\alpha]_D^{24} - 140°$ (c 1.0, EtOH) and $- 140°$ (c 1.1, $CHCl_3$). The hydrochloride crystallizes as colourless needles, m.p. 140–2°C; the picrate, m.p. 203°C; methiodide, m.p. 227°C and the benzoyl derivative, m.p. 232°C. The last named behaves as a neutral compound. The alkaloid itself is a secondary base and does not react with either 2:4-dinitro-phenylhydrazine or hydroxylamine. With methyl iodide it gives N-methylgel-semicine hydriodide, m.p. 227°C. On hydrogenation with PtO_2 in dry AcOH it yields a hexahydro derivative.

Chou., *Chem. Abstr.*, **25**, 4085 (1931)
Forsyth, Marrian, Stevens., *J. Chem. Soc.*, 579 (1945)
Przyblska, Marion., *Can. J. Chem.*, **39**, 2124 (1961)
Przyblska., *Acta Cryst.*, **15**, 301 (1962)

GELSEMINE

$C_{20}H_{22}O_2N_2$

M.p. 178°C

The major constituent of *Gelsemium sempervirens*, Ait., this alkaloid crystallizes from Me_2CO with 1 mole of solvent which is lost at 120°C. It has $[\alpha]_D + 15.9°$ ($CHCl_3$) and forms a hydrochloride, m.p. 333°C (*dec.*); $[\alpha]_D + 2.6°$ (H_2O); hydrobromide, m.p. 325°C (*dec.*); nitrate, m.p. 288°C; methobromide, m.p. 313–4°C; methiodide, m.p. variable from 284–301°C (*dec.*); picrate, m.p. 203°C; dibromo-derivative, m.p. 309°C and the benzoyl derivative which forms a crystalline hydrochloride, m.p. 303°C. Several workers have reported the failure of gelsemine to react with Ac_2O to form an acetyl derivative although one has been described with m.p. 111–113°C; $[\alpha]_D^{18} + 26°$ ($CHCl_3$), forming a crystalline hydrochloride, m.p. 290°C.

On boiling with HCl, the base takes up 1 mole of H_2O to form *apo*gelsemine, $C_{20}H_{24}O_3N_2$, an amorphous solid giving a crystalline methiodide, m.p. 295°C (*dec.*); $[\alpha]_D + 12.4°$ (H_2O), and *isoapo*gelsemine which has m.p. 310°C. A third product in which HCl has been added, namely chloro*isoapo*gelsemine, is also formed during this reaction.

Hydrogenation with PtO_2 yields the dihydro derivative which crystallizes from Me_2CO with 1 mole of solvent, m.p. 224–5°C; $[\alpha]_D^{17} + 78.5°$ ($CHCl_3$) forming crystalline salts, e.g. the hydrochloride, m.p. 318–320°C (*dec.*); hydrobromide, m.p. 328–330°C (*dec.*); nitrate, m.p. 285°C (*dec.*) and the methiodide, m.p. 301–2°C (*dec.*). Hydrogenation with the same catalyst in dry

AcOH gives the hexahydro-compound, m.p. 170°C yielding a crystalline methiodide, m.p. 296°C. Distillation with Zn dust yields skatole (3-methylindole) and two basic products, $C_{14}H_{11}N$ (picrate m.p. 218–220°C) and $C_{11}H_{11}N$ (picrate, m.p. 185–7°C).

Pharmacologically, the alkaloid exhibits a strychnine-like action. Raymond-Hamet has recorded that a dosage of 0.2 mgm per kilo of the hydrochloride, given intravenously, produces a prolonged fall in blood pressure in dogs together with increased respiration. A dose of 8 mgm per kilo augments the pressor action of adrenaline and virtually abolishes the apnoea brought about by the latter.

Gerrard., *Pharm. J.*, **13**, 641 (1883)
Spiegel., *Ber.*, **26**, 1045 (1893)
Göldner., *Ber. deut. pharm. Ges.*, **5**, 330 (1895)
Moore., *J. Chem. Soc.*, **99**, 1231 (1911)
Witkop., *J. Amer. Chem. Soc.*, **70**, 1424 (1948)
Kates, Marion., *ibid*, **72**, 2308 (1950)
Prelog *et al., Helv. Chim. Acta,* **34**, 1962 (1951)
Lovell, Pepinsky, Wilson., *Tetrahedron Lett.*, **4**, 1 (1959)
Conroy, Chakrabarti., *ibid*, **4**, 6 (1959)
Teuber, Rosenberger., *Chem. Ber.*, **93**, 3100 (1960)
Roe, Gates., *Tetrahedron,* **11**, 148 (1960)

Pharmacology:
Cushny., *Ber.*, **26**, 1725 (1893)
Cushny., *Arch. exp. Path. Pharm.*, **31**, 49 (1893)
Dale., *J. Chem. Soc.*, **97**, 2223 (1910)
Dale., *ibid*, **99**, 1231 (1911)
Raymond-Hamet., *Compt. rend.*, **205**, 1449 (1937)
Chen., *J. Amer. Pharm. Assoc.*, **32**, 178 (1943)

GELSEMININE

This amorphous alkaloid was reported as being present in the rhizomes of *Gelsemium sempervirens,* Ait. No physical constants nor chemical information has been given and it appears likely that the base is a mixture of alkaloids, or possibly identical with sempervirine (q.v.).

Thompson., *Pharm. J.,* **17**, 803 (1887)

GELSEMOIDINE

This amorphous fraction of the extracts of *Gelsemium sempervirens,* Ait. was isolated by Stevenson and Sayre. A crystalline methiodide was obtained by Forsyth *et al.,* m.p. 296–7°C (*dec.*); $[\alpha]_D + 3.9°$ (H_2O) which, although possessing a different specific rotation, has the same composition and melting point as *apo*gelsemine methiodide (q.v.).

Stevenson, Sayre., *Pharm. J.,* **32**, 242 (1911)
Forsyth, Marrian, Stevens., *J. Chem. Soc.,* 579 (1945)

GELSEVERINE

$C_{21}H_{24-26}O_3N_2$

B.p. 130–150°C/0.0001 mm

Obtained from *Gelsemium sempervirens* Ait., this alkaloid is a colourless oil which forms crystalline derivatives, e.g. the perchlorate, m.p. 250–2°C and the methiodide, m.p. 259–262°C (*dec.*). The structure has not yet been fully elucidated.

Schwartz, Marion., *Can. J. Chem.*, **31**, 958 (1953)
Wenkert, Reid., *Chem. & Ind.*, 1390 (1953)

GENESERINE

$C_{15}H_{21}O_3N_3$

M.p. 128–9°C

First obtained from the seeds of *Physostigma venenosum,* Balf., after previous soaking in NaOH solution with Et_2O, this alkaloid forms orthogonal crystals. It is paevorotatory with $[\alpha]_D - 175°$ (EtOH) or $- 188°$ (dilute H_2SO_4). Being only a weak base, it does not yield crystalline salts with mineral acids but does form a crystalline methiodide, m.p. 215°C; a picrate, m.p. 175°C and a salicylate, m.p. 89–90°C. When heated at 160°C it evolves methylcarbimide and yields geneseroline, $C_{13}H_{18}O_2N_2$, on decomposition with sodium in EtOH. Zn dust and AcOH in EtOH reduce the alkaloid to physostigmine (q.v.), the reverse reaction being brought about by hydrogen peroxide. On these grounds, Polonovski regarded the base as the amine oxide of physostigmine. The structure has, however, been modified recently by Hootele to that given above. The absolute configuration has been deduced by the application of the nuclear Overhauser effect in the NMR spectrum.

The alkaloid is not as potent as eserine (q.v.) in its action on the parasympathetic nervous system.

Polonovski, Nitzberg., *Bull. Soc. Chim. Fr.,* **17**, 244 (1915)
Polonovski, Nitzberg., *ibid,* **19**, 27 (1916)
Polonovski., *ibid,* **21**, 191 (1917)
Hootele., *Tetrahedron Lett.,* 2713 (1969)

Absolute configuration:
Robinson, Moorcroft., *J. Chem. Soc., C,* 2077 (1970)

GENISTEINE

$C_{16}H_{28}N_2$

M.p. 60.5°C;
B.p. 139.5–140.5°C/5 mm

This volatile base occurs in *Cytisus scoparius* L. and is isolated from the mother liquors after the removal of (−)-spartein sulphate. It forms a crystalline hydrate, m.p. 117°C; $[\alpha]_D$ − 52.3° (EtOH) and a picrate, m.p. 215°C.

Valeur., *J. Pharm. Sci.*, **8**, 573 (1913)
Valeur., *Compt. rend.*, **167**, 26 (1918)
Winterfield, Nitzsche., *Arch. Pharm.*, **278**, 393 (1940)

GENTIABETINE

This uncharacterized base has been obtained from *Gentiana asclepiadea*. So far, no salts or derivatives have been reported.

Rulko, Nadler., *Diss. Pharm. Pharmacol.*, **22**, 329 (1970)

GENTIALUTINE

A further uncharacterized alkaloid found in *Gentiana asclepidea*, the structure of which is not known with certainty.

Rulko, Nadler., *Diss. Pharm. Pharmacol.*, **22**, 329 (1970)

GENTIANADINE

$C_8H_7O_2N$

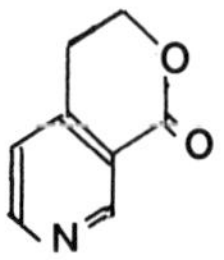

This alkaloid has been found in *Gentiana macrophylla* and *G. olgae*. The structure given above has been confirmed by synthesis.

Liang Xioa-tian, De-quan, Feng-yung., *Sci. Sinica* (Peking), **14**, 869 (1965)

GENTIANAINE

$C_6H_7O_3N$

M.p. 149−150°C

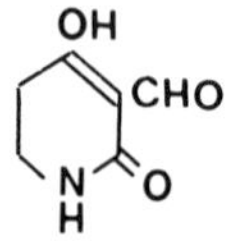

A tetrahydropyridone alkaloid, this base is present in *Gentiana olgae, G. olivieri* and *G. turkestanorum*. The alkaloid is characterized as the 2:4-dinitrophenylhydrazone, m.p. 221−2°C. The structure has been established from spectroscopic data.

Rakhmatullaev, Akramov, Yunusov., *Khim. Pir. Soedin*, **5**, 32 (1969)

GENTIANIDINE

$C_9H_9O_2N$

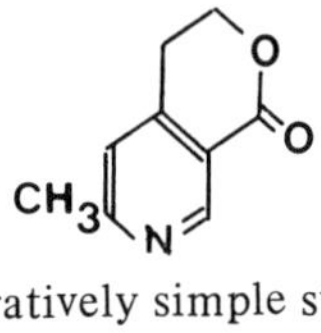

A pyridine alkaloid of comparatively simple structure, this base occurs in

Erythraea centaurum, Gentiana asclepiadea and *Swertia japonica.* The structure has been confirmed by synthesis.

Liang Xioa-tian, De-quan, Feng-yung., *Sci. Sinica* (Peking), 14 (1965)
Inouye, Ueda, Shinokawa., *J. Pharm. Soc., Japan,* **86**, 1202 (1966)
Marekov, Popov., *Tetrahedron,* **24**, 1323 (1968)
Marekov, Popov., *Compt. Rend. Acad. Bulg. Sci.,* **21**, 435 (1966)
Marekov, Arnaudov, Popov., *ibid,* **23**, 81 (1970)
Marekov, Mondeshky, Arnaudov., *ibid,* **23**, 803 (1970)
Rulko, Nadler., *Diss. Pharm. Pharmacol.,* **22**, 329 (1970)

GENTIANINE

$C_{10}H_9O_2N$

M.p. 82–3°C

First obtained from *Gentiana kirilowi*, this alkaloid also occurs in *Anthocleista procera* and *Enicostemma littorale*. The occurrence of the alkaloid in *A. procera* is somewhat doubtful since it has been discovered that this plant contains a precursor of this base and the isolation of gentianine may be spurious when aqueous ammonia is used as the extracting agent.

The alkaloid forms colourless crystals from EtOH and the ultraviolet spectrum has absorption maxima at 218 and 285 mμ with an inflexion at 245 mμ. Several crystalline salts have been prepared, e.g. the hydrochloride, m.p. 171–2°C (*dec.*); hydrobromide, m.p. 178°C; nitrate, m.p. 113°C (*dec.*); picrate, m.p. 123–4°C; oxalate, m.p. 156°C; methiodide, m.p. 193°C and the (+)-tartrate, m.p. 138°C. Catalytic hydrogenation yields the dihydro derivative, m.p. 75–6°C and forming a crystalline picrate, m.p. 140–2°C. Oxidation with $KMnO_4$ in Me_2CO furnishes an acid, $C_9H_7O_4N$, m.p. 260–2°C (*dec.*) which gives pyridine-3:4:5-tricarboxylic acid on further oxidation with alkaline $KMnO_4$. When warmed with aqueous NaOH, the alkaloid forms sodium gentianate, m.p. 132–4°C, being converted back into the alkaloid on acidification. Distillation with Zn dust yields pyridine. The structure has been established as 4-2'-hydroxyethyl-5-vinylnicotinic lactone.

Proskurnina., *J. Gen. Chem., USSR,* **14**, 1148 (1944)
Proskurnina, Shpanov., *ibid,* **26**, 936 (1956)
Govindachari, Nagarajan, Rajappa., *J. Chem. Soc.,* **551**, 2725 (1957)
Plat *et al., Bull. Soc. Chim.,* 1302 (1963)
Lavie, Taylor-Smith., *Chem. & Ind.,* 781 (1963)

GENTIATIBETINE

M.p. 161°C

An alkaloid isolated from the dried leaves of *Menyanthes trifoliata* L., the base is prepared from the total alkaloidal extract by thin-layer, preparative-layer and column chromatography.

Rulko., *Rocz. Chem.,* **43**, 1831 (1969)

GENTIOCRUCINE

$C_6H_7O_3N$

M.p. 139–140°C

This simple base from *Gentiana cruciana* has been identified by NMR, mass spectrometry and chemical methods as 4-carbamoyl-2:3-dihydro-6*H*-pyran-6-one.

Popov, Marekov., *Chem. Ind.*, 2, 49 (1969)
Marekov, Popov., *Izv. Otd. Khim. Nauki, Bulg. Akad. Nauk.*, 2, 575 (1970)

GENTIOFLAVINE

$C_{10}H_{11}O_3N$

M.p. 218–220°C (*dec.*).

This alkaloid is found in several species of *Gentiana* and crystallizes from $CHCl_3$ as pale yellow prisms. It is freely soluble in H_2O, pyridine and EtOH, only sparingly so in $CHCl_3$ and insoluble in hexane or C_6H_6. It contains an aldehydic group, an imino group and a six-membered lactone ring. The semicarbazone has m.p. 221–3°C (*dec.*) and the oxime, m.p. 203–5°C (*dec.*). The structure, that of a dihydropyridine lactonic alkaloid has been established on the basis of infrared and NMR spectral evidence and chemical conversion into gentianidine (q.v.).

Mollov *et al.*, *Compt. rend. Acad. bulg. Sci.*, 18, 947 (1965)
Structure:
Marekov, Popov., *Tetrahedron*, 24, 1323 (1968)

GEOFFROYINE (*Surinamine*)

$C_9H_{11}O_3N$

This base has been isolated from several species, including *Andira inermis, A. retusa, Ferreira spectabilis, Geoffroea surinamensis* and *Krameria triandra*. It is described in the literature under several names, e.g. angeline, andirine, surinamine and rhatinine. The structure has been established as N-methyltyrosine (β-*p*-hydroxylphenyl-α-methyl-aminopropionic acid).

Hiller-Bombien., *Arch. Pharm.*, 230, 513 (1892)
Blau., *Zeit. Physiol. Chem.*, 58, 153 (1908)
Friedmann, Guthmann., *Biochem. Zeit.*, 27, 491 (1910)
Johnson, Nicolet., *Amer. Chem. J.*, 47, 459 (1912)
Goldschmeidt., *Monatsh.*, 33, 1379 (1912)
Goldschmeidt., *ibid,* 34, 659 (1913)

Synthesis:
Kanevskaja., *J. pr. Chem.*, 124, 48 (1929)
Deulofue, Mendwelzua., *Ber.*, 68, 783 (1935)

GERALBINE

$C_{22}H_{33}O_2N$

M.p. 221–3°C

A steroidal alkaloid isolated from *Veratrum album,* the base forms colourless plates when crystallized from Et_2O-AcOEt or as prisms from aqueous Me_2CO. It may be characterized as the crystalline hydrochloride, colourless needles, m.p. 270°C. The alkaloid gives a deep yellow colour with concentrated H_2SO_4.

Stoll, Seebeck., *J. Amer. Chem. Soc.,* 74, 4728 (1952)

GERMANITRINE

$C_{39}H_{59}O_{11}N$

M.p. 228–9°C

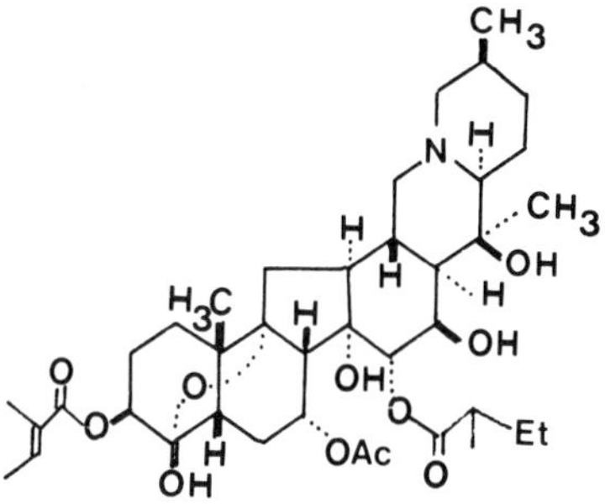

A further *Veratrum* alkaloid, this hypotensive base is found in *V. fimbriatum* and forms colourless crystals from aqueous Me_2CO. It is laevorotatory in pyridine with $[\alpha]_D^{24} - 61°$ (c 1.0, pyridine) but optically inactive in $CHCl_3$. The crystalline picrate forms colourless plates from aqueous Me_2CO, m.p. 240–1°C (*dec.*). The structure has been established on the basis of spectroscopic evidence and chemical degradation as germine-3-angelate-7-acetate-15-[(−)-2-methyl-butyrate]. When hydrolyzed by heating with NaOH it furnishes germine, AcOH, tiglic acid and (−)-α-methylbutyric acid. With MeOH it forms germanidine.

Klohs *et al., J. Amer. Chem. Soc.,* 74, 4473 (1952)
Klohs *et al., ibid,* 75, 4925 (1953)
Kupchan, Afonso., *J. Amer. Pharm. Assoc., Sci.,* 48, 731 (1959)

GERMBUDINE

$C_{37}H_{59}O_{12}N$

M.p. 160–4°C

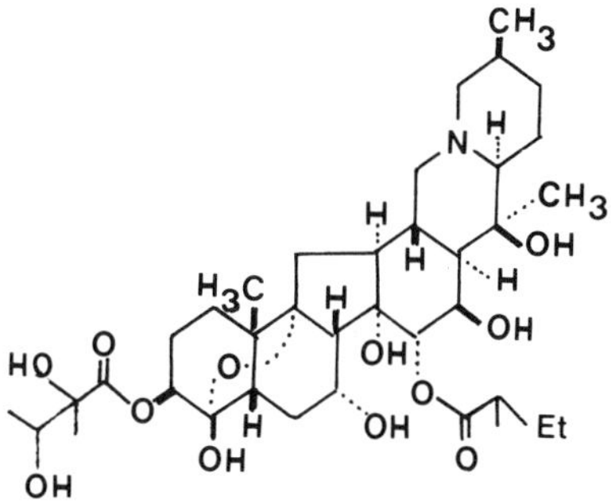

This hypotensive alkaloid occurs in *Veratrum viride.* It is best crystallized from

C_6H_6 when it is obtained as colourless prisms. It has $[\alpha]_D^{24} - 7°$ (c 1.0, pyridine). It contains eight hydroxyl groups, three methyl groups and two methylbutyrate groups in the molecule. Alkaline hydrolysis yields germine, α-methylbutyric acid and $\alpha\beta$-dihydroxy-α-methylbutyric acid.

Myers *et al., J. Amer. Chem. Soc.*, **74**, 3198 (1952)
Myers *et al., ibid*, **77**, 3348 (1955)
Kupchan, Gruenfeld., *J. Amer. Pharm. Assoc., Sci.*, **48**, 737 (1959)

GERMERINE

$C_{37}H_{59}O_{11}N$

M.p. 193–5°C

This alkaloid was first isolated from *Veratrum album* by Poetke who assigned to it the empirical formula $C_{36}H_{57}O_{11}N$ which was modified to that given above following the new formula given for germine by Craig and Jacobs. It crystallizes well from C_6H_6 but is extremely hygroscopic in the anhydrous form. It has $[\alpha]_D^{20} - 14.2°$ (c 1.0, pyridine) or $+ 10.8°$ (c 1.0, $CHCl_3$). The alkaloid is only sparingly soluble in Et_2O, moderately so in Me_2CO, EtOH or AcOEt and dissolves readily in $CHCl_3$ or MeOH. With strong H_2SO_4 it initially gives a colourless solution that changes to a carmine red on warming or even on standing. Fröhde's reagent slowly produces a red-violet colour, differentiating it from protoveratridine which is instantly coloured a deep violet by this reagent.

The following crystalline salts have been prepared: the hydrochloride, dihydrate, m.p. 215°C; hydrobromide dihydrate, m.p. 212–3°C, thiocyanate, m.p. 221–3°C (*dec.*) and the monopicrate (monohydrate), m.p. 186–7°C (*dec.*). Alkaline hydrolysis furnishes germine, *l*-methylethylacetic acid and methylethylglycollic acid. When allowed to stand in $Ba(OH)_2$ solution it is converted into protoveratridine, with the elimination of 1 molecule of methylethylglycollic acid.

Poethke., *Arch. Pharm.*, **275**, 571 (1937)
Myers *et al., J. Amer. Chem. Soc.*, **74**, 3198 (1952)
Kupchan., *ibid*, **81**, 1921 (1959)

GERMIDINE

$C_{34}H_{53}O_{10}N$

M.p. 202-3°C

and 242-4°C

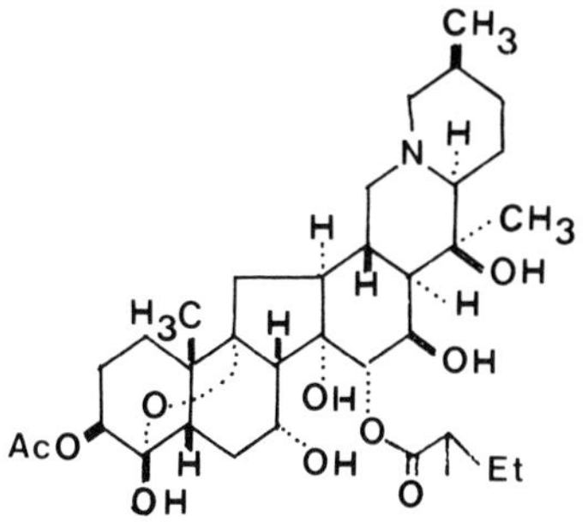

Present in *Veratrum viride,* this alkaloid exists in two crystalline forms when purified from aqueous MeOH having the melting points given above. In CHCl₃ it has $[\alpha]_D^{25} + 13°$ while in pyridine it is − 11°. The O-acetate has been prepared as colourless crystals, m.p. 248−9°C. From the nature of the alkaline hydrolysis products, viz. germine, acetic acid and (−)-2-methylbutyric acid, the structure is established as germine-3-acetate-15 (−)-2-methylbutyrate. Pharmacologically, the alkaloid acts as a depressant of blood pressure.

Fried, White, Wintersteiner., *J. Amer. Chem. Soc.,* 71, 3260 (1949)
Weisenborn, Bolger., *ibid,* 76, 5543 (1954)
Kupchan, Narayanan., *Chem. & Ind.,* 1092 (1956)
Kupchan, Narayanan., *J. Amer. Chem. Soc.,* 81, 1921 (1959)

GERMINALINE

$C_{39}H_{61}O_{12}N$

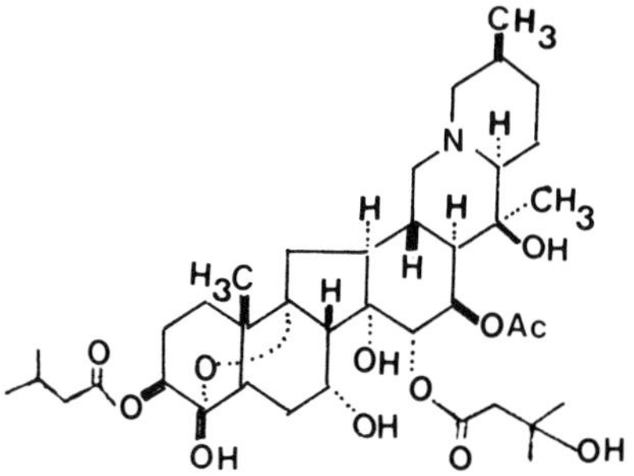

This alkaloid has recently been discovered in *Veratrum lobelianum.* Like all of these bases, it contains the basic germine structure and is germine 3-(2-methyl-butyrate)-15-[-(2-hydroxy-2-methylbutyrate)]-16-acetate.

Samikov, Shakirov, Yunusov., *Khim. Prir. Soedin.,* 7, 790 (1971)

GERMINE

$C_{27}H_{43}O_8N$

M.p. 220°C

This very potent hypotensive alkaloid is formed by the hydrolysis of all of the foregoing *Veratrum* alkaloids and protoveratridine (q.v.) and is also found naturally in *Veratrum album, V. viride* Ait and certain species of *Zygadenus*. It is obtained as colourless crystals from MeOH which contain 2 moles of solvent. On heating, the crystals effervesce at 163–173°C and finally melt at 220°C. The alkaloid has $[\alpha]_D^{25} + 5°$ (95% EtOH) or $+ 21.1°$ (dilute AcOH). The aurichloride forms golden-yellow leaflets; the picrate sinters at 175°C and finally decomposes at 205°C. The amino oxide has been prepared as colourless needles, m.p. 249°C (*dec.*) while the monoacetate has m.p. 219–221°C; $[\alpha]_D^{23} + 10°$ (EtOH). A tetraacetate, m.p. 260–1°C; $[\alpha]_D^{23} - 98°$ (pyridine) and a pentaacetate, m.p. 257.5–258.5°C; $[\alpha]_D^{24} - 88.8°$ (pyridine) have also been obtained. In the presence of HCl, the alkaloid combines with Me₂CO to yield acetonylgermine hydrochloride, m.p. 275°C (*dec.*) after forming a resin above 255°C. The free acetonylgermine may be obtained from this salt, m.p. 235–9°C. Germine cannot be hydrogenated but with sodium in boiling BuOH it gives the dihydro derivatine which resinifies above 258°C and melts at 265°C. This derivative still contains the eight replaceable hydrogens of the original alkaloid and forms a crystalline hydrochloride, m.p. > 265°C (*dec.*).

NaOH in aqueous MeOH furnishes a base, *iso*germine which crystallizes from MeOH without solvent and has m.p. 260°C; $[\alpha]_D^{?} - 46.5°$ (EtOH). In the presence of PtO₂, this base forms the dihydro derivative, m.p. 277–8°C (*dec.*); $[\alpha]_D^{28} - 61°$ (pyridine).

Selenium dehydrogenation of germine yields 5-methyl-2-ethylpyridine, cevanthrol and cevanthridine.

Germine, in common with other *Veratrum* alkaloids, has a characteristic effect upon the heart which includes a moderate change in sinus rate, a positive inotropic action, the production of irregularities and prolongation of the beat. It also renders certain tissues responsive to brief stimuli in a characteristically prolonged manner. Instead of a single all-or-none impulse, these tissues show a repetitive response, long outlasting the initial stimulus, and similar in some respects to the after discharge observed in certain reflex systems.

Although alkaloidal extracts of *Veratrum viride* have long been employed as insecticides, particularly against the American cockroach, *Periplaneta americana,* germine itself is only moderately toxic in this respect and the most potent agent appears to be germerine (q.v.).

Poethke., *Arch. Pharm.*, **275**, 571 (1937)
Craig, Jacobs., *J. Biol. Chem.*, **148**, 57 (1943)
Craig, Jacobs., *ibid*, **149**, 451 (1943)

Heubner, Jacobs., *ibid,* **170**, 181 (1947)

Jacobs, Sato., *ibid,* **175**, 57 (1947)

Klohs *et al., J. Amer. Chem. Soc.,* **75**, 4925 (1953)

Weisenbirn, Bolger., *ibid,* **76**, 5543 (1954)

Pharmacology:

Sieferle, Johns, Richardson., *J. Econ. Entom.,* **35**, 35 (1942)

Krayer, Acheson., *Physiological Review,* **26**, 383 (1946)

Jagues., *Rev. Can. biol.,* **5**, 246 (1946)

GERMINITRINE

$C_{39}H_{57}O_{11}N$

M.p. 175°C

A further hypotensive alkaloid present in *Veratrum fimbriatum,* this base crystallizes from aqueous Me_2CO as colourless prisms. It has $[\alpha]_D^{24} + 7.8°$ (c 1.35, $CHCl_3$) or $- 36°$ (c 1.12, pyridine). It forms a crystalline picrate as yellow plates, m.p. 238°C (*dec.*). Alkaline hydrolysis furnishes germine, acetic acid, tiglic acid and angelic acid.

Klohs *et al., J. Amer. Chem. Soc.,* **74**, 4473 (1952)

Klohs *et al., ibid,* **75**, 4925 (1953)

GERMITETRINE

$C_{41}H_{63}O_{14}N$

M.p. 229–230°C

This, and the following alkaloid, occur as minor constituents in *Veratrum album.* Germitetrine is laevorotatory with $[\alpha]_D^{25} - 12°$ (c 1.0, $CHCl_3$) or $- 74°$ (c 1.0, pyridine). Alkaline hydrolysis yields germine, acetic acid, 2-methylbutyric acid and 2:3-dihydroxy-2-methylbutyric acid. The structure is germine 3-[(2-hydroxy-2-methyl-3-acetylbutyrate)]-7-acetyl-15-[(2-methylbutyrate)].

Glen *et al., Nature,* **170**, 932 (1952)

Nash, Brooker., *J. Amer. Chem. Soc.,* **75**, 1942 (1953)

Kupchan, Deliwala., *ibid,* **75**, 4671 (1953)

Myers *et al., ibid,* **78**, 1621 (1956)

Kupchan, Ayres., *Chem. & Ind.,* 1594 (1958)

Morgan, Barltrop., *Quart. Rev.,* **12**, 34 (1958)

GERMITETRINE B

$C_{42}H_{63}O_{14}N$

M.p. 233–4°C

A minor component of *Veratrum album*, this alkaloid crystallizes from aqueous Me_2CO or butyl chloride as colourless crystals. It is laevorotatory having $[\alpha]_D^{25} - 17°$ (c 1.0, $CHCl_3$) or $- 70°$ (c 1.0, pyridine). Alkaline hydrolysis yields the same products as germitetrine, viz. germine, acetic acid, 2-methylbutyric acid and 2:3-dihydroxy-2-methylbutyric acid. If it is not identical with the previous base, and the physical constants are all very similar, it must be closely related to it.

Nash, Brooker., *J. Amer. Chem. Soc.*, **75**, 1942 (1953)
Kupchan, Deliwala., *ibid*, **75**, 4671 (1953)

GERMITRINE

$C_{42}H_{67}O_{22}N$

M.p. 197–9°C

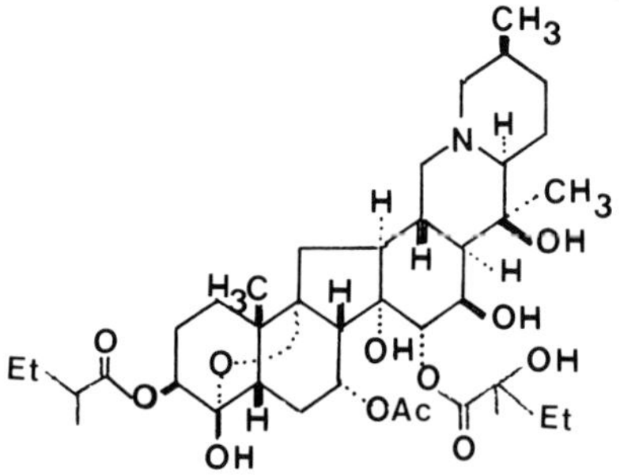

Found in *Veratrum viride*, this alkaloid forms colourless crystals from aqueous EtOH and has $[\alpha]_D^{25} + 11°$ (c 1.0, $CHCl_3$). On alkaline hydrolysis it gives germine, (−)-2-methylbutyric acid and (+)-2-hydroxy-2-methylbutyric acid. Pharmacologically, it acts by lowering the blood pressure.

Fried, White, Wintersteiner., *J. Amer. Chem. Soc.*, **71**, 3260 (1949)
Kupchan., *ibid*, **81**, 1921 (1959)

GERRARDINE

$C_{11}H_{19}O_2NS_4$

M.p. 180°C

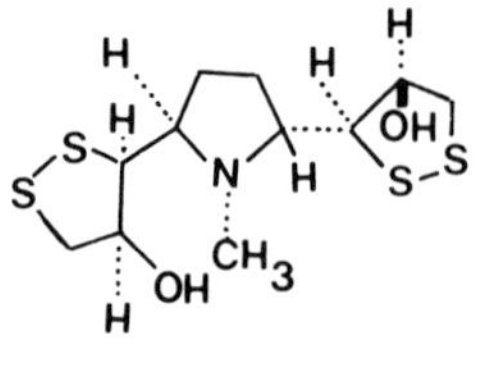

A sulphur-containing alkaloid occurring in *Cassipourea gerrardii* Alston., this base is obtained as yellow orthorhombic crystals which have the above melting point in the anhydrous form. It normally crystallizes with solvent, e.g. as an unstable compound from C_6H_6 with 1 mole of solvent and similarly from EtOH when it exists as two forms with m.p. 90°C and 178°C respectively. The hydrochloride crystallizes from H_2O as triangular plates which sublime at 197°C and then melt at 207°C with decomposition. This salt is laevorotatory with $[\alpha]_D^{23}$ − 172° (c 1.0, H_2O). The alkaloid also forms a sulphite as a dense white precipitate. The four sulphur atoms have been shown to be present in two dithiolane rings linked in the 2:5 positions to a pyrrolidine ring.

Wright, Warren., *J. Chem. Soc., C,* 283, 284 (1967)

GERRARDOLINE

$C_8H_{15}O_2NS_2$

This alkaloid is a minor constituent of *Cassipourea gerrardii*. The structure has been determined by chemical and spectroscopic techniques.

Wright, Warren., *J. Chem. Soc., C,* 283 (1967)

GIGANTINE

$C_{13}H_{19}O_3N$

M.p. 151–2°C

An *isoquinoline* alkaloid found in *Carnegia gigantea* (Engelm.), this dextrorotatory base has $[\alpha]_D^{25}$ + 27.1° (c 2.0, $CHCl_3$). Two methoxyl groups, a methyl group, a hydroxyl and a methylimino group are present. The hydroxyl group was originally placed at C-4 but has now been changed to C-5 in the benzene ring of the molecule. This revised structure has recently been confirmed by synthesis of the alkaloid.

Hodgkins, Brown, Massingill., *Tetrahedron Lett.,* 1322 (1967)

Revised structure:
Kapadia *et al., Chem. Commun.,* 856 (1970)

Synthesis:
Kapadia *et al., Chem. Ind.,* 1593 (1970)

GINDARICINE

$C_{18}H_{19}O_3N$

M.p. 193°C (*dec.*).

Chaudry and Siddiqui have isolated this alkaloid from the tubers of *Stephania glabra*. It is best crystallized from C_6H_6 when it forms colourless prisms. It yields well crystallized salts, e.g. the hydrochloride, m.p. 232°C; platinichloride, m.p. 230°C (*dec.*) and the picrate as yellow needles, m.p. 150°C (*dec.*).

Chaudry, Siddiqui., *J. Sci. Ind. Res.,* (India), **9B**, 79 (1950)

GINDARINE

$C_{21}H_{25}O_4N$

M.p. 147°C

A further alkaloid isolated from the tubers of *Stephania glabra,* the base yields a series of crystalline salts and derivative, e.g. the hydrochloride, m.p. 245°C (*dec.*); hydrobromide, m.p. 240°C (*dec.*); hydriodide, m.p. 228°C (*dec.*); nitrate, m.p. 222°C (*dec.*); sulphate, m.p. 218°C (*dec.*); platinichloride, m.p. 212°C (*dec.*); picrate, m.p. 188°C (*dec.*) and the methiodide, m.p. 248–9°C (*dec.*).

Chaudry, Siddiqui., *J. Sci. Ind. Res.,* (India), **9B**, 79 (1950)

GINDARININE

$C_{21}H_{21}O_4N$

This alkaloid is found in the tubers of *Stephania glabra* as the nitrate, m.p. 248°C (*dec.*). It yields a hydrochloride, m.p. 215°C (*dec.*); hydriodide, m.p. 245°C (*dec.*); platinichloride, m.p. 276°C (*dec.*) and a picrate, m.p. 200°C (*dec.*).

Chaudry, Siddiqui., *J. Sci. Ind. Res.,* (India), **9B**, 79 (1950)

GIRGENSONINE

$C_{13}H_{16}ON_2$

M.p. 147–8°C

This alkaloid occurs with N-methylpiperidine in *Girgensohnia oppositiflora* Pall. It is optically inactive and forms a crystalline hydrochloride, m.p. 145–8°C and a picrolonate, m.p. 192–4°C. On hydrolysis with alkali it furnishes piperidine, hydrocyanic acid and *p*-hydroxybenzaldehyde suggesting that its structure is N-piperidyl-*p*-hydroxyphenylacetonitrile. This has been confirmed by mixed melting point determination with an authentic specimen.

Juraschevski, Stepanova., *J. Gen. Chem., USSR,* **16**, 141 (1946)

GIRIMBINE

$C_{18}H_{17}ON$

M.p. 173–6°C

A carbazole alkaloid present in the leaves and roots of *Murraya koenigii* Spreng., this base forms colourless prisms when crystallized from $CHCl_3$-hexane. The ultraviolet spectrum has been recorded in EtOH solution and has absorption maxima at 222, 237, 278, 287, 314, 328, 342 and 358 mμ. The structure has been confirmed by several independent syntheses.

634

Chakraborty, Barman, Bose., *Sci. Cult.*, (Calcutta), **30**, 445 (1964)
Chakraborty., *J. Ind. Chem. Soc.*, **46**, 177 (1969)
Dutta, Quasim., *Ind. J. Chem.*, **7**, 307 (1969)
Joshi, Kamat, Gawad., *Tetrahedron*, **26**, 1475 (1970)
Synthesis:
Kureal, Kapil, Popli., *Chem. Ind.*, 1262 (1970)
Narasimhan, Paradkar, Gokhale., *Tetrahedron Lett.*, 1665 (1970)
Chakraborty, Islam., *J. Ind. Chem. Soc.*, **48**, 91 (1971)

GLAUCAMINE

$C_{21}H_{23}O_6N$

M.p. 222–3°C

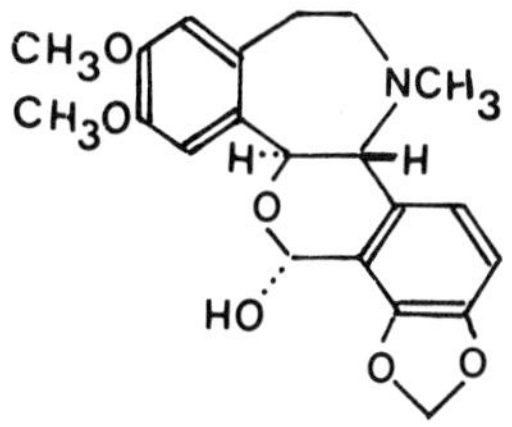

This alkaloid occurs in *Papaver glaucum* Boiss. et Hauskn. It forms colourless crystals from EtOH and is strongly dextrorotatory with $[\alpha]_D^{22} + 298°$ (c 0.25, $CHCl_3$). The ultraviolet spectrum in EtOH shows absorption maxima at 238 and 286 mμ. With mineral acids, it forms a series of crystalline salts including the hydrochloride, m.p. 201–3°C; hydriodide, m.p. 203–5°C and the oxalate, m.p. 160°C. Two methoxyl groups, one hydroxyl, a methylenedioxy and a methylimino group are present. The O-methyl ether is identical with Glaudine (q.v.).

Pfeifer., *Pharmazie*, **19**, 724 (1964)
Slavik *et al.*, *Collect. Czech. Chem. Commun.*, **30**, 2864 (1965)
Cross, Slavik., *ibid*, **31**, 1425 (1966)
Dolejs, Hanus., *Tetrahedron*, **23**, 2997 (1967)

Stereochemistry:
Shamma *et al.*, *Chem. Commun.*, 212 (1968)

epi-GLAUCAMINE

$C_{21}H_{23}O_6N$

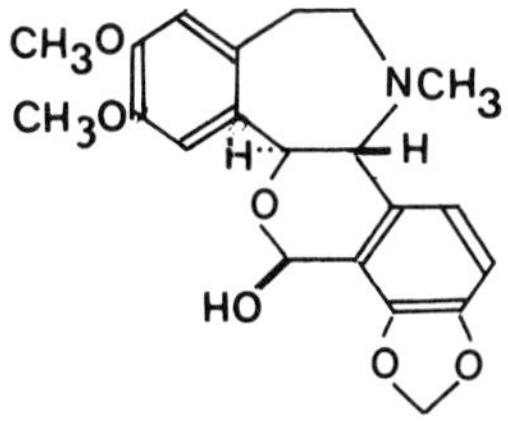

This epimer of the preceding alkaloid also occurs in *Papaver glaucum*. It is dextrorotatory with $[\alpha]_D^{22} + 126° \pm 3°$ ($CHCl_3$).

Slavik, Appelt., *Collect. Czech. Chem. Commun.*, **30**, 3687 (1965)

GLAUCENTRINE

$C_{20}H_{23}O_4N$

M.p. 148°C

An aporphine alkaloid occurring in *Dicentra eximia* (Ker) Torr., *D. formosa* Walp. and *D. oregana* Eastwood. The base forms crystalline salts such as the hydrochloride, m.p. 236−7°C and the hydrobromide, m.p. 239°C. The methiodide, m.p. 225°C, has also been prepared and the ethyl ether (−)-tartrate, m.p. 189°C. Treatment with CH_2N_2 yields (+)-glaucine indicating that the alkaloid is O-demethylglaucine. The solution in cold H_2SO_4 is colourless but becomes a greenish-blue and finally a deep mauve on heating.

Manske., *Can. J. Res.*, **8**, 592 (1933)

Manske., *ibid*, **10**, 521, 765 (1934)

Manske., *ibid*, **16B**, 81 (1938)

Manske, Charlesworth, Ashford., *J. Amer. Chem. Soc.*, **73**, 3751 (1951)

GLAUCINE

$C_{21}H_{25}O_4N$

M.p. 119−120°C

This aporphine alkaloid is wide-spread among the species of the natural order Rhoedales, occurring in *Corydalis ternata* Nakai, *C. tuberosa* DC., *Dicentra eximia* (Ker) Torr., *D. formosa* Walp., *D. oregana* Eastwood, *Glaucium flavum* Crantz and *G. serpieri* Heldr. The base was first obtained by Probst but obtained in the pure form many years later by Fischer. The natural alkaloid is the (+)-form with $[\alpha]_D + 115.4°$ (aqueous EtOH). It is readily soluble in EtOH, $CHCl_3$ or MeOH, sparingly so in C_6H_6 or hot H_2O and insoluble in cold H_2O or petroleum ether. The hydrochloride forms colourless crystals, m.p. 243−6°C (*dec.*) and the hydrobromide, pale pink crystals, m.p. 235°C.

Although the alkaloid is tasteless, the salts are intensely bitter. The solution in H_2SO_4 is colourless becoming bright blue or violet on standing or warming. Fröhde's reagent yields a green colour changing to blue while HNO_3 yields a transient green tint.

The (−)-form of the alkaloid, obtained from (±)-glaucine on recrystallization of the *l*-hydrogen tartrates has m.p. 124−5°C and $[\alpha]_D - 115.4°$ (aqueous EtOH). It forms a hydrochloride trihydrate, m.p. 243−5°C; hydrobromide, m.p. 241°C (*dec.*); $[\alpha]_D^{17} - 98.04°$ (H_2O); methiodide, m.p. 224−5°C; $[\alpha]_D^{17} - 72.46°$; (+)-hydrogen tartrate, m.p. 216−7°C; $[\alpha]_D^{18} - 44.12°$ and the (−)-hydrogen tartrate, m.p. 165°C. The (±)-form of the base has m.p. 137−9°C.

Glaucine brings about slight narcosis in animals which is interrupted by epileptiform convulsions. It also acts as a depressant of the heart and blood vessels and can damage striated muscle.

Probst., *Annalen*, **31**, 241 (1839)
Fischer., *Arch. Pharm.*, **239**, 426 (1901)
Gadamer., *Chem. Zentr.*, **I**, 151 (1912)
Gorter., *ibid*, **III**, 345 (1921)
Girardet., *J. Chem. Soc.*, 2630 (1931)
Faltis, Adler., *Arch. Pharm.*, **284**, 281 (1951)
Corrodi, Hardegger., *Helv. Chim. Acta*, **39**, 889 (1956)

GLAUDINE

$C_{22}H_{25}O_6N$

M.p. $103-5°C$

Isolated from *Papaver glaucum* Boiss et Hauskn. this alkaloid forms colourless crystals from EtOH and is strongly dextrorotatory with $[\alpha]_D + 455°$ (c 0.5, $CHCl_3$). The ultraviolet spectrum has two absorption maxima at 237 and 287 $m\mu$. Several crystalline salts and derivatives have been prepared, e.g. the hydrochloride, m.p. $185-7°C$; hydriodide, m.p. $180-2°C$; perchlorate, m.p. $178-181°C$; oxalate, m.p. $152°C$ and the methiodide, m.p. $173-4°C$. The alkaloid contains three methoxyl groups, one methylenedioxy and one methylimino group. Alkaline hydrolysis yields Glaucamine (q.v.). The structure has been determined from spectroscopic evidence and comparison with glaucamine.

Pfeifer., *Pharmazie*, **19**, 724 (1964)
Cross, Mann, Pfeifer., *ibid*, **21**, 181 (1966)
Pfeifer, Mann., *ibid*, **20**, 643 (1965)
Dolejs, Hanus., *Tetrahedron*, **23**, 2997 (1967)

Stereochemistry:
Shamma *et al.*, *Chem. Commun.*, 212 (1968)

GLAZIOVINE

$C_{18}H_{19}O_3N$

M.p. $235-7°C$ (*dec.*).

A spiroisoquinoline alkaloid present in *Ocotea glaziovii*, the base is obtained in the form of colourless needles from EtOH and has $[\alpha]_D + 7°$ (c 1.0, $CHCl_3$). It

contains one hydroxyl group, a methoxyl and a methylimino group and forms
a crystalline picrate, m.p. 199–203°C.

Gilbert *et al., J. Amer. Chem. Soc.,* **86**, 694 (1964)
Haynes *et al., Proc. Chem. Soc.,* 261 (1964)

GLOCHIDICINE

$C_{15}H_{25}ON_3$

M.p. 103–5°C

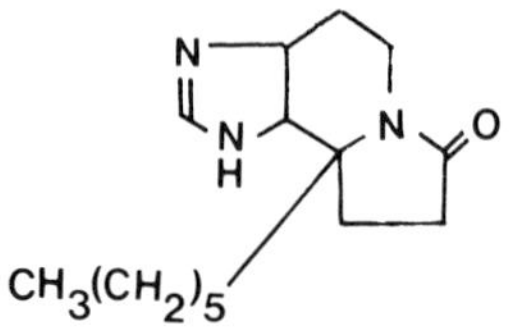

$CH_3(CH_2)_5$

Two isomeric alkaloids have been obtained from the leaves of a species of
Glochidon which has been tentatively identified as *G. philippicum* (Cav.) C.B.
Rob. This alkaloid forms colourless crystals from Me_2CO which contain 0.5 mole
of solvent. The base is optically inactive.

Johns, Lamberton., *Austral. J. Chem.,* **20**, 555 (1967)

GLOCHIDINE

$C_{15}H_{23}ON_3$

M.p. 65–7°C

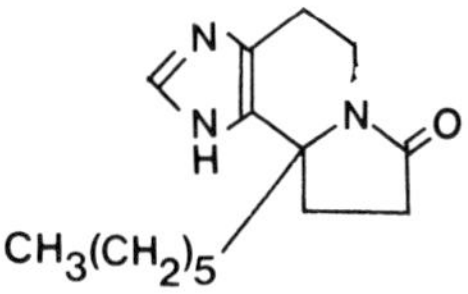

$CH_3(CH_2)_5$

Also present in the leaves of *Glochidion philippicum* (Cav.) C.B. Rob., this
isomer of glochidicine crystallizes from Me_2CO with 0.5 mole of solvent. Like
the preceding base it is optically inactive.

Johns, Lamberton., *Chem. Commun.,* 312 (1966)
Johns, Lamberton., *Austral. J. Chem.,* **20**, 555 (1967)

GLOMERINE

$C_{10}H_{10}ON_2$

M.p. 208°C

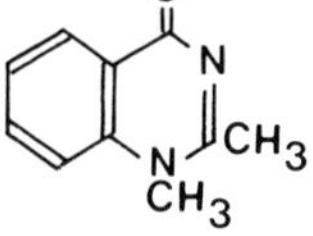

A quinazolone alkaloid obtained from the arthropod *Glomeris marginata.*
Glomerine crystallizes in colourless needles from either H_2O or AcOEt. In
neutral solution (EtOH), the ultraviolet spectrum has absorption maxima at 215,
228, 266, 275, 304 and 312 mμ. In acid solution (1.0 N/HCl), the absorption
maxima occur at 235, 270, 293 and 303 mμ. The structure, as 1:2-dimethyl-4-
quinazolone, has been confirmed by synthesis.

638

Schildknecht *et al.*, *Zeit. Naturforsch.*, **21B**, 121 (1966)

Schildknecht, Wenneis., *ibid*, **21B**, 552 (1966)

Synthesis:

Weddige., *J. prakt. Chem.*, **36**, 154 (1887)

Chakravarti *et al.*, *Tetrahedron*, **16**, 224 (1961)

Biosynthesis:

Schildknecht, Wenneis., *Tetrahedron Lett.*, 1815 (1967)

GLORIOSINE

$C_{22}H_{25}O_6N$

M.p. 248–250°C

An alkaloid found in the tubers of *Gloriosa superba*, this base is laevorotatory with $[\alpha]_D^{34}$ − 200.5° (c 1.172, $CHCl_3$). On demthylation it gives Colchiceine (q.v.).

Subbaratnam., *J. Sci. Ind. Res.*, (India), **11B**, 446 (1952)

10-β-D-GLUCOSYLOXYVINCOSIDE LACTAM

$C_{32}H_{40}O_{12}N$

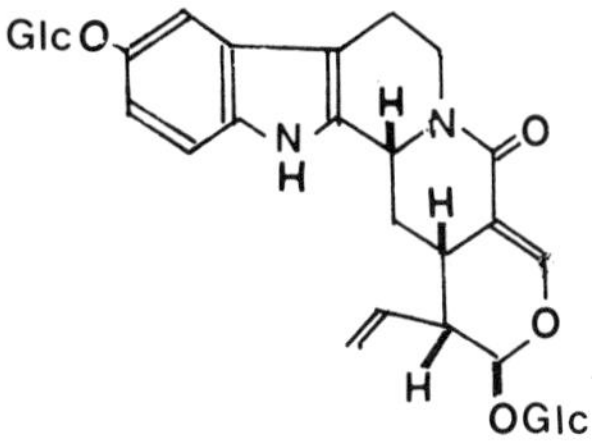

Recently discovered in the roots of *Adina rubescens*, this glucoalkaloid has been characterized as the octaacetate which has $[\alpha]_D^{24}$ − 85.8°.

Brown, Blackstock., *Tetrahedron Lett.*, 3063 (1972)

GLYCORINE

$C_9H_8O_2N$

M.p. 145–7°C

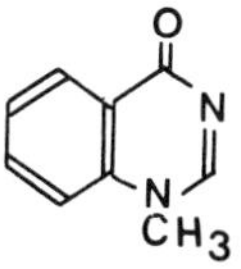

An alkaloid found in the leaves of *Glycosmis arborea* (Roxb.). DC. The base gives an ultraviolet spectrum with absorption maxima at 269, 278, 306 and 317 mμ. It yields a crystalline hydrochloride, m.p. 242°C (*dec.*) and a picrate, m.p. 249°C (*dec.*). The alkaloid has been shown to possess the structure of 1-methyl-4-quinazolone.

Pakrashi *et al.*, *Tetrahedron*, **19**, 1011 (1963)

GLYCOSINE

$C_{15}H_{12}ON_2$

M.p. 155–6°C

This base occurs in *Glycosmis pentaphylla* and crystallizes as the solvate from EtOH, AcOEt, C_6H_6 and $CHCl_3$, retaining all but EtOH after treatment at 140°C *in vacuo* for 8 to 10 hours. It is a monoacidic base and gives a hydro- ʹ chloride, m.p. 209–210°C (*dec.*); platinichloride, m.p. 175–7°C (*dec.*) and the picrate, m.p. 171–2°C (*dec.*). The ultraviolet spectrum has absorption maxima at 231, 268, 277 and 306 mμ.

Chatterjee, Majumder., *Sci. Cult.* (Calcutta), **18**, 505, 604 (1953)

GLYCOSMICINE

$C_9H_8O_2N_2$

M.p. 270–1°C

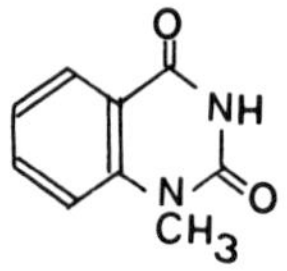

This simple quinazolone alkaloid has been isolated from the leaves of *Glycosmis arborea* (Roxb.) DC. It gives an ultraviolet spectrum with absorption maxima at 219, 244 and 311 mμ. The structure has been shown to be 1:2-dihydro-1-methyl-2-oxo-4-quinazolone.

Pakrashi *et al., Tetrahedron*, **19**, 1011 (1963)

GLYCOSMININE (*Glycosmine*)

$C_{15}H_{12}ON_2$

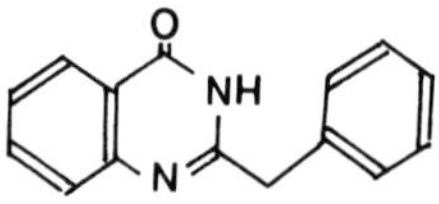

This alkaloid is a minor constituent of *Glycosmis arborea*. The structure has been established, from spectroscopic data, as 2-benzyl-4-quinazolone.

Pakrashi *et al., Tetrahedron*, **19**, 1011 (1963)

GLYCOZOLIDINE

$C_{15}H_{15}O_3N$

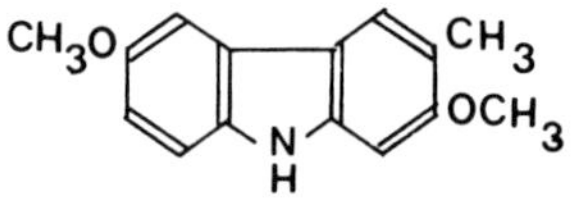

A carbazole alkaloid present in *Glycosmis pentaphylla* D.C., the structure of the base has been shown from spectroscopic measurements to be 2:6-dimethoxy-3-methylcarbazole.

Kureel, Kapil, Popli., *Chem. Ind.*, 1262 (1970)
Islam, Bhattacharyya, Chakraborty., *Chem. Commun.*, 537 (1972)

GLYCOZOLINE

$C_{14}H_{13}ON$

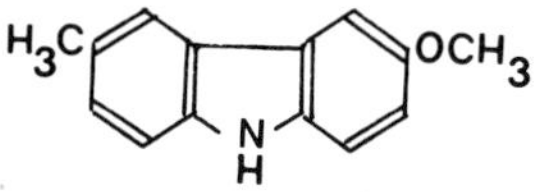

M.p. 182–2°C

A further constituent of the roots of *Glycosmis pentaphylla* D.C., this alkaloid has been characterized as the crystalline picrate, m.p. 182°C. The ultraviolet spectrum exhibits absorption maxima at 227, 252, 264 and 304 mμ. The structure, of 3-methoxy-6-methylcarbazole, has been confirmed by synthesis.

Chakraborty., *Tetrahedron Lett.*, 661 (1966)

Synthesis:

Chakraborty, Das, Chowdhury., *Sci. Cult.*, (Calcutta), **32**, 245 (1966)

Chakraborty, Das, Chowdhury., *Chem. Ind.*, 1684 (1966)

Carruthers., *Chem. Commun.*, 272 (1966)

GOMANDO BASE A

M.p. 199°C

One of several minor alkaloids isolated from *Aconitum subcuneatum,* this base is dextrorotatory with $[\alpha]_D^{20} + 76.6°$. The structure has not yet been determined.

Ochiai, Okanoto, Sasaki., *J. Pharm. Soc., Japan,* **75**, 550 (1955)

GOMANDO BASE B

An uncharacterized alkaloid obtained from *Aconitum subcuneatum*. The base is present in such small quantities that insufficient has yet been isolated to yield any physical constants.

Ochiai, Okanoto, Sasaki., *J. Pharm. Soc., Japan,* **75**, 550 (1955)

GOMANDO BASE C

M.p. 320°C (*dec.*).

A further minor constituent of *Aconitum subcuneatum*. The structure has not yet been elucidated since the alkaloid is present in such minute quantities.

Ochiai, Okanoto, Sasaki., *J. Pharm. Soc., Japan,* **75**, 550 (1955)

GOZILINE

$C_{43}H_{50}O_5N_4$

M.p. 260°C (dec.).

This complex dimeric alkaloid is present in the root bark of *Hedranthera barteri* Pichon. It forms colourless crystals from MeOH or EtOH and is laevorotatory with $[\alpha]_D^{25} - 337°$ (c 0.0196, CHCl$_3$). It contains one methoxyl, one methoxycarbonyl and one imino group. The remaining three nitrogen atoms are tertiary.

   Agwada *et al., Helv. Chim. Acta,* **53**, 1567 (1970)

GRAMINE (*Donaxine*)

$C_{11}H_{14}N_2$

M.p. 138–9°C

First obtained from barley mutants and subsequently discovered in *Arundo donax* by Orekhov and Norkina who named it donaxine and characterized it, the alkaloid crystallizes as flat needles or leaflets. It is optically inactive and furnishes a perchlorate, m.p. 150–1°C; platinichloride as bright red needles, m.p. 180–1°C (*dec.*); a picrate, m.p. 144–5°C and the methiodide, m.p. 176–7°C. Treatment with methyl iodide in MeOH yields trimethylamine, tetramethylammonium iodide and 3-hydroxymethylindole. With ethyl iodide in Me$_2$CO it furnishes a normal ethiodide, m.p. 176°C.

   von Euler and Erdtman proposed the structure 2-dimethylamino-3-methylindole for the alkaloid and also suggested its identity with donaxine. The proposed structure was later found to be erroneous when Wieland and Hsing obtained the alkaloid by the reaction of magnesium 3-indolyl iodide with dimethylaminoacetonitrile, showing that it must be 3-dimethylaminomethylindole. The base has also been synthesized by the reaction of formaldehyde, dimethylamine and indole in AcOH at room teperature.

   Pharmacologically, the alkaloid, in the form of the somewhat unstable hydroxhloride, elevated the blood pressure in anaesthetized cats in small doses. On raising the doe, however, the blood pressure is lowered although a secondary rise is often noted. It has the effect of reducing the main effects of adrenaline without reversal and, in mammals, excites the central nervous system although in larger doses it causes paralysis. At a concentration of only 1 in 25,000 it brings

642

about contraction of the isolated uterus. It is moderately toxic, the toxic dose for rats being of the order of 65 mgm per kilo.

von Euler, Hellström., *Zeit. physiol. Chem.*, **208**, 43 (1932)
von Euler, Hellström., *ibid*, **217**, 23 (1933)
von Euler, Hellström, Löfgren., *ibid*, **234**, 151 (1935)
Orekhov, Norkina., *Ber.*, **68**, 436 (1935)
Orekhov, Norkina., *J. Gen. Chem.*, *USSR*, **7**, 673 (1937)
Madinaveitia., *Nature*, **139**, 27 (1937)
Wieland, Hsing., *Annalen*, **526**, 188 (1936)
Kuhn, Stein., *Ber.*, **70**, 567 (1937)

Pharmacology:
Powell, Chen., *Proc. Soc. exp. Biol. Med.*, **58**, 1 (1945)
Supniewski, Serafinowna., *Bull. Acad. Polon.*, 479 (1937)

GRAMINIFOLINE

$C_{18}H_{23}O_5N$

M.p. 236°C

A hepatotoxic alkaloid isolated from *Senecio graminifolius* Jacq. This is one of the less clearly defined of these bases and the structure has not yet been fully determined.

de Waal., *Onderstepoort J.*, **16**, 149 (1941)

GRANDIFLORINE

A highly toxic *Solanum* alkaloid isolated from *Solanum grandiflorum* var. *pulverulentem,* this base has, so far, not been characterized.

Freire., *Compt. rend.*, **105**, 1074 (1887)

GRANDIFOLINE

$C_{36}H_{52}O_{12}N$

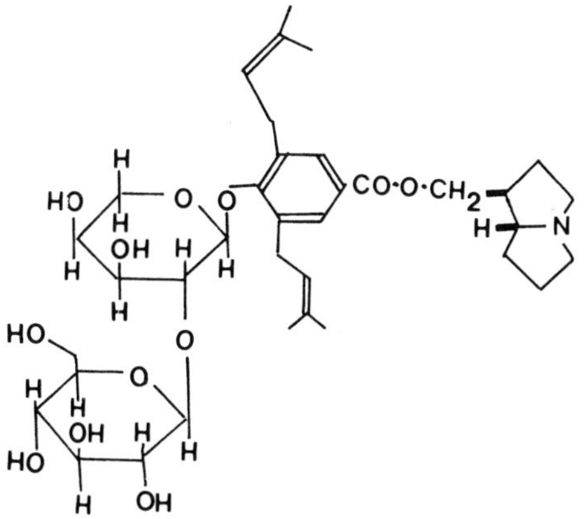

A complex pyrrolizidine alkaloid present in *Malaxis grandifolia* Schltr., this base is amorphous with no definite melting point. It has $[\alpha]_D^{23} - 7°$ (c 0.69, EtOH) and the ultraviolet spectrum exhibits one absorption maximum at 246 mμ.

Lindstrom, Luning, Siirala-Hansen., *Acta Chem. Scand.*, **25**, 1900 (1971)

GRANTIANINE

$C_{18}H_{23}O_7N$

M.p. 204–5°C

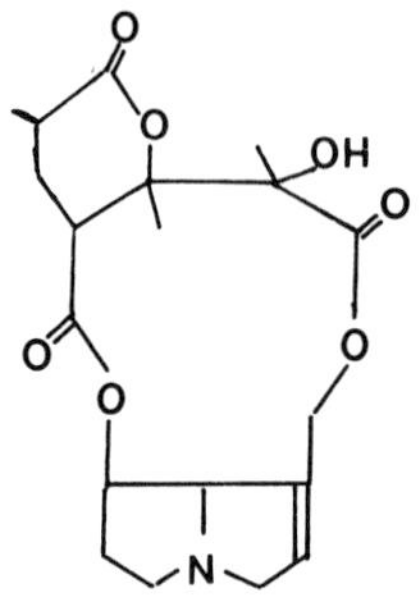

This pyrrolizidine alkaloid occurs in the seeds of *Crotalaria grantiana* and is dextrorotatory with $[\alpha]_D^{27} + 50.6°$ (c 1.0, CHCl$_3$). It forms a hydrochloride, m.p. 221–2°C (*dec.*); methiodide, m.p. 242–3°C and a picrate, m.p. 225–8°C (*dec.*). The base can be hydrogenated without cleavage to form tetrahydro-grantianine, m.p. 242.5°C (*vac.*), giving a crystalline picrate, m.p. 156–7°C (*dec.*). Alkaline hydrolysis furnishes retronecine and grantianinic acid which is difficult to obtain in the pure state.

Adams, Carmack, Rogers., *J. Amer. Chem. Soc.*, **64**, 571 (1942)
Adams, Gianturco., *Angew. Chem.*, **69**, 5 (1957)
Adams, Gianturco., *J. Amer. Chem. Soc.*, **78**, 4458 (1956)

GRAVEOLINE

$C_{17}H_{13}O_3N$

M.p. 204–5°C

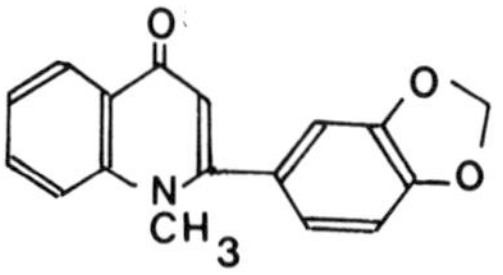

A quinolone alkaloid found in *Ruta graveolens*, this base forms colourless needles from MeOH or EtOH. It forms no salts with mineral acids.

Goodwin, Smith, Horning., *J. Amer. Chem. Soc.*, **79**, 2239 (1957)
Arthur, Cheung., *Austral. J. Chem.*, **13**, 510 (1960)
Arthur, Loh., *J. Chem. Soc.*, 4360 (1961)

GRAVEOLININE

$C_{17}H_{13}O_3N$

M.p. 115–6°C

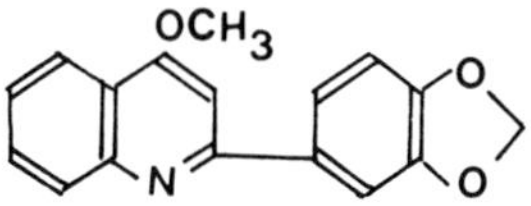

Isomeric with the preceding base and also present in *Ruta graveolens*, this alkaloid has subsequently been discovered in *Lunasia amara* Blanco. It yields clusters of colourless crystals from AcOET. The ultraviolet spectrum has absorption maxima at 236, 275 and 311 mμ. Spectroscopic and chemical degradative experiments have demonstrated that the structure is 4-methoxy-2-(3':4'-methylenedioxyphenyl)quinoline.

Goodwin *et al., J. Amer. Chem. Soc.*, **81**, 6209 (1959)
Beyerman, Rooda., *Proc. Kon. Nederland Akad. Wetensch.*, **62B**, 181 (1959)
Beyerman, Rooda., *ibid*, **63B**, 427 (1960)
Chatterjee, Deb., *Chem. & Ind.*, 1982 (1962)

C-GUAIANINE

$C_{21}H_{25}O_2N^+$

A quaternary alkaloid found in the bark of *Strychnos toxifera*, the base has been isolated as the crystalline picrate with a melting point above 305°C.

Asmis *et al., Helv. Chim. Acta*, **37**, 1968 (1954)
Geisbrecht *et al., ibid*, **37**, 1974 (1954)

GUAIPYRIDINE

$C_{15}H_{21}N$

An oily alkaloid present in *Pogostemon patchouli* Pellet, this laevorotatory base has $[\alpha]_D^{25.5} - 34.5°$ (c 2.69, EtOH). The ultraviolet spectrum exhibits absorption maxima at 278 mμ with shoulders at 215 and 273 mμ. The alkaloid yields a perchlorate as a waxy, crystalline solid from Et$_2$O-MeOH, m.p. 105–105.5°C; $[\alpha]_D^{29} - 17°$ (c 8.0, EtOH). The original structure has recently been revised and confirmed by synthesis.

Büchi, Goldman, Mayo., *J. Amer. Chem. Soc.*, **88**, 3109 (1966)

Revised structure:
Van Der Gren, Van Der Linde, Witteveen., *Rev. trav. Chim.*, **91**, 1433 (1972)

GUAN-FU BASE A

$C_{24}H_{31}O_6N$

M.p. 198°C

The Chinese drug 'Guan-Bai-Fu-Tzu', derived from *Aconitum koreanum*, yields Hypaconitine (q.v.) and five new alkaloids which have been provisionally designated Guan-Fu bases A to E. This particular alkaloid has $[\alpha]_D^{22.8} + 49°$ (CHCl$_3$) and yields crystalline salts and derivatives including the hydrochloride, m.p. 290°C; hydrobromide, m.p. 293°C; nitrate, m.p. 265°C; perchlorate, m.p. 272–3°C; methiodide, m.p. 284.5–285.5°C and the diacetate, m.p. 154.5–

155°C. When hydrolyzed in KOMe, acetic acid and an alkamine, $C_{20}H_{27}O_4N$, m.p. 243–4°C are formed. Oxidation with acid $KMnO_4$ yields two crystalline products, $C_{22}H_{27}O_7N$, m.p. 204°C and $C_{23}H_{29}O_8N$, giving a perchlorate, m.p. 286°C (dec.). Hydrogenation with PtO_2 as catalyst yields the dihydro derivative, m.p. 200°C.

Kao, Yo, Chu., *Yao Hseuh Hseuh Pao.*, **13**, 186 (1966)

GUAN-FU BASE B

$C_{22}H_{29}O_5N$

M.p. 204°C

The second alkaloid isolated from *Aconitum koreanun* is also slightly dextro-rotatory with $[\alpha]_D^{26.6} + 16°$ ($CHCl_3$). It yields a hydrobromide, m.p. 257–8°C; perchlorate, m.p. 255–6°C; methiodide, m.p. 317–8°C and the triacetate, m.p. 154–5°C. The monoacetate is identical with the preceding alkaloid.

Kao, Yo, Chu., *Yao Hseuh Hseuh Pao.*, **13**, 186 (1966)

GUAN-FU BASE C

$C_{22}H_{33}O_2N$

M.p. 150°C

Also present in *Aconitum koreanum,* this alkaloid is laevorotatory having $[\alpha]_D^{16.4} - 21.2°$ (EtOH). It gives crystalline salts and derivative, e.g. the hydro-bromide, m.p. 235°C; nitrate, m.p. 222°C and the diacetate hydrochloride, m.p. 222.5–224°C. It contains two hydroxyl groups, a methyl group and an ethylimino group in the molecule.

Kao, Yo, Chu., *Yao Hseuh Hseuh Pao.*, **13**, 186 (1966)

GUAN-FU BASE D

$C_{24}H_{35}O_3N$

The fourth alkaloid to be isolated from *Aconitum koreanum,* the free base has not yet been obtained in the crystalline form. It has been characterized as the crystalline nitrate, m.p. 210–1°C.

Kao, Yo, Chu., *Yao Hseuh Hseuh Pao.*, **13**, 186 (1966)

GUAN-FU BASE E

$C_{29}H_{43}O_7N$

Like the preceding base, this alkaloid from *Aconitum koreanum* has not been obtained crystalline but yields a perchlorate as colourless needles, m.p. 272°C.

Kao, Yo, Chu., *Yao Hseuh Hseuh Pao.*, **13**, 186 (1966)

(+)-GUATAMBUINE (*u-Alkaloid C*)

$C_{18}H_{20}N_2$

M.p. 245–8°C

This alkaloid occurs in several species of *Aspidosperma,* particularly in *A. australe* Müll. Agrov. It is obtained as colourless crystals from EtOH and has $[\alpha]_D^{29}$ + 113° (c 0.485, pyridine). The ultraviolet spectrum shows several absorption maxima occurring at 240, 250, 262, 299 and 330 mμ. Selenium dehydrogenation furnishes Olivacine (q.v.). The alkaloid contains two methyl groups, one imino and one methylimino group.

Schmutz, Hunziker, Hirt., *Helv. Chim. Acta,* **40**, 1189 (1957)
Schmutz, Hunziker, Hirt., *ibid,* **41**, 288 (1958)
Ondetti, Deulofeu., *Tetrahedron,* **15**, 160 (1961)

(–)-GUATAMBUINE

$C_{18}H_{20}N_2$

M.p. 247–8°C

This enantiomorph of the alkaloid is found in the root bark of *Aspidosperma australe* Müll. Agrov. It has $[\alpha]_D^{26} - 107°$ (pyridine). Its other characteristics are identical with those given for the (+)-form above.

Schmutz, Hunziker, Hirt., *Helv. Chim. Acta,* **40**, 1189 (1957)
Schmutz, Hunziker, Hirt., *ibid,* **41**, 288 (1958)
Ondetti, Deulofeu., *Tetrahedron,* **15**, 160 (1961)

(±)-GUATAMBUINE

$C_{18}H_{20}N_2$

M.p. 224–5°C

Found in the aerial bark of *Aspidosperma australe* Müll. Agrov., this optically inactive alkaloid yields a crystalline methiodide, m.p. 299–301°C. On selenium dehydrogenation it gives Olivacine (q.v.).

Schmutz, Hunziker, Hirt., *Helv. Chim. Acta,* **40**, 1189 (1957)
Schmutz, Hunziker, Hirt., *ibid,* **41**, 288 (1958)
Carvalho-Ferreira, Marini-Bettolo, Schmutz., *Experientia,* **15**, 179 (1959)
Carvalho-Ferreira, Marini-Bettolo, Schmutz., *Ann. Chim.,* **49**, 869 (1959)
Ondetti, Deulofeu., *Tetrahedron,* **15**, 160 (1961)

GUVACINE

$C_6H_9O_2N$

M.p. $271-2°C$ (*dec.*).

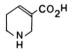

This is the simplest of the alkaloids found in the seeds of *Areca catechu* (betel nut) and crystallizes from H_2O or aqueous EtOH in small, lustrous prisms. A somewhat higher melting point than that given above, m.p. $293-5°$ has been recorded by Winterstein and Weinhagen. The base is optically inactive, neutral to litmus and is insoluble in all solvents except H_2O and aqueous EtOH. The hydrochloride crystallizes in prisms, m.p. $316°C$ (*dec.*); the aurichloride in broad, flattened prisms, m.p. $197-9°C$ (*dec.*) and the platinichloride, m.p. $233°C$ (*dec.*). The alkaloid behaves as a secondary amine, yielding an acetyl derivative, m.p. $189-190°C$ and a nitroso compound, m.p. $167-8°C$, the methyl ester of which, in treatment with liquid ammonia gives N-nitroso-4-aminopiperidine-3-carboxylamide, m.p. $172°C$. Distillation with Zn dust yields 3-methylpyridine. The suggestion that the structure might be Δ^1-tetrahydro-pyridine-3-carboxylic acid was first put forward by Trier although it was Freudenberg who first called attention to the similarity of the two and subsequently demonstrated their identity. The methyl ester of the alkaloid is identical with guvacoline (q.v.).

The alkaloid is not markedly toxic, being a moderate central stimulant. Comparatively recently, it has been shown that it is also as powerful a growth factor for certain bacteria as nicotinic acid.

Jahns., *Ber.*, **21**, 3404 (1888)
Jahns., *ibid*, **23**, 2972 (1890)
Jahns., *ibid*, **24**, 2665 (1891)
Jahns., *Arch. Pharm.*, **229**, 669 (1891)
Trier., *Zeit. physiol. Chem.*, **85**, 372 (1913)
Winterstein, Weinhagen., *ibid*, **104**, 48 (1918)
Freudenberg., *Ber.*, **51**, 976, 1669 (1918)
Chemnitius., *J. pr. Chem.*, **117**, 147 (1927)
von Euler *et al.*, *Helv. Chim. Acta*, **27**, 382 (1944)

*iso*GUVACINE

$C_6H_9O_2N$

M.p. $220°C$

This optically inactive alkaloid occurs with guvacine as a minor constituent of *Areca catechu*. It is slightly acid to litmus and furnishes crystalline salts, e.g. the hydrochloride, m.p. $231°C$, aurichloride, m.p. $198-200°C$ and the platini-chloride, m.p. $235°C$. It also yields a dimethyl derivative, the platinichloride of which has m.p. $252°C$. Trier regarded the alkaloid as Δ^2-tetrahydropyridine-3-carboxylic acid which other workers have suggested that it may be a mixture, consisting mainly of arecaidine (q.v.). However, on Zn dust distillation it yields a substance giving the typical pyrrole reactions and it may be a simple pyrrole derivative isomeric with guvacine.

Jahns., *Ber.*, **21**, 3404 (1888)
Jahns., *ibid*, **24**, 2665 (1891)
Trier., *Zeit. physiol. Chem.*, **85**, 372 (1913)
Winterstein, Weinhagen., *ibid*, **104**, 48 (1918)

GUVACOLINE

$C_7H_{11}O_2N$

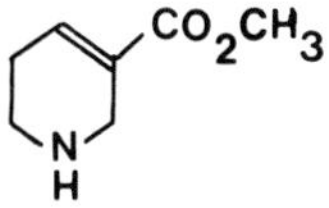

B.p. 114°C/13 mm

Also present in *Areca catechu,* this alkaloid forms a colourless oil which discolours on prolonged exposure to air. It yields crystalline salts and derivatives: the hydrochloride, m.p. 121–2°C; hydrobromide, m.p. 144–5°C and platinichloride, m.p. 211°C. With methyl iodide, it gives a mixture of arecoline iodide and arecoline methiodide. The hydrobromide has been identified as guvacine methyl ester hydrobromide, thereby establishing guvacoline as the methyl ester of givacine.

Hesse., *Ber.*, **51**, 1004 (1918)

GYMNAMINE

$C_{19}H_{26}O_3N_2$

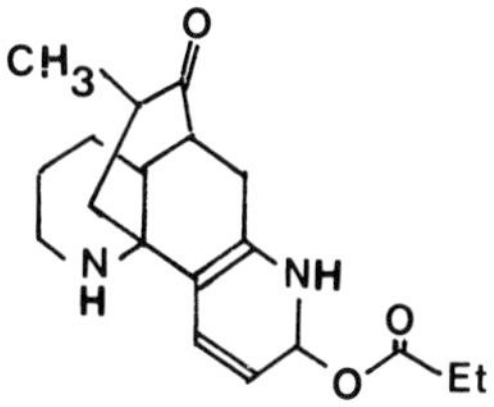

M.p. 60–70°C

This alkaloid is present as a minor component of the extract from the leaves of *Gymnema sylvestre* R. Br. and is obtained as an amorphous solid which has not yet been obtained in the crystalline form. The ultraviolet spectrum in ethanol shows absorption maxima at 231, 281 and 288 mμ with a shoulder at 250 mμ. It may be characterized as the picrate, forming pale yellow needles, m.p. 260°C. The alkaloid contains a methyl group, two imino groups and a propionyl group.

Rao, Sinsheimer, McIlhenny., *Chem. Ind.*, 537 (1972)

H

HABRANTHINE

$C_{17}H_{21}O_4N$

M.p. 198–9°C

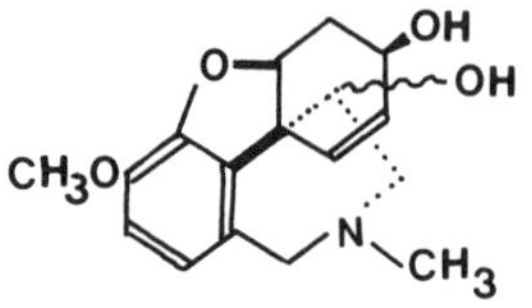

This novel Amaryllidaceae alkaloid has been isolated from *Habranthus brachy-andrus* in 0.006 per cent yield. It is strongly laevorotatory with $[\alpha]_D^{25} - 320°$ and forms a dihydro derivative and the O,O-diacetyl compound. Successive treatment of the dihydro compound with $SOCl_2$ and $LiAlH_4$ has established the basic ring structure as that of galanthamine (q.v.). The evidence obtained from the NMR spectrum and the fragmentation pattern of the mass spectrum confirm the given structure.

Wildman, Brown., *Tetrahedron Lett.*, 4573 (1968)

HAEMANTHAMINE (*Natalensine*)

$C_{17}H_{19}O_4N$

M.p. 203–203.5°C

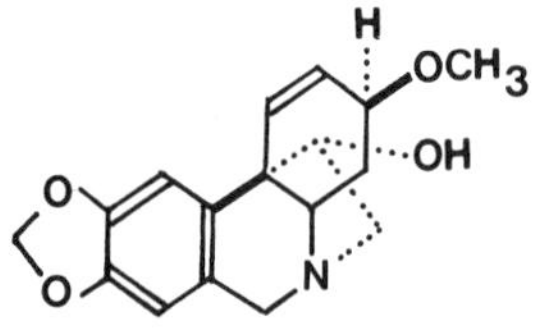

A further alkaloid found in several of the Amaryllidaceae species, this base is dextrorotatory having $[\alpha]_D^{25} + 33°$ (c 1.25, CHCl₃) or + 19.66° (c 3.77, MeOH). The ultraviolet spectrum shows two absorption maxima at 240 and 297 mμ. Among the crystalline derivatives that have been prepared are the methiodide, m.p. 190–2°C; methoperchlorate, m.p. 244–5°C (*dec.*); the m-nitrobenzoyl derivative, m.p. 153–4°C and the O-acetate which yields a crystalline perchlorate having m.p. 209°C. The alkaloid contains one hydroxyl group, a methylenedioxy group and one methoxyl. The structure has been determined by spectroscopic methods and is similar to that of the preceding alkaloid but without the oxygen bridge between the aromatic and hydroaromatic rings.

Boit., *Chem. Ber.*, **87**, 1339 (1954)
Wildman, Kaufman., *J. Amer. Chem. Soc.*, **77**, 1248 (1955)
Fales, Wildman., *Chem. & Ind.*, 561 (1958)
Fales, Wildman., *J. Amer. Chem. Soc.*, **82**, 197, 3368 (1958)

Mass spectrum:
Duffield *et al.*, *J. Amer. Chem. Soc.*, **87**, 4902 (1965)

epi-HAEMANTHAMINE

$C_{17}H_{19}O_4N$

M.p. 205°C

This epimer of haemanthamine occurs in *Haemanthus katherinae* and forms colourless prisms from Me$_2$CO. It is laevorotatory with $[\alpha]_D^{25} - 24°$ (c 0.2, CHCl$_3$). The stereochemistry has been determined mainly from NMR data.

Nogueiras *et al., Tetrahedron Lett.*, 2743 (1971)

HAEMANTHIDINE

$C_{17}H_{19}O_5N$

M.p. 189–190°C

An Amaryllidaceae alkaloid which yields colourless crystals from Me$_2$CO or CHCl$_3$, this base is laevorotatory having $[\alpha]_D^{22} - 41°$ (c 1.0, CHCl$_3$). It readily forms a picrate as yellow crystals from H$_2$O, m.p. 208°C (*dec.*). The O,O-diacetate has m.p. 200–4°C (*dec.*) and the N-methyl derivative is characterized as the methiodide, m.p. 228–9°C (*dec.*) or the methoperchlorate, m.p. 244°C (*dec.*). Two hydroxyl groups, a methylenedioxy and a methoxyl group are present. The nitrogen atom is tertiary. According to King *et al*, the alkaloid exists as a mixture of the C-6 epimers when in solution.

Boit., *Chem. Ber.*, **87**, 1339 (1954)
Uyeo *et al., J. Amer. Chem. Soc.*, **80**, 2590 (1958)
King, Murphy, Wildman., *ibid*, **87**, 4912 (1965)

Mass spectrum:
Duffield *et al., J. Amer. Chem. Soc.*, **87**, 4902 (1965)

epi-HAEMANTHIDINE

$C_{17}H_{19}O_5N$

This alkaloid occurs in *Haemanthus natalensis* and forms colourless prisms, m.p. 211°C when crystallized from Me$_2$CO-ligroine. It has $[\alpha]_D^{20} + 44°$ (c 1.0, CHCl$_3$). A stable hydrate, m.p. 146°C has been prepared by crystallization from aqueous Me$_2$CO. The ultraviolet spectrum exhibits absorption maxima at 242 and 293 mμ. The alkaloid forms a methiodide, m.p. 174°C; $[\alpha]_D^{23} + 57°$ (c 1.0, MeOH) and a methopicrate, m.p. 146°C. With Ac$_2$O in pyridine, an amorphous O,O-diacetate is formed, m.p. 182–4°C.

When heated with HCl, the alkaloid forms apohaemanthidine while oxidation with manganese dioxide yields oxoepihaemanthidine.

Goosen *et al., J. Chem. Soc.*, 1088 (1960)

HAEMULTINE

$C_{16}H_{17}O_3N$

M.p. 174–5°C

An alkaloid of the *Amaryllidaceae*, this dextrorotatory base has $[\alpha]_D + 147°$ (c 1.0, $CHCl_3$). Some crystalline salts have been described, the hydriodide, m.p. 102°C; picrate, m.p. 208–210°C; methiodide, m.p. 263–4°C and the perchlorate of the O-acetyl derivative, m.p. 192°C (*dec.*). The above testative structure has been suggested for this alkaloid which may be a mixture of α- and β-demethoxy-haemanthamines.

Boit, Döpke., *Naturwiss.*, **45**, 262 (1958)

Boit, Döpke., *Chem. Ber.*, **91**, 1965 (1958)

Fales, Wildman., *J. Org. Chem.*, **26**, 1617 (1961)

HALFORDAMINE

$C_{12}H_{13}O_4N$

M.p. 240–1°C

Isolated from *Halfordia kendack,* this alkaloid forms colourless crystals from a mixture of C_6H_6 and light petroleum. It contains three methoxyl groups and one imino group and has been shown by spectroscopic methods and synthesis to be 4:6:8-trimethoxy-2-quinolone. The alkaloid has been synthesized by reaction of 2:4-dimethoxyaniline and $CH_2(CO_2Et)_2$ followed by hydrolysis to the acid and then cyclization in polyphosphoric acid. Treatment of the resulting 4:6-dimethoxy-8-hydroxy-2-quinolone with CH_2N_2 gave the alkaloid.

Crow, Hodgkin., *Austral. J. Chem.*, **21**, 2075 (1968)

Revised structure by synthesis:

Storer, Young., *Tetrahedron Lett.*, 1555 (1972)

Alternate synthesis:

Venturella, Bellino, Piozzi., *Chem. Ind.*, 887 (1972)

HALFORDANINE

M.p. 240–1°C

A minor constituent of *Halfordia scleroxyla,* a member of the Australian Rutaceae. The structure is not yet known with certainty.

Crow, Hodgkin., *Austral. J. Chem.*, **21**, 3075 (1968)

HALFORDINE

$C_{19}H_{20}O_4N_2$

M.p. 164°C

A further alkaloid found in the bark of *Halfordia scleroxyla,* this base is obtained in the form of pale yellow needles when crystallized from MeOH. The O-acetate forms colourless crystals from Me$_2$CO-light petroleum.

Crow, Hodgkin., *Tetrahedron Lett.,* **85** (1963)
Crow, Hodgkin., *Austral. J. Chem.,* **17**, 119 (1964)
Mass spectrum:
Crow, Hodgkin, Shamma., *Austral. J. Chem.,* **18**, 1433 (1965)

HALFORDININE

M.p. 150–1°C

A minor alkaloid isolated from the bark of *Halfordia scleroxyla,* this base is separated from the accompanying alkaloids by column chromatography.

Crow, Hodgkin., *Austral. J. Chem.,* **21**, 3075 (1968)

HALFORDINOL

$C_{14}H_{10}O_2N_2$

M.p. 255–6°C

A further alkaloid occurring in *Halfordia scleroxyla* which also forms pale cream needles from MeOH. The O-acetate has a similar appearance and m.p. 167–180°C; the N-methyl derivative forms a crystalline hydrochloride as brown-yellow needles, m.p. 258°C and a picrate as orange-brown needles, m.p. 316–320°C. The O-methyl compound is obtained as colourless crystals from light petroleum with m.p. 99–100°C.

Crow, Hodgkin., *Austral. J. Chem.,* **17**, 119 (1964)

HALFORDINOL-3:3-DIMETHYLALLYL ETHER

$C_{19}H_{18}O_2N_2$

M.p. 109–111°C

This alkaloid is present in *Aeglopsis chevalieri* Swing and yields colourless crystals from a mixture of AcOEt and hexane. The ultraviolet spectrum in EtOH has absorption maxima at 248, 260 and 325 mμ. The structure has been determined from spectroscopic data and comparison with Halfordinol.

Dreyer., *J. Org. Chem.,* **33**, 3658 (1968)

HALFORDINONE

$C_{19}H_{18}O_3N_2$

M.p. 132–3°C

A minor constituent of *Halfordia scleroxyla*, this alkaloid is obtained in the form of colourless crystals from a mixture of Me_2CO and light petroleum. It contains a carbonyl group in the side chain attached to the benzene ring. The structure has been determined on the basis of its infrared, NMR and mass spectra.

Crow, Hodgkin., *Austral. J. Chem.*, **17**, 119 (1964)

HALOSALINE

$C_{10}H_{21}ON$

This alkaloid from *Haloxylon salicornicum* is difficult to obtain in a crystalline form and the melting point is somewhat indefinite. It has $[\alpha]_D - 19.5°$ (c 0.6, EtOH) or $+ 3.3°$ (c 1.0, $CHCl_3$). The structure has been determined as 2-(2-hydroxypentyl)piperidine from spectroscopic and chemical degradation data.

Michel *et al.*, *Acta Pharm. Suecia.*, **4**, 97 (1967)

Absolute configuration:
Michel *et al.*, *Acta, Chem. Scand.*, **23**, 3479 (1969)

HALOSTACHINE

$C_9H_{13}ON$

M.p. 43–5°C

This alkaloid has been isolated from *Halostachis caspica* (sometimes given in the literature as *Halostachys caspia*), a member of the family Chenopodiaceae. The crystalline hydrochloride has m.p. 113–4°C; the methiodide, m.p. 230–1°C. The N-methyl derivative is an oil, b.p. 125–7°C/20 mm; $[\alpha]_D - 65°$ and with $SOCl_2$ yields the chloride hydrochloride, $C_{10}H_{14}NCl.HCl$, m.p. 202–3°C. A similar reaction with the free base yields the corresponding chloride hydrochloride, $C_9H_{12}NCl.HCl$, m.p. 168–9°C. On oxidation with $KMnO_4$ the alkaloid yields benzoic acid. The alkaloid has been synthesized and resolved into its (+)- and (−)-forms, the latter giving a hydrochloride, $[\alpha]_D - 52.46°$ and an acid tartrate, having $[\alpha]_D - 18.73°$. Pharmacologically, the alkaloid is said to resemble ephedrine in its action.

654

Men'shikov, Rubinshtein., *J. Gen. Chem., USSR,* **13**, 801 (1943)
Synthesis:
Men'shikov, Borodina., *J. Gen. Chem., USSR,* **17**, 1569 (1947)
Pharmacology:
Syrneva., *Farmakol i Toksikol.,* **4**, 105 (1941)

HAMADINE

Stated to occur in the roots of *Convolvulus hamadae,* this alkaloid was isolated by Lazur'evskii. No detailed description has yet been given of this base.

Lazur'evskii., *Trudy Uzbekskogo Gos. Univ. Sbornik Rabot Khim.,* **15**, 43 (1939)
Lazur'evskii., *Chem. Abstr.,* **35**, 4029 (1941)

HAMMARBINE

$C_{27}H_{39}O_9N$

M.p. Indefinite

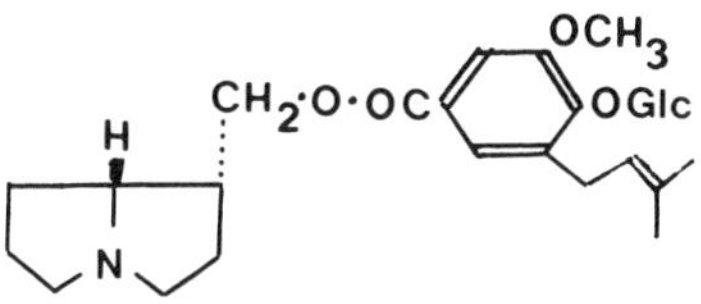

An amorphous pyrrolizidine alkaloid present in *Hammarbya paludosa,* the base is dextrorotatory with $[\alpha]_D^{23} + 9°$ (c 0.31, EtOH). The sugar moiety has been identified as D-glucose.

Lindström, Lüning., *Acta Chem. Scand.,* **26**, 2963 (1972)

HANADAMINE

$C_{21}H_{24}O_4N$

M.p. 187°C

This alkaloid occurs in *Ourouparia Kawakamii* Hayata and is laevorotatory with $[\alpha]_D^{18} - 123.7°$. It forms a crystalline aurichloride, m.p. 156°C (*dec.*); and an amorphous platinichloride, m.p. 228—9°C. The complete structure has not yet been determined but it has been established that the base contains one hydroxyl group and one methoxycarbonyl group in the molecule.

Kondo, Oshima., *J. Pharm. Soc., Japan,* **52**, 63 (1932)

HANFANCHINE A

$C_{38}H_{42}O_6N_2$

M.p. 218°C

This alkaloid isolated from the Chinese drug 'Han-fang-Chi', the source of which appears to be *Stephania tetrandra,* has $[\alpha]_D^{18} + 268.7°$ (CHCl₃) and has been shown to be identical with tetrandrine (q.v.).

Hsü., *J. Chin. Chem. Soc.*, **3**, 260, 365 (1935)
Hsü., *ibid*, **5**, 14 (1937)
Hsü., *ibid*, **7**, 123 (1940)

HANFANCHINE B

$C_{36}H_{40}O_6N_2$

M.p. $241-2°C$

A non-phenolic alkaloid also present in the drug 'Han-fang-Chi', this base is dextrorotatory with $[\alpha]_D^{23.5} + 272.4°$ ($CHCl_3$).

Hsü., *J. Chin. Chem. Soc.*, **3**, 260, 365 (1935)
Hsü., *ibid*, **5**, 14 (1937)
Hsü., *ibid*, **7**, 123 (1940)

HANFANCHINE C

$C_{32}H_{42}O_{12}N$

M.p. $215-7°C$ (*dec.*).

A third alkaloid found in 'Han-fang-Chi' from *Stephania tetrandra*, this alkaloid crystallizes as colourless prisms of the octahydrate. It is laevorotatory with $[\alpha]_D^{23} - 12.9°$ (H_2O) and forms a crystalline hydrochloride, m.p. $220-2°C$ (*dec.*) and a methiodide, m.p. $182-4°C$.

Hsü., *J. Chin. Chem. Soc.*, **3**, 260, 365 (1935)
Hsü., *ibid*, **5**, 14 (1937)
Hsü., *ibid*, **7**, 123 (1940)

HAPLOCIDINE

$C_{21}H_{26}O_3N$

M.p. $183-4°C$

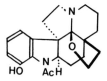

Obtained from *Haplophyton cimicidum*, a member of the Apocynaceae family, this dextrorotatory alkaloid has $[\alpha]_D + 231°$ ($CHCl_3$) and the ultraviolet spectrum exhibits absorption maxima at 218.5, 258 and 291 mμ. The alkaloid contains an N-acetyl group and forms a crystalline O-acetyl derivative, m.p. $196-7°C$. The structure has been determined on the basis of spectroscopic data.

Cava *et al.*, *Chem. & Ind.*, 1242 (1963)

Stereochemistry:
Cava, Nomura, Talapatra., *Tetrahedron*, **20**, 581 (1964)

HAPLOCINE

$C_{22}H_{28}O_3N_2$

M.p. 186–7°C

A further base present in *Haplophyton cimicidum*, this alkaloid is also dextro-rotatory having $[\alpha]_D + 196°$ (CHCl$_3$). The ultraviolet spectrum is very similar to that of the preceding base with absorption maxima occurring at 219.5, 258 and 292 mμ. It also forms a crystalline O-acetyl derivative, m.p. 194–5°C. It contains one hydroxyl and one N-propionyl group.

Cava *et al., Chem. & Ind.,* 1242 (1963)

HAPLOPHYLLIDINE

$C_{18}H_{21}O_4N$

M.p. 110–1°C

A furoquinoline alkaloid found in the seeds of *Haplophyllum perforatum,* this base has $[\alpha]_D^{20} - 16°$ (c 1.477, Me$_2$CO). Two methoxyl groups, one methyl group and a hydroxybutyl group are present. A crystalline O-acetyl compound has been reported, m.p. 147–8°C.

Shakirov, Sidyakin, Yunusov., *Dokl. Akad. Nauk. Uzbek SSR,* **9,** 40 (1960)
Shakirov, Sadyakin, Yunusov., *ibid,* No. 8, 47 (1961)

HAPLOPHYTINE

$C_{37}H_{40}O_7N_4$

M.p. 288–292°C (*dec.*).

The major constituent of *Haplophyton cimicidum*, this alkaloid forms colourless crystals from EtOH-CHCl$_3$. The earlier formula of $C_{27}H_{31}O_5N_3$ has been shown to be incorrect by high resolution mass spectrometry. The base has $[\alpha]_D^{25} + 109°$ (c 1.3, CHCl$_3$) and the ultraviolet spectrum has absorption maxima at 220, 265 and 305 mμ. The picrate is obtained as a yellow microcrystalline powder, m.p. 140–160°C (*dec.*); the dihydrochloride, m.p. 208–218°C (*dec.*); the hydro-bromide, a hygroscopic yellow powder, m.p. 200–6°C (*dec.*).
Treatment with CH$_2$N$_2$ furnishes the O-methyl derivative as a microcrystalline

powder, m.p. 288–291°C (dec.); $[\alpha]_D^{24} + 12°$ (c 4.37, CHCl$_3$). Ac$_2$O in
pyridine gives the O-acetyl derivative which has m.p. 187–9°C followed by
solidification and remelting at 242–6°C. When reduced over PtO$_2$, the alkaloid
yields tetrahydrohaplophytine I as colourless needles, m.p. 206.8°C while
reduction with NaBH$_4$ gives tetrahydrohaplophytine II as a white solid with an
indefinite melting point. When reduced with Zn and HCl, the base forms
canthiphytine, $C_{15}H_{16}O_2N_2$, as colourless crystals yielding a hydrochloride,
m.p. 302°C (dec.). Boiling with 6N HCl gives aspidophytine, $C_{22}H_{26}O_4N_2$, again
as colourless needles, m.p. 201–3°C.

Roger, Snyder, Fischer., *J. Amer. Chem. Soc.,* **74**, 1987 (1952)
Snyder *et al., ibid,* **76**, 2819, 4601 (1954)
Snyder, Strohmayer, Mooney., *ibid,* **80**, 3708 (1958)

Revised structure:
Yates *et al., J. Amer. Chem. Soc.,* **95**, 7842 (1973)

Absolute configuration:
Rae *et al., J. Amer. Chem. Soc.,* **89**, 3061 (1967)

HARMALINE

$C_{13}H_{15}ON_2$

M.p. 248–250°C (dec.).

First isolated by Goebel from the seeds and roots of *Peganum harmala,* this is
the major alkaloid of this plant. It crystallizes in colourless, or pale yellow,
prisms and is optically inactive. The hydrochloride forms yellow needles of the
dihydrate, m.p. 212°C (*dry*) while the platinichloride is obtained as a microcrystalline powder. The methochloride, m.p. 277°C; methiodide, m.p. 260°C,
methosulphate, m.p. 170–2°C and a crystalline benzylidene derivative, m.p.
245°C have also been prepared. The picrate, yellow needles, has m.p. 246°C. The
base may also be characterized as the mercurichloride or the acid chromate, the
latter being insoluble in H$_2$O. A precipitate of the hydrocyanide is formed when
solutions of the salts of the alkaloid are treated with HCN.

An N-acetyl derivative has been prepared as colourless needles, m.p. 204–5°C,
and with methyl iodide the alkaloid yields a mixture of N-methylharmaline
iodide and dimethylharmaline iodide, m.p. 220°C. By the action of Ba(OH)$_2$ on
the former, N-methylharmaline, m.p. 162°C, may be obtained as colourless
needles. Oxidation of harmaline gives harmine (q.v.) while reduction yields the
tetrahydro derivative, m.p. 199°C. On demethylation, the alkaloid furnishes the
phenolic base harmalol (q.v.).

Harmaline is almost twice as toxic as harmine and in moderate doses causes
tremors and clonic convulsions but with no increase in spinal reflex excitability.
Lethal doses bring about the convulsions which are soon followed by motor
paralysis owing to the marked depressant action upon the central nervous
system. The respiration is paralyzed and a decrease in body temperature occurs,
particularly in mammals. The perfused heart in diastole is arrested and the
contractions of most kinds of smooth muscle are diminished with the notable
exception of the uterus which may be made to contract powerfully. Over a wide
range of dosage there is a reduction in the blood pressure due to a pronounced
weakening of the cardiac muscle.

Some interest has been shown in this, and the related harmala alkaloids, as possible therapeutic agents, particularly as coronary dilators, ecbolics, and protozooicidal agents.

Goebel., *Annalen,* **38**, 363 (1841)
Fischer., *Ber.,* **30**, 2482 (1897)
Perkin, Robinson., *J. Chem. Soc.,* **101**, 1778 (1912)
Perkin, Robinson., *ibid,* **115**, 967 (1919)
Manske, Perkin, Robinson., *ibid,* 1 (1927)
Späth, Lederer., *Ber.,* **63**, 122 (1930)

Synthesis:
Kermack, Perkin, Robinson., *J. Chem. Soc.,* **119**, 1617 (1921)

Crystal structure:
Ahmed, Rizvi., *Pak. J. Sci. Ind. Res.,* **12**, 157 (1969)

Pharmacology:
Gunn *et al., Arch. int. Pharmacodyn.,* **50**, 379 (1935)
Sato., *Tohuku J. Exp. Med.,* **26**, 161 (1935)
Beer., *Arch. exp. Path. Pharm.,* **193**, 377, 393 (1939)
Raymond-Hamet., *Compt. rend.,* **212**, 408 (1941)
Raymond-Hamet., *C. r. Soc. biol.,* **135**, 69, 328 (1941)
Raymond-Hamet., *Compt. rend.,* **221**, 387 (1945)

HARMALOL

$C_{12}H_{12}ON_2$

M.p. 212°C (*dec.*).

Also occurring in *Peganum harmala,* this alkaloid crystallizes from H_2O as the trihydrate. It is freely soluble in hot H_2O, Me_2CO or $CHCl_3$ but only sparingly so in C_6H_6. The alkaloid is unstable when exposed to air. One hydroxyl group is present capable of etherification, the ethyl ether having m.p. 247–9°C; the *iso*propyl ether, m.p. 196–7°C, forming a crystalline hydrochloride, m.p. 232–4°C. The methyl ether is harmaline (q.v.).

Fischer., *Ber.,* **30**, 2483 (1897)
Perkin, Robinson., *J. Chem. Soc.,* **115**, 933 (1919)
Manske, Perkin, Robinson., *ibid,* 1 (1927)
Späth, Lederer., *Ber.,* **63**, 120 (1930)

HARMAN

$C_{12}H_{10}N_2$

M.p. 238°C

Present in the bark of *Arariba rubra,* indigenous to Brazil, this alkaloid crystallizes from several organic solvents as colourless prisms. It is readily soluble in MeOH, EtOH, Me_2CO, $CHCl_3$ or Et_2O but only moderately so in hot H_2O or ligroin. It dissolves in mineral acids and exhibits a marked blue-violet fluorescence.

The hydrochloride has m.p. 292–5°C; the methobromide, m.p. 298–300°C (*dec.*) and the methiodide, m.p. 275°C (*dec.*). It forms two N-methyl derivatives, the N(2)-compound having m.p. 180°C (*dec.*) and the corresponding N(9)-methyl derivative, m.p. 100–2°C.

Späth., *Monatsh.*, **41**, 401 (1920)
Kermack, Perkin, Robinson., *J. Chem. Soc.*, **119**, 1603, 1612 (1921)
Späth, Lederer., *Ber.*, **63**, 120 (1930)
Akabori, Saiot., *ibid*, **63**, 2245 (1930)
Gray, Spinner, Cavallito., *J. Amer. Chem. Soc.*, **76**, 2792 (1954)

HARMAN-3-CARBOXYLIC ACID

$C_{13}H_{10}O_2N_2$

This alkaloid has recently been identified in the bark extract of *Aspidosperma exalatum* Monachino. The structure has been elucidated from chemical degradation and spectroscopic evidence.

Sanchez *et al.*, *An. Acad. Brasil Cienc.*, **43**, 603 (1971)

HARMANINE

An alkaloid of this name has been obtained from *Calligonium minimum* and characterized as the picrate, m.p. 239–240°C (*dec.*). No further details have been reported.

Abdusalanov, Sadykov, Aslanov., *Nauchn. Tr. Tashkentsk. Gos. Univ.*, **263**, 3 (1964)

HARMIDINE

$C_{13}H_{14}ON_2$

M.p. 257–8°C

This alkaloid from *Peganum harmala* has recently been identified as harmaline. The chemical constants are very similar to those of the latter base, e.g. hydrochloride, m.p. 236°C; hydriodide, m.p. 242°C; platinichloride, m.p. 259–260°C; picrate, m.p. 246°C; methiodide, m.p. 269–270°C and methosulphate, m.p. 170°C.

Siddiqui., *Chem. & Ind.*, 356 (1962)

Crystal structure:
Ahmed, Rizvi., *Pak. J. Sci. Ind. Res.*, **12**, 157 (1969)

Identity with harmaline:
Robinson., *Chem. Ind.*, 605 (1965)

HARMINE (*Banisterine*)

$C_{13}H_{12}ON_2$

M.p. 266°C

Present in *Peganum harmala* and in some species of *Banisteria*, viz., *B. caapi,* Spruce., *B. lutea* and *B. metallicolor,* this alkaloid has also been variously designated as telepathine and yageine although it now seems certain that only the one alkaloid is concerned. The alkaloid is optically inactive and forms colourless rhombic prisms from MeOH. It is only slightly soluble in EtOH, Et_2O or H_2O. Solutions of the salts show a pronounced deep blue fluorescence. The melting point of the hydrochloride has been recorded as 269.5−270.5°C and as 321°C. Harmine behaves as a monoacidic base and among the other salts and derivatives that have been prepared are the platinichloride, m.p. 264−6°C; nitrate; acid chromate; oxalate; picrate, m.p. 249−250°C (*dec.*); methiodide, m.p. 305−7°C; methosulphate, m.p. 220°C; benzylidene derivative, m.p. 191− 2°C and the N-methyl compound, m.p. 124−5°C forming a crystalline mono-hydrate, m.p. 114−8°C and a hydrochloride monohydrate, m.p. 280°C (*dec.*). On demethylation, the base furnishes harmol, $C_{12}H_{10}ON_2$, m.p. 321°C. The dihydro-derivative is harmaline (q.v.).

On oxidation, the alkaloid gives harminic acid which, when heated *in vacuo* loses the two carboxyl groups in two stages to give *apo*harmine, m.p. 183°C, a secondary base giving well-crystallized salts, e.g. the aurichloride, m.p. 240°C and picrate, m.p. 247°C. Oxidation with concentrated HNO_3 yields, in addition to harminic acid, *m*-nitroanisic acid. On further oxidation with dilute HNO_3, harminic acid yields pyridine-4-carboxylic acid (*iso*nicotinic acid) indicating that the alkaloid contains a methoxybenzene and a pyridine ring. When condensed with benzaldehyde, harmine forms the benzylidene derivative, the formation of which is characteristic of compounds containing a pyridine ring with a methyl group in the α-position.

Pharmacologically, the alkaloid resembles harmaline in its actions but is less toxic. The hydrochloride has been found to be highly active against *Mycobacterium tuberculosis.*

Fischer., *Ber.,* **30**, 2483 (1897)
Perkin, Robinson., *J. Chem. Soc.,* **115**, 933 (1919)
Reinburg., *J. Soc. d'Amer. Paris.,* **13**, 25, 197 (1921)
Rusby., *J. Amer. Pharm. Assoc.,* **13**, 98 (1924)
Villalba., *J. Soc. Chem. Ind.,* **44**, 205T (1925)
Elger., *Helv. Chim. Acta,* **11**, 164 (1927)
Manske, Perkin, Robinson., *J. Chem. Soc.,* 1 (1927)
Lewin., *Arch. exp. Path. Pharm.,* **129**, 133 (1928)
Lewin., *Compt. rend.,* **186**, 469 (1928)
Späth, Lederer., *Ber.,* **63**, 120 (1930)

Pharmacology:
Gunn *et al., Arch. int. Pharmacodyn.,* **50**, 379 (1935)
Sato., *Tohuku J. Exp. Med.,* **26**, 161 (1935)
Beer., *Arch. exp. Path. Pharm.,* **193**, 377, 393 (1939)
Raymond-Hamet., *Compt. rend.,* **212**, 408 (1941)
Raymond-Hamet., *C. r. Soc. biol.,* **135**, 69, 328 (1941)
Raymond-Hamet., *Compt. rend.,* **221**, 387 (1945)

HARRINGTONINE

$C_{28}H_{37}O_9N$

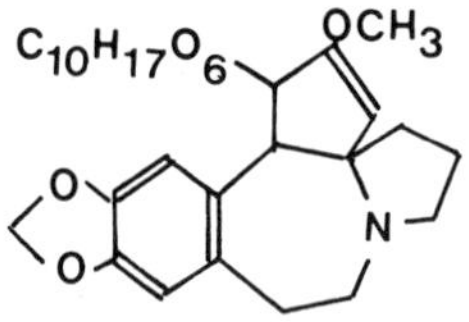

Recently isolated from *Cephalotaxus harringtonia* var. *drupacea*, the partial structure given above has been deduced from spectroscopic evidence, particularly the mass spectrum.

Powell *et al.*, *Tetrahedron Lett.*, 4081 (1969)

Structure:

Powell *et al.*, *Tetrahedron Lett.*, 815 (1970)

HASLERINE

M.p. 237°C

This uncharacterized alkaloid has been reported as occurring in the bark of *Aspidosperma quirandy* Hassler, together with aspidospermine and aspidosamine (q.v.).

Floriani., *Ann. Farm. Bioquim.*, **1**, 135 (1930)

Floriani., *Rev. Cent. Estud. Farm. Bioquim.*, **25**, 373, 423 (1935)

HASTACINE

$C_{18}H_{27}O_5N$

M.p. 170–1°C

A hepatotoxic alkaloid of the pyrrolizidine group obtained from *Cacalia hastata*, this base is laevorotatory with $[\alpha]_D - 72.34°$. On alkaline hydrolysis it yields hastanecinic acid, $C_9H_{15}O_3$, m.p. 148–9°C; $[\alpha]_D + 4.6°$ containing one hydroxyl and one carboxyl group and hastanecine, $C_8H_{15}O_2N$, m.p. 113–4°C; $[\alpha]_D - 9:07°$ which has been shown to be 7β-hydroxy-1α-hydroxylmethyl-8Hα-pyrrolizidine. The alkaloid is said to possess spasmolytic properties.

Konovalova, Men'shikov., *J. Gen. Chem., USSR*, **15**, 328 (1945)

Aasen, Culvenor, Smith., *J. Org. Chem.*, **34**, 4137 (1969)

HASUBANONINE

$C_{21}H_{27}O_5N$

M.p. 116°C

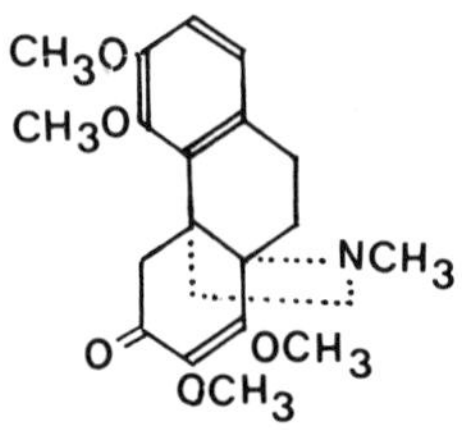

A phenanthrene type alkaloid occurring in *Stephania japonica* Miers., the base contains four methoxyl groups and one methylimino group. On reduction with $NaBH_4$ it gives quasi-axial dihydrohasubanonine and the quasi-equatorial dihydro derivative. On treatment with activated MnO_2 in $CHCl_3$, the former yields the original alkaloid and the lactam whereas the latter gives only hasubanonine. Hofmann degradation gives finally the methine base, m.p. 158–9°C (*dec.*) which, on treatment with Ac_2O and AcONa yields 3-acetoxy-1:5:6-trimethoxyphenanthrene, crystallizing from EtOH, m.p. 120–1°C. The total synthesis of the (±)-form of the alkaloid has been reported.

Kondo *et al., Ann. Rep. Itsuu Lab.,* 2, 35 (1951)
Kondo *et al., ibid,* 3, 37 (1953)
Kondo *et al., ibid,* 8, 41 (1957)

Structure:
Ibuka, Kitano., *Chem. Pharm. Bull.* (Tokyo), 15, 1809 (1967)
Ibuka *et al., J. Pharm. Soc., Japan,* 87, 1014 (1967)

Synthesis:
Ibuka, Tanaka, Inubushi., *Tetrahedron Lett.,* 4811 (1970)

(+−)(SR)-HAYATIDIN

$C_{37}H_{40}O_6N_2$

M.p. 179–180°C

Found in the roots of *Cissampelos pareira* L., this alkaloid is laevorotatory with $[\alpha]_D$ − 109° (pyridine). The ultraviolet spectrum in EtOH has an absorption maximum at 280 mμ which is shifted to 287 mμ in alkaline solution (4:1-EtOH:N/NaOH). It contains three methoxyl groups, two methylimino groups and one hydroxyl group in the molecule and forms an O-ethyl ether as an amorphous solid with no definite melting point. The structure, as a member of the bisbenzyl*iso*quinoline group of alkaloids, has been determined from chemical and spectroscopic data.

Bhatnagar, Popli., *Experientia,* 23, 242 (1967)

HAYATIN (*Alkaloid CP-1*)

$C_{36}H_{38}O_6N_2$

M.p. 303°C (*dec.*).

Also present in the roots of *Cissampelos pareira* L., this alkaloid crystallizes as colourless prismatic rods from a mixture of MeOH and pyridine. It is readily soluble in pyridine and aqueous Me_2CO, sparingly so in EtOH, MeOH, Me_2CO, $CHCl_3$ or AcOEt and insoluble in petroleum ether. It is optically inactive in both pyridine and HCl and gives no colour reaction with $FeCl_3$. It has been suggested that the structure is that of the $(++)(--)$ recemate of curine (q.v.).

Hayatin forms a series of crystalline salts and derivatives, e.g. the hydrochloride as colourless, prismatic rods, m.p. 286°C (*dec.*); aurichloride, m.p. 190—5°C (*dec.*); platinichloride, m.p. 320°C after sintering at 285°C; picrate, yellow needles, m.p. 234—5°C (*dec.*); methochloride, m.p. 306°C (*dec.*); methiodide, m.p. 281°C (*dec.*); methoplatinate, m.p. 285°C; butiodide, m.p. 249—250°C (*dec.*) and the triacetyl derivative, m.p. 183—4°C. The O-methyl ether forms a crystalline methiodide as small needles, m.p. 270—2°C (*dec.*).

Bhattacharji, Sharma, Dhar., *Bull. Nat. Inst. Sci. India*, 4, 39 (1955)

Mass spectra:
Milne, Plimmer., *J. Chem. Soc., C,* 1966 (1966)

HEDRANTHERINE

$C_{21}H_{24}O_4N_2$

M.p. Indefinite

An amorphous alkaloid which occurs in the leaves of *Hedranthera barteri,* this base is strongly laevorotatory with $[\alpha]_D^{24} - 459°$ (c 1.0, dimethylformamide). One hydroxyl, one methylimino and one methoxycarbonyl group are present.

Naranjo, Hesse, Schmid., *Helv. Chim. Acta,* 55, 1849 (1972)

HEDYOTINE

$C_{16}H_{22}O_3N_2$

A minor constituent of *Hedyotis auricularia* Linn., this alkaloid has been characterized as the crystalline hydrochloride, m.p. 245°C; nitrate, m.p. 252°C (*dec.*); aurichloride, m.p. 305—310°C (*dec.*) and the picrate, m.p. 265°C (*dec.*).

Dey, Lakshminarayanan., *Arch. Pharm.,* 271, 485 (1933)

HEIMIDINE

$C_{26}H_{31}O_6N$

This minor alkaloid of *Heimia salicifolia* has been shown to possess the same structure as Lythridine (q.v.) but with a *cis*-fuzed quinolizidine system.

El-Olemy *et al.*, *Lloydia*, **34**, 439 (1971)

HEIMINE

$C_{26}H_{29}O_6N$

M.p. 247.5–249°C

This alkaloid has also been isolated from *Heimia salicifolia*. It forms colourless crystals from EtOH and has $[\alpha]_D^{25} + 43°$ (c 0.205, CHCl$_3$). The ultraviolet spectrum shows two absorption maxima at 260 and 285 mμ. A crystalline hydrochloride, m.p. 326°C (*dec.*), has been prepared.

Blomster, Schwarting, Bobbitt., *Lloydia*, **27**, 15 (1964)

HELERITRINE

Bocconia cordata yields this alkaloid as a minor constituent. The base is probably at its maximum concentration in the foliage of the plant during the blossoming period and may be separated from the accompanying alkaloids by chromatography on neutral alumina.

Kiryakov, Kitova, Georgieva., *Compt. Rend. Acad. Bulg. Sci.*, **20**, 189 (1967)

HELEURINE

$C_{16}H_{27}O_4N$

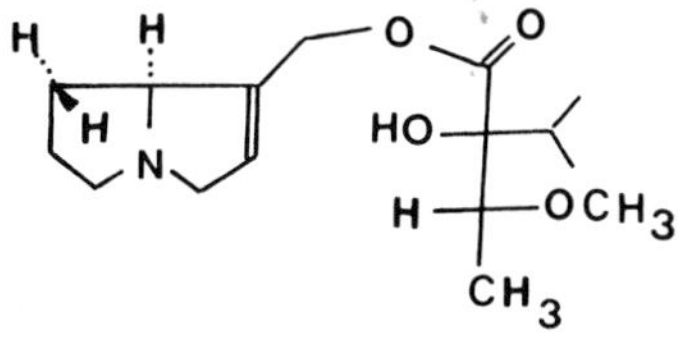

This alkaloid has been isolated from several *Heliotropium* species and the structure, as one of the pyrrolizidine bases, determined from the infrared, NMR and mass spectra.

Culvenor., *Austral. J. Chem.*, **7**, 287 (1954)

HELIOSUPINE

$C_{20}H_{31}O_7N$

M.p. Indefinite

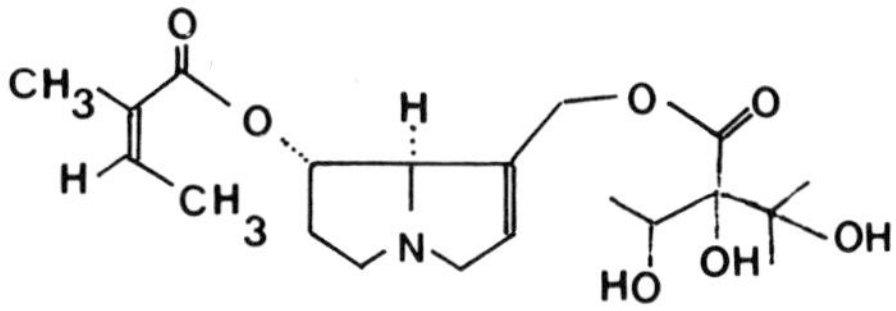

Present in both *Cynoglossum officinale* L. and *Heliotropium supinum* L., this base is obtained in the form of a gum which cannot be crystallized. It has $[\alpha]_D^{20} - 4.3°$ (c 5.10, EtOH) and is characterized as the picrate which forms a crystalline monohydrate, m.p. 97–100°C. Although the water of crystallization may be removed in a vacuum at 80°C, the resulting product is a non-crystallizable resin. Alkaline hydrolysis of the alkaloid furnishes heliotridine, Me_2CO and angelic acid. Catalytic hydrogenation yields echimidinic acid. The (+)-form of the alkaloid is Echimidine (q.v.).

Denisova, Men'shikov, Utkin., *Dokl. Akad. Nauk, SSSR*, **93**, 59 (1953)
Culvenor., *Austral. J. Chem.*, **9**, 512 (1956)
Crout., *J. Chem. Soc., C*, 1968 (1966)

HELIOTRINE

$C_{16}H_{27}O_5N$

M.p. 125–6°C

A pyrrolizidine alkaloid found in *Heliotropium lasiocarpum* F and M., the base is obtained in the form of colourless prisms from Me_2CO. It has $[\alpha]_D^{20} - 3.75°$ (EtOH) or $- 75°$ ($CHCl_3$). It is soluble in EtOH, $CHCl_3$ or H_2O but only slightly so in petroleum ether and Et_2O. It yields a crystalline methiodide, m.p. 108–111°C and contains a methoxyl group, two hydroxyl groups and a tertiary nitrogen atom. Alkaline hydrolysis yields heliotridine, m.p. 116.5–118°C; $[\alpha]_D + 31°$ (MeOH), forming a hydrochloride, m.p. 122–4°C and an acid, heliotric (heliotrinic) acid, m.p. 92.5–94.5°C; $[\alpha]_D - 12°$ (H_2O). On hydrogenation in the presence of PtO_2 it absorbs two molecules of hydrogen giving, as scission products, heliotric acid and hydroxyheliotridane, m.p. 60–5°C, b.p. 126–8°C/12 mm; $[\alpha]_D - 14.5°$ (H_2O).

Men'shikov., *Ber.*, **65**, 974 (1932)
Men'shikov., *ibid*, **66**, 875 (1933)
Men'shikov., *ibid*, **68**, 1051 (1935)
Men'shikov, Schdanowitsch., *ibid*, **69**, 1110 (1936)
Men'shikov, Kuzovkov., *Chem. Abstr.*, **44**, 1113 (1950)

HELIOTRINE N-OXIDE

$C_{16}H_{27}O_6N$

M.p. 171–2°C

The seeds of *Heliotropium europeum* have been found to contain this alkaloid. The structure follows from the spectroscopic evidence.

Culvenor, Drummond, Price., *Austral. J. Chem.*, **7**, 277 (1954)
Culvenor., *ibid*, **7**, 287 (1954)

HEMITOXIFERINE I

$C_{20}H_{25}O_2N_2^+$

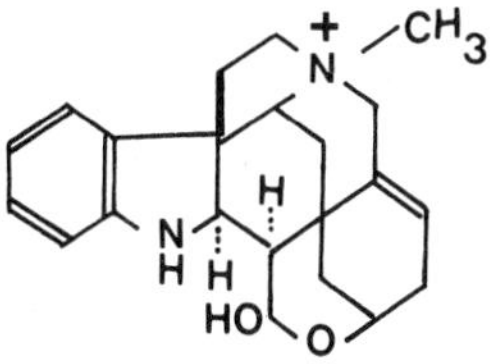

A quaternary alkaloid of the curare type isolated from the bark of *Strychnos toxifera* obtained from British Guiana, this base may also be obtained by the action of mineral acids on Toxiferine I (q.v.). It is characterized as the chloride which is laevorotatory with $[\alpha]_D^{24} - 43°$ (c 1.0, H_2O) and the picrate, yellow prisms from aqueous Me_2CO, m.p. 233–5°C. The alkaloid gives a characteristic orange colour with $Ce(SO_4)_2$.

Asmis *et al.*, *Helv. Chim. Acta*, **38**, 1661 (1955)
Battersby, Hodson., *J. Chem. Soc.*, 736 (1960)
Battersby *et al.*, *ibid*, 412 (1961)

HENNINGSAMINE (*Acetyldiaboline*)

$C_{23}H_{26}O_4N_2$

M.p. 205–6°C

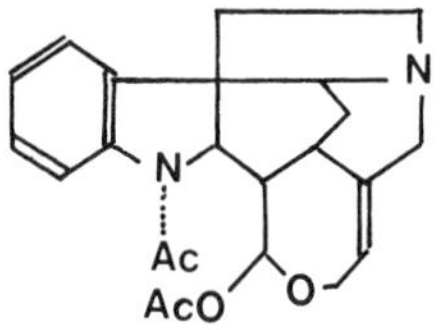

The bark of *Strychnos henningsii* Gilg. yields this crystalline alkaloid which forms colourless needles when crystallized from a mixture of AcOEt and light petroleum. The ultraviolet spectrum in EtOH shows two absorption maxima at 208 and 252 mμ. It contains one N-acetyl group and one O-acetyl group and gives a crystalline picrate, m.p. 229–231°C and a methiodide, m.p. 231–3°C. The structure has been determined primarily from the fragmentation pattern of the mass spectrum.

Grossert *et al.*, *J. Chem. Soc.*, 2812 (1965)

Structure:
Biemann *et al.*, *J. Chem. Soc.*, 2814 (1965)

HENNINGSOLINE

$C_{22}H_{26}O_5N_2$

M.p. 207–9°C

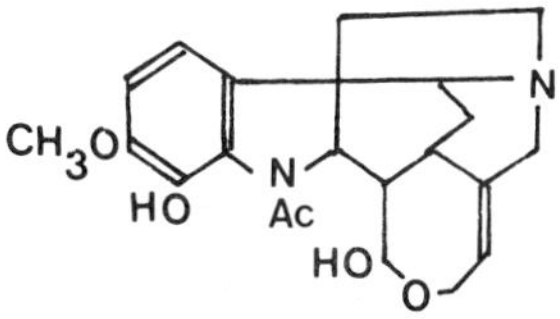

A further strychnine type alkaloid present in the bark of *Strychnos henningsii* Gilg, this laevorotatory base has $[\alpha]_D^{20} - 200°$ (c 1.0, $CHCl_3$). The ultraviolet spectrum in EtOH exhibits an absorption maximum at 256 mμ and an inflexion at 285 mμ. It yields several crystalline salts and derivatives, e.g. the perchlorate, m.p. 253–4°C (*dec.*); picrate, m.p. 167–8°C; oxime, m.p. 254–5°C; reineckate, decomposing above 200°C; the monobenzoyl derivative, m.p. 180–2°C, yielding a hydrochloride, m.p. 175–7°C; the dibenzoyl compound, m.p. 214–220°C and the *p*-toluenesulphonyl derivative, m.p. 233–4°C. The 17-acetyl derivative also occurs naturally (q.v.).

Grossert *et al., J. Chem. Soc.,* 2812 (1965)

Structure:
Biemann *et al., J. Chem. Soc.,* 2818 (1965)

HEPTAPHYLLINE

$C_{18}H_{17}O_2N$

M.p. 170–1°C

This weakly basic alkaloid is obtained from the hexane extract of the roots of *Clausena heptaphylla* Wt. & Arn. The ultraviolet spectrum has absorption maxima at 234, 278, 298 and 346 mμ. A crystalline 2:4-dinitrophenylhydrazone, m.p. 315–6°C has been prepared. With FeCl$_3$ the base gives a deep blue colour and also reduces ammoniacal silver nitrate. When treated with polyphosphoric acid, ring closure of the ortho hydroxyl and dimethylallyl groups occurs giving the corresponding chromane, cycloheptaphylline. The structure has been determined mainly from the infrared and NMR spectra. The alkaloid has been synthesized from 2-hydroxycarbazole and N-methylformanilide followed by reaction with γ,γ-dimethylallyl bromide, giving the base in an overall yield of 5 per cent.

Joshi *et al., Tetrahedron Lett.,* 4019 (1967)

Synthesis:
Joshi, Rane., *Chem. Ind.,* 685 (1968)

HEPTAZOLINE (*8-hydroxyheptaphylline*)

$C_{18}H_{17}O_3N$

M.p. 213–4°C

A further alkaloid present in the stem bark of *Clausena heptaphylla* Wt. & Arn., the structure has been elucidated by chemical and spectroscopic analysis and comparison with heptaphylline.

Chakraborty, Das, Islam., *J. Ind. Chem. Soc.,* **47**, 1197 (1970)

668

HERBACEINE

$C_{23}H_{30}O_5N_2$

M.p. 144°C (*dec.*).

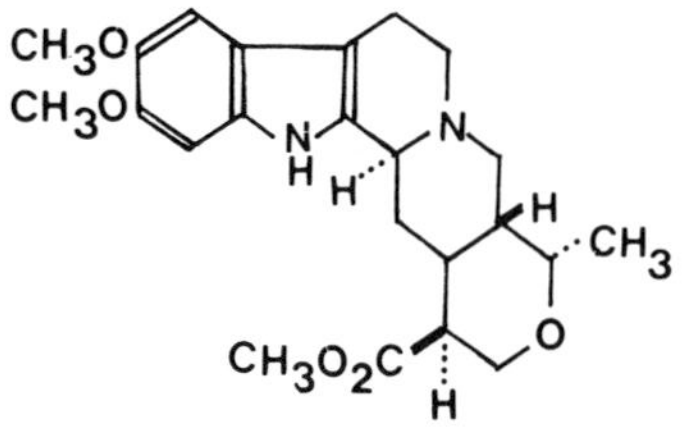

A strychnine type alkaloid isolated from *Vinca herbacea* W.K., the base yields colourless crystals from MeOH and has $[\alpha]_D^{22} - 219°$ (c 0.544, pyridine). The ultraviolet spectrums shows two absorption maxima at 226 and 300 mμ. Two methoxyl groups, a methoxycarbonyl group, a methyl group and a methylimino group are present. The alkaloid yields a methiodide as deep orange crystals, m.p. 219–223°C. The structure has been determined from spectroscopic data together with the stereochemistry.

Mollov *et al., Compt. Rend. Acad. Bulg. Sci.,* **14**, 43 (1961)
Ognyanov, Pyuskyulev., *Chem. Ber.,* **99**, 1008 (1966)
Stereochemistry:
Ognyanov *et al., Chem. Commun.,* 579 (1967)

HERBALINE

$C_{23}H_{30}O_6N_2$

M.p. 276–8°C (*dec.*).

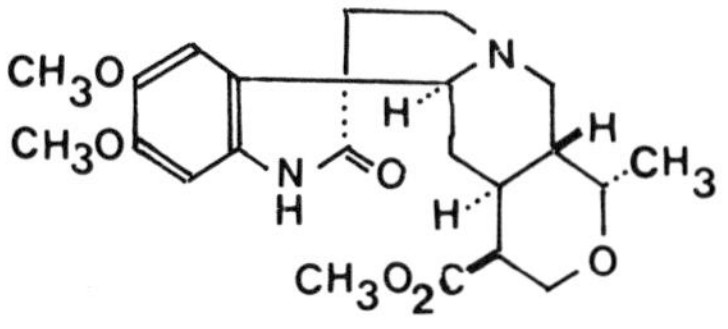

This alkaloid is also present in *Vinca herbacea* W.K. and forms colourless crystals from EtOH or MeOH. It is laevorotatory with $[\alpha]_D^{20} - 147°$ (c 1.5, pyridine) and the ultraviolet spectrum exhibits absorption maxima at 215, 273 and 305 mμ. By means of the infrared, NMR and mass spectra, the above structure has been established.

Ognyanov., *Chem. Ber.,* **99**, 2052 (1966)
Stereochemistry:
Ognyanov *et al., Chem. Commun.,* 579 (1967)

HERBAVINE

$C_{23}H_{28}O_4N_2$

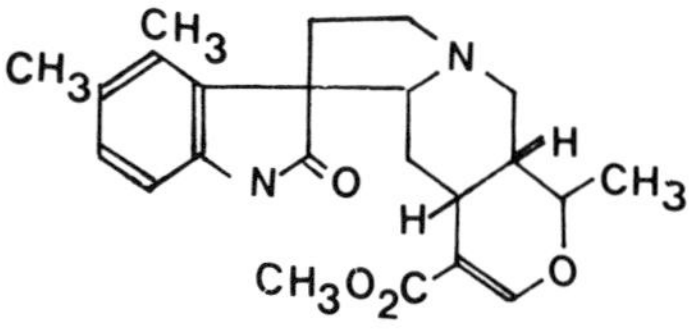

An indole alkaloid present as a minor constituent in *Vinca herbacea* grown in

Georgia SSR. Infrared, NMR and mass spectrometry show the alkaloid to have the probable structure given above.

Dzhakeli, Mudzhiri., *Soobshch. Akad. Nauk. Gruz. SSR,* **57**, 353 (1970)

HERNANDALINE

$C_{29}H_{31}O_7N$

M.p. 170–171.5°C

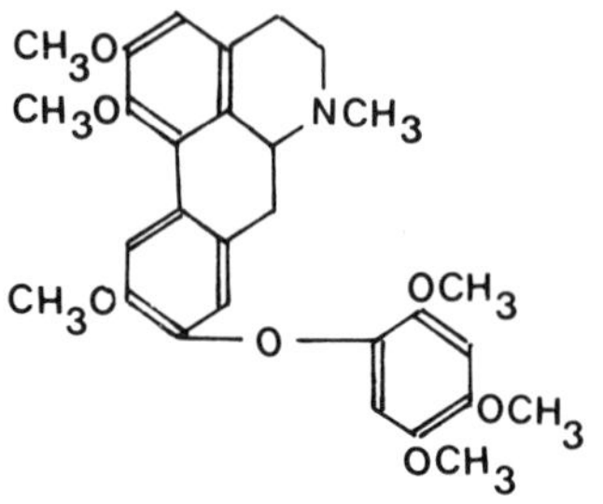

Isolated from *Hernandia ovigera* L. (Lauriceae), this alkaloid is obtained as colourless needles when crystallized from EtOH. It is dextrorotatory with $[\alpha]_D^{25} + 35.6°$ (c 0.10, $CHCl_3$). In EtOH, the ultraviolet spectrum shows absorption maxima at 216, 278 and 304 mμ. The alkaloid contains five methoxyl groups, one formyl group and one methylimino group and has the basic aporphine skeleton.

Cava *et al., Tetrahedron Lett.,* 4279 (1966)

Synthesis:
Cava., *U.S. Patent,* 3,376,305 April 2, 1968
Kupchan, Liepa., *Ger. Offen.,* 2,161,187 June 14, 1973

HERNANDEZINE

$C_{39}H_{44}O_7N_2$

M.p. 192–3°C

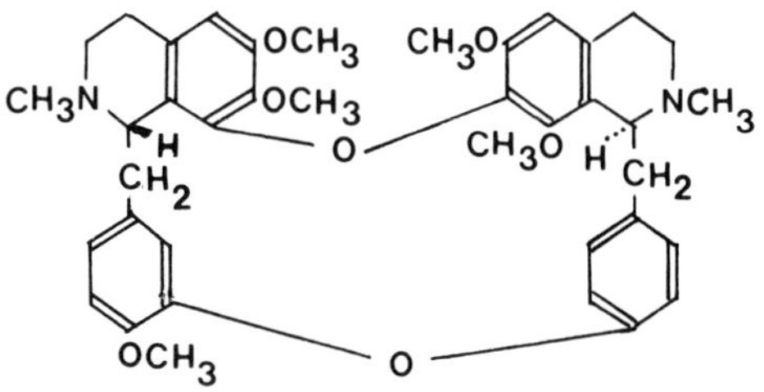

A bisbenzyl*iso*quinoline alkaloid present in *Tralictrum hernandezii* where it is found mainly in the roots. The base forms colourless crystals from cyclohexane which are anhydrous. It may also be crystallized from Me_2CO, MeOH or Et_2O but in each case it forms solvates which have lower melting points than that given above. The alkaloid is strongly dextrorotatory with $[\alpha]_D^{20} + 250°$ (c 0.2, $CHCl_3$). There are two absorption maxima present in the ultraviolet spectrum occurring at 209 and 283 mμ. Five methoxyl groups and two methylimino groups are present in the molecule.

Padilla, Herran., *Tetrahedron,* **18**, 427 (1962)

670

HERNANDINE

$C_{19}H_{19}O_5N$

M.p. 240–1°C

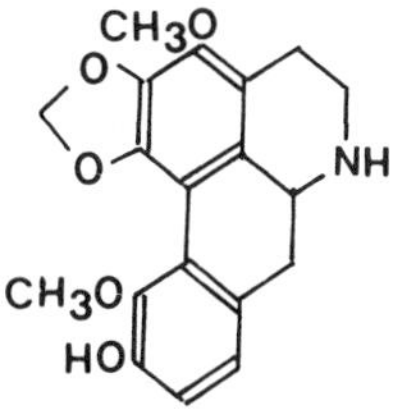

A noraporphine alkaloid found in *Hernandia bivalvis* Benth., this base gives colourless crystals from MeOH or EtOH and is dextrorotatory having $[\alpha]_D^{27} +$ 347°. A crystalline hydrochloride is known, m.p. 260–1°C (*dec.*) and the O,N-dimethylhernandine methiodide, m.p. 234–6°C; $[\alpha]_D + 95°$. The structure has been confirmed by the synthesis of the (±)-form, m.p. 227–8°C (*dec.*).

Greenhalgh, Lahey., *Current Trends in Heterocyclic Chemistry*, Butterworth, London, 100, (1966)

Revised structure:
Soh, Lahey, Greenhalgh., *Tetrahedron Lett.*, 5279 (1966)

Synthesis:
Soh, Lahey., *Tetrahedron Lett.*, 19 (1968)

HERNANDOLINE

$C_{20}H_{25}O_5N$

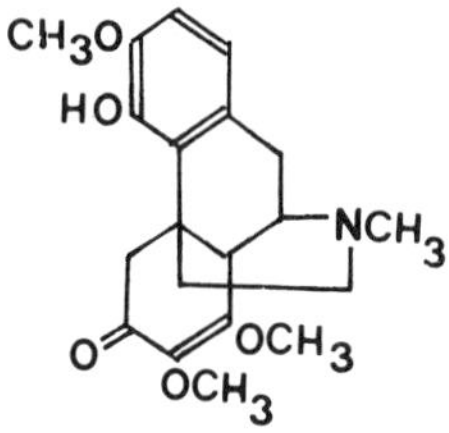

This alkaloid has been isolated from *Stephania hernandifolia* and characterized as the O-methyl ether, m.p. 192–3°C. The structure has been determined from spectroscopic data and contains three methoxyl, one hydroxyl and one methylimino group.

Fadeeva *et al.*, *Farmatsiya*, **19**, 28 (1970)

HERNANDOLINOL

$C_{20}H_{27}O_5N$

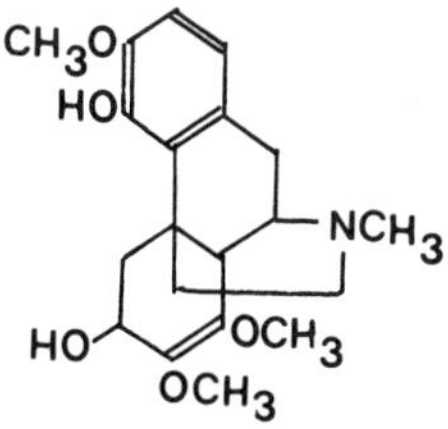

Also present in *Stephania hernandifolia*, this alkaloid is the secondary alcohol corresponding to hernandoline as the ketone.

Fadeeva *et al.*, *Khim. Prir. Soedin.*, **6**, 492 (1970)

HERNANDONINE

$C_{18}H_9O_5N$

M.p. $> 280°C$

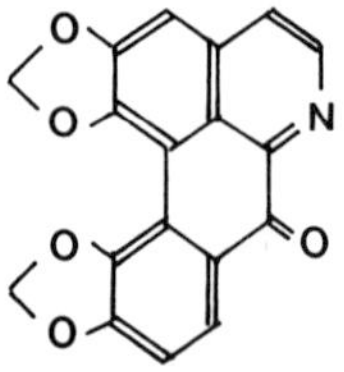

A dibenzoquinolinone alkaloid obtained from the trunk bark of *Hernandia ovigera* L., this base is purified by crystallization from $CHCl_3$ when it forms orange-yellow crystals, the colour being due to the high degree of conjugation in the molecule. It contains two methylenedioxy groups and gives an ultraviolet spectrum having absorption maxima at 222, 265, 364 and 426 mμ.

Ito, Furukawa., *Tetrahedron Lett.*, 3023 (1970)

HERNOVINE

$C_{18}H_{19}O_4N$

M.p. $234-6°C$ (*dec.*).

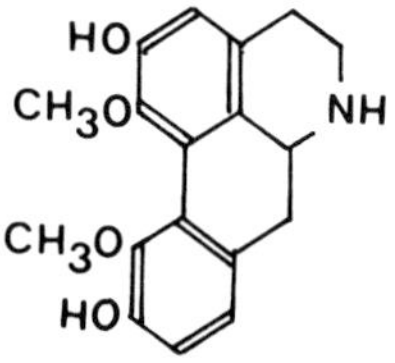

A second alkaloid found in the trunk bark of *Hernandia ovigera* L., this phenolic noraporphine base yields colourless plates from MeOH. The ultraviolet spectrum has absorption maxima at 221, 272 and 306 mμ. The base contains two methoxyl groups and two hydroxyl groups, forming an O,O'-dimethyl ether identical with catalpifoline (q.v.).

Cava *et al.*, *Tetrahedron Lett.*, 1577 (1966)
Cava *et al.*, *ibid*, 4279 (1966)

HERPESTINE

$C_{34}H_{46}O_6N_2$

M.p. $116-8°C$

The leaves and roots of *Monniera cuneifolia* Michx. (*Herpestis monniera* HB and K. yield this base as the major component of the alkaloidal extract. It forms colourless crystals and yields the following crystalline salts: sulphate, decomposing at 120°C; aurichloride, m.p. $210-3°C$ (*dec.*); platinichloride, decomposing at 242°C and the tartrate, m.p. $209-210°C$. The alkaloid behaves as a diacidic base.

Basu, Walia., *Ind. J. Pharm.*, **6**, 85, 91 (1944)
Basu, Pabrai., *Quart. J. Pharm. Pharmacol.*, **20**, 137 (1947)

672

HERVINE

$C_{23}H_{27}O_4N_2$

M.p. 173–5°C

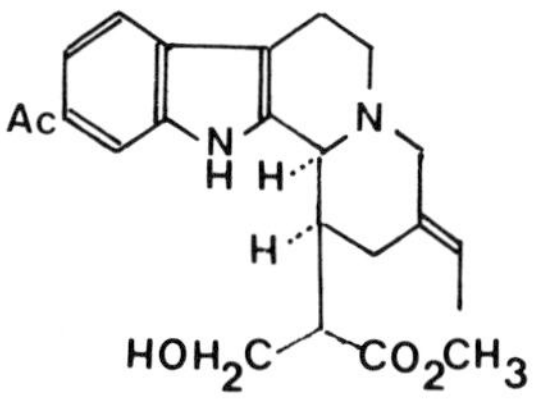

This alkaloid from *Vinca herbacea* is laevorotatory with $[\alpha]_D - 93°$ (c 0.2, EtOH). Treatment with $LiAlH_4$ or $NaBH_4$ gives hervinol while acetylation with Ac_2O in pyridine yields the O-acetate. The structure given has been proposed on the basis of spectroscopic evidence.

Ognyanov *et al.*, *Monatsh.*, **97**, 857 (1966)
Pgnyanov *et al.*, *Helv. Chim. Acta*, **50**, 754 (1967)

HESPERIDINE

$C_{20}H_{19}O_5N$

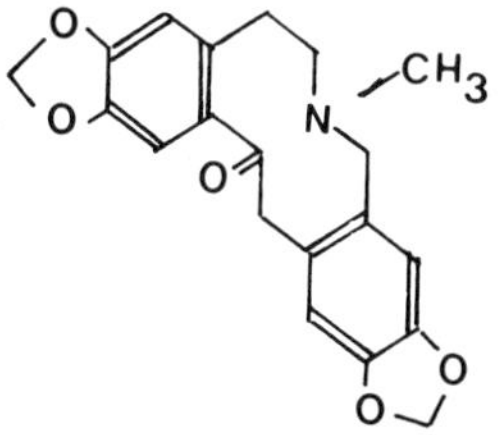

An isomer of Protopine (q.v.), this alkaloid occurs in the bark of *Zanthoxylum conspersipunctatum*. The structure has been established from chemical and spectroscopic data.

Johns *et al.*, *Austral. J. Chem.*, **22**, 2233 (1969)

HETERATISINE

$C_{22}H_{33}O_5N$

M.p. 267–8°C (*dec.*).

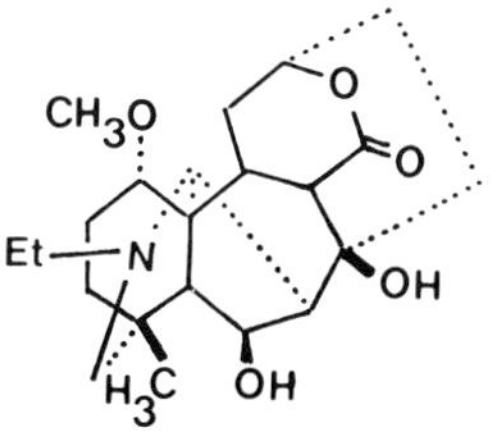

An atisine alkaloid obtained from the mother liquors which accumulate during the isolation of Atisine (q.v.) from *Aconitum heterophyllum*, this base has $[\alpha]_D^{27} + 40°$ (MeOH). It contains a lactone ring which is opened by alkali and reformed on acidification. The alkaloid yields a hydrochloride, m.p. 265–270°C (*dec.*); a hydrobromide as the monohydrate from H_2O; the perchlorate, colourless needles, m.p. 252–6°C (*dec.*); an acetyl derivative, m.p. 161.5–167°C; $[\alpha]_D + 16°$ (c 1.66, $CHCl_3$) and the benzoyl compound, m.p. 213–4°C;

$[\alpha]_D^{25}$ + 73° (EtOH), giving a crystalline hydrochloride, m.p. 218–221°C (*dec.*). The last compound is readily hydrolyzed to benzoic acid and the parent alkaloid and Jacobs and Craig have suggested that heteratisine does not occur naturally in the plant but is produced from the benzoyl derivative during the extraction process.

Jacobs, Craig., *J. Biol. Chem.*, **143**, 605 (1942)
Jacobs, Craig., *ibid*, **147**, 571 (1943)
Przybylska., *Can. J. Chem.*, **41**, 2911 (1963)
Aneja, Pelletier., *Tetrahedron Lett.*, 669 (1964)
Edwards, Ferrari., *Can. J. Chem.*, **42**, 172 (1964)

Mass spectra:
Pelletier, Aneja., *Tetrahedron Lett.*, 557 (1967)

Absolute configuration:
Aneja, Pelletier., *Tetrahedron Lett.*, 215 (1965)

HETEROPHYLLIDINE

$C_{21}H_{31}O_5N$

M.p. 269–272°C

The rhizomes of *Aconitum heterophylla* yields this atisine alkaloid which is dextrorotatory with $[\alpha]_D$ + 42.3° (c 1.26, MeOH). Since the base contains a γ-lactone ring it may be recovered from hot aqueous alkaline solutions on acidification. The 1-methyl ether is identical with Heteratisine (q.v.).

Pelletier, Aneja., *Tetrahedron Lett.*, 557 (1967)

HETEROPHYLLINE

Two alkaloids of this name have been described in the literature and their characteristics are given below.

$C_{21}H_{31}O_4N$

M.p. 221.5–223°C

An atisine alkaloid present in the rhizomes of *Aconitum heterophyllum*, this base is slightly dextrorotatory with $[\alpha]_D$ + 10.5° (c 2.0, MeOH). Like the preceding alkaloid, it contains a γ-lactone ring which is opened by alkali and reformed on acidification. The structure has been determined primarily from the mass spectrum.

Pelletier, Aneja., *Tetrahedron Lett.*, 557 (1967)

$C_{21}H_{26}O_4N_2$

M.p. 186.5–187.5°C

One of the *Rauwolfia* alkaloids, this base occurs in *R. heterophylla* and has $[\alpha]_D^{25} - 89°$ (CHCl$_3$) or $- 66°$ (pyridine). It yields crystalline salts, e.g. the hydrochloride as colourless needles, m.p. 239–241°C (*dec.*); nitrate, m.p. 258.1–259.5°C; oxalate as fine needles, m.p. 233–5°C (*dec.*); tartrate, crystals from EtOH, m.p. 197–200°C; picrate as yellow cubic crystals, m.p. 213–5°C (*dec.*) and the diacetyl derivative, m.p. 152–5°C; $[\alpha]_D^{25} - 69°$ (CHCl$_3$). With concentrated HNO$_3$ the alkaloid gives a stable orange colour.

Hochstein, Murai, Boegemann., *J. Amer. Chem. Soc.*, 77, 3551 (1955)

HETEROPHYLLISINE

$C_{22}H_{33}O_4N$

M.p. 178–9°C

A further atisine alkaloid isolated from the rhizomes of *Aconitum heterophyllum*, this base has $[\alpha]_D + 15.5$ (c 0.9, MeOH). It is also a lactone alkaloid, the ring being opened by alkali and closed by acid. The structure has been determined spectroscopically, particularly from the mass spectrum.

Pelletier, Aneja., *Tetrahedron Lett.*, 557 (1967)

HETISINE

$C_{20}H_{27}O_3N$

M.p. 253–6°C (*dec.*).

An atisine alkaloid present in the mother liquors of the extract from the roots of *Aconitum heterophyllum* after the removal of atisine, this base crystallizes from C_6H_6 with solvent and effervesces at 145°C before melting. When heated under vacuum, the alkaloid sublimes at 190–210°C/0.1 mm. It is dextrorotatory with $[\alpha]_D^{25} + 13.7°$ (EtOH). The crystalline hydrochloride changes at 320°C and ceases to be doubly refractive at 328–335°C. This salt has $[\alpha]_D^{25} + 12.7°$ (EtOH). Stable to alkalies, the base furnishes a dihydro derivative on hydrogenation, m.p. 136–9°C followed by solidification and remelting at 250–5°C, yielding a crystalline hydrochloride, m.p. 333°C (*dec.*). The methiodide melts above 300°C and may be decomposed by silver oxide, followed by pyrolysis, to give desmethylhetisine, $C_{21}H_{29}O_3N$, m.p. 122–4°C, forming a hydrochloride, m.p. 303–5°C; a methiodide, m.p. 245–250°C and a methochloride, m.p. 285–290°C. Selenium dehydrogenation yields a mixture of products, two neutral hydrocarbons, pimanthrene and $C_{34}H_{60}$, b.p. 260°C and three basic products isolated as their picrates with m.p. 225–230°C (*dec.*), 235–245°C (*dec.*) and 320–5°C respectively, of which the first two may be identical. Like the majority of the atisine alkaloids, hetisine is relatively non-toxic compared with the corresponding aconitines.

Jacobs, Craig., *J. Biol. Chem.*, **143**, 605 (1942)
Jacobs, Craig., *ibid*, **147**, 571 (1943)
Jacobs, Heubner., *ibid*, **170**, 189 (1947)
Przybylska., *Can. J. Chem.*, **40**, 566 (1962)

HETISINONE (*Dehydrohetisine*)

$C_{20}H_{25}O_3N$

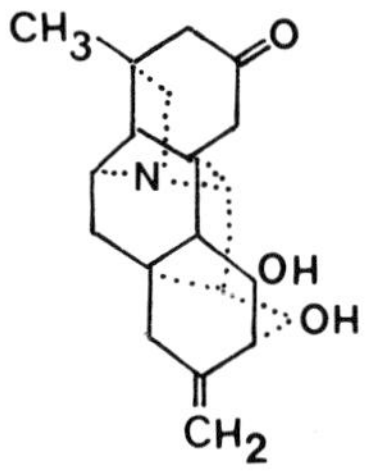

First obtained as a transformation product of hetisine, this alkaloid has been found to occur naturally in *Delphinium denudatum* and subsequently in *D. cardinalis*. The structure has been confirmed by spectroscopic methods.

Aplin *et al.*, *Can. J. Chem.*, **46**, 2635 (1968)

HEXADECANOYLSEVERINE

$C_{41}H_{63}O_5N$

M.p. 113–4°C

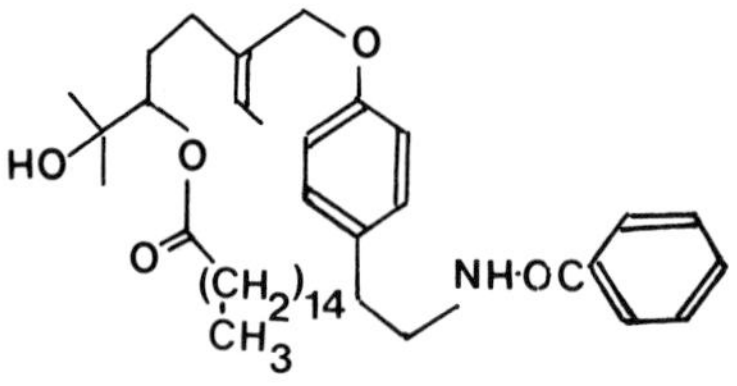

This alkaloid from *Severina buxifolia* (Poir) Ten., crystallizes as colourless prisms from C_6H_6. The ultraviolet spectrum shows absorption maxima at 226, 272 and 282 mμ. Alkaline hydrolysis yields severine, m.p. 141–3°C and hexadecanoic acid.

Dreyer., *Tetrahedron*, **23**, 4613 (1967)

HIMANDRAVINE

$C_{22}H_{35}O_2N$

M.p. 119°C

One of several alkaloids isolated from the bark of *Himantandra* (*Galbulimina*) *belgraveana*, this base has $[\alpha]_D^{18} + 23°$ (c 1.89, CHCl$_3$) and contains no N-methyl group. It yields a crystalline hydrochloride from EtOH-Me$_2$CO, m.p. 238–240°C and an N-methyl derivative, m.p. 129°C; $[\alpha]_D - 7.5°$ (c 0.94, CHCl$_3$). It has been shown to be a stereoisomer of himbeline (q.v.).

Brown *et al.*, *Austral. J. Chem.*, 9, 283 (1956)
Pinhey, Ritchie, Taylor., *ibid*, 14, 106 (1961)

HIMANDRELINE

$C_{32}H_{41}O_3N$

M.p. 189–190°C

This alkaloid from *Himantandra baccata* forms colourless crystals from a mixture of C$_6$H$_6$ and light petroleum. It has $[\alpha]_D^{14} - 12°$ (c 1.01, CHCl$_3$) and has been shown to be a polymorphous form of himandridine (q.v.).

Brown *et al.*, *Austral. J. Chem.*, 9, 283 (1956)
Binns *et al.*, *ibid*, 18, 569 (1965)

HIMANDRIDINE

$C_{30}H_{37}O_7N$

M.p. 204–5°C

A constituent of *Himantandra baccata* bark, this alkaloid may be crystallized from aqueous MeOH, C$_6$H$_6$-hexane or AcOEt-light petroleum. It has $[\alpha]_D^{18} - 22°$ (c 2.0, CHCl$_3$). The ultraviolet spectrum in EtOH has absorption maxima at 230, 272 and 280 mμ, while in acid solution (HCl-EtOH), the maxima occur at 228, 273 and 280 mμ. The alkaloid forms a crystalline hydriodide, m.p. 194–5°C and a 13-acetyl and 20-acetyl derivative which are Galbulimina alkaloids G.B.6 and G.B.7 respectively.

Brown *et al.*, *Austral. J. Chem.*, 9, 283 (1956)

Structure:
Mander, Ritchie, Taylor., *Austral. J. Chem.*, 20, 981, 1021 (1967)

HIMANDRINE

$C_{30}H_{37}O_6N$

M.p. 185–6°C

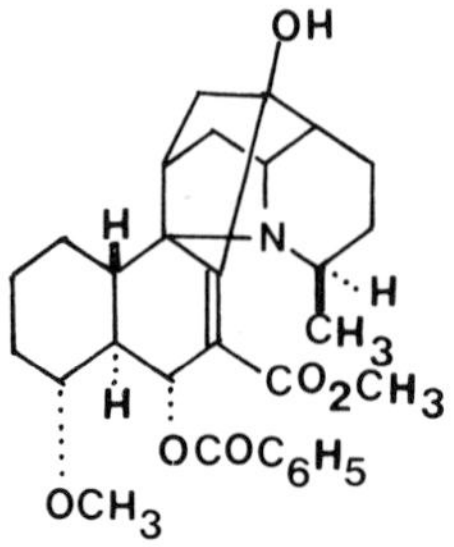

This alkaloid from the bark of *Himantandra baccata* and also from *H. belgraveana*, crystallizes from EtOH and has $[\alpha]_D^{20} - 38°$ (c 1.22, $CHCl_3$). The EtOH solution gives an ultraviolet spectrum with absorption maxima at 230, 272 and 280 mμ, while in HCl-EtOH solution, these occur at 228, 272 and 280 mμ. The base forms crystalline salts and derivatives, of which the following have been prepared: hydrochloride, m.p. 222°C (*dec.*); hydriodide, m.p. 201–2°C and methosulphate, m.p. 202°C.

Brown *et al., Austral. J. Chem.,* **9**, 283 (1956)

Structure:
Guise *et al., Austral. J. Chem.,* **20**, 1029 (1967)

HIMBACINE

$C_{22}H_{35}O_2N$

M.p. 132°C

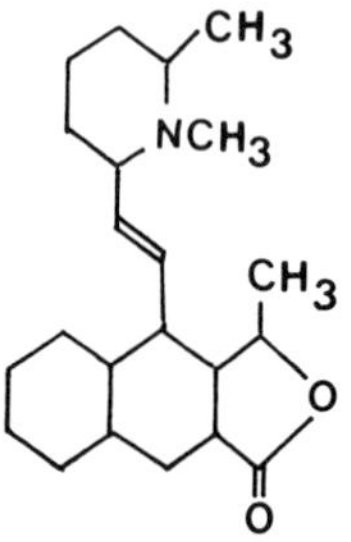

Obtained from the bark of *Himantandra baccata* and *H. belgraveana,* this base forms colourless crystals from n-heptane and has $[\alpha]_D^{14} + 63°$ (c 1.04, $CHCl_3$). It contains one N-methyl group and forms a crystalline hydrochloride monohydrate, m.p. 267°C; the hydrobromide, m.p. 192–3°C and the aurichloride, m.p. 125–7°C.

Brown *et al., Austral. J. Chem.,* **9**, 283 (1956)
Pinhey, Ritchie, Taylor., *ibid,* **14**, 106 (1961)
Fridrichsons, Mathieson., *Acta Cryst.,* **15**, 119 (1962)

HIMBADINE

$C_{21}H_{31}O_2N$

M.p. 110–4°C

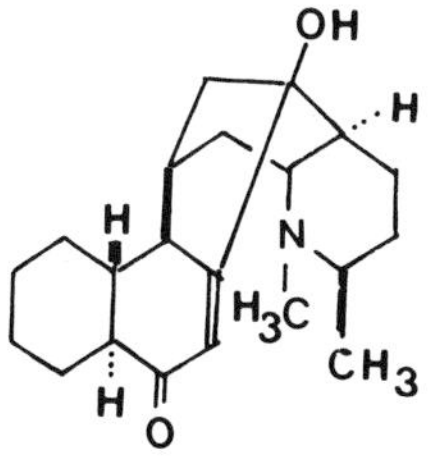

The bark of *Himantandra baccata* yields this alkaloid which is usually obtained in the form of the hemihydrate. It has $[\alpha]_D^{25} - 42°$ (c 1.43, CHCl$_3$) and yields crystalline salts, e.g. the hydrochloride, m.p. 233–5°C; perchlorate, m.p. 239°C; methiodide, m.p. 247–9°C and the methosulphate, m.p. 237–8°C. It also forms an oxime, m.p. 200–4°C as yellowish crystals; a 2:4-dinitrophenylhydrazone, orange needles, m.p. 148°C (perchlorate, orange plates, m.p. 234°C *dec.*) and an O-acetyl derivative, m.p. 120°C; $[\alpha]_D^{20} - 27°$ (c 1.51, CHCl$_3$). The alkaloid contains one methyl, one hydroxyl and one methylimino group.

Brown *et al.*, *Austral. J. Chem.*, **9**, 283 (1956)
Structure:
Mander *et al.*, *Austral. J. Chem.*, **20**, 1473 (1967)

HIMBELINE

$C_{21}H_{33}O_2N$

M.p. 100°C

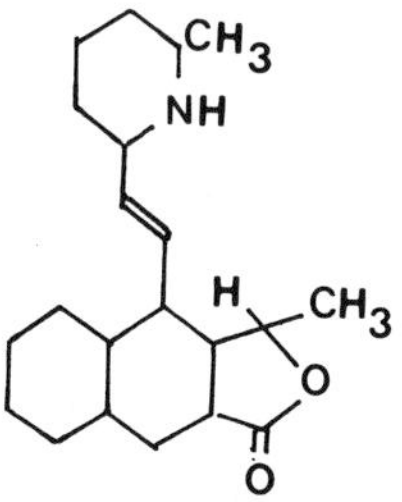

An alkaloid present in the bark of *Himantandra belgraveana*, the base yields colourless crystals from petroleum ether and has $[\alpha]_D^{18} + 19°$ (c 2.4, CHCl$_3$). It furnishes a hydrochloride monohydrate, m.p. 265–6°C.

Brown *et al.*, *Austral. J. Chem.*, **9**, 283 (1956)
Pinhey, Ritchie, Taylor., *ibid*, **14**, 106 (1961)

HIMBOSINE

$C_{35}H_{41}O_{10}N$

M.p. 262°C

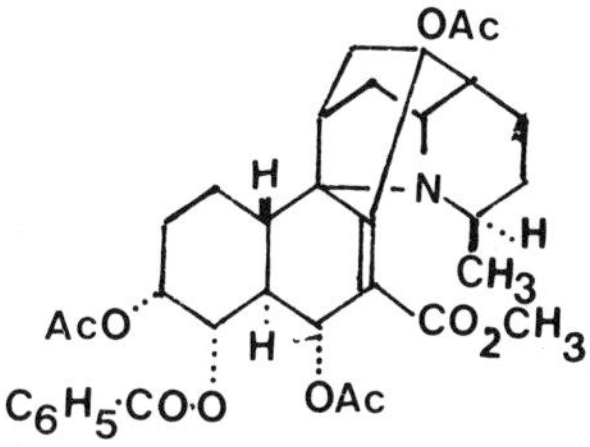

This base is obtained in the form of colourless, rectangular prisms from CHCl$_3$-

MeOH and was originally assigned the empirical formula $C_{35}H_{41}O_{13}N$. It is present in the bark of *Himantandra baccata* and is dextrorotatory with $[\alpha]_D^{15} + 55°$ (c 0.89, CHCl$_3$) or $[\alpha]_D^{25} + 28°$ (c 1.1, CHCl$_3$). The ethanol solution gives an ultraviolet spectrum with absorption maxima at 229, 273 and 280 mμ. That in HCl-EtOH solution, has the absorption maximum in exactly the same positions. A crystalline hydrobromide has been prepared as colourless needles, m.p. 228°C, this being used to determine the crystal structure.

Brown *et al., Austral. J. Chem.*, **9**, 283 (1956)

Crystal structure:

Lovell., *Proc. Chem. Soc.*, 58 (1964)

HIMDRELINE

$C_{32}H_{41}O_7N$

M.p. 189–190°C

Present in the bark of *Himantandra belgraveana*, this alkaloid has $[\alpha]_D^{14} - 12°$ (c 1.01, CHCl$_3$). It yields colourless crystals from a mixture of C_6H_6 and light petroleum.

Brown *et al., Austral. J. Chem.*, **9**, 283 (1956)

HIMGALINE

$C_{20}H_{31}O_2N$

M.p. 222–4°C

Present in several *Himantandra* species, this alkaloid is obtained as silky needles when crystallized from C_6H_6. It forms several crystalline salts with mineral acids, e.g. the hydrochloride, m.p. 311°C; hydrobromide, m.p. 320°C; $[\alpha]_D^{20} - 60°$ (c 1.05, H$_2$O), hydriodide, m.p. 325°C and the picrate as pale yellow needles, m.p. 136–7°C. The methiodide is obtained as the monohydrate, m.p. 178°C or 245–6°C (*dry*); $[\alpha]_D^{20} - 59°$ (c 0.8, MeOH) and the methosulphate, m.p. 213°C; $[\alpha]_D^{20} - 47°$ (c 0.8, MeOH). The alkaloid contains a tertiary nitrogen, a secondary and a tertiary hydroxyl and yields a monoacetyl derivative, m.p. 214–5°C; $[\alpha]_D^{25} - 67°$ (c 1.1, CHCl$_3$); a diacetyl compound, m.p. 143–5°C; $[\alpha]_D^{20} - 95°$ (c 3.1, CHCl$_3$); the p-toluenesulphonyl derivative, m.p. 183–4°C; $[\alpha]_D^{25} - 81°$ (c 0.95, CHCl$_3$) and the monobenzoyl compound, m.p. 267–8°C; $[\alpha]_D^{25} - 98°$ (c 0.93, CHCl$_3$).

Binns *et al., Austral. J. Chem.*, **18**, 569 (1965)

Structure:

Mander *et al., Austral. J. Chem.*, **20**, 1705 (1967)

HIMGRAVINE

$C_{22}H_{33}O_2N$

M.p. $120°C$

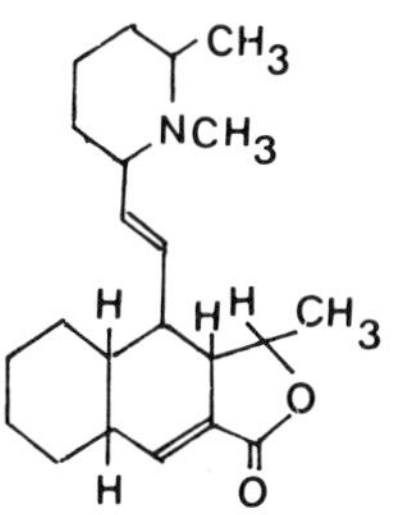

This alkaloid has been isolated from the bark of *Himantandra baccata* and yields colourless crystals from petroleum ether. It has $[\alpha]_D^{18} + 47°$ (c 1.5, $CHCl_3$) and gives a crystalline methiodide as the monohydrate, m.p. $191-2°C$.

Brown *et al.*, *Austral. J. Chem.*, **9**, 283 (1956)
Abraham, Bernstein., *ibid*, **14**, 64 (1961)
Pinhey, Ritchie, Taylor., *ibid*, **14**, 106 (1961)

HIMGRINE

$C_{22}H_{33}O_3N$

An amorphous alkaloid present in the bark of *Himantandra belgraveana*, this base has been isolated and characterized as the crystalline perchlorate, m.p. $143-4°C$. The methiodide, m.p. $222-3°C$ has also been prepared as crystals from EtOH. The base contains one methylimino group.

Brown *et al.*, *Austral. J. Chem.*, **9**, 283 (1956)

HIERACIFOLINE

$C_{18}H_{25}O_5N$

M.p. $227°C$

A pyrrolizidine alkaloid obtained from *Erechtites hieracifolia* (L), Raf, this base has $[\alpha]_D^{26} - 89.7°$ ($CHCl_3$). On alkaline hydrolysis it furnishes retronecine and hieracinecic acid, $C_{10}H_{16}O_5$, m.p. $132°C$.

Manske., *J. Can. Res.*, **17B**, 8 (1939)

HIPPEASTRINE

$C_{17}H_{17}O_5N$

M.p. $214-5°C$

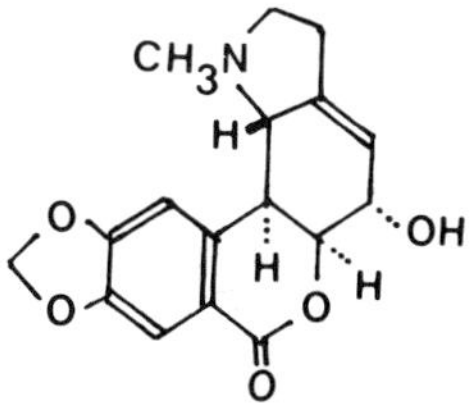

One of the *Amaryllidaceae* alkaloids, this base yields colourless prisms from

Me$_2$CO. It is dextrorotatory with $[\alpha]_D^{22} + 160°$ (c 0.3, CHCl$_3$). It has been characterized as the methopicrate, m.p. 234–6°C (*dec.*). One hydroxyl group, a methylendioxy group and a methylimino group are present in the molecule.

Boit., *Chem. Ber.*, **89**, 1129, 2093, 2462 (1956)

Kitagawa, Uyeo, Yokoyama., *J. Chem. Soc.*, 3741 (1959)

HIPPODAMINE

C$_{13}$H$_{23}$N

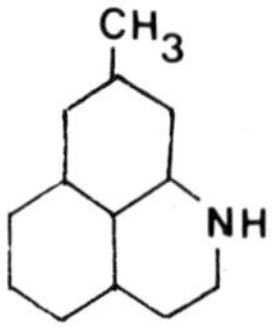

An alkaloid obtained from the American ladybird (*Hippodamia convergens*), the structure has been shown to be (±)-2-methyl-trans, cis, cis,-perhydro-9b-azaphenalene.

Tursch *et al.*, *Bull. Soc. Chim. Belg.*, **81**, 649 (1972)

HIRSUTINE

C$_{22}$H$_{28}$O$_3$N$_2$

M.p. 101°C

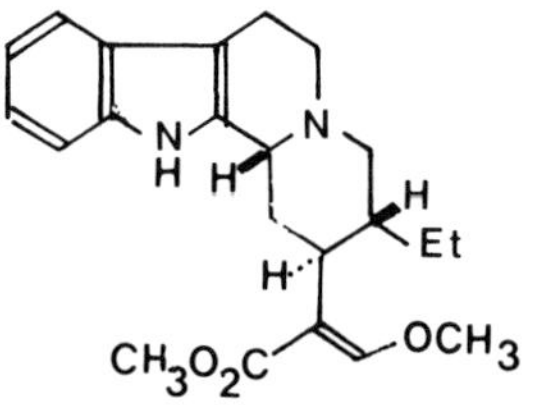

A carboline alkaloid present in *Mitragyna hirsuta* Havil., the base forms colourless crystals from Et$_2$O and has $[\alpha]_D^{23} + 68.6°$ (c 0.32, CHCl$_3$). The ultraviolet spectrum exhibits absorption maxima at 226, 282 and 290 mμ. A crystalline methiodide, m.p. 254°C has been prepared. The structure has been assigned mainly on the NMR data.

Shellard *et al.*, *J. Pharm. Pharmacol.*, **18**, 553 (1966)

Absolute configuration:

Trager *et al.*, *Tetrahedron*, **23**, 1043 (1967)

HODGKINSINE

C$_{33}$H$_{38}$N$_6$

M.p. Indefinite

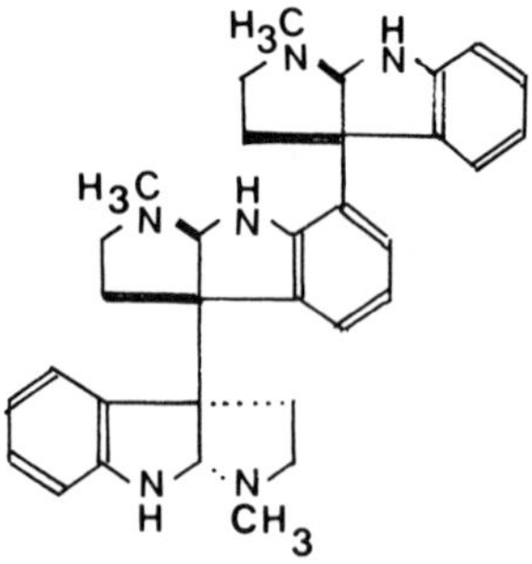

An amorphous alkaloid isolated from *Hodgkinsonia frutescens,* this base was originally given the empirical formula $C_{22}H_{26}N_4$, subsequently altered to that given above. It is dextrorotatory with $[\alpha]_D^{23} + 60°$ (c 1.0, 0.3 N/HCl). When crystallized from C_6H_6, it yields a crystalline adduct, m.p. 128°C. The ultraviolet spectrum shows absorption maxima at 232, 252, 310 and 326 mμ. The alkaloid has a trimeric structure as deduced from spectroscopic evidence and molecular weight determinations.

Anet, Hughes, Ritchie., *Austral. J. Chem.*, **14**, 173 (1961)

Crystal structure:
Fridrichsons, Mackay, Mathiseon., *Tetrahedron Lett.*, 3521 (1967)

HODORINE

$C_{19}H_{31}O_5N$

M.p. Indefinite

An amorphous base obtained from *Stemona sessilifolia* Miq. A crystalline hydrochloride, m.p. 244−5°C (*dec.*) and the hydrobromide, m.p. 258−9°C have been prepared.

Furuya., *Chem. Zent.*, 1823 (1913)

HOERHAMMERICINE

$C_{21}H_{24}O_4N_2$

M.p. 140−4°C

A *Catharanthus* alkaloid obtained from the roots of *C. lanceus,* the base crystallizes in fine, colourless needles from C_6H_6. It has $[\alpha]_D^{25} - 403°$ (c 2.04, $CHCl_3$) and the ultraviolet spectrum shows two absorption maxima at 299 and 327 mμ. The ultraviolet spectrum and the high negative optical rotation are typical of the α-methyleneindoline chromophore and comparison of the physical data for this alkaloid and those of hoerhammerinine show the two alkaloids to be very similar. Subsequently it has been shown that the base is demethoxyhoer-hammerinine.

Blomster, Farnsworth, Abraham., *Naturwiss.*, **55**, 298 (1968)

HOLADYSAMINE

$C_{22}H_{35}ON$

M.p. 173°C

This alkaloid has been isolated from a species of *Holarrhena antidysenterica* grown in Vietnam. It is laevorotatory with $[\alpha]_D - 78°$ (CHCl$_3$). It contains a methylamino group and a hydroxyethyl group.

Janot, Longevialle, Goutarel., *Bull. Soc. Chim. Fr.*, 2158 (1964)

HOLADYSINE

$C_{22}H_{35}ON$

M.p. 120°C

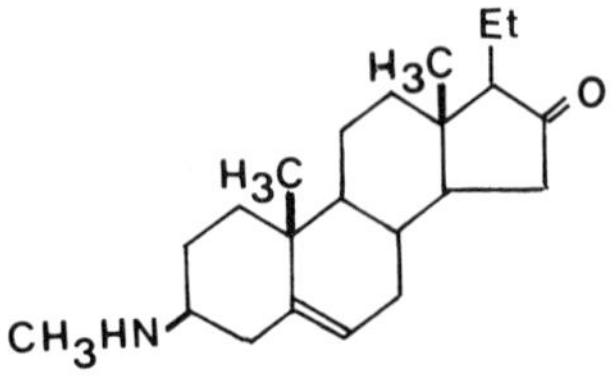

Also present in the Vietnamese specimen of *Holarrhena antidysenterica,* this alkaloid has $[\alpha]_D - 199°$ (CHCl$_3$). It contains a methylamino group, an ethyl group and a ketonic oxygen.

Janot, Longevialle, Goutarel., *Bull. Soc. Chim. Fr.*, 2158 (1964)

HOLAFEBRINE

$C_{21}H_{35}ON$

M.p. 177°C

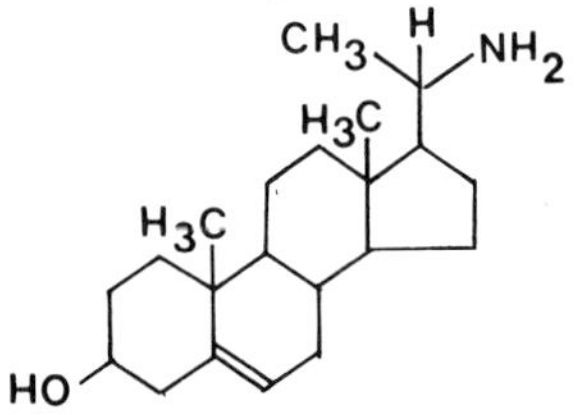

A pregnene type alkaloid, this base has been obtained from *Holarrhena febrifuga* and *Kibatalia arboren.* It yields colourless crystals from AcOEt and is laevorotatory with $[\alpha]_D - 61.5°$ (c 0.85, CHCl$_3$). The hydrochloride crystallizes from MeOH with 1 mole of solvent, m.p. > 310°C. The diacetyl derivative has m.p. 250°C; $[\alpha]_D - 56.6°$ (c 0.7, CHCl$_3$).

Janot *et al., Bull. Soc. Chim. Fr.*, 285 (1962)

HOLAFRINE

$C_{28}H_{44}O_2N_2$

M.p. 116–7°C

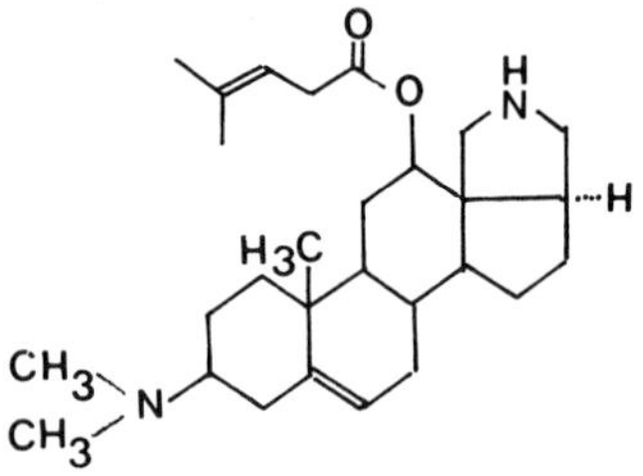

This steroidal alkaloid occurs in *Holarrhena africana* A. DC. and crystallizes as colourless, flat plates from aqueous Me$_2$CO. It has $[\alpha]_D^{20} - 19.1°$ (c 0.93, CHCl$_3$) or − 5.1° (c 0.98, EtOH). A crystalline diperchlorate, m.p. 180–1°C has been prepared. Acid hydrolysis furnishes 12-hydroxyconessimine and 4-methyl-3-pentenoic acid.

Rostock, Seebeck., *Helv. Chim. Acta,* **41**, 11 (1958)

HOLALINE

$C_{24}H_{42}ON_2$

M.p. 267°C

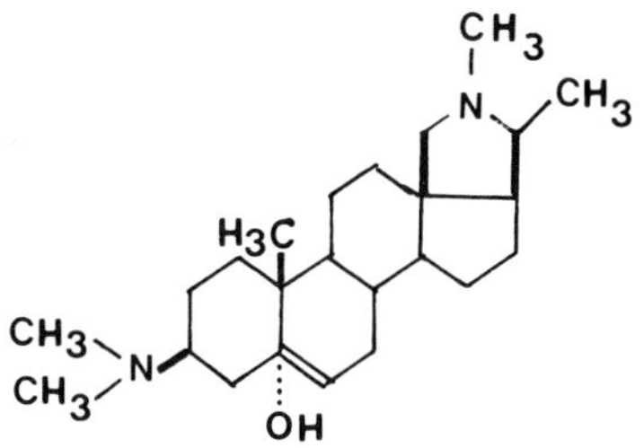

A further steroidal *Holarrhena* alkaloid found in *H. floribunda* (G. Dom) Dur et Schinz., this base has $[\alpha]_D + 36°$ (CHCl$_3$:MeOH, 1:1). A hydroxyl group, a methylimino group and a dimethylamino group are present.

Janot *et al., Ann. Pharm. fr.*, (1967)
Janot *et al., C.R. Acad. Sci.*, **260**, 6631 (1965)
Janot *et al., Bull. Soc. Chim. Fr.*, 4315 (1967)

HOLAMINE

$C_{21}H_{33}ON$,

M.p. 135°C

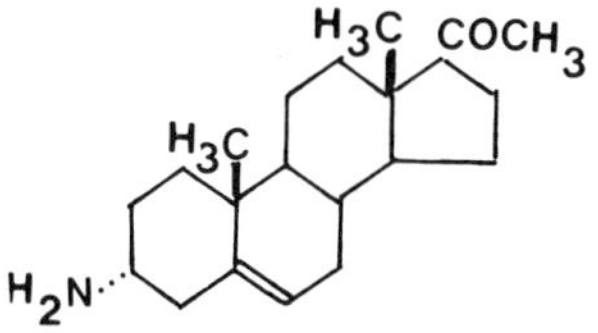

A further alkaloid isolated from *Holarrhena floribunda* (G. Don) Dur et Schinz., this pregnene base has $[\alpha]_D + 23°$ (CHCl$_3$). The structure has been shown by spectroscopic determinations to be 3α-amino-20-oxo-4-pregnene.

Janot, Cave, Goutarel., *Compt. rend.*, **251**, 559 (1960)

HOLANTOSINE A

$C_{28}H_{47}O_6N$

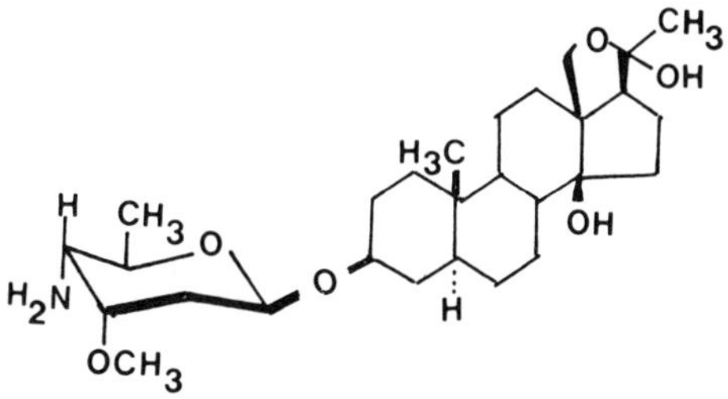

An amorphous alkaloid isolated from *Holarrhena antidysenterica* Wall., this pregnane base is characterized as the N-acetyl derivative, m.p. 260–1°C; $[\alpha]_D^{20} - 28°$ (CHCl$_3$). The structure has been elucidated from chemical degradation and spectroscopic studies.

Janot *et al., Tetrahedron*, **26**, 1695 (1970)

HOLANTOSINE B

$C_{28}H_{45}O_5N$

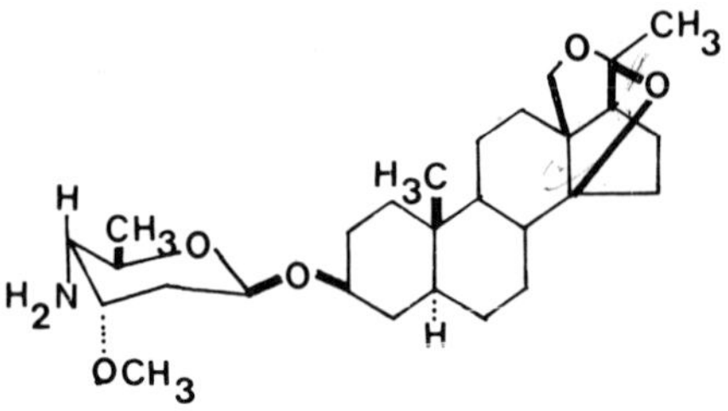

A further amorphous base present in *Holarrhena antidysenterica* Wall, the alkaloid forms a crystalline N-acetyl derivative, m.p. $> 290°C$; $[\alpha]_D^{20} - 29°$ (CHCl$_3$).

Janot *et al.*, *Tetrahedron*, **26**, 1695 (1970)

HOLANTOSINE C

$C_{28}H_{47}O_6N$

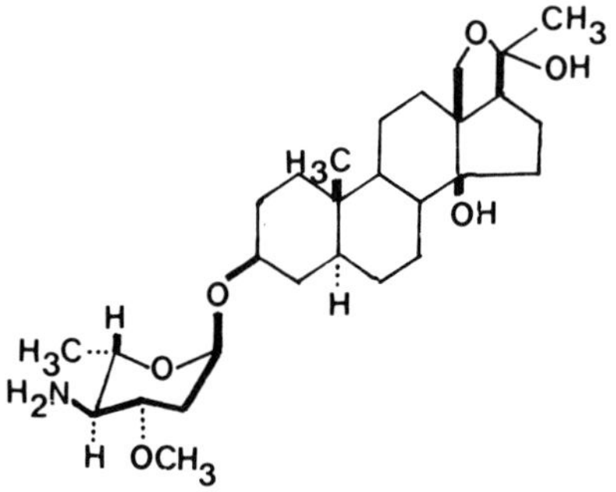

A third amorphous base isolated from the leaves of *Holarrhena antidysenterica* Wall., this alkaloid is possibly stereoisomeric with holantosine A. The N-acetyl derivative has m.p. $245°C$; $[\alpha]_D - 73°$ (MeOH:CHCl$_3$, 3:7). On alkaline hydrolysis, it yields holantosamine, $C_7H_{15}O_3N$.

Khuong-Huu *et al.*, *Bull. Soc. Chim. Fr.*, 864 (1971)

HOLANTOSINE D

$C_{28}H_{45}O_5N$

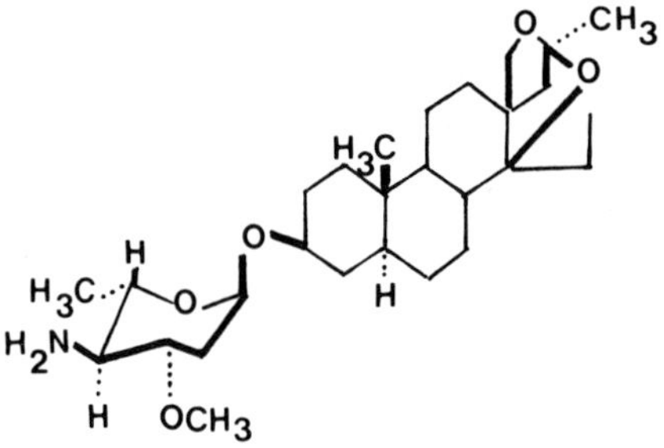

This constituent of the leaf extract of *Holarrhena antidysenterica* Wall, is a

686

stereoisomer of holantosine B. It is laevorotatory with $[\alpha]_D - 67°$ (c 6.0, CHCl$_3$). It yields an N-acetyl derivative, m.p. 262–3°C; $[\alpha]_D - 74°$ (CHCl$_3$). Like the preceding alkaloid, it furnishes holantosamine on alkaline hydrolysis.

Khuong-Huu et al., Bull. Soc. Chim. Fr., 864 (1971)

HOLANTOSINE E

$C_{30}H_{47}O_6N$

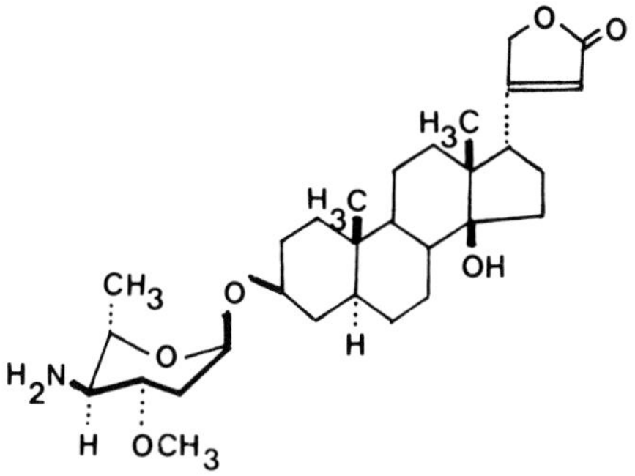

An amorphous alkaloid isolated from the leaves of *Holarrhena antidysenterica* Wall., this base resembles the four preceding alkaloids but contains a furanone ring as a substituent.

Khuong-Huu et al., Bull. Soc. Chim. Fr., 864 (1971)

HOLAPHYLLAMINE

$C_{21}H_{33}ON$

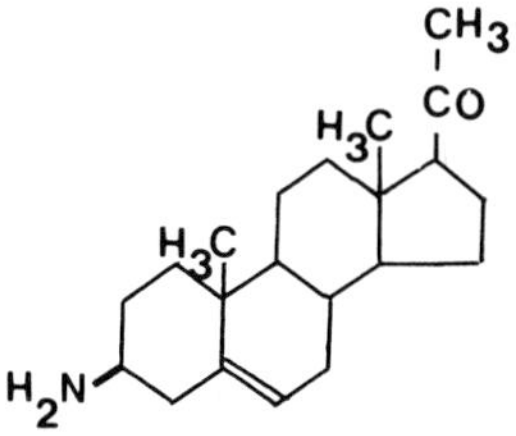

An amorphous alkaloid from *Holarrhena floribunda* (G. Don) Dur et Schinz., the base has been characterized as the crystalline hydrochloride, m.p. 260°C; $[\alpha]_D + 33°$ (c 0.68, MeOH). The structure has been established as 3α-amino-20-oxo-5-pregnene (cf. holamine). The N-methyl derivative is identical with holaphylline (q.v.).

Janot, Cave, Goutarel., *Bull. Soc. Chim. Fr.*, 896 (1959)
Janot, Cave, Goutarel., *Compt. rend.*, **251**, 559 (1960)

Partial synthesis:
Goutarel et al., *Bull. Soc. Chim. Fr.*, 4575 (1967)
Hodosan, Serban., *Experientia*, **24**, 881 (1968)

HOLAPHYLLINE

$C_{22}H_{35}ON$

M.p. 128°C

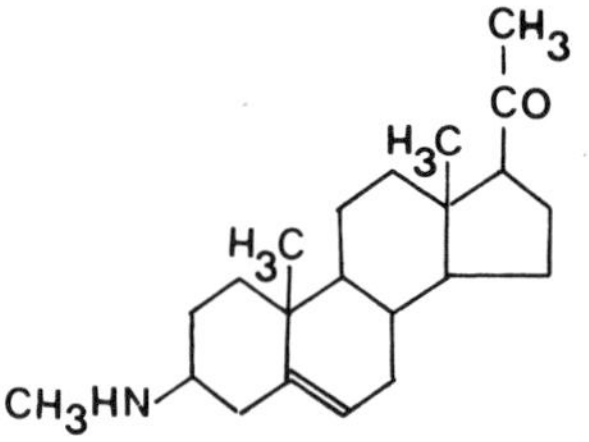

A crystalline alkaloid from *Holarrhena floribunda* (G. Don) Dur et Schinz., this alkaloid has $[\alpha]_D + 23.7°$ (CHCl$_3$). It forms the N-acetyl derivative, m.p. 205–6°C; $[\alpha]_D + 16.7°$ (c 1.2, CHCl$_3$) and with CH$_2$N$_2$ gives the N-methyl compound, m.p. 121°C; $[\alpha]_D + 30.5°$ (c 0.86, CHCl$_3$).

Janot, Cave, Goutarel., *Bull. Soc. Chim. Fr.*, 896 (1959)

HOLAROSINE A

$C_{30}H_{47}O_6N$

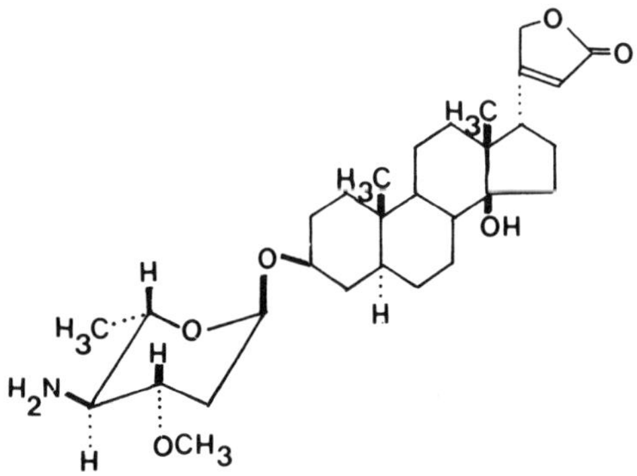

An amorphous base present in the leaf extract of *Holarrhena antidysenterica* Wall., this alkaloid is characterized as the N-acetyl derivative, m.p. 268–270°C; $[\alpha]_D - 39°$ (c 0.87, CHCl$_3$). Alkaline hydrolysis yields holarosamine.

Khuong-Huu *et al.*, *Bull. Soc. Chim. Fr.*, 864 (1971)

HOLARRHENINE

$C_{24}H_{38}ON_2$

M.p. 197–8°C

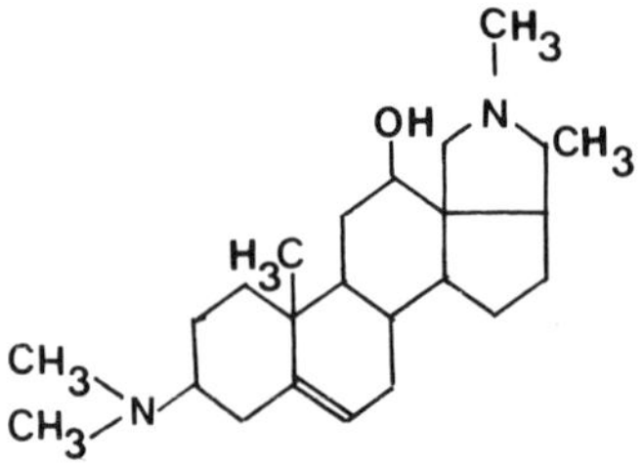

Obtained from the bark of *Holarrhena congolensis*, this alkaloid crystallizes from

AcOEt as silky white needles and has $[\alpha]_D - 7.1°$ (CHCl$_3$). Although only sparingly soluble in Me$_2$CO, Et$_2$O or cold AcOEt, it dissolves readily in CHCl$_3$ and EtOH. The hydrobromide forms flat needles of the trihydrate from H$_2$O, m.p. 265–8°C (*dry*) and has $[\alpha]_D + 11.0°$ (H$_2$O). A methiodide has also been prepared, m.p. 275–280°C and the oxygen is present as a hydroxyl group since the base forms an O-acetyl derivative, oblong plates from Me$_2$CO, m.p. 180°C which is still diacidic.

Pyman., *J. Chem. Soc.*, **115**, 163 (1919)
Uffer., *Helv. Chim. Acta*, **39**, 1834 (1956)

HOLARRHESSIMINE

$C_{22}H_{36}ON_2$

M.p. 160–4°C

A further alkaloid from *Holarrhena antidysenterica* Wall., found mainly in the bark, this base has $[\alpha]_D^{18} - 31°$ (c 0.775, CHCl$_3$). It forms a crystalline hydrobromide, m.p. 293–4°C; a methiodide, m.p. 279–280°C and a picrate, m.p. 250–5°C (*dec.*).

Tschesche, Petersen., *Chem. Ber.*, **87**, 1719 (1954)

HOLARRHETINE

$C_{29}H_{46}O_2N_2$

M.p. 74–5°C

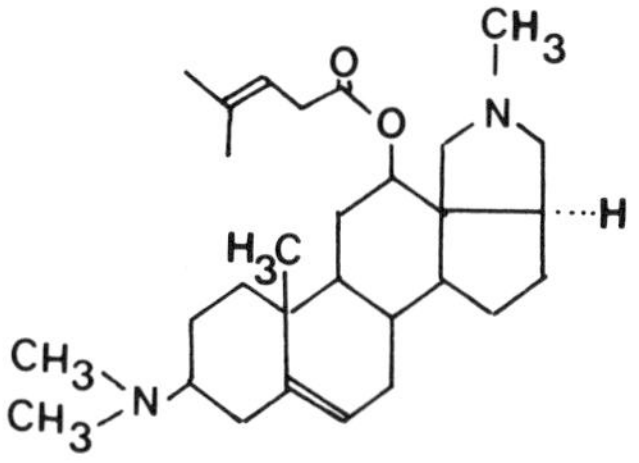

This alkaloid which occurs in *Holarrhena africana* A. DC., forms colourless cubic crystals from Me$_2$CO and is laevorotatory with $[\alpha]_D - 14.9°$ (c 1.12, CHCl$_3$) or $- 4.6°$ (c 1.12, EtOH). It forms a crystalline dithiocyanate as the hemihydrate, crystallizing in colourless prisms from H$_2$O, m.p. 148–150°C. The alkaloid may be hydrolyzed with dilute acid to yield holarrhenine and 4-methyl-3-pentenoic acid.

Rostock, Seebeck., *Helv. Chim. Acta*, **41**, 11 (1958)

HOLARRHIDINE

$C_{21}H_{36}ON_2$

M.p. 180–1°C

Isolated from the trunk bark of *Holarrhena antidysenterica* Wall, this alkaloid is best purified by crystallization from aqueous tetrahydrofuran. It is laevorotatory with $[\alpha]_D^{20} - 23°$ (c 2.8, $CHCl_3$). It contains two amino groups and yields a crystalline tetramethyl derivative, m.p. 163–4°C; $[\alpha]_D^{20} - 34°$ (c 1.97, $CHCl_3$).

Lubler, Cerny, Sorm., *Collect. Czech. Chem. Commun.*, **24**, 370, 378 (1959)

HOLLARHIMINE

$C_{21}H_{36}ON_2$

M.p. 183°C

A pregnene alkaloid from the bark of *Hollarrhena antidysenterica* Wall, this laevorotatory base has $[\alpha]_D^{25} - 22.8°$ (MeOH) or $- 14.19°$ ($CHCl_3$). It behaves as a diacidic base, yielding a hydrochloride, m.p. 345°C (*dec.*); $[\alpha]_D^{25} - 22.8°$ (MeOH); hydrobromide, m.p. 358–360°C (*dec.*); sulphate, m.p. 337°C; picrate, m.p. 198–200°C (*dry*) and a platinichloride as a yellow powder which discolours at 270°C and chars, without melting, above 300°C. With formaldehyde and formic acid, it yields the tetramethyl derivative, m.p. 233–5°C which occurs naturally in *Holarrhena antidysenterica* Wall (q.v.).

With excess BzCl in pyridine, the alkaloid furnishes the tribenzoyl derivative, m.p. 269–270°C while methyl iodide in $CHCl_3$ yields the dimethiodide, m.p. 279°C which may be converted by alkalies into methylholarrhimine, m.p. 170°C (hydrochloride, m.p. 266°C *dec.*, picrate, m.p. 205°C). The alkaloid also forms a disalicylidene derivative, m.p. 246–7°C.

Siddiqui, Pillay., *J. Ind. Chem. Soc.*, **9**, 561 (1932)
Siddiqui., *ibid*, **11**, 283 (1934)
Siddiqui., *Proc. Ind. Acad. Sci.*, **3A**, 249, 257 (1936)
Cerny, Sorm., *Chem. Listy*, **49**, 723, 1389 (1955)
Labler, Cerny, Sorm., *Chem. & Ind.*, 1119 (1955)
Favre *et al.*, *J. Chem. Soc.*, 1115 (1953)

HOLARRHINE

$C_{20}H_{38}O_3N_2$

M.p. 240°C

An alkaloid present in the leaves of *Holarrhena antidysenterica* Wall, the base is laevorotatory, having $[\alpha]_D^{25} - 17.01°$ (MeOH). It is insoluble in Et_2O, AcOEt or petroleum ether, slightly soluble in $CHCl_3$ and dissolves readily in MeOH, EtOH. A platinichloride has been prepared as yellow needles which darken at 270°C and char, without melting, at 300°C. The picrate behaves similarly, darkening at 275°C and melting above 320°C.

Siddiqui, Pillay., *J. Ind. Chem. Soc.*, **9**, 562 (1932)

HOLONAMINE

$C_{21}H_{27}O_2N$

M.p. 257–9°C

A further alkaloid from the bark of *Holarrhena antidysenterica* Wall, this base crystallizes well from C_6H_6 as colourless needles, and has $[\alpha]_D^{21} - 14.8°$ (c 1.1, MeOH). Two methyl and one hydroxyl group are present in the molecule.

Tschesche, Ockenfels., *Chem. Ber.*, **97**, 2316, 2326 (1964)

HOLSTIINE

$C_{22}H_{26}O_4N_2$

M.p. 247–8°C (*dec.*).

There is still some doubt as to whether the above empirical formula, of $C_{23}H_{28}O_4N_2$, is the correct one for this alkaloid from *Strychnos helotii* var. *reticulata*. It is a crystalline solid and is strongly dextrorotatory with $[\alpha]_D + 268°$ ($CHCl_3$). It is readily soluble in $CHCl_3$ and only sparingly so in Et_2O, EtOH or C_6H_6. It gives a blue violet colour with ferric sulphate in H_2SO_4. In H_2SO_4 with a crystal of potassium dichromate, it yields a blue colour, gradually becoming violet.

Janot, Goutarel., *Compt. rend.*, **232**, 852 (1951)
Bosly., *J. pharm. Belg.*, **6**, 150, 243 (1951)

HOMALINE

$C_{30}H_{42}O_2N_4$

M.p. 134°C

This spermine type alkaloid is the main component of the leaf extract of *Homalium pornyense*, being also present in lesser amounts in other *Homalium* species. It has $[\alpha]_D - 34°$ (CHCl$_3$) and the structure has been determined by chemical studies and investigation of the NMR and mass spectra. When treated with LiAlH$_4$ in tetrahydrofuran, the alkaloid yields a deoxy base, $C_{30}H_{46}N_4$ which forms a crystalline dipicrate, m.p. 140°C. With methyl iodide, the base furnishes a mixture of the mono- and dimethiodides. Hofmann degradation of the former gives a methine base, $C_{31}H_{44}O_2N_4$, $[\alpha]_D - 20°$ (CHCl$_3$) while the latter yields a corresponding methine, $C_{32}H_{46}O_2N_4$, forming a hydrochloride, m.p. 231°C. Acid hydrolysis of the alkaloid gives *trans*-cinnamic acid.

Pais *et al.*, *Compt. Rend.*, **266C**, 37 (1968)
Pais *et al.*, *ibid*, **267C**, 82 (1968)

Structure:
Pais *et al.*, *Compt. Rend.*, **272C**, 1729 (1971)
Pais *et al.*, *Tetrahedron*, **29**, 1001 (1973)

HOMOAROMOLINE

$C_{38}H_{42}O_6N_2$

M.p. 238–240°C

This bisbenzyl*iso*quinoline alkaloid occurs in the rhizomes of *Cyclea barbata*. It forms colourless needles when crystallized from CHCl$_3$. Treatment with CH$_2$N$_2$ yields O-methoxyacanthine.

Tomita, Kozuka, Satomi., *J. Pharm. Soc., Japan*, **87**, 1012 (1967)

HOMOBATRACHOTOXIN (*Isobatrachotoxin*)

$C_{32}H_{44}O_6N_2$

An amorphous alkaloid present in the skin secretions of *Phyllobates aurotaenia*, a species of frog found in Columbia, the poison of which has been used in the past to tip arrow heads. The ultraviolet spectrum in acid solution (HCl-MeOH) has absorption maxima at 233 and 264 mμ. The complex structure of this alkaloid has been determined from chemical degradations and spectroscopic studies.

Tokuyama, Daly, Witkop., *J. Amer. Chem. Soc.*, **91**, 3931 (1969)

692

HOMOCHASMANINE

$C_{26}H_{43}O_6N$

M.p. 105–7°C

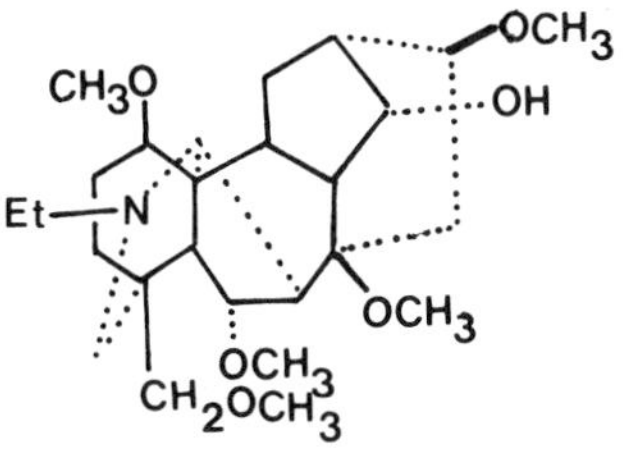

As atisine alkaloid present in *Aconitum chasmanthum* Stapf., this base yields colourless prisms when crystallized from hexane. It is dextrorotatory with $[\alpha]_D^{25} + 19.2°$ (c 2.4, EtOH). It contains five methoxyl groups, one hydroxyl and an ethylimino group. The structure has been determined as chasmanine 8-methyl ether. It yields an O-acetyl derivative as a colourless gum which cannot be crystallized.

Achmatowicz, Marion., *Can. J. Chem.*, **43**, 1093 (1965)

α-HOMOCHELIDONINE

$C_{21}H_{23}O_5N$

M.p. 182°C

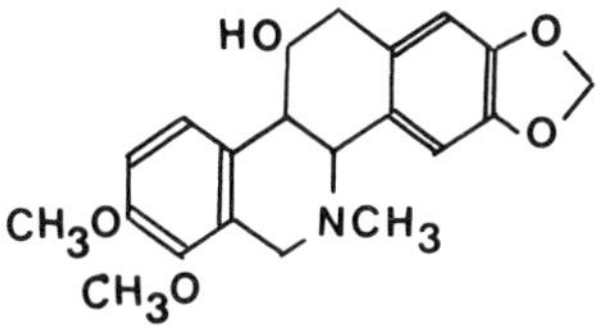

Isolated from *Chelidonium majus,* this base is obtained as colourless prisms from AcOEt. It dissolves freely in $CHCl_3$ or EtOH but is only sparingly soluble in Et_2O.

Schmidt, Selle., *Arch. Pharm.*, **228**, 441 (1890)
Späth, Kuffner., *Ber.*, **64**, 1123 (1931)

β-HOMOCHELIDONINE

See α-Allocryptopine

γ-HOMOCHELIDONINE

See β-Allocryptopine

HOMOCINCHONIDINE

$C_{19}H_{22}ON_2$

M.p. 207.5°C

A minor constituent of the bark of *Cinchona Calisaya* Ledger and *C. succirubra,* the alkaloid forms colourless prisms from EtOH and has $[\alpha]_D - 107.3°$ (EtOH).

It is insoluble in H_2O, slightly soluble in Et_2O and readily so in $CHCl_3$ and EtOH. It forms a crystalline hydrochloride as the dihydrate, $[\alpha]_D - 138°$ (EtOH). When oxidized with $KMnO_4$ it yields cinchonetidine, m.p. 256°C.

Pharmacologically, the alkaloid resembles Cinchonine (q.v.) and is active against *Plasmodium lophurae* in ducklings and *P. gallinaceum* in chicks.

Hesse., *Annalen*, **205**, 203 (1880)
Hesse., *Ber.*, **14**, 1891 (1881)

HOMOGLOMERINE

$C_{11}H_{12}ON_2$

M.p. 149°C

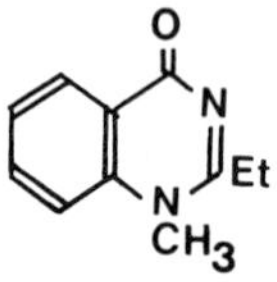

A quinazolone alkaloid isolated from the arthropod *Glomeris marginata*. The base may be purified by crystallization from AcOEt or by sublimation when it yields pale yellow prisms. The structure has been deduced from spectroscopic determinations and confirmed by synthesis.

Schildknecht, Maschwitz, Wenneis., *Naturwiss.*, **54**, 196 (1967)
Chakravarti *et al.*, *Tetrahedron*, **16**, 224 (1961)
Biosynthesis:
Schildknecht, Wenneis., *Tetrahedron Lett.*, 1815 (1967)

HOMOHARRINGTONINE

$C_{29}H_{38}O_9N$

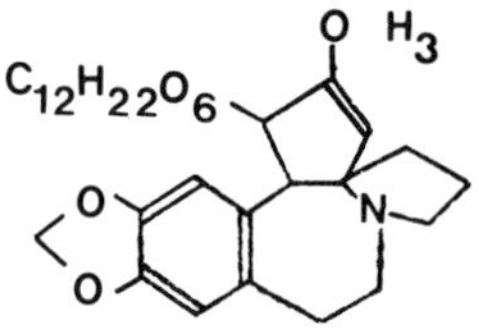

A complex alkaloid isolated from various species of *Cephalotaxus*, the structure of this base has been determined from the reaction products forms on treatment with NaOMe in MeOH.

Powell *et al.*, *Tetrahedron Lett.*, **11**, 815 (1970)

HOMOLINEARISINE

$C_{18}H_{19}O_3N$

M.p. 218–9°C (*dec.*).

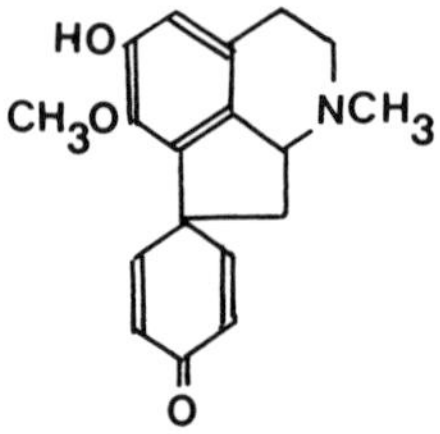

This spiroisoquinoline alkaloid occurs in *Papaver caucasicum*. The structure has been confirmed by synthesis of the optically inactive form utilizing the Pschorr reaction of 8-amino-1:2:3:4-tetrahydro-7-methoxy-1-(4-methoxybenzyl)-2-methyl-6-isoquinolinol under alkaline conditions. It is noteworthy that the base cannot be synthesized by the phenolic oxidative coupling method.

Ishiwata, Itakura., *Chem. Pharm. Bull.*, **18**, 1841 (1970)

HOMOMOSCHATOLINE

$C_{19}H_{15}O_4N$

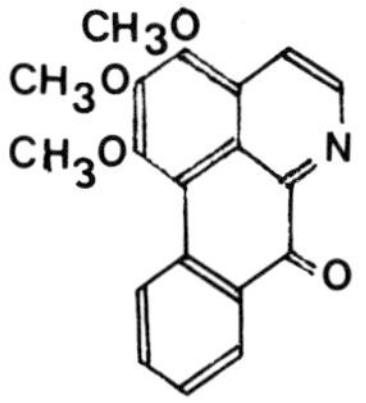

The bark of *Guatteria subsessilis* yields this oxo-proaporphine alkaloid, the structure of which has been established by chemical and spectroscopic evidence.

Hasegawa *et al.*, *Acta Cient. Venez.*, **23**, 165 (1972)

HOMOPHLEINE

$C_{56}H_{90}O_9N_2$

M.p. Indefinite

An amorphous base found in *Erythrophleum guineense* bark, this alkaloid has not yet been characterized. It is stated to resemble Erythrophleine (q.v.) in appearance and physical characteristics.

Dalma., *Ann. Chim. Appl.*, **25**, 569 (1935)
Dalma., *Helv. Chim. Acta*, **22**, 1497 (1939)

HOMOSTEPHANOLINE

$C_{39}H_{44}O_6N_2$

M.p. 233°C

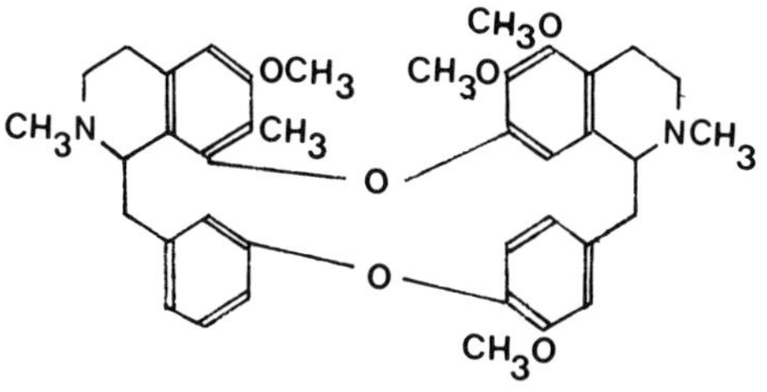

This base occurs in the phenolic fraction obtained from *Stephania japonica* and is separated from the associated alkaloids by chromatography. The structure and absolute stereochemistry have been elucidated from infrared, ultraviolet, NMR and mass spectrometry.

Tomita *et al.*, *J. Pharm. Soc., Japan*, **76**, 686 (1956)

Structure:
Ibuka, Kitano., *Chem. Pharm. Bull.*, **15**, 1939 (1967)

HOMOTHERMOPSINE

This alkaloid is stated to be present in the leaves, flowers and seeds of *Thermopsis lanceolata* and has been identified by paper electrophoresis and paper chromatography.

Jarzebinska., *Diss. Pharm. Pharmacol.*, **18**, 399 (1966)

HOMOTRILOBINE

See Isotrilobine

HOPROMALINOL

This spermine type alkaloid has recently been isolated from the leaves of *Homalium pornyense* together with homaline (q.v.).

Pais *et al.*, *Tetrahedron*, **29**, 1001 (1973)

HOPROMINE

A further spermine alkaloid present in the leaves of *Homalium pornyense*, this alkaloid is present only in small amounts in the alkaloidal extract.

Pais *et al.*, *Tetrahedron*, **29**, 1001 (1973)

HOPROMINOL

The third minor constituent of the leaf extract of *Homalium pornyense*, this alkaloid is apparently of the spermidine class.

Pais *et al.*, *Tetrahedron*, **29**, 1001 (1973)

HORDENINE (*Anhaline*)

$C_{10}H_{15}ON$

M.p. 117°C;
B.p. 173–4°C/11 mm

This alkaloid was first isolated from barley malt germs by Leger and has subsequently been discovered in other grass embryos and various *Anhalonium* species, particularly in *A. fissuratum*, indigenous to Mexico. The base yields colourless prisms and sublimes at 140–150°C. It is strongly alkaline and will liberate ammonia from solutions of its salts. It behaves as a monoacidic, tertiary base and forms a series of crystalline salts, e.g. the hydrochloride, m.p. 176.5–177.5°C; sulphate, m.p. 209–211°C (*dry*); reineckate (as the pentahydrate), m.p. 176–8°C; picrate, m.p. 139–140°C; picrolonate, m.p. 219–220°C; methiodide, m.p. 229–230°C; methopicrate, m.p. 165°C; benzoyl derivative, m.p. 47–8°C and the diphenylsulphimide, m.p. 146°C. The O-acetyl derivative is oxidized by $KMnO_4$ to p-acetoxybenzoic acid while exhaustive methylation furnishes trimethylamine and p-vinylanisole. These observations led Leger to propose that the alkaloid is p-hydroxy-β-phenylethyldimethylamine and this structure has been confirmed by the synthesis of the base from phenylethyl alcohol.

Hordenine is said to possess a comparatively low toxicity although large doses cause death by paralysis of the respiration. The methiodide possesses a marked nicotine-like action and this effect is also shown by the alkaloid although to a slightly lesser extent. The hydrochloride of hordenine dimethylcarbamic ester possesses an anticholine-esterase action *in vitro* and is similar to physostigmine in action although markedly less potent. This stimulant action upon the central nervous system is absent in the alkaloid itself which is a central depressant.

Leger., *Compt. rend.,* **142**, 108 (1906)
Leger., *ibid*, **143**, 234, 916 (1906)
Leger., *ibid*, **144**, 208, 488 (1907)
Barger., *J. Chem. Soc.,* **95**, 2193 (1909)
Voswinckel., *Ber.,* **45**, 1004 (1912)
Späth., *Monatsh.,* **40**, 129 (1919)
Raoul., *Compt. rend.,* **199**, 425 (1934)
Raoul., *ibid,* **204**, 74 (1937)
Kirkwood, Marion., *J. Amer. Chem. Soc.,* **72**, 2522 (1950)
Badger, Christie, Rodda., *Austral. J. Chem.,* **16**, 734 (1963)

Pharmacology:
Camus., *Compt. rend.,* **142**, 110, 237, 350 (1906)
Barger, Dale., *J. Physiol.,* **41**, 19 (1910)
Schweitzer, Wright., *ibid,* **92**, 422 (1938)
Raymond-Hamet., *Compt. rend.,* **209**, 67 (1939)

HUNNEMANNINE

$C_{20}H_{21}O_5N$

M.p. 208–9°C

This alkaloid, isolated from *Hunnemannia fumariaefolia* Sweet, forms colourless crystals from propan-2-ol and contains a methylenedioxy, a methoxyl, a hydroxyl and a methylimino group in the molecule. The ultraviolet spectrum has two absorption maxima at 233 and 285 mμ. With CH_2N_2 it yields the O-methyl ether, m.p. 159–160°C, identical with α-allocryptopine (q.v.) thereby establishing the structure as O-demethyl-α-allocryptopine. The O-ethyl ether, m.p. 168°C, may be degraded to 4-methoxy-3-ethoxy-o-toluic acid, m.p. 175°C, thus confirming that the hydroxyl group is at C-9.

Manske, Marion, Ledingham., *J. Amer. Chem. Soc.,* **64**, 1659 (1942)
Slavikova, Slavik., *Collect. Czech. Chem. Commun.,* **31**, 1355 (1966)
Synthesis:
Giacopello, Deulofeu., *Tetrahedron,* **23**, 3265 (1967)

HUNTABRINE

$C_{20}H_{26}O_2N_2^+$

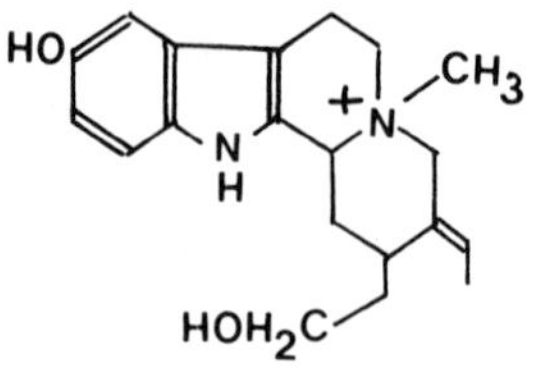

A quaternary base present in the roots of *Pleiocarpa mutica,* the alkaloid is isolated as the methochloride, m.p. $282-6°C$ which forms colourless crystals from aqueous MeOH; $[\alpha]_D^{26} + 56°$ (c 0.585, H_2O). The methopicrate is also crystalline, as yellow needles, m.p. $104-5°C$ *(dec.).*

Khan, Hesse, Schmid., *Helv. Chim. Acta,* **48**, 1957 (1965)

HUNTERACINE

$C_{18}H_{23}ON_2^+$

M.p. $343-4°C$ *(dec.).*

(Chloride)

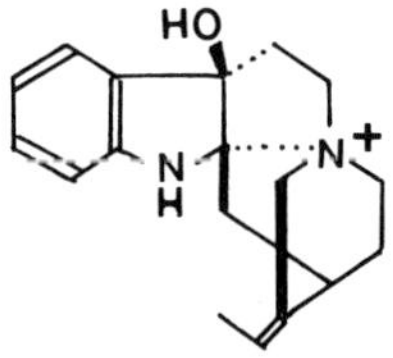

This quaternary alkaloid occurs in *Hunteria eburnea* and has been obtained as the chloride with the above melting point. This salt crystallizes from EtOH and has $[\alpha]_D - 91°$ (aqueous MeOH) and an ultraviolet spectrum showing two absorption maxima at 234 and 291 mμ. The structure has been determined from spectroscopic determinations, particularly the NMR and mass spectra.

Bartlett *et al., J. Org. Chem.,* **28**, 1445 (1963)

Structure:
Burnell *et al., Chem. Commun.,* 772 (1970)

HUNTERIAMINE

$C_{39}H_{48}O_2N_4$

A hypotensive alkaloid occurring in *Hunteria eburnea,* this base is characterized as the hydrochloride, m.p. $310-315°C$ *(dec.);* $[\alpha]_D^{23} + 27.3°$ (c 1.0, MeOH; the hydriodide, m.p. $> 300°C$ and the perchlorate, m.p. $278-281°C$; $[\alpha]_D^{23} + 29.6°$ (c 1.0, MeOH).

Renner., *Z. physiol. Chem.,* **331**, 105 (1963)

698

HUNTERBURNINE

$C_{19}H_{24}O_2N_2$

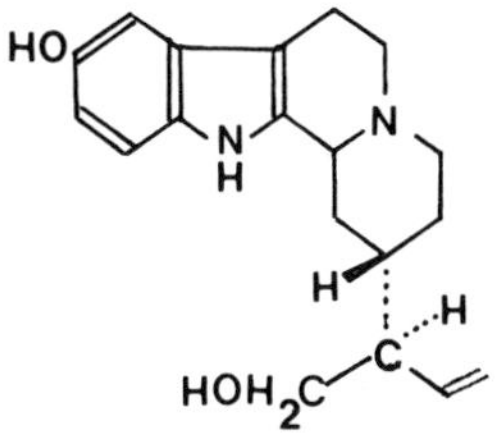

A carboline alkaloid present in *Hunteria eburnea,* the base yields crystalline derivatives, e.g. the α-methochloride (q.v.), m.p. 335°C; β-methochloride (q.v.), m.p. 307–8°C; α-methiodide, m.p. 322–4°C (*dec.*); and the β-methiodide, m.p. 277–280°C. It contains a hydroxyl group, a hydroxymethyl group and a vinyl group in the molecule.

Asher *et al., Proc. Chem. Soc.,* 72 (1962)
Scott, Sim, Robertson., *ibid,* 355 (1962)

Absolute configuration:
Sawa, Matsumura., *Tetrahedron,* 25, 5319 (1969)

HUNTERBURNINE α-METHOCHLORIDE

$C_{20}H_{27}O_2N_2Cl$

M.p. 335°C

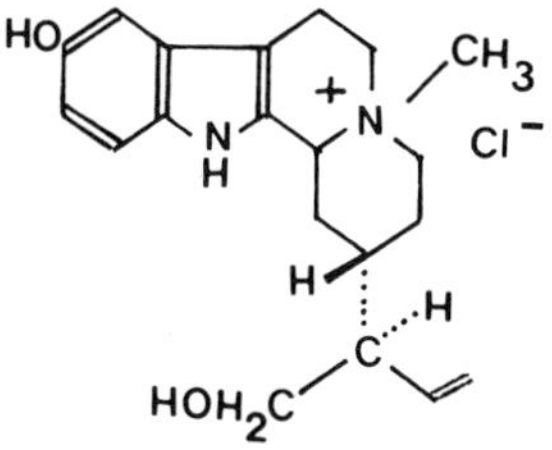

This derivative of hunterburnine occurs in *Hunteria eburnea* and *Ochrosia sandwicensis* A. Gray. It crystallizes from MeOH as slender white needles and is dextrorotatory with $[\alpha]_D^{22} + 44.1°$ (c 0.6, aqueous pyridine) or $[\alpha]_D^{21} + 10.1°$ (c 0.25, aqueous MeOH). The ultraviolet spectrum in neutral solution (MeOH) shows absorption maxima at 274 and 302 mμ with shoulders at 268 and 311 mμ. In 0.25 N/NaOH solution, there is an absorption maximum at 269 mμ and a shoulder occurring at 323 mμ.

Bartlett *et al., J. Org. Chem.,* 28, 1445 (1963)
Jordan, Scheuer., *Tetrahedron,* 21, 3731 (1965)

HUNTERBURNINE β-METHOCHLORIDE

$C_{20}H_{27}O_2N_2Cl$

M.p. 307–8°C

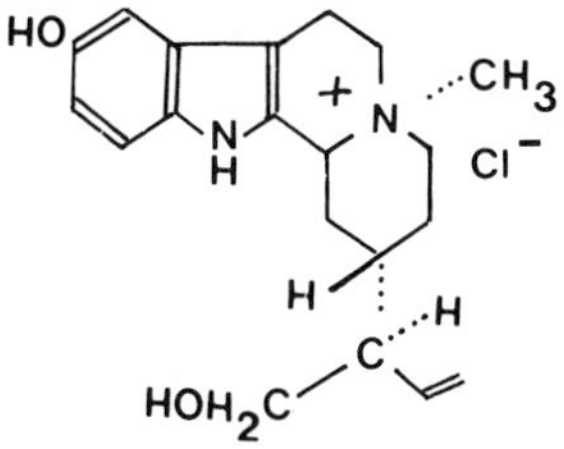

A minor constituent of *Hunteria eburnea* and *Ochrosia sandwicensis* A. Gray, this alkaloid yields colourless crystals from aqueous Me_2CO and has $[\alpha]_D$ + 105° (aqueous MeOH).

Bartlett *et al.*, *J. Org. Chem.*, **28**, 1445 (1963)
Jordan, Scheuer., *Tetrahedron*, **21**, 3731 (1965)

HUNTERINE

$C_{42}H_{52}O_4N_4$

M.p. 264–5°C (*dec.*).

The root barks of *Hunteria eburnea* yields this alkaloid which, when recrystallized from MeOH, forms colourless rectangular plates. The alkaloid is strongly laevorotatory with $[\alpha]_D^{27}$ − 205.1° (c 1.0, $CHCl_3$). The ultraviolet spectrum in ethanol solution exhibits absorption maxima at 228, 293 and 350 mμ.

Neuss, Cone., *Experientia*, **16**, 302 (1960)

β-(−)-HYDRASTINE

$C_{21}H_{21}O_6N$

M.p. 132°C

First isolated by Perrins from *Hydrastis canadensis*, the alkaloid also occurs in *Berberis laurina*. It forms colourless, rhombic prisms from EtOH, is alkaline to litmus and possesses an intensely bitter taste. It has $[\alpha]_D^{20}$ − 67.8° ($CHCl_3$), − 49.8° (absolute EtOH) or + 115° (aqueous EtOH). The salts do not crystallize well and are unstable in aqueous solution. The hydrochloride is a microcrystalline powder, m.p. 116°C; $[\alpha]_D$ + 127.3° (dilute HCl) and is obtained by passing dry HCl through an ethereal solution of the alkaloid. The picrate forms yellow needles, m.p. 184°C but the platinichloride is an amorphous yellow powder with no definite melting point. A solution of iodine precipitates the characteristic periodide as a dark, chocolate-brown powder. With dilute HNO_3 the base undergoes hydrolytic oxidation giving opianic acid and hydrastinine, $C_{11}H_{13}O_3N$, m.p. 116–7°C and optically inactive. The latter base forms crystalline salts with the simultaneous elimination of H_2O, e.g. the chloride as pale yellow needles, m.p. 212°C and the iodide, m.p. 233–4°C. It also forms an oxime, m.p. 145–6°C.

The epimer of the alkaloid, α-(−)-hydrastine, has m.p. 162°C; $[\alpha]_{546}^{18}$ − 163° (c 1.2, $CHCl_3$). So far, this base has not been found to occur naturally.

The alkaloid causes strychnine-like convulsions in the frog which are sometimes succeeded by paralysis when large doses are given. In mammals, the spinal and bulbar centres are stimulated, convulsions occur, and again there may be paralysis following large doses. It has sometimes been employed medicinally as an internal styptic in uterine haemorrhage. From the evidence available, the base appears to be excreted, unchanged, in the urine.

Perrins., *Pharm. J.*, **3**, 546 (1862)
Mahla., *Silliman's J.*, **36**, 57 (1863)
Power., *Pharm. J.*, **15**, 297 (1884)
Eykman., *Rec. trav. Chim.*, **5**, 291 (1886)
Freund, Will., *Ber.*, **20**, 88 (1887)
Mirza, Robinson., *Nature*, **166**, 271 (1950)
Haworth, Pinder., *J. Chem. Soc.*, 1776 (1950)
Ohta, Tani, Morozumi., *Tetrahedron Lett.*, 859 (1963)
Safe, Moir., *Can. J. Chem.*, **42**, 160 (1964)

HYDROALKAMINE S

$C_{27}H_{45}O_8N$

M.p. 248–250°C

An alkaloid from *Sabadilla minor*, this base has $[\alpha]_D - 45°$ (EtOH) and gives a crystalline hydrochloride, m.p. 240–5°C and a nitrate, m.p. 255°C. It is not reduced catalytically with Pt or Raney Ni.

Auterhoff., *Arch. Pharm.*, **288**, 549 (1955)

HYDROCINCHONIDINE (*Cinchamidine*)

$C_{19}H_{24}ON_2$

M.p. 229°C

A component of the bark of *Cinchona* species, this alkaloid was first obtained from commercial cinchonidine by Forst and Böhringer but it is more readily obtainable by the hydrogenation of pure cinchonidine. It crystallizes from EtOH in hexagonal leaflets and has $[\alpha]_D^{20} - 95.8°$ (c 0.377, EtOH) or $- 144.6°$ (c M/40, 0.1 N/H_2SO_4). It is readily soluble in EtOH but only slightly soluble in other organic solvents and insoluble in H_2O. The hydrochloride dihydrate forms colourless prisms, m.p. 202–3°C (*dry*); $[\alpha]_D - 89.4°$ (c 1.19, H_2O); the dihydrobromide dihydrate has $[\alpha]_D^{25} - 92.9°$ (c 0.4, H_2O); the sulphate forms the crystalline heptahydrate as colourless needles which are very soluble in H_2O; the acid sulphate pentahydrate yields colourless leaflets, $[\alpha]_D^{15} - 106.8°$ (c 0.4, H_2O) and the methiodide has m.p. 248°C.

The alkaloid exhibits an antipyretic action in rats.

Forst, Böhringer., *Ber.*, **14**, 1270 (1881)
Skita, Nord., *ibid*, **45**, 3312 (1912)
Emde., *Helv. Chim. Acta*, **15**, 557 (1932)

HYDROCOTARNINE

$C_{12}H_{15}O_3N$

M.p. 55.5–56.5°C

This alkaloid is one of the basic hydrolytic products from narcotine (q.v.) and also occurs in the latex of *Papaver somniferum*. It is soluble in most organic solvents but insoluble in H_2O or alkalies. It yields well crystallized salts, e.g. the hydrobromide, m.p. 236–7°C; hydriodide, colourless needles, m.p. 195–6°C and the methiodide, m.p. 206–7°C. Oxidation with $KMnO_4$ yields cotarnine while reduction with sodium in EtOH furnishes hydrohydrastinine by elimination of a methoxyl group.

Hesse., *Annalen*, Suppl., **8**, 326 (1872)
Beckett., *J. Chem. Soc.*, **28**, 577 (1875)
Bandow, Wolffenstein., *Ber.*, **31**, 1577 (1898)
Steiner., *Compt. rend.*, **176**, 224 (1923)
Dey, Kantam., *J. Ind. Chem. Soc.*, **12**, 421 (1935)

HYDROIPECAMINE

This uncharacterized alkaloid has been obtained from the roots of *Cephaelis Ipecacuanha* (Brot) A. Rich. It is said to occur along with a further base of unknown constitution, ipecamine (q.v.).

Pyman., *J. Chem. Soc.*, **111**, 428 (1917)

HYDROMENISARINE

$C_{36}H_{36}O_6N_2$

M.p. 164°C

Kondo and Tomita have isolated this alkaloid from *Cocculus sarmentosus* Diels. It is dextrorotatory with $[\alpha]_D^{15} + 265.8°$ ($CHCl_3$) and yields a blue colour with a mixture of H_2SO_4 and HNO_3 which is characteristic of dibenzodioxans. When oxidized with $KMnO_4$ it furnishes 6-methoxyphenyl ether-3:4'-dicarboxylic acid. It gives a positive Liebermann nitroso reaction.

Kondo, Tomita., *J. Pharm. Soc., Japan,* **55**, 100, 637 (1935)

HYDRORHOMBININE

$C_{16}H_{30}O_2N_2$

B.p. 140°C/0.2 mm

This liquid alkaloid is said to be obtained from various *Thermopsis* species, yielding a crystalline perchlorate, m.p. 213°C; $[\alpha]_D - 40.9°$ (H_2O).

Manske, Marion., *Can. J. Res.,* **20B**, 265 (1942)
Manske, Marion., *ibid*, **21B**, 144 (1943)

702

6-HYDROXYBUPHANIDRINE

$C_{18}H_{21}O_5N$

M.p. 95–6°C

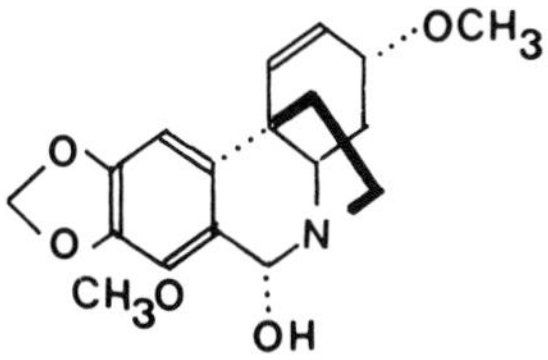

Isolated from *Nerine bowdenii* W. Wats., this alkaloid forms colourless prisms when crystallized from $CHCl_3$. It is laevorotatory, having $[\alpha]_D^{24} - 63°$ (c 0.19, MeOH). The ultraviolet spectrum in EtOH shows absorption maxima at 215, 238 and 285 mμ. Two methoxyl groups, a methylenedioxy group and a hydroxyl group are present. The alkaloid yields a crystalline O-acetate, m.p. 165–8°C.

Slabaugh, Wildman., *J. Org. Chem.*, **36**, 3202 (1971)

10-HYDROXYCAMPTOTHECIN

$C_{20}H_{16}O_5N_2$

M.p. 268–270°C

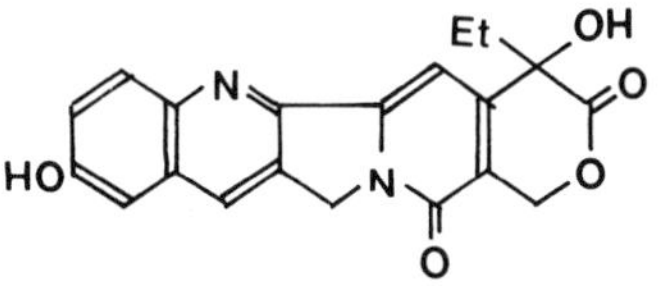

This alkaloid occurs in *Camptotheca acuminata* and forms colourless crystals from a mixture of MeOH, $CHCl_3$ and AcOEt. The ultraviolet spectrum in MeOH has absorption maxima at 222, 267, 330 and 382 mμ. The 10-O-acetyl derivative has m.p. 255–7°C and the diacetate, m.p. 270–3°C. The 10-methyl ether also occurs naturally in this plant.

Wani, Walls., *J. Org. Chem.*, **34**, 1364 (1969)

19-HYDROXYCASSAINE

$C_{24}H_{39}O_5N$

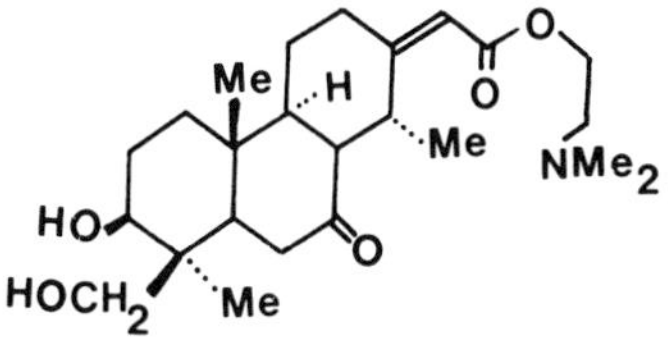

A recently discovered alkaloid from the bark of *Erythrophleum ivorense*. The structure has been determined primarily from the NMR and mass spectra.

Cronlund., *Acta Pharm. Suec.*, **10**, 507 (1973)

16-HYDROXY-α-COLUBRINE

$C_{22}H_{23}O_4N_2$

M.p. 225–7°C

This alkaloid, and the following base, have been obtained from the alkaloidal extract of *Strychnos nux-vomica*. They occur in the mother liquors after the removal of strychnine sulphate and may be separated by countercurrent distribution methods. This alkaloid has $[\alpha]_D^{20} - 54°$ (CHCl$_3$). When oxidized with H_2O_2, the base yields N-oxy-α-colubrine which may then be further oxidized with potassium chromate, followed by treatment with aqueous sodium bicarbonate to give a mixture of the original alkaloid and 18-oxo-α-colubrine (α-colubrone). The structure has been established from the infrared, NMR and mass spectra.

Marini-Bettolo *et al.*, *Ann. Chim.* (Rome), **60**, 444 (1970)
Villar del Fresno *et al.*, *Atti. Accad. Naz. Lincei, Cl. Sci. Fis. Mat. Natur. Rend.*, **48**, 250 (1970)

16-HYDROXY-β-COLUBRINE

$C_{22}H_{23}O_4N_2$

M.p. 140–3°C

A positional isomer of the preceding base, this alkaloid also occurs in the mother liquors following the removal of strychnine sulphate from the seed extract of *Strychnos nux-vomica*. It is also laevorotatory with $[\alpha]_D^{20} - 56°$ (CHCl$_3$). On oxidation with H_2O_2 it gives the isomeric N-oxo-β-colubrine which may then be further oxidized with potassium chromate and treated with sodium bicarbonate to yield 18-oxo-β-colubrine (β-colubrone). The structure has been determined in a like manner from spectroscopic data.

Marini-Bettolo *et al.*, *Ann. Chim.* (Rome), **60**, 444 (1970)
Villar del Fresno *et al.*, *Atti. Accad. Naz. Lincei, Cl. Sci. Fis. Mat. Natur. Rend.*, **48**, 250 (1970)

12β-HYDROXYCONESSIMINE

$C_{23}H_{38}ON_2$

M.p. 197–8°C

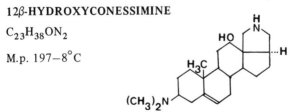

Present in minute quantities in various *Holarrhena* species, this alkaloid has

$[\alpha]_D^{20} + 13°$ (c 1.08, EtOH). It yields a diacetyl derivative as colourless prisms from light petroleum, m.p. 122–4°C. The 4-methyl-3-pentenoyl ester is identical with Holafrine (q.v.) while the N-methyl compound is Holarrhenine (q.v.).

Rostock, Seebeck., *Helv. Chim. Acta*, **41**, 11 (1958)

α-HYDROXYCONESSINE

$C_{24}H_{40}ON_2$

M.p. 157°C

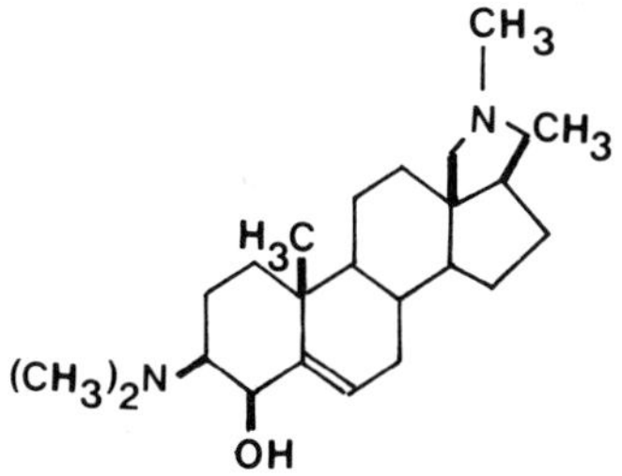

This base is a minor constituent of various *Holarrhena* species and has $[\alpha]_D + 20°$ (c 0.8, $CHCl_3$-EtOH). It contains a dimethylamino group, a methylimino group and a hydroxyl group in the molecule and forms a crystalline O-acetate, m.p. 127°C; $[\alpha]_D - 75°$ (c 1.1, $CHCl_3$).

Bertho., *Annalen*, 557, 220 (1947)
Bertho., *ibid*, 561, 1 (1950)
Bertho., *ibid*, 619, 96 (1957)
Howarth, Michael., *J. Chem. Soc.*, 4973 (1957)
Goutarel, Conreur, Parello., *Bull. Soc. Chim. Fr.*, 2401 (1963)

7α-HYDROXYCONESSINE

$C_{24}H_{40}ON_2$

M.p. 176–8°C

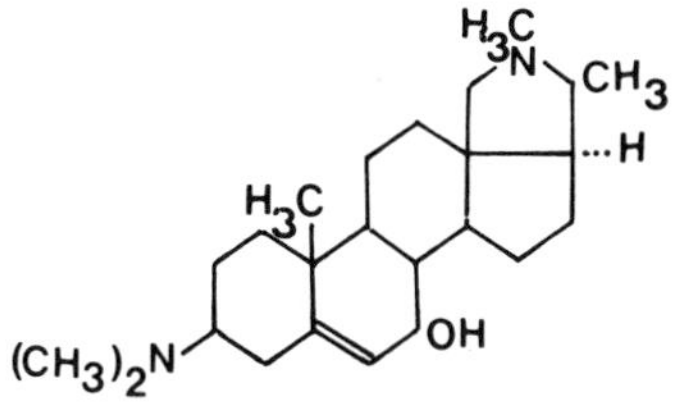

This alkaloid found in *Holarrhena antidysenterica* Wall is laevorotatory with $[\alpha]_D^{20} - 61° \pm 1°$ (c 0.95, $CHCl_3$). It is obtained as colourless crystals from C_6H_6 and forms a monoacetate, m.p. 148–150°C.

Tschesche, Ockenfels., *Ber.*, **97**, 2316 (1964)

6-HYDROXYCRINAMINE (*epiHaemanthidine*)

$C_{17}H_{19}O_5N$

M.p. 209–211°C

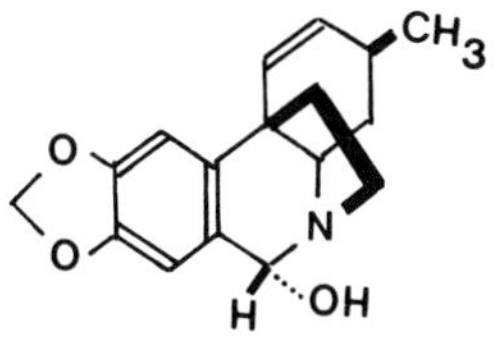

This alkaloid occurs in several *Crinum* species, particularly in *C. erubescens, C.*

705

fribriatulum and *C. zeanicum*. It is also present in *Ammocharis coranica* (Ker-Gaul) Herb and *Haemanthus natalensis*. When crystallized from aqueous Me_2CO it forms colourless crystals of the hemihydrate, m.p. 146°C. Colourless prisms of the anhydrous base are obtained from a mixture of Me_2CO and light petroleum. The alkaloid has $[\alpha]_D^{25} + 46°$ (c 1.0, $CHCl_3$) or $[\alpha]_D^{14} + 47°$ (c 0.446, $CHCl_3$). The ultraviolet spectrum shows absorption maxima at 240 and 294 mμ. In solution, the base is believed to exist as a tautomeric mixture of the C-6 epimers. The methiodide is obtained as colourless prisms from H_2O, m.p. 174°C; $[\alpha]_D^{23} + 57°$ (c 1.0, EtOH) and the methopicrate has m.p. 146°C. The diacetyl derivative is normally found as an amorphous solid although it has been obtained in the crystalline form, m.p. 182–4°C. The structure has been established from the NMR and mass spectra.

Fales, Horn, Wildman., *Chem. Ind.*, 1415 (1959)
Goosen *et al.*, *J. Chem. Soc.*, 1088 (1960)
Hauth, Stauffacher., *Helv. Chim. Acta*, **45**, 1307 (1962)
King, Murphy, Wildman., *J. Amer. Chem. Soc.*, **87**, 4912 (1965)

Crystal structure:
Karle, Estlin, Karle., *J. Amer. Chem. Soc.*, **89**, 6510 (1967)

Spectra:
Haugwitz, Jeffs, Wenkert., *J. Chem. Soc.*, 2001 (1965)
Duffield *et al.*, *J. Amer. Chem. Soc.*, **87**, 4902 (1965)

HYDROXY-DE-N-METHYL-α-OBSCURINE

$C_{16}H_{24}O_2N_2$

M.p. 300–5°C

This alkaloid is a minor constituent of *Lycopodium flabelliforme* and may be purified by recrystallization from MeOH-Me_2CO when it forms fine colourless needles. The ultraviolet spectrum exhibits one absorption maximum at 255 mμ. The structure has been established primarily from the fragmentation pattern of the mass spectrum.

Alam, Adams, MacLean., *Can. J. Chem.*, **42**, 2456 (1964)

2-HYDROXYDENDROBINE

$C_{16}H_{25}O_3N$

M.p. 103–4°C

A minor alkaloid from *Dendrobium findlayanum* Par. et Rchb., this base is laevorotatory with $[\alpha]_D^{26} - 45°$ (c 0.73, CHCl$_3$). A methyl group, hydroxyl group, methlimino and *iso*propyl group are present together with a lactam ring.

Granelli, Leander, Luning., *Acta Chem. Scand.*, 24, 1209 (1970)

6-HYDROXY-2:3-DIMETHOXY-9:11:12:13:13a:14-HEXAHYDRO DIBENZO-[f,h PYRROLO 1,2-b]ISOQUINOLINE

$C_{22}H_{23}O_3N$

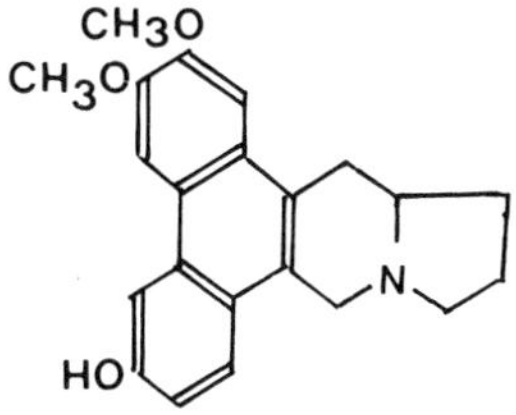

Cynanchum vincetoxicum yields this minor alkaloid together with Tylophorine (q.v.). The structure follows from the infrared, ultraviolet, NMR and mass spectra.

Wiegrebe *et al., Justus Liebig's Ann. Chem.*, 721, 154 (1969)
Synthesis:
Wiegrebe *et al., ibid*, 733, 125 (1970)

1-HYDROXY-2:3-DIMETHOXY-N-METHYLACRIDONE

$C_{16}H_{15}O_4N$

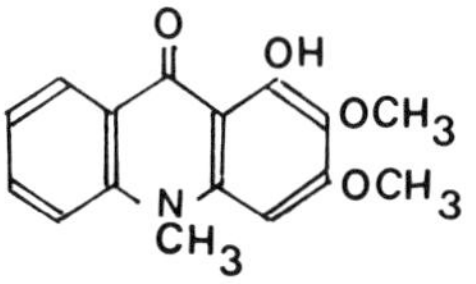

This 9-acridone alkaloid has been isolated by C_6H_6 extraction from the neutral fraction of the MeOH extract of the bark of *Fagara leprieurii*. It also occurs in a Nigerian species of *F. rubescens*. The structure has been confirmed by methylation to the known trimethoxy derivative, m.p. 168—170°C.

Fonzes, Winternitz., *Compt. Rend.*, 266C, 930 (1968)
Fish, Waterman., *J. Pharm. Pharmacol.*, 23, 1325 (1971)

9-HYDROXY-3:10-DIMETHOXY-1:2-METHYLENEDIOXYNORAPORPHINE

$C_{19}H_{19}O_5N$

M.p. 217—9°C (*dec.*).

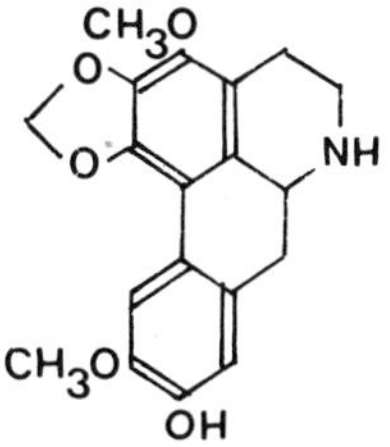

This alkaloid from *Cassytha filiformis* L. is also known as Cassyfiline or

Cassythine. It forms colourless crystals from a mixture of EtOH and CHCl$_3$. It has $[\alpha]_D$ + 24° (c 0.56, CHCl$_3$) and the ultraviolet spectrum has absorption maxima at 218, 283 and 303 mμ. It forms the O-methyl ether as colourless needles, M.p. 150–1°C, giving a crystalline hydrochloride, m.p. 260–1°C and also the N-methyl derivative, m.p. 208°C which yields an O-acetate as colourless crystals, m.p. 195–6°C. The O,N-dimethyl derivative is Ocoteine (q.v.).

Tomita, Lu, Wang., *J. Pharm. Soc., Japan*, 85, 827 (1965)

Johns, Lamberton., *Austral. J. Chem.*, 19, 297 (1966)

Johns, Lamberton, Sioumis., *ibid*, 19, 2331, 2339 (1966)

6-HYDROXY-2:3-DIMETHOXYPHENANTHRO-[9,10-f]INDOLIZIDINE

C$_{22}$H$_{23}$O$_3$N

M.p. 226–8°C

The above-ground parts of *Cynanchum vincetoxicum* yield this alkaloid which forms colourless crystals from EtOH. It is strongly laevorotatory with $[\alpha]_D^{22}$ − 125° ± 6° (c 1.05, pyridine) and gives an ultraviolet spectrum in MeOH with absorption maxima at 260, 287, 344 and 362 mμ.

Wiegrabe *et al.*, *Annalen*, 721, 154 (1969)

7-HYDROXY-3:6-DITIGLOYLTROPANE

C$_{18}$H$_{27}$O$_5$N

From certain species of Datura grown in Egypt, e.g. *D. arborea, D. Metel* and *D. meteloides*, this alkaloid has been isolated from the root extract. It occurs to the extent of 0.18–0.25 per cent.

Karawya, Balbaa., *Bull. Fac. Pharm., Cairo Univ.*, 6, 9 (1967)

11-HYDROXYERYSOTRINE

C$_{19}$H$_{23}$O$_4$N

This *Erythrina* alkaloid has been isolated from *E. arborescens* Roxb. The structure has been determined from chemical and spectroscopic data.

Ito, Furukawa, Harina., *J. Pharm. Soc., Japan*, 93, 1617 (1973)

N-2-HYDROXYETHYLCINNAMIDE

$C_{11}H_{13}O_2N$

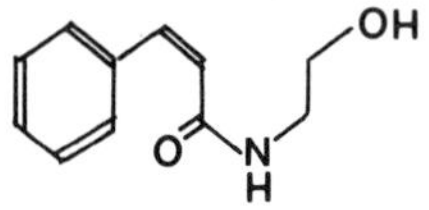

A recently discovered constituent of the leaves of *Erythrophleum chlorostachys,* the structure of this alkaloid has been proved by synthesis. It is possibly an artifact of isolation.

Griffen *et al., Phytochem.,* **10**, 2793 (1971)

N-2-HYDROXYETHYL-N-METHYLCINNAMIDE

$C_{12}H_{15}O_2N$

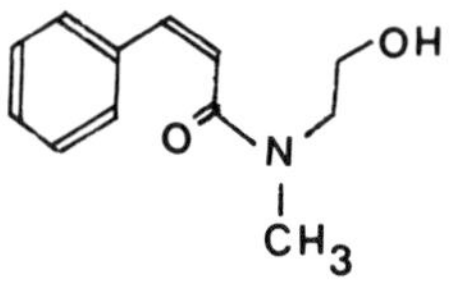

Also present in the leaf extract of *Erythrophleum chlorostachys,* this base has been synthesized and, like the preceding alkaloid, may be an artifact produced during the isolation process.

Griffen *et al., Phytochem.,* **10**, 2793 (1971)

HYDROXYGARDNUTINE

$C_{20}H_{22}O_3N_2$

M.p. $311-2°C$

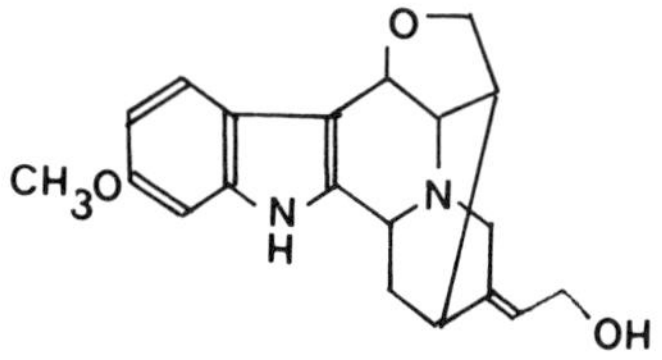

An alkaloid present in the stem and roots of *Gardneria nutans* Sieb et Zucc., this base has $[\alpha]_D^{25} + 36.2°$ and the ultraviolet spectrum shows absorption maxima at 223, 260.5, 295 and 301 mμ. It contains a methoxyl group, a hydroxyallyl and a methylimino group in the molecule, the structure having been determined from the infrared, NMR and mass spectra.

Sakai, Kubo, Haginiwa., *Tetrahedron Lett.,* 1485 (1969)

14-HYDROXYGELSEMICINE (*Alkaloid C*)

$C_{20}H_{24}O_5N_2$

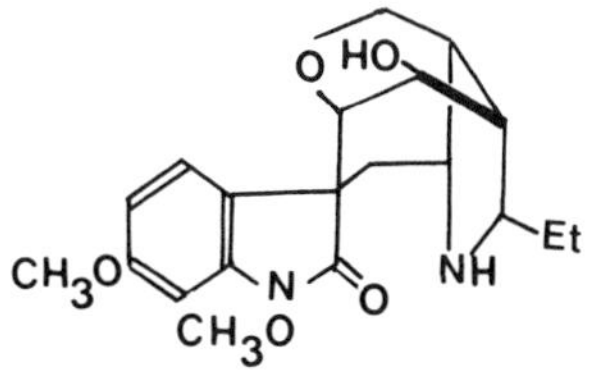

Formerly known as Alkaloid C, this alkaloid has been obtained from Gelsemium sempervirens and its structure determined from NMR and mass spectroscopic determinations. It contains two methoxyl groups, one hydroxyl and an imino group.

Wichtl *et al.*, *Monatsh.*, **104**, 87 (1973)

17-HYDROXYHEDRANTHERINE

$C_{21}H_{24}O_5N_2$

M.p. 245°C (*dec.*).

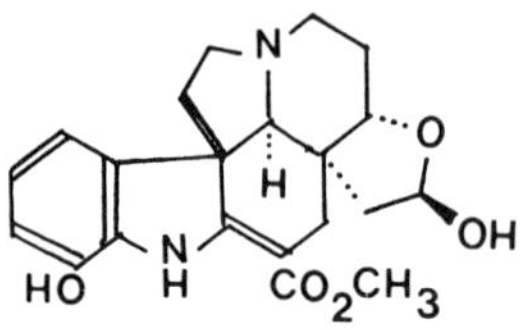

An imidazolidinocarbazole alkaloid present in the leaf extract of *Hedranthera barteri*, this alkaloid forms colourless crystals from MeOH-CHCl$_3$. The ultraviolet spectrum has absorption maxima at 235, 290 and 336 mμ. It forms an O,N-diacetyl derivative, m.p. 75°C and the 17-methyl ether which is an amorphous solid that cannot be crystallized.

Naranjo, Hesse, Schmid., *Helv. Chim. Acta*, **55**, 1849 (1972)

6-HYDROXYHYOSCYAMINE

$C_{17}H_{23}O_4N$

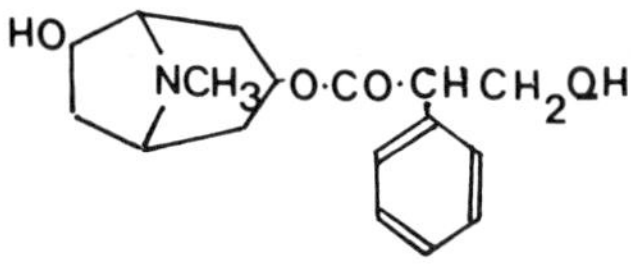

Isolated from the roots of *Physochlaina dubia*, this alkaloid is laevorotatory with $[\alpha]_D^{20} - 13.5°$ (c 1.9, MeOH). The structure has been determined from spectroscopic data and comparison with hyoscyamine.

Mirzamatov *et al.*, *Khim. Prir. Soedin.*, **8**, 493 (1972)

6-HYDROXYHYOSCYAMINE DIACETATE

$C_{21}H_{27}O_6N$

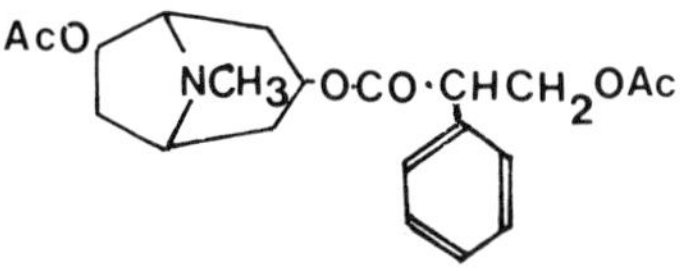

This base occurs together with the previous alkaloid in the root extract of *Physochlaina dubia*. The structure has been established by comparison with similar bases.

Mirzamatov *et al.*, *Khim. Prir. Soedin.*, **8**, 493 (1972)

6-HYDROXY-N-ISOPENTENYLDENDROXINE

$C_{22}H_{34}O_4N^+$

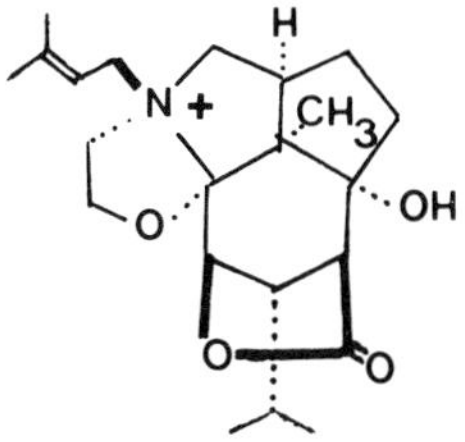

A quaternary alkaloid, this base is found in several *Dendrobium* species and is usually isolated as the chloride which forms colourless needles from EtOH, m.p. 144–156°C (*dec.*). This salt is laevorotatory with $[\alpha]_D^{22} - 30°$ (c 0.5, MeOH).

Hedman, Leander, Lüning., *Acta Chem. Scand.*, **25**, 1142 (1971)

(−)-7-HYDROXY-β-ISOSPARTEINE

$C_{15}H_{26}ON_2$

M.p. 103.5–104.5°C

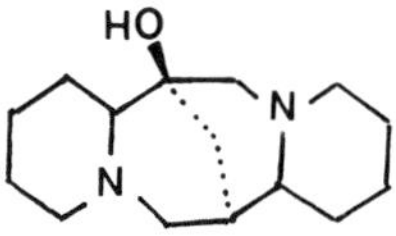

This sparteine alkaloid is present in *Lupinus sericeus* Pursh. It gives crystalline salts, e.g. the hydriodide, m.p. 258.5–260°C and the perchlorate, m.p. 207.5–208.5°C. On acetylation with AcOCl, it yields the acetyl derivative which is not crystallizable and has $[\alpha]_D^{25.2} + 23.5°$ (c 0.66, EtOH) and yielding a crystalline diperchlorate, m.p. 231–236.5°C; $[\alpha]_D^{24.2} + 4.5°$ (c 0.32, CHCl$_3$).

Carmack, Goldberg, Martin., *J. Org. Chem.*, **32**, 3045 (1967)

6β-HYDROXYKOPSININE (*Hydroxylkopsinine I*)

$C_{21}H_{26}O_3N_2$

M.p. 190–6°C

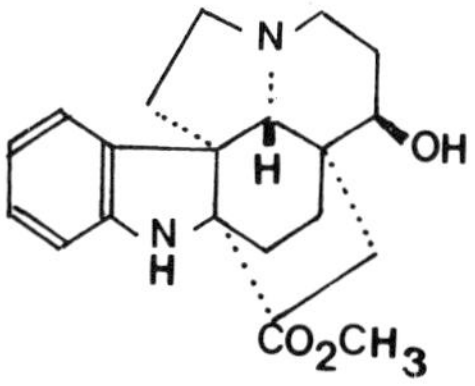

Melodinus australis yields two very similar alkaloids, sometimes referred to as hydroxykopsinines I and II. This particular base yields fine, colourless prisms from a mixture of Et$_2$O and CHCl$_3$ and has $[\alpha]_D^{23} - 62°$ (c 1.14, CHCl$_3$). It gives an ultraviolet spectrum showing absorption maxima at 242 and 294 mμ.

Linde., *Helv. Chim. Acta*, **48**, 1822 (1965)
Linde., *Pharm. Acta Helv.*, **45**, 248 (1970)

14α-HYDROXYKOPSININE (*Hydroxykopsinine II*)

$C_{21}H_{26}O_3N_2$

M.p. 187–192°C

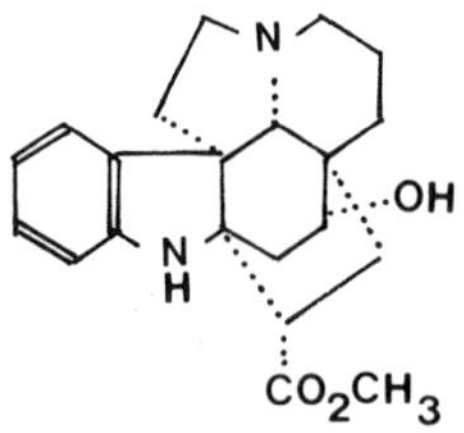

This second isomeric alkaloid from *Melodinus australis* has a similar optical rotation to the previous base being $[\alpha]_D^{23} - 63°$ (c 1.03, CHCl$_3$). The ultraviolet spectrum in EtOH is also identical with absorption maxima at 242 and 294 mμ.

Linde., *Helv. Chim. Acta,* **48**, 1822 (1965)
Linde., *Pharm. Acta Helv.,* **45**, 248 (1970)

(−)-HYDROXYLUNINE

$C_{16}H_{17}O_5N$

M.p. 228–230°C

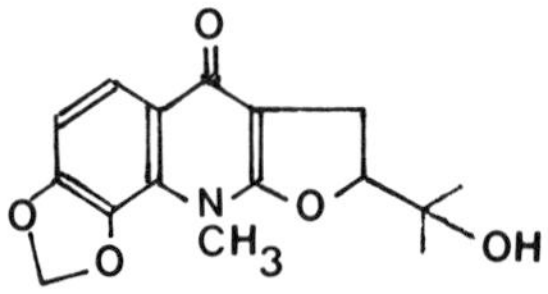

A furoquinolone alkaloid found in the leaves of *Lunasia amara* Blanco, the base has $[\alpha]_{436}^{25} - 13.8°$ (c 0.276, EtOH) and $[\alpha]_{589}^{25} - 5.9°$ (c 0.276, EtOH). The ultraviolet spectrum shows four absorption maxima at 220, 246, 320 and 330 mμ with a shoulder at 268 mμ. The structure has been established from spectroscopic data.

Goodwin *et al., J. Amer. Chem. Soc.,* **81**, 6209 (1959)

(+)-HYDROXYLUNINE

$C_{16}H_{17}O_5N$

M.p. 224–7°C

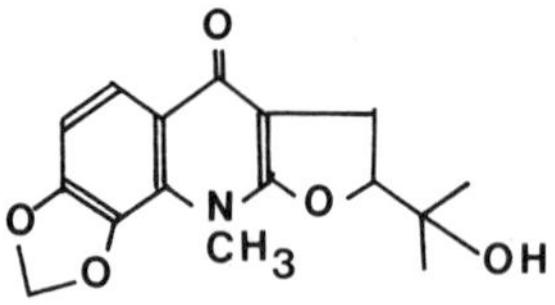

The enantiomorph of the preceding alkaloid occurs in the leaf extract of *Ptelea trifoliata* and forms colourless crystals from MeOH. It has $[\alpha]_{436}^{25} + 21°$ (c 0.59, EtOH) and $[\alpha]_{589}^{25} + 6°$ (c 0.59, EtOH). The ultraviolet spectrum is identical to that of the previous alkaloid.

Goodwin *et al., J. Amer. Chem. Soc.,* **81**, 6209 (1959)

712

13-HYDROXYLUPANINE (*Octalupine*)

$C_{15}H_{24}O_2N_2$

M.p. 172–4°C

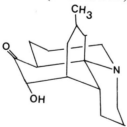

This lupanine alkaloid has been isolated from the seeds of *Lupinus albus, L. perennis*, L., *L. wyethii* and other species of this family. It occurs in the high-boiling fraction of the alkaloidal extract. It forms a stable dihydrate as colourless rhombic prisms, m.p. 76–7°C and has $[\alpha]_D^{32}$ + 51.8° (c 1.0, EtOH) or + 74.1° (c 3.59, H_2O). It yields a series of well crystalline salts and derivatives: the hydrochloride, m.p. 296–8°C; hydriodide hydrate, m.p. 91–3°C or 234–8°C (*dry*); aurichloride, m.p. 205–6°C; methiodide existing in two forms, m.p. 236–9°C and 238–9°C respectively; picrolonate, m.p. 174–5°C and the benzoyl derivative, m.p. 202–3°C.

The presence of a primary alcoholic hydroxyl is shown by the formation of an aldehyde on oxidation, giving an oxime, m.p. 217–8°C and a semicarbazone, m.p. 221–3°C. With Hi it is reduced to d-lupanine, m.p. 40–4°C, b.p. 185–6°C/ 0.08 mm. Concentrated H_2SO_4 dehydrates the alkaloid to the anhydro-base, $C_{15}H_{22}ON_2$, which again gives d-lupanine on catalytic hydrogenation.

Bergh., *Arch. Pharm.*, **242**, 416 (1904)
Beckel., *ibid*, **248**, 451 (1910)
Beckel., *ibid*, **250**, 691 (1912)
Ueno., *J. Pharm. Soc., Japan*, **50**, 435 (1930)
Couch., *J. Amer. Chem. Soc.*, **58**, 686, 1296 (1936)
Couch., *ibid*, **59**, 1471 (1937)
Deulofeu, Gatt., *J. Org. Chem.*, **10**, 179 (1945)
Marion, Douglas., *Can. J. Chem.*, **29**, 721 (1951)
Turcotte, Leduc, Marion., *ibid*, **31**, 387 (1953)
Bohlmann, Winterfeldt, Brackel., *Chem. Ber.*, **91**, 2194 (1958)
Wie'wiorowski, Bartz, Wysocka., *Bull. Acad. Polon. Sci., Ser. Sci. Chim.*, **9**, 715 (1961)
Goosen., *J. Chem. Soc.*, 3067 (1963)

6-α-HYDROXYLYCOPODINE (*Alkaloid L-20*)

$C_{16}H_{25}O_2N$

M.p. 258–9°C

A *Lycopodium* alkaloid present in *L. lucidulum* Michx., this base yields colourless needles from light petroleum. The ultraviolet spectrum contains one absorption maximum at 296 mμ. A crystalline O-acetate has been obtained by the action of Ac_2O at low temperatures, m.p. 143–4°C.

Manske, Marion., *Can. J. Res.*, **24B**, 57 (1946)
Ayer, Berezowsky, Law., *Can. J. Chem.*, **41**, 649 (1963)

12-HYDROXYLYCOPODINE (*Alkaloid L-23*)

$C_{16}H_{25}O_2N$

M.p. 163–4°C

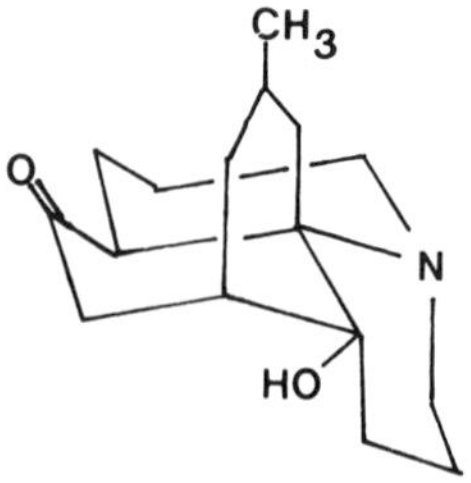

This isomer of the preceding alkaloid, also obtained from *Lycopodium lucidulum* Michx., was originally designated alkaloid L-23 by Manske and Marion during their investigation of the bases of *Lycopodium* species. It has $[\alpha]_D$ − 43° (c 0.13, EtOH).

Manske, Marion., *Can. J. Res.*, **24B**, 57 (1946)
Ayer *et al.*, *Can. J. Chem.*, **47**, 449 (1969)

2-HYDROXY-1-METHOXYAPORPHINE

$C_{18}H_{19}O_2N$

M.p. 195–6°C

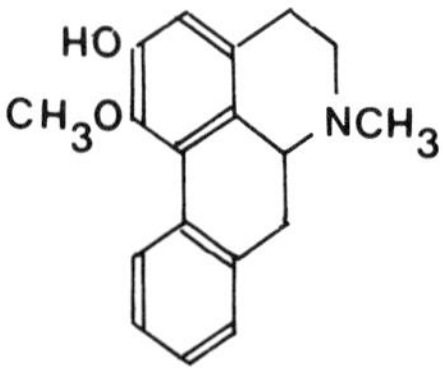

This simple aporphine alkaloid occurs in *Nelumbo nucifera* and is laevorotatory with $[\alpha]_D$ − 265° (CHCl$_3$). The early name of nornuciferine is no longer in use for this alkaloid having been given to the des-N-methyl derivative. The O-methyl ether is identical with nuciferine (q.v.).

Tomita, Watanabe, Furukawa., *J. Pharm. Soc., Japan,* **81**, 469, 492, 1644 (1961)

1-(3-HYDROXY-4-METHOXYBENZYL)-6:7-DIMETHOXYISOQUINOLINE

See Palaudine

7-HYDROXY-4-METHOXYFURO(2,3-b)QUINOLINE

$C_{12}H_9O_3N$

M.p. 240–2°C

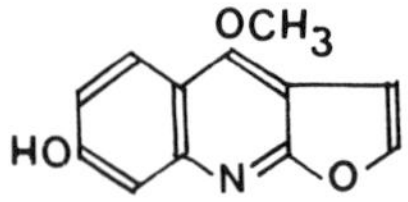

The leaves of *Evodia elleryana* F. Muell. yield this furoquinoline alkaloid which may be purified by recrystallization from MeOH when it forms pale yellow needles. The ultraviolet spectrum in EtOH has absorption maxima at 245, 310,

325 and 335 mμ with an inflexion at 296 mμ. The base contains one phenolic hydroxyl group and yields a crystalline O-acetate as colourless needles, m.p. 156–7°C. The O-methyl ester is identical with Evolitrine (q.v.).

Johns, Lamberton, Sioumis., *Austral. J. Chem.*, **24**, 1897 (1968)

1-HYDROXY-3-METHOXY-10-METHYLACRID-9-ONE

$C_{15}H_{13}O_3N$

A minor alkaloid of a Nigerian species of *Fagara rubescens,* the structure has been determined from chemical reactions and spectroscopic evidence.

Fish, Waterman., *J. Pharm. Pharmacol.*, **23**, 1325 (1971)

7α-HYDROXY-1-METHOXYMETHYL-1:2-DEHYDRO-8α-PYRROLIZIDINE

$C_9H_{15}O_2N$

M.p. 54°C;
B.p. 90–4°C/0.3 mm

Two comparatively simple alkaloids of the pyrrolizidine type are present in *Crotalaria aridicola* Domin. and *C. trifoliastrum* Willd. This particular base has $[\alpha]_D^{20}$ + 25.2° (c 1.78, EtOH) and yields a crystalline picrate as pale yellow needles, m.p. 161–161.5°C. The structure has been established from the infrared and NMR spectra.

Sethi, Atal., *Ind. J. Pharm.*, **25**, 159 (1963)
Culvenor, O'Donovan, Smith., *Austral. J. Chem.*, **20**, 757 (1967)

7β-HYDROXY-1-METHOXYMETHYL-1:2-DEHYDRO-8α-PYRROLIZIDINE

$C_9H_{15}O_2N$

M.p. 35–40°C;
B.p. 77°C/0.4 mm

The stereoisomer of the preceding base also occurs in *Crotalaria aridicola* Domin. and *C. trifoliastrum* Willd. It has $[\alpha]_D^{18}$ + 38° (c 2.3, EtOH). The alkaloid furnishes a crystalline hydrochloride, m.p. 159–160°C; $[\alpha]_D^{18}$ − 19.2° (c 1.12, EtOH) and a picrate as slender yellow needles, m.p. 185–6°C; $[\alpha]_D^{18}$ − 9° (c 1.99, Me$_2$CO).

Culvenor, Smith., *Austral. J. Chem.*, **15**, 121 (1962)
Culvenor, O'Donovan, Smith., *ibid*, **20**, 757 (1967)

12-HYDROXY-11-METHOXYSPERMOSTRYCHNINE

$C_{22}H_{28}O_4N_2$

M.p. 272–3°C

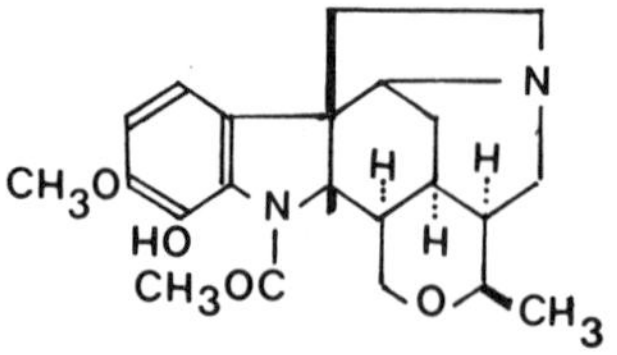

One of the *Strychnos* alkaloids, this base is found in *S. brasiliensis* Mart and forms colourless plates from EtOH. It is laevorotatory with $[\alpha]_D^{25} - 217°$ (c 0.58, CHCl$_3$) and gives an ultraviolet spectrum in ethanol with absorption maxima at 225, 255 and 290 mμ. The structure has been determined from spectroscopic evidence and comparison with similar *Strychnos* bases.

Iwataki, Comin., *Tetrahedron*, **27**, 2541 (1971)

12-HYDROXY-11-METHOXYSTRYCHNOBRASILINE

$C_{23}H_{28}O_5N_2$

M.p. 229–230°C

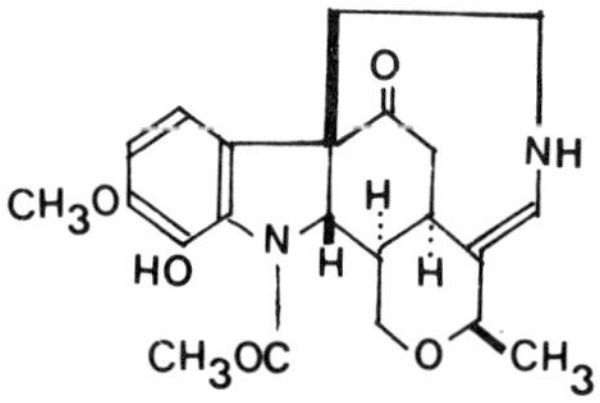

A further alkaloid of *Strychnos* species, this base occurs in *S. brasiliensis* Mart. When crystallized from MeOH it yields clusters of fine, colourless needles. It is laevorotatory, having $[\alpha]_D^{18} - 31°$ (c 0.57, CHCl$_3$). The ultraviolet spectrum in ethanol shows an absorption maximum at 227 mμ and shoulders at 263 and 290 mμ.

Iwataki, Comin., *Tetrahedron*, **27**, 2541 (1971)

1-HYDROXY-N-METHYLACRIDONE

$C_{14}H_{11}O_2N$

M.p. 192–4°C

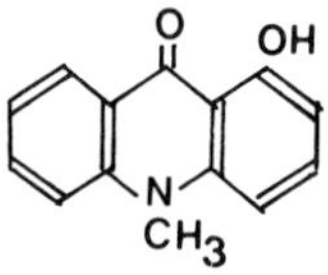

This simple acridone alkaloid is found in the root extract of Ruta graveolens. It contains one phenolic hydroxyl but no crystalline salts have yet been reported.

Reisch *et al.*, *Experientis*, **27**, 1005 (1971)

1-HYDROXYMETHYL-β-CARBOLINE

$C_{12}H_{10}ON_2$

This alkaloid has recently been isolated from the stems of *Picrasima cilanthoides*. Few details have been reported of any salts or derivatives. The structure has been determined mainly from spectroscopic evidence.

Kondo, Takamoto., *Chem. Pharm. Bull.*, **21**, 837 (1973)

10-HYDROXY-1,2-METHYLENEDIOXYAPORPHINE

$C_{18}H_{17}O_3N$

M.p. 220–2°C

The CHCl₃ extract of the leaves of *Phoebe clemensii* Allen contains this alkaloid which yields glistening prisms when recrystallized from CHCl₃. The base darkens at about 208°C before melting. It has $[\alpha]_D$ – 76.5° (c 0.366, CHCl₃). The ultraviolet spectrum shows absorption maxima at 265, 275 and 308 mμ. It yields a crystalline hydrochloride as colourless needles from H₂O, darkening around 250°C but not melting below 330°C. This salts has $[\alpha]_D$ – 28.3° (c 0.315, H₂O). The methiodide is also crystalline, m.p. 237–9°C; $[\alpha]_D$ – 58° (c 0.27, MeOH). The alkaloid contains a methylimino group, a methylene-dioxy group and a phenolic hydroxyl, the latter yielding the O-acetate as a colourless gum which cannot be crystallized. The O-methyl ether is identical with laureline (q.v.).

Johns, Lamberton., *Austral. J. Chem.*, **20**, 1277 (1967)

7α-HYDROXY-1-METHYLENE-8β-PYRROLIZIDINE

$C_8H_{13}ON$

M.p. 34–6°C;
B.p. 62°C/0.03 mm

A simple pyrrolizidine alkaloid occurring in *Crotalaria goreensis* Guill et Perr. The base yields colourless needles when purified by recrystallization from EtOH and has $[\alpha]_D^{18}$ + 36.1° (c 1.39, EtOH). The alkaloid forms a picrate as yellow needles, m.p. 173.5–174.5°C; a picrolonate, also as yellow needles, m.p. 234–234.5°C and the phenylurethane, m.p. 135.5–136°C; $[\alpha]_D^{20}$ – 20.5° (c 0.77, EtOH). With KMnO₄ in Me₂CO, it gives formaldehyde, indicative of the exocyclic methylene group.

Culvenor, Smith., *Austral. J. Chem.*, **14**, 284 (1961)

1β-HYDROXYMETHYL-8Hβ-PYRROLIZIDINE
(*Larurnine*)

$C_8H_{15}ON$

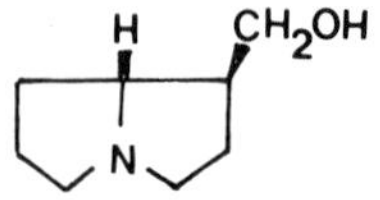

The seeds of *Cytisus laburnum* yield this alkaloid as a colourless oil which is non-crystallizable and has $[\alpha]_D + 15.4°$ (c 1.44, MeOH). Several crystalline derivatives have been prepared, including the methiodide, m.p. 307–9°C; the picrate, m.p. 174–5°C and the picrolonate, m.p. 181–2°C.

Galinovsky, Goldberger, Pohm., *Monatsh.*, **80**, 550 (1949)
Galinovsky, Vogl, Nesvadba., *ibid*, **85**, 913 (1954)
Hart, Lamberton., *Austral. J. Chem.*, **19**, 1259 (1966)

5-HYDROXY-1-METHYL-2-PHENYL-4-QUINOLONE

$C_{16}H_{15}O_4N$

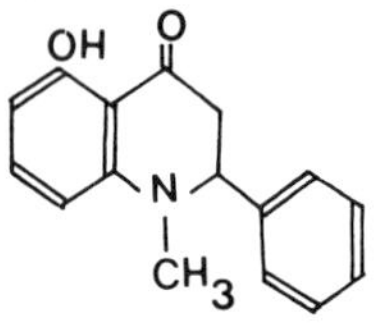

A minor constituent of the leaves of *Lunasia quercifolia,* this alkaloid occurs in the non-phenolic alkaloidal fraction. The structure has been determined by its preparation from (+)-lunidine by heating with aqueous HCl.

Hart *et al.*, *Austral. J. Chem.*, **21**, 1389 (1968)

13-HYDROXYMULTIFLORINE

$C_{15}H_{22}O_2N_2$

An alkaloid obtained from the high boiling fraction of the extract of *Lupinus albus,* followed by chromatography on alumina. The ultraviolet spectrum shows a single absorption maximum at 315 mμ.

Wieiorowski, Bartz, Wysocka., *Bull. Acad. Polon. Sci., Ser. Sci. Chim.*, **9**, 715 (1961)

6-HYDROXYNOBILINE

$C_{17}H_{27}O_4N$

M.p. 158–159.5°C

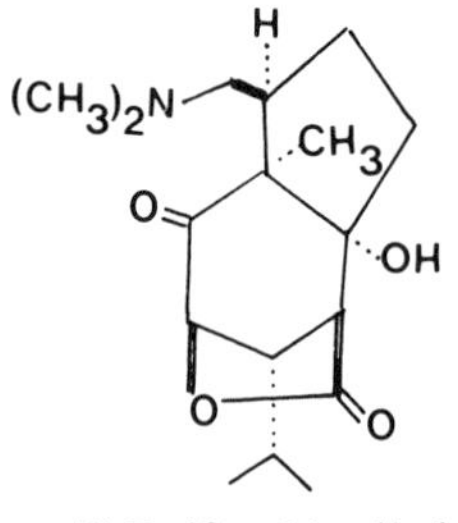

Present in *Dendrobium hildebrandii* Rolfe, this alkaloid yields colourless needles from C_6H_6 and has $[\alpha]_D^{23} + 62°$ (c 0.58, CHCl$_3$). An *iso*propyl group, a dimethylaminoethyl group and a hydroxyl group are present in the molecule, together with a lactam ring.

Elander, Leander., *Acta Chem. Scand.*, **25**, 717 (1971)

14-HYDROXYNOVACINE

$C_{24}H_{28}O_6N_2$

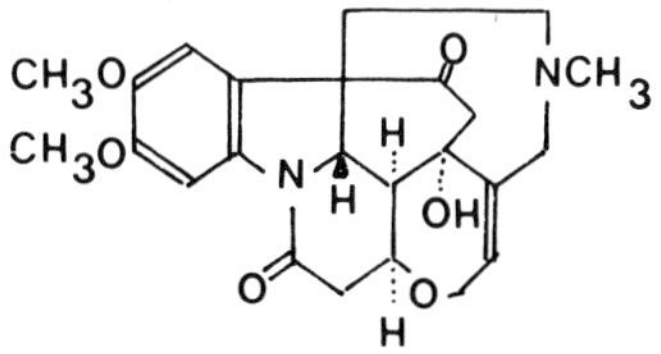

This minor alkaloid of the leaves of *Strychnos wallechiana* has only recently been isolated. No salts or derivatives have been reported.

Bisset, Chaudry., *Phytochem.*, **13**, 259 (1974)

20-HYDROXY-19-OXOCORONARIDINE

$C_{21}H_{24}O_5N_2$

M.p. Indefinite

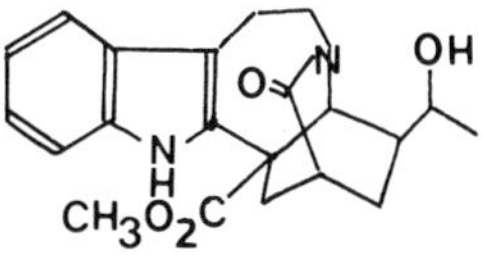

An amorphous alkaloid present as a minor constituent of the bark of *Conopharyngia jollyana*, the base contains a secondary hydroxyl group and a methoxycarbonyl group in the molecule.

Hootele, Pecher., *Chimia*, **22**, 245 (1968)

7α-HYDROXYPARAVALLARINE

$C_{21}H_{31}O_3N$

M.p. 213°C

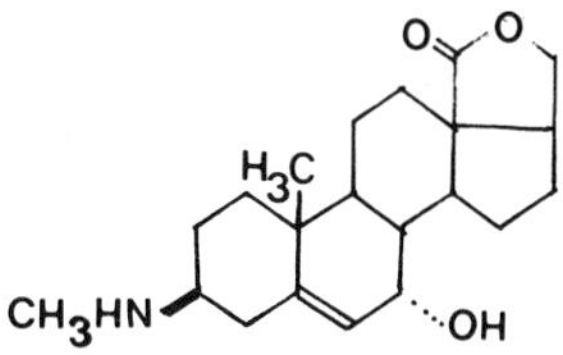

The leaves of *Paravallaris microphylla* yield this steroidal alkaloid which is stereoisomeric with the following base. The alkaloid forms colourless crystals from EtOH and is laevorotatory with $[\alpha]_D^{20} - 113°$ (CHCl$_3$).

Husson *et al., Bull. Soc. Chim. Fr.*, 3162 (1969)

7β-HYDROXYPARAVALLARINE

$C_{21}H_{31}O_3N$

M.p. 210°C

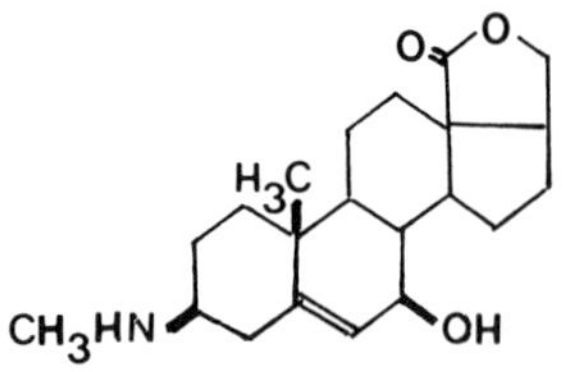

The stereoisomer of the preceding alkaloid also occurs in the leaves of *Paravallaris microphylla* Pirard and has $[\alpha]_D - 13.5°$ (CHCl$_3$).

Husson *et al.*, *Bull. Soc. Chim. Fr.*, 3162 (1969)

11α-HYDROXYPARAVALLARINE

$C_{21}H_{31}O_3N$

M.p. 235°C

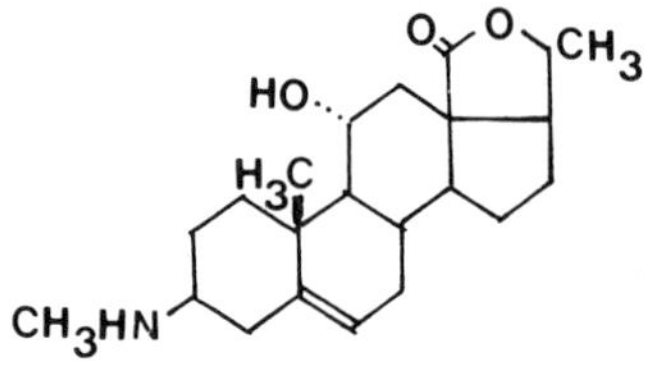

This isomer of the two alkaloids just mentioned has been isolated from the leaf extract of *Paravallaris microphylla* Pirard. It is laevorotatory with $[\alpha]_D^{20} - 55°$ (CHCl$_3$).

Husson *et al.*, *Bull. Soc. Chim. Fr.*, 3162 (1969)

11-HYDROXYPLEIOCARPAMINE

$C_{20}H_{22}O_3N_2$

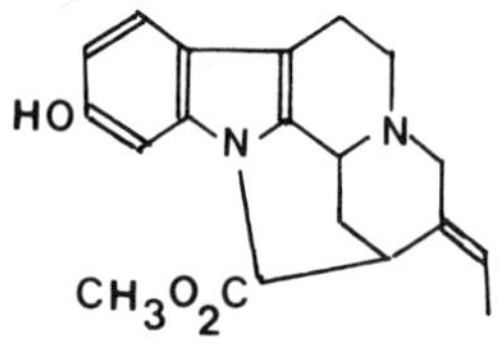

An alkaloid recently obtained from the aerial parts of *Vinca erecta*, this base contains a hydroxyl group, a methoxycarbonyl group and two tertiary nitrogens.

Il'yasova, Malikov, Yunusov., *Khim. Prir. Soedin.*, **6**, 717 (1970)

6-HYDROXYPOWELLINE

$C_{17}H_{19}O_5N$

M.p. 233–5°C

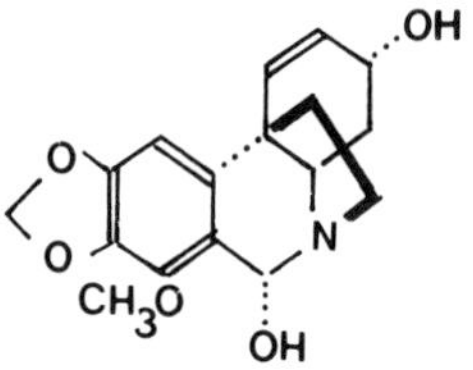

Present in *Nerine bowdenii* W. Wats, this alkaloid is obtained as colourless prismatic crystals from Me_2CO. It has $[\alpha]_D^{24} - 36°$ (c 0.19, MeOH) and the ultraviolet spectrum exhibits absorption maxima at 218, 235 and 286 $m\mu$. It contains one methoxyl group, a metylenedioxy group and two non-phenolic hydroxyl groups, yielding the 3-acetate which is an amorphous solid and the 3:6-diacetate, colourless crystals, m.p. 114—7°C. The 3-methyl ether is 6-hydroxy-buphanidrine (q.v.).

Slabaugh, Wildman., *J. Org. Chem.*, **36**, 3202 (1971)

HYDROXYSENKIRKINE

$C_{19}H_{27}O_7N$

M.p. 124—5°C

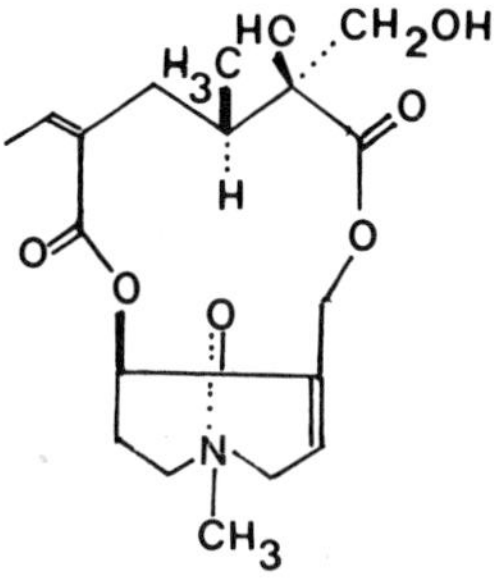

A member of the hepatotoxic alkaloids, this base occurs in *Crotalaria laburnifolia* L. and is obtained as colourless crystals from Me_2CO. It is slightly dextrorotatory with $[\alpha]_D^{26} + 5.3°$ (c 0.682, EtOH). The alkaloid furnishes a crystalline hydrochloride as colourless needles, m.p. 229—230°C (*dec.*) and a picrate as pale yellow plates from EtOH, m.p. 242°C (*dec.*).

Crout., *J. Chem. Soc., Perkin I*, 1602 (1972)

4(a)-HYDROXYSKYTANTHINE

$C_{11}H_{21}ON$

M.p. 91—2°C

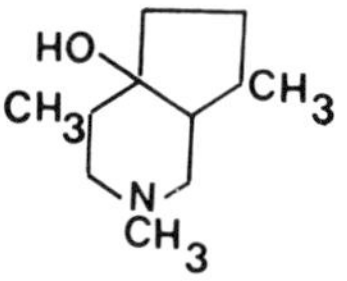

This alkaloid has been obtained by Dickinson and Jones from *Tecoma stans*. Under reduced pressure, the base sublimes at 110°C/0.25 mm. It gives crystalline derivatives, e.g. the methiodide, m.p. 293—5°C; picrate, m.p. 170—170.5°C and the benzoyl derivative, m.p. 60—5°C. Two further isomers of this base are known and described below.

Dickinson, Jones., *Tetrahedron*, **25**, 1523 (1969)

HYDROXYSKYTANTHINE I (*Alkaloid D*)

$C_{11}H_{21}ON$

M.p. 94–5°C

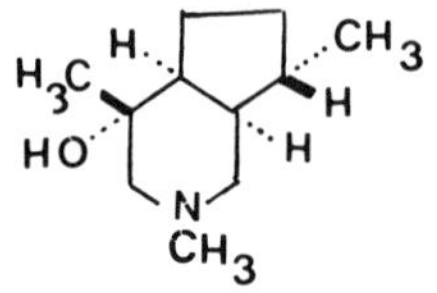

This isomeric alkaloid is a minor component found in the leaf extract of *Skytanthus acutus* Meyen and may be purified by crystallization from cyclohexane or by sublimation. It is dextrorotatory with $[\alpha]_D^{19} + 38.5°$ (c 1.5, cyclohexane). The stereochemistry has been determined mainly from the NMR spectrum.

Appel, Müller., *Scientia* (Valparaiso), **115**, 3 (1961)
Adolphen *et al.*, *Tetrahedron*, **23**, 3147 (1967)

HYDROXYSKYTANTHINE II

$C_{11}H_{21}ON$

M.p. 119–120°C

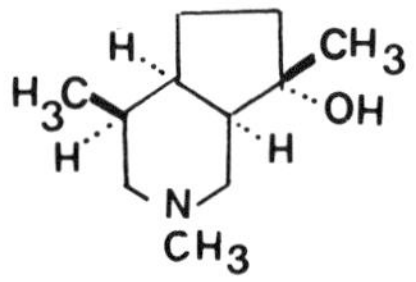

An isomer of the preceding two alkaloids, this base also occurs in the leaves of *Skytanthus acutus* Meyen and may be obtained pure by the same methods of sublimation or crystallization. It is laevorotatory with $[\alpha]_D^{19} - 38.5°$ (c 1.0, MeOH). The stereochemistry has again been deduced from the NMR spectrum.

Adoplhen *et al.*, *Tetrahedron*, **23**, 3147 (1967)

15α-HYDROXYSOLADULCIDINE

$C_{27}H_{45}O_3N$

M.p. 156–9°C

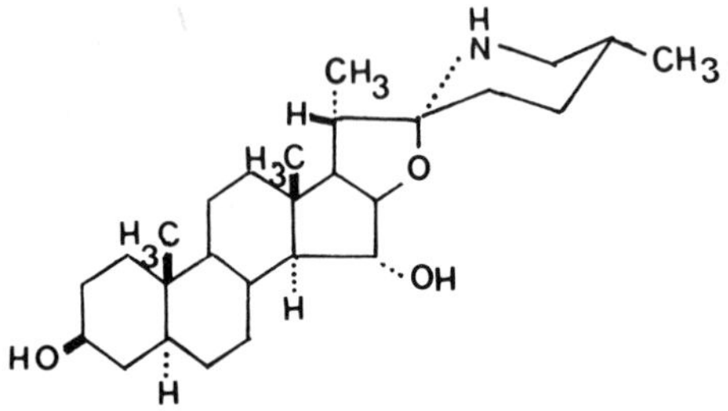

The roots of *Solanum dulcamara* L. yield this steroidal alkaloid which forms colourless prismatic crystals from aqueous MeOH corresponding to the monohydrate. The base has $[\alpha]_D^{21} - 38.9°$ (c 1.0, CHCl₃). It contains two hydroxyl groups and an imino group and yields the O,O,N-triacetyl derivative as a crystalline mass, m.p. 168–170°C; $[\alpha]_D^{17} - 12.7°$ (CHCl₃). The alkaloid also furnishes the N-notroso compound, m.p. 218–223°C (*dec.*); $[\alpha]_D^{21} + 59.6°$ (CHCl₃).

Rönsch, Schreiber., *Tetrahedron Lett.*, 1947 (1965)

3α-HYDROXYSOPHORIDINE

$C_{15}H_{24}O_2N_2$

M.p. 214–5°C

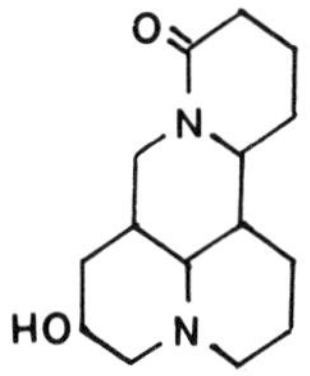

This alkaloid has recently been identified as a minor component of the alkaloidal extract from the above ground parts of *Sophora alopecuroides*. It has been characterized by infrared, NMR and mass spectroscopy and shown to possess the above structure.

Monakhova *et al., Khim. Prir. Soedin.*, **9**, 59 (1973)

7-HYDROXYSPARTEINE

$C_{15}H_{26}ON_2$

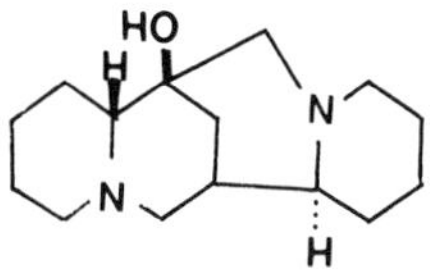

A minor constituent of *Cytisus hirsutus*, the structure of this alkaloid has been established from spectroscopic and chemical data and comparison with sparteine (q.v.).

Mollov, Ivanov, Panov., *Dokl. Bolg. Akad, Nauk.*, **24**, 1657 (1971)

4-HYDROXYSTRYCHNINE

$C_{21}H_{22}O_3N_2$

M.p. 275–6°C

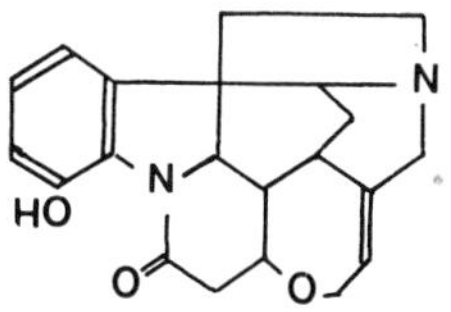

A *strychnos* alkaloid present in *S. icaja* Baill., this base gives colourless crystals when crystallized from absolute EtOH. It has $[\alpha]_D^{20} - 8°$ (c 0.7, CHCl₃). Spectroscopic evidence has shown the hydroxyl to be at C-4 in the molecule.

Sandberg *et al., Tetrahedron Lett.*, 6217 (1968)
Sandberg *et al., ibid*, 227 (1969)

11-HYDROXY-(−)-TABERSONINE

This base has recently been identified as a minor component of the leaf extract of *Melodinus balansae*. No further details of its chemical or physical properties have been reported.

Mehri *et al., Ann. Pharm. Fr.*, **30**, 643 (1972)

16-HYDROXYTHEBAINE

C$_{19}$H$_{21}$O$_4$N

M.p. 126–8°C (capillary)

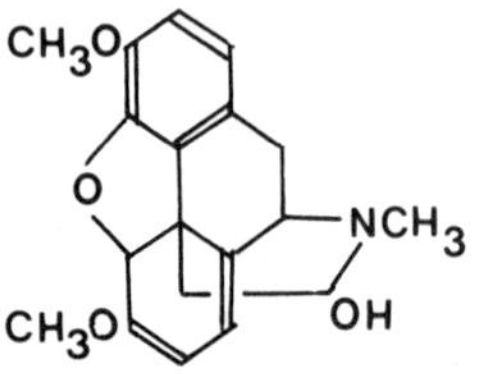

A minor alkaloid from the latex of *Papaver somniferum* L., the base may be purified by recrystallization from Me$_2$CO-light petroleum when it yields light yellow crystals. It contains two methoxyl groups and a methylimino group in addition to the hydroxyl group.

Brochmann-Hansenn, Leung, Richter., *J. Org. Chem.*, **37**, 1881 (1972)

6-HYDROXYTHIOBINUPHARIDINE

C$_{29}$H$_{40}$O$_2$N$_2$S

M.p. Indefinite

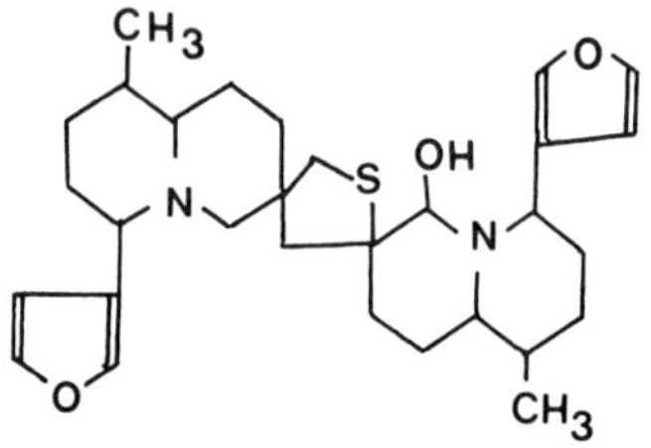

This alkaloid from the rhizomes of *Nuphar luteum* forms a colourless glass which cannot be obtained crystalline. It has $[\alpha]_D^{25} + 38°$ (c 0.36, CH$_2$Cl$_2$). It forms a crystalline perchlorate, m.p. 238–242°C and a diperchlorate, liquifying at 265°C and decomposing at 273°C. On reduction with NaBH$_4$ it furnishes thiobinupharidine.

Achmatowicz, Wrobel., *Tetrahedron Lett.*, **129**, 927 (1964)

15α-HYDROXYTOMATIDINE

C$_{27}$H$_{45}$O$_3$N

M.p. 150–5°C

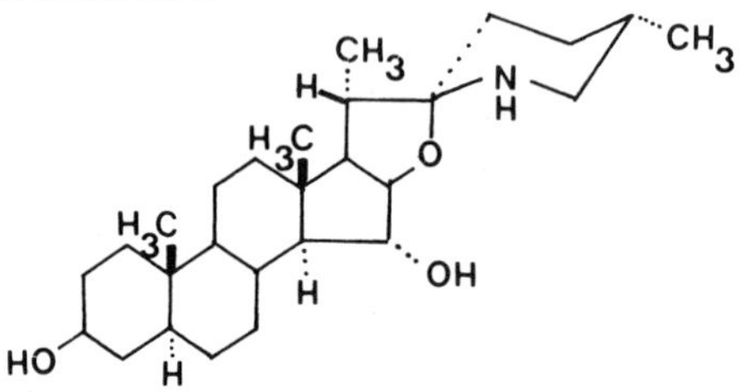

A minor alkaloid from the root extract of *Solanum dulcumara* L., the base gives clusters of colourless needles from MeOH and has $[\alpha]_D^{18} + 17.8°$ (c 1.0, CHCl$_3$). With Ac$_2$O in pyridine it yields the O,O,N-triacetyl derivative, m.p. 203.5–204.5°C; $[\alpha]_D^{18} - 3.1°$ (CHCl$_3$). The N-nitroso compound has also been prepared, m.p. 242.4–244°C; $[\alpha]_D^{18} - 87.7°$ (CHCl$_3$).

Rönsch, Schreiber., *Tetrahedron Lett.*, 1947 (1965)

1-HYDROXY-2:9:10-TRIMETHOXYAPORPHINE
(Alkaloid GF-B)

$C_{19}H_{17}O_4N$

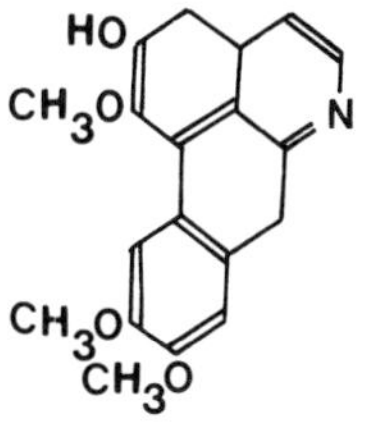

A minor constituent of this name has been isolated from *Glaucium flavum* and identified by thin-layer chromatography. On the accepted numbering of this basic alkaloidal skeleton, the name should strictly be 2-hydroxy-1:9:10-trimethoxyaporphine and even with this modification, the name is still a misnomer since the isoquinoline ring is fully unsaturated.

Duchevska, Orahovats., *Dokl. Bolg. Akad. Nauk.*, **26**, 899 (1973)

2-HYDROXY-1:9:10-TRIMETHOXYAPORPHINE

$C_{20}H_{23}O_4N$

M.p. Indefinite

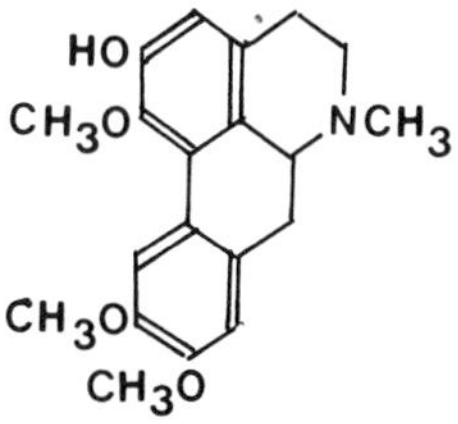

This alkaloid, more correctly described by this name (see the preceding entry), has been obtained from the leaves of *Beilschmiedia podagrica* Kostermans as the crystalline hydrobromide, forming colourless needles, m.p. 200–5°C (*dec.*); $[\alpha]_D + 97°$ (c 0.2, EtOH). The ultraviolet spectrum has absorption maxima at 283 and 302 mμ.

Johns *et al.*, *Austral. J. Chem.*, **22**, 1277 (1969)

10-HYDROXY-1:2:9-TRIMETHOXYAPORPHINE

$C_{20}H_{23}O_4N$

M.p. 180–3°C

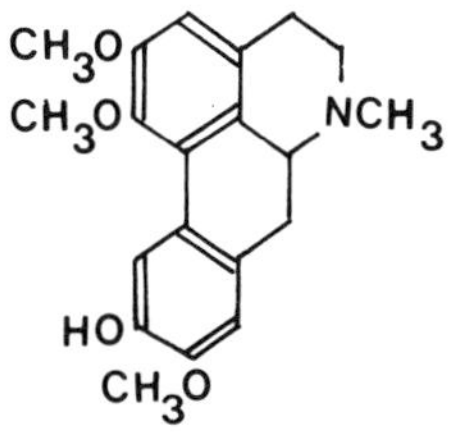

Probably present in small amounts in the leaves of *Beilschmiedia podagrica* Kostermans, this base yields colourless crystals from a mixture of C_6H_6 and light petroleum.

It may be characterized as the yellow crystalline picrate, m.p. 240–1°C (*dec.*).

Clezy, Lau., *Austral. J. Chem.*, **19**, 437 (1966)

1-HYDROXY-2:9:10-TRIMETHOXY-N-METHYLAPORPHINIUM

$C_{21}H_{26}O_4N^+$

Present in *Fagara rhoifolia* Lam. and *F. tinguassoiba* Hoehne, this quaternary alkaloid is usually isolated as the crystalline chloride, m.p. 215–9°C (*dec.*); $[\alpha]_D^{25} + 30.2°$ (c 2.16, H_2O). The solution in EtOH gives an ultraviolet spectrum containing absorption maxima at 228, 281, 307 and 321 mμ with a shoulder at 271 mμ. The salts yields an O-acetate, m.p. 234–8°C. The iodide has m.p. 226–9°C and forms the O-methyl ether, m.p. 216–8°C. The aporphinium base yields a picrate which exists in two crystalline modifications, as yellow prisms from aqueous Me_2CO, m.p. 148–151°C and light yellow needles from EtOH, m.p. 118–124°C. In the original structure, according to the accepted method of numbering, the hydroxyl group was placed at C-2, later revised to that given above.

Riggs, Antonaccio, Marion., *Can. J. Chem.*, **39**, 1330 (1961)
Calderwood, Fish., *Chem. Ind.*, 237 (1966)

Revised structure:
Tschesche, Welzel, Legler., *Tetrahedron Lett.*, 445 (1965)

1-HYDROXY-2:9:10-TRIMETHOXYNORAPORPHINE

$C_{19}H_{21}O_4N$

M.p. 108–110°C

The bark of several species of *Popowia*, indigenous to the Australian continent, yields this noraporphine alkaloid which, on recrystallization from Me_2CO forms colourless needles. The base is dextrorotatory with $[\alpha]_D + 47°$ (c 0.13, MeOH). The (±)-form of the alkaloid is wilsonirine (q.v.).

Johns *et al.*, *Austral. J. Chem.*, **23**, 363 (1970)

1-HYDROXY-2:10:11-TRIMETHOXYNORAPORPHINE

$C_{19}H_{21}O_4N$

This base accompanies the preceding alkaloid in the bark of *Popowia* species. It is an amorphous solid which is non-crystallizable. The structure has been determined from spectroscopic examination.

Johns *et al.*, *Austral. J. Chem.*, **23**, 363 (1970)

2-HYDROXY-1:9:10-TRIMETHOXYNORAPORPHINE

$C_{19}H_{21}O_4N$

This alkaloid from the leaves of *Beilschmiedia podagrica* Kostermans, is an amorphous powder which has not been obtained in the crystalline form. It furnishes a crystalline N-acetyl derivative, m.p. 133–5°C; $[\alpha]_D + 406°$ (c 0.1, $CHCl_3$) and gives an ultraviolet spectrum in ethanol solution with two absorption maxima at 282 and 302 mμ.

Johns *et al.*, *Austral. J. Chem.*, **22**, 1277 (1969)

20-HYDROXYVINCAMINE

$C_{21}H_{26}O_4N_2$

M.p. 222–5°C

A carboline type alkaloid present in *Vinca minor*, the structure has been established from infrared, NMR and mass spectroscopy. In addition to the hydroxyl group, a hydroxyethyl and a methoxycarbonyl group are also present.

Mokry, Kompis., *Lloydia*, **27**, 428 (1964)

(–)-HYGRINE

$C_8H_{15}ON$

B.p. 193–5°C

First obtained by Lossen from the Et_2O extract of a slightly alkaline percolate of the leaves of *Erythroxylon truxillense* Rusby from Peru, this alkaloid is also present in *Dendrobium chrysanthemum* Wall and *D. primulinum* Lindl, while Lazur'evskii has reported its presence in *Convolvulus hamadae*. The alkaloid is a strongly alkaline liquid that absorbs CO_2 from the air and decomposes on exposure to light. It is slightly laevorotatory with $[\alpha]_D - 1.3°$. It yields an aurichloride and a crystalline picrate, m.p. 158°C; an oxime, m.p. 116–120°C and the D(+)-bitartrate, m.p. 69°C (as the dihydrate) or 130°C (*dry*); $[\alpha]_D^{18}$ –

1.8° (H_2O). Chromic acid oxidizes the alkaloid to hygric acid (1-methylpyrroli-dine-2-carboxylic acid), m.p. 164°C. The structure of the alkaloid has been confirmed by various independent syntheses.

Lossen., *Annalen,* **121**, 374 (1862)
Liebermann, Kühling., *Ber.,* **24**, 407 (1891)
Liebermann, Cybulski., *ibid,* **28**, 578 (1895)
Hess., *ibid,* **46**, 3113, 4104 (1913)
Lazur'evskii., *Trudy Uzbeksk. Gos. Univ. Sbornik Rabot Khim.,* **15**, 43 (1939)
Sorm., *Collect. Czech. Chem. Commun.,* **12**, 245 (1947)
Anet, Hughes, Ritchie., *Nature,* **163**, 289 (1949)
Galinovsky, Wagner, Wieser., *Monatsh.,* **82**, 551 (1951)

Mass spectrum:
Luning, Leander., *Acta Chem. Scand.,* **19**, 1607 (1965)

β-HYGRINE

$C_{14}H_{24}ON_2$

B.p. 215°C/50 mm

Liebermann *et al.,* were able to show that the alkaloid isolated by Lossen as hygrine could be separated into two components by distillation under reduced pressure. The second fraction decomposes when distilled at atmospheric pressure but has the above boiling point at reduced pressure. It yields a crystalline aurichloride and a dimethiodide. On oxidation with chromic acid, a small quantity of hygrine is formed.

Liebermann, Kühling., *Ber.,* **24**, 407 (1891)
Liebermann, Cybulski., *ibid,* **28**, 578 (1895)

HYGROLINE

$C_8H_{17}ON$

M.p. 33–4°C;
B.p. 78–82°C/12 mm

This alkaloid accompanies cocaine in the leaves of *Erythroxylon coca* Lam and E. truxillense Rusby. The natural base is laevorotatory with $[\alpha]_D^{23} - 63.2°$ (c 11.4, H_2O) and is freely soluble in H_2O and most organic solvents. With benzoyl chloride, it yields an oily benzoyl derivative which forms characteristic crystalline salts, e.g. the aurichloride, m.p. 114–5°C; platinichloride, m.p. 150–2°C and the 3:5-dinitrobenzoate, m.p. 65°C. When oxidized with chromic acid it yields hygrine, the latter being optically inactive possibly due to racemization, identified as the crystalline picrate, m.p. 153–4°C and the oxime, m.p. 124–5°C. The alkaloid is therefore the secondary alcohol corresponding to the ketone, hygrine. The (+)-form has m.p. 34°C; $[\alpha]_D^{17} + 84.1°$ (H_2O) and the (±)-form has m.p. 24–5°C.

Späth, Kittel., *Ber.,* **76**, 942 (1943)
Galinovsky, Zuber., *Monatsh.,* **84**, 798 (1953)

HYGROPHYLLINE

$C_{18}H_{27}O_6N$

M.p. 173–4°C

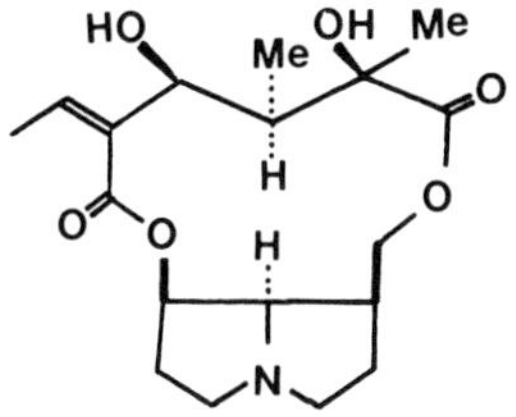

A pyrrolizidine alkaloid present in *Senecio hydgrophylus* Dyet and Sm., this base yields colourless prisms when crystallized from Me_2CO and is laevorotatory with $[\alpha]_D^{20} - 67.3°$ (c 2.9, EtOH). Alkaline hydrolysis furnishes platynecine and hygrophyllinecic acid, the latter being obtained in the form of the monolactone.

Schlosser, Warren., *J. Chem. Soc.*, 5707 (1965)

HYMENOCARDINE

$C_{37}H_{50}O_6N_6$

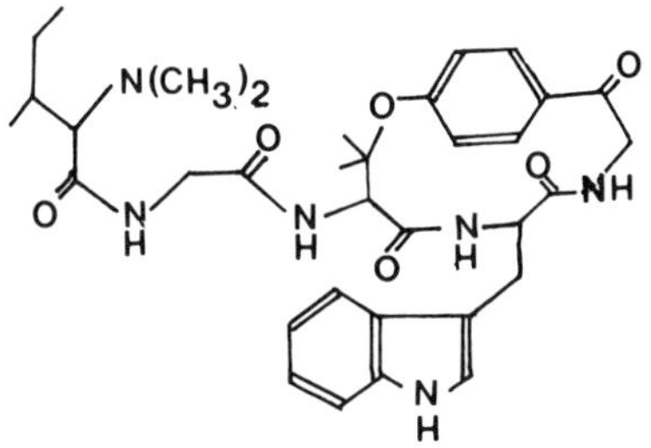

This complex indole alkaloid has been isolated from *Hymenocardia acida* Tul. It belongs to the peptide group of alkaloids and contains four nitrogen atoms in the form of amide groups, the two remaining nitrogens being present, one in the indole nucleus and the other as a dimethylamino group.

Pais *et al.*, *Bull. Soc. Chim. Fr.*, **29**, 79 (1968)

HYOSCINE (*Atroscine, Scopolamine*)

$C_{17}H_{21}O_4N$

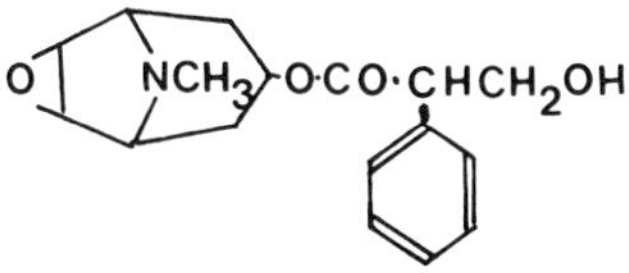

A Solanaceous alkaloid obtained from *Datura Metel*, but also present in *D. alba* Nees, *D. arborea, D. fastuosa, D. meteloides, D. quercifolia, D. Stramonium* Linn (roots), *Hyoscyamus albus, H. niger, Mandragora vernalis* and the rhizomes of *Scopolia carniolica*. The free base is a colourless syrup and has $[\alpha]_D^{20} - 28°$ (H_2O) or $- 18°$ (EtOH). With alkalies it is recemized to the (±)-form (q.v.). It forms a series of crystalline salts and derivative: the hydrochloride, m.p. 200°C; hydrobromide trihydrate, m.p. 193–4°C (*dry*); $[\alpha]_D - 15.72°$ (EtOH) or $- 25.9°$ (H_2O); aurichloride, m.p. 208–9°C (*dec.*); auribromide, rectangular chocolate-red needles, m.p. 191–2°C and methobromide, m.p. 214–7°C (*dec.*). The picrate exists in two crystalline forms, as slender yellow needles from EtOH, m.p. 187–8°C and irregular hexagonal scales from boiling H_2O, m.p. 191–2°C (*corr.*).

With dilute acids or alkalies, the base yields (−)-tropic acid and (±)-scopoline. The (+)-form is also a colourless syrup, furnishing a crystalline aurichloride, m.p. 204–5°C (*dec.*); a hydrobromide trihydrate, m.p. 193–4°C (*dry*) and a picrate, m.p. 187–8°C (*dec.*). The base has $[\alpha]_D^{20} + 27.8°$ (H_2O).

Pharmacologically, the alkaloid has a similar action to that of atropine (q.v.) upon the peripheral, cholinergic, autonomic nervous system, but one which is more transitory. It has found some use in medicine as a sedative and in particular in treatment of motion sickness. Although there may be some preliminary excitement in small doses, the normal reaction is one of fatigue passing into sleep.

Ladenburg., *Annalen,* **206**, 299 (1880)
Schmidt., *Arch. Pharm.,* **232**, 409 (1894)
Jowett., *J. Chem. Soc.,* **71**, 680 (1897)
Carr, Reynolds., *ibid,* **101**, 950 (1912)
King., *ibid,* **115**, 476 (1919)
Dobo *et al., ibid,* 3461 (1959)

(±)-HYOSCINE

$C_{17}H_{21}O_4N$

The optically inactive form of this alkaloid occurs naturally in *Duboisia Leichhardtii* von Muell. The alkaloid is a syrup but it forms two stable, crystalline hydrates, the monohydrate, m.p. 56–7°C and the dihydrate, m.p. 37–8°C. It also yields crystalline salts, e.g. the hydrobromide trihydrate, m.p. 181–2°C (*dry*); aurichloride, m.p. 214–5°C; auribromide, m.p. 209–210°C and the picrate, m.p. 173.5–174.5°C.

Mitchell., *J. Chem. Soc.,* 480 (1944)

(−)-HYOSCYAMINE

$C_{17}H_{21}O_3N$

M.p. 108.5°C

This is the most widely-spread of the tropane alkaloids and has been isolated from such species as *Anthotroche pannosa, Atropa belladonna* Linn, *A. boetica, Datura alba* Nees, *D. arborea, D. fastuosa, D. Metel, D. meteloides, D. quercifolia, D. Stramonium* Linn, *Duboisia Leichhardtii* von Muell, *D. myoporoides, Hyoscyamus albus, H. muticus* (seeds), *H. niger, Hyposcyamus reticulatus, Mandragora scopoliae, M. vernalis, Scopolia carniolitica, S. japonica* and *S. lurida* (roots).

730

The alkaloid crystallizes from aqueous EtOH as silky needles and is laevo-rotatory with $[\alpha]_D - 22°$ (50% EtOH). It is freely soluble in EtOH, CHCl$_3$ or C$_6$H$_6$ but less so in cold H$_2$O or Et$_2$O. In EtOH it racemizes slowly but very rapidly on the addition of acids or alkalies, or even on melting. With H$_2$O, it is hydrolyzed to (−)-tropic acid and (±)-tropine. It yields several crystalline salts; the hydrobromide, m.p. 151.8°C is deliquescent and is usually obtained as the dihydrate; the sulphate dihydrate is also deliquescent and has m.p. 206°C (*dry*); the oxalate, m.p. 176°C; aurichloride, m.p. 165°C; auribromide, dark red needles, m.p. 115–120°C; platinichloride, orange prisms, m.p. 206°C; metho-bromide, m.p. 210–2°C and the picrate, m.p. 165°C. The optically inactive form is atropine (q.v.).

The (−)-form of the alkaloid acts more powerfully upon the peripheral nerves than the (+)-form. Both closely resemble atropine in their bitter taste and mydriatic action.

Ladenburg., *Annalen,* **206**, 282 (1880)
Gadamer., *Arch. Pharm.,* **239**, 294 (1901)
Carr, Reynolds., *J. Chem. Soc.,* **97**, 1329 (1910)
Marion, Spenser., *Can. J. Chem.,* **32**, 1116 (1954)
Marion, Thomas., *ibid,* **33**, 1853 (1955)
Bremner, Cannon., *Austral. J. Chem.,* **21**, 1369 (1968)

Biosynthesis:
Baralle, Gros., *Chem. Commun.,* 721 (1969)

HYPACONITINE

C$_{33}$H$_{45}$O$_{10}$N

M.p. 197.5–198.5°C

This aconitine alkaloid occurs in numerous *Aconitum* species, e.g. in *A. calliantum* Koidzumi, *A. grossedentatum* Nakai, *A. hakusanense* Nakai, *A. ibukiense* Nakai, *A. kamtschaticum* Willd et Reichb., *A. senanense* Nakai, *A tortuosum* Willd., and *A. Zuccarini* Nakai. The alkaloid crystallizes in colourless prisms from MeOH or Et$_2$O and has $[\alpha]_D^{17} + 22.7°$ (CHCl$_3$). It forms crystalline salts: hydrochloride (3.5 H$_2$O), m.p. 242–4°C (*dry*); $[\alpha]_D^{13} - 6.5°$ (H$_2$O); hydrobromide (2.5 H$_2$O), m.p. 178–9°C (*dry*); $[\alpha]_D^{17} - 19.7°$ (H$_2$O); perchlorate, m.p. 178–180°C (*dec.*); $[\alpha]_D^9 - 11.2°$ (EtOH); aurichloride, m.p. 243–5°C (*dec.*) and the O-acetate, m.p. 197–200°C. With boiling dilute H$_2$SO$_4$, the alkaloid is hydrolyzed to acetic acid and benzhypaconine, C$_{31}$H$_{43}$O$_9$N, which is amorphous but yields a crystalline hydrochloride, m.p. 242–4°C. When hydrolyzed with H$_2$O in a sealed tube, the alkaloid furnishes hypaconine together with acetic and benzoic acids. Hypaconine is characterized as the tetracetyl derivative, m.p. 182–4°C (*dec.*). The alkaloid yields pyrohypaconitine on heating, C$_{31}$H$_{41}$O$_8$N, m.p. 119–120°C; $[\alpha]_D^{13} + 21.7°$ (CHCl$_3$) while oxidation with KMnO$_4$ in Me$_2$CO gives formaldehyde and hypoxonitine, m.p. 267–8°C (*dec.*); $[\alpha]_D^{15} - 63.1°$ (CHCl$_3$). Unlike aconitine or mesaconitine, this alkaloid is scarcely affected by chromic or nitric acids and the latter, in particular, fails to yield a crystalline oxidation product.

Majima, Morio., *Annalen,* **476**, 171, 210 (1929)
Majima, Tamura., *ibid,* **526**, 116 (1936)
Majima, Tamura., *ibid,* **545**, 1 (1940)

HYPAPHORINE

$C_{14}H_{18}O_2N_2$

M.p. 255°C (dec.).

First isolated by Greshoff from the seeds of *Erythrina subumbrans* (Hassk) Merr (syn. *E. hypaphorus* Boerl), this alkaloid has subsequently been discovered in numerous *Erythrina* species. It yields monoclinic crystals of the dihydrate from H_2O and although soluble in H_2O and EtOH is insoluble in most other organic solvents. It has $[\alpha]_D^{27} + 113.1°$ (H_2O) and yields crystalline salts, e.g. the nitrate, m.p. 223.5−224.5°C; $[\alpha]_D + 94.7°$; hydrochloride, m.p. 234−5°C; $[\alpha]_D^{20} + 89.2°$ (H_2O); hydrobromide, m.p. 225°C and the hydriodide, m.p. 220−1°C.

Heating the alkaloid with KOH gives indole and trimethylamine, while hypaphorine may be synthesized from tryptophan and methyl iodide in the presence of NaOH in MeOH, the resulting methylhypaphorine iodide, m.p. 200.5−201.5°C, being heated at 100°C with very dilute NaOH to avoid hydrolysis of the alkaloid as it is formed.

Hypaprohine causes increased reflex irritability and ensuing tetanic convulsions in frogs although it exhibits little action on other animals. The methylester iodide has curarizing properties.

Greshoff., *Meded uit's Lands Plant.*, **7**, 29 (1890)
Maranon, Santos., *Philippine J. Sci.*, **48**, 563 (1932)
Romburgh, Barger., *J. Chem. Soc.*, **99**, 2069 (1911)
Rao *et al.*, *Proc. Ind. Acad. Sci.*, **7A**, 179 (1938)

Pharmacology:
Plugge., *Arch. exp. Path. Pharm.*, **32**, 313 (1893)
Folkers, Koniuszy., *J. Amer. Chem. Soc.*, **61**, 1232 (1939)

HYPECORINE

$C_{20}H_{19}O_5N$

M.p. 154−6°C

This spiroisoquinoline alkaloid has been isolated from *Hypecorum erectum* during the flowering season. It contains two methylenedioxy groups and one methylimino group. The structure has been determined by spectroscopic investigations.

Yakhontova *et al.*, *Khim. Prir. Soedin.*, **5**, 624 (1972)

HYPECORININE

$C_{20}H_{17}O_6N$

M.p. 197–8°C

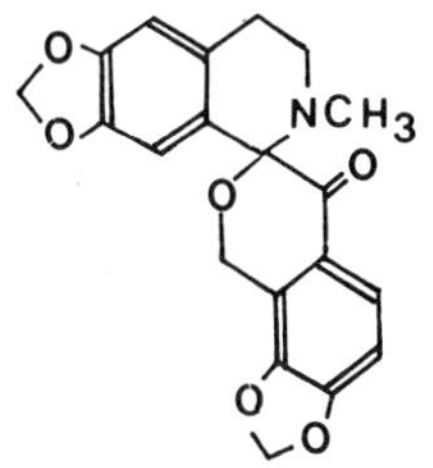

Also present in flowering *Hypecorum erectum,* the structure of this oxo-base closely resembles that of the preceding alkaloid. The structure has likewise been elucidated from the infrared, NMR and mass spectra.

Yakhontova *et al., Khim. Prir. Soedin.,* **5**, 624 (1972)

HYPOEPISTEPHANINE

M.p. 256.7°C

This alkaloid occurs in the phenolic portion of the extract from *Stephania japonica* and is separated from the accompanying bases by chromatography on alumina. It has $[\alpha]_D^{15.5} + 183.8°$.

Tomita *et al., J. Pharm. Soc., Japan,* **76**, 686 (1956)
Tomita, Ibuka., *ibid,* **83**, 996 (1963)

HYPOGNAVINOL

$C_{20}H_{27}O_4N$

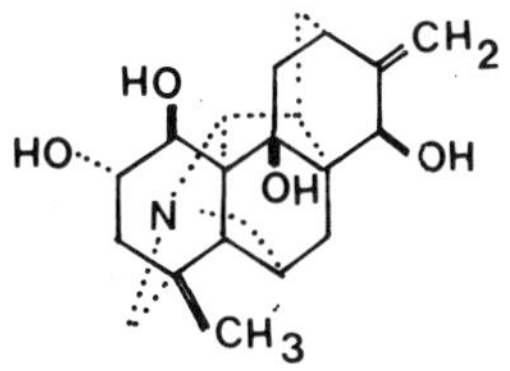

This alkaloid occurs in *Aconitum sanyoense* and forms colourless crystals which are orthorhombic with a − 13.69, b = 14.41, c = 10.0 Å; Z = 4. The structure has been solved by the heavy atom method of X-ray crystallography using the methiodide.

Pelletier *et al., Tetrahedron Lett.,* **11**, 795 (1971)

HYPOQUEBRACHINE

This alkaloid has been reported from the bark of *Aspidosperma quebracho* by Hesse but according to Ewins it is possibly a decomposition product of aspidospermine, formed during the extraction process.

Hesse., *Annalen,* **211**, 249 (1892)
Ewins., *J. Chem. Soc.,* **105**, 2738 (1914)

HYSCYAMINE

$C_{17}H_{23}O_3N$

M.p. 102–5°C

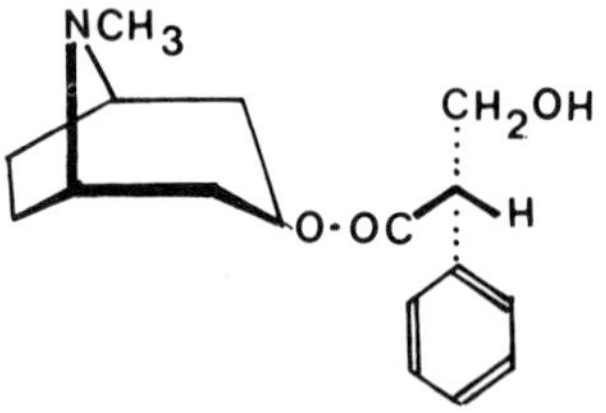

This tropine alkaloid occurs in several *Anthoceris* species and yields colourless needles when crystallized from Et_2O-C_6H_6. It has $[\alpha]_D^{24} - 5°$ (c 1.9, EtOH). A picrate has been prepared as yellow needles, m.p. 165–6°C.

Cannon *et al., Austral. J. Chem.*, **22**, 221 (1969)

HYSTRINE

$C_{10}H_{16}N_2$

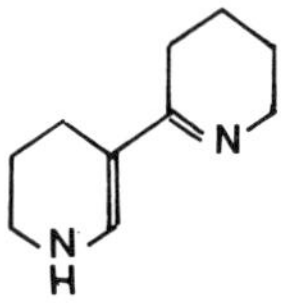

This alkaloid has been obtained from *Genista hystrix*. It forms a characteristic crystalline N-nitroso derivative. By chemical and spectroscopic studies the structure has been demonstrated to be 3-(2:3:4:5-tetrahydro-6-pyridyl)-1:4:5:6-tetrahydropyridine. This has been confirmed by the preparation of the alkaloid by the introduction of a double link into the piperidine nucleus of synthetic ammodendrine, followed by deacetylation.

Steinegger, Moser, Weber., *Phytochem.*, **7**, 849 (1968)
Steinegger, Weber., *Helv. Chim. Acta.*, **51**, 206 (1968)